the complete guide to
natural homemade
beauty products
& treatments

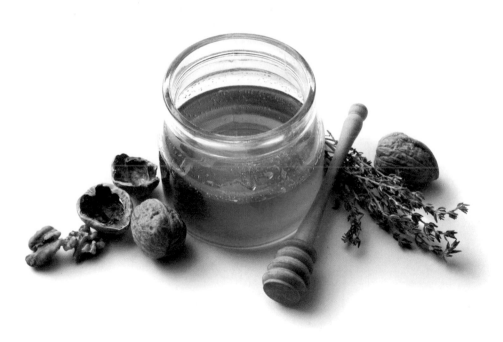

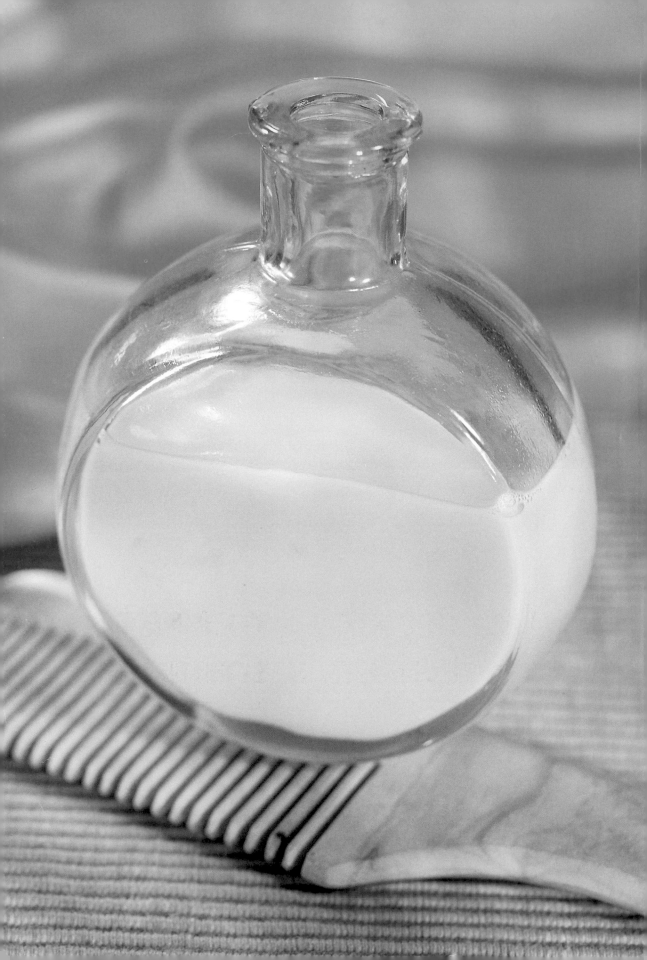

Contents

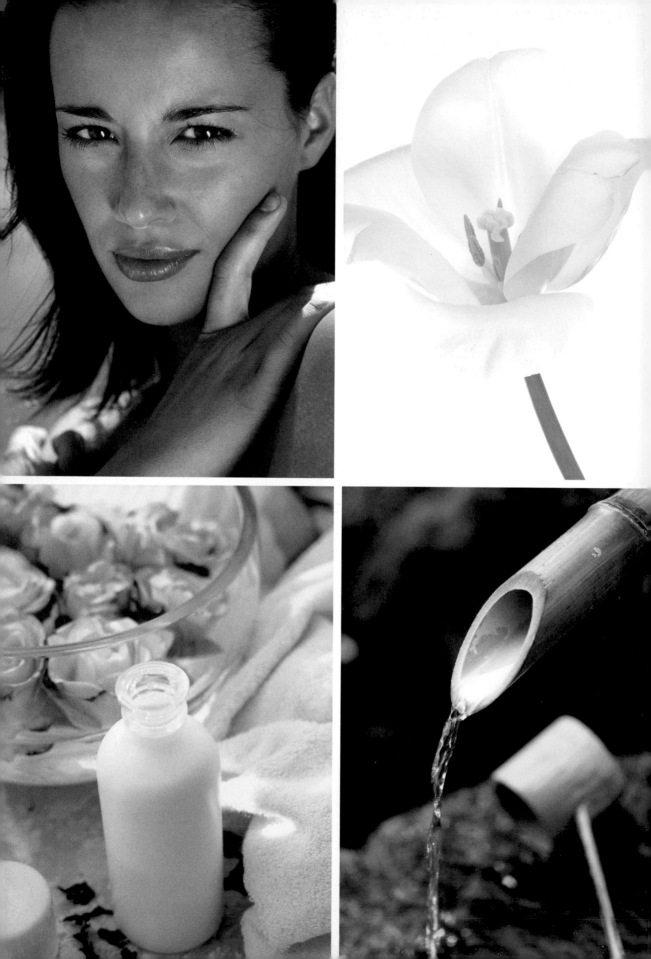

the complete guide to
natural homemade
beauty products
& treatments

175 recipes
from scrubs & masks to
moisturizers & shampoos

Amelia Ruiz

For complete cataloguing information, see page 368.

Disclaimer: The author and the publisher are not responsible for any adverse effects or consequences resulting from the use of the information in this book. It is the responsibility of the reader to consult a physician or other qualified health-care professional regarding his or her personal care.

To the best of our knowledge, the recipes or formulas in this book are safe for ordinary use and users. For those people with allergies or health issues, please read the suggested contents of each recipe or formula carefully and determine whether or not they may create a problem for you. All recipes or formulas are used at the risk of the consumer.

We cannot be responsible for any hazards, loss or damage that may occur as a result of any recipe or formula use.

For those with special needs, allergies, requirements or health problems, in the event of any doubt, please contact your medical adviser prior to the use of any recipe or formula.

Design and production: Daniella Zanchetta/PageWave Graphics Inc.
Editor: Tina Anson Mine | Copy editor/proofreader: Marnie Lamb | Indexer: Beth Zabloski

Cover image: Soap with flowers © fotosearch.com
Original interior images: Becky Lawton, M&G Studios, Stock Photos, AGE Fotostock, Archivo Océano Ámbar
Additional interior images: p.1 © iStockphoto.com/Floortje; p.6 Top right © iStockphoto.com/_Vilor; p.15 Clockwise from top left © iStockphoto.com/ElenaGaak, © iStockphoto.com/andresr, © iStockphoto.com/tycoon751, © iStockphoto.com/PeopleImages; p.19 Clockwise from top left © iStockphoto.com/Mariha-kitchen, © iStockphoto.com/OlgaMiltsova, © iStockphoto.com/bhofack2, © iStockphoto.com/Elenathewise; p.22 © iStockphoto.com/Creativeye99; p.26 Clockwise from top left © iStockphoto.com/servickuz, © iStockphoto.com/PeopleImages, © iStockphoto.com/WillSelarep, © iStockphoto.com/XiXinXing; p.30 Clockwise from top left © iStockphoto.com/Elenathewise, © iStockphoto.com/agitons, © iStockphoto.com/LOVE_LIFE; p.36 Clockwise from top left © iStockphoto.com/haoliang, © iStockphoto.com/Olha_Afanasieva, © iStockphoto.com/digitalskillet, © iStockphoto.com/matka_Wariatka; p.42 Top right © iStockphoto.com/Elenathewise, Bottom © iStockphoto.com/Beboy_ltd; p.47 Clockwise from top left © iStockphoto.com/Thomas_EyeDesign, © iStockphoto.com/baibaz, © iStockphoto.com/Floortje, © iStockphoto.com/v777999; p.50 Clockwise from top left © iStockphoto.com/kerdkanno, © iStockphoto.com/Sohadiszno, © iStockphoto.com/taragovcom, © iStockphoto.com/yangna; p.54 © iStockphoto.com/heibaihiu; p.60 © iStockphoto.com/Bubble1502; p.62 Clockwise from top left © iStockphoto.com/prudkov, © iStockphoto.com/XiXinXing; p.69 Clockwise from top left © iStockphoto.com/Yuri_Arcurs, © iStockphoto.com/mediaphotos, © iStockphoto.com/Antonio_Sanchez, © iStockphoto.com/junial; p.72 © iStockphoto.com/Magone; p.74 © iStockphoto.com/4kodiak; p.78 © iStockphoto.com/anna1311; p.87 © iStockphoto.com/yonel; p.88 © iStockphoto.com/Ciungara; p.90 © iStockphoto.com/eAlisa; p.92 © iStockphoto.com/kaanates; p.96 © iStockphoto.com/Olgaorly; p.98 © iStockphoto.com/DanielaAgius; p.100 © iStockphoto.com/HandmadePictures; p.102 © iStockphoto.com/deliormanli; p.103 Mashed Potato © iStockphoto.com/creacart; p.114 © iStockphoto.com/Floortje; p.115 © iStockphoto.com/miss_j; p.117 Clockwise from top left © iStockphoto.com/smusselm, © iStockphoto.com/hammett79, © iStockphoto.com/martinedoucet, © iStockphoto.com/Juanmonino; p.119 © iStockphoto.com/daffodilred; p.124 © iStockphoto.com/robynmac; p.130 © iStockphoto.com/anna1311; p.133 © iStockphoto.com/eyewave; p.134 © iStockphoto.com/srekapi; p.136 Clockwise from top left © iStockphoto.com/dlewis33, © iStockphoto.com/PeopleImages, © iStockphoto.com/markos86; p.142 Cucumber © iStockphoto.com/fcafotodigital, p.149 © iStockphoto.com/narcisa; p.152 Clockwise from top left © iStockphoto.com/Yuri, © iStockphoto.com/knape, © iStockphoto.com/Yuri_Arcurs; p.163 Sage © iStockphoto.com/Zoryanchik; p.166 Clockwise from top left © iStockphoto.com/matka_Wariatka, © iStockphoto.com/ValuaVitaly, © iStockphoto.com/Ingalvanova, © iStockphoto.com/MorePixels; p.169 © iStockphoto.com/Indric; p.172 © iStockphoto.com/atoss; p.179 © iStockphoto.com/RedHelga; p.182 © iStockphoto.com/keithferrisphoto; p.187 © iStockphoto.com/bergamont; p.190 Clockwise from top left © iStockphoto.com/Velniux, © iStockphoto.com/Stockphoto4u, © iStockphoto.com/PeopleImages, © iStockphoto.com/Fitzer; p.194 Clockwise from top left © iStockphoto.com/Yuri_Arcurs, © iStockphoto.com/Nastia11, © iStockphoto.com/Maridav; p.196 © iStockphoto.com/masa44; p.198 © iStockphoto.com/ptlee; p.199 © iStockphoto.com/robynmac; p.200 © iStockphoto.com/anna1311; p.201 © iStockphoto.com/Okssi68; p.202 © iStockphoto.com/chengyuzheng; p.204 © iStockphoto.com/UroshPetrovic; p.208 © iStockphoto.com/andsem; p.212 © iStockphoto.com/ValentynVolkov; p.226 Clockwise from top left © iStockphoto.com/EduLeite, © iStockphoto.com/AnnaOmelchenko, © iStockphoto.com/IS_ImageSource; p.230 Clockwise from top right © iStockphoto.com/andresr, © iStockphoto.com/PeopleImages, © iStockphoto.com/Yuri_Arcurs; p.234 © iStockphoto.com/dianazh; p.238 © iStockphoto.com/enter89; p.240 © iStockphoto.com/Eivaisla; p.250 © iStockphoto.com/morningrage; p.255 Top right © iStockphoto.com/naumalex, Bottom Left © iStockphoto.com/ValuaVitaly; p.260 © iStockphoto.com/DrPAS; p.262 Clockwise from top right © iStockphoto.com/redtea, © iStockphoto.com/twinsterphoto, © iStockphoto.com/PetrePlesea; p.266 Top left © iStockphoto.com/Wavebreakmedia; p.269 Clockwise from top right © iStockphoto.com/Sveti, © iStockphoto.com/ElenaTa, © iStockphoto.com/PeopleImages; p.272 © iStockphoto.com/posteriori; p.276 Clockwise from top right © iStockphoto.com/PeopleImages, © iStockphoto.com/daffodilred, © iStockphoto.com/stevecoleimages, © iStockphoto.com/OlgaMiltsova; p.278 © iStockphoto.com/Eliza317; p.279 © iStockphoto.com/Elenathewise; p.280 © iStockphoto.com/Denira777; p.282 © iStockphoto.com/swkunst; p.284 © iStockphoto.com/elf911; p.290 Dried Linden © iStockphoto.com/serjiunea; p.291 © iStockphoto.com/eAlisa; p.294 © iStockphoto.com/republica; p.304 © iStockphoto.com/AlexRaths; p.310 © iStockphoto.com/fcafotodigital; p.311 © iStockphoto.com/abadonian; p.313 Almonds © iStockphoto.com/Kaleidoscope_; p.314 © iStockphoto.com/Imo; p.316 © iStockphoto.com/Natikka; p.318 © iStockphoto.com/supermimicry; p.322 © iStockphoto.com/nanka-stalker; p.323 © iStockphoto.com/kaanates; p.324 Clockwise from top right © iStockphoto.com/GlobalStock, © iStockphoto.com/Elenathewise, © iStockphoto.com/Maridav; p.330 © iStockphoto.com/tfazevedo; p.332 Jasmine © iStockphoto.com/bonchan; p.335 © iStockphoto.com/frytka; p.339 © iStockphoto.com/KieselUndStein; p.354 © iStockphoto.com/Floortje; p.355 © iStockphoto.com/Buriy

The publisher gratefully acknowledges the financial support of our publishing program by the Government of Canada through the Canada Book Fund.

Published by Robert Rose Inc. | 120 Eglinton Avenue East, Suite 800 | Toronto, Ontario, Canada M4P 1E2 |
Tel: (416) 322-6552 Fax: (416) 322-6936 | www.robertrose.ca

Printed and bound in Canada

1 2 3 4 5 6 7 8 9 TCP 22 21 20 19 18 17 16

Part 1
The Fundamentals of Natural Beauty

Pamper Yourself Nature's Way

For millennia, the dream of eternal youth and beauty has led people to try endless numbers of personal-care treatments and remedies. In many cases, these natural products have been refined over time, and many are still in use today. A variety of medicinal plants, fruits and oils are used in modern natural cosmetic products with excellent results.

The good news is that it's never too late to start a beauty regimen that takes advantage of the infinite possibilities Mother Nature offers. It's time to let her pamper you.

Nature Is Your Ally

The natural world provides us with all sorts of ingredients for making facial masks, tonics, lotions, deodorants and beauty products that are a treat for the body. With these gifts from the Earth, we can nourish ourselves both inside and out.

Chemical-Free Alternatives Are on the Rise

The cosmetics industry has become highly profitable, and companies have become very successful by appealing to the vanity of both men and women. It seems like every day new beauty products appear on the market, promising eternal youth, permanent good looks and miraculous results. Unfortunately, many of these cosmetics contain chemicals, have been tested on animals and come in ultra-sophisticated packaging, all of which make them the opposite of beauty that's created in harmony with nature and other human beings. Many of these products also contain synthetic substances that can provoke allergic skin reactions.

In recent years, a trend toward nature-derived cosmetics and body-care products has emerged. Many companies are getting into this new market, which is great for consumers. However, you don't need to buy these treatments. You can create homemade beauty products from herbs, plants, oils and other natural ingredients that have been used throughout history.

By avoiding synthetic ingredients and chemical additives, you will protect your body's harmonic balance. Unlike industrial cosmetic products, natural cosmetics rarely cause allergic reactions or rashes, even on the most sensitive skin. In this book, you will find delightful recipes for making your own beauty and body-care products based on delectable (edible!) ingredients, such as cucumber, avocado, honey, fruit juices and more. These will be the base for many of the creams, facial masks and shampoos you will learn how to make.

Health Begins with Nutritious Food

Before you begin creating natural beauty products, there's one concept that's crucial to learn: eating right is vital for maintaining beauty through the years. When it comes to food, the most important thing to keep in mind is that quality, not quantity, counts. In this book, we will explore an integrated approach to eating that helps maintain beauty, and learn which vitamins, minerals and trace elements promote attractiveness and health. Remember: if you eat a healthy, balanced diet, your skin and your whole body will stay more youthful and fit.

Q: Other than diet, how can I improve my well-being?

A: Another element that is essential for good health and a radiant appearance is exercise. Regular physical activity improves circulation, eliminates toxins and helps tone the body by firming up the muscles and increasing flexibility. It is highly advisable to swim or take walks several times per week, because these two activities use almost every muscle in the body.

Rest is also closely related to physical beauty, although it is true that sleep is an individual matter; not everyone needs the same number of hours per night. Each person should get the amount of rest that's necessary to feel good and have adequate energy. Lack of sleep makes you feel tired and irritable, and it also shows on your face. The eyes become dull and lackluster, and bags can form beneath them.

The final element needed to create outer beauty is actually the most beneficial and necessary element the body depends on: clean, fresh air. Proper breathing, done deeply and evenly, stimulates circulation by increasing the flow of oxygen in the body. For this reason, it's important to make sure your house and workplace are well ventilated, and that the air you breathe is not too dry in winter, when buildings are heated.

Milestones in Natural Cosmetics

- **Ancient China.** The beginnings of natural cosmetics have been dated to more than 4,000 years ago. The *Shen Nung Pen Ts'ao Ching,* written around 2800 BCE by the legendary Chinese emperor Shen Nung, describes the medicinal properties of herbs and their use in body treatments.

- **Ancient Egypt.** The pharaohs of Ancient Egypt were mummified and buried with their belongings, which included perfumes, balms and cosmetics such as kohl, henna powder and eye shadow.

- **Roman Empire.** Baths became a part of daily life in Ancient Rome, and people began to use water-based perfumes scented with lavender, roses or marjoram. Milk baths were also customary. The use of soap did not begin until around 100 AD; until then, a mixture of oil and pumice had been used. After bathing, women whitened their faces with lead dust and chalk.

- **Middle Ages.** Cosmetics and caring for one's body were seen as sinful for European women in the Middle Ages; vanity was considered the mother of all vices. However, by the 15th century, women of the French court let go of their fears and objections, and the use of cosmetics began to spread throughout the courts of Europe. Women whitened their faces with lead powder, sulfur, boric acid, alabaster powder and starch mixed with egg white.

- **Age of Enlightenment.** In 1709, Eau de Cologne was invented and named for the famous city in Germany. A mixture of alcohol and citrus oils (including bergamot, lemon and orange), it is still sold today and has essentially the same composition. Its name, or simply cologne, is now used as a generic term in perfumery.

This book will also highlight a number of substances that are enemies of beauty. You'll learn why these substances — such as alcohol, coffee, certain fats, refined foods and excess animal protein — should be eliminated from your daily diet. By limiting or avoiding exposure to them, you can avoid building up the toxic, long-lasting residues they leave behind and the damage they cause to your body. You'll also discover information on nutrients that help purify the organs (such as the kidneys, liver, skin and lungs) and help them function properly. Detoxification can be an important first step toward enjoying a pleasingly healthy body.

Men Need to Take Care Too

Modern men have discovered that caring for their bodies is good for their health and their confidence. It can also keep them looking great as they age. Traditionally, men had no idea what type of skin they had or which shampoo worked best on their hair, but today, more and more men are interested in these issues and make the time to take care of their appearance.

Many men are still primarily concerned with the effects of daily shaving, because it can cause skin irritation. However, they are gradually becoming aware that aging, stress and external factors (such as ultraviolet light exposure and overly dry environments) can also rob their skin of moisture and elasticity, increasing its sensitivity. And while women have traditionally attended to them more, many of the problems that detract from beauty are not exclusive to females.

Women and men have different skin; therefore, they require different care. In general, men's skin produces more fat, so wrinkles tend to form later in life, but when they appear, they are deeper and more pronounced than women's wrinkles. Prevention is the best tool for men to keep their skin in good condition; this may mean following a shave with a massage. Men also have a more pronounced tendency to baldness, which requires special attention.

The recipes and beauty tips in this book will benefit men as much as they will women. Men will find treatments that can help solve, or at least soothe, many appearance-related problems. In these pages, they can find complete regimens to keep them looking healthy and attractive.

What Is True Beauty?

The natural beauty we talk about in this book has nothing to do with the beauty standards imposed on us by big companies selling cosmetics, perfumes and clothing. Their products promise to help us look like models or film stars, in a useless pursuit of the beauty laws laid down by movies and advertising. That is not natural beauty but rather a fleeting, superficial beauty based on the application of chemicals, which often produce more dissatisfaction and feelings of failure than improvement.

True physical beauty cannot be dissociated from inner beauty. By exercising, eating a nutritious diet, getting restful sleep and living a balanced life without excesses, you ensure you will remain beautiful, agile and mentally vigorous throughout your life. According to this rational, harmonious concept of beauty, the point at which youth ends and aging begins is not clearly defined. True beauty is ageless.

Love Yourself First

True beauty comes from within, not just by having a healthy body but also by having a balanced mind and a positive way of looking at life with optimism, joy and fulfillment. One key to that positive thinking is to learn to like yourself. The first step is to stop commenting on your bad points and focus on your good points. Start by appreciating what you like best about your body, and then extend your love to include the aspects that you don't like as much. By doing this, you learn to feel at ease with your body as it is, creating an image of yourself that you can love in spite of your perceived flaws.

Aging is, to some extent, a result of your state of mind and physical well-being. Many symptoms of it occur due to neglect, sometimes even a lifetime of neglect. In this book, you will find that what matters is not the physical beauty of youth. Rather, you will learn how you can improve your appearance and maintain a state of natural beauty regardless of age.

Clearly, adults won't be able to maintain the perfectly soft, smooth skin of a baby. But that is not the goal. A young person who neglects his or her skin, doesn't get enough sleep and eats poorly can have a dull, grayish complexion despite his or her youth. Meanwhile, an elderly person who eats a nutritious diet and cares for his or her skin by moisturizing and pampering it can have a beautiful appearance.

Treating Obesity

Obesity is a dangerous condition that negatively affects cardiovascular function. It can also be a barrier to feeling comfortable in your own body. Carrying excess weight erodes self-confidence for many people.

In cases of severe obesity, the best strategy is to consult with a specialist, who can help you find a diet and exercise program that best suits your metabolism. Once you have reached a healthy weight, it is important to keep in mind that permanent lifestyle changes, such as consistent exercise and substituting nutritious foods for junk foods, are the keys to maintaining it.

The Right Diet Is Key

If you want to lose weight, it's important to avoid overly strict or extreme diets. They initially help you drop weight, but can cause you to lose your good health along with the pounds. Drastic diets that forbid all but one or two foods are never recommended for long-term well-being. They can cause nutritional deficiencies and, besides being hazardous to your health, simply don't work. Your body gets used to the restrictiveness. Then, when you return to normal, healthy eating, you quickly and easily regain the weight that you lost through such miserable sacrifice.

Practically All Diets Are Aging

It's ironic. We go on diets motivated by the desire to look younger and more beautiful, but instead, we age faster. Crash diets add years to our appearance in a short time. This is because we don't understand our cells' metabolic processes.

The body can burn different forms of fuel to give energy to your muscles and organs. Generally, it uses up glucose (a readily available form of sugar in carbohydrates) first, then glycogen (a stored form of sugar present in the liver), then fat. Early on in a diet, the weight you lose consists almost entirely of water and glycogen. Your body thinks you have fallen on hard times, and holds on to the cells in your fatty tissue as a reserve against further deprivation. Before burning fat, it will use up the glycogen stored in your liver and any stored protein in your body. That's why the first fat molecules do not start burning off until about the second week of a diet. As a result of this starvation mode, the metabolism becomes keener than ever to replenish the body's depleted reserves; the slightest slip — an extra snack or a cookie — speeds through the digestive tract and the bloodstream and is converted straight into fat.

Q: **Why are most weight-loss diets harmful to health and beauty?**

A: Most diet plans are based on caloric reduction and limiting or eliminating certain foods. Many popular ones are based on eating excessive amounts of protein or eating insufficient amounts of fat, which can result in blood acidification and the accumulation of toxins in the body. These diets are not nutritionally balanced, and this imbalance is the enemy of beauty. It promotes disease and aging, because cells cannot cope with attacks by free radicals. This situation is further aggravated by the absence of certain essential fatty acids and vitamin E, minerals and other elements that help strengthen cells against these attacks. Plus, an overload of toxins can contribute to the formation of cellulite.

So what's the solution? Restrict calories gently, by eating sensibly and naturally every day rather than ruling out whole groups of foods. Consume a wide variety of whole, organic foods in reasonable amounts: fruits, vegetables, whole grains and grain products (such as breads and pastas), fresh cheeses and tofu.

Eating Well Is Better than Dieting

Virtually all of today's popular diets are quite far from the original concept of diet; the word comes from the Middle English *diete*, meaning "manner of living." Some are the opposite of this principle of balanced living. Eating should be a pleasure — to the eyes, the nose and the palate — that lasts your whole life. When you finish a meal, you should feel full and satisfied. Food should also provide you with energy and enable your body to replace damaged or aged cells.

Q: Why do most diets fail?

A: Fortunately, failing a diet is actually a good thing, nutritionally and psychologically speaking. There are a number of reasons people can stay on diets only so long:

- **Lack of variety.** Some diets omit higher-calorie, nutritionally important foods, such as nuts. Others recommend consuming excessive protein in order to restrict calories from carbohydrates. But the human body (and the cells within it) needs certain vital substances in these foods that it cannot manufacture itself. Missing out on these foods means missing out on these nutrients as well.

- **Mental anguish.** Leaving the table still hungry causes an unpleasant feeling of deprivation. You feel starved all the time. This feeling of negativity and prohibition makes you able to maintain the diet only temporarily. Eating, rather than being a pleasant and satisfying activity, becomes a daily source of trauma.

- **Cravings.** The body needs certain nutrients in tiny amounts (measured in milligrams or even micrograms): for example, vitamins, essential fatty acids and trace elements. It is not unusual for the daily food intake on a restrictive diet to lack the required amounts of these substances. As cells become malnourished, their membranes weaken and let in free radicals or attacking viruses. When you lack these substances, your survival instinct kicks in, in the form of cravings, which result in the desire to eat more. This leads to a vicious circle: the body lacks the necessary vital substances, which leads to increased hunger, which leads to increased eating of food without these substances, which leads to increased feelings of deprivation and hunger.

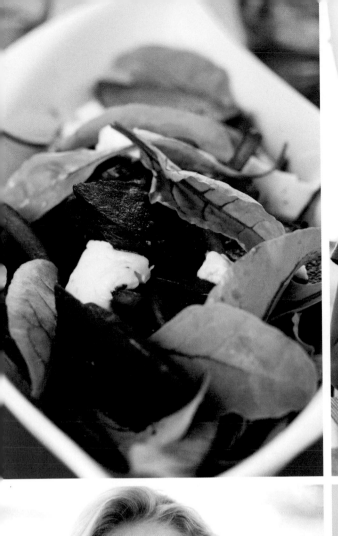
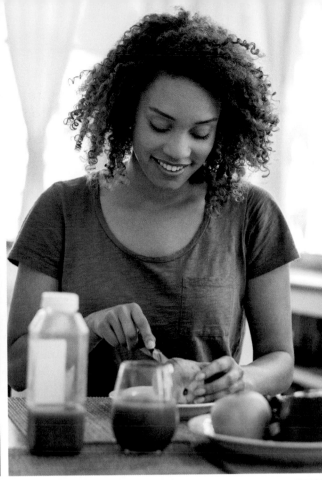
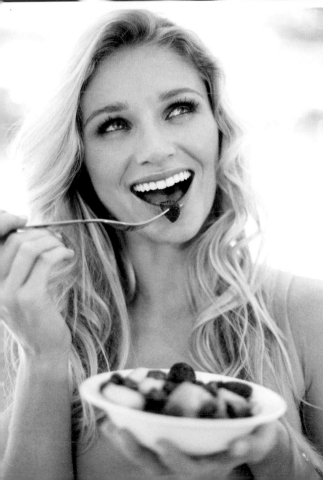
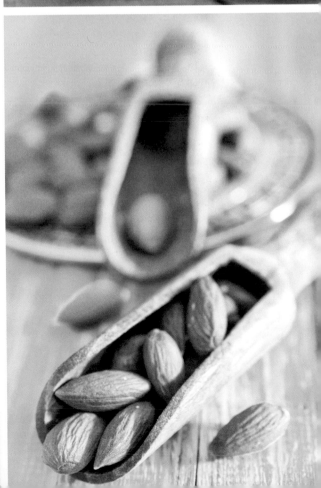

Why Calories Can Be Misleading

It is a serious mistake to judge the value of a food only in terms of its calorie content. Why? Calories aren't always absorbed the same way. Logically, according to calorie charts, it should be more fattening to eat an apple and a piece of chocolate cake than to eat just the cake; the combination contains more calories. However, in reality, it is more fattening to eat the cake alone because the fiber in the apple slows down the absorption of the carbohydrates and fats in the cake. This keeps glucose in the blood from spiking as quickly and decreases the amount of fat the body will store as it digests these foods.

If you learn to eat in a balanced way, your relationship with food will flourish. You do not need to suffer through any unpleasant feelings. Highly restrictive diets act against your best interest, whereas your healthy, natural instincts will help you make good choices in terms of the quality, quantity and combination of foods you eat.

Nine Rules for Healthy Eating

Here are nine guidelines that promote smart eating and help you maintain a lean, well-nourished body:

1. **Drink water or fresh fruit juice half an hour before each meal.** Doing this means you'll start off feeling fuller, which helps you to eat more slowly. In addition, drinking sufficient liquid is important for proper intestinal and kidney function, which are essential for maintaining a healthy weight and body. Taking a tablet of spirulina (see page 24) along with your glass of water will further increase the feeling of fullness and satiety.

2. **Chew thoroughly and savor every bite.** This is essential for both good digestion and for weight loss and maintenance. It helps in a number of ways. First, chewing well allows you to appreciate the flavors of your food better. Your taste buds will fully experience the freshness and the subtle contrasts that each ingredient lends to a dish. You will begin to appreciate new flavors and textures, and eventually, you will not want to eat highly processed foods anymore.
   Second, chewing promotes good digestion by breaking down foods so that their nutrients can be absorbed properly in the gut. Digestion

actually begins in the mouth for carbohydrates. By thoroughly mixing foods with enzyme-containing saliva, you ensure that important nutrients are released from breads, pastas and other grain-based foods.

Third, chewing food thoroughly helps prevent compulsive or rapid eating. By slowing down and taking your time with each bite, you will feel full and stop before you've had the chance to overeat.

3. **Eat a nutritious breakfast.** A balanced breakfast of fruit, whole-grain bread or oatmeal, and dairy or soy milk will provide a stable source of energy to fuel your body throughout the morning — and that's just what you need to do your normal daily activities.

A breakfast of coffee and refined carbs (such as white bread or a pastry) won't do that. If you consume these, by midmorning you will feel the classic energy slump and increased appetite that follow a less-nutritious breakfast. The reason is simple: refined carbohydrates are rapidly broken down, making them an explosive calorie bomb. Not long after you eat these foods, they release a large number of glucose molecules into your bloodstream, flooding your body with energy it can't use all at once (see box, page 18). Any extra glucose your body can't use is stored as fat. After that, the glucose level drops swiftly, robbing you of energy.

4. **Eat healthy snacks if you feel hungry between meals.** If you are truly hungry and it is still too early for lunch or dinner, it is a good idea to eat a healthy snack to keep you going. If you don't, you might find yourself ravenous at mealtime and prone to overeating (or eating too fast). By sitting down to a meal when you're not starving, you will be more selective about what you eat.

Replace Sugar...Gradually

Avoid using refined sugar to make homemade baked goods or to sweeten tea or yogurt. Start by switching to brown sugar, and then substitute honey for it once you get used to the taste. There are many types of honey made from the nectar of different flowers, and each has a unique flavor and consistency that your palate will learn to appreciate. Always choose raw, unfiltered honey. For variety, try maple syrup, grain-based syrup (such as brown rice syrup, sorghum syrup or malt syrup), molasses or apple concentrate. In baking or muesli, try adding dried fruit, such as raisins, apricots or figs.

When you have a snack, make sure it is easy to digest and gives you something satisfying to chew on. Some good snacks are fruit and yogurt, whole-grain cookies or crackers (made with grain-based sweeteners or, better yet, without added sugar), or whole-grain toast topped with grilled tofu or unsweetened nut butter.

5. **Replace cereals, white flour and refined sugar with organic whole-grain foods, honey, molasses and grain-based syrups.** Grains contain nutrients and vital elements that are mostly lost during the refining process. These include the germ (the protein-rich part of the grain kernel), vitamins (especially B and E), minerals (such as magnesium) and trace elements (such as selenium), which are very important for health.

   In addition, whole grains provide dietary fiber, which helps food move along the intestinal tract and prevents stagnation of toxins. Whole grains are also more satisfying and filling, making it easier to control the amount of food you eat. Another important effect is that they decrease the assimilation of fat molecules, absorb fat (and cholesterol in the case of soluble fiber) and slow down the absorption of sugars and refined carbohydrates in the intestines.

Why Sugar Causes Energy Spikes

Easily digestible carbohydrates, such as white bread, pastries or refined sugar, initially supply the body with a quick jolt of energy. Nature invented the glucose molecule as an emergency vehicle for energy transport. The intestines break it down quickly from refined sugar and refined grains and send it into the bloodstream right away, spiking your blood glucose level. At the same time, the pancreas releases large amounts of insulin into the bloodstream; this hormone helps cells use sugar to generate quick energy or convert it into glycogen for longer storage.

Once the insulin has taken care of all that glucose, your blood sugar level quickly falls. So that means you get a quick boost from a sugary breakfast only to have the bottom drop out an hour later. At this point, your energy level decreases rapidly, triggering sleepiness, hunger or even dizziness in some cases.

When you replace refined carbohydrates with whole fruits and whole grains, you combat this roller coaster. Whole grains are full of slow-burning carbohydrates; they offer a stable source of energy and consistent blood sugar levels.

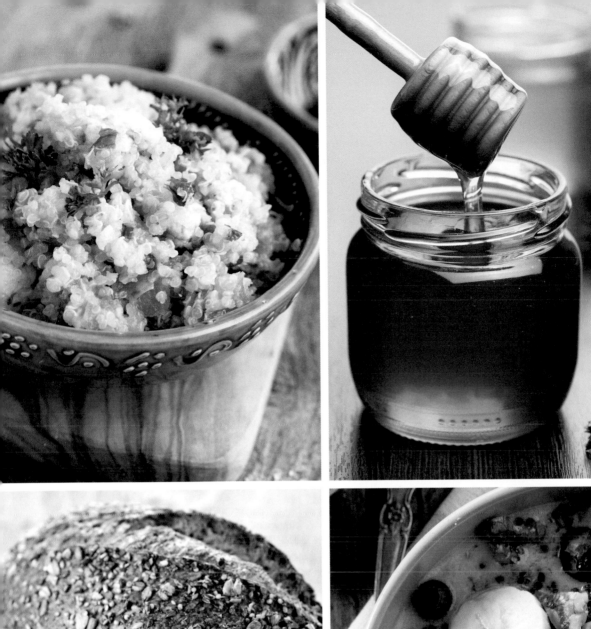
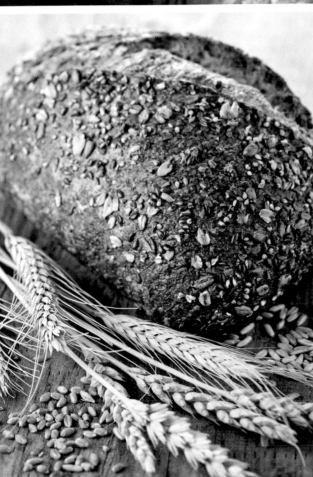
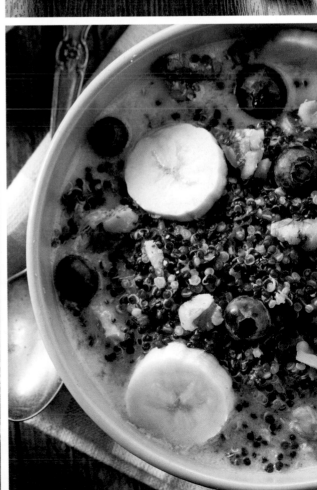

Naturally Sweet

People who love sweets often feel frustrated at the idea of eating well because they think sweet treats are not allowed. But there is good news: you can indulge in natural, good-quality foods that satisfy your cravings.

When you have a strong desire for cookies or candies, try organic cereal bars made with whole grains. Other good choices are cookies made with whole-grain flour, or carob bars (the perfect substitute for chocolate). Look for these in natural food stores.

Another piece of good news is that by including more fresh, whole foods in your diet — even if you introduce them gradually — your cravings and "need" for sweet foods will diminish naturally without any effort. Once you begin to appreciate the natural sweetness of foods that have not been devitalized, you will come to love their varied, more delicate flavors. After a while, a cake that once looked and tasted delicious will lose its appeal and taste cloyingly sweet. This is how your tastes can evolve in a healthier direction.

6. **Start meals with raw fruit or a hearty salad.** Raw foods are the ideal way to start a meal because they contain digestive enzymes, which are inactivated when foods are cooked. What's more, within minutes of your eating raw foods, a bevy of essential vitamins and minerals will reach your bloodstream. The richer in vital substances a food is, the greater the amount of energy generated in the cells, making you feel fresher, more alive and younger.

Salads and fruits have a stimulating and purifying effect on the body too, because they alkalize the blood and neutralize toxins. They are rich in vital elements, such as enzymes, vitamins, minerals and antioxidants, that promote cell metabolism and strengthen the body's defenses. These raw foods also contain fiber and water, which reduce intestinal absorption of subsequent, fattier courses of a meal. This helps reduce the impact of high-fat or high-carbohydrate foods. Salads and fruits also promote regularity.

Raw foods have more substance than cooked foods, so you have to chew them well, which increases salivation. They help you avoid the temptation to gulp your food quickly or to keep eating after you feel full. In contrast, cooked foods can be too easy to chew and swallow, leading you to eat more than you need.

For all these reasons, raw foods help awaken the natural instincts that signal when you truly *need* food. Once you try some raw recipes, you'll realize how rich and varied their tastes are, and you'll benefit from their superior nutritional content.

7. Avoid fried foods and animal fats. Completely eliminating fat from your diet in the hope that it will lead to weight loss is a serious mistake. Fortunately, there is no food that is totally fat free (even fruits contain a small amount) because fats are essential for the absorption of fat-soluble vitamins (vitamins that dissolve in fat), such as vitamins A, D and E. In addition, fats provide essential fatty acids, which are necessary for a number of vital processes, including protecting cell membranes (by keeping their viscosity at the right level in order to provide resistance, flexibility and permeability) and ensuring proper brain and nervous system function.

Instead of eliminating fats completely, choose the most beneficial ones. The good fats — cold-pressed plant oils made from seeds and nuts — are essential for good health. Bad fats — saturated and animal fats and deep-fried foods — have been linked to higher blood viscosity, which can impede healthy circulation.

Over the course of the last century, fat consumption (especially from animal sources) has increased while physical activity levels have decreased significantly. Plus, homes in the developed world are warmer and more comfortable than ever, so their residents don't burn as much body fat for thermoregulation. This delicately balanced body mechanism keeps a person's core temperature stable at about 98.6°F (37°C), and you need to burn more fat when the outside temperature is cold to keep it in the correct range.

The best plan: don't overdo it on fats. You can cover your daily needs by eating some salad dressing made with good-quality olive oil and a few nuts (or some fresh cheese or an egg). If you eat too much fat, too much refined sugar and too many refined carbohydrates (such as white pasta, bread and rice), you put too much stress on your liver, which makes it produce large amounts of lipoproteins and cholesterol. In fact, excess fat can come both from eating fatty foods, and from the accumulation of triglycerides synthesized by the liver itself due to excessive consumption of carbohydrates.

Educate Your Palate

You can train yourself to like whole, natural foods. They have different, more subtle flavors, but they are more varied and rewarding than the concentrated, single-note tastes of refined sugar, refined flour or artificial flavorings. It just takes time to get used to them. As you practice, your food preferences and choices will change.

Why You Need Fats

You need fat in your diet to counteract dry skin and hair and to help you use fat-soluble vitamins. People with oily skin or hair should limit their fat intake but not eliminate fats completely; they are vital for maintaining healthy skin and cell structures.

8. **Reduce your animal protein consumption.** Many popular diets tell you to reduce or eliminate bread and pasta, and increase your consumption of red meat and cheese. This myth needs to be debunked.

   There's no guarantee that eating large amounts of protein won't make you gain weight. The body needs a set amount of protein (or rather its building blocks, called amino acids), to construct tissue and to replace aged or damaged cells and tissues. The average adult needs 0.5 to 1 g of protein per each 2.2 lbs (1 kg) of body weight per day. Where you fall in that range depends on your eating habits and your body's ability to use the nutritional content of food.

   Typically, the body uses protein for building and uses sugars and fats for energy production. When you eat more protein than you need, especially when you're consuming few carbohydrates and perhaps few fats, the body can transform excess protein into energy as well. It adapts to this "emergency" situation but at a certain cost: metabolizing protein produces waste products. Excess waste turns into toxins, which become a serious burden on certain organs, especially the kidneys. This is why it is important to consume sufficient carbohydrates. It will ensure the proper metabolism of the protein in your food, and will create the energy your body needs to feed your muscles, nervous system and brain.

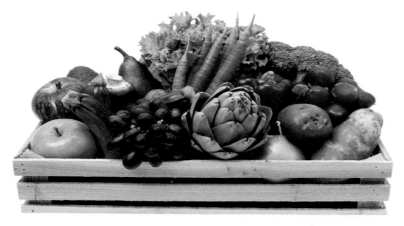

9. **Combine dishes appropriately.** Eating the right foods is great, but eating them to ensure optimal digestion is even smarter. By combining them in specific ways, you can help aid digestion. Each type of nutrient requires a different enzyme, and each enzyme works best in a particular environment.

Starches or carbohydrates — such as potatoes, bananas, bread, grains and pasta — need a slightly alkaline environment for digestion (the enzymes for these foods are secreted in the salivary glands and pancreas). This makes them incompatible with, for example, acidic fruits, which kill the effectiveness of these enzymes.

Proteins — such as cheese, tofu or meat — require an acidic environment for digestion (the enzyme for this, called pepsin, is produced in the stomach). It makes sense to combine cheese with an acidic fruit but not with something sweet, which creates an alkaline environment that destroys pepsin.

Fats can be combined with carbohydrates or proteins. However, people with a tendency to gain weight easily should not eat carbohydrates in the same meal with fats. It is also important not to eat something sweet after a meal that contains fat. The glucose in the sweet food is absorbed quickly, and encourages the body to store the fat in rich, high-calorie foods, which are digested more slowly. It is best to combine high-fat foods with vegetables.

Remember not to overdo it with any single category. Avoid eating two different carbohydrate foods (such as rice and potatoes) in the same meal or two different proteins (such as soy and cheese).

Cooking with Less Fat

Try grilling, or cook foods in a nonstick skillet, substituting water (or vegetable cooking water) for butter or oil. Fats that are high in omega-3 fatty acids are transformed by heat and can encourage free radical attacks in the body, so save these for cold dishes. For lunch or dinner, eat a salad and/or vegetables with an oil dressing. Add seasonings but avoid prepared condiments. Keep it simple: try a mix of good cold-pressed extra-virgin olive oil, a pinch of sea salt, a little lemon juice or cider vinegar, and some fragrant, fresh herbs.

Healthy Weight-Loss Aids

There are lots of weight-loss aids out there. The good news is that there are some natural ones that can help build good health from the inside:

- **Natural, plant-based dietary supplements** are not weight-loss formulas but rather superfood extracts that help regulate metabolism. The ingredients "swell" in the stomach when taken with water and help create a sensation of fullness. If you take them half an hour before each meal, they will dull your hunger and discourage you from eating compulsively. If you feel dizzy or light-headed after changing your diet, that could signal a nutritional deficiency. These substances are rich in vitamins and minerals and can help your body achieve an optimal balance.

- **Korean ginseng** (*Panax ginseng*), like Siberian ginseng (*Eleutherococcus senticosus*) and garlic, helps tonify the body and boosts concentration and immune defenses. Korean ginseng also increases physical endurance, promotes antibody production and increases glucose tolerance.

- **Spirulina** is a blue-green algae that stimulates elimination of stored fat. It contains iodine, which has a stimulating effect on the thyroid gland, increasing the production of thyroxine, which induces cells to burn fat (in effect, it is the spark that ignites fat combustion, stepping up metabolism and energy expenditure). This algae is considered one of the richest, most complete food sources in nature: it offers about 60 g of protein per $3\frac{1}{3}$ oz (100 g), as well as vitamins, minerals, chlorophyll, enzymes and antioxidants. Moreover, taken before meals with plenty of water, it can curb your appetite. You can find spirulina powder in health food stores; if you don't like its strong taste, it's also available in pill form.

- **Glucomannan** is a fiber extracted from the konjac plant (*Amorphophallus konjac*), which grows in Asia. It expands when it comes into contact with water, absorbing as much as 200 times its dry weight. Using it regularly can help create a feeling of fullness and satisfaction, which keeps you from overeating. Taking about 1 g dissolved in a glass of water half an hour before sitting down to a meal is recommended for most people, but consult your doctor or naturopath to find your optimal dosage.

Beauty and Health Come from Within

You won't find these two in salons, but you will find them if you have a healthy diet and lifestyle. By learning how cell metabolism functions, you can adapt your dietary choices to recapture and preserve your natural beauty. When your cells receive all the nutrients they need (that is, when the blood that supplies them is rich in vital substances), you'll radiate energy and look youthful and healthy. A blood supply rich in nutrients is a fountain of youth and health for cells.

When you eat poorly and lead a chaotic life with abundant stress, your blood tends to lack most of the essential bioactive substances that your cells need. Refined foods don't contain these vital components; they contribute only calories, acidify the blood and steal minerals, leaving blood with as little as 8 to 15% of the optimum amounts of magnesium, calcium, copper, chromium, phosphorus and sulfur it should have, as well as reduced levels of certain vitamins and fatty acids. This makes the blood excessively acidic and toxic. As a result, cell membranes and the immune system become increasingly weak, allowing bacteria, viruses, fungi, toxins, pollutants and free radicals to invade and do serious damage.

The best way to rejuvenate your cells isn't with injections or treatments. Refresh them with vitamins consumed in whole grains, salads, fruits, tofu and nuts. The richer in nutrients your diet is, the more energy your cells will generate, and the fresher, more vital and younger you will feel.

Keep Your Cells Young

Of course, eating well can help you achieve an optimal weight and shape. It can also give you smooth, silky skin; thick, shiny hair; lively eyes; and sparkling teeth. Thanks to modern testing equipment, biochemists and researchers have been able to study cell metabolism in detail, even observing it directly. It may seem incredible, but some scientists say that a 50-year-old can indeed look 30.

What's incredible is that the body does not age as a whole; rather, its individual cells (all 70 billion of them!) do. This happens when you fail to protect them against the effects of free radicals and other pathogens, and do not feed them properly. When you learn to nourish your cells — by making sure the blood that feeds them is rich in bioactive vitamins, minerals, trace elements, carbohydrates, proteins, fatty acids and water — your whole body will age much more slowly.

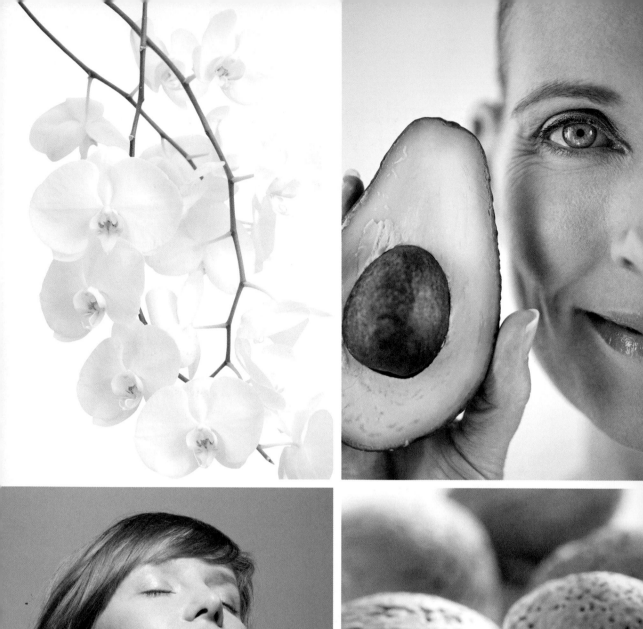

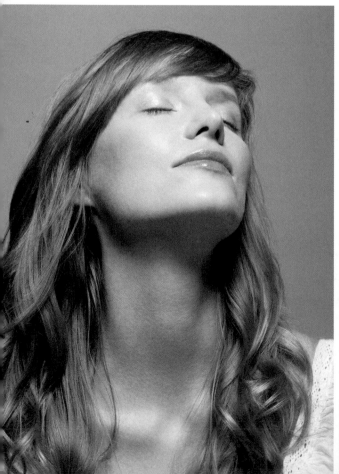

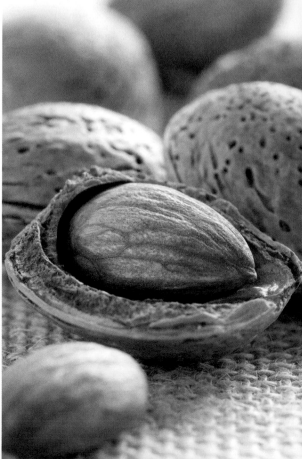

Beauty's Friends and Enemies

If your goal is to stay radiant throughout the years, good health is your best ally. And the most natural way to achieve good health is to eat a proper, balanced diet. Let the nutrients and vitamins that are your friends care for your body and defend it from its enemies.

Vitamins and Minerals for Beauty

Of all the nutrients in food, it is vitamins and minerals that work most actively to maintain your physical condition. Vitamins are essential for metabolism to work properly. They do not build tissue or provide energy; rather, they are catalysts for vital processes in the body.

In addition to vitamins, minerals — especially calcium, iron, copper, zinc, magnesium and selenium — are another important group of components that are involved in the body's growth and functions. Mineral deficiencies can cause brittle bones, anemia and heart disease, among other conditions. Let's look at what role each nutrient plays in making your body beautiful.

Teamwork Is Crucial

Vitamins and minerals are micronutrients, or nutrients that exist in very small quantities. Trace elements are simply minerals needed in minuscule amounts. Minerals and trace elements work in tandem with vitamins, and some have no effect when their vitamin partners are not present.

Vitamin A

Vitamin A plays an important role in nourishing the hair and skin, by increasing the stability of cell wall tissue. This helps prevent premature aging and contributes to better oxygenation of body tissues. Vitamin A also has an important role in epidermis cell differentiation and regulates epithelial tissues.

Without vitamin A, the skin becomes dry and brittle. Vitamin A deficiency can also be a cause of brittle nails and hair. Moreover, this micronutrient is essential for vision; a lack of it can cause twilight blindness, also called night blindness (poor vision after dark or in low light). Vitamin A also strengthens the immune system, so a deficiency can increase your risk of infections, such as measles. It can also cause dry eyes and corneal ulcers.

One note of caution: too much vitamin A isn't good for you either. Excessive amounts can be harmful to the hair and skin, causing dry skin, inflammation of the hair follicles and hair loss. You can get what you need easily from natural sources in your diet. Vitamin A is abundant in yellow, orange and dark green fruits and vegetables, such as sweet potatoes, pumpkins, carrots, Swiss chard, spinach, apricots, cantaloupe and kale; and goat cheese, eggs and milk.

B Vitamins

This group of vitamins is the most important for beautiful skin and hair. They help your body produce energy, maintain its reserves and keep the nervous system healthy. They contribute to the prevention of premature aging, and help regulate skin secretions, which are vital for the maintenance of healthy hair and skin. The B complex consists of a number of different vitamins, including thiamine (B_1), riboflavin (B_2), niacin (B_3), pyridoxine (B_6), cyanocobalamin (B_{12}) and folate. Foods rich in B vitamins are helpful for fighting stress, which has a very harmful effect on the appearance.

Good Nutrition: The Pathway to Beauty

Just as diet and health are closely related, so are diet and beauty. The appearance of your skin, hair and nails reveals your overall health and dietary deficiencies. In many cases, nails that break easily or fragile, thinning hair are the result of a diet low in B vitamins.

Poor eating habits detract not only from your physical well-being but also from your appearance. It's worth noting that many diseases, including some skin conditions, arise due to chronic constipation, which contributes to digestive disorders and a continuous self-poisoning that results in skin and face problems.

Eating a diet rich in whole foods and raw, fresh vegetables and fruits will help you stay healthy and maintain your natural beauty for the long term. Unless you have celiac disease or an allergy that prevents you from consuming it, whole wheat should always be a part of your diet because it is rich in vitamins, protein, unsaturated fats and fiber. Consume other whole grains as well, as they also contain an abundance of vitamins and minerals.

The Bs You Need

Each of the B vitamins plays a unique role in your physical well-being and appearance. Here is a little more about some of the key players:

- **Vitamin B_1 (thiamine).** This vitamin makes an essential contribution to your metabolism by helping your body unlock the energy in food. By enabling you to metabolize carbohydrates and proteins, vitamin B_1 keeps the brain, heart and nervous system in good condition. A deficiency can lead to weakness, fatigue, headaches and nausea. A severe deficiency causes beriberi, a disease that is characterized by confusion, fluid buildup in the lungs and nerve damage. Fortunately, many common foods are excellent sources of this vitamin, including brewer's yeast and yeast extract, wheat germ, fortified whole-grain products, legumes and soy products.

- **Vitamin B_2 (riboflavin).** This is one of the vitamins responsible for maintaining healthy skin, and it aids in the production of other B vitamins. Vitamin B_2 helps metabolize carbohydrates, proteins and fats. It has been linked with potentially reducing the risk of esophageal cancer too. Deficiency can result in sore throats, cracks at the corner of the mouth, anemia and seborrheic dermatitis (an uncomfortable, itchy condition of the skin, often on the scalp). Some natural sources of vitamin B_2 are milk and dairy products, eggs, mushrooms, spinach, broccoli, brewer's yeast or yeast extract, and whole grains.

- **Vitamin B_3 (niacin).** This vitamin plays a large role in keeping the digestive system, nervous system and especially the skin functioning properly. Some of the conditions caused by a vitamin B_3 deficiency include indigestion, vomiting, tiredness and canker sores in the mouth. A serious deficiency causes the condition pellagra; symptoms include a burning sensation in the mouth, redness of the tongue, cracked skin and diarrhea. High doses of this vitamin in supplement form aren't necessary and shouldn't be taken without consulting your doctor. It's easy to eat enough vitamin B_3 in your diet: healthy sources include brewer's yeast and yeast extract, portobello mushrooms, potatoes, fortified whole-grain products, soy foods, legumes, peanuts, almonds and sunflower seeds.

- **Vitamin B_6 (pyridoxine).** The body needs vitamin B_6 to be able to create and use proteins, make red blood cells and ensure proper nervous and immune system function. It's also a key player in keeping skin and hair healthy. Consumption of sufficient amounts of this vitamin has been linked to reducing asthma symptoms and lowering the risk of cardiovascular disease, but more studies are needed to confirm this. A vitamin B_6 deficiency can cause rashes, itchy and/or cracked skin, a swollen tongue, muscle weakness, irritability, reduced ability to concentrate and depression. Again, it's easy to get what you need of this vitamin from food sources such as potatoes, bananas, brewer's yeast and yeast extract, wheat bran, chickpeas and pistachios.

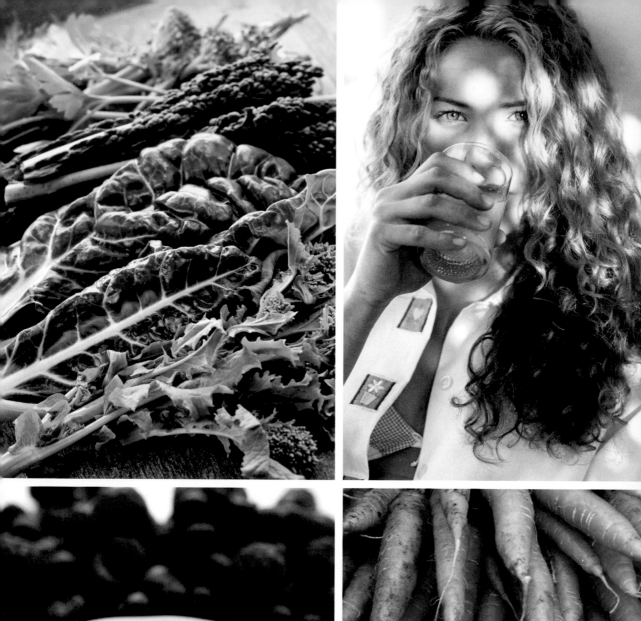
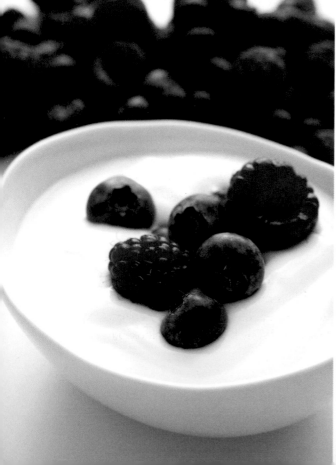
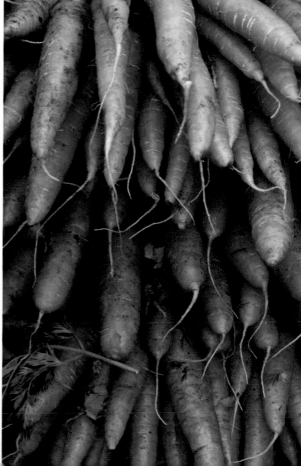

Deficiencies in the B complex vitamins can cause a number of appearance-related problems, including oily hair, dandruff, dry skin, redness and irritation, wrinkles and poor hair growth. To get B vitamins from your diet, make sure to eat a wide variety of whole foods, such as brewer's yeast, whole grains, nuts and seeds. For more details on specific B vitamins, see box, page 29.

Vitamin C

Also called ascorbic acid, this is perhaps the most important vitamin for healthy skin, because it helps purify and revitalize the blood and is very important for the formation of collagen. Among other things, vitamin C keeps tissues healthy, aids in healing and strengthens the body's resistance to disease. It also contributes to healthy blood circulation and oxygen use, and its antioxidant properties help it defend the body against aging.

A severe deficiency can result in a condition called scurvy, which is characterized by bleeding, swollen gums; tooth loss; scaly skin; muscle weakness; and brittle nails. This is rare, since many common foods contain vitamin C. The vegetables and fruits that provide the most are cabbage, broccoli, bell peppers (especially red ones), leafy greens, guava, papaya, kiwifruit, citrus fruits, cherries, pineapple, cantaloupe and strawberries.

Vitamin D

Vitamin D is known primarily for its role in the formation and maintenance of healthy bones and teeth; it helps the body absorb calcium and phosphorus, ensuring the proper development of these structures. A diet low in vitamin D can lead to tooth decay and bone problems. Vitamin D is found naturally in egg yolks, and is present in milk and butter that have been fortified. It is also produced by the skin when it is exposed to direct sunlight; this is why it's often called "the sunshine vitamin."

Vitamin E

Lately, vitamin E has garnered a reputation for defeating the effects of time. It is closely related to beauty, and is commonly used to heal scar tissue and reduce wrinkles, thanks to its antioxidant action. It also helps prevent skin dryness, age spots and dandruff. For healthy, good-looking skin, eating foods high in vitamin E is a must. Wheat germ is particularly rich in it, and it is also found in spinach, dandelion greens, turnip greens and cooked red bell peppers. Wheat germ oil, sunflower oil, safflower oil and oils made from other whole grains and nuts are other sources of vitamin E.

To heal abrasions or reduce the look of scars, you can use vitamin E topically. Simply pierce a supplement capsule and rub the oil over the skin.

Zinc

A mineral closely related to skin beauty, zinc plays an important role in preventing and treating acne. There is also anecdotal evidence that zinc can help prevent baldness. Zinc is used by the bones, hair and skin. It also aids in blood clotting and strengthens the immune system. You need only a small amount of this mineral, so dietary sources are sufficient. Some healthy sources are wheat germ, raw green pumpkin seeds (pepitas), sunflower seeds, brewer's yeast, milk and eggs.

Sulfur

When it comes to minerals that make you attractive, sulfur holds a top spot. Often called "the beauty mineral," it is essential for healthy hair, nails and skin. Hair contains a large amount of sulfur, upwards of 4%. Its task in the hair is to ensure that keratin fibers cohere, increasing strength and promoting growth. A sulfur deficiency increases the probability that hair will turn gray. Overuse of certain chemicals, such as hair permanent solutions, ammonia or hydrogen peroxide, depletes the sulfur in the hair. Vegetables such as radishes, onions, Brussels sprouts, celery and watercress contain a considerable amount of sulfur and can replenish your reserves.

Iodine

Iodine promotes physical and mental energy and helps the body synthesize thyroid hormones. It can also be used externally as an antiseptic. Eating foods rich in iodine helps prevent wrinkles and rough skin and keeps your thyroid functioning normally. Some good natural sources of iodine are seaweed, lima beans, garlic, green peas, soybeans, milk and dairy products, eggs and legumes.

Copper

Besides sulfur, iodine and zinc, tiny amounts of copper are essential in the diet. This micronutrient keeps hair healthy and helps preserve its natural color. Copper is an important trace element for iron absorption. It also acts as a catalyst in the early stages of red blood cell formation and assists in the production of melanin (natural skin pigment). You can consume sufficient copper in healthy, natural foods such as whole grains, nuts, legumes and leafy dark green vegetables.

Silica

Like copper, silica is linked to healthy hair growth, and is often recommended to strengthen skin and nails. It is important for skin cell metabolism and has a protective effect on connective tissue. Green beans and bananas are two widely available foods that contain easily absorbable silica.

How Fasting Can Boost Beauty

If you have never fasted before, this concept might sound challenging. You might worry about being very hungry and uncomfortable. But the truth is that anyone who has tried fasting knows that after a couple of days, hunger disappears completely and you feel light. And feeling better inside leads to looking better outside.

You will probably lose some weight during a period of fasting, but that's not the true purpose of this undertaking. Rather, fasting is a respite for the body, allowing it to take a break from the continuous process of building new tissues using nutrients in food. In addition, fasting helps cleanse your insides of metabolic wastes and toxins ingested with foods. One way fasting helps is that it removes excess protein accumulated in the smallest blood vessels, which can result from overconsumption. When you fast, this buildup is removed more quickly via the kidneys.

Fasting — under the supervision of a medical professional — can also be an excellent therapeutic treatment for people who suffer from obesity, diabetes, rheumatism, gout, early heart attacks, allergies and acne; poor diet is often one of the factors in developing these conditions. Fasting is also a way to purify the spirit. As you go without food, thoughts — both pleasant and unpleasant — can be put in perspective. As a result, you may find it easier to acknowledge repressed feelings. Fasting can bring you one step closer to inner balance.

Apart from the beneficial effects it has on body and mind, fasting is an excellent beauty treatment. At first, fluid loss causes the skin to appear loose, and blemishes may also appear as toxins are eliminated. Soon, however, tissues firm up again, and the complexion becomes clear and radiant. Fasting helps get the body into shape by giving it a few days to eliminate contaminants, thereby renewing strength and energy.

Tips for Healthy Fasting

Your first fast should not last more than a week; when you have more experience, you can fast for up to three weeks. It is best to schedule your fast when you're on vacation or able to indulge in a period of rest or low activity and focus on yourself. You can spend some of the time walking, reading or meditating.

Drink plenty of water throughout the fast: 8 to 12 cups (2 to 3 L) per day is enough. When the fasting period ends, you have to restore your digestive juices slowly and gradually, so let your body get reacquainted with food little by little. Eat small, easy-to-digest meals and take it slow.

Types of Fasts

There are several different ways to fast. It's easy to design a plan tailored to your needs, your goals and the amount of time you have. As with all dietary regimens, it's a good idea to consult with your doctor or naturopath before you start.

Complete Fast

The strictest type of fasting is to abstain from food completely. For this fast, drink 8 to 12 cups (2 to 3 L) of water or unsweetened herbal teas daily, and do not eat any solid food. If you like, you can replace the water with unsweetened, natural fruit juices. Drinking unsalted vegetable broth five times a day is also an ideal component of a healing, purifying, fasting diet. If you can't go without any solids, substitute some plain, warm, cooked vegetables or oatmeal porridge for some of the liquid. Divide these foods into small portions and eat them periodically during the day.

Weekly One-Day Detox

If you lead a fast-paced life, it may be difficult to do a complete fast for a week or more, but there is an alternative: a once-a-week one-day detox. Try one of the options in the boxes below and on page 37, spending a full day eating a single type of food rich in vital substances. This will give your digestive system a considerable rest from its usual routine. Plus, vital foods have detoxifying properties that help cells regenerate and rid the body of impurities.

Fruits and vegetables are excellent tonics that alkalize and clean the blood. Germinated sprouts are also a rich source of vital and detoxifying substances; eat them often. Infusions of nettle, dandelion, thyme and yarrow have an excellent cleansing effect as well.

Wild plants with purifying properties, including nettle, dandelion and purslane, are particularly abundant in spring. This is no coincidence: this is when we especially need to rid ourselves of the toxins that have accumulated over the winter. Pick the tender leaves of these plants, add them to your salads and dress them with good-quality cold-pressed vegetable oil. Their slightly spicy and/or sour flavors add a subtle contrast to the usual greens. They are delicious, and many chefs have rediscovered these humble wild plants and made them stars in their standout dishes.

Fruit-Based One-Day Detox

This is a simple detox plan: just eat a single type of fruit all day. At the height of cherry season, this is no hardship for many people! Peaches also lend themselves deliciously to an all-fruit day, especially if they are local and freshly picked. During the autumn apple season (not the rest of the year, when apples come out of long-term cold storage), alternate fresh apples, cooked apples and freshly squeezed apple juice. A day of only grapes is popular around the world as a cleansing diet, and you can enjoy it as the season changes from summer to fall.

One handy tip: during a fruit detox day, let your appetite guide you. Rather than sticking to fixed mealtimes, eat a small portion of fruit whenever you feel like it. Although fruit contains a lot of water, you should still hydrate from time to time during the day, taking small sips between meals only. If you like fresh fruit salads, feel free to eat them, but do not add sugar of any kind.

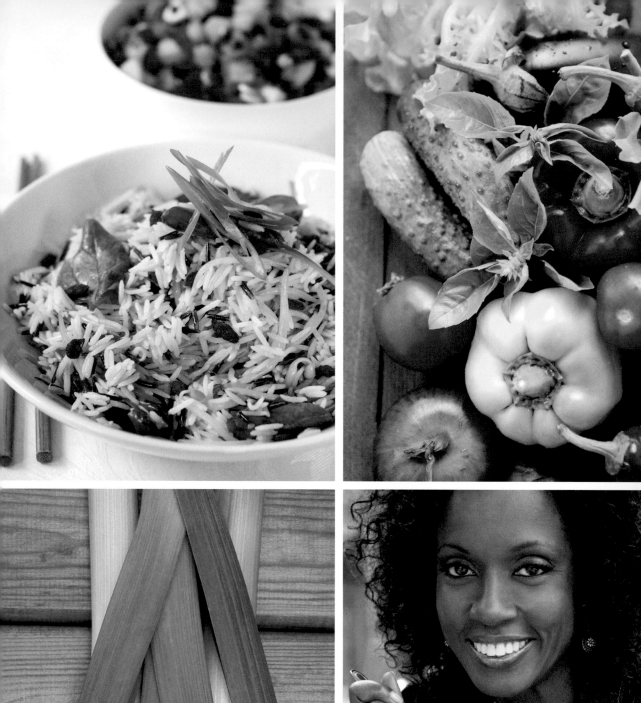
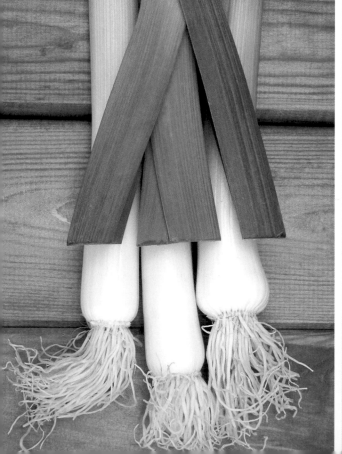
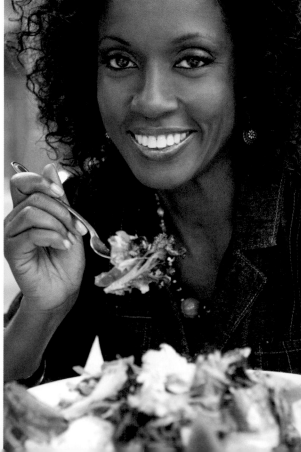

Veggie-Based One-Day Detox

A whole day of nothing but one kind of vegetable is another delicious way to detoxify your body. In the spring, treat yourself to a whole day of steamed asparagus. In the fall, eat just carrots: grate then dress them with a squeeze of lemon juice and a spoonful of olive oil (just don't add salt). Or alternate meals of raw carrots with meals of cooked carrots or freshly squeezed carrot juice.

A potato-based one-day detox is highly recommended for people who suffer from water retention and those who find it difficult to eat less-substantial vegetables or fruits all day. You can eat a cooked potato whenever you feel hungry. Use organic potatoes, and boil or roast them in their skins with no added salt. You will find that a good potato is delicious even when served plain.

A day of nothing but mixed salads is a less strict alternative to a single-food one-day detox. Eat raw, fresh greens and vegetables dressed with only lemon juice and cold-pressed extra-virgin oil. Eat only two salads: one for lunch and one for dinner. Throughout the day, drink water to stay hydrated.

Rice-Based One-Day Detox

Consuming nothing but rice for a day can be very soothing to the gut and offers excellent cleansing provided that you are consuming organically grown brown rice. Boil the rice in more water than usual — use a ratio of 4 to 5 cups (1 to 1.25 L) of water to 1 cup (250 mL) of rice — and cook it longer that you normally would, about $1\frac{1}{2}$ hours. Do not drain the rice when it is finished cooking; rather, eat it soupy, like a rice porridge, to ensure you get all the nutrients in the liquid.

Fast in the Spring and the Fall

Many ancient religions and cultures provided for regular periods of purification, during which people followed precise rules, which limited food to that which was simple and easily digested. The timing of these periods was not accidental: the body is more receptive to a thorough inner cleansing during certain seasons and specific lunar cycles. The start of spring and autumn are two times when it is especially useful to undertake a few days of fasting or cleansing.

Beauty Food Superstars

Variety is wonderful when it comes to eating a healthy diet. By eating a wide array of different fruits, vegetables, protein sources and fats, you ensure you consume the most complete assortment of nutrients. However, some foods deserve a little extra attention in a beauty-boosting diet. Here are a number of superstar ingredients to stock up on.

Lecithin

Lecithin is a fatty compound found in egg yolks, some vegetable oils and especially in soybeans. You can consume it in these food sources, but it is also extracted from them and made into supplements sold in different forms (oil, capsules or granules).

Soy lecithin's amazing properties have made it popular with fans of healthy, natural foods. It is an emulsifier, meaning it binds fat with liquid to keep the mixture from separating. Lecithin is often used to produce chocolate, making it flow more easily. By emulsifying fat, lecithin helps the body eliminate excess fats and reduce dietary cholesterol. It is also an excellent natural diuretic.

Lecithin is an important source of two relatives of the B vitamin family that are among the most difficult to consume in sufficient quantities: choline and inositol, which make hair look strong, shiny and silky. Lecithin also contains vitamin E, a vitamin whose antioxidant properties help prevent premature aging. It also helps tighten and tone the muscles, so you can get great results reducing flab if you combine lecithin consumption with regular, vigorous exercise.

Seaweed

An important health-enhancing characteristic of seaweed is its high iodine content. Iodine makes the metabolism run faster and therefore burn fat faster. The Japanese diet contains a large amount of seaweed, and therefore, the population consumes a relatively large amount of iodine. The Japanese diet also contains plenty of simple carbohydrates, in the form of rice, but the population there suffers fewer heart attacks than in other countries. Iodine plays a part in this protection of the cardiovascular system. It also helps hair grow and stay soft and shiny, so it is a terrific nutrient that will help you look your best.

Wheat Germ

This familiar grain product isn't an everyday food on many tables, but it has extraordinary nutritional and therapeutic value. It contains up to 35% protein, the essential fatty acids and many different vitamins, especially B vitamins. Wheat germ is also a major source of iron, calcium, phosphorus and magnesium. It's delicious sprinkled over oatmeal or on peanut butter–topped toast. You can also mix 1 tsp (5 mL) of wheat germ into fruit juice or sprinkle it over salads or vegetables.

Cider Vinegar

This age-old remedy is one of those beauty secrets that gets passed from generation to generation — and for good reason because it's so effective as a hair rinse and face wash. It's great as a dietary supplement as well, because it contains many of the nutrients in whole apples, such as potassium. A popular folk remedy suggests that taking 1 tsp (5 mL) of cider vinegar in a glass of water after every meal is the secret to losing weight and increasing beauty. If you do try this, be sure to rinse your mouth out with water and/or brush your teeth afterwards, because vinegar can damage tooth enamel.

Relaxation: The Best Prescription

As we have learned, inner beauty influences and determines outer beauty. Just as the lack of certain nutrients in your daily diet can take a toll on your physical appearance, so can a lack of relaxation time in your life. Vitamins and minerals are some of the best natural "cosmetics" to keep you in shape, both inside and out — and so is stress reduction.

There is no such thing as good-looking and bad-looking people; each and every one is attractive in a unique way. If you respect yourself and devote time to taking care of your body, your thoughts can easily focus on the positive parts of life. On the other hand, if you dwell on negative feelings, such as envy, fear and insecurity, you will not only undermine your physical health but also mar your natural beauty.

It is important to look after your physical, mental and spiritual well-being to enhance and preserve your natural beauty. No matter how sophisticated the cosmetics you apply, they will not have the slightest effect if your face is marked by excessive stress or a lack of self-esteem. The key is to learn to relax and let go, embracing the good in yourself.

Stress Changes Your Appearance

Nervousness and tension leave deep marks on the skin, tense up your muscles and impair circulation. As a result, skin becomes pale, itchy and red, and some people suffer from chronic allergic reactions. Dermatologists agree that a considerable proportion of skin disorders are linked with psychological problems and stressors. It is therefore extremely important to your appearance to be relaxed and get sufficient rest. See the box, below, for some strategies you can use to relax and rejuvenate.

Stress-Busting Strategies

1. **Eat right.** Many foods have a calming effect on the body and are essential for controlling the anxiety and stress that affect your overall balance. Avoid processed foods, particularly carbohydrates and simple sugars, and choose whole grains, fruits, vegetables and lean proteins. As you know, following a healthy, balanced diet that avoids the use of stimulants (such as caffeine) is a great way to keep the mind and body in top condition.

2. **Sleep enough.** Sleep has always been said to have a beautifying effect — the lack of it can lead to unsightly dark circles or bags under the eyes. On average, a person needs six to eight hours of sleep daily. Not everyone requires the same amount; some people can function well on less while others need more than eight hours to recharge their batteries.
   Make sure your sleep environment is dark and quiet, and don't allow stimuli, such as televisions, tablets or cell phones, in your bedroom as you're winding down for the night.

3. **Cultivate calmness.** You can do this formally by learning yoga or other stress-reduction techniques, or casually by taking a few minutes of quiet periodically throughout the day. Either way, taking time to wind down reduces stress hormones and tension.

4. **Exercise.** It doesn't matter if you like to work out on your own at the gym or prefer to join a sports team. Just get out there and be active. Regular physical activity is yet another health-promoting way to eliminate stress and boost your mood.

5. **Meditate.** Meditation helps combat stress by helping you experience a general feeling of calm. As you become experienced in its many techniques, your health will improve and you will feel more satisfied with your appearance.

Nutrients That Build Nerves of Steel

Choline and inositol are essential for inducing a calm state. These substances are highly concentrated in the brain cell membranes, nerve cells and lenses of the eyes. These two relatives of the B vitamin family act together and complement each other, preventing tension, anxiety and insomnia. Both are found in soy lecithin (see page 38); eat tofu every day or take a lecithin supplement to boost your level.

You can also strengthen your nervous system with magnesium and B vitamins, which are noted for their stress-reducing effect. To get them through food, choose a variety of organic whole grains and nuts.

Remember, refined carbohydrates are energy bombs that are high on the glycemic index (GI). Foods that are high on this scale flood the body with glucose, making the blood sugar rise, then fall again very quickly. Eating high-GI foods can make you feel faint, exhausted or irritable after an initial burst of energy.

Cut refined sugar and refined flour out of your meals; instead, consume small amounts of grain-based sweeteners and honey (go easy on them), and add plenty of whole-grain foods to your diet. Organic whole-grain foods are great for maintaining a steady energy level and preventing mood fluctuations produced by blood sugar highs and lows. These foods provide constant, slow-release energy that your nerves need.

Herbal Infusions for Sleep and Relaxation

There are a number of medicinal herbs that help relax the body. Infusions (also known as herbal teas) made from them can help you wind down and get you ready for sleep.

To prepare the soothing herbal teas below and on page 43, avoid metal teapots, because they can react with some herbs. Instead, use a glass, enamel or china teapot. Generally, use a ratio of 1 tsp (5 mL) of herbs (chopped or whole fresh herbs, or dried, are fine) to 1 cup (250 mL) of boiling water. Always cover infusions as they're steeping, to keep the beneficial volatile compounds in the cup.

Hops Tea

Hops, in addition to being a common ingredient in beer, are a medicinal herb that promotes sleep. To prepare tea, in a small saucepan, combine 1 cup (250 mL) of cold water and 2 tsp (10 mL) of dried hops; bring to a boil. Reduce heat, cover and simmer for 2 minutes. Strain the infusion and drink before bedtime.

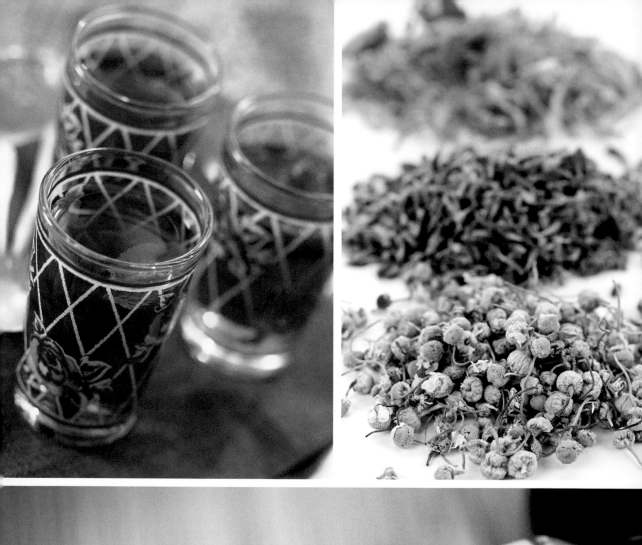
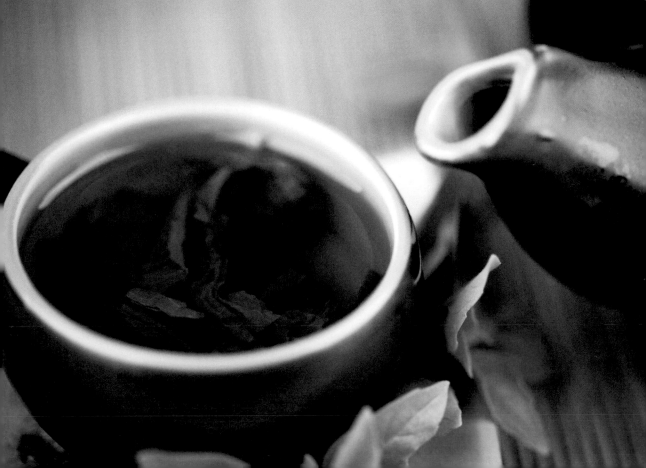

Lavender Tea

Lavender leaves and flowers make a fragrant, sleep-inducing tea. To prepare tea, place 1 tsp (5 mL) of fresh or dried lavender leaves or flowers in a cup; pour 1 cup (250 mL) of boiling water over top. Cover and let stand for 10 minutes. Strain the infusion and drink before bedtime.

Elderflower Tea

Elderflowers are often used in home remedies and made into a sweet cordial that's particularly popular in Europe. They make a delicious tea that helps you relax and fall asleep. To prepare tea with fresh flowers, in a small bowl or saucepan, combine 1 cup (250 mL) of flowers with 1 cup (250 mL) of boiling water; cover and let stand for 10 minutes. To prepare tea with dried flowers, reduce the flowers to 1 tsp (5 mL) and follow the same procedure. Strain the infusion and sweeten it with 1 tsp (5 mL) of honey if you like; drink before bedtime.

Chamomile Tea

Chamomile has been a common medicinal plant for millennia. Although it is usually used to aid digestion, it is excellent for soothing and calming the nervous system. To prepare tea, place 1 tsp (5 mL) of dried chamomile flowers in a cup; pour 1 cup (250 mL) of boiling water over top. Cover and let stand for 5 minutes. Strain the infusion and sweeten it with 1 tsp (5 mL) of honey if you like; drink before bedtime.

Lemon Balm Tea

Lemon balm has a minty, lemony flavor and is perfect for encouraging calm and relaxation. To prepare tea, place 1 tsp (5 mL) of dried lemon balm or 3 fresh lemon balm leaves in a cup; pour 1 cup (250 mL) of boiling water over top. Cover and let stand for 10 minutes. Strain the infusion and drink before bedtime. This tea is tasty hot and delightfully refreshing when served chilled.

Lemon Verbena Tea

The dried leaves of this shrubby herb make a relaxing tea with a pleasant lemon flavor. To prepare tea, place 2 tsp (10 mL) of dried lemon verbena leaves in a cup; pour 1 cup (250 mL) of boiling water over top. Cover and let stand for 5 minutes. Strain the infusion and drink before bedtime. Like lemon balm tea, this infusion is good served hot or cold.

Meditate for Beauty

Meditation, like yoga and other relaxation techniques, releases tension and stress, and helps you achieve inner peace and well-being. The best part is that you can see this calmness and serenity clearly on your face.

Stress wears you down in many ways, from etching wrinkles on your face to giving you gray hair. Meditation can stop or slow down these processes; it has a proven beneficial effect on mental and physical health and therefore on genuine beauty. One way meditation improves your physical appearance is by teaching you to breathe more deeply and evenly, which results in more oxygen pumping into your blood. Blood circulation to the cerebellum portion of your brain is improved, decreasing skin tension.

Before starting your meditation practice, it is important to spend about five minutes relaxing and getting yourself ready to enter the meditative state. When you begin the practice, sit in an upright position, with erect posture. You can meditate sitting in a chair, or on a comfortable mat on the floor with your legs crossed or folded in the lotus position. Keep your eyes half closed and unfocused, or close them gently.

Some meditation techniques concentrate only on breathing. In others, attention is directed using sounds, words or imagery. Experiment with a few types to find the one you're most comfortable with; many community centers offer classes, and there are lots of free resources on the Internet. Through meditation, you can discover the answers to many questions. You will feel much more in touch with the world, and you'll uncover an intuitive knowledge of yourself. You will be at peace, feeling more relaxed and receptive to situations and people.

The Free Radical Aging Theory

You know that viruses, bacteria and fungi can be threats to your health and well-being. But there is also a well-known theory about another type of pathogen that can cause disease and aging: the free radical. Certain free radicals can be extremely aggressive, destructive substances. Most live for only fractions of a second, but this short period is enough for them to destroy the nuclei of cells and age the body.

What They Are

You might need a little refresher on high school chemistry to understand free radicals. Electrons are the negatively charged parts of an atom or molecule. Stable molecules have an even number of electrons. Free radicals are molecules or atoms that have a single free electron, which makes them unstable, meaning they are always trying to steal an electron from the nearest molecule to create an even number.

When a cell is weak, perhaps due to lowered defenses or exposure to toxins, its electron bonds can be broken, allowing a free radical to bind with it. This creates a new free radical from the molecule that had its electron stolen, which in turn will attack another healthy cell to grab one of its electrons. This starts a chain reaction that can destroy entire colonies of cells in the body (it can occur in minutes or even seconds in some cases). In extreme situations, excessive free radicals in the body can damage cells and cause tumors to form — and these can become malignant cancers.

Where They Come From

Free radicals occur in the body all the time and come in very different types. Some may be small molecules, like oxygen, or may form part of a macromolecule, such as a protein. Some free radicals are aggressive, and others are relatively unreactive. They can arrive in the body in the food you've eaten or the air you've breathed. Free radicals are also produced inside the body when it's exposed to radiation (such as solar radiation, or sun exposure), contaminants, poisons or decay.

What They Do

Cell death, which ages the body, is caused mainly by the oxidizing action of free radicals. When a free radical has penetrated a cell membrane, it heads toward the cell nucleus, which contains the chromosomes. These structures contain the genes (which consist of our DNA, the long rows of nucleotides coiled into a double helix), which are the blueprints for building proteins in the body. If free radicals manage to reach the chromosomes, they can alter or destroy genes, leading to an increased risk of disease.

How to Fend off Free Radical Attacks

Luckily, your body's cells can defend against attacks by free radicals, thanks to bioactive substances that work as part of the immune system. These are called antioxidants, a term that seems to be everywhere these days.

To stop excessive aggressive free radicals from attacking, it's critical to have fewer oxidants (that is, free radicals) than antioxidants in your cells. These immunity boosters — particularly vitamins A, C and E and the trace element selenium — form the cell's defense system. Antioxidants are therefore indispensable for preventing premature aging due to free radical damage. Ultimately, it is impossible to prevent free radicals, as well as other pathogens, from invading the body, but antioxidants can help keep them from inflicting too much damage.

Antioxidant Cocktail for Youth

So how do you slow down aging or even reverse it? Eat organic whole grains, sprouts, nuts, seeds, tofu and cheese daily to help the nuclei of damaged cells regenerate and prevent further attacks. Or give your system a (good) shock by making sure you get enough of four important antioxidants: vitamins A, C and E and the trace element selenium. Speak with your doctor or naturopath first to ensure you're getting the right dose and not exceeding the daily intake limit.

- **Vitamin A and beta-carotene** (provitamin A) effectively neutralize oxidizing radicals. They protect cells from becoming damaged, which can protect against cancer. Some good sources are leafy greens; and deep yellow, orange and red vegetables and fruits, such as carrots, pumpkins, bell peppers, squash, zucchini, apricots and cantaloupe.

- **Vitamin C** protects the fluid inside cells, rejuvenates and cleanses the fatty acids of cell membranes and regenerates vitamin E molecules used up in the fight against free radicals. Vitamin C and bioflavonoids are plant substances that help protect flowers, herbs, fruits and leaves against aggression from free radicals, bacteria and fungi. Try to eat fresh fruits, preferably acidic ones, such as kiwifruit, oranges and lemons. It is better to eat whole fruit than to drink juice, because the pulp contains a good portion of the active ingredients.

- **Vitamin E** destroys damaging free radicals at the cell membrane level. An easy way to incorporate this into the diet is by dressing dishes with cold-pressed vegetable and seed oils, and eating plenty of raw seeds and nuts, such as walnuts and hazelnuts.

- **Selenium** is another excellent antioxidant that acts within the cell to expel or destroy free radicals. Selenium is showing promise as a cancer fighter too. To get your quota, it's a good idea to have brewer's yeast and whole grains or whole-grain products (such as bread) every day. Brazil nuts, garlic and eggs also contain abundant selenium.

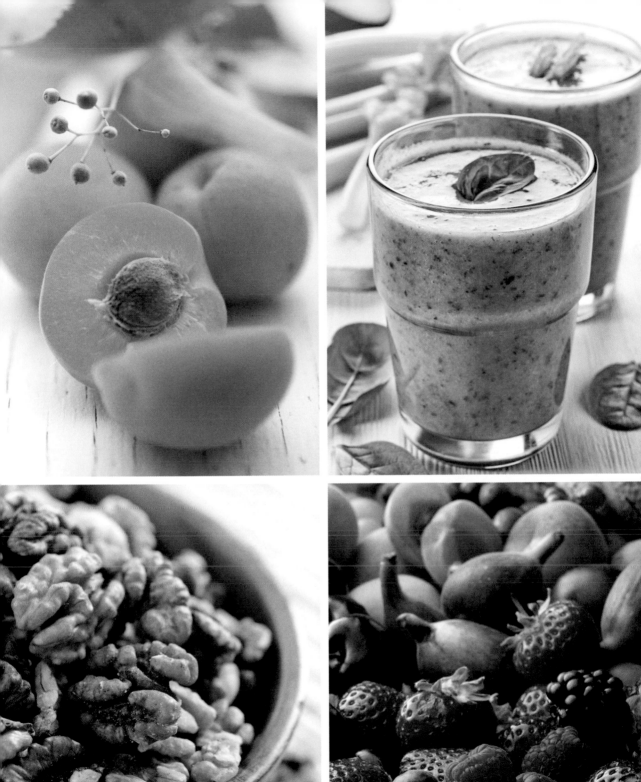
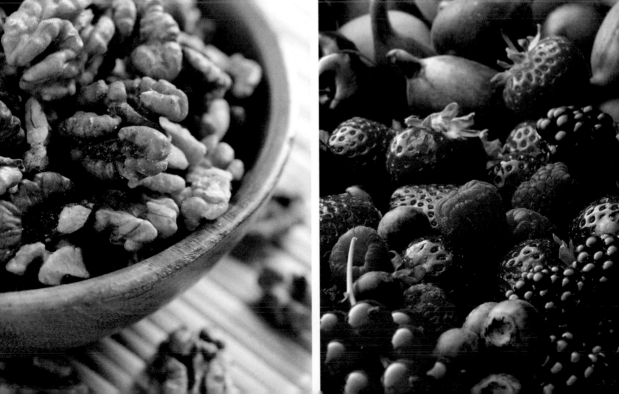

Beauty Thieves

These are the culprits that work hard to take away glowing skin, bright eyes, shiny hair and overall health. Some you can't avoid, like certain medications, but some are easy to banish from your daily life so you can feel beautiful outside and inside.

Refined Sugar

This villain detracts from the health of hair because it robs the body of B vitamins and minerals, such as calcium, which it needs. Without them, the body can't counteract cell acidity, which causes demineralization of the bones, hair, teeth and nerves. Fortunately, there are wonderful alternatives to refined sugar, such as honey, apple concentrate, raisins and dates. They are delicious and are a source of vitamins and minerals.

Smoking

Smoking is the worst enemy of good skin. It causes facial wrinkles to form, in part for mechanical reasons: the muscles around the mouth repeat a specific set of movements over and over when you pucker your lips around a cigarette, inhale and exhale. These nearly unconscious, repeated movements form wrinkles, which are especially noticeable in people with delicate skin.

Moreover, each cigarette you consume robs the body of a considerable amount of vitamin C, a vital antioxidant. Studies have shown that smokers have particularly low blood levels of vitamin C, which they must compensate for with a higher intake through food or supplements. In addition, tobacco smoke introduces toxic substances, such as arsenic and carbon monoxide, into the body, which contribute to wear and tear on the skin, cell damage and therefore premature aging.

Medications

Many medicines alter the chemical functions of the body, which affects the skin. The main reason is that generally drugs tend to drain the body of certain essential nutrients, such as B vitamins, vitamin C and zinc.

Antibiotics can be especially irritating. While their healing properties are worth it, the skin tends to pay an enormous price. Often, a course of antibiotic treatment will provoke allergic skin reactions or worsen acne.

Hormone-based prescriptions also tend to produce side effects that take a toll on skin. In women, certain hormonal therapies can cause facial hair growth, which is annoying and unsightly. Birth control pills are another common medication that affects hormone balance in the body. Abnormal hair loss can be one of the side effects of taking certain pill formulations.

Alcohol

Alcohol depletes levels of B vitamins in the body, which play an important role in maintaining physical beauty. Drinking too much can also literally scar your face by causing a buildup of fibrous veins that are almost impossible to eradicate. Excess alcohol consumption invariably ends up showing in your complexion, because it gradually destroys vitamins, minerals, trace elements, amino acids and other nutrients essential for health.

The most direct consequence of alcohol consumption is dehydration of the skin. The body requires a large amount of fluid to metabolize alcohol and other toxic substances, so it uses up a portion of the water that would otherwise hydrate the skin. Even if you have a glass or two of wine with dinner, you might wake up the next morning with dry, tight facial skin and/or red spots, both of which are results of dehydration.

Abstaining from alcohol may be one of the best things you can do to care for your body, although it is tough to avoid in social situations in many societies. By skipping wine, beer and cocktails, you'll be doing both your physical and mental well-being a favor.

Coffee

Coffee is a powerful stimulant that takes a toll on physical appearance and well-being. Coffee drinkers who are constantly nervous and excited increase their chances of getting blemishes and suffering from eczema. Moreover, coffee is a potent diuretic and can dehydrate the body when consumed in excess. Coffee also reduces iron absorption; if you drink coffee and your diet is deficient in this mineral, you may find yourself with anemia, which can be a serious health problem.

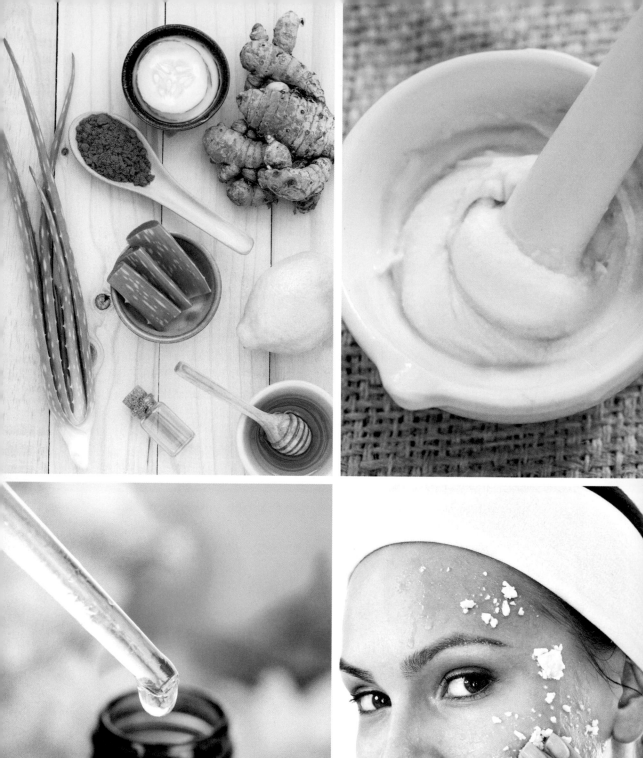
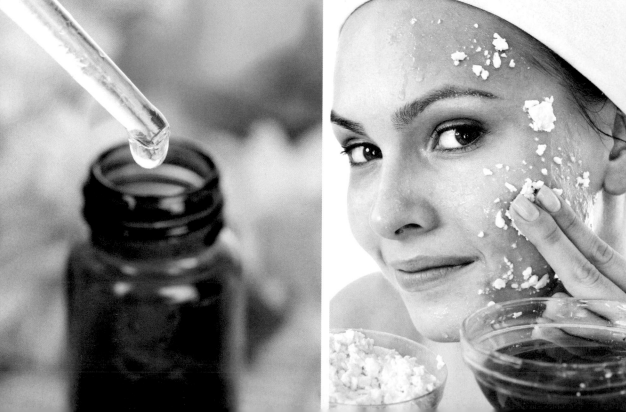

Making Homemade Beauty Products

There's no need to buy beauty products when you can make such a huge array of them at home, including creams, lotions, shampoos, conditioners, perfumes and bath oils. The best part is that you determine the type and quality of the ingredients you use. And you can customize your selection to the exact needs of your skin, hair or whatever body part you want to pamper.

Basic Vocabulary

There's a specific vocabulary used to describe beauty products, their components and their properties. Here are terms you'll run across as you're preparing the recipes in this book:

- **Astringent:** A substance that produces a drying effect on the skin. Some ingredients commonly added to astringent creams are lemon and cucumber, which are used to treat excessively oily skin.
- **Balm:** A skin treatment normally applied in the form of an ointment. It is used to soften and heal the skin.
- **Body oil:** A transparent, oil-based liquid, which may be scented, used to lubricate the skin after bathing.
- **Cream:** A thick, opaque, spreadable mixture used to treat the skin. Its purpose varies depending on the ingredients: it may be moisturizing or nourishing or serve an entirely different purpose.
- **Decoction:** A liquid prepared by boiling plant parts in liquid, generally water, to extract the active ingredients.
- **Deodorant:** A personal hygiene product used to prevent body odor.
- **Emollient:** A substance used to soften the outer layers of the skin. The most widely used emollients are glycerin, vegetable oil (often sweet almond or olive oil) and mineral oil (or petroleum jelly).

- **Emulsion:** A milky fluid in which oil is combined with water using an emulsifier to keep the mixture from separating. This is a common form for many facial preparations because it facilitates absorption of ingredients by the skin.

- **Extract:** A liquid made using evaporation or a solution produced with the help of a solvent. The vital substances in some herbs or other plants are made into extracts.

- **Friction massage:** A technique that involves pressing on the skin with the hands, making the skin slide underneath them while the hands stay in the same place. Pressure can be applied with the fingertips, knuckles, palms or fists. Friction works to release adhesions and mobilize fluids in the tissues.

- **Infusion:** A liquid made by steeping herbs, flowers, leaves or other plant parts in boiling water for a few minutes to extract their medicinal or vital components.

- **Lanolin:** A yellowish, fatty substance extracted from the wool of sheep. It is used as a moisturizing base for many different creams and has a distinctive aroma.

- **Lotion:** A solution with a liquid consistency and that is spread over the skin or hair. There are many types of lotions, and the action of each is determined by its active components.

- **Mask:** A thick but pliable or creamy substance applied to the skin to supply it with specific active substances. Masks may be used to hydrate skin or to remove excess oil and impurities.

- **Milk:** A synonym for an emulsion.

- **Perfume:** An aromatic preparation used to scent the body. Perfume comes in a variety of forms, including liquid, oil and cream. It is usually composed of natural essences.

- **Shampoo:** A soap-like mixture used to clean hair. There are many different types, which can be used to treat everything from dry to oily hair.

- **Soap:** A foamy cleansing agent used to remove debris and contaminants from the body. Soap comes in liquid, solid and gel forms. It is produced by combining a fatty ingredient, such as oil or melted fat, with a base (or alkaline) ingredient, such as sodium hydroxide or potassium hydroxide.

- **Tisane:** An infusion (see above), or tea, made from medicinal or nutritional herbs.

- **Tonic:** A cleansing preparation made in the form of a lotion. It generally refreshes the skin, finishes cleansing the area where it is applied (after washing) and tones the skin. The function depends on its formulation and ingredients.

Tools You Need

Many of the tools you need for making your own beauty products are easy to find in kitchen and houseware stores. It's best to have a separate set of these tools — even a separate electric hand mixer — for making creams, lotions and other beauty products. (You don't want your food to taste like face cream!) Here are the basics you'll need:

- Electric hand mixer, for beating creams
- Blender, for puréeing fruits and vegetables
- Mortar and pestle, for crushing and grinding spices, herbs and other ingredients
- Heatproof container or bowl, for heating ingredients in a hot-water bath (special tempered glass, such as Pyrex, is ideal)
- Scale, for weighing solid ingredients (see box, below)
- Measuring spoons in assorted sizes
- Metal or plastic measuring cups, for measuring dry ingredients

- Glass measuring cups with graduated markings and a spout, for measuring liquid ingredients
- Plastic syringe with graduated markings on the side, for measuring very small amounts of liquids
- Ceramic bowl, for mixing oils
- Wooden spoons, spatulas and stirring rods
- Glass bottles with airtight lids, in assorted sizes
- Glass jars with airtight lids, in assorted sizes
- Colanders and fine-mesh sieves

The Right Scale

An accurate digital scale is an ideal tool for making beauty products. Here's what to look for when you're buying:

Increments: If you're using imperial measurements, a scale that reads in increments of 0.1 oz is good, but one that reads in increments of 0.01 oz is even better for these recipes, which sometimes require very tiny amounts of ingredients. For metric measurements, look for a scale that reads in 1 g increments.

Accuracy: Precision is important. When choosing an imperial scale, look for one that is accurate to within 0.1 oz (0.01 oz is even better). If you are buying a metric scale, it should be accurate to within 1 g (0.5 g is even better).

Tare button: A tare button allows you to place a bowl or other receptacle on the scale, then "zero" the scale so that it weighs only the contents. It's very handy to have.

Tips for Making Homemade Beauty Products

- Always start by washing and completely drying all tools and equipment you will be using.

- Read through the recipe and assemble all of the ingredients before you begin.

- Follow the recipe, using the exact amounts called for. Substitutions will change the properties of whatever you are making, and the results will not be the same.

- When heating ingredients in a hot-water bath, fill a saucepan with water to a depth of about 2 inches (5 cm) and bring it to a simmer. Then, set your bowl of ingredients on the saucepan above the simmering water.

Keep Your Products Fresh

- Masks made with fruit and fresh ingredients should be used immediately after they are prepared.

- Creams should be stored in a cool place. They can be kept for 4 to 6 weeks unless otherwise specified.

- Powders should be stored in clean, dry airtight jars to keep them dry and prevent clumping.

- Essential oils, tinctures and facial lotions should be kept in dark or opaque glass bottles to prevent light from damaging their therapeutic components.

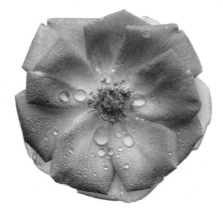

Ingredients A to Z

There is a broad selection of ingredients you can use to make your own custom beauty products. Choose good-quality ingredients, and buy them from a reputable seller with high product turnover to ensure freshness. There are many retailers online (see page 360) that sell herbs, waxes, soap bases and oils. Fruits, herbs and many other additions are available at your local natural food store or supermarket.

Many of the herbs and plants below have their Latin name listed in parentheses after their common name. Many common names apply to multiple plants that are not of the same genus and species, so the Latin name will help you know what to choose if you're faced with more than one option when purchasing.

Almond (*Prunus amygdalus var. dulcis*): Almond flour can be used as a facial cleanser for oily skin with pimples. Almond milk is healing, softening and slightly astringent; it is an ingredient in countless recipes for tonics and lotions. See also sweet almond oil, page 60.

Apple: Apples contain iron, calcium, phosphorus, magnesium and vitamins A, B and C, which help invigorate nerve and muscle fibers. Apples are an excellent tooth cleanser and strengthen the gums.

Apricot kernel oil: The properties of apricot kernel oil are very similar to those of sweet almond oil (see page 60). It is a pleasant-smelling oil that can be used as a night lotion to protect the face and neck from dehydration.

Arrowroot (*Maranta arundinacea*): The starchy white powder made from arrowroot soothes the skin, especially when mixed with liquid to form a gel (though you can also apply the powder directly).

Avocado: This tropical fruit is rich in vitamins A, B, C, D and E. The pulp can be mashed and used as a soothing facial mask.

Avocado oil: This brown-hued vegetable oil is extracted from avocado pulp. It is used to make treatments for dry, flaky and combination skin, and restores firmness and elasticity. Its oil is valued for its ability to heal skin and to reduce the depth of wrinkles.

Basil (*Ocimum basilicum*): This herb is said to be native to India and has been cultivated since ancient times throughout Asia Minor and Greece. This aromatic, refreshing plant is ideal for making infusions.

Bay (*Laurus nobilis*): A native of the Mediterranean, the bay, or laurel, tree is appreciated not only for its uses in the kitchen, but also for its properties as an ingredient in natural cosmetics. It also makes an excellent infusion that can be added to all sorts of beauty products.

Beeswax: Beeswax, a natural wax produced by honeybees, has long been used to emulsify and bind ingredients in cosmetics, creams and lip balms.

Beet: Beets contain beta-carotene, B vitamins, vitamin C, magnesium, phosphorus, potassium, zinc and sulfur. They are nutritious, provide energy and help prevent constipation and varicose veins. The beta-carotene and other nutrients they contain help keep cells in working order.

Benzoin: This reddish-brown resin is extracted from a tree that grows in southeast Asia. It can be used as a preservative in homemade cosmetics, and is useful for emulsifying solid shea butter when making cosmetic creams without having to melt it first. Benzoin has a tonic effect on the skin, a beauty secret shared for centuries by women in the Middle East, where it is also used to make perfumes and medicines.

Bergamot (*Citrus bergamia*): The essential oil extracted from the pulp of the bergamot fruit has a pleasant citrus fragrance. Added to bathwater, it is a gentle moisturizing treatment for the skin. It also has an antiseptic, refreshing and toning effect.

Borage (*Borago officinalis*): The spiny leaves and attractive bluish-purple or pink flowers from this plant can be used to prepare an infusion to bathe irritated eyes. It acts as a tonic and reduces swelling. Borage tea is also very beneficial as a mild sedative.

Calendula (*Calendula officinalis*): Originally from India, this plant (also known as marigold) has excellent healing properties and can be used on the face or added to bathwater. It acts as an emollient, a decongestant and an anti-inflammatory on the skin.

Carrot: Carrots are often used to treat blemished skin because they smooth and firm it. They are very gentle, so a mixture of grated carrot and vegetable oil can be used in skin creams, facial masks and treatments for children.

Castor oil: This oil is obtained from the castor bean. It soothes the skin and helps promote healthy hair. Among its properties is the ability to extract harmful substances from the skin, making it useful for medical as well as cosmetic purposes.

Chamomile (*Matricaria chamomilla*): Chamomile tea calms the nerves and has a soothing effect on facial skin. It also strengthens facial tissues. Chamomile flowers can be added to shampoos and rinses for blond hair to make it shiny and beautiful.

Cider vinegar: Cider vinegar restores the acid balance of the topmost layer of skin, helping it stay healthy. It is good for balancing oils in the skin, and is also beneficial for dry skin because it softens it and reduces flaking. Cider vinegar is an excellent hair rinse, leaving the hair soft and shiny. Used to give friction massages (see page 52), it strengthens and restores body tissues.

Cinnamon (*Cinnamomum* spp.):
This familiar spice contains tannins and essential oils, and in phytocosmetics (ones that are based on plants rather than chemicals), it is used as a tonic for facial muscles.

Clay: This is a dense, sticky type of earth that retains its properties even when wet. It is a blend of many minerals, such as silica, titanium, aluminum, iron, calcium, magnesium, potassium and sodium. It can be used in both hot and cold treatments, mainly to stimulate the circulation and absorb toxins. See also kaolin, page 58.

Clove (*Syzygium aromaticum*):
This common spice is the flower bud of the clove tree. An aromatic essential oil containing eugenol is extracted from the buds. Cloves and clove oil are widely used in perfumes and in phytocosmetics for their antiseptic and healing powers.

Cocoa butter: This is a solid fat, yellowish in color, that is extracted from roasted cocoa beans. It is frequently used in cosmetics for its emollient and lubricating properties.

Coconut (*Cocos nucifera*): This fruit of the coconut palm tree contains minerals and fats, which make it a very suitable ingredient for nourishing creams for dry skin.

Comfrey (*Symphytum officinale*):
Comfrey belongs to the same family as borage (see opposite) and is one of the most balancing, emollient and astringent plants, making it useful for treating dry skin. Comfrey preparations can be used for face, eye and hair treatments and in the bath.

Cucumber: Cucumber juice is especially good for improving oily skin; it is refreshing and mildly astringent. It also helps prevent sunburn and can be used to bleach freckles. Cucumber-based lotions and creams soften facial skin.

Dandelion (*Taraxacum officinale*):
Both dandelion flowers and leaves are used in cosmetics and body products. Dandelion also can be used as a tonic and cleanser for face and body. It contains calcium, potassium, phosphorus, beta-carotene, B vitamins and vitamin C.

Egg yolk: This rich yellow sac that floats in the center of an egg nourishes skin, making it smooth and soft. It is a common ingredient in shampoos and facial masks. Masks that contain egg yolk don't last and are usually applied immediately after they are made.

Elderflower (*Sambucus nigra*):
The elder is one of the most-used medicinal plants in cosmetics, thanks to its toning and protective properties. Traditionally, it was used to heal burns and lighten freckles.

Essential oils: These pure oils are distilled from the flowers, leaves or stems of medicinal plants. Typically, a large amount of plant material is needed to produce a single bottle of oil, so it tends to be expensive. But it is worth the price in terms of purity and effectiveness. Essential oils have intense aromas, and many have slight disinfectant and bactericidal effects. Because they can cause irritation in their concentrated form, they should not be used in large doses or applied directly to the skin (dilute them in a gentle vegetable oil first).

Fennel (Foeniculum vulgare): The seeds of this delicious vegetable make a great skin tonic due to their strengthening properties, and they can be used to make treatments for tired, sore eyes as well.

Honey: Honey has superb healing and softening properties for the skin. It moisturizes dry skin and can be added to any cream, lotion or oil to make it easier to rub in.

Horsetail (Equisetum arvense): This plant has healing and anti-inflammatory powers and helps strengthen connective tissue. It is often used as an ingredient in creams to treat stretch marks, sagging breasts and flabby skin.

Kaolin: This fine white clay (see page 57) is used in the manufacture of a variety of products, such as soap, cloth, paper and even porcelain. It has oil-fighting and astringent properties when applied to the skin.

Lavender (Lavandula angustifolia): Made into an infusion and taken internally, lavender has a calming, sedative effect. Used externally, it is stimulating and has antiseptic properties, so it can be used as a skin tonic for treating oily skin and pimples. Lavender oil is very good for keeping hair healthy.

Lemon (Citrus limon): Lemon juice is excellent for treating dry, chapped skin. It counteracts the alkalinity of soap, helping the skin stay moisturized and smooth.

Lemon verbena (Aloysia citriodora): This shrubby herb, also called lemon beebrush, is an astringent and is used primarily to treat hair and the skin around the eyes.

Licorice (Glycyrrhiza glabra): Licorice extract contains an acid that inhibits the synthesis of collagen fibers, which helps increase elasticity in the skin.

Madonna lily (Lilium candidum): This plant is an excellent moisturizer, soothes irritated skin and can be used to discourage the growth of unwanted hair. It is a useful remedy for dull skin and pimples, and it is good for decreasing wrinkles and crow's-feet, especially when used in conjunction with massage.

Mint (Mentha spicata): Mint is a generic term applied to members of the Lamiaceae family, but it's often used to mean spearmint (Mentha spicata) specifically. Tea made from the leaves has a soothing effect on the stomach. Mint is also used in creams and lotions for its stimulating properties on the skin.

Oat (Avena sativa): Oats have long been appreciated in beauty products due to their soothing and healing actions on the skin. They can also be used to make gentle, soap-free cleaners.

Olive oil: Olive oil makes an excellent cleanser for dry skin. It is a wonderful neutral base in which to steep herbs to create herbal oils. Olive oil makes a useful emollient for skin and hair and acts as a muscle relaxant. It is also a nourishing oil that should be included in the diet.

Orange: Originally from Asia, the orange was later brought to the Mediterranean region and the southern United States, where it has thrived. Both sweet oranges *(Citrus sinensis)* and bitter oranges *(Citrus aurantium)* are used in body-care products. Orange blossom essential oil, also called neroli essential oil, is often used in facial moisturizing lotions and rinses, both for its scent and its astringent properties.

Parsley *(Petroselinum crispum)*: Used as a cosmetic, parsley has soothing and cleansing properties for the face, hair and eyes. It also makes a good deodorant.

Poppy *(Papaver somniferum)*: The oil pressed from the seeds of this flower reduces wrinkles on the forehead and around the eyes. It is particularly suitable for skin that has been overexposed to the sun and for swollen eyes.

Potassium alum: Also known as potassium aluminum sulfate, this water-soluble white powder is used to make shaving lotions. It is also used as a nail hardener and for its astringent and styptic (blood clotting) effects. It is not soluble in alcohol and must always be dissolved in water.

Potato: Potato juice can be used all over the body. It is soothing and anti-inflammatory when applied externally, and it reduces swelling.

Pumpkin seed oil: This oil extracted from the seeds of the pumpkin *(Curcubita pepo)* is rather dark and thick, and it has considerable healing properties. For cosmetic purposes, it is mixed with lighter, flavorless oils, such as apricot kernel oil (see page 55).

Rose water: This fragrant liquid is made by steam-distilling rose petals. It contains the same active substances as rose essential oil but in lower concentrations. It is a well-known, popular ingredient in cosmetics because it moisturizes and cleanses the skin and is also an astringent. Rose water makes a lovely base for creams and facial toners. It can be used on both the face and the body, because it is gentle, well tolerated by the skin and pleasantly aromatic.

Rosemary *(Rosmarinus officinalis)*: For use in homemade body-care products, rosemary leaves can be made into an infusion or rosemary essential oil can be added. Rosemary has stimulating, regenerative and cleansing properties, making it an ideal ingredient in shampoos, hair rinses and deodorants.

Sage *(Salvia officinalis)*: This herb is used as a perfume fixative, because it blends well with other herbal aromas. The leaves can be used to prepare facial lotions or baths, and sage seeds can be used to make an eye lotion. It inhibits sweating and heals inflammation.

Salt: Salt is an ingredient in bath salts, for both whole-body and foot baths. It is suitable for treating oily skin and excessively sweaty feet.

Stearic acid: This natural acid is obtained from certain waxes; it is white and has a greasy, grainy consistency. It is usually well tolerated by the skin, so it is a common ingredient in creams and cleansers, in which it enhances the emulsifying properties of beeswax. Products that contain stearic acid usually have a slightly pearly shine.

Sweet almond oil: This oil is pressed from almonds (see page 55). It has long been used as an effective beauty agent. It reduces the appearance of reddened veins on sensitive skin, softens the skin and makes it appear plumper and smoother. Apply to dry skin and leave overnight for a simple treatment.

Sweet violet (*Viola odorata*): This flower was used by the Ancient Romans to make perfumes, cosmetics and medicines. It soothes and cleanses the skin and has a mild astringent effect.

Walnut oil: This oil acts as a sunscreen and is used in the preparation of natural sunscreen products. It is well tolerated by all skin types.

Witch hazel: Astringent and styptic properties are attributed to this solution, which contains about 15% alcohol. Its benefits to the skin are due to its alcohol content and the tannin extracted from the witch hazel plant.

Yogurt: Yogurt is an excellent food for the skin and can also be used in facial masks and smoothing treatments.

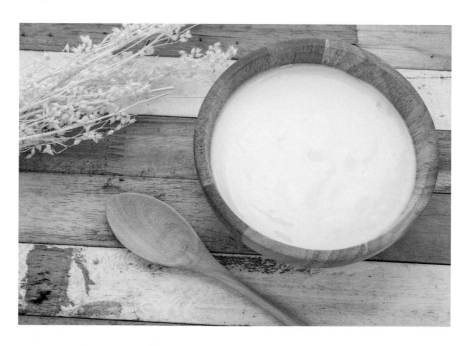

Part 2

Recipes for the Whole Body

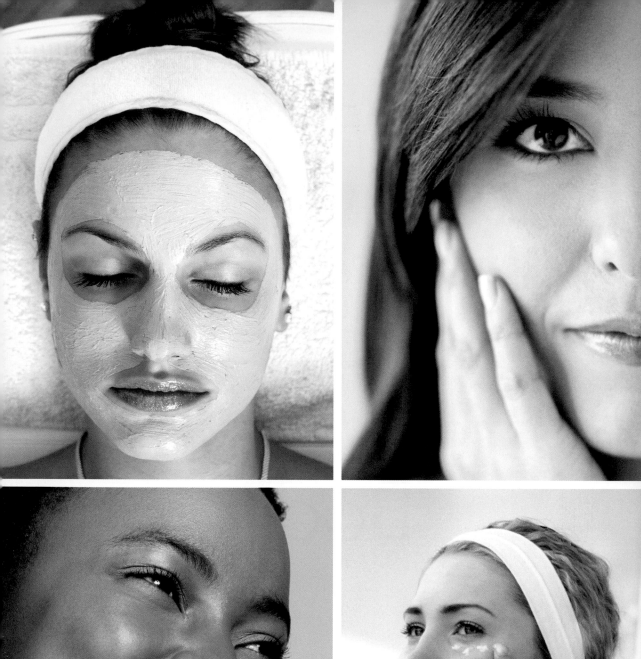
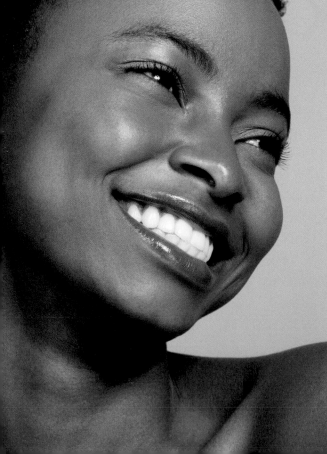
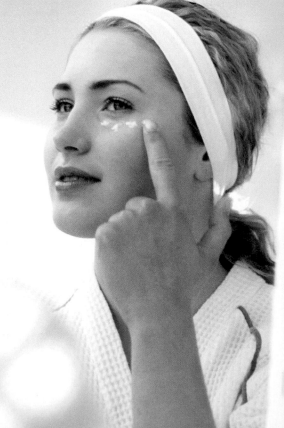

Face Products and Treatments

Your face says a lot about you. In this chapter, we will examine the facial skin, its requirements and the recipes you can create that will cater to its unique needs and enhance your natural beauty.

Love Your Face

Caring for your skin has something in common with caring for your health: you may start to be concerned only when you begin to notice signs of deterioration and neglect. One day, you look in the mirror and suddenly see wrinkles or unsightly spots starting to appear. You decide it's time to pay more attention to your neglected face.

The good news is that it's never too late to start pampering your skin. It may take a little more effort if you've neglected it for a long time, but you can help reduce and reverse damage. In beauty as in health, prevention is easier and less costly than cure. By taking care of your facial skin, you can prevent common problems, such as the acne and oily skin associated with puberty and young adulthood, and the chronic dryness that comes on later in life.

What Is Your Skin Type?

There are four basic types of skin. The most common is combination skin; according to experts, upwards of 70% of people have this skin type. The table on page 64 explains the characteristics of each skin type and recommends ways to care for its particular needs.

Skin: The Inside Story

Skin consists of three layers: the epidermis, the dermis and the hypodermis. The terms *skin* and *epidermis* are commonly used interchangeably, but they are actually two different things.

The epidermis is the outer layer of skin. Its role is to act as a barrier, both to protect the body from external attacks and to protect the vital substances within the body from escaping. When the epidermis is sick,

Find Your Skin Type

	Characteristics	Recommendations
Oily skin	• Secretes too much oil. • Pimples and blackheads often appear, especially around the nose. • Firm, smooth appearance thanks to a thick fatty tissue layer. • The face readily becomes shiny.	• Reduce intake of fats, and refined sugar and flour. • Eliminate stress. • Cleanse the face several times a day. • Use moisturizing lotions and masks designed for oily skin.
Dry skin	• Delicate with fine pores. • Peels and flakes easily. • Feels tight after washing with soap. • Reddens when exposed to cold; sensitive to changes in temperature. • Sometimes reddened and swollen with dilated veins showing on the cheeks as a result of internal or external factors.	• Massage the face with a rich moisturizing cleanser and remove with cotton pads. • Avoid using tap water directly on the face. • Use moisturizing creams to keep skin from drying out even more. • Deeply moisturize the face with a treatment or mask once a week. • Eat plenty of foods rich in B vitamins and vitamins A, C and E.
Normal skin	• Healthy looking. • Appearance changes appropriately with age. • May be somewhat oily during adolescence. • Dries over time.	• Maintain the skin's natural equilibrium with a balanced diet. • Use masks, cosmetics and natural treatments to prevent drying.
Combination skin	• Has traits of both oily and dry skin. • Driest areas are usually around the eyes, mouth, neck and cheeks. • The chin, nose and forehead tend to secrete more oil.	• Dry areas are more sensitive and therefore require more attention. • Treat dry areas with moisturizing creams that contain oils. • Treat oily areas with moisturizers and creams for oily skin.

dehydrated or weakened (either by injuries that break the skin or by aggressive exfoliation), its permeability increases.

The dermis lies below the epidermis. It is a connective tissue that contains the blood and lymphatic vessels that nourish and remove wastes from the skin. It also contains nerves, sweat glands and sebaceous glands, which secrete the oils necessary for healthy skin. The lower part of the dermis is where intertwined collagen and elastin fibers are located; these give the skin tone, elasticity and a youthful appearance.

The third level, below the dermis, is the hypodermis. It forms a padded cushion of fat, which not only gives the skin its rounded shape but also protects underlying muscles, bones and organs.

Working in tandem with the deeper dermis layer of the skin, the epidermis is essential to keep the body hydrated. It also transports old, dead skin cells to the surface, where they form a thin layer called the stratum corneum. These outermost dead cells are flattened and filled with a protein called keratin. The body constantly renews its epidermal cells (the life cycle is 25 to 45 days from creation to death), so it's important to get rid of this keratin buildup at the surface to promote healthy skin function.

Finally, the epidermis contains and manufactures melanin. When this pigment accumulates in the skin, it results in tanning, freckles, age spots, skin pigmentation changes during pregnancy and some birthmarks.

Collagen and Elastin

Collagen is a shiny white connective tissue made of long chains of fibrous molecules containing thousands of amino acids. It's what gives the skin its smooth, healthy appearance; wrinkles start to form when collagen is in poor condition. Collagen gives skin firmness and serves as a temporary reserve of amino acids that the body can tap into when it needs more proteins or other essential nutrients (especially zinc or vitamin C).

Collagen is exceptionally strong and pliable. In fact, collagen fibers are stronger than steel fibers of the same thickness. Nature's secret is

Epidermis Thickness Varies

In delicate areas, such as the eyelids, the epidermis is no more than 0.00157 inches (0.04 mm) thick. In tougher areas, such as the soles of the feet and the palms of the hands, the epidermis can be upwards of 40 times thicker, or about 0.063 inches (1.6 mm). This explains why the skin around the eyes is so vulnerable to damage, while the skin on the extremities can take a beating.

to twist these macromolecules into left-handed spirals, and then twist those spirals together into larger right-handed spirals. These collagen fibers are reinforced by a network of yellow elastin fibers, which are also pliable and resistant to tearing. This combination produces a firm, smooth layer below the epidermis. It yields to pressure and stretching and helps structures snap back into place; for example, when you laugh, your eyes scrunch up and your mouth opens wide, and then, everything immediately returns to its previous configuration when you stop.

Every 24 hours, the connective tissues in your skin undergo a cycle of destruction and regeneration. Most of this process happens at night; this explains why your skin can feel much firmer in the morning than in the evening. Collagen production is influenced by diet: its formation requires copper (a medium-sized bowl of muesli daily usually provides a sufficient amount), iron (found in soy yogurt, blackstrap molasses, oats and spinach), zinc (supplied by whole grains, brewer's yeast and wheat germ), sulfur (in onions, radishes and Brussels sprouts), proteins (readily available in soy foods, such as tofu, cheese and eggs) and vitamin C (found in citrus fruits, cabbage and many other fruits and vegetables). Consuming plenty of these nutrients provides you with all the biological elements your connective tissues need to rejuvenate themselves.

Skin and Aging

Scientists debate why and how we age. Many claim that exposure to high levels of contamination or pollution, both inside and outside the body, can accelerate the process and cause premature aging of the skin.

The toxic substances that we breathe, such as carbon monoxide, decompose through oxidation processes in the body and form free radicals (see page 44) that are responsible for damaging tissues. Oxidation is a normal process, and it is virtually impossible to prevent free radicals from penetrating our cells and tissues; even sunlight emits them.

Under normal conditions, every cell in the body receives some 10,000 free radical attacks every day. But when you consume a diet heavy in processed food; breathe stale air; ingest too much alcohol, nicotine, coffee or drugs; get insufficient sleep; and receive excessive sun exposure, the number of daily free radical attacks can increase to 80,000 or more per cell! Under these conditions, the body's cells age up to 40 times faster. Free radicals proliferate and spread quickly, which is what makes them so dangerous and likely to cause damage. There are two categories of factors you need to examine to help reduce your risk of prematurely aging.

Hydration Is Key

Children have beautiful skin that hardly needs any care and stays hydrated. This is because cell regeneration is rapid; their skin cells are always young and filled with water, making their skin smooth and soft. However, as the years pass, cell regeneration slows down. Aging skin needs to be hydrated (both through drinking fluids and using moisturizing products) to keep it from drying out and showing signs of damage. In addition to this natural type of skin aging, there are many other factors that can increase the sensitivity of facial skin. That's another vital reason to take care of what you have.

External Factors That Cause Skin to Age

You are exposed to a large array of potentially damaging substances from the external world. There is a long list of compounds that can come into daily contact with skin. Here are some that are especially problematic:

- **Air pollution** has come to be one of the main agents that ages skin. It is virtually impossible for people who live in large cities or industrial areas to avoid contaminants in the air, and they can reach extremely high concentrations in some urban centers.

- **Chemicals** are present in everyone's daily environment. They can come from industrial chemicals released into the atmosphere, secondhand tobacco smoke, acid rain or even everyday items you use at home, such as detergents, cleaning products and cosmetics.

- **Poor-quality indoor air** can contribute to skin aging. Whether you are heating or cooling your house, this less-than-optimal air can circulate contaminants that can make you look older.

- **Temperature extremes** can take their toll on skin. In summer, the skin tends to dry out due to excessive heat and sun exposure. In the winter, cold air and especially wind can do the same. Naturally dry skin is more sensitive to temperature changes in either direction, although it generally suffers more from the dryness and cold of winter.

- **Ultraviolet (UV) rays from the sun** are another factor that damages skin considerably. Without adequate protection, the skin can develop blemishes and dark spots. Exposure to solar radiation stimulates the creation of free radicals in the body. Free radicals prefer skin cells because they are the most abundant in fatty acids.

Internal Factors That Cause Skin to Age

The body is bombarded with damaging substances from the outside, but they can also come from the inside. Here are some to watch for:

- **Alcohol** consumption can have a negative effect on your youthful appearance. It causes dehydration and can make the skin look less fresh and resilient.

- **Smoking** harms the skin via two routes. First, tobacco smoke in the air comes into direct contact with the skin. Second, the toxic substances from inhaled smoke circulate in the blood. Smoking causes dehydration of the epidermis and destruction of the elastic fibers of the dermis, resulting in wrinkles and premature skin aging. In addition, it contributes to dry hair. It also leaches vitamin C, a vital antioxidant, from the body; this means you need to ingest even more vitamin C than the normal daily amount to counteract the effects of the tar and nicotine assaulting your body's defenses.

- **Stress, fatigue and insufficient sleep** also have a negative effect on the skin and can make you look older than your biological age. By making time to practice stress-reduction techniques, such as yoga or meditation, and to get enough sleep every night, you'll help eliminate bags and dark circles under your eyes.

- **Vitamin and mineral deficiencies** can damage skin considerably, because the body lacks the tools it needs to build fresh, healthy skin cells. A diet low in vitamins and minerals can also contribute to the dehydration of skin cells.

Four Steps to Beautiful Skin

There are four basic steps to keeping your skin healthy, glowing and in good condition. In the following pages, you will learn how to prepare all the natural beauty products you need to complete each step: cleansing and toning (see box, page 70), moisturizing (see box, page 80), nourishing (see box, page 88) and exfoliating and fine-tuning skin with a facial mask (see box, page 94). With these tools and techniques in hand, you can enjoy healthy, glowing skin for years to come.

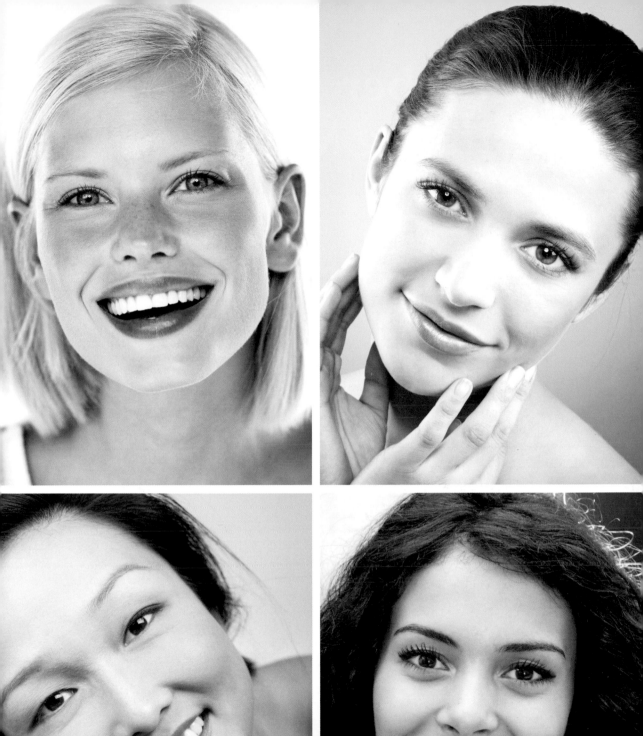
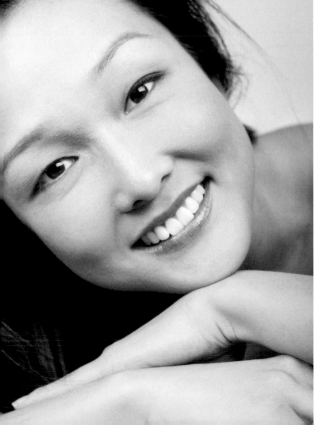
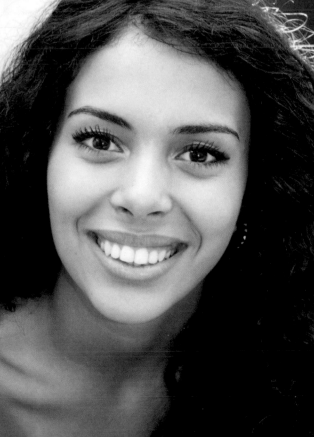

Cucumber Cleansing Milk

This creamy cleanser contains cucumber, a gentle, natural astringent, which helps clean up excess oil in the skin.

Best for: Combination or oily skin

Tip: Buy essential oils sold in dark bottles. Exposure to light can reduce the potency of their medicinal herbal components. Store the bottles in a cool, dark place to keep them fresh.

Note: Always measure accurately when you're making homemade beauty products. See page 53 for tips.

- Blender

1	small cucumber (unpeeled), coarsely chopped	1
1 cup	milk	250 mL
3	drops chamomile essential oil (see tip, at left)	3

1. In blender, purée cucumber until smooth. Pour into a small bowl.

2. Stir in milk and chamomile essential oil until well combined.

3. Dip a cotton ball or pad into cucumber mixture. Apply gently all over face.

4. Rinse off cucumber mixture with warm water. Gently pat face dry with a towel.

Step One: Cleansing and Toning

Getting rid of dirt and impurities is the first step toward building healthy, beautiful skin. There is a cleansing cream for every skin type: choose a heavier one if you have dry skin and a lighter one if you have oily skin. Toners and astringents, applied after cleansing, help further remove impurities and balance the skin, especially in excessively oily areas. Proper cleansing removes the dust, makeup and dirt that accumulate on your face. It also keeps your sebaceous glands, which secrete oil, from getting clogged and forming blackheads and pimples.

Apply cleansers to the face using gently upward and outward strokes. This prevents the skin from stretching in the wrong direction and stimulates nourishing blood flow. Pat toners on gently without rubbing.

If you're using a soapy cleanser, rub it to form a lather (if you have one, a shaving brush works well for this step). Cream cleaners don't contain soap, so they won't bubble; just apply them gently with a cotton ball or pad. Rinse off the cleanser with warm water, and then gently pat your face dry with a towel. Apply a toner if desired and move on to the next step: moisturizing (see box, page 80).

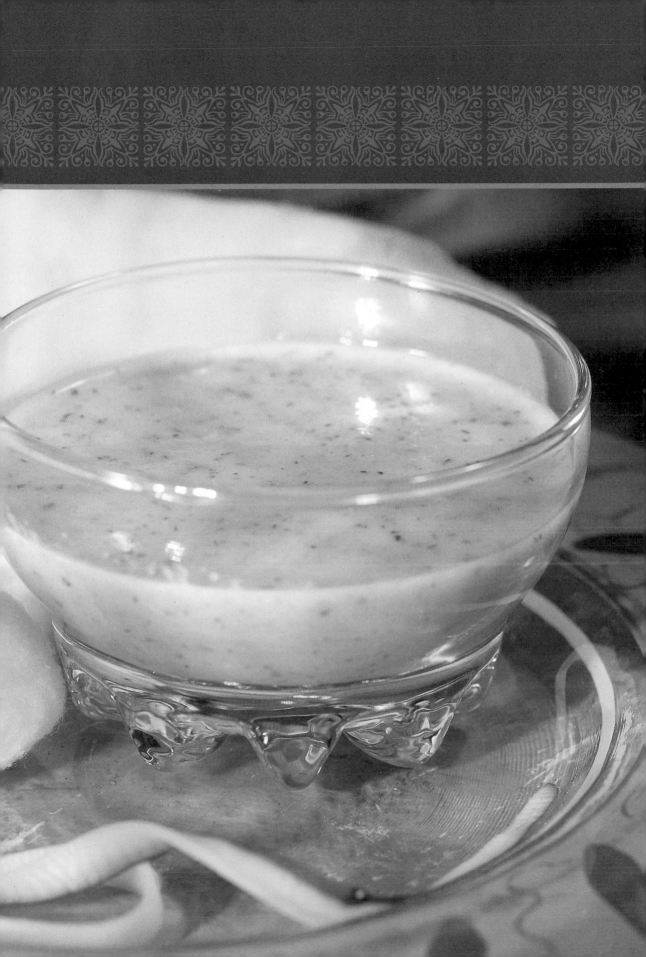

Yogurt Cleansing Cream

Yogurt contains lactic acid, which helps dead skin cells slough off. This cleanser will remove any dullness and reveal glowing, fresh skin.

Best for: All skin types

Tip: Rosemary honey is a light-colored honey made by bees who feed on the nectar of rosemary plants. It has a lovely herbal flavor, so it's terrific for eating as well as using in beauty products. If you can't find it, use another light golden honey, such as clover or lavender.

Note: Always measure accurately when you're making homemade beauty products. See page 53 for tips.

¼ cup	plain yogurt	60 mL
2 tsp	liquid rosemary honey (see tip, at left)	10 mL
3	drops chamomile essential oil (see tip, page 70)	3

1. In a small bowl, combine yogurt, honey and chamomile essential oil. Stir until well combined.

2. Using fingers, spread yogurt mixture all over face, avoiding eye area. Let stand on skin for about 5 minutes.

3. Rinse off yogurt mixture with warm water. Gently pat face dry with a towel.

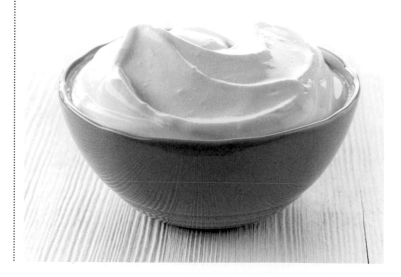

Apple Cleansing Lotion

Apples, milk and oats — sounds like breakfast, doesn't it? But this combination also makes a lovely cleanser for naturally well-balanced skin.

Best for: Normal skin

Tip: You can buy ground oats, but it's very simple to make them at home. Spoon rolled oats into a food processor and grind them until they're fine and powdery.

- Juicer or blender
- Fine-mesh sieve (optional)

1	large apple	1
1 tbsp	finely ground oats or oat flour (see tip, at left)	15 mL
1 tbsp	milk	15 mL
3	drops chamomile essential oil (see tip, page 70)	3

1. In juicer, juice apple, discarding solids. Pour apple juice into a small bowl. (Or in blender, purée apple until smooth. Place fine-mesh sieve over a small bowl; strain juice into bowl, discarding solids.)

2. Stir in oats, milk and chamomile essential oil until well combined.

3. Dip a cotton ball or pad into apple juice mixture. Apply gently all over face.

4. Rinse off apple juice mixture with warm water. Gently pat face dry with a towel.

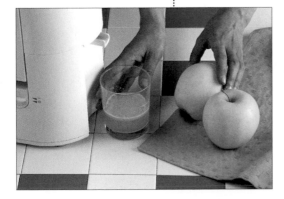
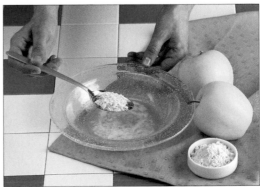

Avocado Cleansing Cream

Avocados are a source of beneficial fats in the diet, and their oil is a wonderful moisturizing ingredient in facial treatments. It helps lock much-needed moisture into dry skin.

Best for: Dry skin

Tips: Shea butter is a rich emollient that's ideal in dry-skin treatments. Look for tubs or bags of it at cosmetic-supply stores or online.

Avocado oil is becoming increasingly popular for cooking. Look for cold-pressed avocado oil that has not been extracted using solvents. It's the most natural, least processed choice.

Raw beeswax often comes in large blocks. Break off a small chunk and grate what you need right before melting. Or substitute small, easy-to-measure beeswax pearls.

Note: Always measure accurately when you're making homemade beauty products. See page 53 for tips.

2 tbsp	shea butter (see tips, at left)	30 mL
1 tbsp	grated raw beeswax (see tips, at left)	15 mL
¼ cup	avocado oil (see tips, at left)	60 mL
¼ cup	distilled water (see tip, page 86)	60 mL
3	drops chamomile essential oil (see tip, page 70)	3

1. In a small heatproof bowl, combine shea butter and beeswax. Set aside.

2. Pour enough water into a small saucepan to come about 2 inches (5 cm) up the side; bring to a simmer.

3. Set bowl on saucepan so that bottom of bowl is not touching simmering water; stir until shea butter mixture is melted and smooth. Remove bowl from heat.

4. Stir avocado oil into shea butter mixture. Let cool slightly.

5. Pour distilled water into another small bowl; stir in avocado oil mixture and chamomile essential oil.

6. Whisk until mixture is completely cooled and well combined.

7. Dip a cotton ball or pad into cleansing cream. Apply gently all over face.

8. Rinse off cleansing cream with warm water. Gently pat face dry with a towel.

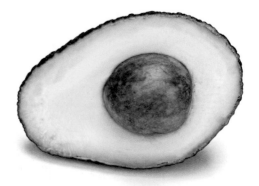

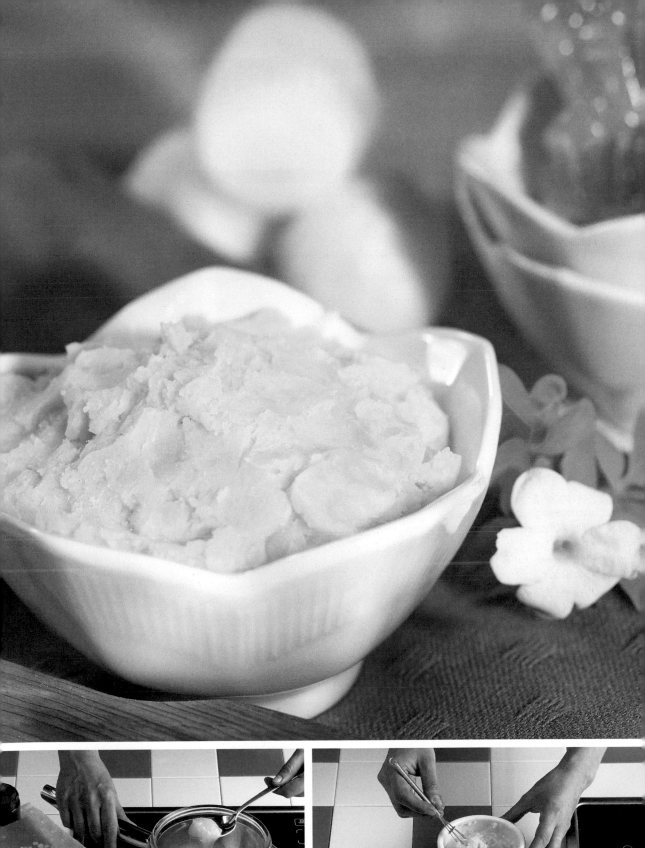
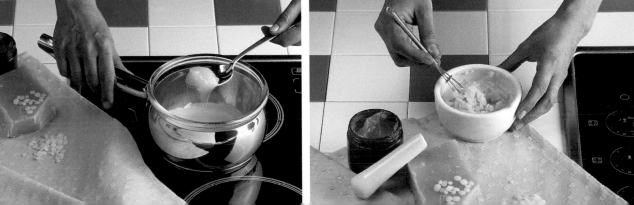

Soothing Chamomile Toner

Chamomile is great for reducing inflammation; it also calms and decongests the skin. The flowers have a delicate herbal smell that makes this treatment pleasant and relaxing.

Best for: All skin types

Tip: Dried chamomile is easy to find at stores that sell medicinal herbs. It's also a very undemanding plant to grow in your garden, so you can grow, harvest and dry your own organic flowers with a minimal amount of effort.

Note: Always measure accurately when you're making homemade beauty products. See page 53 for tips.

- Fine-mesh sieve

1 cup	water	250 mL
1 tbsp	dried chamomile flowers (see tip, at left)	15 mL

1. In a small saucepan, combine water and chamomile flowers. Bring to a boil; remove from heat. Cover and let steep for 5 minutes.

2. Place fine-mesh sieve over a small heatproof bowl; strain infusion into bowl, discarding solids. Let cool to room temperature.

3. Soak a cotton ball or pad in infusion. Pat lightly onto face after cleansing.

Undernourished Skin

An average adult has a total skin surface area of between 12.9 and 23.7 square feet (1.2 and 2.2 square meters). Millions of epithelial cells make up each square inch (6.5 square centimeters) of skin on the body. If your diet contains a lot of convenience foods, refined ingredients, fast foods, junk foods and coffee, these cells may be receiving only a fraction of the protein, vitamins, minerals and trace elements they need to stay in optimal condition. Elements necessary for strengthening connective tissues, such as vitamin B_6, vitamin C and zinc, may be barely present under these circumstances. And some substances that play a special role in protecting the skin, such as vitamin A, vitamin E and selenium, may be entirely absent. So it's not surprising that dietary deficiencies cause the epithelial cells to ring the alarm bells in the form of blemishes, irritation and dryness.

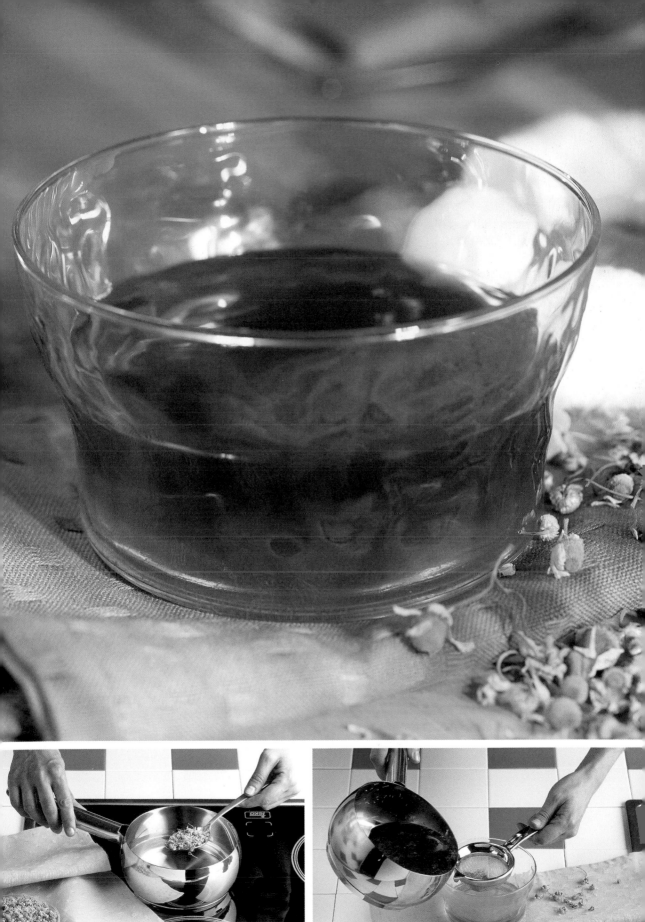

Mint Astringent

This mix of mint and vinegar is refreshing and will give your skin a lift, whether it's dry, oily or somewhere in between.

Best for: All skin types

Tip: In recipes, the generic term *mint* is typically used to mean spearmint rather than peppermint or other members of that herb family. Spearmint is wonderful not only in cooking but also in homemade beauty treatments. It can run wild in the garden, so plant a pot of it instead. That way, you'll always have fresh leaves ready to go into recipes.

Note: Always measure accurately when you're making homemade beauty products. See page 53 for tips.

- 2 glass jars with lids
- Fine-mesh sieve

1 tbsp	coarsely chopped fresh mint (see tip, at left)	15 mL
2 tsp	cider vinegar	10 mL
1 cup	distilled water (see tip, page 86)	250 mL

1. In jar, combine mint and vinegar. Seal tightly and let stand for 1 week in a cool, dry place.
2. Place fine-mesh sieve over clean jar; strain liquid into jar, discarding solids.
3. Stir in distilled water until well combined.
4. Soak a cotton ball or pad in vinegar mixture. Pat lightly onto face after cleansing.

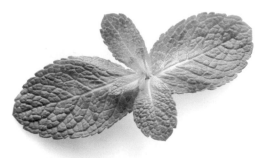

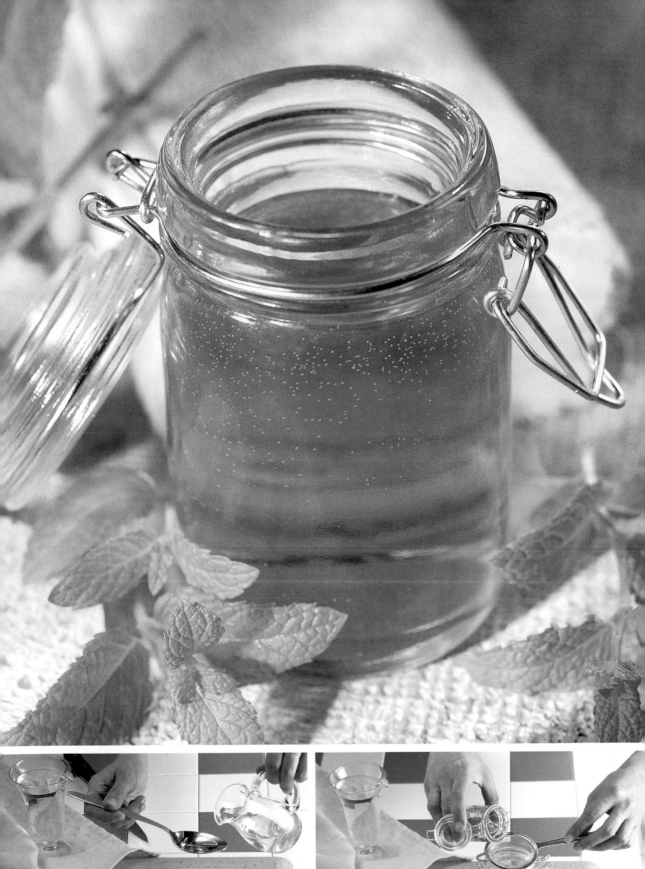

Wheat Germ Moisturizing Cream

Wheat germ oil is full of antioxidant vitamin E and is terrific at delivering moisture to parched skin. Rose water and rose essence give this cream a pretty floral scent.

Best for: Dry skin

Tips: Choose 100% natural cocoa butter for homemade creams like this. You can buy chunks of this creamy, yellowish substance made from cocoa beans at cosmetic-supply stores and online. It is also sold in uniform-size wafers. Either form will work fine in this recipe.

Rose and neroli (orange blossom) essential oils are expensive, because it takes so many flowers to make just a single drop of oil. This recipe substitutes less-expensive rose or orange blossom essence to give the cream a divine scent without the hefty price tag.

Note: Always measure accurately when you're making homemade beauty products. See page 53 for tips.

2 tbsp	rose water (see tips, page 84)	30 mL
1 tbsp	grated raw beeswax (see tips, page 74)	15 mL
1 tbsp	cocoa butter (see tips, at left)	15 mL
1 tbsp	shea butter (see tips, page 74)	15 mL
3 tbsp	wheat germ oil (see tips, page 149)	45 mL
3	drops rose essence or orange blossom essence (see tips, at left)	3

1. In a small saucepan, warm rose water over low heat (do not boil). Keep warm.

2. In a small heatproof bowl, combine beeswax, cocoa butter and shea butter. Set aside.

3. Pour enough water into another small saucepan to come about 2 inches (5 cm) up the side; bring to a simmer.

4. Set bowl on saucepan so that bottom of bowl is not touching simmering water; stir until beeswax mixture is melted and smooth. Remove bowl from heat.

5. Stir rose water and wheat germ oil into beeswax mixture. Using a wooden spoon, beat for 1 to 2 minutes or until lukewarm. Stir in rose essence. Let cool completely.

6. Smooth cream gently over face.

Step Two: Moisturizing

Moisturizing products contain large amounts of (often) water-based substances that are easy to spread across the face. The main purpose of moisturizing products is to restore the water lost by the skin, both through regular day-to-day living and through cleansing and toning (see box, page 70). They also help restructure the skin via the vital substances they contain, such as vitamins, minerals and trace elements. Smooth moisturizers over the face using a delicate touch.

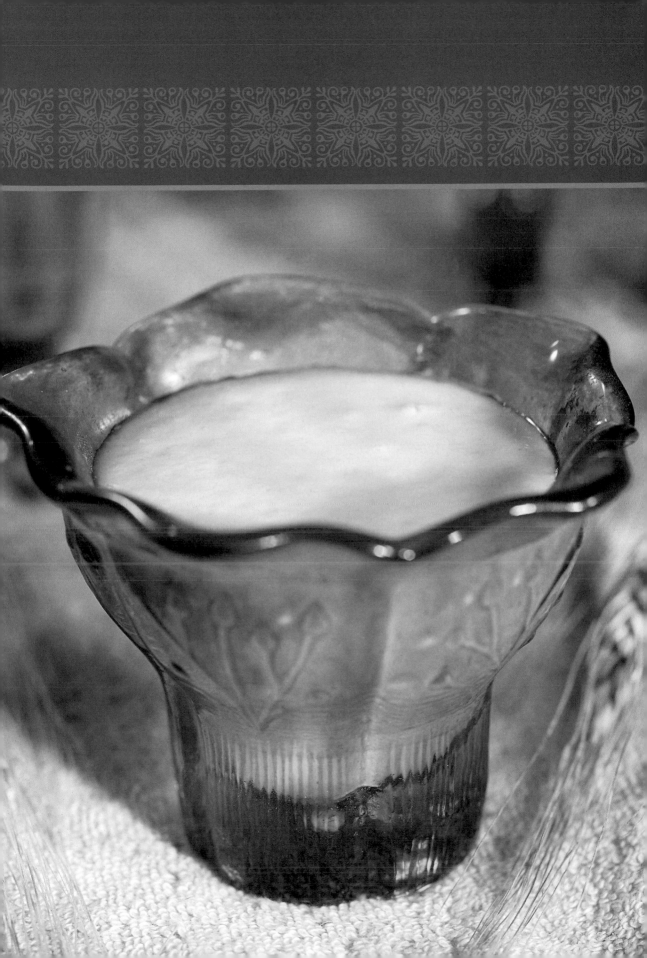

Cucumber Moisturizing Cream

Oily skin needs moisture too. This cream contains astringent ingredients (cucumber and bergamot essential oil) to balance the oiliness of the skin as it hydrates.

Best for: Oily skin

Tips: You don't need a lot of cucumber to make the small amount of juice for this cream. Chop a small handful of chunks in the blender until liquid, and then strain the juice through a fine-mesh sieve into a small bowl. If you have any juice leftover, enjoy it as a refreshing drink.

The bergamot orange is a citrus fruit; oil derived from its rind is used to give Earl Grey tea its distinctive aroma. Bergamot essential oil gives this cream its fresh scent and acts as a light moisturizer and toner at the same time.

Note: Always measure accurately when you're making homemade beauty products. See page 53 for tips.

2 tbsp	cucumber juice (see tips, at left)	30 mL
1 tbsp	cocoa butter (see tips, page 80)	15 mL
1 tbsp	rose water or distilled water (see tip, page 86)	15 mL
1 tsp	grated raw beeswax (see tips, page 74)	5 mL
3	drops bergamot essential oil (see tips, at left)	3

1. In a small heatproof bowl, combine cucumber juice, cocoa butter, rose water and beeswax. Set aside.

2. Pour enough water into a small saucepan to come about 2 inches (5 cm) up the side; bring to a simmer.

3. Set bowl on saucepan so that bottom of bowl is not touching simmering water; stir until cocoa butter mixture is melted and smooth. Remove bowl from heat.

4. Stir bergamot essential oil into cocoa butter mixture. Let cool completely.

5. Smooth cream gently over face.

Using Double Boilers

A double boiler heats ingredients gently, so it's handy for melting waxes and butters so they don't burn. A simple heatproof bowl set over a saucepan (shown below and opposite) works fine in its place.

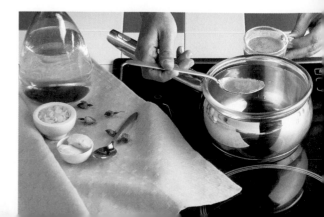

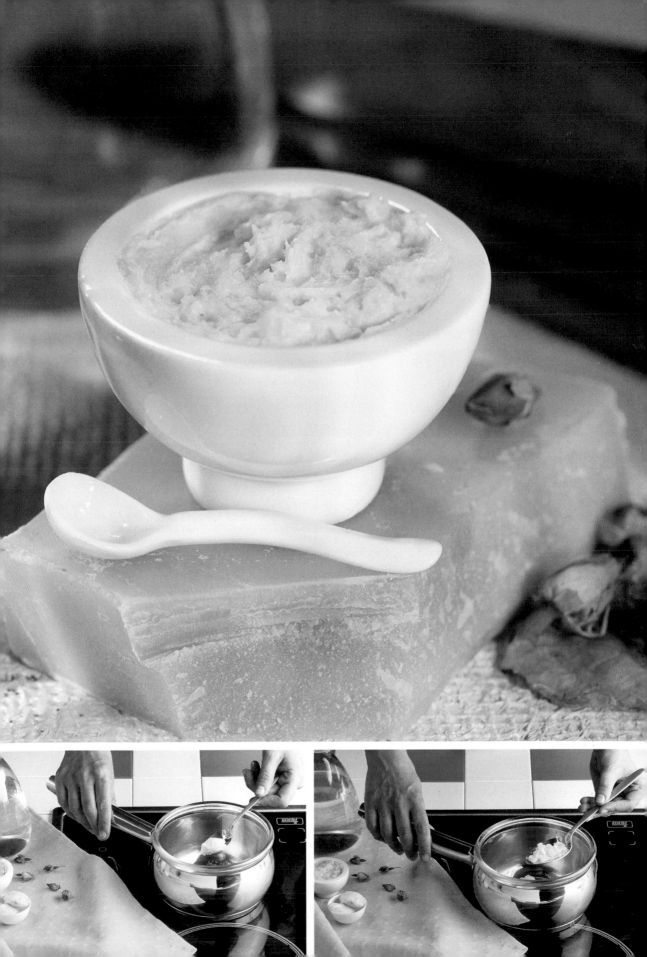

Honey Moisturizing Lotion

Natural comb honey (also called honeycomb) contains beeswax and honey, which are both wonderful for softening the skin.

Best for: All skin types

Tips: Rose water is commonly used in Middle Eastern, Mediterranean, Indian and North African cuisine, so look for bottles of this fragrant essence at specialty grocery stores.

Look for packages of natural comb honey at farmer's markets, natural food stores and some larger supermarkets. Better yet, support local beekeepers and buy it directly from an apiary near you.

Note: Always measure accurately when you're making homemade beauty products. See page 53 for tips.

- Small glass bottle with lid

2 tbsp	rose water (see tips, at left)	30 mL
1½ tsp	comb honey (see tips, at left) or liquid honey	7 mL
3 tbsp	witch hazel	45 mL

1. In a small saucepan, warm rose water over low heat until hot (do not boil). Remove from heat.
2. Stir honey into rose water until melted and smooth. Let cool.
3. Stir in witch hazel until well combined. Pour into bottle.
4. Moisten a cotton ball or pad with water; press to remove excess moisture. Pour a small amount of lotion onto cotton ball. Smooth gently over face. Store bottle in a cool, dark place between uses.

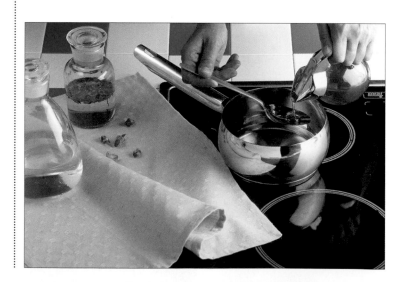

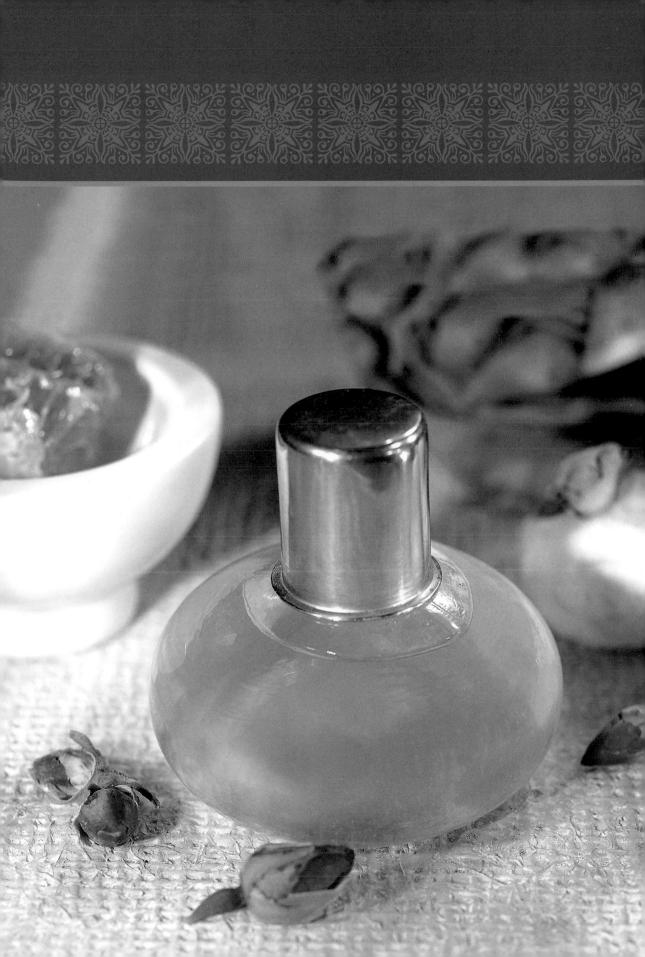

Lettuce Lotion

This leafy green isn't just for salads anymore. It's also a refreshing, moisturizing ingredient that will make your face radiant.

Best for: All skin types

Tip: Distilled water has been purified through the process of distillation; in other words, the water is boiled, and the condensation (which is free of impurities) is collected in a clean vessel. Bottles of it are readily available in supermarkets.

Note: Always measure accurately when you're making homemade beauty products. See page 53 for tips.

- Fine-mesh sieve
- Large glass jar with lid

2 cups	distilled water (see tip, at left)	500 mL
1	head lettuce, separated into leaves and coarsely chopped if large	1

1. In a large saucepan, bring distilled water to a boil.
2. Add lettuce leaves; cover and boil for 10 minutes. Remove from heat. Let cool completely, covered.
3. Place fine-mesh sieve over jar; strain liquid into jar, discarding solids.
4. Soak a cotton ball or pad in lettuce mixture. Smooth gently over face.

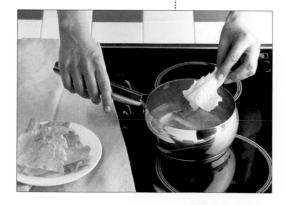
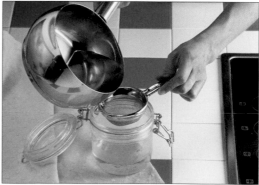

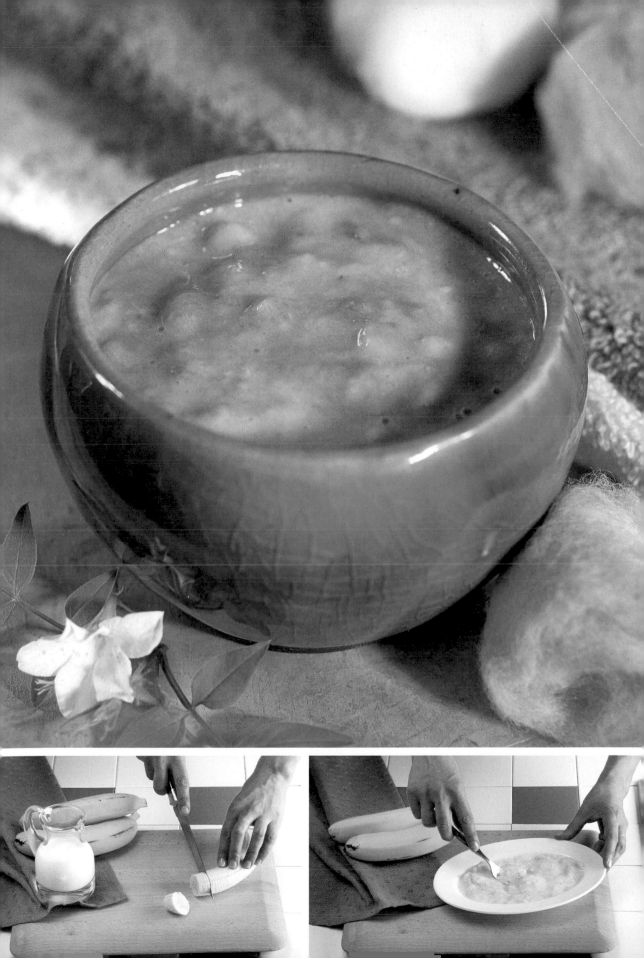

Honey Night Cream

Make this super-moisturizing cream a part of your nighttime ritual as you wind down for bed.
You'll wake up with dewy, fresh skin in the morning.

Best for: All skin types

Tips: This recipe contains raw egg and not enough natural preservatives to make the mixture shelf stable (that's why this makes just one batch). Discard any leftovers and make a fresh batch each time.

Sweet almond oil, like other nut oils, can perish quickly if stored in a warm place or exposed to direct sunlight. Keep the bottle in a dark, cool cupboard and use it up within a couple of months of opening.

Note: Always measure accurately when you're making homemade beauty products.
See page 53 for tips.

- Hand mixer

1	egg white (see tips, at left)	1
2 tsp	liquid honey (see tips, page 96)	10 mL
2 to 4	drops sweet almond oil (see tips, at left)	2 to 4

1. In a medium bowl and using hand mixer, beat egg white until stiff peaks form.
2. Stir in honey and almond oil until well combined.
3. Using fingers, immediately apply egg white mixture to face. Discard any leftovers.
4. Rinse off egg white mixture with lukewarm water. Gently pat face dry with a towel.

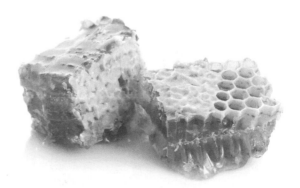

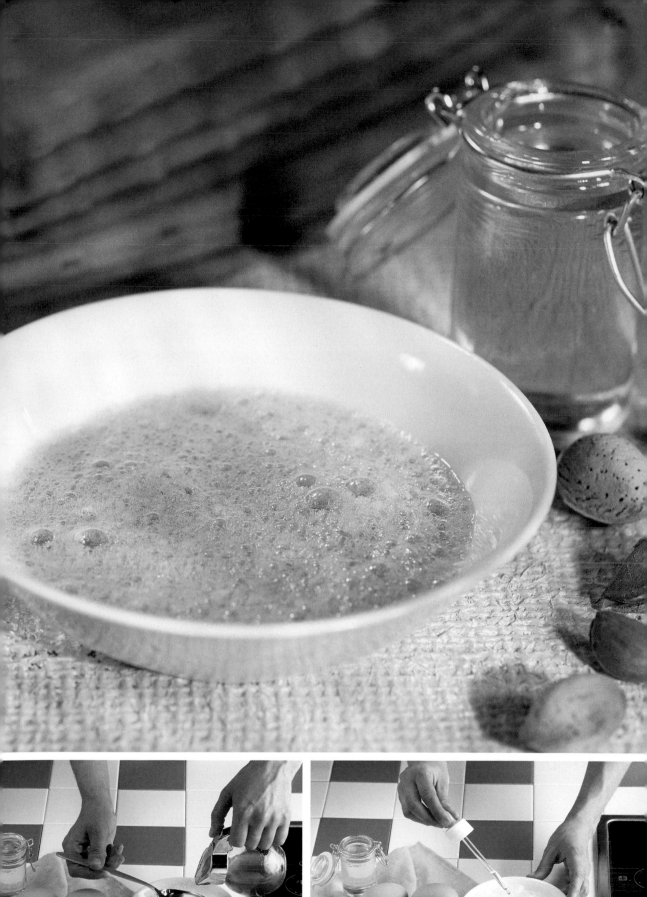

Nourishing Almond Oil Cream

Rose water, vanilla and geranium essential oil are a heavenly scented combination in this creamy moisturizer.

Best for: Dry skin

Tips: Vanilla powder is simply ground dried vanilla beans. Look for a 100% natural version at gourmet stores. It should contain no starches, sugars or other additives.

Buy essential oils sold in dark bottles. Exposure to light can reduce the potency of their medicinal herbal components. Store the bottles in a cool, dark place to keep them fresh.

Note: Always measure accurately when you're making homemade beauty products. See page 53 for tips.

¼ cup	sweet almond oil (see tips, page 90)	60 mL
1 tbsp	grated raw beeswax (see tips, page 74)	15 mL
2 tbsp	rose water	30 mL
½ tsp	vanilla powder (see tips, at left)	2 mL
3	drops geranium essential oil (see tips, at left)	3

1. In a small heatproof bowl, combine sweet almond oil and beeswax. Set aside.

2. Pour enough water into a small saucepan to come about 2 inches (5 cm) up the side; bring to a simmer.

3. Set bowl on saucepan so that bottom of bowl is not touching simmering water; stir until beeswax mixture is melted and smooth. Remove bowl from heat.

4. Stir rose water, vanilla and geranium essential oil into beeswax mixture until well combined and creamy. Let cool.

5. Smooth cream gently over face.

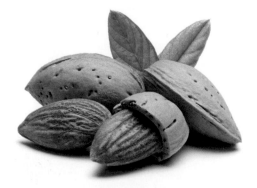

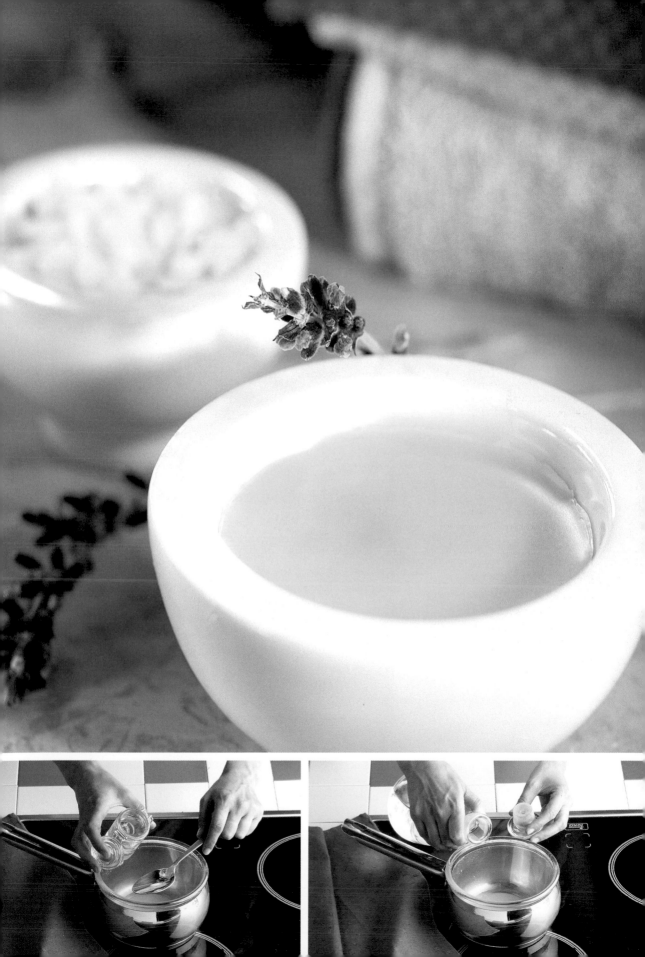

Pear Facial Mask

Pears contain antioxidant vitamins A and C, along with plenty of other vitamins and minerals, and they're just as good for your skin if you apply them directly to it. This mask has a nourishing and softening effect on dry, sensitive skin.

Best for: Dry skin

Tip: Use your fingers and nose to test pears for ripeness. One that's ready will yield to a little pressure from your fingers, and it will have a fresh, strong aroma.

Note: Always measure accurately when you're making homemade beauty products.
See page 53 for tips.

- Hand blender

¼	ripe pear, peeled and cored	¼
2 tbsp	plain yogurt	30 mL
1 tsp	cornstarch	5 mL

1. In a large cup and using hand blender, purée together pear, yogurt and cornstarch.

2. Using fingers, spread pear mixture all over face and neck, avoiding eye area. Let stand on skin for 20 minutes.

3. Rinse off pear mixture with warm water. Gently pat face and neck dry with a towel.

Step Four: Exfoliating and Fine-Tuning with a Facial Mask

Exfoliation renews the epidermis, gently removing dead skin cells and impurities from the surface. It also prevents blackheads by keeping pores free of clogs. Exfoliation is essential to prepare the skin before it receives a facial mask or other treatment. It is a good idea to exfoliate once a week after cleansing the skin. This helps fight wrinkles, makes the skin glow and reduces blemishes.

An easy, natural way to exfoliate your face is to add a pinch of granulated sugar to your regular cleansing cream. As you gently rub this mixture over your face, the sugar granules will deep-clean, oxygenate, smooth and refine the skin, and close pores for a flawless appearance.

Following exfoliation with a facial mask is a terrific way to relax. You can lie down with your eyes closed for a few minutes and indulge in some deep breathing while the mask does its job. A good mask has three features: it must have a creamy consistency, it must cling to the skin and it must be easy to remove. Masks have different purposes depending on their ingredients; they may cleanse, moisturize, nourish or firm skin, or act as an astringent. Choose the one that's right for your skin type.

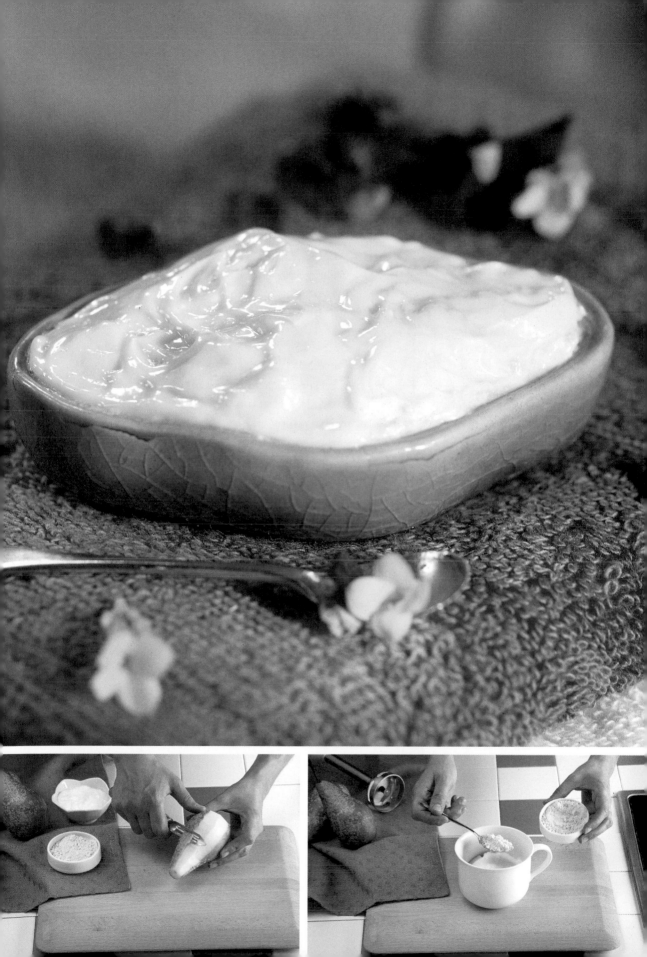

Clay Facial Mask

Clay is excellent at removing oil, dirt and impurities. It also stimulates blood flow to the skin, making it radiant.

Best for: Normal skin

Tips: There are many different types of clay available for making homemade facial masks. Kaolin, a pure white type of clay, is one of the most common and easy to use. French green clay is also popular for its oil-absorbing powers.

Liquid honey often crystallizes in the jar when it's stored in a warm place. There's nothing wrong with it in this state, and you can easily reliquefy it. Just pop the uncovered jar into a saucepan of warm water and heat it gently, stirring it until the crystals dissolve and the honey turns clear again.

Note: Always measure accurately when you're making homemade beauty products. See page 53 for tips.

- Mortar and pestle

2 tbsp	clay (see tips, at left)	30 mL
1 tbsp	plain yogurt	15 mL
1 tbsp	liquid honey (see tips, at left)	15 mL
1	egg (see tips, page 90)	1
½	ripe banana, chopped	½

1. In mortar using pestle, mash together clay, yogurt, honey, egg and banana until a smooth, creamy paste forms.

2. Using fingers, spread clay mixture all over face and neck, avoiding eye area. Let stand on skin for 20 minutes, periodically stretching and relaxing the facial muscles.

3. Rinse off clay mixture with lukewarm water. Gently pat face and neck dry with a towel.

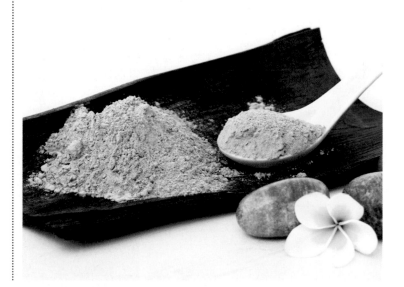

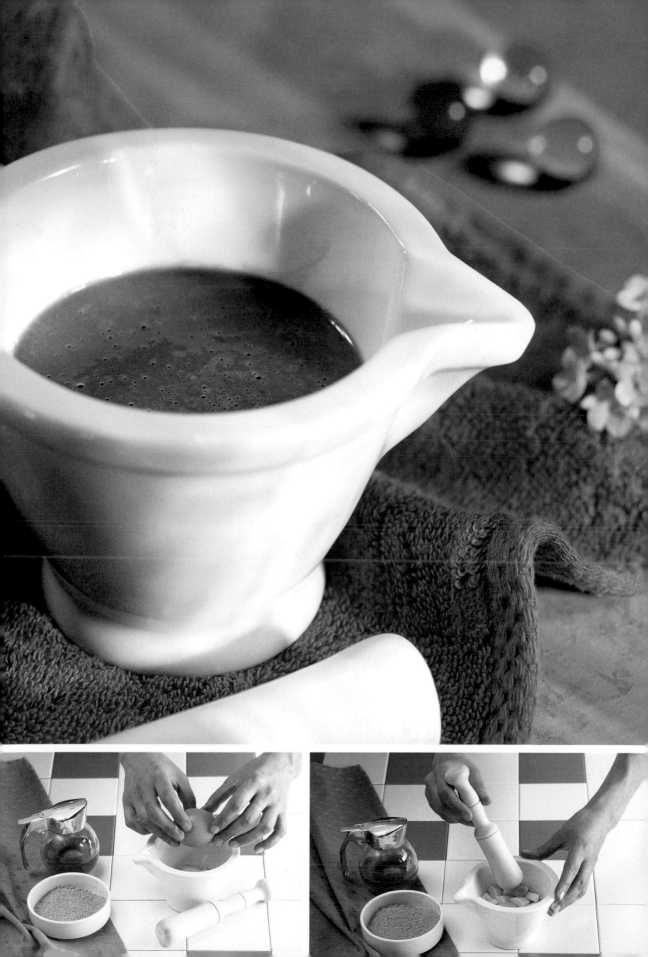

Egg and Olive Oil Facial Mask

This emulsion is similar to mayonnaise and delivers vitamins, minerals and emollients directly to the places on your face that need them most.

Best for: Combination skin

Tip: Cold-pressed extra-virgin olive oil is the purest and most unadulterated type you can buy for making homemade facial treatments. The best part: you can enjoy it on salads to boost nutrition from the inside too.

Note: Always measure accurately when you're making homemade beauty products. See page 53 for tips.

1	egg yolk (see tips, page 90)	1
3 tbsp	olive oil (see tip, at left)	45 mL
1 tbsp	lemon juice	15 mL

1. Place egg yolk in a small bowl. Add oil gradually, whisking constantly, until mixture is thickened and emulsified.

2. Whisk in lemon juice.

3. Using fingers, spread egg yolk mixture all over face and neck, avoiding eye area. Let stand on skin for 20 minutes.

4. Rinse off egg yolk mixture with warm water. Rinse again with cold water. Gently pat face and neck dry with a towel.

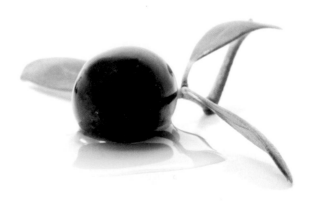

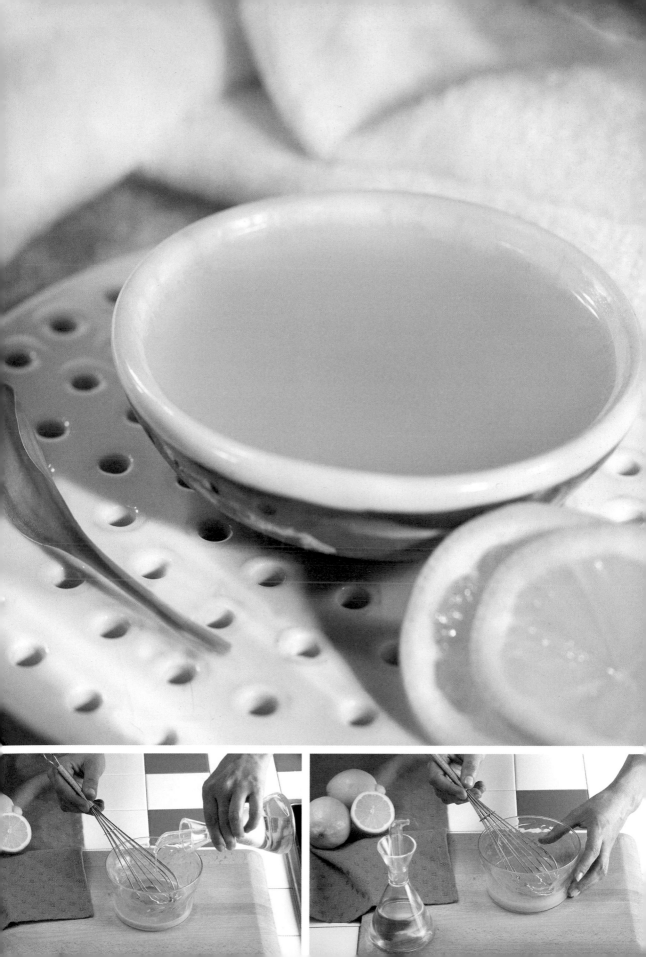

Oatmeal Facial Mask

Oats are ideal for soothing and healing skin. They make an effective, but not harsh, mask that balances oily skin. This mask makes enough for a number of treatments.

Best for: Oily skin

Tips: Brewer's yeast is a potent source of B vitamins. It is a nutritious addition to beauty treatments and to food. Look for it in health food and nutritional supplement stores.

Orange essential oil is just one of the essential oils made from the orange tree; it is extracted from the zest of the fruit. Neroli essential oil is made from the flowers, and petitgrain essential oil is made from the leaves and twigs of the plant.

Note: Always measure accurately when you're making homemade beauty products. See page 53 for tips.

- Small glass jar with lid

2 tbsp	soybean oil	30 mL
3 tbsp	finely ground oats or oat flour (see tip, page 73)	45 mL
1 tsp	brewer's yeast (see tips, at left)	5 mL
3	drops orange essential oil (see tips, at left)	3

1. Pour soybean oil into a small bowl. Gradually stir in oats to form a paste.

2. Stir in brewer's yeast and orange essential oil until well combined.

3. Spoon mixture into jar.

4. Place a little bit of mask in palm and mix with an equal amount of hot (not scalding) water. Using fingers, spread all over face and neck, avoiding eye area. Let stand on skin for 20 minutes.

5. Rinse off mask with warm water. Gently pat face and neck dry with a towel. Store jar in a cool, dark place between uses.

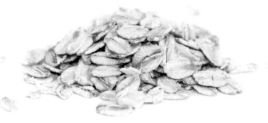

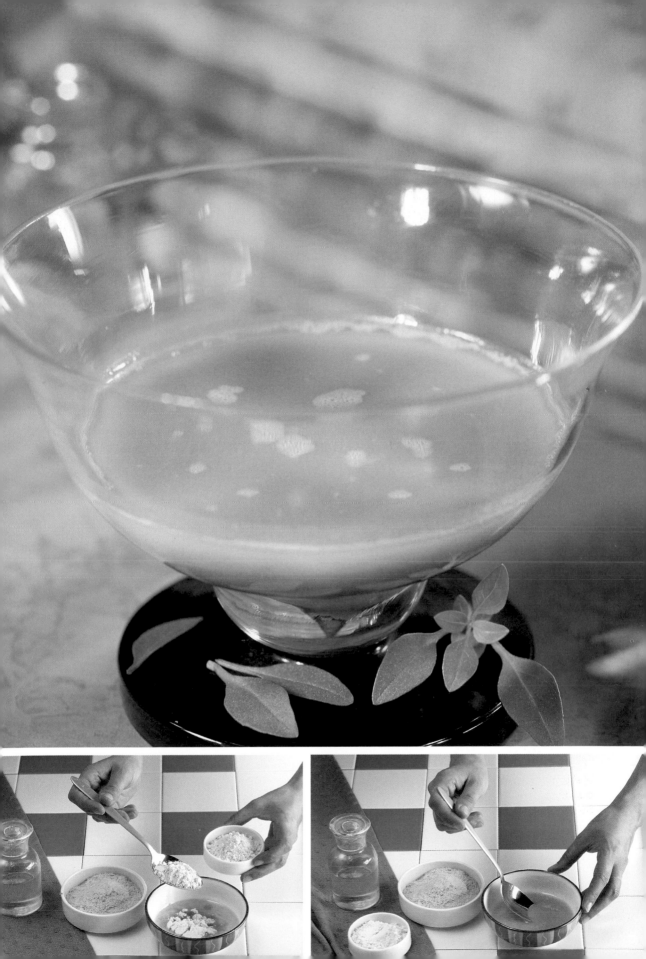

Potato, Honey and Milk Facial Mask

This is a lovely healing mask that soothes irritations and burns. Even sunburns will quickly feel better when treated with this gentle mixture.

Best for: Treating blemishes or burns

Tip: Powdered milk (also called dry milk) is commonly found in the baking aisle at the supermarket. You can store it in a tightly sealed airtight container in a cool, dark place for up to a year. If you keep it in the freezer, it will last even longer.

Note: Always measure accurately when you're making homemade beauty products. See page 53 for tips.

• Vegetable peeler

1	potato (unpeeled), scrubbed	1
2 tbsp	powdered milk (see tip, at left)	30 mL
1 tbsp	liquid honey (see tips, page 96)	15 mL

1. In a medium saucepan, cover potato with water; bring to a boil. Boil until fork-tender, 10 to 20 minutes. Drain potato and let cool enough to handle.

2. Using vegetable peeler, peel skin off potato and discard; in a medium bowl and using a fork, mash potato. Mash in powdered milk and honey until well combined.

3. Pat skin to remove any moisture. Using fingers, spread potato mixture all over face and neck, avoiding eye area. Let stand on skin for 20 to 30 minutes.

4. Rinse off potato mixture with lukewarm water, without rubbing skin. Gently pat face and neck dry with a towel.

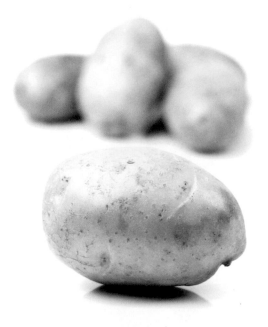

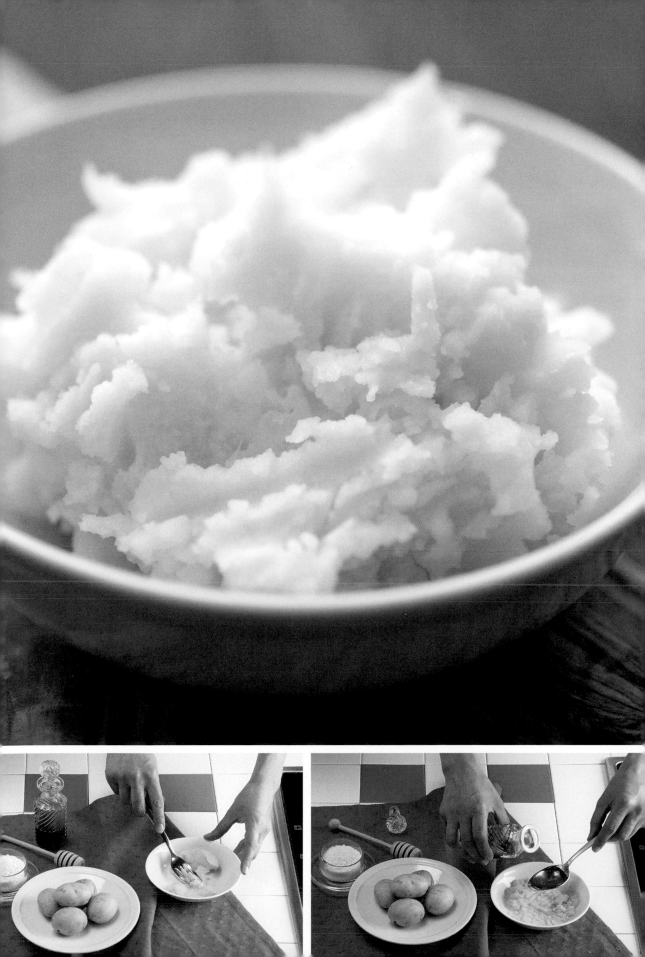

Nourishing Peach Facial Mask

Ripe peaches deliver a healthy dose of vitamins and minerals to the skin, and they give this mask a fresh, fruity scent.

Best for: All skin types

Tip: Ripe peaches are not overly soft but will give a little if you press them with your fingers. They also have a strong, fresh aroma. Avoid rock-hard peaches, which will never ripen well; they have usually been picked too early.

Note: Always measure accurately when you're making homemade beauty products. See page 53 for tips.

- Blender

1	ripe peach (see tip, at left)	1
⅓ cup	plain yogurt	75 mL
1 tsp	cornstarch	5 mL

1. Using a sharp knife, peel and pit peach.

2. In blender, combine peach and yogurt. Blend until a thick purée forms. Pour into a small bowl; stir in cornstarch.

3. Using fingers, spread peach mixture all over face, avoiding eye area. Let stand on skin for 20 minutes.

4. Rinse off peach mixture with lukewarm water. Gently pat face dry with a towel.

Stronger Skin in 60 to 90 Days

Biochemists who specialize in dermatology have determined a plan that can help you regenerate weakened skin from within in three months or less:

• **Eat fresh fruit several times a day.** Vitamin C, found in abundance in lemon and orange pulp and juice, activates cell growth, facilitates renewal of connective tissues, destroys free radicals and helps generate vitamin E.

• **Get enough vitamin E.** Vitamin E helps block free radical chain reactions that break down skin. Vitamin E is found in cold-pressed oils, nuts and the germ of whole grains.

• **Eat your muesli.** Start each day with ½ cup (125 mL) of this delicious mixture of raw rolled oats, dried or fresh fruit, nuts, seeds, and yogurt or milk. It increases the vitamin E concentration in skin cell membranes and contains selenium, which strengthens the immune system.

• **Stockpile sulfur.** The sulfur that your skin (and hair) needs to stay beautiful is found in egg yolks. It is advisable to eat one every other day.

• **Always eat this trio of health enhancers.** Eating tofu (or taking a soy lecithin supplement), brewer's yeast and plenty of salad every day will ensure your body gets the lecithin, B vitamins and minerals it needs to build healthy skin, nails and hair.

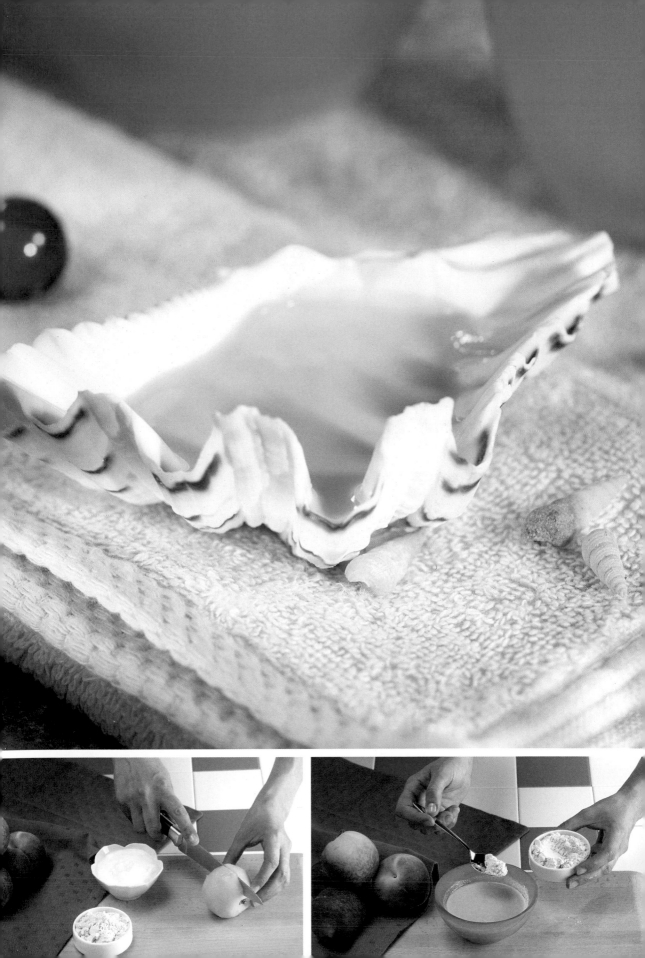

Cream and Herb Facial Mask

Adding a bit of cream to this herbal oil mixture gives it extra skin-softening power.

Best for: Normal skin

Tips: Cold-pressed extra-virgin oils are the purest and most unadulterated type you can buy for making homemade beauty treatments. They are worth the higher price tag.

Calendulas, or marigolds, are versatile medicinal plants that have many healing properties, especially for the skin. They are really easy to grow in the garden or in pots, and they love just about any location, from sunny to shady.

Note: Always measure accurately when you're making homemade beauty products. See page 53 for tips.

- ½-cup (125 mL) canning jar with lid
- Fine-mesh sieve
- Small dark glass bottle with lid

3 tbsp	soybean oil (see tips, at left)	45 mL
2 tsp	sweet almond oil (see tips, page 90)	10 mL
2 tsp	avocado oil	10 mL
1 tsp	fresh rosemary leaves	5 mL
1 tsp	chopped fresh calendula leaves (see tips, at left)	5 mL
	Heavy or whipping (35%) cream	

1. In jar, combine soybean oil, sweet almond oil, avocado oil, rosemary leaves and calendula leaves. Seal tightly and let stand for 3 weeks in a cool, dry place.

2. Place fine-mesh sieve over a small bowl; strain oil into bowl, discarding solids. Pour into bottle.

3. Mix 1 tbsp (15 mL) of herbed oil with 1 tsp (5 mL) cream. Using fingers, spread all over face, avoiding eye area. Let stand on skin for 10 to 20 minutes.

4. Rinse off cream mixture with lukewarm water. Gently pat face dry with a towel. Store bottle in a cool, dark place for up to 1 month.

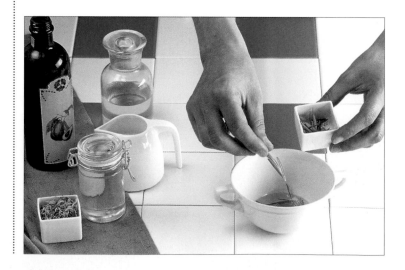

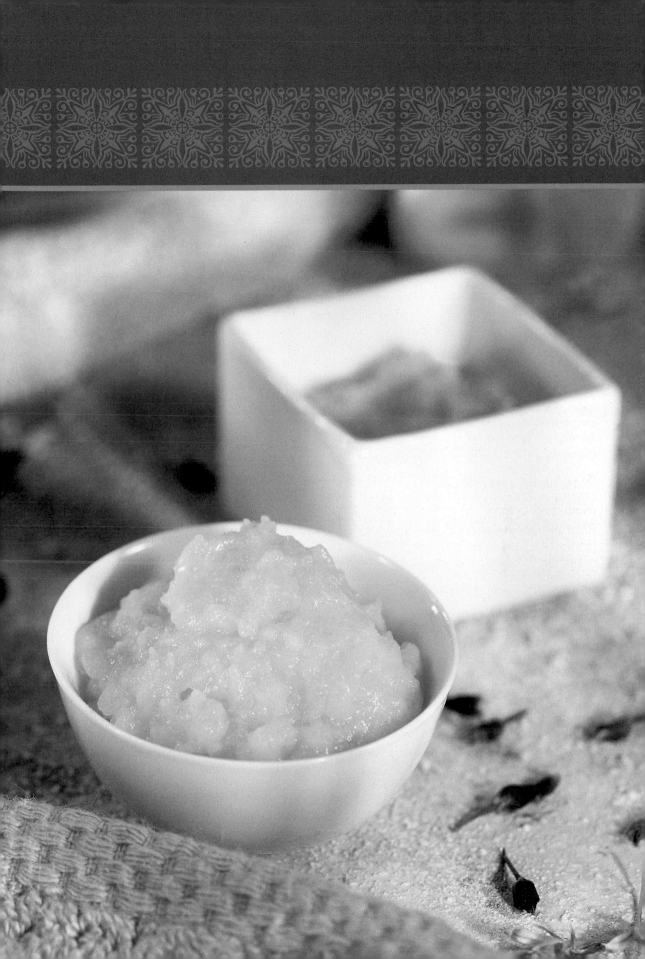

Horsetail Aftershave Lotion

Soothe skin after a close shave with this astringent lotion. It has a fresh citrusy aroma that's clean and masculine.

Best for: Treating razor burn and skin tightness after shaving

Tip: Ethyl alcohol is the type of alcohol in spirits and other alcoholic beverages. It is not the same as isopropyl alcohol, the type you find at the drugstore for disinfecting wounds. You can get high-proof grain alcohol from the liquor store (look for the brand name Everclear). In a pinch, substitute unflavored vodka or brandy.

Note: Always measure accurately when you're making homemade beauty products. See page 53 for tips.

- Fine-mesh sieve
- Dark glass bottle with lid

2 tsp	dried horsetail (see tips, page 272)	10 mL
¼ cup	boiling water	60 mL
2 tbsp	ethyl alcohol (see tip, at left)	30 mL
2 tbsp	witch hazel	30 mL
5	drops lemon essential oil (see tips, page 92)	5

1. Spoon horsetail into a small heatproof bowl; pour boiling water over top. Cover and let steep for 8 minutes.
2. Place fine-mesh sieve over another small heatproof bowl; strain liquid into bowl, discarding solids.
3. Stir in alcohol, witch hazel and lemon essential oil. Pour into bottle.
4. Soak a cotton ball or pad in horsetail mixture. Pat gently over face after shaving. Store bottle in a cool, dark place for up to 2 months.

For Him: Aftershave Care

Men's skin needs special care and moisturizing, just like women's skin. Shaving puts continual stress on men's faces and can cause dryness or tightness. While it is true that shaving cleans and exfoliates the skin, it also removes surface cells and the hydrolipidic film that protects the skin from damaging external aggressors. In addition, shaving can result in nicks and cuts, which make the skin more vulnerable to germs and infection. The solution is a good homemade aftershave treatment, like the ones on this page and pages 110 to 114. They ease tight skin and soothe uncomfortable razor burn.

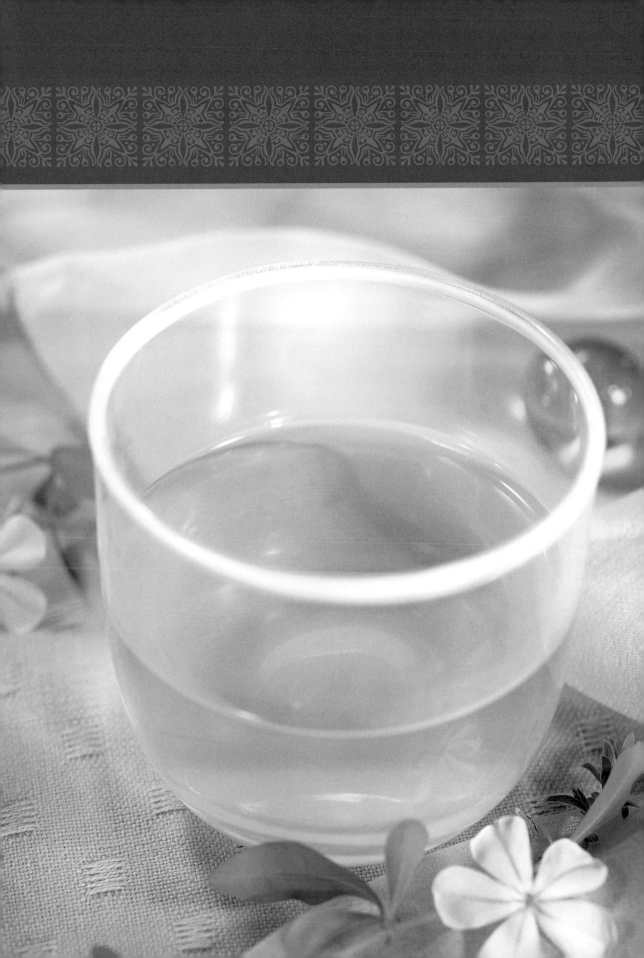

Almond Aftershave Cream

Horsetail is a healing grass that is used to reduce skin inflammation. Look for the chopped dried leaves at herbalists' shops or online.

Best for: Treating razor burn and skin tightness after shaving

Tips: Choose 100% natural cocoa butter for homemade creams like this. You can buy chunks of this creamy, yellowish substance made from cocoa beans at cosmetic-supply stores and online. It is also sold in uniform-size wafers. Either form will work fine in this recipe.

Stearic acid crystals are commonly added to mixtures that contain beeswax, to help boost the wax's emulsifying powers. Look for them at cosmetic-supply stores or online.

Note: Always measure accurately when you're making homemade beauty products. See page 53 for tips.

- Fine-mesh sieve
- Hand blender
- Small glass jar with lid

2½ tbsp	water	37 mL
1 tsp	dried horsetail	5 mL
1 tbsp	soybean oil (see tips, page 106)	15 mL
1 tbsp	sweet almond oil (see tips, page 90)	15 mL
1 tsp	grated raw beeswax (see tips, page 74)	5 mL
1 tsp	cocoa butter (see tips, at left)	5 mL
1 tsp	stearic acid (see tips, at left)	5 mL
3	drops rosemary essential oil (see tips, page 92)	3

1. In a small saucepan, combine water and horsetail; bring to a boil. Remove from heat; cover and let steep for 5 minutes.

2. Place fine-mesh sieve over a small heatproof bowl; strain liquid into bowl, discarding solids. Set aside.

3. In another small heatproof bowl, combine soybean oil, sweet almond oil, beeswax, cocoa butter and stearic acid. Set aside.

4. Pour enough water into a small saucepan to come about 2 inches (5 cm) up the side; bring to a simmer.

5. Set bowl with soybean oil mixture on saucepan so that bottom of bowl is not touching simmering water; stir until melted and mixture turns a lighter color. Remove bowl from heat.

6. Add horsetail infusion. Using hand blender, beat for 1 to 2 minutes or until mixture is milky. Beat in rosemary essential oil. Beat for 1 to 2 minutes or until mixture is thickened and has a creamy consistency.

7. Spoon cream into jar.

8. Smooth over face after shaving. Store jar in the refrigerator for 4 to 6 weeks.

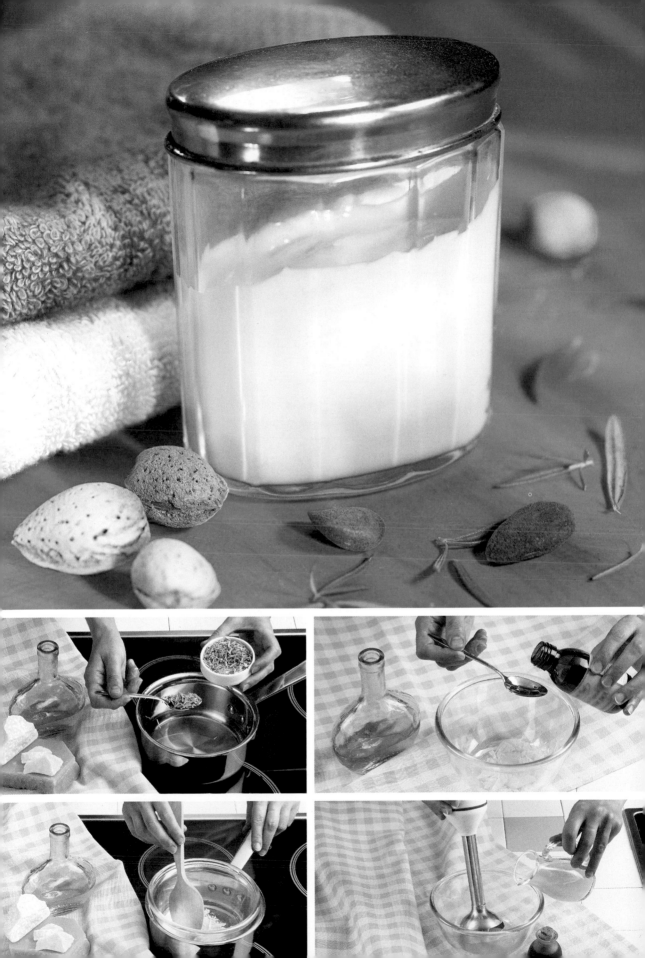

Sage and Rosemary Aftershave Lotion

With a fresh, nutty herbal scent, this lotion is a balm for facial skin that's tired and weakened by daily shaving.

Best for: Treating razor burn and skin tightness after shaving

Tip: Look for bottles of pure hazelnut extract in gourmet stores or online. Avoid imitation extracts, because they are made with artificial fragrances and flavorings.

Note: Always measure accurately when you're making homemade beauty products.
See page 53 for tips.

- Fine-mesh sieve
- Dark glass bottle with lid

1 cup	cider vinegar	250 mL
1 tbsp	crumbled dried sage leaves	15 mL
1 tbsp	dried rosemary leaves	15 mL
	Hazelnut extract (see tip, at left)	

1. Pour vinegar into a small bowl; add rosemary and sage. Cover tightly and let stand for 1 week in a cool, dry place.

2. Place fine-mesh sieve over a glass measuring cup; strain liquid into measuring cup, discarding solids.

3. Check measurement of liquid in cup; add an equal amount of hazelnut extract. Pour into bottle.

4. Soak a cotton ball or pad in vinegar mixture. Pat gently over face after shaving. Store bottle in a cool, dark place for up to 1 month.

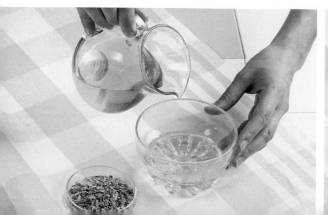

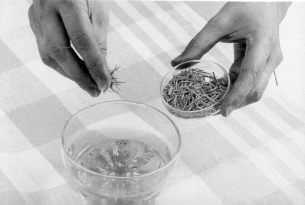

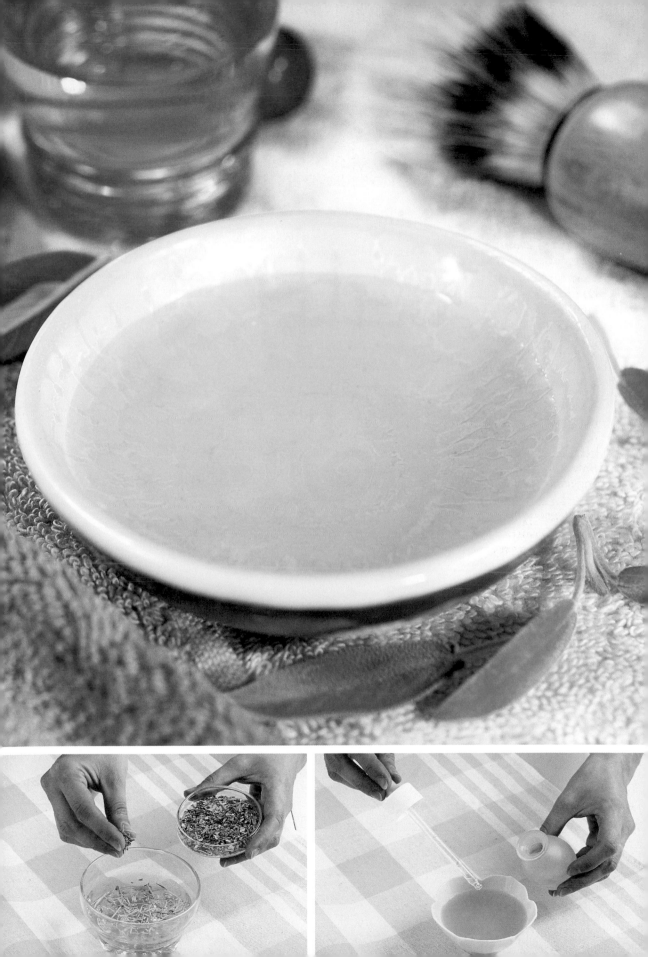

Hibiscus Flower Aftershave Lotion

This lotion is terrific for treating tender shaved skin, but it can also serve as an astringent to return a healthy glow to pale, lackluster skin.

Best for: Treating razor burn and skin tightness after shaving

Tip: Look for dried hibiscus flowers (called *flor de jamaica* in Spanish) in Mexican or Latin American grocery stores. They are often used to make beverages, so look for them near the teas.

Note: Always measure accurately when you're making homemade beauty products. See page 53 for tips.

- Dark glass bottle with lid

8 oz	dried hibiscus flowers (see tip, at left)	250 g
1 cup	rose water (see tips, page 84)	250 mL

1. Place hibiscus flowers in a medium heatproof bowl. Set aside.

2. In a small saucepan, bring rose water just to boil; pour over hibiscus flowers. Cover and let steep for 10 minutes.

3. Uncover and let cool completely. Pour into bottle.

4. Soak a cotton ball or pad in hibiscus mixture. Pat gently over face after shaving. Store bottle in a cool, dark place for up to 1 month.

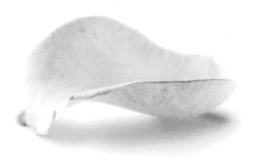

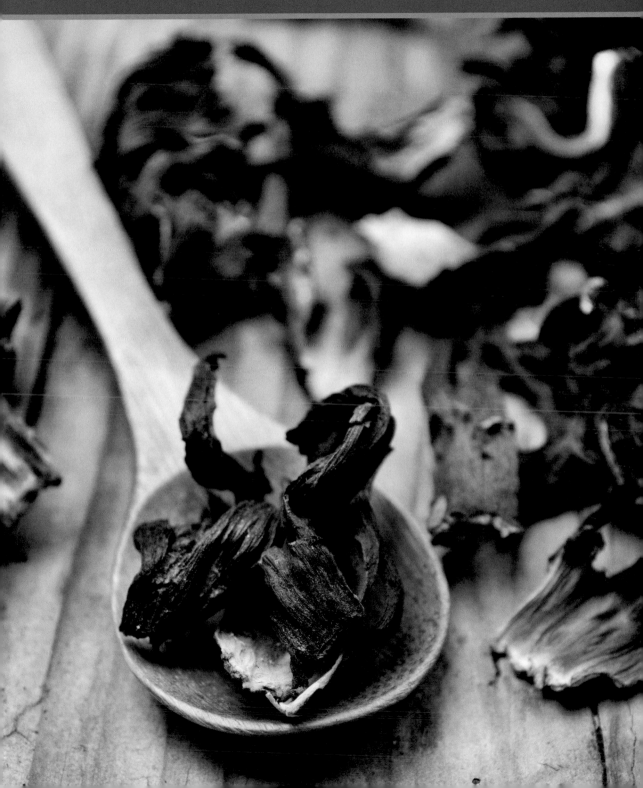

Acne: The Scourge of Adolescence

An estimated three-quarters of all young people suffer from acne to some extent. It is most common during adolescence because so many hormonal changes take place during this stage of life. However, acne's characteristic blemishes or pimples can appear at any age — even in people who had perfectly clear skin during their teenage years.

Acne often disappears of its own accord. It is not a serious disorder, but it feels like one. It appears just as teenagers are already suffering through the normal identity crisis that comes with adolescence. Cosmetic companies offer a large variety of products that promise miraculous results in a short time, the perfect relief from the anxiety over breakouts. But treating acne is not that easy, and nothing will cure it overnight.

What Causes Pimples and Blackheads?

To understand how acne forms, you have to remember that the skin is made up of layers of cells, among which lie many hair follicles. Around these follicles are many sebaceous glands, which secrete a type of fat called sebum. Sebum helps keep the skin moisturized, repels water and acts as a sort of protective lubricant.

Sebum, dead skin cells and dirt can build up in the hair follicles, where the oil travels upward to the surface of the skin. When the follicles get plugged, the sebum hardens and can be a host to bacteria, which can inflame the follicle. If the plug ulcerates, it will push out a pimple above the surface of the skin. If the plug doesn't ulcerate, the topmost part that comes into the contact with the air will oxidize and turn brown or black, producing a blackhead.

Natural Acne Treatments

The most important step in avoiding acne breakouts is to keep your skin scrupulously clean. Cleanse your face two or three times a day using a natural cleanser, followed by a pure soap if your skin is extremely oily. After cleansing, apply an astringent, and then, carefully apply a light moisturizing fluid to counter any tendency toward flakiness.

There are two other important acne-fighting strategies to try. First, give up makeup for a time to avoid adding more substances that can clog pores and exacerbate acne. Second, avoid the temptation to squeeze pimples. Touch the affected area as little as possible to avoid spreading bacteria and contaminating the skin.

Acne can also be treated and prevented with dietary changes. Avoid starchy, fried and refined foods; coffee; alcoholic beverages; and soft drinks, which can all aggravate the condition. Your best allies for eliminating acne are fresh vegetables and fruits that are rich in B vitamins and vitamin C. Unsweetened natural yogurt is an excellent choice — both to eat and to apply externally — because it contains abundant nutrients, particularly zinc (see box, page 124).

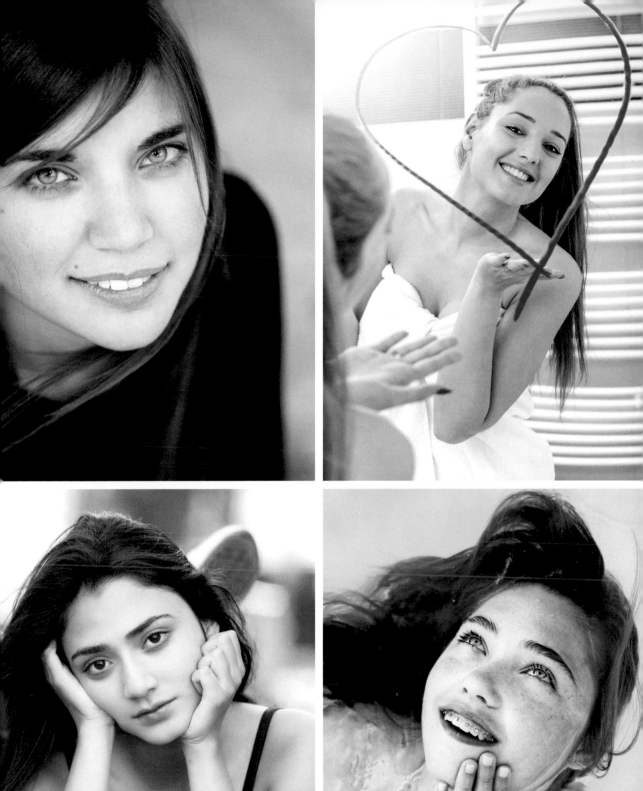
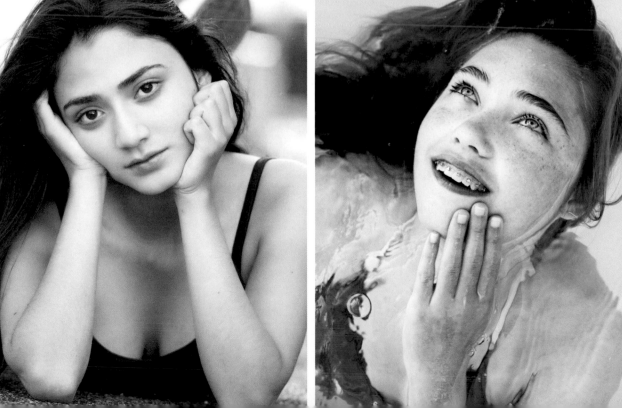

Anti-Acne Salt Massage Treatment

Salt is a good exfoliant and a natural bacteria fighter. Rub very gently and let the granules of salt do the work for you.

Best for: Acne-prone skin

Tips: Large-flake kosher sea salt is easy to find and a good texture for this recipe.

The bergamot orange is a citrus fruit; oil derived from its rind is used to give Earl Grey tea its distinctive aroma.

Note: Always measure accurately when you're making homemade beauty products. See page 53 for tips.

2	handfuls coarse salt (see tips, at left)	2
1 cup	water	250 mL
2	drops bergamot essential oil (see tips, at left)	2

1. Place salt in a medium bowl; moisten with water and bergamot essential oil, gently stirring to combine (do not let mixture form a liquidy paste).

2. Using hands and making circular massaging movements, gently rub salt mixture over face for 1 to 2 minutes.

3. Rinse off salt mixture with plenty of cold water. Gently pat face dry with a towel.

What Is Cystic Acne?

Cystic acne usually occurs in teenagers and young adults. It starts like regular acne, but pockets of bacteria and infection form much deeper inside the skin. They cause large dark red cysts to form on the face (and often the chest, upper arms and shoulders), which are painful and itchy. The cysts may ooze pus or a pinkish fluid, and can leave deep scars.

During puberty, masculinizing hormones called androgens begin to form in both men and women. These hormones help stimulate the development of certain secondary sexual characteristics, and in some adolescents, they cause the sebaceous glands to make more sebum. The problem is not actually excessive androgen secretion, but that some people's sebaceous glands are overly sensitive to these hormones.

This condition can become a nightmare for the sufferer. If you have cystic acne, find a good dermatologist and get professional treatment to help minimize discomfort, infections and scarring. To make treatments more effective, avoid saturated fats and sugar.

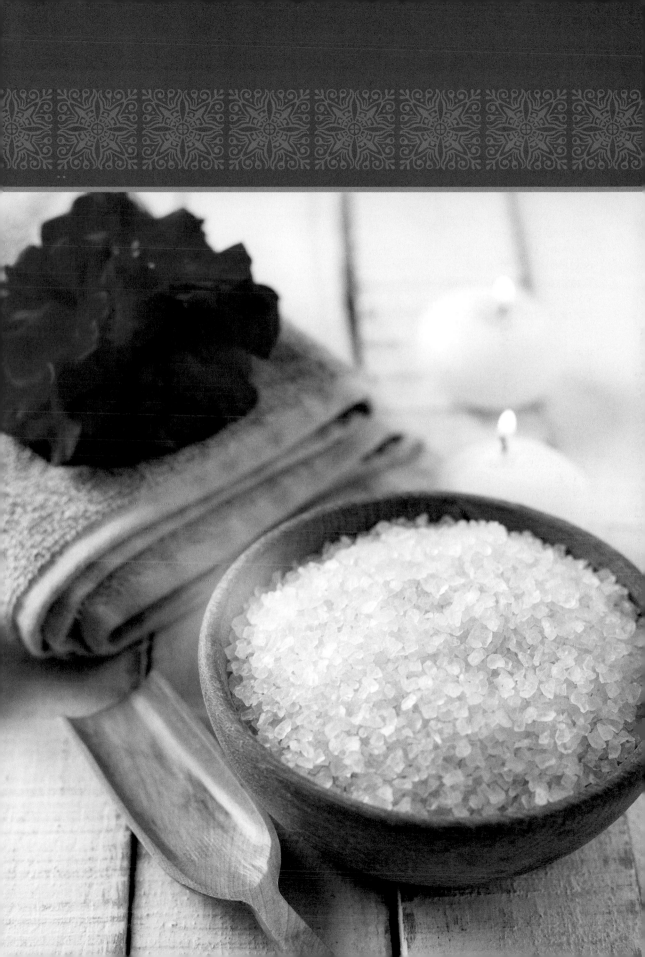

Acne-Fighting Steam Treatment

Steam baths like this are great for opening the pores and purifying the skin. They're also relaxing, so they can help reduce stress.

Best for: Acne-prone skin

Tip: Sempervivum (*Sempervivum tectorum*) is a succulent plant whose leaves have been traditionally used to soothe inflamed skin, due to their astringent properties. It is also known by the names common houseleek, and hens and chicks. There are many types of sempervivum available; choose this one for its specific medicinal powers.

Note: Always measure accurately when you're making homemade beauty products. See page 53 for tips.

1 tbsp	fresh sempervivum leaves (see tip, at left)	15 mL
1 tbsp	fennel seeds	15 mL
1 tbsp	dried comfrey root (see tip, page 148)	15 mL
4 cups	boiling water	1 L

1. In a large heatproof bowl, combine sempervivum leaves, fennel seeds and comfrey root; pour boiling water over top. Cover and let stand for 5 minutes.

2. Cover your head and the bowl with a towel; hold your face over the bowl and inhale the steam for 15 minutes. Keep a safe distance away from the surface of the water to avoid scalding yourself.

3. Wet a washcloth in cold water and wring out the excess. Wipe face with towel to help close pores and restore normal skin temperature. Pat face dry with another towel.

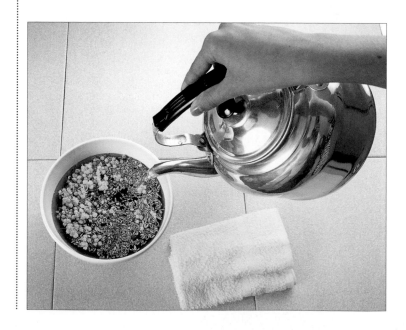

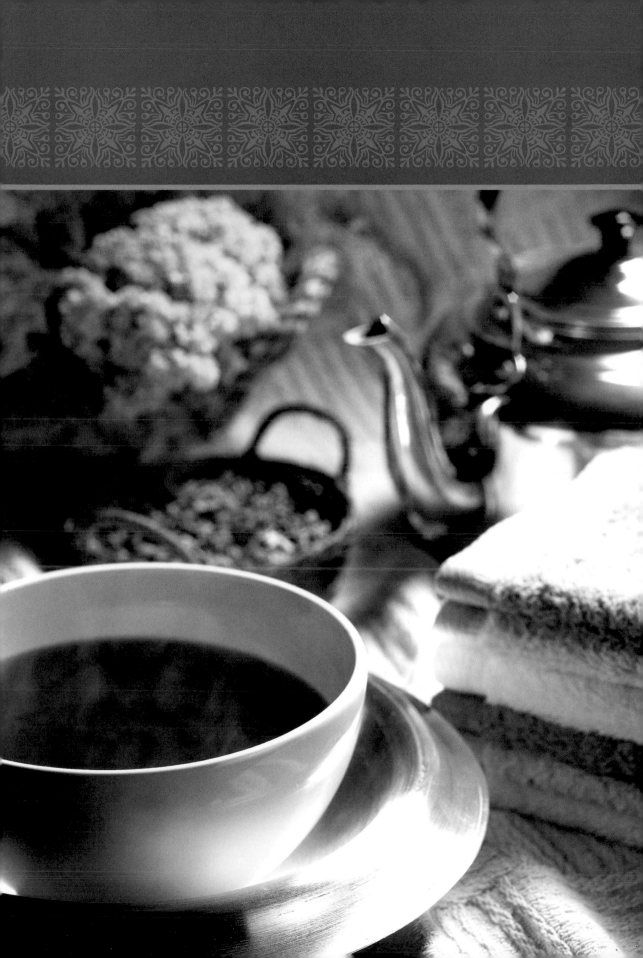

Q&A: Acne

There are lots of myths and truths out there about acne. Here are the top questions people ask about this common skin problem:

Q: Does stress cause acne?

A: No, but stress probably makes acne worse because it lowers resistance to infection.

Q: Does chocolate cause acne?

A: Not generally. Some people have a chemical sensitivity to chocolate, which can make them break out after consuming it. In these cases, try replacing chocolate with carob, a healthy and nutritious substitute that does not contain cocoa butter (the possible culprit).

Q: Can losing weight make acne flare up?

A: Yes, because dieting makes the body burn off accumulated fat, which can have the same negative effect on skin as eating a diet high in saturated fats.

Q: Does sweating make acne worse?

A: Yes, it can. Sweat can clog pores and aggravate inflammation.

Q: Does popping pimples cause scars?

A: Not always. Scars are usually produced by cysts, which get infected, forming pus and destroying underlying tissues. Still, it's not a good idea to pop pimples, as this can transfer harmful bacteria to weakened skin.

Q: Can I use makeup if I have acne?

A: You can use cosmetics if you like, but be sure to choose products that are noncomedogenic; this means they will not clog pores.

Q: Should I take a vitamin A supplement if I have severe acne?

A: Many natural health experts recommend this. It seems that vitamin A is best for fighting cystic acne (see box, page 118), and helps patients with large, painful nodules and many keratin plugs blocking their pores.

Q: Should I treat my acne with antibiotics?

A: Dermatologists often prescribe tetracycline to treat acne. It works, but keep in mind that when antibiotics are taken for a prolonged period of time, they kill beneficial bacteria and gut flora along with acne-causing bacteria. This can upset intestinal balance. If you choose this therapy, make sure to eat plenty of probiotic foods (such as yogurt and fermented foods like sauerkraut and miso) to boost the good bacteria in your gut.

Q: Is there a miracle cure?

A: Unfortunately, there isn't. Don't trust people or products that promise to cure acne in just one month. If it sounds too good to be true, it is.

Herbal Steam for Acne

A facial steam bath smells wonderful and helps your body remove impurities naturally.

Best for: Acne-prone skin

Tip: Look for a reliable source of dried medicinal herbs, such as an herbalist's shop or a reputable online dealer. Make sure it's a business with high turnover, to ensure you're getting the freshest, most effective herbs possible.

Note: Always measure accurately when you're making homemade beauty products. See page 53 for tips.

1 tbsp	dried licorice root (see tip, at left)	15 mL
1 tbsp	dried violet leaves	15 mL
1 tbsp	dried comfrey root	15 mL
1 tbsp	dried dandelion leaves	15 mL
1 tbsp	white willow bark	15 mL
1 tbsp	chopped rhubarb	15 mL
	Boiling water	

1. In a large heatproof bowl, toss together licorice root, violet leaves, comfrey root, dandelion leaves, white willow bark and rhubarb.

2. Pour in enough boiling water to cover herbs and fill bowl about halfway.

3. Cover your head and the bowl with a towel, hold your face over the bowl and inhale the steam for 15 minutes. Keep a safe distance away from the surface of the water to avoid scalding yourself.

4. Uncover your head. Using cotton balls or pads, or a soft, clean washcloth, gently wipe your face to remove any impurities.

5. Rinse face with cold water. Gently pat face dry with a towel.

Oat and Almond Mask

Rinsing with cold water after removing a mask closes pores and stimulates circulation.

Best for: Oily or acne-prone skin

Tip: You can buy ground oats, but it's very simple to make them at home. Spoon rolled oats into a food processor and grind them until they're fine and powdery.

1 tbsp	finely ground oats or oat flour (see tip, at left)	15 mL
1	egg white	1
10	drops sweet almond oil (see tips, page 90)	10
3	drops myrrh essential oil (see tips, page 92)	3
	Milk	

1. In a medium bowl, stir together oats, egg white, sweet almond oil and myrrh essential oil. Mix in enough milk to give the mask a creamy consistency.

2. Using fingers and making upward motions, spread oat mixture all over face and neck. Let stand on skin for 20 minutes.

3. Rinse off oat mixture with cold water. Gently pat face dry with a towel.

Carrot Anti-Acne Mask

The results of this mask are amazing: the yogurt nourishes, softens and combats infections; the carrot absorbs contaminants; and the cornstarch softens, clears and firms up the skin. Use it immediately after cleansing for best results.

Best for: Acne-prone skin

Tip: Use the smaller holes on a box grater to grate the carrot for this recipe. You want tiny flecks of carrot that will distribute evenly in the yogurt mixture.

Note: Always measure accurately when you're making homemade beauty products. See page 53 for tips.

½ cup	plain yogurt	125 mL
1 tbsp	finely grated carrot (see tip, at left)	15 mL
1 tsp	cornstarch	5 mL

1. In a small bowl, stir together yogurt, carrot and cornstarch until well combined.

2. Using fingers, spread carrot mixture all over face and neck, avoiding eye area. Let stand on skin for 20 minutes.

3. Rinse off carrot mixture with cold water. Gently pat face and neck dry with a towel.

The Link Between Acne and Zinc

Recent studies have shown that most cases of acne are associated with zinc deficiency. Try taking soy lecithin every day, because this dietary supplement acts as an emulsifier; that is, it disperses fats and helps break them down. You also need to improve circulation and increase blood flow to the surface of the skin, so make sure you get enough sleep, exercise and fresh air too.

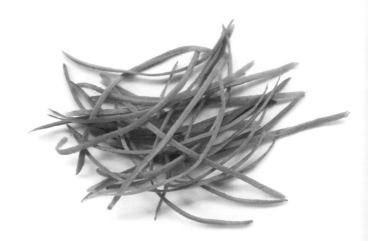

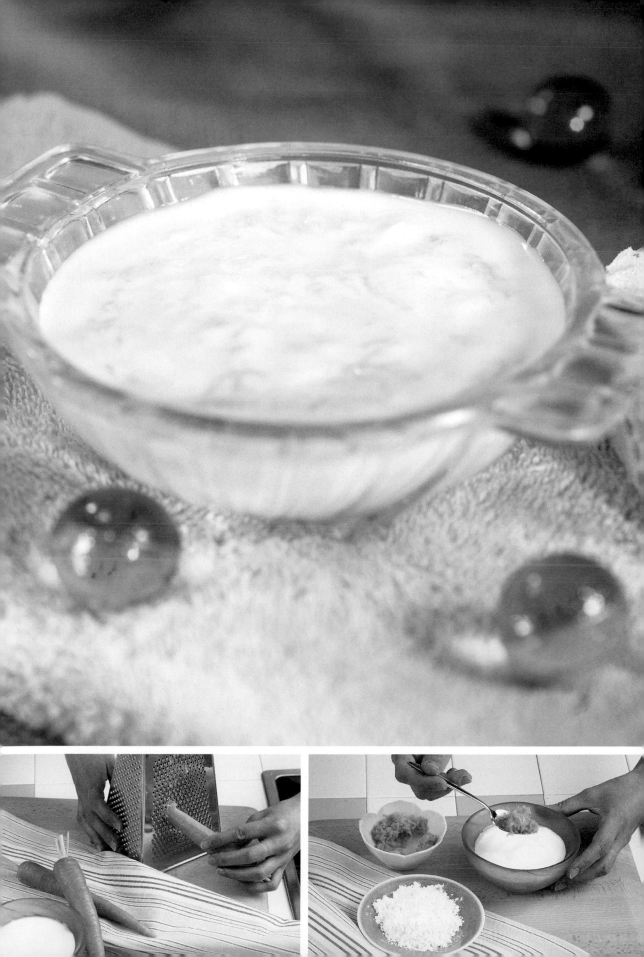

Easy Guava Mask

It doesn't get simpler than this mask. Guavas contain natural astringents that help tone and tighten the skin. They are juicy, delicious and full of health-enhancing compounds, so buy extra and snack on them too. As with all masks, this one works best when applied to cleansed skin.

Best for: Oily or acne-prone skin

Tip: Choose guavas the same way you choose avocados. They should have unblemished skin and be slightly soft to the touch; ripe fruit will yield to gentle pressure when you press it. Guavas perish quickly, so use or eat them within a day or two of purchase.

- Potato masher
- Fine-mesh sieve

| 1 | guava (see tip, at left), halved | 1 |

1. Using a spoon, scoop out guava flesh; chop. In a medium bowl and using potato masher, mash guava flesh. Set fine-mesh sieve over a small bowl; scoop mashed guava flesh into sieve and press with the back of a spoon to release juice. Set guava juice aside.

2. Scrape remaining guava pulp in sieve into another medium bowl; using a potato masher, mash well to make a paste.

3. Using fingers, spread guava paste immediately all over face and neck, avoiding eye area. Let stand on skin for 15 minutes.

4. Rinse off guava paste with warm water. Soak cotton balls or pads in reserved guava juice. Smooth over face and neck.

5. Rinse off face and neck with cold water. Gently pat dry with a towel.

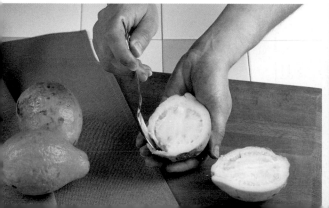

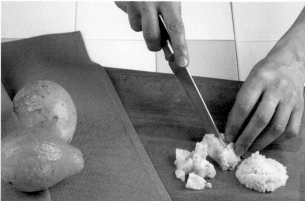

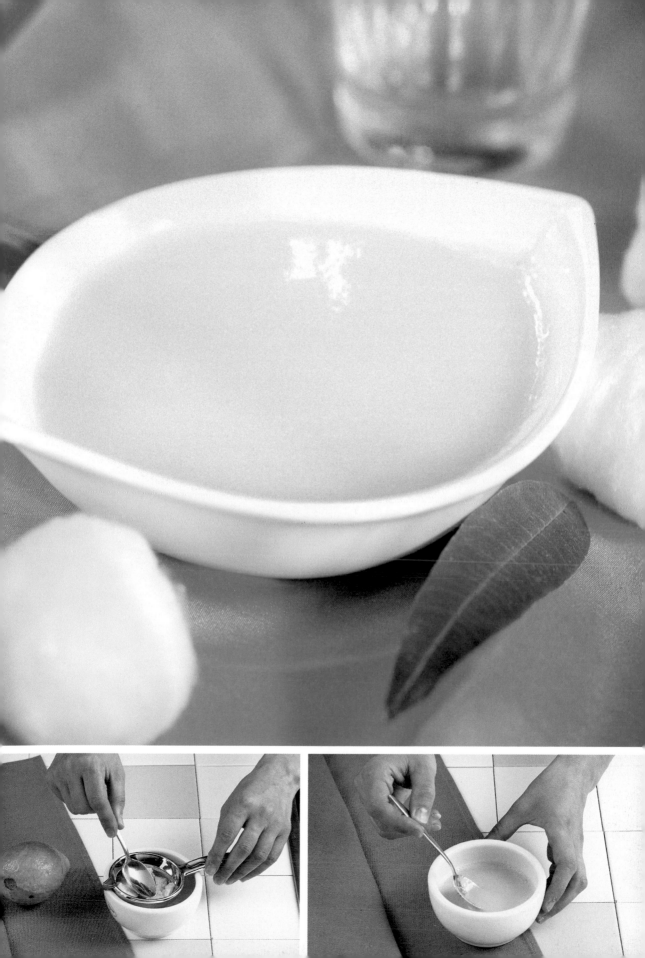

Wrinkles, the Fingerprints of Time

Throughout life, the skin undergoes changes, just as the rest of the body does. As the years pass, the soft, velvety skin of childhood becomes drier and loses elasticity. Its regenerative capacity is reduced, and the supply of oxygen and nutrients diminishes as blood flow through the skin decreases.

There are a few things to keep in mind as your skin becomes more sensitive and begins to lose the freshness of youth. On pages 130 to 134, there are some excellent recipes that will help you combat the aging process so that you look your very best. There are a number of products you can create at home that will slow down the formation of wrinkles and keep skin healthy if you do have them.

Wrinkles are an inevitable consequence of the passage of time. It's important to remember that they aren't signs of deterioration but rather of experience: the mark of years of smiling, frowning and having emotions. Wrinkles are just a new and evolving feature of your appearance, and having them doesn't give you an excuse to neglect your skin. On the contrary, you need to pamper it to highlight your natural beauty.

Where Wrinkles Come From

Your genes significantly influence the development of wrinkles and crow's-feet (those pesky furrows at the outer corners of the eyes), but they can also be signs of an unhealthy diet. Wrinkles form at the points where collagen thins; in some places, it can lose up to 20% of its original thickness. When connective tissues are malnourished, their cells are destroyed by free radicals and die. Enzymes are unable to break down these masses of dead protein and stale cholesterol and remove them via the bloodstream, so they form plaques that clump together into large deposits under the skin. This results in the hills and valleys in skin that we call wrinkles.

What Is Photoaging?

This term is used to describe premature aging of the skin caused by excessive sun exposure. Ultraviolet radiation increases the formation of oxygen free radicals, which damage the skin and cause it to lose its elasticity. The resulting condition, characterized by yellowing of the skin and deep wrinkle formation, is called solar elastosis. This type of aging is not related to chronoaging, or the natural aging process that occurs as a result of the passage of time.

Sun lovers are particularly at risk for photoaging. The best prevention strategy is simply to avoid prolonged exposure to the sun. But if you do choose to tan, take larger amounts of antioxidants to help your body counteract some of the damage. The most helpful supplement you can take is vitamin A (or beta-carotene), but make sure you get plenty of vitamins C and E and selenium as well. See pages 350 to 358 for some sunscreens and treatments to try if you love the sun.

Nature's Contribution to Wrinkle Prevention

The emergence of wrinkles with advancing age is inevitable. And while you can't avoid them completely, you can delay their appearance and diminish their impact. Wrinkle prevention treatments nourish and hydrate the skin to help offset the loss of moisture and fat that comes with aging. The formulas on the following pages will make skin softer and boost elasticity to make skin look beautiful in spite of wrinkles.

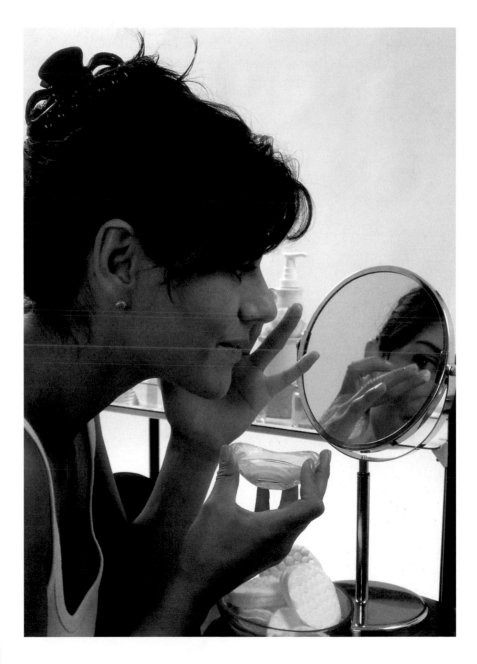

Rich Coconut Mask

This hydrating mask provides the oils necessary to combat dry skin associated with aging.

Best for: Dry and/or wrinkled skin

Tip: Fresh coconut is particularly good for this mask, because it is plump and moist with hydrating coconut oil. You can freeze grated fresh coconut with great results, so freeze any leftovers to make more masks later.

Note: Always measure accurately when you're making homemade beauty products. See page 53 for tips.

| ⅓ cup | plain yogurt | 75 mL |
| 1 tbsp | finely grated coconut (see tip, at left) | 15 mL |

1. In a small bowl, stir yogurt with coconut until well combined.

2. Using fingers, spread coconut mixture all over face and neck, avoiding eye area. Let stand on skin for 30 minutes.

3. Rinse off coconut mixture with lukewarm water. Rinse again with cold water. Gently pat face dry with a towel before applying your favorite moisturizing lotion.

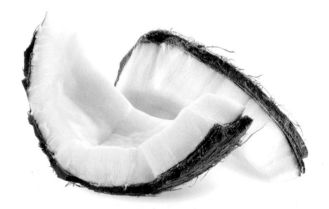

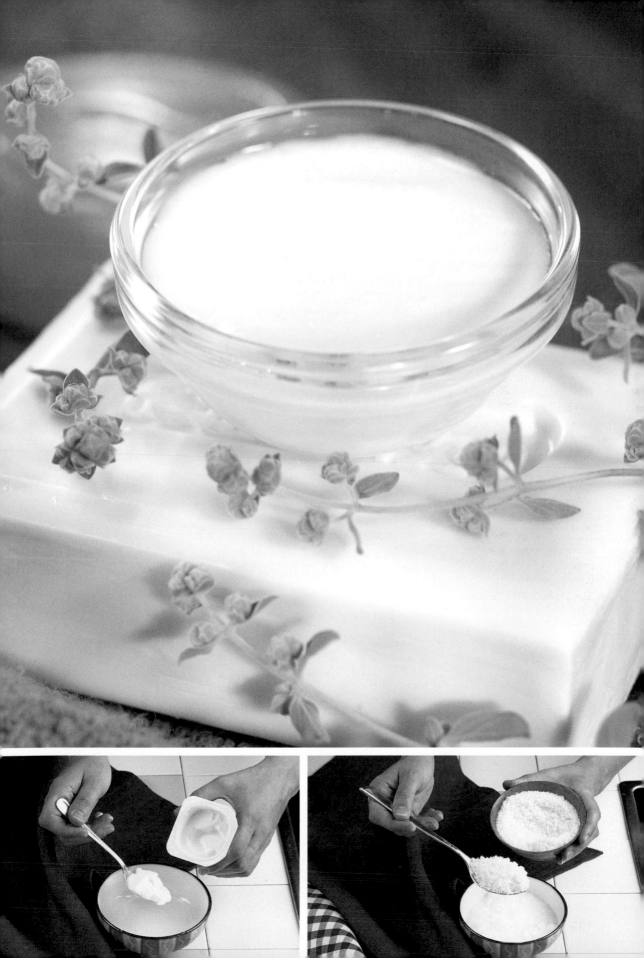

Herbal Anti-Wrinkle Lotion

This floral lotion is soothing and hydrating, and works with beaten egg white to smooth wrinkles.

Best for: Wrinkled skin

Tips: Lemon balm (*Melissa officinalis*) is a member of the mint family but has a lovely lemon scent. It's an easy-to-grow garden plant, and it attracts honeybees.

Also known as tilia flowers, linden flowers are a common ingredient in herbal teas. An infusion made with them is a powerful wrinkle fighter.

Note: Always measure accurately when you're making homemade beauty products. See page 53 for tips.

- Fine-mesh sieve

1¾ oz	fresh or dried lemon balm leaves (see tips, at left)	50 g
1¾ oz	fresh or dried chamomile flowers	50 g
1¾ oz	fresh or dried linden flowers (see tips, at left)	50 g
1 cup	boiling water	250 mL
1	egg white, lightly beaten (see tips, page 90)	1

1. Place lemon balm, chamomile flowers and linden flowers in a medium heatproof bowl; pour boiling water over top. Cover and let steep for 5 minutes.

2. Set fine-mesh sieve over small heatproof bowl; strain liquid into bowl, discarding solids. Let cool to room temperature.

3. Using fingers, spread egg white over most-wrinkled areas of face; let stand for about 2 minutes or until skin is slightly firmed up. Rinse off egg white with lukewarm water. Pat skin dry with a towel.

4. Soak a cotton ball or pad in infusion. Pat lightly onto face.

Natural Wrinkle-Fighting Strategies

If you want to escape the effects of premature aging, it is essential to eat a healthy diet rich in fresh, whole foods, and to avoid refined and processed foods. Smoking is one of the most harmful habits for skin. The free radicals generated by the smoke accelerate aging by damaging the genes that are responsible for regulating cell development. The same is true of alcohol and stimulants; they are harmful to your health and accelerate the formation of wrinkles. Maintaining a healthy weight, getting plenty of outdoor exercise and having a positive attitude can also go a long way toward slowing down wrinkle formation.

Avocado Wrinkle Cream

Rich in healthy fats, avocados are good for your skin, whether you eat them or apply them topically. Here, avocado oil works with other emollients to help smooth out dry, tired skin.

Best for: Wrinkled skin

Tips: Raw beeswax often comes in large blocks. Break off a small chunk and grate what you need right before melting. Or substitute small, easy-to-measure beeswax pearls.

Choose 100% natural cocoa butter for homemade creams like this. You can buy chunks of this creamy, yellowish substance made from cocoa beans at cosmetic-supply stores and online. It is also sold in uniform-size wafers. Either form will work fine in this recipe.

- Hand mixer
- Small glass jar with lid

1 tbsp	avocado oil (see tips, page 179)	15 mL
1 tbsp	soybean oil	15 mL
1 tsp	grated raw beeswax (see tips, at left)	5 mL
1 tsp	cocoa butter (see tips, at left)	5 mL
2 tbsp	water	30 mL
3	drops geranium essential oil	3

1. In a small heatproof bowl, combine avocado oil, soybean oil, beeswax and cocoa butter. Set aside.

2. Pour enough water into a small saucepan to come about 2 inches (5 cm) up the side; bring to a simmer.

3. Set bowl on saucepan so that bottom of bowl is not touching simmering water; stir until beeswax mixture is melted, smooth and lighter in color. Remove bowl from heat.

4. Using hand mixer, beat for 2 to 3 minutes or until mixture is cooled and has a milky consistency. Add water and geranium essential oil; beat for 1 minute or until creamy. Let cool.

5. Spoon into jar.

6. Smooth gently over face. Store jar in the refrigerator for 4 to 6 weeks.

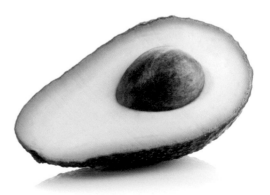

Wrinkle-Fighting Massage Cream

Combining a simple moisturizing treatment with a gentle massage helps improve circulation, which also improves the skin's appearance.

Best for: Wrinkled skin

Tip: Glycerin is an effective moisturizer that is often added to facial treatments and cosmetics. Look for bottles of it at cosmetic-supply stores or online.

Note: Always measure accurately when you're making homemade beauty products. See page 53 for tips.

2 tbsp	finely ground oats or oat flour (see tip, page 123)	30 mL
1 tbsp	liquid glycerin (see tip, at left)	15 mL
	Rose water	

1. In a small bowl, stir oats with glycerin until combined.
2. Adding rose water a few drops at a time, stir until mixture has a creamy consistency.
3. Using fingers and upward motions, massage oat mixture over face for 10 minutes.
4. Rinse off oat mixture with lukewarm water. Rinse again with cool water. Pat face dry with a towel.

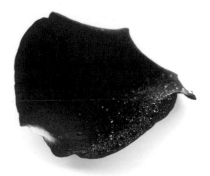

Top Antiaging Tips for Skin

- **Minimize sun exposure.** This is one of the best ways to preserve youthful skin. Even if you spent your teen years tanning, you can prevent further damage. Use a sunscreen with adequate sun protection factor (SPF), and stay out of the sun, especially in the harsh light of the afternoon.

- **Drink plenty of water.** Aim to get a minimum of 8 cups (2 L) of water daily. This is essential for keeping the skin hydrated.

- **Take vitamin E supplements.** Taking 400 IU of vitamin E a day is like putting on SPF 4 sunscreen — it's a small amount of protection that adds up. To avoid the harmful effects of the sun, take wheat germ oil capsules, which are a rich source of vitamin E. Selenium also reduces sun damage and is helpful for people with a history of excessive solar exposure. Take 20 to 50 micrograms of selenium a day.

- **Turn down heating and air conditioning and humidify the air.** Urban dwellers spend around 90% of their time indoors. The humidity is much lower than it is outdoors, due to excessive heating in winter and overuse of air conditioning in summer. Since it is almost impossible to avoid artificial climates, the best remedy is to invest in a humidifier and open the windows from time to time. Remember to follow the instructions on your humidifier for cleaning and sanitizing, and change the filter at the recommended intervals. No humidifier? Leave bowls of water near radiators and allow them to evaporate into the air.

- **Nourish your skin from the inside.** Make sure that your diet is rich in whole foods and fresh vegetables and fruits. These foods purify and revitalize the body and help its natural defense systems neutralize skin-damaging free radicals.

- **Eliminate acidifying foods.** Cut out foods that acidify the blood: refined sugar and flour, fried foods, fats, spicy foods, alcohol and animal protein.

- **Care for your skin regularly.** Every day, without fail, cleanse, moisturize and nourish your skin.

- **Quit smoking.** Smoking is one of your skin's worst enemies. Quitting is the best thing you can do for your skin.

- **Get enough sleep.** Adequate rest is very important to help you look and feel your best. Try to get all the sleep your body needs — for most people, that's six to eight hours every night.

- **Minimize stress.** Take time to relax and get away from day-to-day pressures. Whether that means reading a book in a quiet place, going to a yoga class or spending time in meditation, your body will reward you for stress reduction with glowing skin.

- **Use natural beauty products.** Substitute homemade, natural cosmetics for cosmetics made with chemicals; the former are much safer and more effective. The recipes in this book are a terrific place to start!

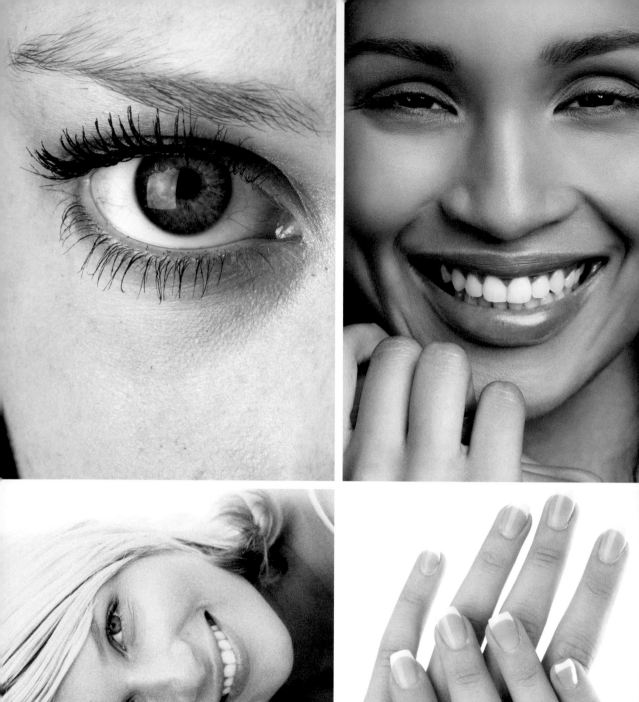
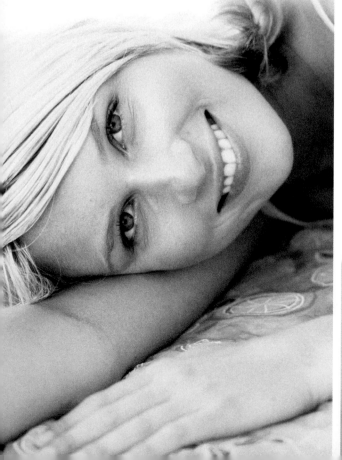
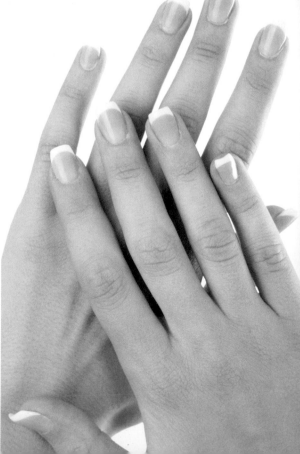

Eye, Mouth, Hand and Nail Treatments

Now that your facial skin is in top condition, it's time to look a little more closely at other areas that reflect natural beauty. The eyes are the window to your soul, but they are also a window to your overall health. The same goes for your teeth and your nails: they can reflect a lifetime of neglect or of tender loving care.

In this chapter, you will discover easy ways to care for your eyes, pamper your lips, keep your smile bright and nourish your hands and nails. You'll learn what these important body parts need and how to make them look their best with simple homemade beauty treatments.

Eyes: Your Best Reflection

Your eyes are an extremely important part of your body. They are well worth caring for and protecting, and they can reflect how your internal systems are working. Plus, the skin around your eyes is very delicate and fine, so it requires a little more special attention than your facial skin. In this section, you will find natural remedies to combat crow's-feet, remedies that minimize dark circles under the eyes, and homemade eye creams and makeup removers.

What Makes Your Eyes Shine

A number of different nervous system and hormonal processes happen in the eyes. When the eyes signal a need for neuropeptides (protein molecules that allow communication between nerve cells), hormones and neurotransmitters, these substances can reach them with incredible speed and activate metabolic processes in the eyes in just a few tenths of a second. Zinc is a crucial mineral for eye health, so the exchange of activated zinc enzymes in the eye can be multiplied by up to 3,000 times within a few minutes. It is precisely these types of reactions that cause

The Eyes' Natural Defenses

Eyes are fairly delicate structures, and they are exposed to extremes in the environment. Wind, cold, heat and pollution are just some of the daily stresses they face. But nature has provided the eyes with enhanced immune defenses. Tears contain high levels of protective substances: up to 400 times more vitamin C and other elements than you'll find in blood plasma. Every time you blink or close your eyes, you bathe the eyeballs in a thin film of nutrient-rich moisture. This keeps your eyes well equipped to fight bacteria, viruses and other pathogens.

a sort of phosphorescence in the eyes. This creates a special light in the gaze of a person who is in love, surprised or pleased.

When your eyes see something that excites sensations of love or passion, your body produces billions of hormone molecules that trigger feelings of well-being. For the nervous system cells to be able to synthesize the required molecules in a split second, a cell messenger called cyclic adenosine monophosphate gets involved. This molecule is the engine of the nervous system, transmitting feelings of passion, love and other strong emotions that course through the body at great speed.

Your eyes also shine during a fight-or-flight situation. When you see something that triggers this stress response, the central nervous system very quickly synthesizes hormones, such as adrenaline (epinephrine) and noradrenaline (norepinephrine), that ready the body for action. Adrenaline speeds up the metabolism of the eyes in a split second, allowing them to dilate and see more clearly. This process is also dependent on the presence of sufficient amounts of the amino acids tyrosine and phenylalanine, as well as vitamins B_6 and C, magnesium and manganese.

Vitamins and Minerals That Nourish Your Eyes

Well-protected, well-nourished eyes are always bright and expressive. Vitamins A, C and E do the most to support the eyes. These three protective vitamins always work in relation to one another in the body, but they are especially united when they work to protect vision. This means that visual acuity depends on the quality of your diet. Making sure you get a wide array of nutrients guarantees well-nourished eyes and the clearest eyesight possible.

To keep your eyes healthy and beautiful, make sure your diet provides plenty of vitamin A, which protects vision and helps with your ability to see in low light. This link goes as far back as Ancient Egypt, where doctors advised their patients to eat liver, which is rich in vitamin A, to protect their eyesight. Liver is not the only food that provides generous amounts of this vitamin; there is plenty in vegetable sources such as sweet potatoes, pumpkins, carrots, leafy greens and squash. Dairy products are often fortified with vitamin A, so they are another good source.

Vitamins C and E are also vital for eye health, and B vitamins play a role too. Turn to pages 28 to 31 for more on these important micronutrients. It's easy to get them from food sources. A particularly rich source of eye-related nutrients is young plants and plant parts designed for growth and reproduction: seeds, nuts, whole grains, sprouts, young leaves, buds and new shoots. Try adding these to your diet for a nutritional boost.

Eye Exercises

A few short workouts for your eyes will go a long way toward making them look and feel good. Try to take a break every few hours during the day and do one of these routines:

- **Palming.** Keeping your eyes open but relaxed, place your palms over your eyes, blocking out all light. Relax in this position for 5 minutes. While your eyes are covered, move them slowly in every direction to stretch the muscles around them.

- **Faraway focusing.** People, especially those who use computers frequently, often stare at the same thing for long stretches of time. Periodically, look up and focus on an object in the distance (it should be the farthest thing you can see). Look at the faraway object as a whole; then, blink and look at it again, this time focusing on some detail.

- **Relaxing deeply.** This routine is ideal for relaxing your vision after an intense day of work and eye strain. Wear comfortable clothing and remove any restrictive footwear. Sit up straight in a quiet place. Take 12 deep breaths. Circle your head 12 times, alternating the direction with each rotation. Now, with a relaxed gaze, look at a distant object located at eye level while swinging your head from side to side 12 times. Palm your eyes (see above) for 5 minutes. Then, breathe slowly and deeply as you gently massage your eyes, using the heel of your hand over your eyeballs. To finish, place compresses soaked in Herbal Eye Soother (page 140) on your eyelids for about 15 minutes.

Herbal Eye Soother

Chamomile is a great anti-inflammatory for the skin, and chamomile tea has a nice soothing effect when you drink it. For best results, enjoy a cup along with this treatment.

Best for: Red, puffy eyes

Tip: Dried chamomile is easy to find at stores that sell medicinal herbs. It's also a very undemanding plant to grow in your garden, so you can grow, harvest and dry your own organic flowers with a minimal amount of effort.

Note: Always measure accurately when you're making homemade beauty products. See page 53 for tips.

- Teapot
- Fine-mesh sieve (optional)

2 tbsp	dried chamomile flowers (see tip, at left)	30 mL
1 tsp	fennel seeds	5 mL
2 or 3	small clusters fresh parsley leaves	2 or 3
2 cups	boiling water	500 mL

1. Place chamomile flowers, fennel seeds and parsley leaves in a teapot; pour boiling water over top. Cover and let stand for 10 minutes or until lukewarm.

2. Place fine-mesh sieve (if using) over a medium heatproof bowl; pour infusion into bowl, discarding solids.

3. Soak a washcloth or cotton pads in infusion. Place on eyelids. Let stand on skin for 10 minutes.

4. Rinse off infusion with warm water. Pat eyelids and face dry with a towel.

Tea Compresses for Red, Puffy Eyes

Fatigue takes a toll on your body and mind, and your eyes show it by becoming puffy, red and irritated. Tea compresses are an old-fashioned and effective remedy. Simply make two cups of black tea using tea bags. Remove the tea bags, squeeze out the excess moisture and refrigerate until cold. Lay the chilled tea bags on your eyelids. Lie back and relax for a few minutes.

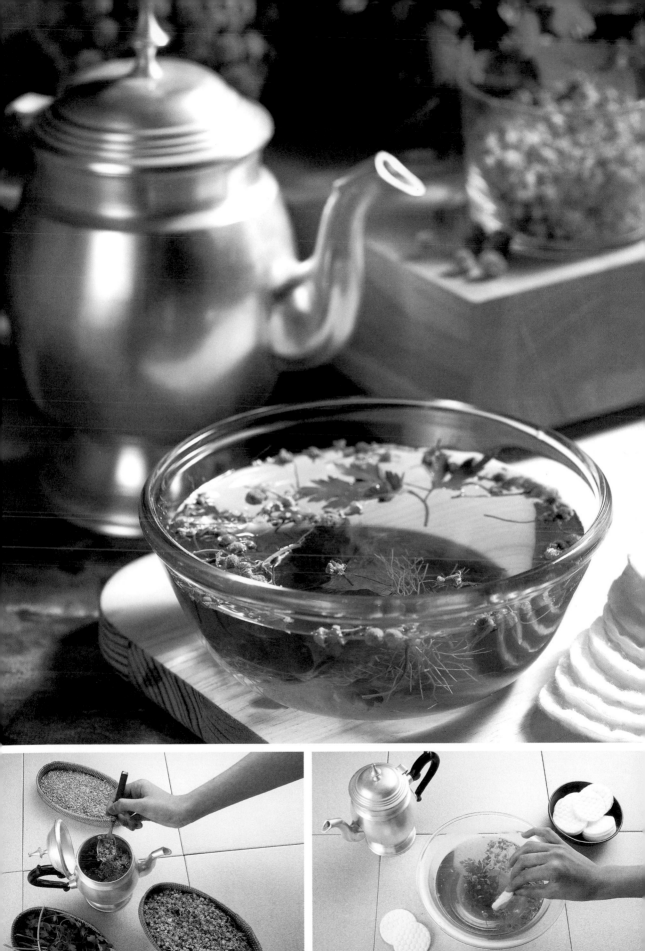

Cucumber Eye Soother

This easy cucumber purée contains natural astringents that reduce swelling and relieve the stinging that comes with tired eyes.

Best for: Red, puffy eyes

Tip: You can also place slices of fresh cucumber directly on your eyelids to help reduce puffiness.

Note: Always measure accurately when you're making homemade beauty products. See page 53 for tips.

- Hand blender with a tall cup, or blender

| ¼ | English cucumber (unpeeled) | ¼ |

1. Cut cucumber into thick slices. Place in tall cup; using hand blender, purée until pasty.

2. Spoon cucumber paste into a small bowl. Soak a cotton pad or ball in cucumber mixture. Gently pat over eyelids. Let stand on skin for 10 minutes.

3. Rinse off cucumber mixture with warm water. Pat eyelids and face dry with a towel.

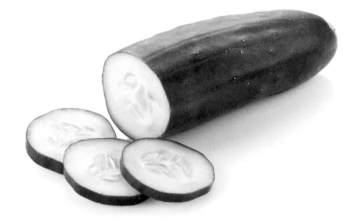

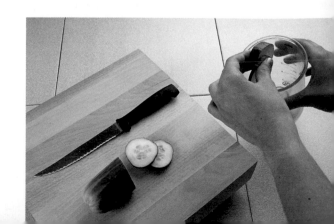

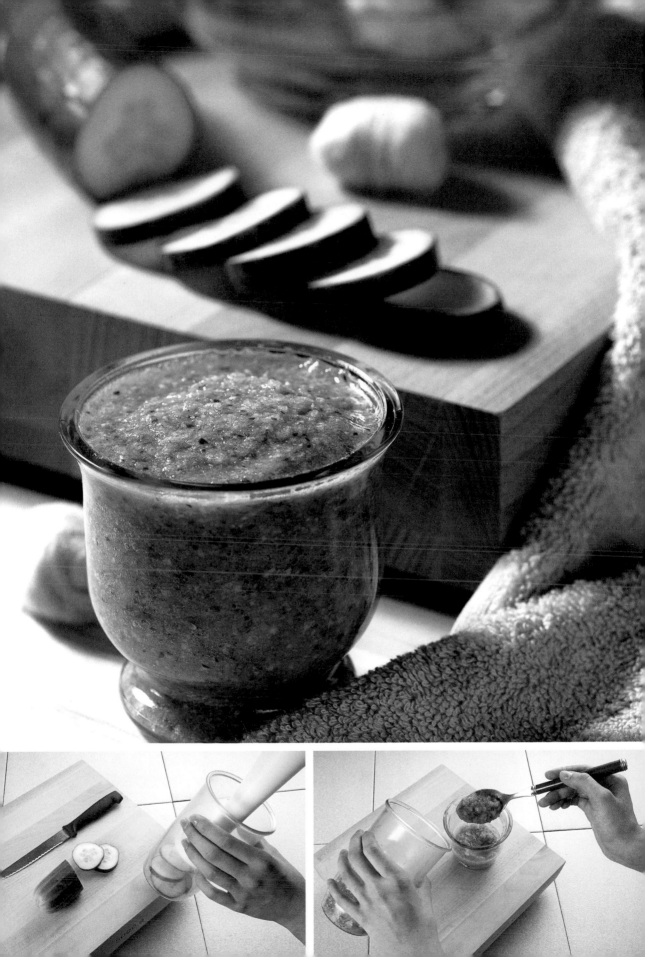

Violet Leaf Toning Lotion

Sweet violet *(Viola odorata)* is a commonly used medicinal herb, and its pretty purple flowers make it a lovely plant to grow in your garden. Plant a little clump so you'll have a steady supply of the leaves to make this gentle cream.

Best for: Delicate eye skin and crow's-feet

Tip: You'll need a handful or so of fresh sweet violet leaves to make the juice for this recipe. Use a juicer or purée the leaves in a blender until liquefied. If using a blender, strain the juice through a fine-mesh sieve into a small bowl, discarding the solids.

Note: Always measure accurately when you're making homemade beauty products. See page 53 for tips.

1	egg white (see tips, page 90)	1
1 tbsp	violet leaf juice (see tip, at left)	15 mL
1 tsp	liquid honey	5 mL
½ tsp	sweet almond oil (see tips, page 149)	2 mL

1. In a small bowl, beat egg white until frothy. Stir violet leaf juice, honey and sweet almond oil into egg white until well combined.

2. Dip finger into lotion and gently smooth over skin under eyes. Rinse off lotion with lukewarm water.

Combat Crow's-Feet

The area around the eyes is covered with some of the finest, most delicate skin on the face. It is usually one of the first areas where wrinkles form, especially if this zone is neglected. Moisturizing Eye Oil (page 146), Eye Cream (page 146) and Violet Leaf Toning Lotion (above) are made with ingredients that are rich in vitamin E, which helps delay and minimize wrinkles. In addition to these treatments, crow's-feet require the use of plenty of toner to firm up tired skin that has lost elasticity.

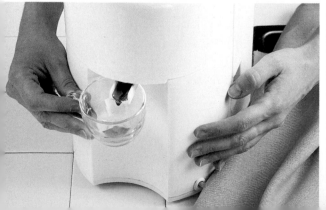

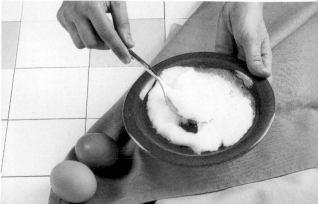

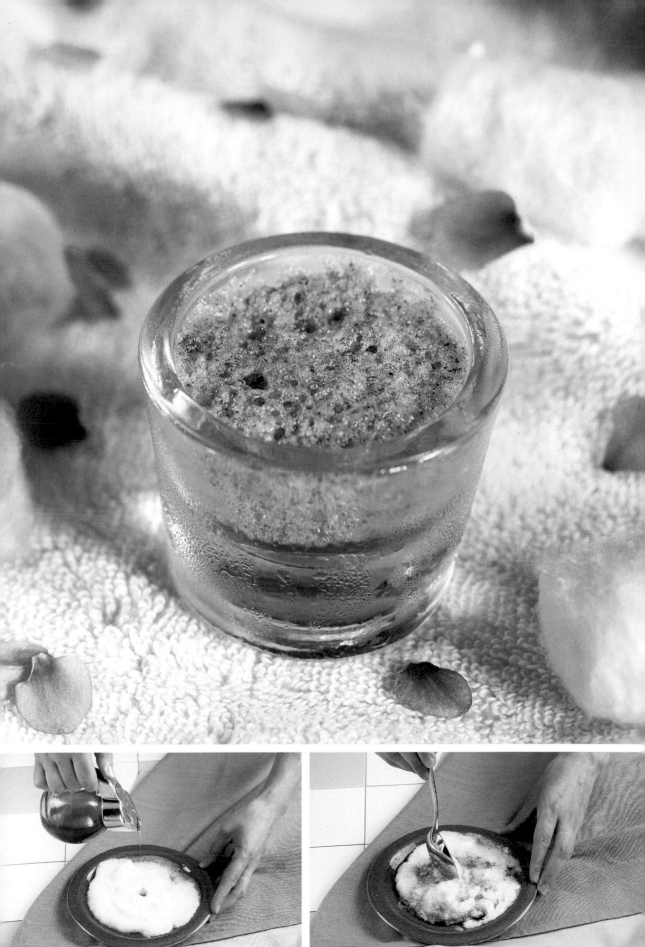

Eye Cream

Wheat germ oil is a terrific source of vitamin E. Look for gel capsules of it in the supplement aisle of the drugstore or supermarket.

Best for: Delicate eye skin and crow's-feet

Tips: Shea butter is a rich emollient that's ideal in dry-skin treatments. Look for tubs or bags of it at cosmetic-supply stores or online.

To extract the wheat germ oil from the capsule, use a large, clean sewing needle. Pierce the capsule over a small dish and squeeze it to extract the oil.

- Small glass jar with lid

1½ tbsp	sweet almond oil (see tips, page 149)	22 mL
1 tbsp	shea butter (see tips, at left)	15 mL
2 tbsp	cold water	30 mL
1	capsule wheat germ oil, oil squeezed out (see tips, at left)	1

1. In a small heatproof bowl, combine sweet almond oil and shea butter. Set aside.

2. Pour enough water into a small saucepan to come about 2 inches (5 cm) up the side; bring to a simmer.

3. Set bowl on saucepan so that bottom of bowl is not touching simmering water; stir until shea butter mixture is melted and smooth. Remove bowl from heat.

4. Whisk cold water and wheat germ oil into shea butter mixture until creamy. Let cool.

5. Spoon into jar. Dip finger into cream and gently smooth over skin under eyes. Store jar in a cool, dark place for up to 1 month.

Moisturizing Eye Oil

Just a tiny dab of this rich oil will keep delicate eye skin hydrated and looking young.

Best for: Delicate eye skin and crow's-feet

Tip: Cold-pressed extra-virgin oils are the purest and most unadulterated type you can buy for making homemade beauty treatments. They are worth the higher price tag.

Note: Always measure accurately when you're making homemade beauty products. See page 53 for tips.

- Small glass jar with lid

2 tsp	soybean oil (see tip, at left)	10 mL
2 tsp	sweet almond oil (see tips, page 149)	10 mL
1 tsp	avocado oil	5 mL

1. In a small bowl, stir together soybean oil, sweet almond oil and avocado oil. Pour oil mixture into jar.

2. Dip tip of finger into oil mixture. Gently massage oil into skin under eyes.

3. Store jar in a cool, dark place for up to 2 months.

Facial Makeup Remover

This smooth, oil-based makeup remover gets rid of all traces of foundation and under-eye concealer without harsh chemicals.

Best for: Removing foundation and other base makeup

Tip: Choose 100% natural cocoa butter for homemade creams like this. You can buy chunks of this creamy, yellowish substance made from cocoa beans at cosmetic-supply stores and online. It is also sold in uniform-size wafers. Either form will work fine in this recipe.

- Small glass bottle with lid

2 tsp	soybean oil (see tip, opposite)	10 mL
1 tsp	cocoa butter (see tip, at left)	5 mL
1 tbsp	water	15 mL

1. In a small heatproof bowl, combine soybean oil and cocoa butter. Set aside.
2. Pour enough water into a small saucepan to come about 2 inches (5 cm) up the side; bring to a simmer.
3. Set bowl on saucepan so that bottom of bowl is not touching simmering water; stir until cocoa butter is melted and smooth. Remove bowl from heat.
4. Stir water into cocoa butter mixture until well combined and creamy. Continue stirring until completely cool. Spoon into bottle.
5. Soak cotton ball or pad in mixture. Wipe over face, repeating until all makeup is removed. Store bottle in a cool, dark place between uses.

Eye Makeup Remover

This simple oil combination is effective at removing mascara, eye shadow and eyeliner.

Best for: Removing eye makeup

Tip: Castor oil is made from castor beans (*Ricinus communis*). It's oily enough to take off makeup but gentle and soothing to skin.

- Small glass bottle with lid

2 tbsp	sweet almond oil (see tips, page 149)	30 mL
2 tbsp	castor oil (see tip, at left)	30 mL

1. In a small bowl, stir sweet almond oil with castor oil. Pour into bottle.
2. Soak cotton ball or pad in mixture. Wipe over eye area, repeating until all makeup is removed. Store bottle in a cool, dark place between uses.

How to Remove Eye Makeup

It's important to get rid of mascara and eye makeup at the end of the day. Always use a makeup remover specifically formulated for the eyes; other types are less gentle and can cause allergic reactions. Apply makeup remover with a cotton ball or pad, gently wiping from the upper lids and eyelashes toward the inner corner of the eye.

Comfrey Toner

When you lighten up dark circles under your eyes, you'll instantly look younger and fresher. This easy toner helps you appear relaxed and well rested.

Best for: Dark under-eye circles

Tip: The comfrey plant (*Symphytum officinale*) contains allantoin, which is very effective for treating skin inflammation, wounds and premature wrinkles. Comfrey is a perennial herb, which means you can plant it once and it will come up every year. If you don't have it in your garden, you can buy dried comfrey leaves at an herbalist's shop or online.

Note: Always measure accurately when you're making homemade beauty products. See page 53 for tips.

- Fine-mesh sieve

4 to 6	fresh comfrey leaves (see tip, at left)	4 to 6
1 cup	boiling water	250 mL
3	drops wheat germ oil (see tips, opposite)	3

1. Place comfrey leaves in a small heatproof bowl or cup; pour boiling water over top. Cover and let steep for 5 minutes.

2. Place fine-mesh sieve over another small heatproof bowl; strain infusion into bowl, discarding solids. Let cool to room temperature. Stir in wheat germ oil.

3. Soak a cotton ball or pad in toner. Pat lightly onto under-eye area.

Goodbye, Dark Circles!

You can add other herbs to a simple comfrey infusion to treat dark under-eye circles and bags. Try parsley, rose hips, lemon verbena leaves or chamomile flowers. Make a weak infusion of your favorite blend, and apply the warm liquid to your skin using a cotton ball or pad. Follow with Dark Circle Cream (opposite).

Dark Circle Cream

This cream treats dark circles gently while lightening them up and nourishing the skin under the eyes.

Best for: Dark under-eye circles

Tips: Sweet almond oil, like other nut oils, can perish quickly if stored in a warm place or exposed to direct sunlight. Keep the bottle in a dark, cool cupboard and use it up within a couple of months of opening.

Wheat germ oil is a good source of vitamin E, but it can go rancid quickly if stored at room temperature. Keep it in the fridge to extend the shelf life.

- Small glass jar with lid

2 tbsp	shea butter (see tips, page 146)	30 mL
1 tbsp	apricot kernel oil	15 mL
1 tbsp	sweet almond oil (see tips, at left)	15 mL
1 tbsp	wheat germ oil (see tips, at left)	15 mL

1. Place shea butter in a small heatproof bowl. Set aside.

2. Pour enough water into a small saucepan to come about 2 inches (5 cm) up the side; bring to a simmer.

3. Set bowl on saucepan so that bottom of bowl is not touching simmering water; stir until shea butter is melted and smooth. Remove bowl from heat.

4. Stir apricot kernel oil, sweet almond oil and wheat germ oil into shea butter until well combined and creamy. Let cool. Spoon into jar.

5. Dip finger into cream and gently smooth over skin under eyes. Store jar in a cool, dark place for up to 1 month.

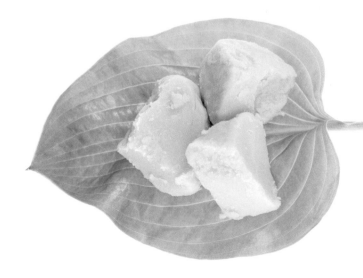

Potato Eye Poultice

Brighten up dark circles with this super-easy treatment. It's gentle on skin and easy on the budget too.

Best for: Dark under-eye circles

Tip: Any regular boiling potato will work fine in this poultice.

Note: Always measure accurately when you're making homemade beauty products. See page 53 for tips.

- Vegetable peeler
- Box grater
- Cheesecloth

| 1 | large potato (see tip, at left) | 1 |

1. Using vegetable peeler, peel skin off potato and discard.

2. Using fine side of box grater, shred potato.

3. Spoon potato shreds onto cheesecloth. Fold cloth up around potato shreds to enclose. Press lightly to soak the cloth with potato juice. Place poultice on eyelids and under-eye area. Let stand on skin for 10 minutes.

4. Rinse off potato juice with warm water. Pat eyelids and face dry with a towel.

Give Tired Eyes a Break

You use your eyes for so many things, all day long: reading, writing, driving and watching. Remember how beneficial it is to give your hard-working eyes a rest at some point during the day. Take periodic breaks, letting your eyes unfocus themselves, before you get back to the task at hand.

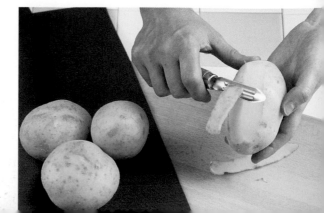

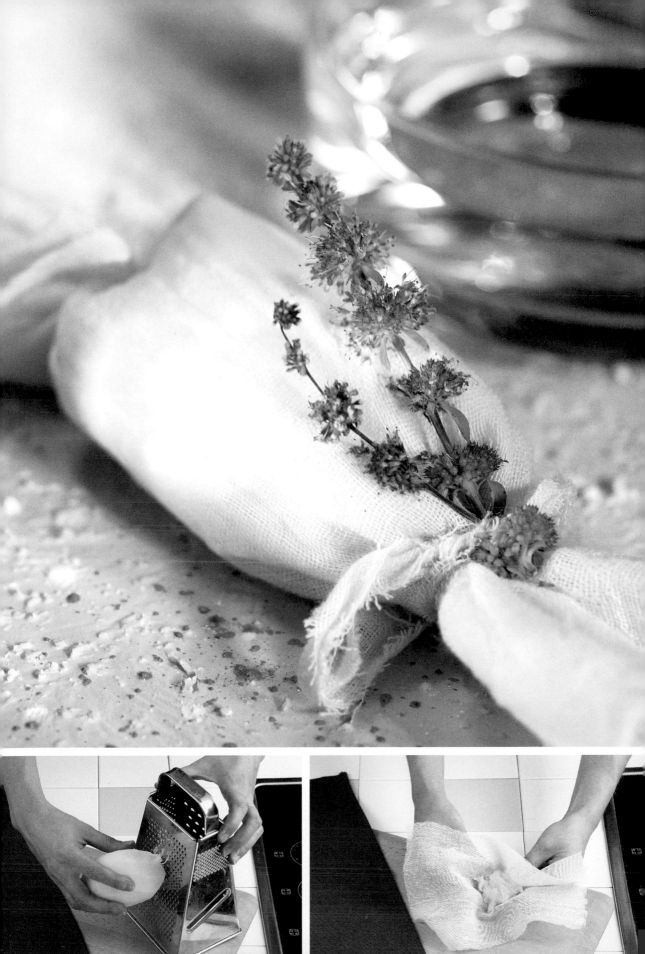

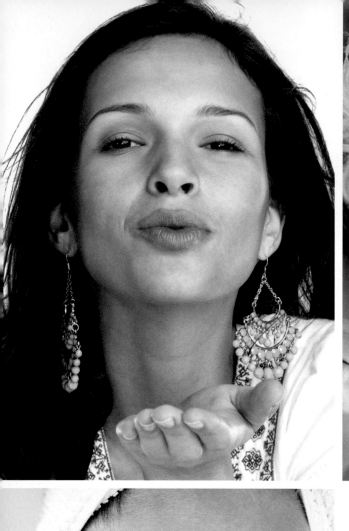
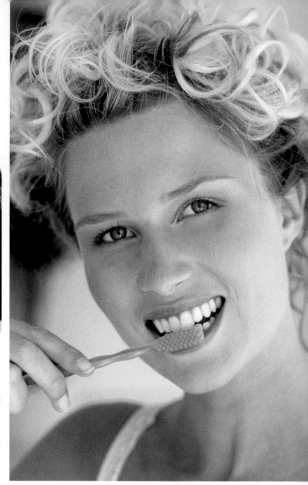
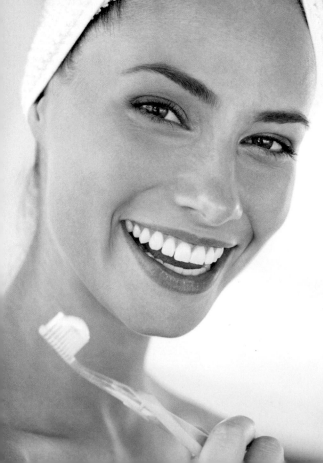
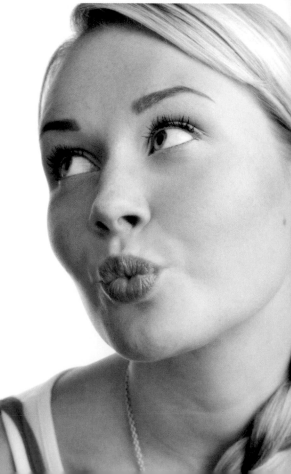

Mouth: Protect Your Smile

A genuine smile is the best way to show off your natural inner beauty. Taking care of your lips and your teeth ensures that you'll always be ready to flash your best grin. And while there are so many easy-to-buy products out there to pamper your mouth, you can make even simpler, more natural products at home.

Nourishment for Lips

Lips are sensitive and delicate, so they need protection and gentle treatment. The skin on them lacks sebaceous glands, so it can maintain only a limited amount of natural moisture. This makes lips prone to drying out and cracking, especially during the winter and when exposed to windy weather. This dehydration happens even more readily if your diet is deficient in B vitamins.

You can nourish and pamper your lips to combat this natural tendency. Add more foods that are sources of B vitamins to your diet, such as oats, wheat germ, bran, brewer's yeast, eggs, yogurt and sprouts. It is also helpful to apply good-quality moisturizing cream or lip balm several times a day. A simple remedy to keep lips soft and smooth is to put a bit of honey on them and then rub them gently with a slice of avocado. It's also delicious!

Nourishment for Teeth

Diet obviously plays an important role in dental health. Modern western diets include a large proportion of foods that contain refined sugar, which leads to a high level of tooth decay in the population.

People who eat a diet based on whole foods, fruits and vegetables enjoy healthier, stronger teeth and tend not to have cavities (or at least have fewer). For strong teeth, choose fresh, whole foods that contain ample amounts of phosphorus, calcium, vitamins A and D and protein. One-third of your diet should consist of raw fruits and vegetables.

Dental Health for Children

Ideally, a dental hygiene regimen should start as soon as a baby's first teeth appear. This gets the child used to having his or her teeth brushed and makes tooth care a regular part of daily life. It also pays to start children on healthy snacks early. Offer bites of fresh fruit, carrots and raw celery instead of sweets and candy.

Another significant shortcoming of today's conventional diets is the lack of cold-pressed virgin oils, which contain a host of healthy fatty acids and other nutrients. Include more of these oils and replace refined oils and margarine with real butter. Either limit your consumption of animal proteins and fats, or replace them with those that come from vegetable sources.

How Tooth Decay Occurs

Also known as cavities, tooth decay starts with plaque. Plaque begins as a dense mass of carbohydrates, saliva proteins, food debris and different kinds of fats. If you don't brush your teeth after a meal, this mixture builds up and spreads to cover all of your teeth.

Plaque is a paradise for bacteria, which feed on its carbohydrate-rich components, transforming them into acids that can erode tooth enamel. The process begins during a meal and may continue for several hours. The pH of the plaque decreases as it remains on your teeth; that is, this sticky, bacteria-laden coating becomes increasingly acidic. It reaches a critical level when it has dropped to a pH of between 5.5 and 5.3; at this point, it becomes destructive and attacks the tooth surface, allowing decay to set in.

Preventing Cavities

According to experts, 70% of people over 14 years old have experienced tooth decay. It is one of the most widespread health challenges experienced by societies around the world.

You can keep plaque from attacking your teeth by starving the bacteria in your mouth. As long as you eat sweet things, you give them food to go on multiplying. If you stop providing sugars for them to

Natural Toothpastes and Breath Fresheners

It is easy to make homemade toothpastes and tooth powders. The recipes on pages 159 to 164, made using medicinal plants that work as disinfectants, offer a few pleasant alternatives to conventional store-bought toothpastes. Most ancient books on herbal medicine praise the qualities of lavender water for protecting teeth and gums; an infusion of this herb makes an excellent mouthwash. Another very good plant for making mouthwash is myrrh. Its disinfectant properties stimulate the mucous membranes of the mouth and cleanse the oral cavity.

consume — and especially if you brush your teeth to remove them — the bacteria no longer have sustenance, the pH in your mouth rises and your teeth are safe from attack.

Pay close attention to the quality of the food you consume. First, eat fewer products that contain refined sugar. Fresh, natural foods, preferably raw ones, should be the focus of your diet. As a matter of fact, chewing fresh, raw vegetables is one of the best ways to fight plaque naturally. Second, avoid eating between meals. Third, brush your teeth within half an hour after eating.

Most people know that they should brush their teeth multiple times a day, but not everyone brushes enough. Ideally, you should brush your teeth after every meal or at least twice a day. Knowing the correct way to brush teeth is the most important part (see box, page 164); toothpaste plays a secondary role in good dental hygiene.

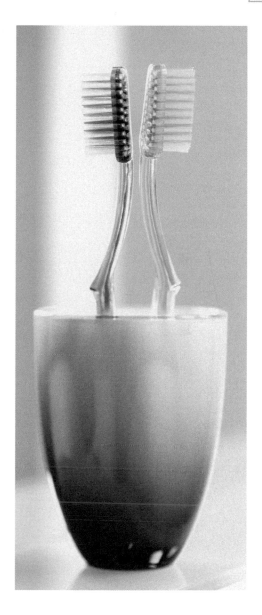

Pumpkin Seed Oil Lip Softener

This mix of natural oils and cocoa butter is gentle on delicate lip skin and offers superior softening powers to prevent cracks and chapping.

Best for: All lips

Tip: The seeds found inside pumpkins (*Cucurbita pepo*) contain a nutrient-rich, dark-colored oil that's prized for both its flavor and its healing properties for the skin. You can add the oil to this lip treatment and drizzle a bit over salads for a nutritional boost.

Note: Always measure accurately when you're making homemade beauty products. See page 53 for tips.

- Small glass jar with lid

1 tbsp	coconut oil	15 mL
1½ tsp	cocoa butter (see tip, page 158)	7 mL
1½ tsp	pumpkin seed oil (see tip, at left)	7 mL

1. In a small heatproof bowl, combine coconut oil, cocoa butter and pumpkin seed oil. Set aside.

2. Pour enough water into a small saucepan to come about 2 inches (5 cm) up the side; bring to a simmer.

3. Set bowl on saucepan so that bottom of bowl is not touching simmering water; stir until coconut oil mixture is melted and smooth. Remove bowl from heat. Let cool completely.

4. Pour into jar. Dip finger into mixture and smooth over lips. Store in a cool, dark place for up to 2 months.

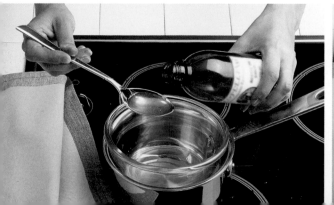
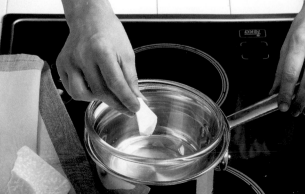

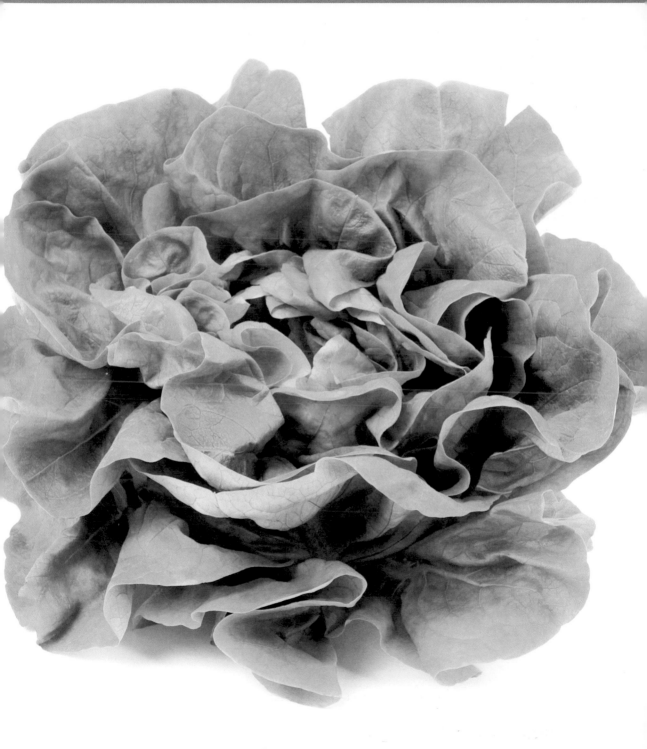

Nourishing Banana Cream

Bananas are good for beauty, both inside and out. They contain a host of vitamins and minerals, including B vitamins, vitamins A, C and E and potassium.

Best for: Normal skin

Tip: Ripe bananas are the most fragrant and easiest to mash. A banana is soft and very ripe when it's yellow all over with a few small brown freckles.

Note: Always measure accurately when you're making homemade beauty products. See page 53 for tips.

| ½ | ripe banana (see tip, at left) | ½ |
| 3 tbsp | milk | 45 mL |

1. Slice banana. In a small bowl and using a fork, mash banana with milk to form a paste.

2. Using fingers, spread banana mixture over face and neck. Let stand on skin for 3 to 4 minutes.

3. Rinse off banana mixture with lukewarm water. Gently pat face and neck dry with a towel.

Step Three: Nourishing

Nourishing creams, also called night creams or regenerative creams, are applied at night to add nutrients to the skin while you sleep. Their higher fat content makes them slick to the touch, and their purpose is to add oil to the skin. They are mainly prescribed for dry skin. Like moisturizers, they should be smoothed over the face using a gentle touch.

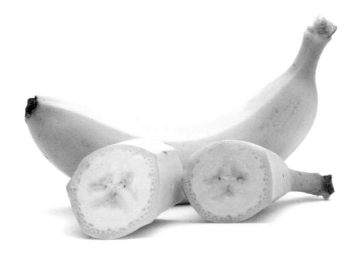

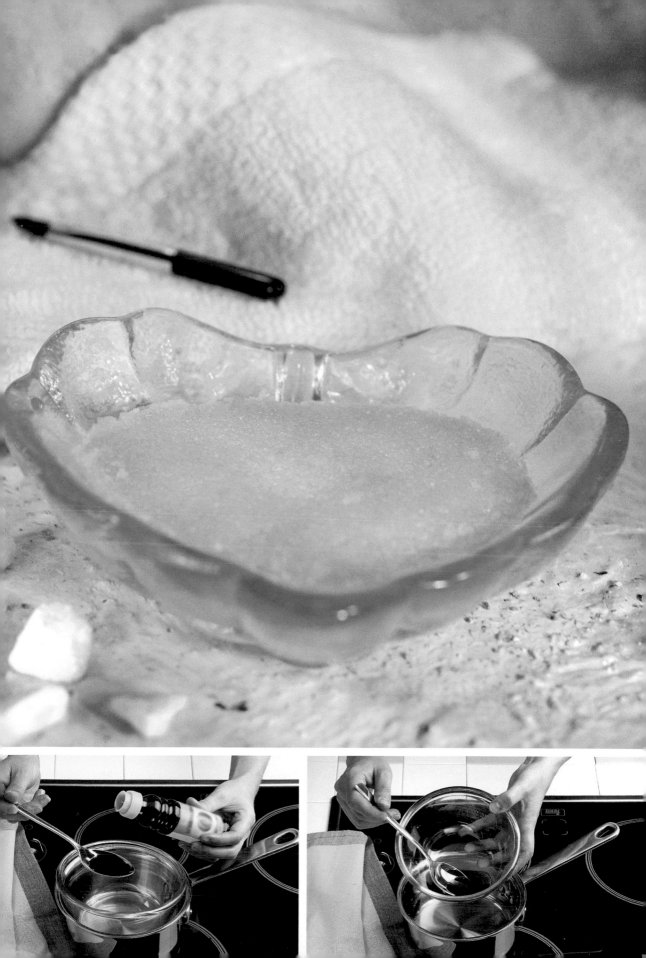

Soy and Cocoa Butter Lip Balm

Soybean oil is easy for skin to absorb and leaves it smooth and hydrated. Keep a pot of the balm in your purse, and apply it anytime your lips start to feel parched.

Best for: All lips

Tip: Raw beeswax often comes in large blocks. Break off a small chunk and grate what you need right before melting. Or substitute small, easy-to-measure beeswax pearls.

Note: Always measure accurately when you're making homemade beauty products. See page 53 for tips.

- Small glass jar with lid

2 tsp	soybean oil (approx), see tip, page 146	10 mL
1 tsp	cocoa butter (see tip, below)	5 mL
½ tsp	grated raw beeswax (see tip, at left)	2 mL

1. In a small heatproof bowl, combine soybean oil, cocoa butter and beeswax. Set aside.

2. Pour enough water into a small saucepan to come about 2 inches (5 cm) up the side; bring to a simmer.

3. Set bowl on saucepan so that bottom of bowl is not touching simmering water; stir until cocoa butter mixture is melted and smooth.

4. Test consistency by spooning a few drops of the warm mixture onto a small plate. Let cool for 30 seconds to 1 minute or until solid. Rub mixture on lips. If it is too hard to spread easily, add more soybean oil to the warm mixture, a drop or two at a time, stirring and testing until desired consistency is reached.

5. Pour into jar. Let cool completely. Dip finger into balm and smooth over lips. Store in a cool, dark place for up to 2 months.

Cocoa Butter Lip Gloss

This simple, all-natural mixture gives lips a pretty shine while protecting them from the drying effects of wind and sun.

Best for: All lips

Tip: Choose 100% natural cocoa butter for lip treatments. You can buy chunks of this creamy, yellowish substance made from cocoa beans at cosmetic-supply stores and online. It is also sold in uniform-size wafers. Either form will work fine in this recipe.

- Small glass jar with lid

2 tbsp	cocoa butter (see tip, at left)	30 mL
½ tsp	grated raw beeswax (see tip, above)	2 mL

1. In a small heatproof bowl, combine cocoa butter and beeswax. Set aside.

2. Pour enough water into a small saucepan to come about 2 inches (5 cm) up the side; bring to a simmer.

3. Set bowl on saucepan so that bottom of bowl is not touching simmering water; stir until cocoa butter mixture is melted and smooth. Remove bowl from heat.

4. Pour into jar. Let cool. Dip finger into gloss and smooth over lips. Store in a cool, dark place for up to 2 months.

Herbal Lip Cream

Calendulas, also known as pot marigolds, are an ornamental plant. The yellow-orange flowers are also good at healing skin irritations and wounds.

Best for: All lips

Tips: Shea butter is a rich emollient that's ideal in dry-skin treatments. Look for tubs or bags of it at cosmetic-supply stores or online.

To make the calendula infusion, steep 1 tbsp (15 mL) dried calendula flowers in 1 cup (250 mL) boiling water for 5 minutes. Strain and measure out what you need for this recipe. Calendula is a wonderful skin healer, so add leftovers of this infusion to bathwater.

● Small glass jar with lid

1 tbsp	shea butter (see tips, at left)	15 mL
1 tbsp	apricot kernel oil	15 mL
2 tbsp	calendula infusion (see tips, at left), cooled	30 mL

1. Place shea butter in a small heatproof bowl. Set aside.

2. Pour enough water into a small saucepan to come about 2 inches (5 cm) up the side; bring to a simmer.

3. Set bowl on saucepan so that bottom of bowl is not touching simmering water; stir until shea butter is melted and smooth. Remove bowl from heat.

4. Immediately stir in apricot kernel oil until well combined. Stir in calendula infusion. Pour into jar and seal tightly. Shake mixture until thickened and creamy. Let cool completely.

5. Dip finger into cream and smooth over lips. Store in a cool, dark place for up to 2 months.

Baking Soda Toothpaste

This is a combination your ancestors might have used to get their teeth clean and white. Salt and baking soda are abrasives, so brush gently, especially at the gum line.

Best for: Healthy teeth and gums

Tip: Large-flake kosher sea salt is easy to find and a good texture for this recipe.

1 tsp	coarse salt (see tip, at left)	5 mL
1 tsp	baking soda	5 mL
	Water	

1. In a small bowl, stir salt with baking soda. Add water, a few drops at a time, and stir until mixture is pasty.

2. Moisten toothbrush with water. Press toothbrush into paste to pick up. Brush teeth. Rinse well with water after brushing.

Strawberry Toothpaste

Strawberry seeds help scour teeth, and antioxidants in the berry fight bacteria. Plus, this simple paste tastes sensational.

Best for: Healthy teeth and gums

Tip: Ripe strawberries are very fragrant. Look for berries without dark spots or discolorations, and use them up as soon as possible after you buy them.

Note: Always measure accurately when you're making homemade beauty products. See page 53 for tips.

2 or 3	ripe strawberries (see tip, at left)	2 or 3

1. Remove leaves from strawberries and discard. Place strawberries on a small plate.
2. Using a fork, mash strawberries until pasty.
3. Moisten toothbrush with water. Press toothbrush into paste to pick up. Brush teeth. Rinse well with water after brushing.

Tips for Healthy Teeth

- Get children used to eating foods that don't contain added sugar. If children do not get used to sweet treats, they are less likely to have a sweet tooth when they are older.
- Eat fresh, raw foods and whole-grain products, and avoid foods rich in refined carbohydrates (all-purpose flour and granulated sugar). If you do have a sweet tooth, you can learn to change your tastes. The more you become accustomed to the flavors of fresh, whole foods, the more treats made with refined sugar and flour will taste unpleasantly sweet.
- Brush your teeth within 30 minutes of eating.
- Practice good brushing technique (see box, page 164). Take your time and brush for 3 minutes. Remember, it's not the design of your toothbrush or your toothpaste that gets your mouth clean; it's the movement of the bristles on teeth and gums.
- Munch on crunchy raw vegetables and fruits, such as carrots and apples, to strengthen teeth and gums. They're also great plaque removers.
- Never use your teeth to cut threads or rip plastic wrap off packages. Keep scissors handy for those tasks.

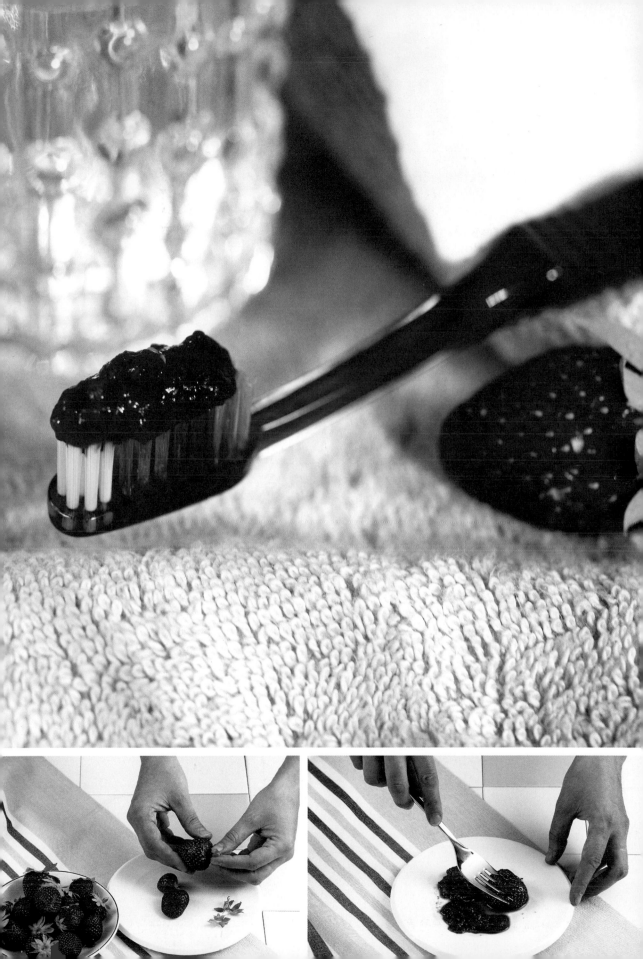

Sage and Mint Tooth Powder

Baking soda is a common ingredient in toothpastes and tooth powders because it has excellent anti-bacterial and tooth-whitening powers.

Best for: Healthy teeth and gums

Tips: Tinctures are liquid extracts made from medicinal plants, such as herbs, resins and roots. The healing properties of the plants are extracted using a solvent such as alcohol or vinegar.

If you have more than one person using this formula in your house, store each person's tooth powder in his or her own container to prevent cross-contamination.

Note: Always measure accurately when you're making homemade beauty products. See page 53 for tips.

- Small glass jar with lid

6 tbsp	baking soda	90 mL
3 tbsp	coarse salt (see tip, page 159)	45 mL
1 tbsp	dried sage leaves, finely crumbled (see tips, page 164)	15 mL
1 tbsp	dried mint leaves, finely crumbled	15 mL
10	drops myrrh tincture (see tips, at left)	10

1. In a small bowl, whisk together baking soda, salt, sage leaves and mint leaves.

2. Stir in myrrh tincture, a drop at a time, until well combined. Pour into jar.

3. Moisten toothbrush with water. Place a small amount of tooth powder in palm. Press toothbrush into powder to pick up. Brush teeth. Rinse well with water after brushing.

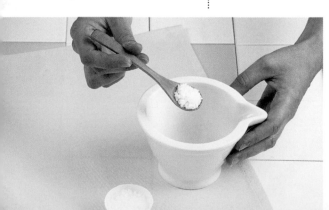
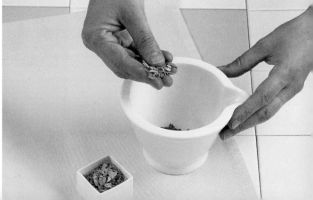

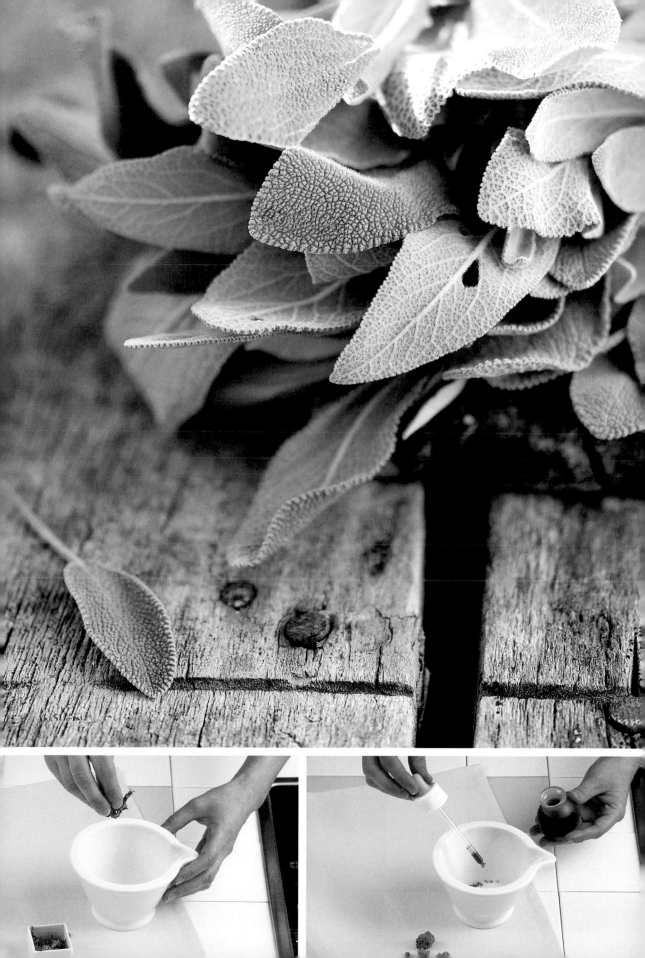

Herbal Tooth Powder

The herbs in this mixture simultaneously clean the teeth and improve gum health. Rosemary and sage are powerful odor fighters as well.

Best for: Healthy teeth and gums

Tips: Look for a reliable source of dried medicinal herbs, such as an herbalist's shop or a reputable online dealer. Make sure it's a business with high turnover, to ensure you're getting the freshest, most effective herbs possible.

This tooth powder is great for taking along on your travels. It doesn't contain liquid, so you can even pack it in your carry-on baggage.

If you have more than one person using this formula in your house, store each person's tooth powder in his or her own container to prevent cross-contamination.

Note: Always measure accurately when you're making homemade beauty products. See page 53 for tips.

- Mortar and pestle
- Fine-mesh sieve
- Small glass jar with lid

1 tbsp	dried rosemary leaves (see tips, at left)	15 mL
1 tsp	dried sage leaves	5 mL
1 tbsp	arrowroot powder	15 mL
½ tsp	licorice root powder	2 mL

1. In mortar and using pestle, crush rosemary and sage leaves into a fine powder. Place fine-mesh sieve over a small bowl; strain to remove any large pieces or fibers.

2. In jar, combine ground rosemary and sage, arrowroot powder and licorice root powder. Seal tightly and shake well to combine.

3. Moisten toothbrush with water. Place a small amount of tooth powder in palm. Press toothbrush into powder to pick up. Brush teeth. Rinse well with water after brushing.

The Right Way to Brush Teeth

The first step is to choose a suitable toothbrush, preferably one with dense, natural bristles. Remember that toothbrushes do not last forever; they should be replaced every three months.

Brush your teeth using vertical strokes, not side-to-side ones. Be sure to brush downward from the gum line on your upper teeth and upward from the gum line on your bottom teeth to remove plaque. Begin with your back teeth and work your way forward, being sure to brush both sides of each tooth. Finish by brushing both sides of your front teeth. Apply a reasonable but gentle amount of pressure. Do not scrub your teeth hard; doing so can irritate the gums and cause unnecessary bleeding.

It is very important to brush not only your teeth but also your gums. This removes plaque from the gum line and gently stimulates the tissue, improving blood circulation.

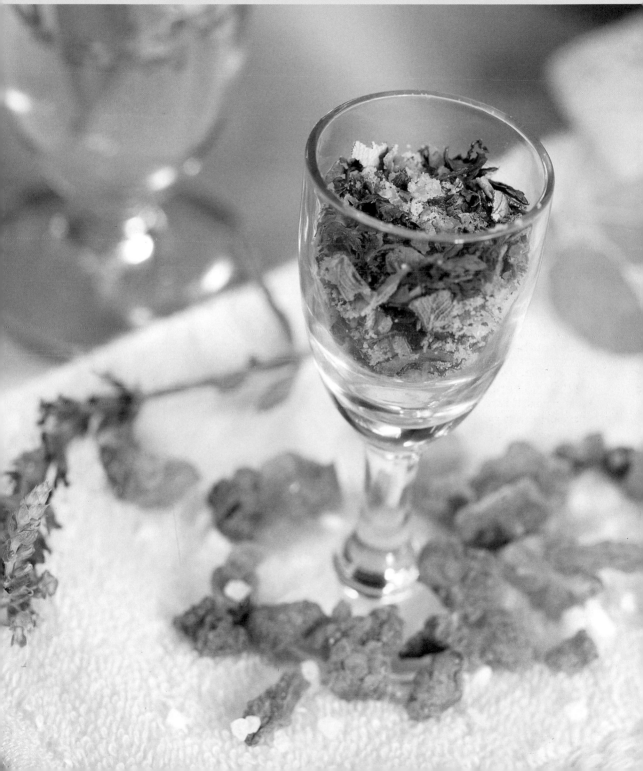

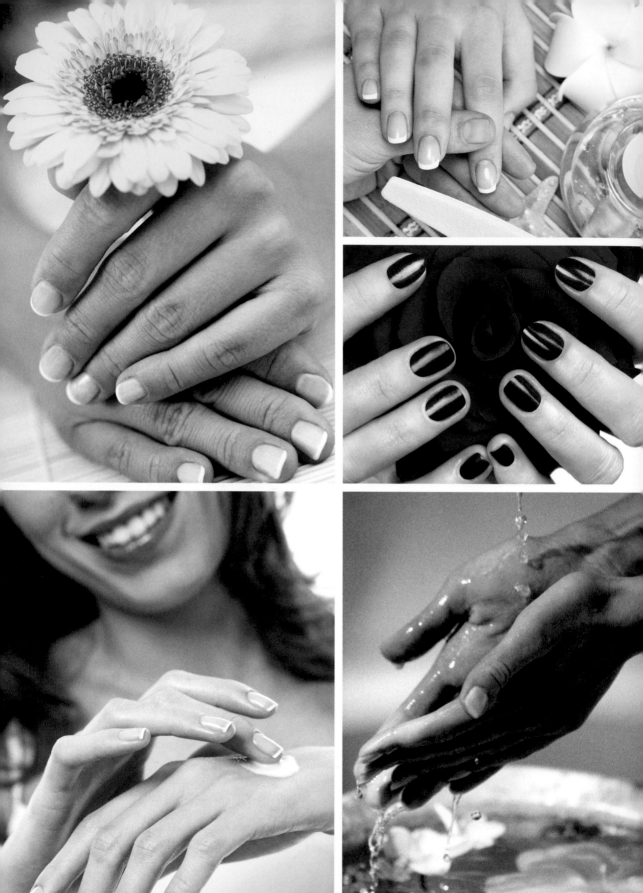

Hands and Nails: Stay Strong

Your hands have a hard time. They are exposed to weather of every type. They regularly get immersed in water that contains chemicals, such as those found in laundry detergent and dish soap. If you neglect your hands for long periods, especially if you do housework without using gloves, they will get dry and rough. It is not surprising then that the hands quickly reveal signs of aging and lack of care.

In this section, you'll discover the best tips for beautiful hands and nails. These suggestions can help you care for them and choose the best pampering products and treatments.

How to Have Silky Hands

The skin on your hands is surprisingly delicate, and it's one of the first places where time takes its toll in the form of age spots and wrinkles. The skin of the hands is thin and fragile because it contains fewer oil glands than skin that covers other parts of the body.

To protect your hands and keep them silky smooth, apply a moisturizing cream at least twice a day year-round. This will keep skin hydrated and crack free, and will also stimulate its natural regeneration processes to help defend it against damaging external factors.

Hand cream is an indispensable product for daily hand care. It comes in a wide variety of styles and can do many different things: fight signs of aging, fade age spots, nourish, moisturize and so on. Choose your hand cream based on what your hands need most. Creams that contain aloe vera and vitamin E are particularly good for general hand nourishment. Apply hand cream to each finger, using circular motions to massage from the fingertips to the knuckles, the back of the hand and the palm. Gently massage the cream up to the wrist until it is completely absorbed.

If your hands are sensitive and tend to turn red, use mild soaps based on glycerin or vegetable fat. Make sure to always reapply hand cream after you wash your hands. At bedtime, apply a coating of hand cream and leave it on overnight.

If your hands are extremely dry or damaged, you can also use a hand mask (turn to page 187 for a homemade one). It will give your hands an extra moisturizing boost, as well as help counter the effects of aging. Weekly exfoliation will also help soften your hands and stimulate blood flow; just mix a little granulated sugar into your usual hand or body cream and massage it in. Rinse off and reapply hand cream. You'll marvel at how smooth your skin will be!

Q: What causes nail problems?

A: All sorts of physiological issues can make your nails weak, brittle or grooved. It's important to consider the potential causes and take steps to correct the underlying problem. Here are a few factors that influence nail appearance:

- **Genetics.** Underlying genetic defects can affect the nails' appearance. Unfortunately, there is no way to change this tendency or correct genetic malformations of the nails.

- **Nutritional deficiencies.** Merely examining your fingernails or toenails can be enough to diagnose these. When a person is iron deficient, the nails are completely flat or too arched. Nails tear easily if there is not enough calcium or magnesium in the diet. When nails take on a marbled appearance, have white spots or are discolored at the edges, you can be sure that there is a zinc deficiency. When they have lengthwise grooves, it indicates a protein deficiency. And when nails flake into layers, there is not enough vitamin A in your diet. In all of these cases, consult your health-care provider and create a dietary plan that addresses these deficiencies.

- **Poor blood circulation.** In some people, blood flow to the extremities is impaired, and nails can look pale to bluish-purple. If you have pale nail beds, consult your doctor to rule out any serious medical conditions.

- **Fungal infections.** These are common and can make nails thick, yellow and brittle. To combat fungi, cut nails short and apply a buttermilk poultice to them overnight: moisten a gauze pad with buttermilk and apply it to the affected nail. Cover with a clean bandage and keep the poultice on overnight. Repeat the treatment until the fungus is gone. A diet rich in calcium and silicic acid is helpful for strengthening the nails' defenses from within while you treat them topically. If the infection doesn't resolve quickly, see your doctor or naturopath for treatment.

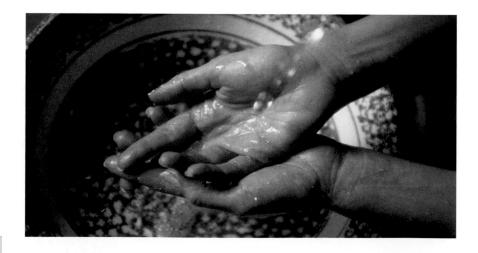

Nail Hardener

If your nails break all the time, this treatment can help you build them up and make them tough again. Plus, the fresh peppermint scent is really nice.

Best for: Weak or brittle nails

Tips: Potassium alum, also known as potassium aluminum sulfate, is a water-soluble white powder with astringent and styptic (blood clotting) effects. It's also an effective nail hardener. You can buy it in cosmetic-supply stores and online shops.

Lactic acid is what gives fermented milk products their distinctive sour taste. It's also a common ingredient in beauty products because it is a potent moisturizer. You can find lactic acid powder online at cosmetic-supply stores and some specialty food purveyors.

Note: Always measure accurately when you're making homemade beauty products. See page 53 for tips.

- Glass bottle with lid
- Small brush or cotton swab

⅓ cup	rose water (see tips, page 178)	75 mL
1 tsp	potassium alum (see tips, at left)	5 mL
½ tsp	lactic acid powder (see tips, at left)	2 mL
2	drops peppermint essential oil (see tips, page 184)	2

1. In a small bowl, combine rose water, potassium alum and lactic acid powder. Stir for 1 to 2 minutes or until the mixture becomes lighter in color.

2. Stir in peppermint essential oil until well combined. Pour mixture into bottle.

3. Dip small brush into oil mixture. Paint onto nails. Store bottle in a cool, dark place for up to 2 months.

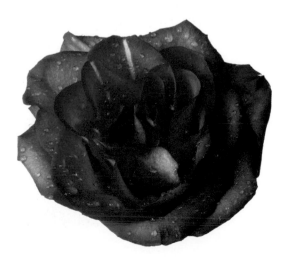

Nail Oil

To keep nails pliable and strong, a good oil treatment is always helpful. This formulation will make the surface of the nail greasy, so polish won't adhere. Use it on bare nails between manicures.

Best for: Healthy nails

Tip: The essential oil made from the leaves of the tea tree (*Melaleuca alternifolia*) is a powerful antifungal and antibacterial agent. It also smells clean and refreshing, so it is added to many natural beauty products.

Note: Always measure accurately when you're making homemade beauty products. See page 53 for tips.

- Small glass bottle with lid
- Small brush or cotton swab

1½ tsp	castor oil (see tips, page 180)	7 mL
1 tsp	soybean oil (see tips, page 186)	5 mL
½ tsp	avocado oil (see tips, page 179)	2 mL
2	drops tea tree essential oil (see tip, at left)	2

1. In a small bowl, combine castor oil, soybean oil and avocado oil. Whisk for 2 minutes or until smooth and well combined. Whisk in tea tree essential oil.

2. Pour mixture into bottle. Dip small brush into mixture. Paint onto nails and let stand for 3 to 5 minutes. Rinse off nails and pat dry. Store bottle in a cool, dark place for up to 2 months.

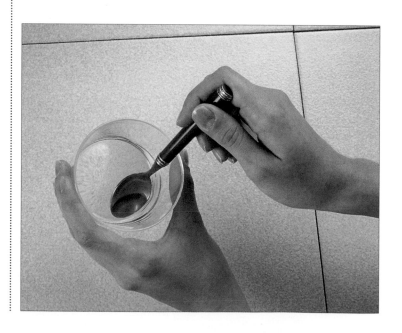

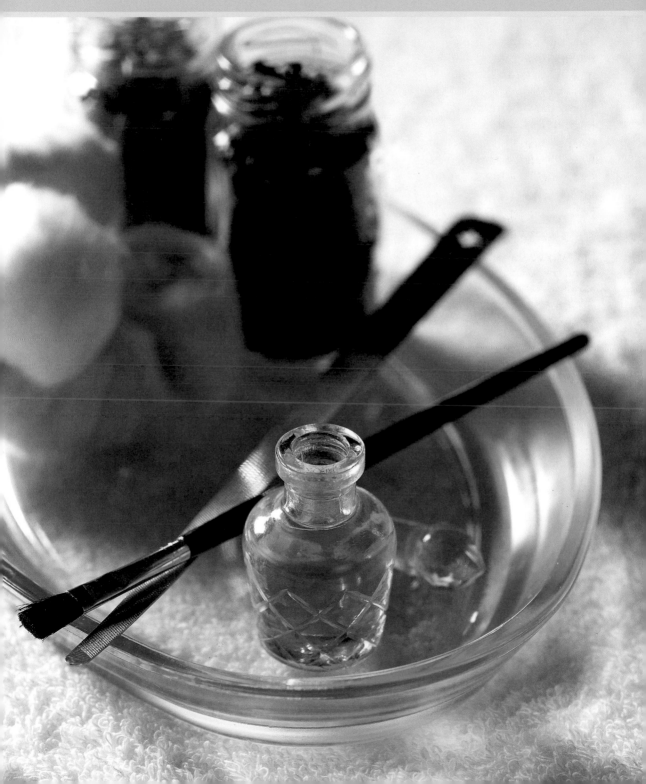

Dill and Oil Nail Treatment

This ultra-simple soak makes nails strong and helps keep them from breaking. The oil rub at the end helps keep nails flexible so they won't tear as easily.

Best for: Dry, brittle nails

Tip: Always cover infusions (or herbal teas) when you're steeping them. This keeps all the volatile compounds from evaporating.

Note: Always measure accurately when you're making homemade beauty products. See page 53 for tips.

- Fine-mesh sieve

2 cups	water	500 mL
1	handful fresh dill sprigs	1
	Olive oil or sweet almond oil (see tip, page 146)	

1. In a medium saucepan, combine water and dill; bring to a boil. Remove from heat, cover and let stand for 10 minutes.

2. Place fine-mesh sieve over a medium heatproof bowl; strain infusion into bowl. Let cool just until warm.

3. Soak nails in infusion for 10 to 15 minutes.

4. Pat nails dry. Massage with a few drops of oil.

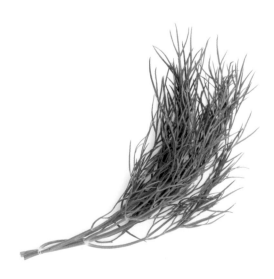

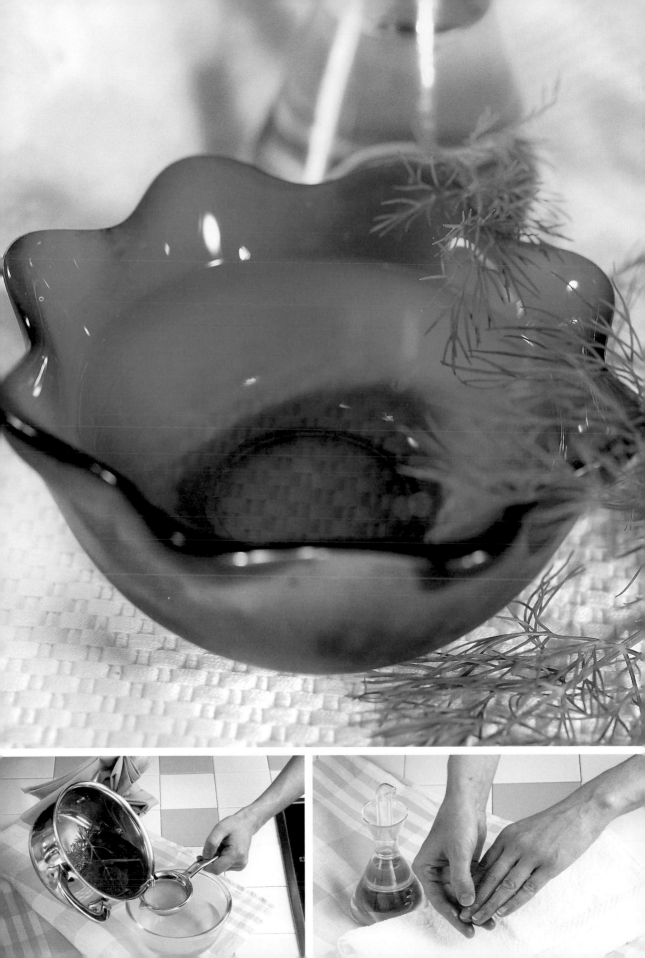

Lemon Nail Rub

The natural oils in lemon zest are a potent cleanser and nail strengthener. They also help lighten nails that have been discolored by nail polish.

Best for: Dry, brittle nails

Tip: Lemon is also excellent for softening rough, dry skin on your hands. Avoid applying it to cracked skin, however; the natural acid in lemons makes broken skin sting.

Note: Always measure accurately when you're making homemade beauty products. See page 53 for tips.

1	lemon	1

1. Using a sharp knife, cut off lemon zest, making large strips. Save lemon for another use.
2. Rub lemon zest all over nails.

Top Tips for Beautiful Nails

Healthy, well-manicured nails complete your overall look. Here are the best things you can do to take care of them:

- **Eat right.** To maintain strong, healthy nails, eat a varied diet that is rich in protein, vitamins and minerals. Drink plenty of milk and eat cheese, eggs and whole grains on a regular basis. Some other especially beneficial foods to include are wheat germ, peas, pumpkins, apples, loquats and salads dressed with cold-pressed oil.

- **Take supplements.** Complement your diet by taking calcium, B complex and vitamin C supplements daily.

- **Exercise your hands.** Open and close your hands and rotate your wrists periodically throughout the day. This improves circulation, stretches tight muscles and helps deliver all those good nutrients to your skin and nails.

- **Cut and file.** Nails grow faster if they are cut and filed with an emery board regularly. File in only one direction to avoid weakening the tips of the nails.

- **Take a polish break.** Nail polish can cause allergies and other adverse reactions in some people. Plus, dark colors can stain nails, making them look yellow and unappealing. Give them a week off here and there, and let your nails breathe.

- **Stop biting.** Nibbling on your nails and cuticles can cause permanent damage. Weakened and injured areas are more susceptible to infection as well. Plus, biting nails can wear down your teeth and cause sensitivity issues. If you find it hard to stop, try to always have something in your hands. Or keep lotion or cuticle oil nearby and rub it onto the area anytime you're tempted to bite.

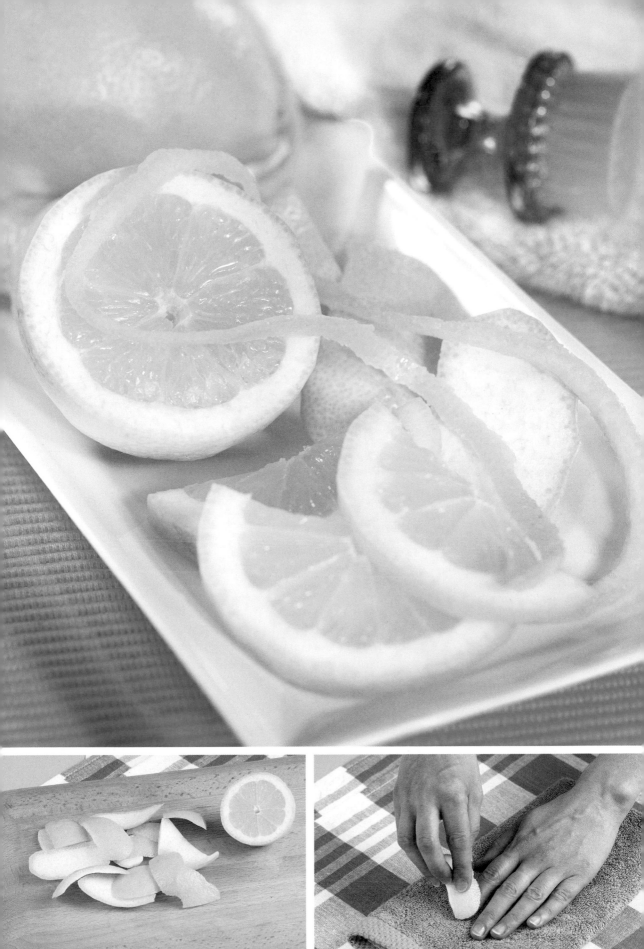

Wart Remover

Onions have excellent antibacterial and antiseptic powers, so they're good at fighting the virus that causes annoying warts on the hands.

Best for: Common warts

Tip: Spring onions are immature onion bulbs that have just started to swell at the root end. They are often sold with their green tops attached, so they look like a fatter version of green onions.

Note: Always measure accurately when you're making homemade beauty products. See page 53 for tips.

- Box grater or flat grater
- Small glass jar with lid

1	spring onion (see tip, at left)	1

1. Trim off green top of spring onion if attached. Peel spring onion.

2. Using coarse side of box grater, grate spring onion until pasty. Spoon onion paste into jar.

3. Using a small spoon or applicator, spread a small amount of paste over wart. Let stand on skin for 5 to 10 minutes.

4. Rinse off paste with warm water. Pat hands dry with a towel. Repeat the treatment daily or every other day until the wart has disappeared.

Remedies for Warts

Warts are small benign skin growths caused by the human papillomavirus. There are many strains of this virus; the one that causes common warts, which tend to form on the hands, is not the same as the virus that causes genital warts or plantar (foot) warts. Common warts appear on the hands in the form of hard, round, raised patches of skin. They are the most common type of warts.

Unfortunately, no remedy is 100% successful; warts can be stubborn and recur repeatedly. Dermatologists often remove them by burning them off. This procedure, called electrocoagulation, is done under local anesthesia. It is rather aggressive and does not necessarily kill the underlying viral infection. Natural medicine offers a larger variety of safe, less-painful treatment options. Sliced garlic and onion juice are two natural wart-fighting substances.

Homeopathy offers a more comprehensive treatment plan. A series of orally administered substances are given to the patient, including Calcarea Carbonica, Causticum, Nitricum Acidum, dulcamara and thuja tincture. Visit a certified homeopathic practitioner for guidance on this and any other homeopathic treatments.

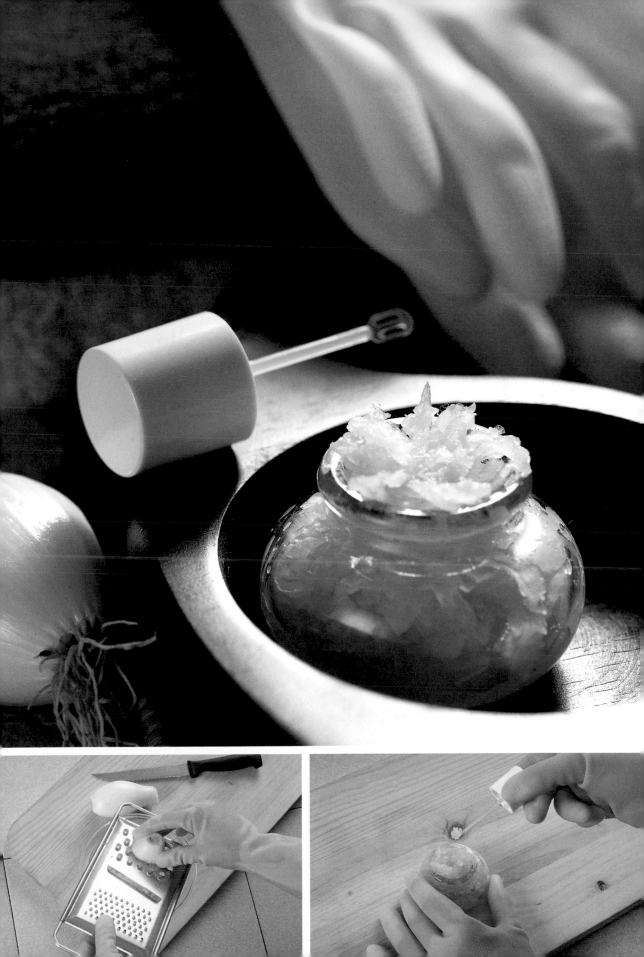

Cucumber Hand Softener

Apply this formula before bed and let it work its magic on chapped hands overnight.

Best for: Dry, rough hands

Tips: Choose 100% natural cocoa butter for homemade creams like this. You can buy chunks of this creamy, yellowish substance made from cocoa beans at cosmetic-supply stores and online. It is also sold in uniform-size wafers. Either will work fine.

Sweet almond oil, like other nut oils, can perish quickly if stored in a warm place or exposed to direct sunlight. Keep the bottle in a dark, cool cupboard and use it up within a couple of months of opening.

- Blender

1	cucumber, peeled and coarsely chopped	1
2 tbsp	cocoa butter (see tips, at left)	30 mL
1 tbsp	sweet almond oil (see tips, at left)	15 mL

1. In blender, purée cucumber until liquefied. Set aside.
2. Place cocoa butter in a small heatproof bowl. Set aside.
3. Pour enough water into a small saucepan to come about 2 inches (5 cm) up the side; bring to a simmer.
4. Set bowl on saucepan so that bottom of bowl is not touching simmering water; stir until cocoa butter is melted and smooth. Remove bowl from heat.
5. Stir sweet almond oil and puréed cucumber into cocoa butter until well combined. Let cool completely.
6. Massage mixture into hands until absorbed.

Almond Hand Cream

This sweetly scented cream makes a thoughtful gift for friends and family.

Best for: Dry or normal hands

Tips: Raw beeswax is yellow and has a light honey aroma. This recipe calls for white beeswax pearls, which have had the color and scent removed. They are easy to find at cosmetic-supply stores.

Rose water is commonly used in Middle Eastern, Mediterranean, Indian and North African cuisine, so look for bottles of this fragrant essence at specialty grocery stores.

- Hand mixer
- Small glass jar with lid

6 tbsp	sweet almond oil (see tips, above)	90 mL
1 tbsp	white beeswax pearls (see tips, at left)	15 mL
3 tbsp	rose water (see tips, at left)	45 mL

1. In a small heatproof bowl, combine sweet almond oil and white beeswax. Set aside.
2. Pour enough water into a small saucepan to come about 2 inches (5 cm) up the side; bring to a simmer.
3. Set bowl on saucepan so that bottom of bowl is not touching simmering water; stir until beeswax mixture is melted and smooth. Remove bowl from heat.
4. Using hand mixer, beat in rose water, a few drops at a time, for 3 to 4 minutes or until mixture is creamy and completely cool. Spoon into jar.
5. Smooth cream all over hands. Store jar in a cool, dark place for up to 2 months.

Avocado Sage Hand Cream

Avocados are terrific at hydrating skin. Here, avocado oil is mixed with other emollients and scented with sage to make a smooth-as-silk cream for tired hands.

Best for: Dry or normal hands

Tips: Avocado oil is becoming increasingly popular for cooking. Buy cold-pressed avocado oil that has not been extracted using solvents. It's the most natural, least processed choice.

Stearic acid crystals are commonly added to mixtures that contain beeswax, to help boost the wax's emulsifying powers. Look for them at cosmetic-supply stores or online.

Note: Always measure accurately when you're making homemade beauty products. See page 53 for tips.

- Hand mixer
- Small glass jar with lid

2 tbsp	avocado oil (see tips, at left)	30 mL
1 tsp	grated raw beeswax (see tips, opposite)	5 mL
1 tsp	cocoa butter (see tips, opposite)	5 mL
1 tsp	stearic acid (see tips, at left)	5 mL
1 tsp	soybean oil	5 mL
2 tbsp	hot water	30 mL
5	drops sage essential oil	5

1. In a small heatproof bowl, combine avocado oil, beeswax, cocoa butter, stearic acid and soybean oil. Set aside.

2. Pour enough water into a small saucepan to come about 2 inches (5 cm) up the side; bring to a simmer.

3. Set bowl on saucepan so that bottom of bowl is not touching simmering water; stir until beeswax mixture is melted and smooth. Remove bowl from heat.

4. Immediately stir in hot water. Using hand mixer, beat for 2 minutes or until creamy.

5. Beat in sage essential oil. Beat for 2 to 3 minutes or until mixture is completely cool. Spoon into jar.

6. Smooth cream all over hands. Store jar in a cool, dark place for up to 2 months.

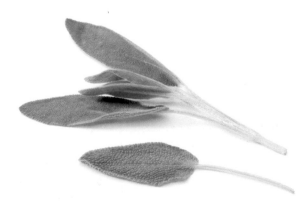

Lemon Hand Cream

Lemon essential oil gives this easy cream a lovely citrusy smell. Make a double batch so you can always have a jar with you to soothe dry, irritated hands.

Best for: Dry or normal hands

Tips: Shea butter is a rich emollient that's ideal in dry-skin treatments. Look for tubs or bags of it at cosmetic-supply stores or online.

Castor oil is made from castor beans (*Ricinus communis*). It's gentle and soothing to skin.

Note: Always measure accurately when you're making homemade beauty products. See page 53 for tips.

- Small glass jar with lid

1 tbsp	shea butter (see tips, at left)	15 mL
1½ tsp	apricot kernel oil (see tips, page 186)	7 mL
1½ tsp	castor oil (see tips, at left)	7 mL
3	drops lemon essential oil	3

1. Place shea butter in a small heatproof bowl (see box, page 82). Set aside.

2. Pour enough water into a small saucepan to come about 2 inches (5 cm) up the side; bring to a simmer.

3. Set bowl on saucepan so that bottom of bowl is not touching simmering water; stir until shea butter is melted and smooth. Remove bowl from heat.

4. Stir apricot kernel oil and castor oil into shea butter until well combined and creamy. Stir in lemon essential oil. Let cool completely.

5. Spoon into jar. Massage cream into hands until absorbed. Store jar in a cool, dark place for up to 1 month.

Nutrients for Strong, Healthy Nails

Nails, like hair, are a surprisingly accurate indicator of a person's general health. When minerals and trace elements are insufficient, nails and hair become fragile and their natural structures become weak (see box, page 168). Also like hair, nails are especially in need of the sulfur-containing amino acids (namely, methionine, taurine, cystine and cysteine) to build proteins. You'll get these mainly from egg yolks; soybeans and soy foods, such as tofu and tempeh; nuts; and seeds.

Also, make sure you eat whole grains every day; they provide you with the zinc you need. Nails also require protein, so eat plenty of tofu, cheese, seitan, nuts and eggs on a regular basis. And always make sure your diet includes a rainbow of vegetables. Dark green or bright yellow or orange flesh indicates that the vegetable contains abundant amounts of vitamin A and magnesium.

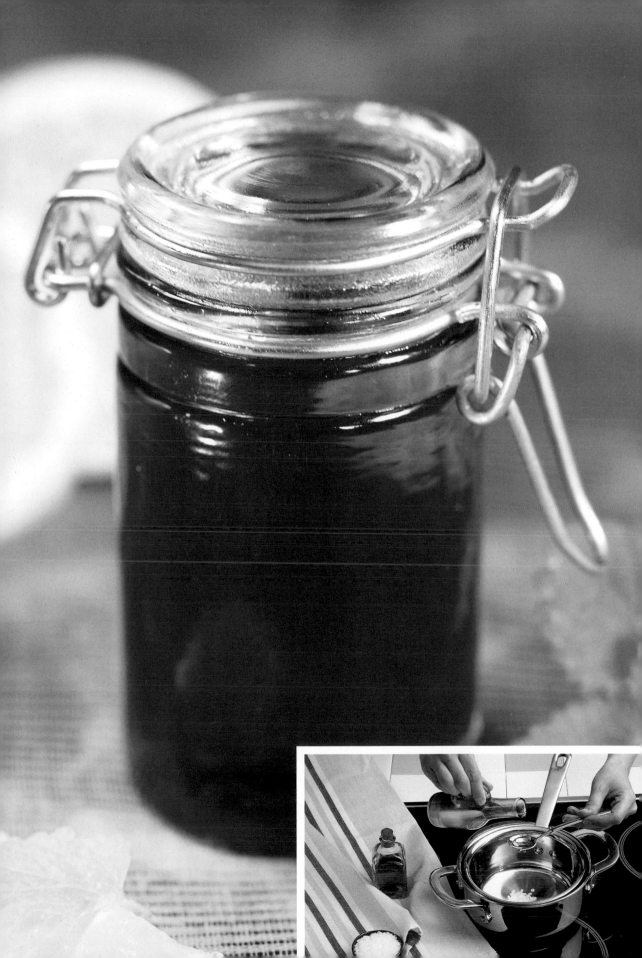

Calendula Vinegar Hand Cleanser

Vinegar is a natural germ fighter that's safer for you than the synthetic antibacterial agents in some commercial hand cleansers. Mixed with gentle soap and medicinal flowers, it becomes a potent clean-up tool for dirty hands.

Best for: Dry or normal hands

Tips: Look for good-quality ready-made soaps at natural food stores. You may also like to support local artisanal soap makers and use their bars to create this cleanser.

Common mallow (*Malva sylvestris*) is frequently used in beauty products to reduce inflammation. It's also great at protecting and nourishing dry skin. Look for these flowers and calendula flowers at your favorite herbalist's shop or online herb store.

Note: Always measure accurately when you're making homemade beauty products. See page 53 for tips.

- Box grater
- 6-cup (1.5 L) canning jar with lid

1	bar natural pH-balanced coconut oil soap (see tips, at left)	1
4 cups	cider vinegar	1 L
1 tbsp	dried calendula flowers	15 mL
1 tbsp	dried common mallow flowers (see tips, at left)	15 mL
1	sprig fresh rosemary	1

1. Using box grater, grate soap into a large bowl. Pour into jar.

2. Stir in vinegar, calendula flowers, mallow flowers and rosemary. Seal tightly and let stand at room temperature for 1 week.

3. Pour a small amount of vinegar mixture into palm. Scrub hands under warm running water. Rinse well. Store jar in a cool, dark place for up to 2 months.

Gentle Hand Washing

To keep your hands in great shape, wash them with the mildest soaps you can find. The best are pH balanced and made with a coconut- or almond-oil base. Avoid highly alkaline soaps; they negatively affect the naturally acidic pH of the skin and progressively damage the tissue, making hands dry, rough and red. Sometimes, this can result in flaking and peeling or even in eczema.

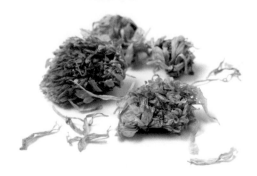

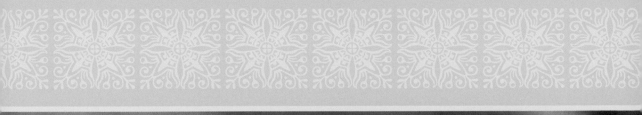

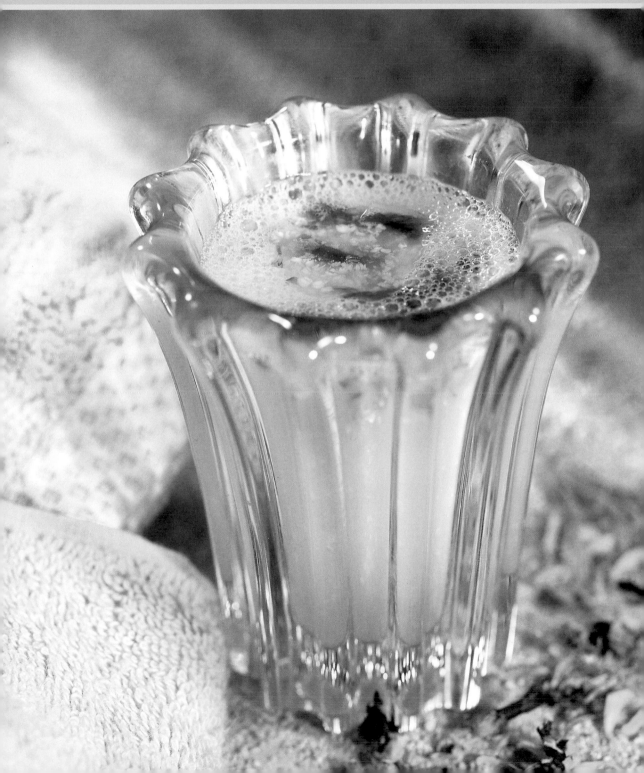

Nourishing Hand Oil

This mixture is wonderful at nourishing tired, dry skin. It can make your hands a little greasy, so make sure to rub it in as much as possible before touching anything.

Best for: Dry or normal hands

Tips: The seeds found inside pumpkins (*Cucurbita pepo*) contain a nutrient-rich, dark-colored oil that's prized for both its flavor and its healing properties for the skin. You can add the oil to this nail treatment and drizzle a bit over salads for a nutritional boost.

Buy essential oils sold in dark bottles. Exposure to light can reduce the potency of their medicinal herbal components. Store the bottles in a cool, dark place to keep them fresh.

Note: Always measure accurately when you're making homemade beauty products. See page 53 for tips.

● Small glass jar with lid

2 tbsp	apricot kernel oil (see tips, page 186)	30 mL
1 tbsp	pumpkin seed oil (see tips, at left)	15 mL
2	drops lavender essential oil (see tips, at left)	2

1. In a small bowl, combine apricot kernel oil, pumpkin seed oil and lavender essential oil. Whisk to combine. Pour into jar; seal tightly and shake well.

2. Smooth oil all over hands, rubbing into skin well. Store jar in a cool, dark place for up to 2 months.

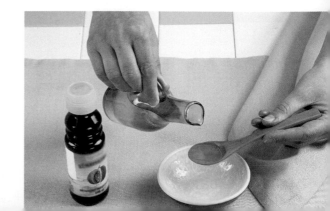

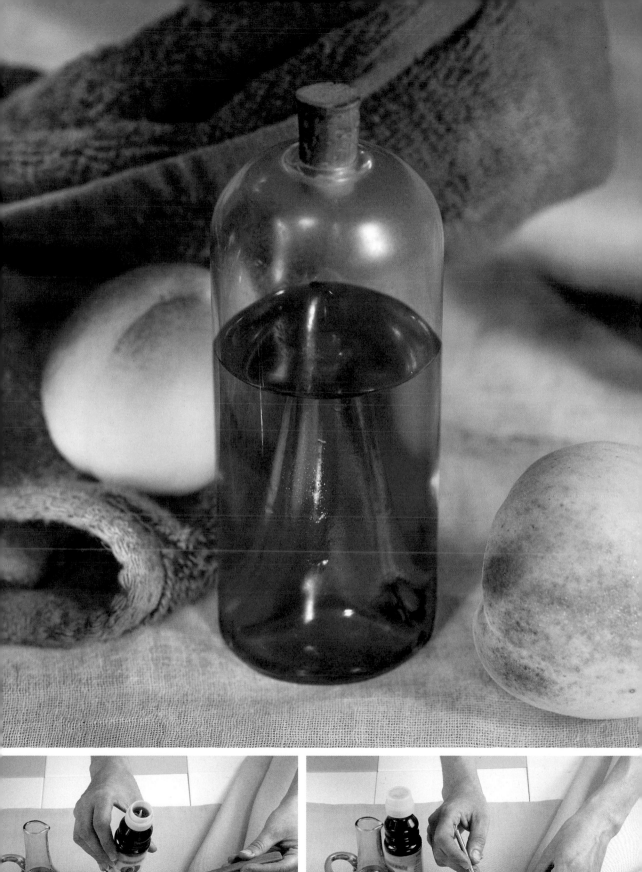

Gentle Scented Hand Lotion

You can choose whatever scent you like for this hydrating lotion. It's so easy to make, you can make a bunch of batches to keep at home, at work and in your purse.

Best for: Dry or normal hands

Tips: Glycerin is an effective moisturizer that is great for softening the hands. Look for bottles of it at cosmetic-supply stores or online.

Baby or child cologne is gentle on skin, and usually made with natural scents derived from flowers, fruits or herbs. Check the label and ensure the ingredients are pure and the formula doesn't contain chemicals.

- Small glass jar with lid

1 tbsp	liquid glycerin (see tips, at left)	15 mL
1 tsp	baby or child cologne (see tips, at left)	5 mL

1. In a small bowl, stir glycerin with baby cologne until well combined.

2. Spoon into jar. Smooth a small amount over hands. Store in a cool, dark place for up to 2 months.

Cream for Chapped Hands

Winter brings biting cold and wind, which can really damage the skin on your hands. This cream will heal the redness and cracked skin that result from this weather.

Best for: Chapped, red, irritated hands

Tips: Cold-pressed extra-virgin oils are the purest and most unadulterated type you can buy for making homemade beauty treatments. They are worth the higher price tag.

Benzoin is a reddish-brown resin extracted from a tree that grows in southeast Asia. The essential oil made from it helps preserve this cream and reduces skin irritation. It also has a pleasant vanilla-like fragrance.

- Glass jar with lid

2 tbsp	cocoa butter (see tips, page 178)	30 mL
2 tbsp	sunflower oil (see tips, at left)	30 mL
1 cup	rose water (see tips, page 178)	250 mL
2	drops benzoin essential oil (see tips, at left)	2

1. Place cocoa butter in a small heatproof bowl. Set aside.

2. Pour enough water into a small saucepan to come about 2 inches (5 cm) up the side; bring to a simmer.

3. Set bowl on saucepan so that bottom of bowl is not touching simmering water; stir until cocoa butter is melted and smooth. Stir in sunflower oil. Remove bowl from heat.

4. Stir in rose water and benzoin essential oil until well combined and creamy. Spoon into jar.

5. Rub a bit of cream on inner wrist to make sure the temperature is comfortable before smoothing cream all over your hands. Store jar in a cool, dark place for up to 2 months.

Hand Mask

Just like a facial mask, a hand mask helps smooth skin and remove impurities.

Best for: Dry or normal hands

Tips: Use rose petals from plants that have not been sprayed with herbicides or fungicides. Choose a fragrant variety of rose for the most enjoyable experience.

The bergamot orange is a citrus fruit; oil derived from its rind is used to give Earl Grey tea its distinctive aroma. Bergamot essential oil gives this mask its fresh scent and acts as a light moisturizer and toner at the same time.

Leftover rose infusion makes a soothing addition to bathwater. Pour it into a clean jar and keep it in the fridge for up to 1 month.

Note: Always measure accurately when you're making homemade beauty products. See page 53 for tips.

- Potato masher
- Fine-mesh sieve

3	apples, peeled and quartered	3
5	whole cloves	5
8 oz	fresh rose petals (see tips, at left)	250 g
2 cups	boiling water	500 mL
2	egg whites (see tips, page 197)	2
2	drops bergamot essential oil (see tips, at left)	2

1. In a large saucepan, combine apples and cloves; pour in enough water to cover. Bring to a boil. Reduce heat and simmer for 20 to 30 minutes or until apples are very tender.

2. Remove pan from heat. Discard cloves. Using a potato masher, mash apples until saucy. Set aside.

3. Place rose petals in a medium heatproof bowl. Pour boiling water over top. Cover and let stand for 5 to 10 minutes.

4. Set fine-mesh sieve over another medium heatproof bowl; strain infusion into bowl, discarding solids. Stir 1 tbsp (15 mL) infusion into apple mixture. Reserve remaining infusion for another use (see tips, at left).

5. Whisk in egg whites and bergamot essential oil until well combined. Rub a bit of mixture on inner wrist to make sure the temperature is comfortable before smoothing mixture all over your hands. Let stand on skin for about 10 minutes. Rinse off mixture with lukewarm water.

Rose Water Lotion

Rose water has such a lovely, old-fashioned aroma. It's especially nice in this effective hand moisturizer.

Best for: Dry or normal hands

Tip: Liquid honey often crystallizes in the jar when it's stored in a warm place. There's nothing wrong with it in this state, and you can easily reliquefy it. Just pop the uncovered jar into a saucepan of warm water and heat it gently, stirring the honey until the crystals dissolve and it turns clear again.

Note: Always measure accurately when you're making homemade beauty products. See page 53 for tips.

- $\frac{1}{2}$-cup (125 mL) canning jar with lid

1 tbsp	rose water (see tips, page 178)	15 mL
2 tsp	liquid glycerin (see tips, page 186)	10 mL
$\frac{1}{2}$ tsp	liquid honey (see tip, at left)	2 mL
$\frac{1}{2}$ tsp	white vinegar	2 mL
20	drops lemon juice	20

1. In jar, combine rose water, glycerin, honey, vinegar and lemon juice. Seal lid tightly and shake vigorously until well mixed and creamy.

2. Smooth lotion all over hands. Store jar in a cool, dark place for up to 2 months.

Handy Tips

There are a few strategies for reducing wear and tear on your hands. Try these and watch how smooth your skin gets:

- **Wear rubber gloves for housework.** Protect your hands with gloves whenever you have to get them wet or expose them to cleaning products.

- **Wear gloves or mittens when it's cold.** In winter, wear a pair of simple woollen gloves or mittens to help prevent cracked, dry hands.

- **Use pH-balanced soaps.** Avoid overly alkaline soaps. Better yet, make your own hand cleanser like the one on page 182.

- **Moisturize your hands daily.** Use a good-quality natural cream or lotion like the ones on pages 178 to 188. And try the popular hand model technique for keeping hands perfectly smooth: before going to bed, apply moisturizer and put on cotton gloves. Sleep with the gloves on, and you'll wake up with perfectly hydrated hands.

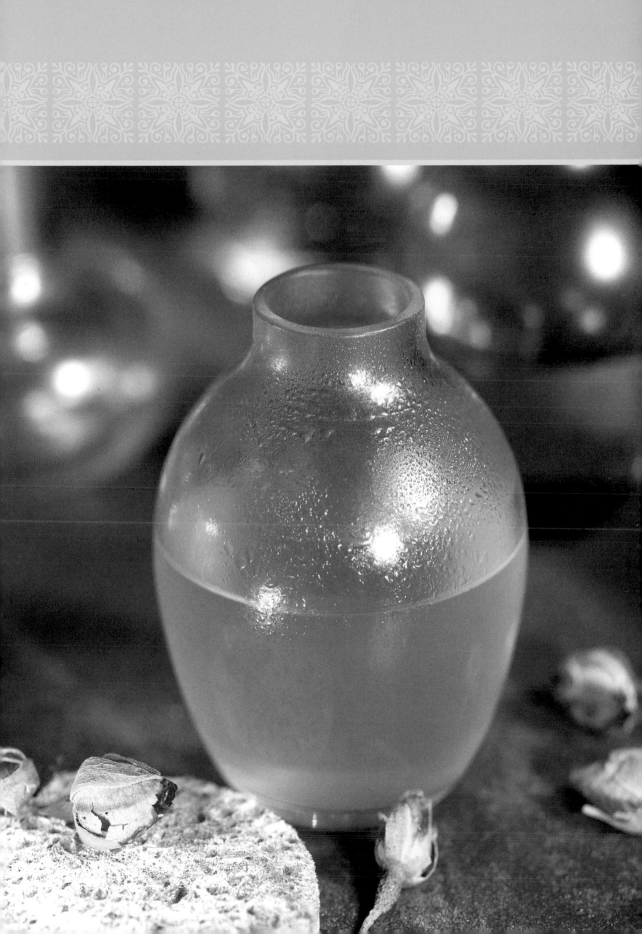

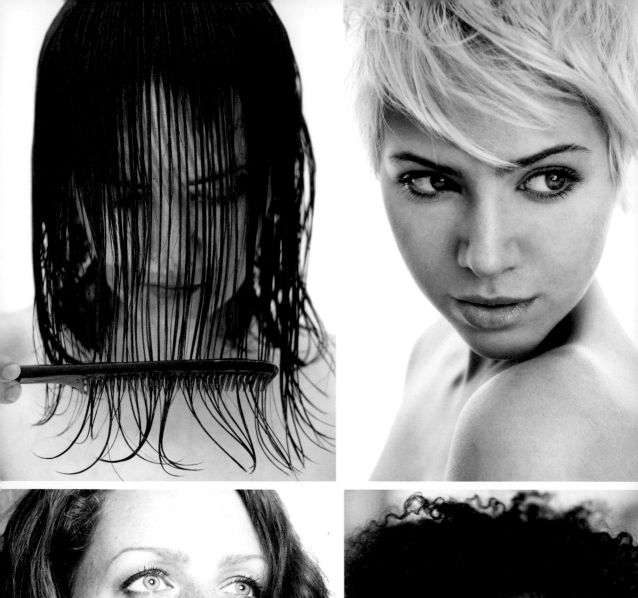
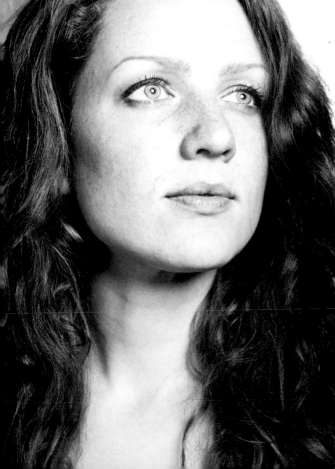
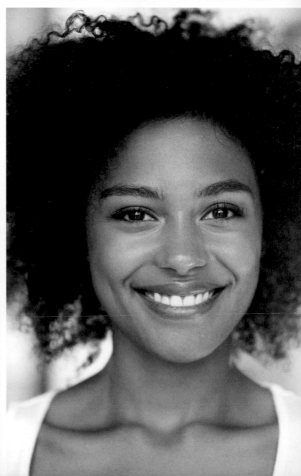

Hair Products and Treatments

Your hair and scalp require as much care as your complexion. The first step before you try any hair treatment is to determine what type of hair you have. Is it oily, dry or right in the middle? Do you have specific issues you'd like to treat, such as dandruff (see page 216) or thinning or brittle hair (see page 222)? Once you determine the challenges you're facing, you can take the proper measures to prevent or address the issues. The recipes in this chapter will help you strengthen and beautify your mane outside while you nourish it inside.

Hair: The Inside Story

Hair is made of a protein called keratin, which is also present in the nails and the outermost layer of the skin. Like skin, hair is made up of three distinct layers. The innermost layer, called the medulla, is composed of spongy tissue that may contain pigment. The medulla is surrounded by the middle layer, or cortex, which consists of long, thin cells that give the hair its elasticity and color. The outermost layer is the cuticle, which is formed by hundreds of thin, overlapping scales.

The hair grows from the follicle, a closed sac beneath the surface of the scalp. Each follicle contains a hair root and is fed by nutrients carried in the blood; this is why good circulation is so important for healthy, attractive hair. Hairs grow a little more than $\frac{1}{2}$ inch (1 cm) per month, but growth is usually faster in summer and decreases with age.

Stress Hampers Hair

Stress has a negative effect on hair. A person living under constant tension constricts his or her neck muscles, which impedes blood flow to the scalp. This can make hair weak and prone to breakage. Practicing stress-reduction techniques, such as yoga, meditation and deep breathing exercises, is a positive way to keep your locks in top condition.

Vitamins and Minerals for Hair

Hair health is a lot like skin health: it depends largely on diet. Hair requires a number of essential nutrients in order to grow. B vitamins encourage hair growth, aid in the production of oils that lubricate hair and help maintain color, so you need an ample supply of these vitamins in your daily diet. Vitamins A and C and several essential minerals (including copper, iron and iodine) are also important for building healthy, beautiful tresses.

Diet for Healthy, Beautiful Hair

To keep your hair at its best, eat fresh fruit, whole grains, muesli and soy lecithin every day. Aim for four servings of fruit per day; ideally, these should be acidic, vitamin C–rich fruits, such as kiwifruit, lemons, grapefruits and oranges. This vitamin is important for regenerating and protecting the arteries. In addition, the bioflavonoids in acidic fruits protect the tiny capillaries in the scalp, which nourish the hair follicles.

Zinc and vitamin B_6, which are abundant in whole grains, are especially important for keeping these tiny blood vessels in good form. Consuming a serving of muesli every day will ensure you get enough of these vital nutrients. Another example of a good breakfast that nourishes the hair is yogurt with oatmeal topped with 1 tsp (5 mL) of wheat germ and a drizzle of molasses. This combination provides a good supply of folic acid and vitamin B_5 (pantothenic acid), two nutrients that help delay the appearance of gray.

Tofu is another food that supports hair growth. It contains lots of protein, one of the raw materials that help hair follicles synthesize keratin. Each hair consists of 97% keratin, a tough, fibrous protein continuously being manufactured in the root of the hair. By eating tofu, you make sure this process continues smoothly, without interruption.

Shiny Hair

A variety of nutrients create glossy hair. Sulfur combines with various amino acids to form proteins; this is the case with cysteine, the amino acid responsible for hair's shiny appearance. Soy products, cottage cheese and eggs contain cysteine and act to fix sulfur ions. It is a good idea to combine these protein-rich foods with foods that contain vitamin C, such as acidic fruits. In general, people who experience high levels of stress and smokers usually have devitalized hair due to a vitamin C deficit.

Nourishing the Roots

When the roots of the hair and the scalp receive sufficient amounts of nutrients, hair retains its body and shine. The only exceptions are gray hair caused by genetic factors and male-pattern hair loss due to hormonal changes — and even these processes can be slowed or halted by consuming the right nutrients.

Hair is fed by fine capillaries, tiny blood vessels that can be as little as $\frac{1}{32}$ inch (1 mm) long and only 0.00012 to 0.0002 inches (0.003 to 0.005 mm) in diameter. They wrap around the hair root and supply it with the nutrients and building blocks it needs to create new hair. Supplying the hair with the bioactive substances it needs revitalizes this system of capillaries.

The main obstacle to hair growth is the formation of plaques inside these minute blood vessels. Plaques can contain cholesterol, calcium or other substances. When this happens, the capillary soon dries up, and the sebaceous glands and nerves starve and atrophy. This is why some experts have linked high cholesterol levels (and the arterial plaque buildup they can cause) with impaired hair growth and hair loss. The best way to avoid this is to take soy lecithin, since it contains up to 40% choline, a relative of the B vitamins, which some studies have identified as having cholesterol-lowering powers.

Gray Hair

Your predisposition to having gray hair is largely determined by heredity; there's nothing you can do to fight your genes unfortunately. In some people, gray or white hairs appear at an early age, while others do not have them until they are elderly; about half of all people over age 45 have some gray hair. Over time, the biological mechanism that gives hair its pigment stops working, and the natural color of the hair disappears. But it's not all genetic: other factors that can contribute to the emergence of gray hair are nervous disorders, strong emotions, stress, mental burnout, insufficient exercise and even obesity.

Fighting Premature Grays

Some people start getting silver strands early in life. While you can't completely prevent premature graying, there is some evidence that you can delay its onset by increasing circulation to the scalp and consuming a super-nutritious diet. To hold off the grays at a young age, eat foods that contain biotin (also known as vitamin H), such as brewer's yeast, egg yolks, whole grains, nuts, fruits and vegetables.

Some research has shown promise in the effort to restore lost hair color. Foods rich in iodine, iron, copper, B vitamins and linoleic acid have been linked with color restoration in gray hair, although it takes several months for the results to show after these are added to the diet.

Pantothenic acid, para-aminobenzoic acid (PABA) and folic acid, all members of the B vitamin family, also seem to help preserve hair color and restore it if it has been lost. All three are found in egg yolks, whole grains, nuts, seeds and sprouts. PABA is the most effective; wheat germ and molasses are good sources of it. The enzymes that activate hair color also need zinc and magnesium. These minerals used to be abundant in whole grains, but today, due to monoculture and the intensive use of pesticides, grains can be deficient in them. For this reason, it is better to buy organic grains.

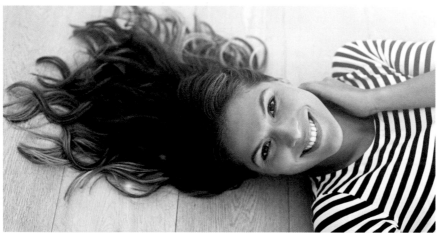

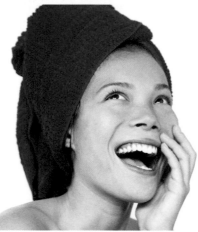

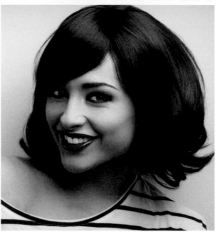

Fennel and Elder Hair Wash

This shampoo cleanses the hair without stripping it of its natural oils. It's a gentle, natural alternative to harsh commercial shampoos.

Best for: Normal or dry hair

Tip: Neutral soap is pH balanced, so it is neither too acidic nor too alkaline. Many commercial soaps are highly alkaline, which can strip too much oil from the hair.

Note: Always measure accurately when you're making homemade beauty products. See page 53 for tips.

- Fine-mesh sieve
- Bottle with lid

1 cup	water (approx)	250 mL
½ oz	fennel bulb, coarsely chopped	15 g
½ oz	elderflowers or red clover	15 g
½ cup	neutral soap (see tip, at left), grated	125 mL

1. In a small saucepan, combine water, fennel and elderflowers. Bring to a boil; boil for 10 minutes.

2. Place fine-mesh sieve over a medium heatproof bowl; strain liquid into bowl, discarding solids.

3. Stir grated soap into liquid until melted and smooth. Add a little more water to thin if desired.

4. Pour into bottle. Let cool completely. Keep in the shower.

Shampoos: Tips for Natural Hair Care

Whatever your hair type, shampoo is important for cleansing the hair and preparing it for conditioning or other treatments. To shampoo, wet hair thoroughly under warm, not hot, running water. Then, place a dollop of shampoo in your palm and, using circular motions, gently massage it into the wet hair. This stimulates circulation in the scalp and ensures that the hair gets completely clean. Don't worry if the shampoo doesn't produce a lot of foam; some of the best and purest shampoos lather very little. Once you're done, rinse hair thoroughly under warm running water, making sure all the shampoo is removed. Finish with a cold-water rinse.

Red Hair Brightening Shampoo

Red hair looks incredible when it reflects light well. This shampoo banishes dullness and brings out the best in this shade.

___

Best for: Normal hair

Tip: You can give this shampoo any scent you like with essential oils. Try lavender, cinnamon, ylang-ylang, orange or another favorite.

___

Note: Always measure accurately when you're making homemade beauty products. See page 53 for tips.

- Fine-mesh sieve
- Large bottle with lid

1 oz	assorted herbs and spices, such as dried calendula flowers, witch hazel bark, henna powder, cloves, red tulip flowers and hibiscus flowers	30 g
2 cups	distilled water (see tips, page 201)	500 mL
1 oz	neutral soap (see tip, page 195), grated	30 g
2	drops essential oil of your choice (see tip, at left)	2

1. Place herbs and spices in a medium saucepan; add distilled water. Bring just to a simmer over medium heat; reduce heat and simmer for 5 to 10 minutes.

2. Remove from heat. Cover and let stand for 10 minutes.

3. Place soap in a medium heatproof bowl. Set aside.

4. Place fine-mesh sieve over another medium heatproof bowl; strain liquid from herbs and spices mixture into bowl, discarding solids. Stir into soap until melted and smooth.

5. Stir in essential oil. Pour into bottle. Let cool completely. Keep in the shower.

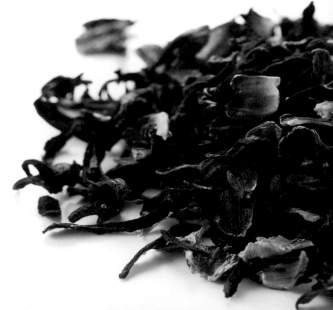

Egg Yolk Cleansing Treatment

This treatment may seem strange at first, but it cleans hair well and no other shampoo is needed after application.

Best for: Normal or dry hair

Tips: If you have long hair, increase the egg yolks to two so you have enough to reach the end of every strand.

This treatment contains raw egg and not enough natural preservatives to make the mixture shelf stable. Discard any leftovers.

The water for this treatment should be hot but not scalding. Once the mixture is complete, rub a bit of it on your inner wrist to make sure the temperature is comfortable before applying it to your scalp.

1	egg yolk (see tips, at left)	1
1 cup	hot water (see tips, at left)	250 mL

1. In a small heatproof bowl, whisk egg yolk with hot water until well combined.
2. Gently massage egg yolk mixture into damp hair. Wrap head in a towel and let stand for 2 to 4 minutes.
3. Rinse off mixture with warm water.

Lemon Rose Hair Lotion

The acid in lemons is a wonderful oil fighter, and rose water is a gentle astringent. This combination is a powerful tool for removing excess oil and toning the scalp.

Best for: Oily hair

Tip: Rose water is commonly used in Middle Eastern, Mediterranean, Indian and North African cuisine, so look for bottles of this fragrant essence at specialty grocery stores.

- Glass jar with lid

1	lemon	1
1 cup	rose water (see tip, at left)	250 mL

1. Juice lemon; discard peel or save for another use.
2. In a small bowl, stir lemon juice with rose water until well combined.
3. Pour into jar.
4. Massage a small amount of lotion into damp, clean hair. Store jar in a cool, dark place for up to 1 month.

Sage Protein Shampoo

Sage has a fantastic herbal scent and is often added to shampoos for its medicinal benefits.

Best for: Normal or dry hair

Tips: Look for a reliable source of dried medicinal herbs, such as an herbalist's shop or a reputable online dealer. Make sure it's a business with high turnover, to ensure you're getting the freshest, most effective herbs possible.

Neutral soap is pH balanced, so it is neither too acidic nor too alkaline. Many commercial soaps are highly alkaline, which can strip too much oil from the hair.

Note: Always measure accurately when you're making homemade beauty products. See page 53 for tips.

- Large fine-mesh sieve
- Large bottle with lid

1 oz	fresh or dried sage leaves (see tips, at left)	30 g
4 cups	boiling water	1 L
1 cup	neutral soap (see tips, at left), grated	250 mL
2	eggs	2

1. Place sage in a large heatproof bowl; pour boiling water over top. Cover and let steep for 5 minutes.

2. Place fine-mesh sieve over a large saucepan; strain infusion into saucepan, discarding solids.

3. Stir in soap and warm over low heat, stirring until soap is melted and smooth. Let cool completely.

4. Whisk eggs into soap mixture until well combined. Pour into bottle. Seal tightly and let stand for 24 hours.

5. Shake well before using. Keep in the shower.

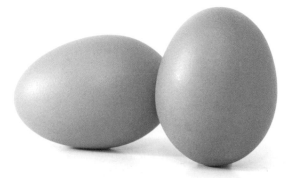

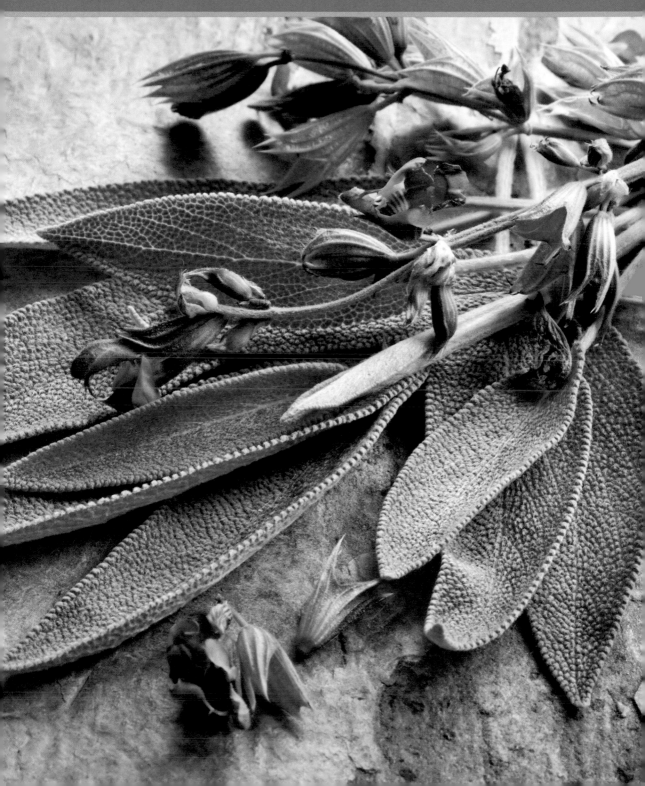

Rosemary Egg Shampoo

Rosemary is a terrific oil-fighting herb to use in shampoos and rinses. It cleanses and balances hair so it looks shiny and healthy.

Best for: Oily hair

Tips: When you use a ready-made neutral shampoo or soap as the base for a cleanser, look for one that is unscented so the aromas of the herbs or other natural ingredients in the formula can be front and center.

This shampoo contains raw egg and not enough natural preservatives to make the mixture shelf stable (that's why this makes just one batch). Discard any leftovers and make a fresh batch each time.

Buy essential oils sold in dark bottles. Exposure to light can reduce the potency of their medicinal herbal components. Store the bottles in a cool, dark place to keep them fresh.

1 tbsp	neutral shampoo (see tips, at left)	15 mL
1	egg yolk (see tips, at left)	1
3	drops rosemary essential oil (see tips, at left)	3

1. In a small bowl, stir together shampoo, egg yolk and rosemary essential oil until combined. Using a wooden spoon, beat until mixture forms a creamy paste.

2. Gently massage egg yolk mixture into hair, discarding any leftovers. Rinse with warm water to remove mixture. Rinse with cold water.

Fixing Oily Hair

Hair can be oily for a variety of reasons. Some people have a scalp that naturally produces more oil, while others might have an infection that revs up oil-producing glands. Oily hair can also result from nutrition-related maladies, such as gout, obesity, diabetes or constipation, or the overconsumption of processed food. To relieve this problem, it is important to follow a healthy, balanced diet that nourishes and purifies the body. If your hair is very oily, don't overuse commercial shampoos designed for oily hair. They are strong and can cause damage. Use a commercial shampoo for normal hair instead.

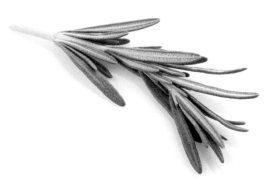

Softening Orange Vinegar Rinse

This is based on a traditional hair remedy your ancestors probably used. A vinegar rinse is a tried-and-true method for making locks shiny and manageable.

Best for: Normal hair

Tips: Distilled water has been purified through the process of distillation; in other words, the water is boiled, and the condensation (which is free of impurities) is collected in a clean vessel. Bottles of it are readily available in supermarkets.

Orange essential oil is just one of the essential oils made from the orange tree; it is extracted from the zest of the fruit. Neroli essential oil is made from the flowers, and petitgrain essential oil is made from the leaves and twigs of the plant.

Note: Always measure accurately when you're making homemade beauty products. See page 53 for tips.

- Large bottle with lid

2 cups	distilled water (see tips, at left)	500 mL
1 tbsp	cider vinegar	15 mL
5	drops orange essential oil (see tips, at left)	5
	Warm water	

1. In a medium bowl, stir together distilled water, vinegar and orange essential oil until well combined.

2. Pour vinegar mixture into bottle.

3. In a large bowl, mix 1 tbsp (15 mL) vinegar mixture with 4 cups (1 L) warm water. Pour slowly over damp, clean hair. Rinse with cold water. Store bottle in a cool, dark place for up to 2 months.

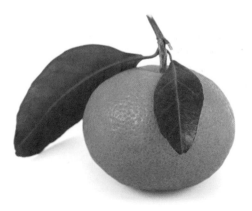

Cinnamon Rum Hair Tonic

Rum is an old-fashioned base for tonics and colognes, and here, it takes on the warm smell of cinnamon to brighten dull locks and give them body.

Best for: Dull hair

Tip: Rum is the traditional liquid used to make bay rum, which is a spicy cologne or aftershave lotion scented with bay leaves. See page 330 for a homemade version.

Note: Always measure accurately when you're making homemade beauty products. See page 53 for tips.

| 3 tbsp | amber or dark rum (see tip, at left) | 45 mL |
| 1 | cinnamon stick | 1 |

1. Pour rum into a small glass; add cinnamon stick, breaking into smaller pieces if necessary to fit. Let stand overnight.

2. Massage mixture into damp, clean hair. Rinse with warm water.

Protecting Hair from the Sun

When summer arrives, so does beach-and-pool season. This is a great time to enjoy outdoor activities, but keep in mind that your hair will dry out and become damaged if you don't protect it. Prolonged sun exposure is harmful to your locks, as are sand, salt and chlorine. Even if you're not swimming, you might take an extra shower to beat the heat, and chlorinated water, found in most swimming pools and some taps, can harm your hair. Cover your hair with a hat if you're out in the sun, and pamper it with a little extra nourishment and care all summer long.

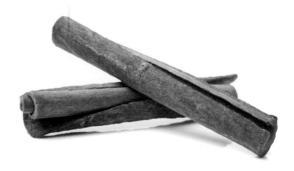

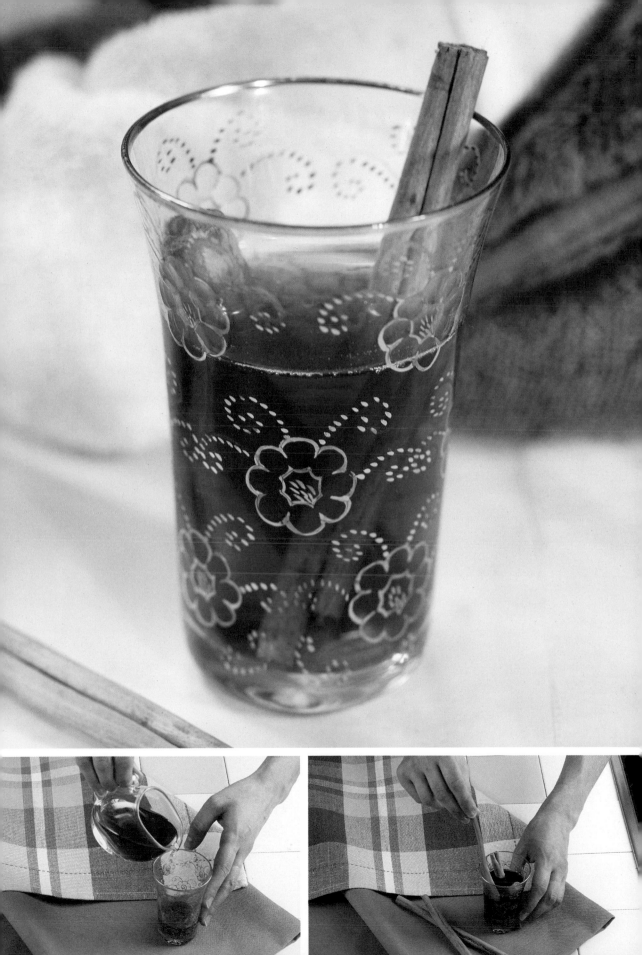

Revitalizing Tonic

Does your hair need a lift? This rosemary-scented tonic will give it a new lease on life.

Best for: Normal hair

Tip: Baker's ammonia is also known as ammonium carbonate. Look for it at supermarkets and gourmet stores.

Note: Always measure accurately when you're making homemade beauty products. See page 53 for tips.

- Large glass bottle with lid

2 cups	amber or dark rum (see tip, page 202)	500 mL
1 cup	ethyl alcohol (see tip, page 208)	250 mL
2 tbsp	castor oil (see tips, page 180)	30 mL
2 tbsp	rosemary essential oil	30 mL
1 tbsp	baker's ammonia (see tip, at left)	15 mL

1. In a large glass measuring cup or bowl, stir together rum, alcohol, castor oil, rosemary essential oil and baker's ammonia until well combined.

2. Pour into bottle. Seal tightly and let stand in a cool, dark place for 8 days.

3. To use, dilute a small amount of tonic with water. Massage into scalp and along the whole length of the hair 2 or 3 times a week after shampooing. Rinse with warm water.

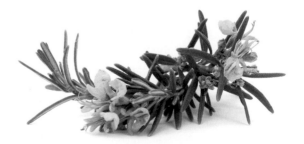

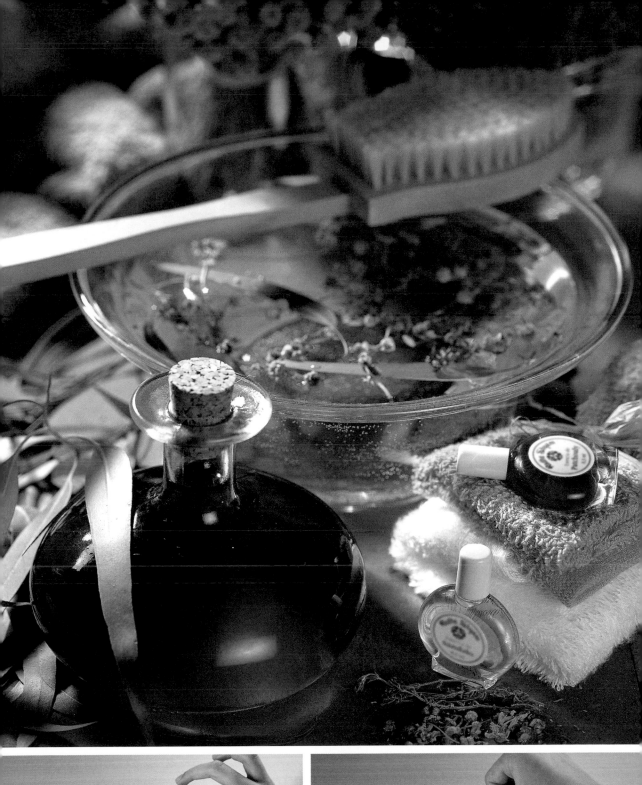
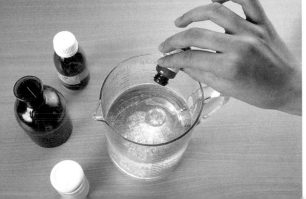
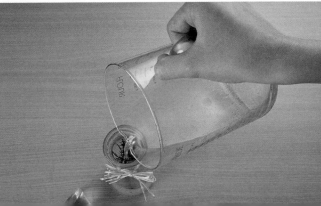

Blond Hair Tonic

Give your locks an even more intense golden hue with this natural color booster.

Best for: Blond hair

Tips: Dried chamomile is easy to find at stores that sell medicinal herbs. It's also a very undemanding plant to grow in your garden, so you can grow, harvest and dry your own organic flowers with a minimal amount of effort.

Note: Always measure accurately when you're making homemade beauty products. See page 53 for tips.

- Two 6-cup (1.5 L) canning jars with lids
- Large fine-mesh sieve

3½ oz	dried white rose petals	100 g
2 oz	dried chamomile flowers (see tips, at left)	60 g
¾ oz	dried marjoram leaves (see tips, page 198)	25 g
4 cups	cider vinegar	1 L

1. In jar, combine rose petals, chamomile flowers and marjoram leaves. Pour in vinegar; stir to combine. Seal jar tightly and let stand in a sunny or warm location for 2 weeks.

2. Place fine-mesh sieve over a large bowl; strain liquid into bowl, discarding solids. Repeat several times to remove all particles. Pour into clean jar.

3. Massage a small amount of tonic into damp, clean hair. Rinse with cold water.

Yogurt Conditioner

Yogurt is a natural at softening hair and making it ultra-glossy. It's also a nutritious food that boosts beauty from the inside.

Best for: Normal or dry hair

Tips: This treatment takes 10 minutes to do its work on your hair, so spend that time relaxing and focusing on deep breathing. This little time-out in a busy day can help reduce stress and build beauty at the same time.

This conditioner contains raw egg and not enough natural preservatives to make the mixture shelf stable (that's why this makes just one batch). Discard any leftovers and make a fresh batch each time.

6 tbsp	plain yogurt	90 mL
1	egg (see tips, at left)	1

1. In a small bowl, stir yogurt with egg until well combined.

2. Using fingers, gently massage yogurt mixture all through damp, clean hair and over scalp for 4 minutes.

3. Wrap head in a hot towel and let stand for 10 minutes.

4. Rinse off mixture with lukewarm water.

Conditioner: Tips for Best Results

Conditioner is great for adding nutrients to hair and making it softer, shinier and more manageable. Always apply conditioner to damp, clean hair. If you have dry hair, use your favorite treatment once a week. For normal hair, use it once every two weeks. For oily hair, use it no more than once a month.

Top Tips for Keeping Hair Healthy

- Make sure that your diet is rich in vitamins and minerals. Eat plenty of whole grains, wheat germ and brewer's yeast to keep hair growth vigorous.

- Brush hair daily with a natural bristle brush or comb to stimulate circulation in the scalp and encourage hair growth.

- Try a daily scalp massage, which also promotes circulation.

- If you wash your hair daily and your tap water is chlorinated, use a water softener or filter. Constant chlorine exposure can damage hair.

- To dry wet hair, pat and gently squeeze it with a towel; rubbing can damage hair and cause frizz. Skip blow-drying and let hair air-dry to minimize damage.

- Trim the ends once every two months. This will keep them tidy and prevent split ends.

- Substitute natural dyes, such as henna, for chemical dyes. These coloring agents are free of ammonia and other harsh substances.

- Reduce stress. It is one of the factors that can directly cause hair problems, such as premature graying or baldness.

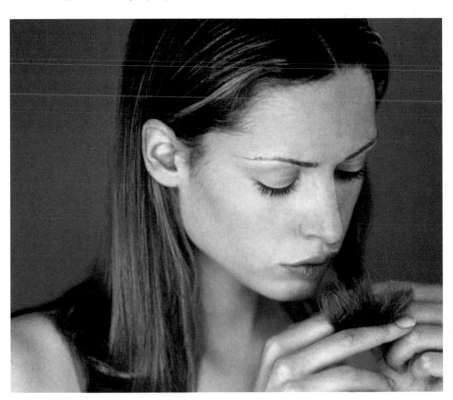

Birch Hair Lotion

Silver birch leaves *(Betula pendula)* are a common medicinal herb used to treat a wide variety of conditions. They strengthen hair and can stimulate growth.

Best for: Normal hair

Tip: Ethyl alcohol is the type of alcohol in spirits and other alcoholic beverages. It is not the same as isopropyl alcohol, the type you find at the drugstore for disinfecting wounds. You can get high-proof grain alcohol from the liquor store (look for the brand name Everclear). In a pinch, substitute unflavored vodka or brandy.

Note: Always measure accurately when you're making homemade beauty products. See page 53 for tips.

- Fine-mesh sieve
- Glass bottle with lid

¼ cup	water	60 mL
4 tsp	dried silver birch leaves (see tips, page 198)	20 mL
3 tbsp	ethyl alcohol (see tip, at left)	45 mL

1. In a small saucepan, combine water and birch leaves. Bring to a boil; boil for 5 to 10 minutes or until liquid is reduced to 3 tbsp (45 mL).

2. Place fine-mesh sieve over a small heatproof bowl; strain liquid into bowl, discarding solids.

3. Stir alcohol into liquid until well combined.

4. Pour into bottle.

5. Massage a small amount of lotion into clean, wet hair. Do not rinse. Store bottle in a cool, dark place for up to 2 months.

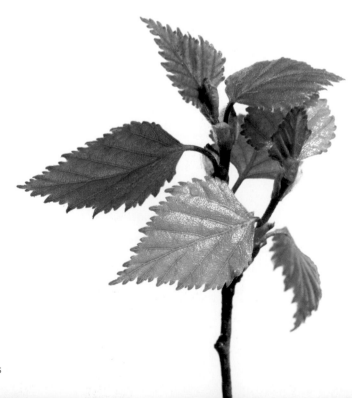

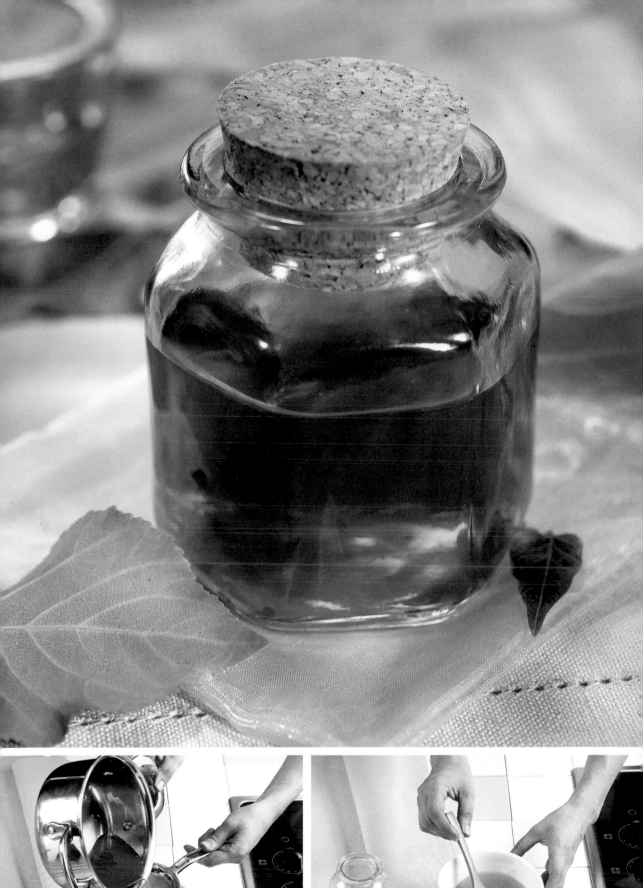

Almond Hair Pack

Sweet almond oil is moisturizing and gentle on skin and hair. Sage essential oil gives this luxe treatment a fresh herbal scent that's invigorating.

Best for: Normal or dry hair

Tip: Sweet almond oil, like other nut oils, can perish quickly if stored in a warm place or exposed to direct sunlight. Keep the bottle in a dark, cool cupboard and use it up within a couple of months of opening.

Note: Always measure accurately when you're making homemade beauty products. See page 53 for tips.

2 tbsp	cognac	30 mL
1	egg yolk (see tips, page 216)	1
1 tsp	sweet almond oil (see tip, at left)	5 mL
5	drops sage essential oil (see tips, page 200)	5

1. In a small bowl, stir cognac with egg yolk until well combined.
2. Stir sweet almond oil and sage essential oil into cognac mixture; stir for 1 minute or until smooth and well combined.
3. Gently massage egg mixture into damp, clean hair. Let stand for 15 minutes.
4. Rinse off egg mixture with lukewarm water.

Protein Hair Pack

Protein is an important component of hair, and it helps to both consume it in food and apply it externally. This treatment softens hair and makes it silky.

Best for: All hair types

Tips: Jojoba oil is a wonderful addition to hair treatments because it is moisturizing and a good scalp cleanser. Choose cold-pressed 100% jojoba oil, which contains the most bioactive substances.

Glycerin is an effective moisturizer that is often added to beauty products. Look for bottles of it at cosmetic-supply stores or online.

2	eggs (see tips, page 216)	2
1 tbsp	jojoba oil (see tips, at left)	15 mL
1 tbsp	liquid glycerin (see tips, at left)	15 mL
1 tsp	cider vinegar	5 mL

1. In a small bowl, whisk together eggs, jojoba oil, glycerin and vinegar until smooth and well combined.
2. Gently massage egg mixture into damp, clean hair. Let stand for 15 minutes.
3. Rinse off egg mixture with lukewarm water.

Hair Coloring

The custom of dyeing hair dates back to the Ancient Egyptians, who used plant extracts and metal compounds to color their locks. Men dyed their beards, and both sexes dyed their hair, using henna to create a red tint and lead salts to make a black one.

The custom did not catch on in Europe until the late 16th and early 17th centuries, when Marguerite de Valois, the queen of France, is said to have changed the color of her hair repeatedly and made dyeing hair popular. During the same era in England, the contemporaries of Queen Elizabeth I imitated the reddish color of her hair by treating their locks with potassium alum and a decoction of rhubarb. In Renaissance-era Italy, people began lightening their hair by soaking it in ash and exposing it to the sun for hours to obtain the famously desirable Venetian strawberry blond.

During the 18th century, upper-class men and women eschewed dyeing for powdering. They whitened their hair by dusting it with starch. Dyeing remained out of fashion and was frowned upon by European and North American people, who favored a traditional, conservative look until the early 20th century. Today, dyeing or bleaching one's hair is entirely acceptable and, in fact, more the rule than the exception.

Chemical Colors Are Harsh

Cosmetics companies offer a variety of permanent and semipermanent hair dyes and temporary color rinses. The chemical compositions of their formulas are based on ammonia and lead salts, which modify the structure of the hair shaft as they deposit pigment.

The chemicals in these commercial colorings leave the hair porous and brittle, and can irritate sensitive scalps. Repeated, prolonged use of chemical dyes is harmful to the skin, increasing the sensitivity of the hair follicles within it. Dyes also make the hair fragile and prone to forming split ends or falling out.

Natural Hair Dyes Are Gentle

Natural dyes prepared at home, on the other hand, do not contain these chemicals and do allow a change in hair color without causing damage. Pigments obtained from natural vegetable or mineral substances, such as henna, walnut, chamomile and radish, revitalize the hair, eliminate oil and give locks a special glow.

For centuries, herbs have been used to color hair, the most common being sage for dark or gray hair and chamomile for light hair. A wide variety of plants and herbs dye and strengthen tresses at the same time. Henna, made from the leaves of the plant *Lawsonia inermis*, is probably the best-known natural dye and has been used for centuries. It is native to Asia, and its use and cultivation has spread across North Africa, where it has become a major crop in Morocco. Henna can be used as the base for healthy all-vegetable hair dyes that give the hair brilliant color.

Brunette Hair Lightener

Chemical bleaches lighten the hair harshly. This gentle chamomile infusion brings out lighter tones that are subtle and natural.

Best for: Dark hair

Tip: Dried chamomile is easy to find at stores that sell medicinal herbs. It's also a very undemanding plant to grow in your garden, so you can grow, harvest and dry your own organic flowers with a minimal amount of effort.

Note: Always measure accurately when you're making homemade beauty products. See page 53 for tips.

• Fine-mesh sieve

¼ cup	dried chamomile flowers (see tip, at left)	60 mL
2 cups	boiling water	500 mL

1. Place chamomile flowers in a medium heatproof bowl; pour boiling water over top. Cover and let stand for 10 minutes or until lukewarm.

2. Place fine-mesh sieve over another medium heatproof bowl; strain infusion into bowl, discarding solids. Let cool completely.

3. Rinse hair with infusion after shampooing.

Minimize Gray Hair

If you can't stop gray hair, at least you can play with the look and minimize it a bit. Infusions of wild grape vine leaves, mulberry, artichoke, oak root, bean pods, poppy flowers, or sage or bay leaves can add a bit of color to graying hair. Make a concentrated infusion by combining your preferred plant with water and boiling the liquid until it is reduced by half. Apply the infusion to damp, clean hair for several consecutive days to increase its effectiveness.

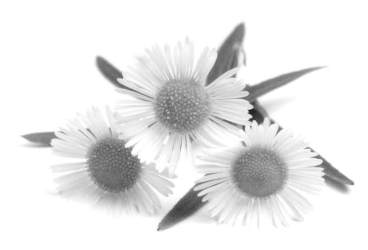

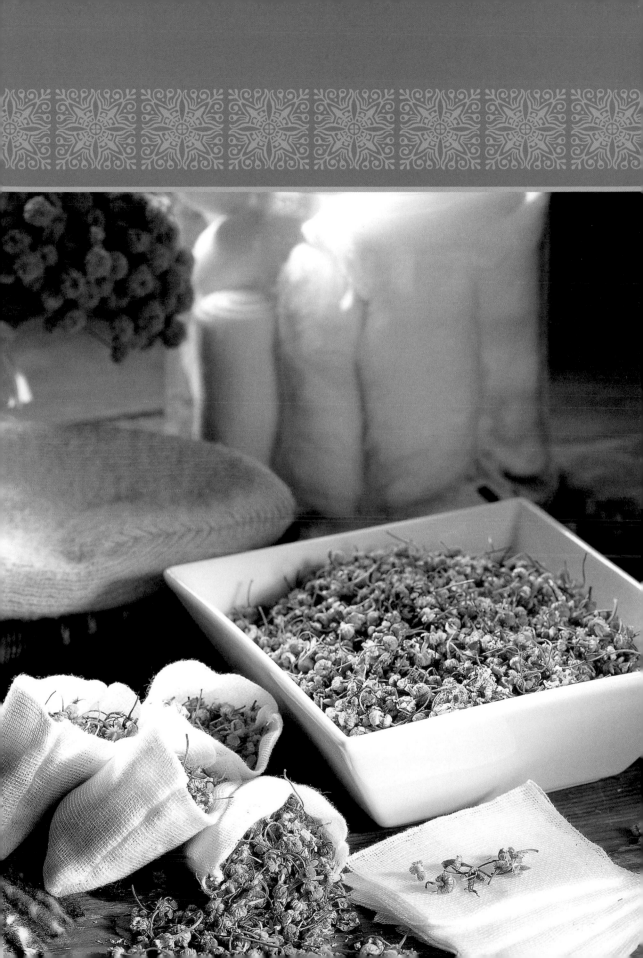

Mahogany Highlight Booster

Dark hair sometimes needs an injection of color too. This simple tea infusion will give it gloss and accentuate its beautiful brown tones.

Best for: Dark hair

Tip: Ceylon tea is a black tea, which means it's fully oxidized for a robust flavor. It's obviously delicious to drink too, and you need only one tea bag to make a strong cuppa.

| 2 or 3 | Ceylon black tea bags (see tip, at left) | 2 or 3 |
| 1 cup | boiling water | 250 mL |

1. Place tea bags in a small heatproof bowl; pour boiling water over top. Cover and let steep for 3 to 5 minutes. Remove tea bags and discard. Let liquid cool slightly.

2. Using a comb, distribute tea through unwashed hair. Let stand for 1 to 2 hours.

3. Shampoo hair as usual.

Blond Highlight Booster

Lemons make your hair look like you've just spent the summer at the beach. This treatment works best for hair that's already on the lighter side.

Best for: Light hair

Note: Always measure accurately when you're making homemade beauty products. See page 53 for tips.

| 2 | lemons | 2 |
| | Lukewarm water | |

1. Juice lemons; discard peel or save for another use.

2. Pour lemon juice into a glass measuring cup. Check measurement of juice in cup; add an equal amount of lukewarm water.

3. Using a comb, distribute lemon juice mixture through damp, clean hair. Let stand for 20 minutes.

4. Rinse out mixture with lukewarm water.

Natural Highlights

Beauty salons use bleaches and artificial dyes to give hair highlights. And while these lighter areas add dimension and depth to your mane, they can also damage your hair and irritate your scalp. Plus, these processes are expensive. Next time, try a much less expensive option: a natural highlight booster, like the ones on these pages. All you need are ingredients from your kitchen to give hair a little more vitality and color.

Red Highlight Booster

Beets are loaded with a natural pigment called betanin, which gives them their deep purplish-red hue. They are safe and effective for giving hair a subtle reddish glow.

Best for: Medium to dark hair

Tip: Beet juice stains the exterior of the hair shaft — and anything else it touches. When you use this treatment, make sure you're wearing an old shirt!

- Colander or sieve

2	beets (see tip, at left)	2
	Cold water	

1. In a medium saucepan, combine beets with enough cold water to cover them. Bring to a boil.
2. Reduce heat and simmer for about 45 minutes or until beets are tender. Set colander over a medium heatproof bowl; drain beets, reserving cooking liquid. (Save beets for eating; they are very nutritious.) Let cooking liquid cool just until warm.
3. Using a comb, distribute liquid through damp, clean hair. Let stand for 20 minutes.
4. Rinse out liquid with lukewarm water.

How to Apply Henna Powder

Henna makes hair shiny and beautiful, and gives it an attractive tone (often reddish, but there are a number of henna colors these days). Do not apply henna to hair that has been colored or permed within the last six months.

To prepare henna hair dye, mix henna powder with hot water to form a thick, sticky paste according to the package directions. Apply paste to damp, unwashed hair (very clean hair makes it harder for the color to penetrate). Use a comb to separate and coat the strands, spreading the henna paste all the way to the ends. Wrap the hair in an old towel soaked in hot water. Let it stand for at least 2 hours. The longer you let it stand, the more intense the color will be. Finish by washing hair as you normally do.

Dandruff-Fighting Avocado Softener

Even if you suffer from dandruff, your scalp still needs a balanced amount of healthy oils. This conditioning treatment delivers exactly what it needs and makes hair shiny and soft.

Best for: Dandruff

Tips: This softener contains raw egg and not enough natural preservatives to make the mixture shelf stable (that's why this makes just one batch). Discard any leftovers and make a fresh batch each time.

Avocado oil is becoming increasingly popular for cooking. Buy cold-pressed avocado oil that has not been extracted using solvents. It's the most natural, least processed choice.

Note: Always measure accurately when you're making homemade beauty products. See page 53 for tips.

1 tbsp	cognac	15 mL
1	egg yolk (see tips, at left)	1
2 tsp	avocado oil (see tips, at left)	10 mL
3	drops rosemary essential oil (see tips, page 200)	3

1. In a small bowl, whisk cognac with egg yolk until well combined.

2. Add avocado oil to cognac mixture; whisk for 1 minute or until smooth and well combined. Whisk in rosemary essential oil.

3. Gently massage egg mixture into damp, clean hair for 1 minute. Let stand for 15 minutes.

4. Rinse off mixture with very warm water.

Dandruff, a Common Complaint

The skin on your scalp is constantly being renewed. Fresh cells push old, dead cells up to the surface, where they form minute, impossible-to-see flakes that slough off. When these tiny bits clump together, they form the large visible flakes we call dandruff.

Dandruff appears on the scalp and behind the ears as small white scales. The latest research associates it with significant hormonal imbalance caused by chemical reactions occurring in the body. Doctors also attribute dandruff to stress, poor diet and improper use of hair products. This condition is generally accompanied by an itchy scalp, but it is not advisable to scratch — this can makes the itch even worse. To banish dandruff, the scalp should be cleaned with special shampoo formulated to fight this condition, like the one on page 218.

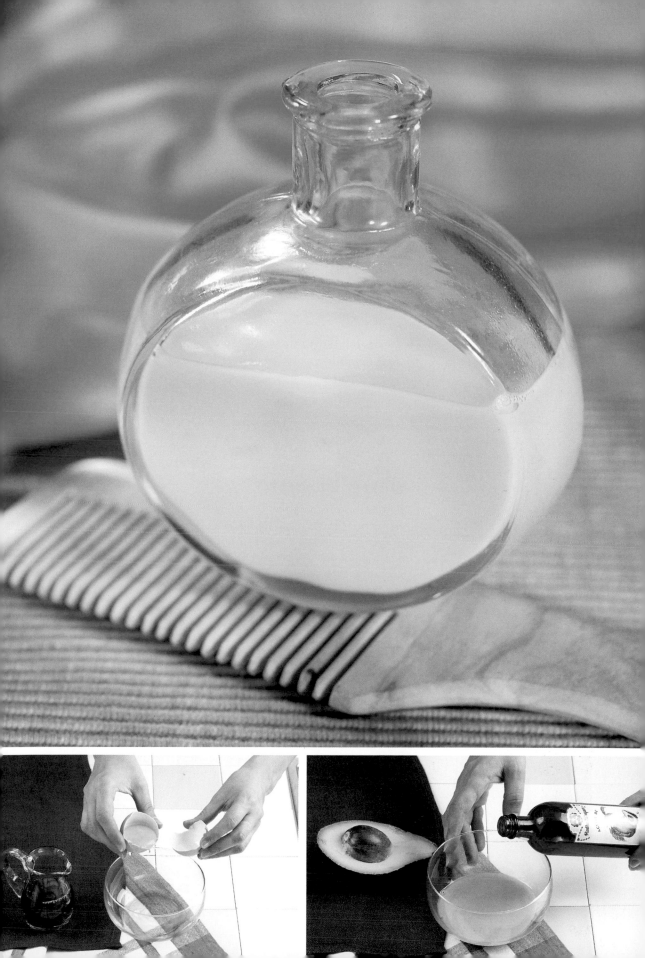

Egg Yolk Dandruff Shampoo

Thyme is a common herb for cooking, but it also has many medicinal uses. Chiefly, it is a potent antibacterial agent.

Best for: Dandruff

Tip: When you use a ready-made neutral shampoo as the base for a cleanser, look for one that is unscented so the aromas of the herbs or other natural ingredients in the formula can be front and center.

Note: Always measure accurately when you're making homemade beauty products. See page 53 for tips.

- Small bottle with lid

1 tbsp	cognac	15 mL
1	egg yolk	1
6 tbsp	neutral shampoo (see tip, at left)	90 mL
3	drops thyme essential oil (see tips, page 200)	3

1. In a small bowl, whisk cognac with egg yolk until well combined.
2. Whisk shampoo and thyme essential oil into egg yolk mixture until creamy.
3. Pour into bottle. Keep in the shower.

What Is Dandruff?

Dandruff is produced by an abnormal increase in secretions from the sebaceous glands, and is often caused by a disturbed or weakened immune system. When the defensive phospholipid barrier in the scalp cells fails, free radicals penetrate and destroy these cells from the inside, causing a protein substance to be shed. This material clumps together, forming dandruff particles.

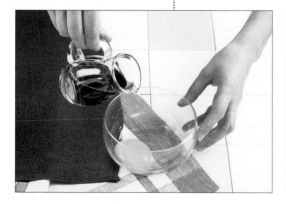
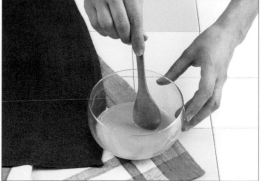

Clay Hair Pack for Dandruff

Clay removes excess oil, which often accompanies dandruff. This pack is an effective cleanser and stimulant for the scalp as well.

Best for: Dandruff

Tip: There are many different types of clay available for making homemade beauty products. Kaolin, a pure white type of clay, is one of the most common and easy to use. French green clay is also popular for its oil-absorbing powers.

3½ oz	clay (see tip, at left)	100 g
4 cups	water	1 L

1. In a large bowl, stir clay with water to form a smooth paste.
2. Using hands and small circular motions, massage clay mixture into scalp after shampooing. Let stand for 15 minutes.
3. Rinse off mixture with lukewarm water. If desired, finish by using Rosemary Anti-Dandruff Rinse (page 220) for the final rinse.

Vinegar Herb Dandruff-Fighting Rinse

Rosemary and mint are a fragrant team, and they are excellent at whisking away oil and dandruff while making hair smell clean and fresh.

Best for: Dandruff

Tip: In recipes, the generic term *mint* is typically used to mean spearmint rather than peppermint or other members of that herb family. Spearmint is wonderful not only in cooking but also in homemade beauty treatments. It can run wild in the garden, so plant a pot of it instead — that way, you'll always have fresh leaves ready to go into whatever you're making.

- Two 6-cup (1.5 L) canning jars with lids
- Large fine-mesh sieve

2 tbsp	fresh rosemary leaves	30 mL
2 tbsp	fresh mint leaves (see tip, at left)	30 mL
4 cups	cider vinegar	1 L

1. In jar, combine rosemary and mint. Pour in vinegar; stir to combine. Seal jar tightly and let stand in a cool, dark place for 2 weeks.
2. Place fine-mesh sieve over a large bowl; strain liquid into bowl, discarding solids. Pour into clean jar. Seal tightly.
3. Dilute a small amount of tonic with an equal amount of water. Rinse hair with mixture after shampooing. Store jar in a cool, dark place for up to 2 months.

Rosemary Anti-Dandruff Rinse

A simple infusion of rosemary makes an effective tonic for dandruff-plagued hair. It's fragrant and gives tresses a clean pine-like scent.

Best for: Dandruff

Tip: Add a sprig of fresh rosemary to the bottle before pouring in the tonic. The fresh herb will release its scent as the mixture stands.

Note: Always measure accurately when you're making homemade beauty products. See page 53 for tips.

- Large fine-mesh sieve
- Large dark glass bottle with lid

4 cups	water	1 L
3 tbsp	fresh rosemary leaves	45 mL

1. In a large saucepan, combine water and rosemary. Bring to a boil. Reduce heat and simmer for 20 minutes.

2. Place fine-mesh sieve over a glass measuring cup; strain infusion into cup, discarding solids. Pour into bottle.

3. Rinse hair with infusion after shampooing. Store bottle in a cool, dark place for up to 2 months.

Fight Dandruff from the Inside Too

The hair follicle, the root of the hair and the scalp are generally very sensitive to antioxidant protection. When the blood level of antioxidants is too low to ensure protection, thousands of hair follicles become clogged. They atrophy and are replaced by sebaceous glands. Vitamins A, C and E and the trace element selenium strengthen the hair's defense mechanisms, provide immune system protection and stimulate hair regeneration. It's important to remember that the body, shine, color and vigor of the hair start with good nutrition and healthy circulation.

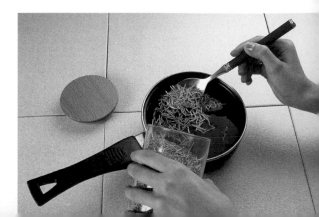

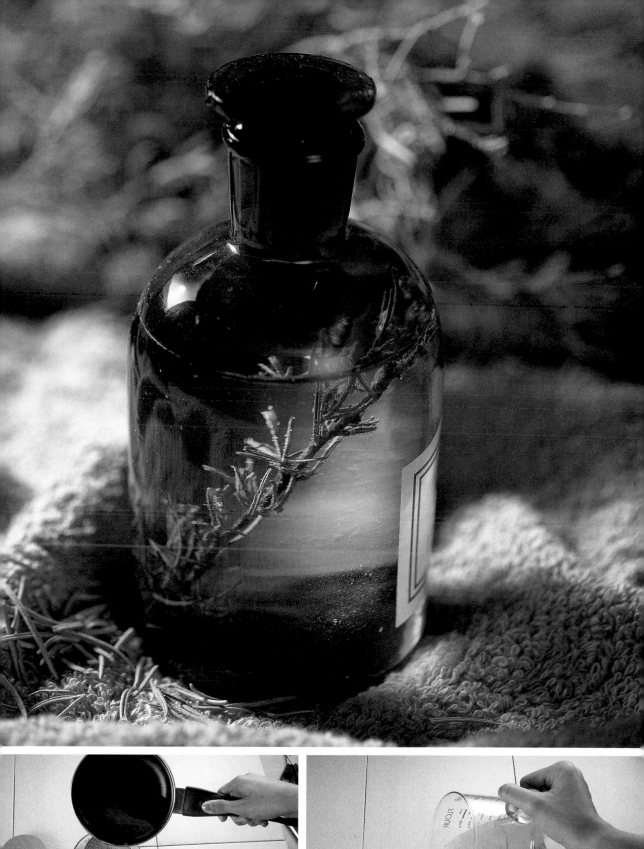
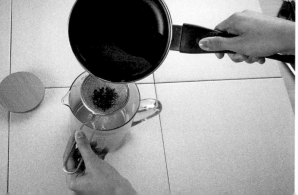
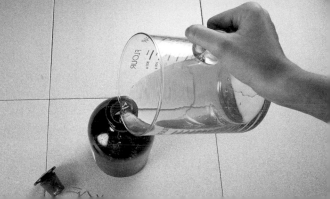

Hair Loss

The average human loses 40 to 100 hairs every day, which normally are replaced by new hairs. However, certain stages of life, such as childbirth or old age, and some diseases can increase hair loss.

Alopecia, or hair loss, traditionally has been associated only with men. Today, its effects are seen and recognized in women as well. Surprisingly, an estimated 50% of women suffer from excessive hair loss at some point in their lives. This can be ascribed to genetic factors as well as the pace of life nowadays; anxiety, overwork, stress and diet have definite influences on weakening and loss of hair.

Alopecia is associated with fibrosis of the hair root. This is a process that begins with the formation of a layer of hard, dense collagen that gradually invades the root and eventually suffocates it completely. The hair is forced out and shed prematurely. The result is a change in the hair life cycle and progressive thinning of the hair that ends in baldness.

Strategies for Treating Thinning Hair

As with most hair and skin conditions, diet is a crucial piece of the treatment puzzle. To minimize hair loss, it is important to eat the right foods. B vitamins are particularly important, so include brewer's yeast, whole wheat bread, wheat germ and whole grains in your daily menu.

When hair starts to fall out, the normal reaction is to avoid touching the scalp out of fear that it could make the problem worse. However, a daily scalp massage can improve circulation and stimulate hair growth — it's one of the best things you can do. You can also supplement the massage with Nettle Tonic (opposite), which stimulates the scalp (it's also great for treating dandruff). If you have long hair, change the location of your part frequently to avoid putting tension on the same portions of the hair roots. Continuous pressure causes the follicles to stop producing new hair.

Nutrients for Fine, Brittle Hair

You may not have alopecia, but hair can look thin if it is fine and brittle and therefore prone to breakage. To boost hair strength, take care to eat a diet rich in vitamins and minerals. Externally, a raw egg applied to the hair and scalp is a great way to help locks grow and make them shine. Eggs contain cholesterol, abundant phosphorus and considerable amounts of vitamins, which all help hair grow strong.

Boost Circulation

Another helpful strategy for thinning hair is to increase blood flow to the head. You can stimulate circulation by aiming pulses of cold water at the back of your neck while showering. A thorough daily brushing of the hair does this as well. A simple vinegar massage can also help: gently massage ¼ cup (60 mL) cider vinegar into the scalp after shampooing.

Nettle Tonic

Nettles are bothersome in the garden because they can sting your hands. But they are an important medicinal herb that is excellent at healing the scalp.

Best for: Thinning hair and dandruff

Tips: You can buy dried nettle leaves (*Urtica dioica*), cinchona bark (*Cinchona succirubra*) and witch hazel leaves (*Hamamelis virginiana*) at many online herb stores.

Some chemical-supply stores sell 90-proof denatured alcohol, but this is definitely not what you want — denaturing chemicals are added to it to make it undrinkable. To make this tonic safe for topical applications, use overproof vodka for the alcohol; it contains a larger percentage of alcohol than regular 80-proof vodka. It will preserve this tonic but is harmless to the skin.

- 4-cup (1 L) canning jar with lid
- Fine-mesh sieve
- Large dark glass bottle with lid

6 oz	dried nettle leaves (see tips, at left)	175 g
3 oz	dried cinchona bark	90 g
3 oz	dried witch hazel leaves	90 g
1 oz	dried sage leaves	30 g
2 cups	90-proof ethyl alcohol (see tips, at left)	500 mL
	Distilled water	

1. In jar, combine nettle leaves, cinchona bark, witch hazel leaves and sage leaves; pour in alcohol. Seal tightly and let stand in a cool, dark place for 2 weeks.

2. Place fine-mesh sieve over a large bowl; strain liquid into bowl, discarding solids. Repeat several times to remove all particles.

3. Pour liquid into bottle.

4. Mix a small amount of tonic with an equal amount of distilled water. Rub gently all over scalp after shampooing and gently towel-drying hair. Store bottle in a cool, dark place for up to 6 months.

Shine Cream Treatment

Brittle, breakable hair can look dull and lifeless. This thick emulsion will build it back up and make it glossier.

Best for: Fine, brittle hair

Tip: This cream contains raw egg and not enough natural preservatives to make the mixture shelf stable (that's why this makes just one batch). Discard any leftovers.

Note: Always measure accurately when you're making homemade beauty products. See page 53 for tips.

1	egg yolk (see tip, at left)	1
2 tbsp	sweet almond oil or olive oil	30 mL
1 tsp	lemon juice	5 mL

1. In a small bowl, whisk egg yolk. Slowly add sweet almond oil, whisking constantly until thickened and creamy. Whisk in lemon juice.

2. Massage egg yolk mixture into damp, clean hair and scalp. Let stand for 1 hour.

3. Rinse off mixture with warm water.

Holm Oak Bark Hair Lotion

Applying this lotion every night will stimulate hair growth and strengthen hair that's already growing.

Best for: Fine, brittle hair

Tips: Holm oak (*Quercus ilex*) is also known as evergreen oak, or *encina* in Spanish. The tree is a common sight in Spain and other Mediterranean countries. Some online retailers sell this bark (or a powder made from it), but it can be a little hard to find in North America.

This lotion contains raw egg and not enough natural preservatives to make the mixture shelf stable (that's why this makes just one batch). Discard any leftovers and make a fresh batch each time.

Note: Always measure accurately when you're making homemade beauty products. See page 53 for tips.

- Mortar and pestle
- Fine-mesh sieve
- Hand mixer

2 tbsp	holm oak bark (see tips, at left)	30 mL
2 cups	distilled water (see tips, page 201)	500 mL
1	egg yolk (see tips, at left)	1

1. In mortar and using pestle, crush holm oak bark into small pieces.

2. In a medium saucepan, combine holm oak bark and distilled water. Bring to a boil. Reduce heat and simmer for 15 minutes.

3. Place fine-mesh sieve over a medium heatproof bowl; strain liquid into bowl, discarding solids.

4. Add egg yolk to liquid. Using hand mixer, beat mixture until well combined. Let cool just until warm.

5. Gently massage egg mixture into damp, clean hair for 1 minute. Let stand for 15 minutes.

6. Rinse off egg mixture with warm water.

Caring for Thinning Hair

When washing thinning hair, it is best to use warm, not hot, water and to avoid strong or harsh shampoos. It's also smart to avoid blow-drying as much as possible. Stress can negatively affect hair growth as well, so it's vital to maintain emotional balance and to work toward building resilience in the face of everyday setbacks.

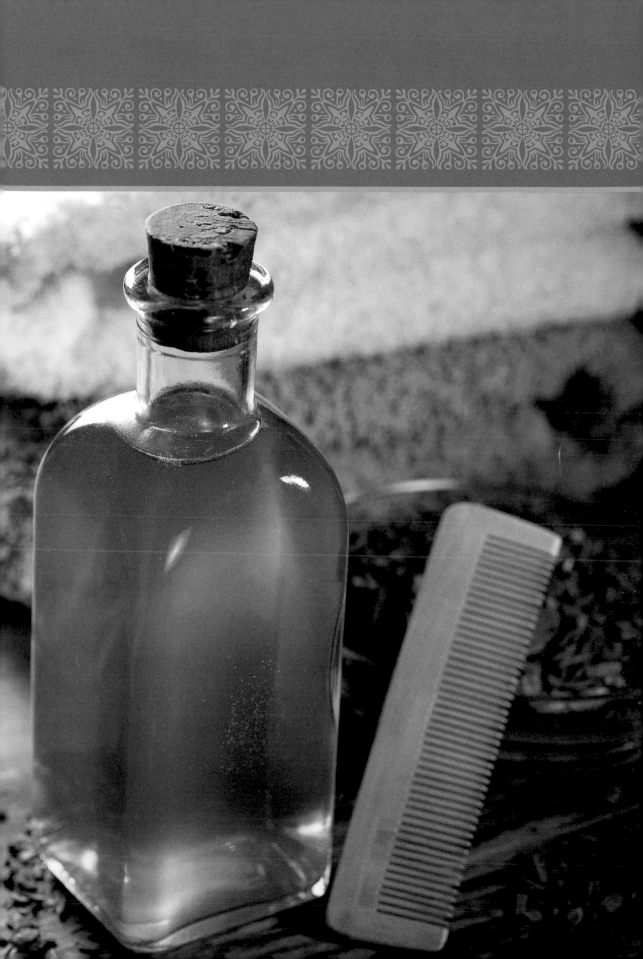

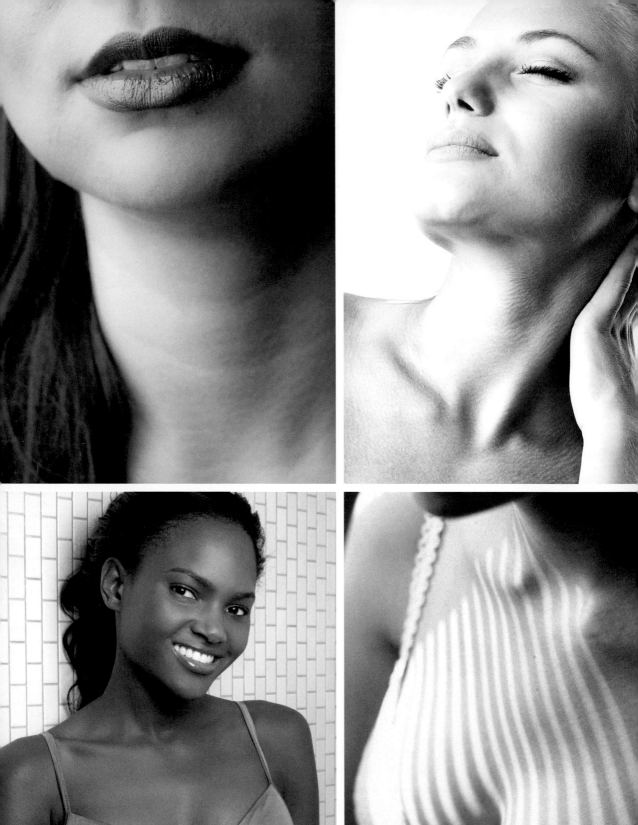
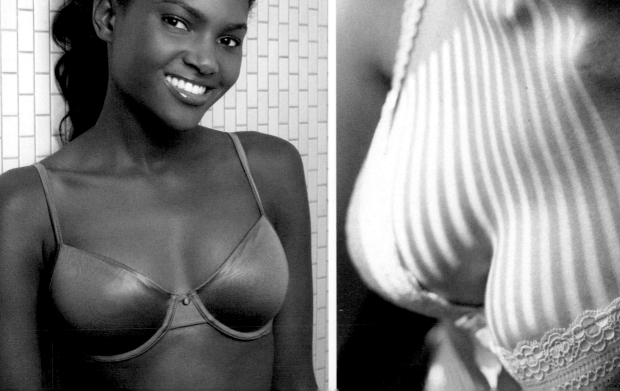

Body Products and Treatments

Weather, diet, stress and the passage of time all make their marks on your skin. And while keeping your face looking youthful may be your first concern, there's much more skin on your body that needs pampering too.

The first step in taking care of your body is learning to accept it as it is. Become best friends with every part of it, and treat each with the same care you dedicate to your hair and face. Each area of the body has unique challenges and needs, and taking a little bit of time every day to fulfill those will ensure you enjoy the health and vitality you deserve. In this chapter, you'll find tips, simple recipes for beauty products and treatments, exercises and advice that will help you look and feel wonderful from your neck to your feet.

Caring for Your Neck

The skin on your neck is delicate and shows signs of aging relatively early. It's an easy part of the body to neglect because the face is usually the focus of antiaging routines. Not giving your neck the same tender care can lead to wrinkling and sagging, which can detract from your otherwise youthful appearance. Pampering your neck with rich hydrating creams and treatments, such as the ones on pages 234 to 236, will keep it looking fresh and well cared for.

Caring for Your Breasts

The skin that covers the breasts, like the skin that covers the neck, is delicate — much more so than facial skin, believe it or not. Women as young as 25 may begin to notice changes in this area, due to both physiological and environmental factors. That means it's never too early to start taking care of your chest. This can start with simply applying the right creams and masks for your skin type (see pages 237 to 239) and staying in good shape. After age 35, when the skin on the breasts begins to get looser, this regimen can be supplemented by applying a special toning mask (see page 240).

Healthy, beautiful breasts are outward signs of good health. And it's not just about the skin that covers them either. To keep your breasts in great shape and looking their best, a number of factors play a role, including proper diet, exercise and the right support garments. For example, did you know that tight bras that impede blood circulation can cause breasts to sag? Maintaining a low-stress lifestyle, reducing your exposure to environmental toxins and eating plenty of vegetables and fruits can all play important roles in caring for this sensitive area. It is also a good idea to do targeted toning exercises (see page 241) and to participate in activities that strengthen the muscles around the breasts, such as swimming.

Q: Why do breasts become loose and saggy?

A: There are a number of reasons. Breasts often droop and become flabby and wrinkled after pregnancy and breastfeeding. Normal aging is another factor; it is a fact of life that your body will change and your skin will lose its youthful elasticity and tautness over time. Sometimes, indifference and neglect of the breast area can result in these changes too. Sagging skin may be the result of consuming a diet that is poor in vitamins and minerals. Rapid and profound weight loss can also cause the breasts to lose their natural firmness.

The good news: you can help slow down and lessen these changes. Women who have given birth and breastfed their children don't have to settle for this satisfying and fulfilling stage of life leaving indelible marks. Even if the underlying chest muscles have become slack and aren't doing their job to hold up breast tissue, you can strengthen them with the right exercise, such as swimming and dance (particularly modern dance and ballet). It's never too late to treat this important area right.

The Right Bra Is Important

Long before the modern bra was invented, women tried to support their busts using garments that were designed without taking women's health and hygiene into account. These devices — such as corsets, stays and complicated boned contraptions — often crushed or squeezed breasts into painful submission. Fortunately, clothing technology has come a long way, and there are properly designed bras in many styles that support the breasts without crushing or squeezing them, or impeding blood flow to the tissues.

Bra opponents think there are more disadvantages than advantages to wearing these garments. Some people think that the breasts can be kept firm and beautiful for years without using a bra. Unfortunately, this won't stop them from sagging eventually. Once a young woman's breasts have developed, the best advice is for her to wear an appropriate bra that does not squeeze the chest or weaken the underlying muscles.

The key is to know how to choose the right bras. Buy them at a reputable store where the salespeople are able to advise you on the proper size and design for the shape of your breasts and figure. Check that the bra does not leave marks or red areas on your skin, and that the straps aren't so thin that they dig mercilessly into your shoulders. If either of these happens, the bra is not the right choice for you.

Avoid the ever-popular push-up bra. Virtually every manufacturer offers some models in this style. This type of bra not only compresses the breasts but also lifts them and squeezes them together for purely aesthetic purposes. It may enhance your bust, but constant compression and blood flow restriction around the breasts can have long-term consequences. It's not worth mortgaging your health for the sake of your appearance.

Bras and Breast Cancer

A heated controversy over bra wearing erupted when anthropologists Sydney Ross Singer and Soma Grismaijer published the book *Dressed to Kill* (ISCD Press, 1995). In it, the pair state that women who wear bras for more than 12 hours a day are 21 times more likely to develop breast cancer than those who do not.

This claim has been widely refuted by scientists and health professionals, who have criticized the unscientific methodology the authors used to develop this hypothesis. There is no scientifically conducted epidemiological research to support the authors' claim, and the few studies that have looked at this issue have found no evidence to link bra wearing with the development of breast cancer. Moreover, these critics note, breast cancer often occurs in the upper part of the breast, in an area where bras do not exert any pressure. There is no evidence that conventional bras compress the tissue to the point of impeding lymphatic drainage, causing a buildup of carcinogenic compounds in the breasts. So don't throw out your bras!

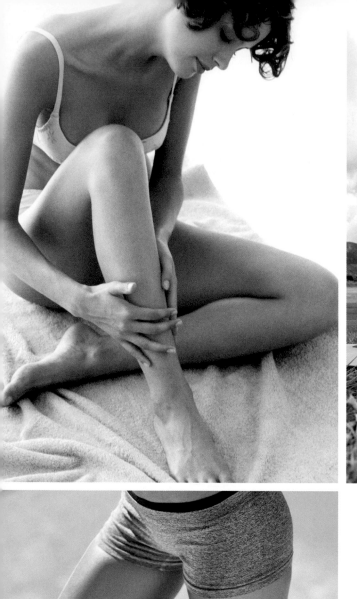
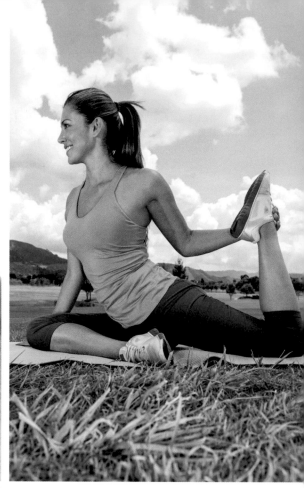
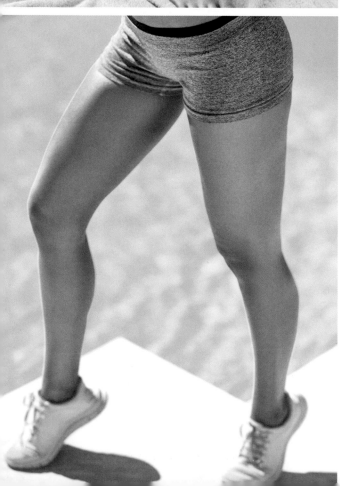
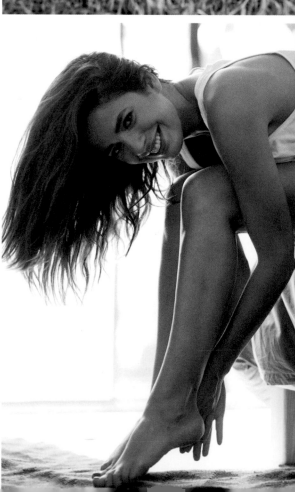

Caring for Your Legs

Do you give your legs the attention they deserve? It's easy to take them for granted. But if you stop and think, you'll realize that they are the pillars that support your body. They do a lot of work every day, carrying you from place to place, and supporting the rest of your frame. They are also a common place for problems to crop up. The smartest way to avoid these issues, such as stretch marks and varicose veins, is to tune in to these important structures and give them the care they need.

Leg Issue #1: Stretch Marks

Although stretch marks can appear on other parts of the body, such as the chest, abdomen or arm, they're arguably most common on the buttocks and inner thighs.

Stretch marks occur when elastic fibers in the dermis layer of the skin rupture. This causes characteristic streak-shaped scars to form. Stretch marks are generally associated with women, especially post-pregnancy or after a major weight gain or loss. However, they also occur in men and adolescents of both sexes. Male stretch marks are more common around the lower back, inner arms, thighs and knees.

The underlying cause of stretch marks is hormonal imbalance, especially related to overactive adrenal glands. This imbalance leads to the destruction of proteins, which in turn increases fluid retention, causing edema (swelling). All this greatly sensitizes the tissues and makes them weak. These imbalances also slow down the production of epidermal cells and fibroblasts in the dermis. Stress has a lot to do with stretch marks, because it causes connective tissues to atrophy.

One natural method for combating stretch marks is acupuncture, which is excellent for regulating metabolism and hormonal balance. A natural, nutrient-rich diet is also crucial for avoiding stretch marks. You can combat them in places where they have already appeared: simply stimulate the skin by gently pinching the affected area. Pinching helps release vasoactive substances in the skin, such as histamine. This treatment is also effective if you have sagging skin.

Leg Issue #2: Varicose Veins

These unsightly dilated veins crop up when pressure is exerted on blood vessels in which blood flow is obstructed. They are common on legs, and the reason is simple: when you stand, the blood in your legs must work against gravity to return to the heart. If this happens for prolonged periods, blood pools in the leg veins and presses on the vessel walls, expanding them. This explains why varicose veins are common in pregnant women, whose legs bear more weight than they are normally accustomed to, and in people who spend most of the day on their feet.

Some people have a genetic predisposition to varicose veins. Other common causes are nutritional imbalance, obesity and constipation. Eating calorie-laden or spicy foods, smoking and consuming excessive alcohol also increase your chances of developing varicose veins. To prevent them, it is important to drink an average of 8 cups (2 L) of water daily and eat foods that are rich in vitamin A (such as nuts and deep yellow or orange vegetables), vitamin C (such as citrus fruits) and vitamin E (such as salmon, carrots and squash).

There are a number of simple varicose vein prevention strategies you can try (see box, page 244). As well, a cup of Mistletoe Infusion for Varicose Veins (page 244) can help encourage healthy circulation in the legs, reducing your chances of developing or exacerbating this uncomfortable condition.

Caring for Your Feet

With healthy, manicured feet, you can take long walks without fatigue or discomfort. On the other hand, neglected feet will tire you out and can be a source of constant problems. Foot care is vital not only because healthy feet look attractive but also because the whole weight of your body rests and balances on those two structures. By keeping your feet in good shape, you will help align your posture and maintain a balanced, comfortable gait.

Help for Sore, Tired Feet

Exhausted, sore feet are normal after a taxing day at work, especially if you have to stand for most of the day. If this describes you, always wear the most comfortable shoes you can find, and make sure they are sized correctly for your feet. They should be breathable and suitable for your feet and your daily activities.

If you come home with tired feet, there are some easy-to-make natural remedies on pages 242 to 248, which you can use to soothe your feet and provide quick relief. Indulge in a relaxing soak, an exfoliating rub and some rich lotion to get your feet back into shape.

Unwanted Hair: A Perennial Problem

Hair was removed in ancient civilizations for a variety of reasons. Some cultures used waxing as part of beauty and body-care routines. Others were religiously motivated to remove excess hair and even considered human hairiness an affront to the divine; sometimes, hair removal was associated with certain rituals. In some places, social norms required hair removal because body hair was considered demeaning.

There have also been countless ways throughout history in which people have rid themselves of unwanted hair. In Turkey, the traditional depilatory was *rusma*, a pasty mixture of quicklime, arsenic sulfide (called orpiment) and starch. The Ancient Greeks and Romans used an array of resins and pastes made with honey or mud, which are the ancestors of modern wax. In the Middle Ages, many Europeans removed hair with their own harsh cream version of Turkish *rusma*, made of quicklime and arsenic sulfide. It was not until the late 19th century that the first hot waxes as we know them today began to appear.

Fortunately, depilatories, waxes and even shaving creams have come a long way from their ancient roots (see box, page 261). The easy home remedies on pages 258 and 260 can help soothe depilated skin, leaving it soft and silky, and slow down regrowth.

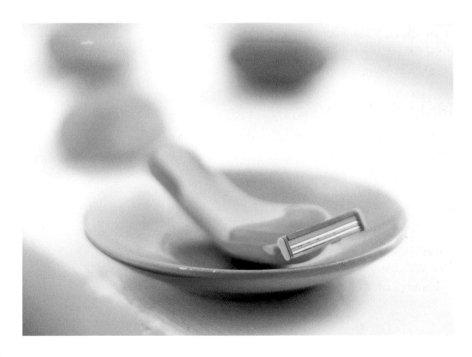

Cocoa Butter Neck Softener

A mix of oil and butters gives this treatment its skin-softening powers. It bathes the skin in nutrients to help it look youthful.

Best for: Delicate neck skin

Tips: Choose 100% natural cocoa butter for homemade creams like this. You can buy chunks of this creamy, yellowish substance made from cocoa beans at cosmetic-supply stores and online. It is also sold in uniform-size wafers. Either form will work fine in this recipe.

Shea butter is a rich emollient that's ideal in dry-skin treatments. Look for tubs or bags of it at cosmetic-supply stores or online.

Note: Always measure accurately when you're making homemade beauty products. See page 53 for tips.

- Jar with lid

½ cup	wheat germ oil (see tips, page 236)	125 mL
1 tbsp	cocoa butter (see tips, at left)	15 mL
1 tbsp	shea butter (see tips, at left)	15 mL
¼ cup	water	60 mL

1. In a small heatproof bowl (see box, page 82), combine wheat germ oil, cocoa butter and shea butter. Set aside.

2. Pour enough water into a small saucepan to come about 2 inches (5 cm) up the side; bring to a simmer.

3. Set bowl on saucepan so that bottom of bowl is not touching simmering water; stir until cocoa butter mixture is melted and smooth. Remove bowl from heat.

4. Immediately stir in water until well combined. Pour into jar. Let cool completely.

5. Smooth a small amount of softener all over neck. Store jar in a cool, dark place for up to 2 months. Shake before each use to recombine.

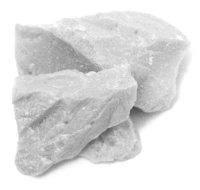

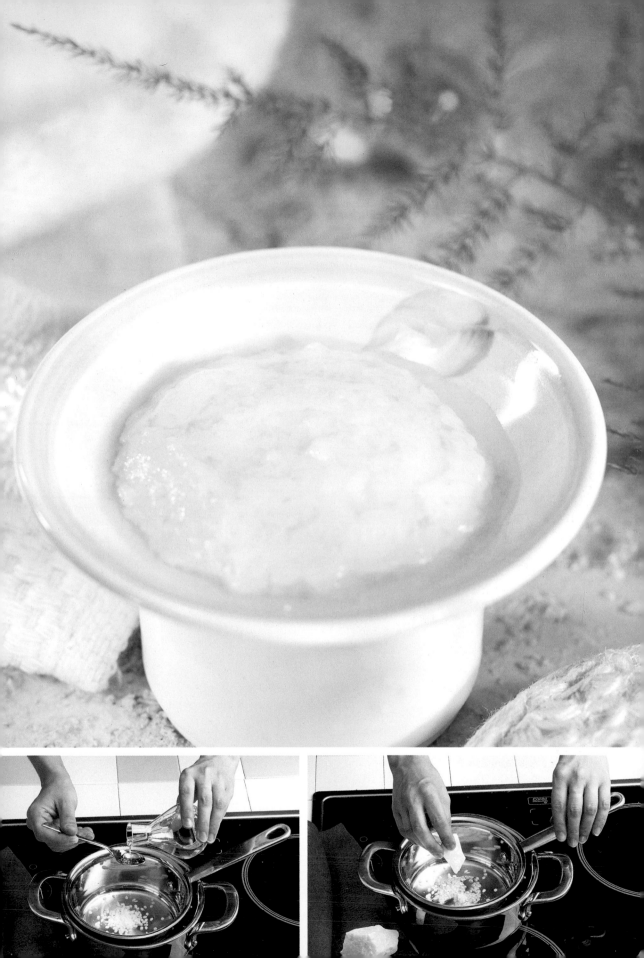

Wheat Germ Neck Mask

Hydrating dry neck skin is important to ensure it looks as dewy and fresh as facial skin. Wheat germ gives this mask a burst of skin-healing vitamin E.

Best for: Delicate neck skin

Tips: Wheat germ and wheat germ oil can go rancid quickly if stored at room temperature. Keep your wheat germ in a tightly sealed container in the freezer and store the oil in the fridge to extend their shelf life.

This mask contains raw egg and not enough natural preservatives to make the mixture shelf stable (that's why this makes just one batch). Discard any leftovers and make a fresh batch each time.

1 tbsp	wheat germ (see tips, at left)	15 mL
1 tbsp	wheat germ oil	15 mL
1	egg yolk (see tips, at left)	1
3	drops patchouli essential oil (see tips, page 248)	3

1. In a small bowl, stir together wheat germ, wheat germ oil, egg yolk and patchouli essential oil until well combined.

2. Using fingers but without rubbing, spread mask all over neck. Let stand on skin for 15 minutes.

3. Rinse off mask with warm water. Gently pat neck dry with a towel.

Milk and Honey Neck Cream

Drench parched neck skin in moisture with this simple but rich hydrating cream. The mint scent makes it an energizing indulgence.

Best for: Delicate neck skin

Tips: Peppermint is a natural antibacterial agent. It acts as an astringent as well, tightening and firming up skin.

The milk and egg white in this formula won't keep at room temperature, even with the honey and peppermint, which are natural preservatives. Keeping the cream in the fridge solves this problem and makes for a cool, refreshing treatment.

- 6-cup (1.5 L) canning jar with lid

1	egg white	1
2 cups	milk	500 mL
2 cups	liquid honey (see tips, opposite)	500 mL
6	drops peppermint essential oil (see tips, at left)	6

1. In a large bowl, whisk egg white until foamy. Whisk in milk, honey and peppermint essential oil until well combined and creamy.

2. Spoon cream into jar. Gently massage a small amount of cream all over neck. Store jar in the refrigerator for up to 2 weeks.

Moisturizing Breast Cream

Onion juice in skin cream? Yes! Onions contain antioxidants and nutrients that are great for making delicate breast skin supple and resilient.

Best for: Breast skin

Tips: Raw beeswax is yellow and has a light honey aroma. This recipe calls for white beeswax pearls, which have had the color and scent removed. They are easy to find at cosmetic-supply stores.

Liquid honey often crystallizes in the jar when it's stored in a warm place. There's nothing wrong with it in this state, and you can easily reliquefy it. Just pop the uncovered jar into a saucepan of warm water and heat it gently, stirring the honey until the crystals dissolve and it turns clear again.

Note: Always measure accurately when you're making homemade beauty products. See page 53 for tips.

- Box grater
- Fine-mesh sieve
- Small glass jar with lid

1	large onion	1
1½ tsp	white beeswax pearls (see tips, at left)	7 mL
2 tbsp	shea butter (see tips, page 234)	30 mL
2 tbsp	sunflower seed oil	30 mL
1 tbsp	liquid honey (see tips, at left)	15 mL
5	drops sandalwood essential oil (see tips, page 248)	5

1. Using small holes on box grater, grate onion into a small bowl. Set fine-mesh sieve over another small bowl. Spoon grated onion into sieve and press with back of spoon or rubber spatula to extract juice. Set onion juice aside, discarding solids or saving them for another use.

2. Place beeswax in a small heatproof bowl. Set aside.

3. Pour enough water into a small saucepan to come about 2 inches (5 cm) up the side; bring to a simmer.

4. Set bowl with beeswax on saucepan so that bottom of bowl is not touching simmering water; stir until beeswax is melted and smooth.

5. Stir shea butter, sunflower seed oil and honey into melted beeswax. Gradually stir in onion juice. Continue stirring until shea butter is melted and smooth. Remove bowl from heat.

6. Adding sandalwood essential oil a drop or two at a time, whisk until mixture is pasty and well combined.

7. Spoon into jar. Seal tightly and let cool. Refrigerate for 2 to 3 hours. Smooth a small amount of cream over breasts. Store jar in the refrigerator for up to 1 month.

Toning Breast Cream

This cream is ideal for breastfeeding mothers because it helps prevent stretch marks and soothes sore, cracked nipples.

Best for: Breast skin

Tips: Rose water is commonly used in Middle Eastern, Mediterranean, Indian and North African cuisine, so look for bottles of this fragrant essence at specialty grocery stores.

Sweet almond oil, like other nut oils, can perish quickly if stored in a warm place or exposed to direct sunlight. Keep the bottle in a dark, cool cupboard and use it up within a couple of months of opening.

Note: Always measure accurately when you're making homemade beauty products. See page 53 for tips.

- Glass jar with lid

1 cup	rose water (see tips, at left)	250 mL
6 oz	shea butter (see tips, page 234)	175 g
2 tbsp	sweet almond oil (see tips, at left)	30 mL
2 tbsp	white beeswax pearls (see tips, page 237)	30 mL
5	drops orange blossom essential oil	5

1. In a medium saucepan, warm rose water over low heat (do not boil). Keep warm.

2. In a medium heatproof bowl, combine shea butter, sweet almond oil and beeswax. Set aside.

3. Pour enough water into another medium saucepan to come about 2 inches (5 cm) up the side; bring to a simmer.

4. Set bowl on saucepan so that bottom of bowl is not touching simmering water; stir until shea butter mixture is melted and smooth. Remove bowl from heat.

5. Add rose water to shea butter mixture; whisk for 1 to 2 minutes or until lukewarm.

6. Whisk in orange blossom essential oil; continue whisking for 3 to 5 minutes or until completely cool.

7. Spoon into jar. Smooth a small amount of cream over breasts. Store jar in a dark, cool place for up to 2 months.

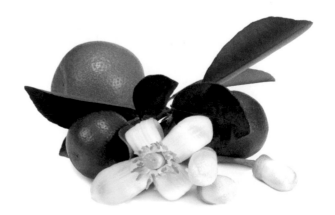

Dry Skin Mask for Breasts

Breast skin, like facial skin, can be dry, oily or a combination of both. This formula is great for skin that gets red, itchy or sensitive due to dryness.

Best for: Dry breast skin

Tips: A juicer is obviously great for making strawberry juice. If you don't have one, just purée strawberries in a blender and strain the juice through a fine-mesh sieve. Add the leftover, fiber-rich strawberry pulp to your morning smoothie or enjoy it over yogurt.

When you use this mask, make sure you have a comfortable place to lie down and relax for the 20 minutes the mixture must stand on the skin.

1 cup	strawberry juice (see tips, at left)	250 mL
2 tbsp	peanut oil or sunflower seed oil	30 mL
1 tbsp	shea butter (see tips, page 234)	15 mL

1. In a small saucepan, warm strawberry juice over low heat just until steaming (do not boil).

2. In a small heatproof bowl, combine peanut oil and shea butter. Slowly add strawberry juice, whisking constantly, until a thick paste forms. Let cool slightly.

3. Rub a bit of mask on inner wrist to make sure the temperature is comfortable before smoothing mask over breasts. Let stand on skin for 20 minutes.

4. Rinse off mask with warm water. Rinse again with cold water. Gently pat skin dry with a towel.

Oily Skin Mask for Breasts

Your face isn't the only place that can get oily and develop pimples. This simple mask helps clear up blemishes and remove excess oil on delicate breast skin.

Best for: Oily breast skin

Tips: There are many different types of clay available for making homemade masks. Kaolin, a pure white type of clay, is one of the most common and easy to use. French green clay is also popular for its oil-absorbing powers.

Freshly squeezed orange juice is best for this recipe. The amount is not specified because it depends how thick you like your mask. Just make sure you don't over-thin with juice; otherwise, the mask won't adhere properly to your skin.

3½ oz	clay (see tips, at left)	100 g
	Orange juice (see tips, at left)	

1. Place clay in a medium bowl. Add orange juice, a little at a time, stirring until a light paste forms.

2. Smooth mask over breasts. Let stand on skin for 15 to 20 minutes.

3. Rinse off mask with warm water. Rinse again with cold water. Gently pat skin dry with a towel.

Astringent Toner for Breasts

Cucumber juice is a natural astringent that tones and tightens skin, making it firm and youthful looking.

Best for: Sagging breast skin

Tip: Distilled water has been purified through the process of distillation; in other words, the water is boiled, and the condensation (which is free of impurities) is collected in a clean vessel. Bottles of it are readily available in supermarkets.

Note: Always measure accurately when you're making homemade beauty products. See page 53 for tips.

- Juicer or blender
- Fine-mesh sieve (optional)

| 2 | cucumbers, peeled and coarsely chopped | 2 |
| | Distilled water (see tip, at left) | |

1. In juicer, juice cucumbers, discarding solids. Pour cucumber juice into a glass measuring cup. (Or in blender, purée cucumber until smooth. Place fine-mesh sieve over a glass measuring cup; strain juice into cup, discarding solids.)

2. Check measurement of liquid in cup; add an equal amount of distilled water.

3. Gently massage toner all over breasts.

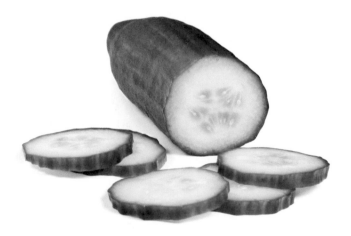

Breast-Toning Exercises

These easy moves help tone the muscles and ligaments that support your breasts. Add them to your regular exercise regimen. The cold-water rinse afterward is refreshing and toning as well.

1. **Setup.** Lie face down on the floor on a mat or blanket. Relax with your body stretched out, legs together and palms flat on the floor at chest level with fingers pointing forward.

2. **First movement.** Pushing up with your hands and arms, raise your upper body as high as possible.

3. **Second movement.** Without moving the rest of your body, bend your feet, tuck your toes under and raise the rest of your body off the floor into a low pushup position.

4. **Third movement.** Tilt your head up and back, making your spine concave and dropping your belly toward the floor.

5. **Reverse.** Repeat all the movements in reverse order, starting with the third and finishing in the setup position.

6. **Cool off.** After finishing these exercises (or at the end of your regular shower or bath), use a handheld sprayer to direct a stream of cold water at your body, moving it from your feet up to your head. If you find the cold water too shocking, start with warm water and gradually turn the temperature down as you go up the body.

Breast Muscle–Strengthening Exercises

Weight lifting is great, but this simple move is another terrific way to build up the muscles that support your chest and your breasts. Do it one or more times a day:

1. **Setup.** Stand up on your toes, with your legs together and your arms stretched downward along the sides of your body.

2. **Lean back.** Raise your arms and cross them in front of you. Bend your elbows and place your hands on your shoulders, near the base of your neck. Inhale deeply as you lean your head and shoulders back as far as you can go.

3. **Reverse.** Slowly exhale as you do the movements in reverse order, returning to the starting position.

Tired Leg and Foot Bath

An infusion of gentle herbs boosts circulation and relieves discomfort on days when you've spent too long standing up.

Best for: Tired, aching legs

Tips: Dried chamomile is easy to find at stores that sell medicinal herbs. It's also a very undemanding plant to grow in your garden, so you can grow, harvest and dry your own organic flowers with a minimal amount of effort.

Sadly, fresh orange leaves are impossible to find if you live in a cold climate. If you can't get them, simply omit them from this recipe. If you are lucky enough to have an orange tree in your backyard, look for glossy unblemished leaves and make sure they have not been sprayed with pesticides or herbicides.

Note: Always measure accurately when you're making homemade beauty products. See page 53 for tips.

- Large fine-mesh sieve

4 cups	water	1 L
3 tbsp	dried chamomile flowers (see tips, at left)	45 mL
3 tbsp	fresh rosemary leaves	45 mL
3 tbsp	fresh mint leaves	45 mL
3 tbsp	fresh orange leaves (see tips, at left)	45 mL
	Warm water	

1. In a large saucepan, combine water, chamomile flowers, rosemary leaves, mint leaves and orange leaves; bring just to a boil. Cover and let steep for 20 minutes.

2. Place fine-mesh sieve over another large heatproof bowl or basin. Strain infusion into bowl, discarding solids. Add more warm water to fill bowl to desired level.

3. Soak feet in infusion for 15 minutes. Gently pat feet dry with a towel.

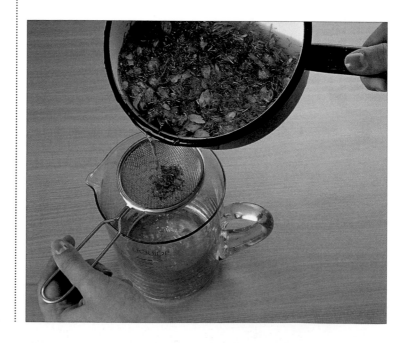

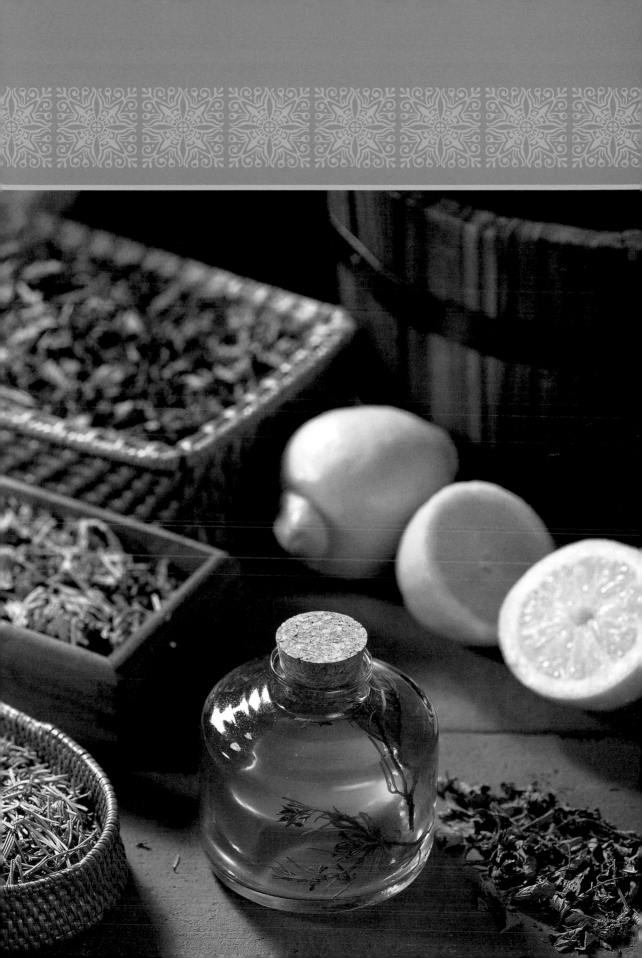

Mistletoe Infusion for Varicose Veins

This infusion works to restore impaired blood circulation, which helps reduce the appearance of varicose veins.

Best for: Varicose veins on the legs

Tips: A teapot with a built-in strainer is a great investment if you make a lot of infusions with loose herbs or teas.

Look for a reliable source of dried medicinal herbs, such as an herbalist's shop or a reputable online dealer. Make sure it's a business with high turnover to ensure you're getting the freshest, most effective herbs possible.

Note: Always measure accurately when you're making homemade beauty products. See page 53 for tips.

- Small teapot with strainer (see tips, at left)
- Teacup

1 tsp	dried mistletoe (see tips, at left)	5 mL
1 tsp	dried yarrow	5 mL
1 tsp	dried lavender flowers	5 mL
1 cup	boiling water	250 mL
	Honey (optional)	

1. In teapot, combine mistletoe, yarrow and lavender. Pour boiling water over top; cover and let stand for 5 minutes.
2. Pour infusion into cup. Sweeten with a little honey (if using) before drinking.

Varicose Veins: Prevention Strategies

- Massaging the legs is a great way to prevent the formation of varicose veins. You can use your hands or special rollers designed for this purpose.
- Walk at least half an hour every day. If you can, take your walk on a beach. Walking on sand is ideal for activating your circulation.
- Keep your legs elevated whenever you're not standing, especially while sleeping.
- Finish your shower with a cold-water rinse. Use a handheld sprayer to direct the water at your body. Start at the ankles and move all the way up to the hips and inner thighs.
- Use elastic compression stockings to improve circulation and keep varicose veins from swelling and causing pain.

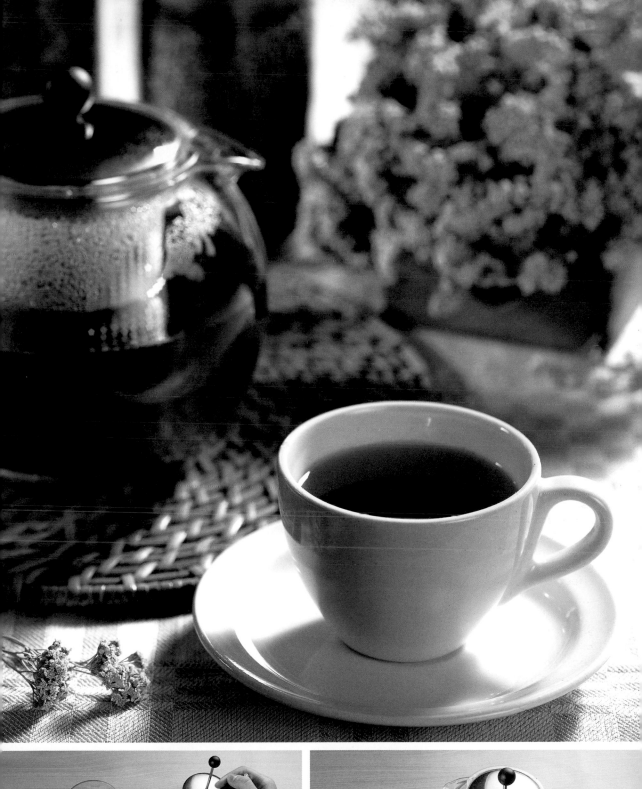
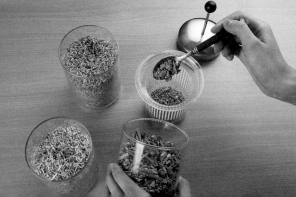
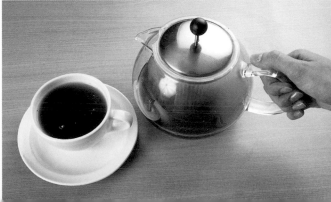

Tired Foot Liniment

Liniments are old-fashioned liquid rubs designed to relieve aches and pains. This one contains camphor spirit, which feels cool as it goes on and helps reduce swelling and irritation in the feet.

Best for: Aching, sore feet

Tip: The arnica plant (*Arnica montana*) produces pretty yellow flowers that are used to reduce inflammation and bruising. Good-quality dried flowers are available online and at herbalists' shops.

Note: Always measure accurately when you're making homemade beauty products. See page 53 for tips.

- Fine-mesh sieve
- Large dark glass bottle with lid

2 cups	water	500 mL
1 tbsp	dried arnica flowers (see tip, at left)	15 mL
2 tbsp	fresh or dried sage flowers	30 mL
1 cup	camphor spirit	250 mL
3	drops rosemary essential oil (see tips, page 248)	3

1. In a medium saucepan, combine water, arnica flowers and sage flowers. Bring to a boil.

2. Remove from heat, cover and let stand for 5 minutes.

3. Place fine-mesh sieve over a large heatproof bowl; strain infusion into bowl, discarding solids. Stir in camphor spirit and rosemary essential oil until well combined. Let cool.

4. Pour into bottle. Rub a small amount of liniment all over feet, massaging gently. Store bottle in a cool, dark place for up to 2 months. Shake well before each use.

Summer Can Be Cruel to Feet

Summer is the hardest season on your feet: you walk more, sweat more and wear shoes that expose heels, soles and toes to the elements. That's why this is the most important time to maintain good foot hygiene. Wash your feet daily (making sure to scrub between your toes), and dry them carefully to eliminate moisture, which can encourage fungal infections. When you're done, don't forget to moisturize your feet and reward them with a relaxing, healing massage.

Leg-Strengthening Exercises

Your legs work hard to support the weight of your body and propel you every day. That's why they need regular exercise. These four easy moves will help stretch and strengthen the muscles in your legs:

Exercise 1: Side-to-Side

1. **Setup.** Stand with legs shoulder width apart. Stretch your arms up and link your hands over your head, keeping your torso straight. Stretch your hands and arms upward as though you're trying to touch the ceiling.

2. **Lean left and right.** Keeping your feet in place and your arms stretched, lean your torso over to the left. Return to the center; then, lean to the right. Return to the center.

3. **Lean back.** Keeping arms stretched toward the ceiling, lean your upper body backward, keeping your head and spine aligned with your arms.

Exercise 2: On Your Toes

1. **Stand on tiptoes.** With your arms at your sides, stand up on your toes, contracting your leg and buttock muscles. Hold for a few seconds.

2. **Lower down.** Relax and lower your heels back down to the floor. Repeat exercise five times.

Exercise 3: Foot Circles

1. **Setup.** Place a sturdy chair to your left. Support yourself by placing your left hand on the back of the chair. Raise your right leg in front of you without bending the knee.

2. **Make circles.** Draw circles in the air with your foot, first to the right, then to the left.

3. **Repeat.** Return to the starting position and repeat the exercise four times. Turn around and repeat on the opposite side.

Exercise 4: One-Leg Crunch

1. **Setup.** Lie on the floor with your legs together and your hands behind your neck.

2. **Crunch.** Bend your right leg and bring it up toward your chest. Hold for a few seconds. Lower leg gently to the ground.

3. **Repeat.** Repeat with the left leg.

Eucalyptus Tired Foot Bath

Menthol-scented eucalyptus enhances this relaxing soak. To revive feet even more, switch them back and forth between this warm bath and a cold one.

Best for: Aching, sore feet

Tips: If you don't have a drawstring bag, place the eucalyptus on a double-thickness square of cheesecloth and tie with cotton string to make a bundle.

Buy essential oils sold in dark bottles. Exposure to light can reduce the potency of their medicinal herbal components. Store the bottles in a cool, dark place to keep them fresh.

Note: Always measure accurately when you're making homemade beauty products. See page 53 for tips.

• Cotton drawstring bag (see tips, at left)		
3½ oz	fresh or dried eucalyptus leaves	100 g
8 cups	cold water	2 L
1¾ oz	baking soda	50 g
3	drops sage essential oil (see tips, at left)	3

1. Place eucalyptus leaves inside drawstring bag and tie tightly. In a large tea kettle or saucepan, combine water and eucalyptus bundle. Bring to a boil. Reduce heat and simmer for 10 minutes. Remove from heat. Discard eucalyptus bundle.

2. Pour infusion into a large heatproof bowl or basin. Stir in baking soda and sage essential oil.

3. Dip toe into infusion to make sure the temperature is comfortable. Soak feet in infusion for 15 to 30 minutes. Gently pat feet dry with a towel.

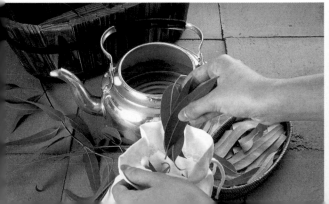
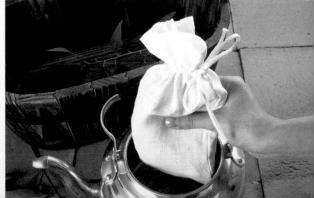

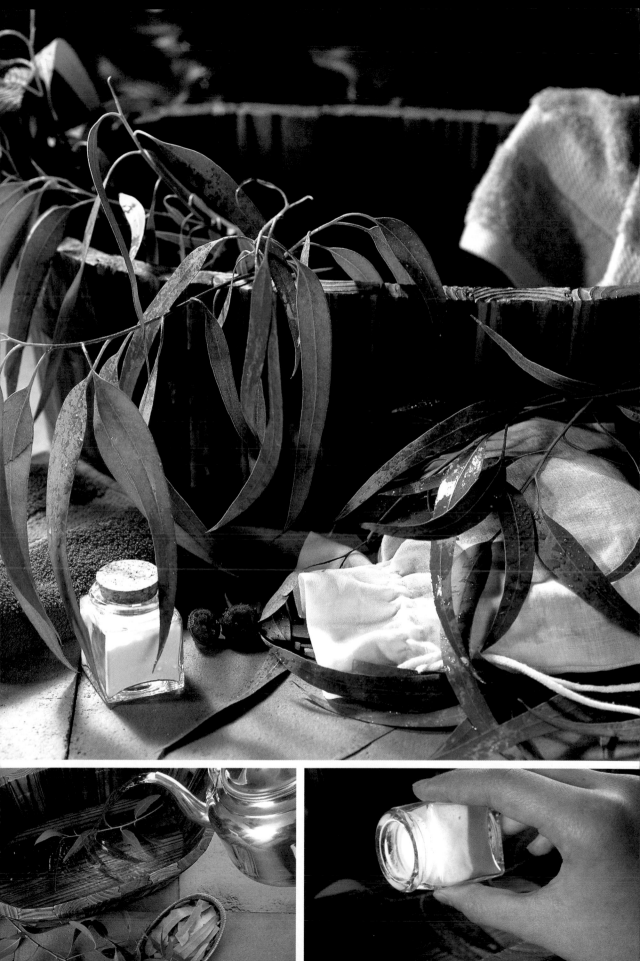

Refreshing Sweaty Foot Solution

When your feet sweat excessively, they can get really stinky. This solution relieves this problem, and the chlorophyll and peppermint essential oil make your soles smell sweet again.

Best for: Excessively sweaty feet

Tips: Chlorophyll is the green pigment in plant leaves that plays a vital role in photosynthesis. It's also a potent odor destroyer that can be used to treat bad breath as well as smelly feet. Liquid chlorophyll is frequently found in health food and nutritional supplement stores.

Iodine tincture (also known as iodine) is an easy-to-find antiseptic solution. It kills bacteria, which are a common cause of smelly feet. Look for it at drugstores.

Note: Always measure accurately when you're making homemade beauty products. See page 53 for tips.

- Two 4-cup (1 L) canning jars with lids
- Small brush

3 cups	liquid chlorophyll (see tips, at left)	750 mL
3 cups	distilled water (see tip, page 240)	750 mL
1 cup	iodine tincture (see tips, at left)	250 mL
3	drops peppermint essential oil (see tips, page 248)	3

1. In a large bowl, stir together liquid chlorophyll, distilled water, iodine tincture and peppermint essential oil until well combined. Divide between jars.

2. Using a small clean brush, brush solution over soles of feet twice a day. Store jars in a cool, dark place for up to 2 months.

Silicon for Sweaty Feet

Before trying special products or treatments to control sweaty feet, check to see whether you are getting enough silicon in your diet. Silicon is found naturally in garlic, barley, onions, parsley, lettuce and celery.

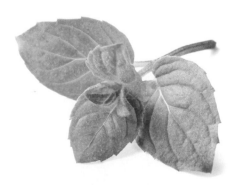

Antiseptic Foot Bath

This lemony, herbal soak contains natural astringents that dry up sweaty feet. Thyme essential oil is a strong antibacterial compound, so it will help keep feet smelling clean and fresh.

Best for: Excessively sweaty feet

Tip: Both spearmint and peppermint are wonderful to grow for use in homemade beauty treatments. They can run wild in the garden, so plant a pot of each instead — that way, you'll always have fresh leaves ready to go into whatever you're making.

- Teapot with strainer (see tips, page 244)

⅓ cup	fresh rosemary leaves	75 mL
⅓ cup	fresh peppermint leaves (see tip, at left)	75 mL
⅓ cup	fresh spearmint leaves	75 mL
4 cups	boiling water	1 L
2	lemons, halved	2
5	drops thyme essential oil (see tips, page 248)	5

1. In teapot, combine rosemary leaves, peppermint leaves and spearmint leaves. Pour boiling water over top; cover and let stand for 20 minutes.

2. Pour infusion into a large heatproof bowl or basin. Squeeze lemon juice into infusion; stir in thyme essential oil.

3. Soak feet in infusion for 10 to 15 minutes. Gently pat feet dry with a towel.

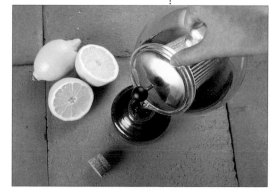
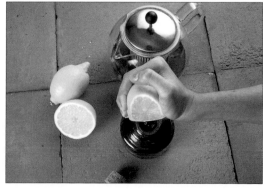

Odor-Reducing Foot Powder

Apply this powder directly to your feet once or twice a day, and sprinkle a little in your shoes to boost its effectiveness.

Best for: Excessively sweaty, smelly feet

Tips: Silk powder is made by grinding the fibrous cocoons spun by silkworms. Silk contains a wide array of amino acids and is a good skin softener. Cosmetic-supply stores often carry this powder.

Tannic acid is a traditional remedy for treating smelly feet. It is the natural astringent found in strong black tea, which is often used as a remedy for excessive sweating. Look for tannic acid powder that is designed for use in food or cosmetics.

Zinc oxide is another powerful astringent and disinfectant that keeps sweaty feet in check. Look for it in cosmetic-supply stores and online.

Note: Always measure accurately when you're making homemade beauty products. See page 53 for tips.

- Glass jar with lid

⅓ cup	silk powder (see tips, at left)	75 mL
1 tbsp	tannic acid powder (see tips, at left)	15 mL
1 tbsp	kaolin clay (see tips, page 239)	15 mL
⅓ oz	zinc oxide powder (see tips, at left)	10 g

1. In a small bowl, stir together silk powder, tannic acid powder, kaolin clay and zinc oxide powder until well combined.

2. Pour into jar. Sprinkle a small amount on feet and/or in shoes. Store jar in a cool, dark place for up to 2 months.

Best Tips for Healthy Feet

- Wear comfortable shoes that are suitable for your feet, especially if you typically spend a lot of time standing or walking.

- Give your feet a break at some point during the day. Put them up for 5 to 10 minutes before continuing your activities.

- Get in the habit of taking foot baths. Alternate between hot and cold water to activate the circulation in your feet.

- To prevent corns and calluses, do toe exercises every day and wear shoes that don't bind feet or cause areas of high friction on the skin.

- Take a barefoot walk on the beach if you're near one. Walking on sand helps strengthen muscles and exfoliates your feet at the same time.

- Avoid fungal infections by keeping your feet clean and dry, and treating fungus immediately if it appears.

- To prevent ingrown toenails, cut your nails straight across and file the corners as little as possible. If you do have an ingrown toenail, experience pain or suspect an infection in your toes, see your doctor or a foot specialist immediately for treatment.

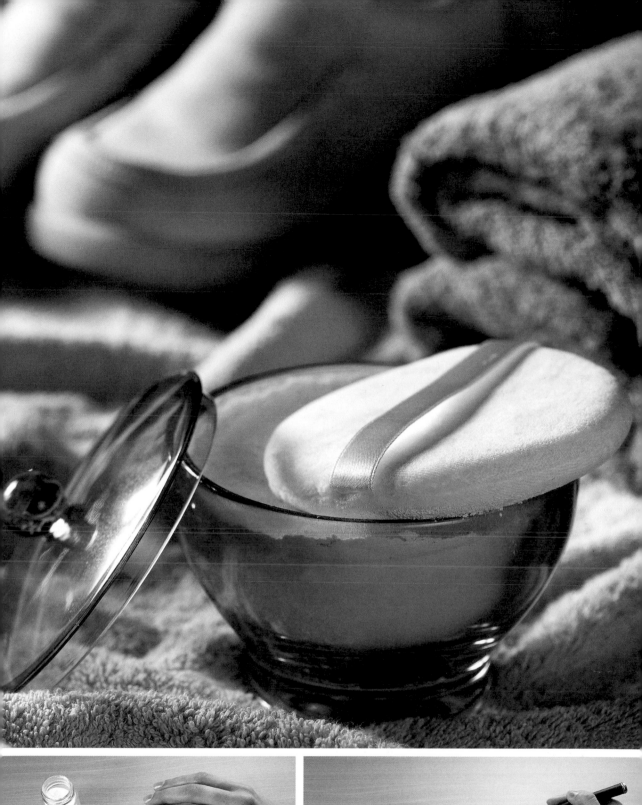
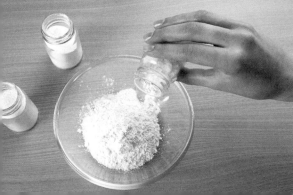
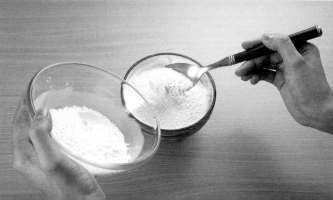

Solutions for Common Foot Troubles

Calluses and athlete's foot are two of the most common problems that affect feet. Fortunately, there are simple home remedies you can try that will effectively treat the causes and soothe the symptoms of these conditions.

Callus Remedies

The first step in fixing a callus is to identify what caused it. Generally, calluses form when you wear poorly fitting, overly narrow shoes for long periods. The shoes may not bother you at first, but over time, they can rub and irritate the skin on your feet, creating painful, bothersome areas. It is better to prevent calluses than to treat them, so buy shoes that fit your feet well and don't cause high-friction points.

Toe exercises are helpful if you tend to get calluses. Move your toes back and forth to activate circulation. Another healthy exercise that will help you prevent callus formation is to walk barefoot on your tiptoes on natural surfaces whenever you can do so safely — for example, on the beach, on trails or on grass.

If you have calluses, you can treat them at home. One option is to remove them mechanically using a special callus plane available at the drugstore; look for it alongside other manicure and pedicure tools. Alternatively, you can remove calluses with a homemade chemical peel. First, wash your feet with warm water and liquid soap made with potassium hydroxide (hard bar soaps are made with sodium hydroxide). As you wash, massage your feet with a natural bristle brush to soften the calluses. Next, crush an aspirin tablet to create powdered acetylsalicylic acid (ASA). Moisten the powder, spread it over the callus and let it stand for a few minutes. Rinse off the ASA paste. Apply a rub made of equal parts camphor spirit and olive oil to the affected area and massage in well. To finish, dust feet with foot powder.

Athlete's Foot Remedies

Whenever you go barefoot, you run the risk of picking up the fungus that causes athlete's foot. It's common in public places where people don't wear shoes, such as pools, saunas, sports facilities and even hotel carpets. The risk is greatest in warm, humid weather, because that is the ideal environment in which the fungus flourishes. Once these microorganisms have made a home in your skin, they are very difficult to get rid of. One of the first athlete's foot symptoms is itching between the toes. As the infection progresses, small blisters or areas of soft, white skin form on the soles of the feet.

One simple way to avoid catching athlete's foot is to always wear sandals in showers, pools and saunas. Another is to always dry the skin between your toes thoroughly; residual moisture in this spot creates a haven for the fungus to grow. Another good tip is to wear cotton socks when you're exercising or doing sports activities, and to let athletic shoes air out thoroughly after taking them off.

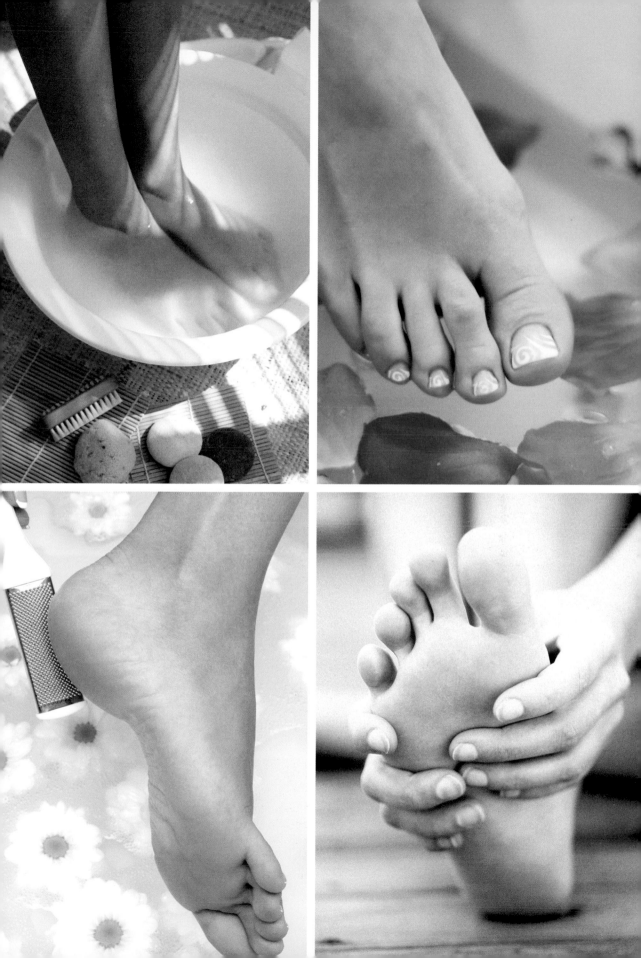

Antifungal Foot Lotion

Tea tree oil gives this lotion a clean herbal aroma, and it adds its antifungal powers to a strong mix of athlete's foot fighters.

Best for: Athlete's foot and other fungal infections of the foot

Tips: In the United States, aspirin is the generic name for painkillers that contain acetylsalicylic acid (ASA); this name is trademarked in Canada and several other countries. No matter what it's called, it comes in a range of concentrations. Look for extra-strength tablets that contain 500 mg of ASA, to make this recipe.

Isopropyl alcohol is often called rubbing alcohol. It disinfects and helps prevent skin infections. Look for bottles of it at the drugstore.

Note: Always measure accurately when you're making homemade beauty products. See page 53 for tips.

- Mortar and pestle
- Small glass jar with lid

2	aspirin tablets (each 500 mg), see tips, at left	2
7 tbsp	isopropyl alcohol (see tips, at left)	100 mL
2 tsp	iodine tincture (see tips, page 250)	10 mL
5	drops tea tree essential oil (see tips, page 248)	5

1. In mortar using pestle, crush aspirin tablets to make a fine powder. Set aside.

2. In a small glass measuring cup, stir together alcohol, iodine and tea tree essential oil. Stir in aspirin powder.

3. Pour into jar. Seal tightly and shake until aspirin powder is dissolved.

4. Soak cotton ball or pad in aspirin mixture. Pat onto areas affected by athlete's foot or nail fungus once or twice daily until infection disappears.

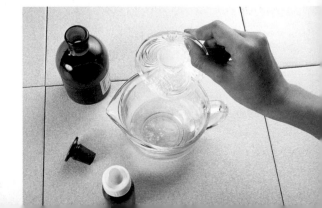

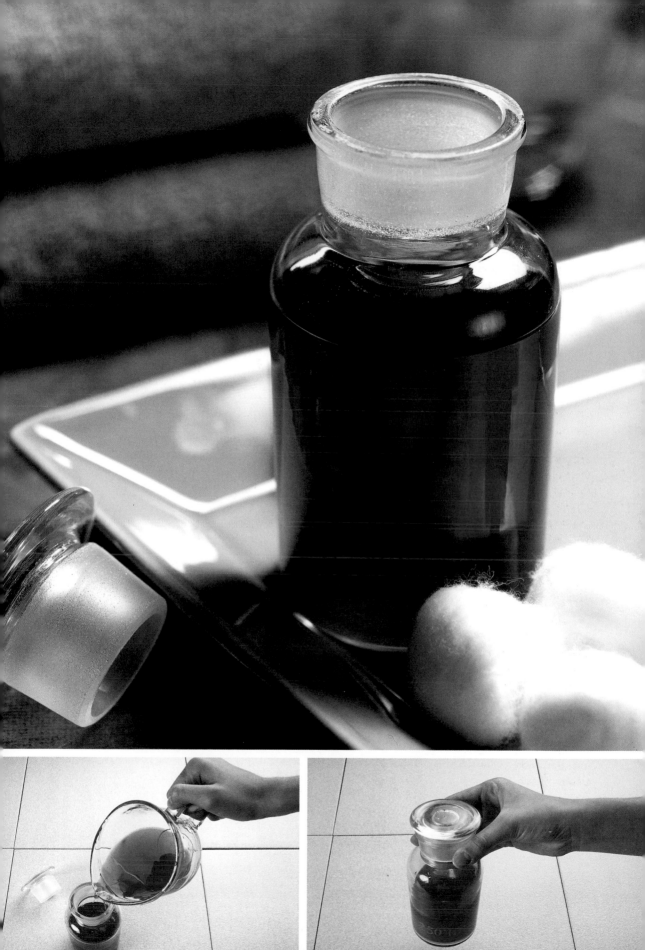

Lily and Honey Hair-Prevention Cream

If you wax your skin to remove unwanted hair (see box, page 261), it may be tender and inflamed afterward. This treatment helps ease any discomfort and reduce irritation. Continuing to apply it will help reduce regrowth of hair.

Best for: Areas with unwanted hair

Tips: Madonna lily bulbs prevent unwanted hair growth and reduce inflammation in the skin. They also produce showy white flowers, so they make a pretty addition to your garden.

Liquid honey often crystallizes in the jar when it's stored in a warm place. There's nothing wrong with it in this state, and you can easily reliquefy it. Just pop the uncovered jar into a saucepan of warm water and heat it gently, stirring the honey until the crystals dissolve and it turns clear again.

Note: Always measure accurately when you're making homemade beauty products. See page 53 for tips.

- Mortar and pestle
- Small glass jar with lid

2	Madonna lily bulbs (see tips, at left)	2
2 tsp	liquid honey (see tips, at left)	10 mL

1. In mortar using pestle, crush lily bulbs to make a paste. Transfer to a small bowl.

2. Stir in honey until well combined. Spoon into jar. Rub a small amount into skin after waxing.

3. Repeat daily if desired for up to 3 months. Store jar in a cool, dark place between uses.

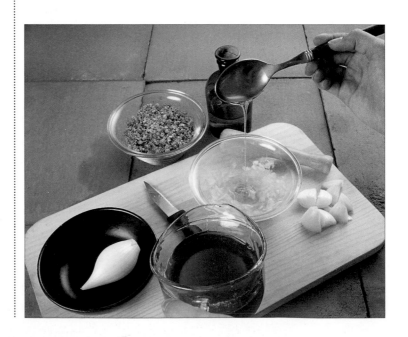

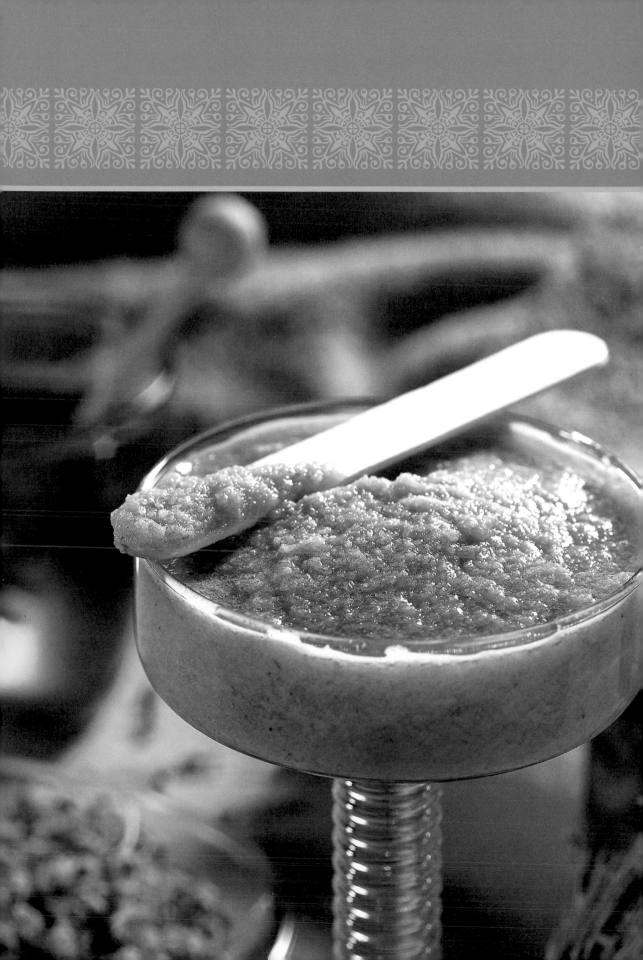

Hair-Weakening Tincture

Alcohol extracts the active components of chamomile flowers, creating an easy-to-use solution for keeping undesired hair at bay.

Best for: Areas with unwanted hair

Tips: Dried chamomile is easy to find at stores that sell medicinal herbs. It's also a very undemanding plant to grow in your garden, so you can grow, harvest and dry your own organic flowers with a minimal amount of effort.

Ethyl alcohol is the type of alcohol in spirits and other alcoholic beverages. It is not the same as isopropyl alcohol, the type you find at the drugstore for disinfecting wounds. You can get high-proof grain alcohol from the liquor store (look for the brand name Everclear). In a pinch, substitute unflavored vodka or brandy.

Note: Always measure accurately when you're making homemade beauty products. See page 53 for tips.

- 6-cup (1.5 L) canning jar with lid

3 tbsp	fresh or dried chamomile flowers (see tips, at left)	45 mL
4 cups	ethyl alcohol (see tips, at left)	1 L

1. Place chamomile flowers in jar. Pour in alcohol and stir to combine. Seal jar tightly. Let stand at room temperature for 1 week.

2. Moisten cotton ball or pad with tincture. Wipe over skin after using Lily and Honey Hair-Prevention Cream (page 258).

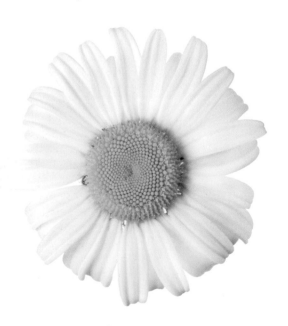

Hair Removal Methods: Pros and Cons

- **Shaving.** Shaving is the usual method of hair removal for many women for both ease and convenience. It has drawbacks, though, especially in sensitive areas such as the underarms and the bikini line. Underarm perspiration can encourage itchy infections and rashes on newly shaved skin. In the bikini area, new hair growth often results in itchy bumps, irritation and ingrown hairs. The main downside of shaving is that hair regrowth happens within a few days.

- **Waxing.** Waxing pulls out entire hairs, including their roots, so regrowth doesn't happen for four to six weeks. **Hot wax** comes in the form of tablets, bars or pearls. It's melted until quite warm (but not hot enough to burn) and applied to the skin with a spatula. A cloth strip is rubbed onto the wax and allowed to cool for a few seconds, then pulled off quickly and firmly so that the hairs are removed along with the wax. **Warm wax** is the same as hot wax but doesn't require as much heating to be effective. **Cold wax** comes on ready-to-use paper sheets. It uses a special wax that melts and adheres to hair using body heat. The strips are applied to the skin, gently pressed to warm them, then pulled off. The main disadvantage to any type of waxing is that it can be quite painful, especially the first time you do it. The legs can stand it most easily, but waxing the underarms and bikini area can be uncomfortable.

- **Depilatory creams.** These creams work by using chemicals to attack the keratin in the hair. They are often used in delicate areas, such as along the bikini line and the underarms, but they are better for the legs, where the skin is less delicate and prone to damage from the chemicals. Sensitive areas can become irritated and inflamed by these creams. Always do a skin test first: apply a bit of the cream to the inside of your elbow; wait a few minutes to see if your skin tolerates it or if you have an allergic reaction. If the latter occurs, discard the cream and try another method of hair removal. After using a depilatory cream, do not apply any product containing alcohol, such as cologne or deodorant, to the area.

- **Electrolysis.** Electrolysis is a permanent hair removal method that destroys the dermal papillae and bulb cells from which the hair follicle grows. A fine, slender needle connected to a device that produces an electrical current is inserted into the follicle along the direction of the hair growth. The current destroys the structures at the base of the hair, preventing it from regenerating. The main drawback is that electrolysis is a slow, cumbersome process: it must be done hair by hair. It can also be quite painful.

- **Laser.** This relatively new technique is considered a permanent hair reduction method. A concentrated beam of laser light is pulsed over the skin. The pigment in the hair follicles absorbs this light energy, which destroys the root of the hair. There are many types of lasers; some work best on dark hair that contrasts with light skin, and some work on many different hair colors. The main disadvantage is that multiple treatments are required, and the technique is quite costly. Laser doesn't work on hair with little to no pigment, so it is not effective for gray or white hair.

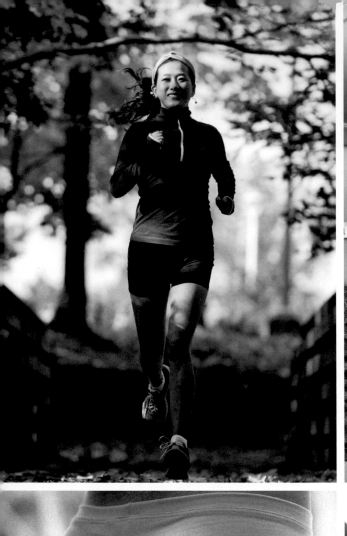
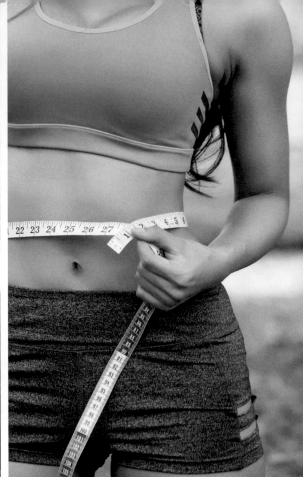
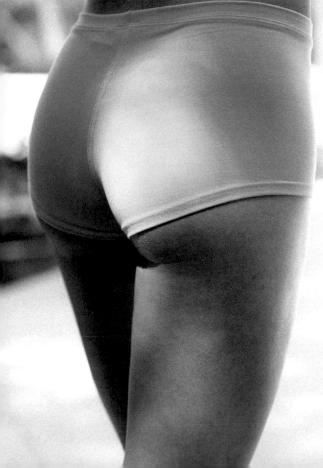
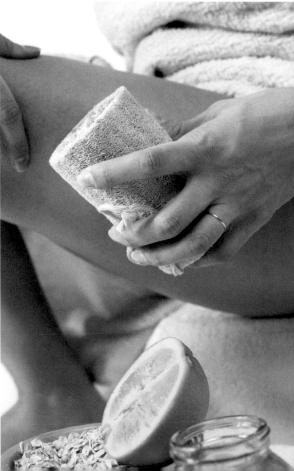

Cellulite: A Common Annoyance

The percentage of women who have cellulite is vastly higher than the percentage of men who have it: about 90% of women versus 10% of men. So cellulite, or fat that's visible through the skin, is often seen as a female issue.

Cellulite is certainly a cause for concern and frustration for most women, who find it unattractive and embarrassing. It takes a lot of patience and perseverance to get rid of cellulite or reduce its appearance, and it's unlikely to disappear without daily treatment. But it's good to know what causes this annoying condition and that there are strategies and homemade remedies, like the ones on pages 265 to 274, that can help.

What Is Cellulite?

Cellulite is located primarily on the hips, thighs, buttocks, knees and legs, but occasionally appears on the arms and the back. Skin affected by it looks dimpled. It is sometimes described as looking like orange peel or cottage cheese, with lumps and dips in the skin overlying fatty deposits.

Cellulite forms when there is an accumulation of fat, toxins and water. The fat cells enlarge, deforming their shape and creating lumps. These lumps are visible through the outermost layer of the skin, called the epidermis, which is thinner than the underlying layers. In some cases, the stretchy elastin fibers in the skin break as a result of this fatty tissue, and the vascular and lymphatic systems become compressed.

What Causes Cellulite

Many factors affect cellulite formation. One is fat accumulation in specific areas. Triglycerides fill up adipocytes, or fat cells, causing them to press on the capillaries, which makes bumps appear on the skin. Decreased blood circulation can also lead to cellulite, because water and toxins build up in these starved areas. Cellulite can also be a genetically inherited tendency. As well, stress can be a causative factor: too much high emotion and certain affective disorders can create imbalances that obstruct peripheral circulation and proper fluid drainage. What's more, stress can contribute to excessive fat storage because of an overabundance of adrenaline in the body.

Leading an unhealthy life — not getting enough exercise and eating foods that lack the proper nutrients — can cause metabolic disorders that lead to the accumulation of fluids, fatty acids and toxins in the body that wind up deposited in the fat cells. Over time, they swell the cells up and cause the typical lumpy texture of cellulite. Insufficient muscle movement also causes decreased blood flow, which reduces the supply of nutrients and oxygen that cells require. As a result, these starved tissues can't remove impurities or excess fluids.

Another factor in the appearance of cellulite is age. The regenerative capacity of collagen and elastin in the skin decreases over your lifetime, and connective tissue becomes looser and less elastic. Eating large amounts of processed foods leads to insufficient nutrient intake, which can also cause connective tissues to lose their shape.

Why Are Women More Prone to Cellulite?

One reason is that women typically have a higher body fat percentage. Women's bodies retain more fat, especially on the legs and buttocks. Cellulite affects the subcutaneous (below the skin) tissues, which are made up of three layers of fat. In women and men, these tissues are structured differently. Men's fat cells are separated by stable layers and crisscrossing fibers, whereas women's fat cells, especially in the hips and thighs, are arranged in vertical columns and separated by flexible layers. This structure allows swollen fat cells to push the skin outward, creating the bumpy appearance of cellulite.

Cellulite also affects women much more frequently than men because of female hormones, namely estrogen and progesterone, which control the distribution and structure of women's fat tissues. These hormones enable female connective tissues to expand considerably when needed, such as in puberty and in pregnancy. But the flexible nature of these connective tissues is precisely what enables the formation of cellulite.

Dr. Karen Burke, author of *Thin Thighs for Life* (Hamlyn, 1995), believes that cellulite formation depends in part on estrogen. She says that women's cells in areas of the body plagued by cellulite are weaker and more easily transformed as a result of excess weight, fluid retention and a sedentary lifestyle. Toxic residues also tend to accumulate in these areas, affecting the health of collagen and elastin in the skin.

Heredity also plays a part. Your chances of developing cellulite depend in part on your genetically determined body composition. If you inherit the tendency to store fat readily, you might be more likely to have cellulite than someone who can eat anything without gaining weight. But even if you have inherited this tendency, you can do something about it with the help of diet and exercise.

Strategies for Fighting Cellulite

Until recently, experts believed that cellulite was simply accumulated fat, so the main treatment recommended was diet, exercise and weight loss. However, it turns out that cellulite has little to do with the normal accumulation of fat or with obesity (a slender woman can have cellulite just as easily as a heavier woman can). An increased number of fat cells in a person's body does not necessarily mean that cellulite will form, although it can increase the probability in some cases.

Cellulite formation involves the lymphatic and circulatory systems, so it requires a comprehensive treatment strategy on several fronts. Getting rid of cellulite starts with a healthy, balanced diet; your best friends for treating cellulite are whole foods, fruits and vegetables. Exercise plays an important role. Natural remedies based on medicinal plants can also exert a positive influence on cellulite. Finally, there are manual techniques, such as dry brushing and lymphatic drainage, that can help ensure the success of these other strategies.

Dietary Changes

Healthy eating prevents the proliferation of the cells that lead to that undesirable orange peel look of cellulite. There are several dietary changes that will reduce the appearance of cellulite.

- **Don't overdo it on protein consumption.** When proteins are digested, they produce toxins that must be eliminated (carbohydrates do not). Nutritionists used to recommend that you consume 1 g of protein per each 2.2 lbs (1 kg) of body weight every day. That number has been revised in recent years. Today, nutrition experts recommend that adults consume 0.8 g of protein per each 2.2 lbs (1 kg) of body weight every day. If you weigh 150 lbs (68 kg), that means you need just over 54 grams of protein per day.

- **Replace refined sugar and refined flour with whole foods.** Refined sugar and flour are simple carbohydrates that the body absorbs rapidly. They give you a short-term energy boost but cause blood sugar levels to spike; the excess energy they provide is then stored as fat. In contrast, whole foods provide carbohydrates that the body absorbs slowly. They are a stable, long-lasting energy source that burns steadily and does not encourage fat formation.

- **Eat plenty of fresh fruits and vegetables.** They are rich in vital elements, such as vitamins, minerals, trace elements, enzymes and antioxidants that protect cells. These micronutrients participate in the elimination of water and contain electrolytes, which are involved in cell osmotic balance. These foods contain bases that alkalize and clean the blood, neutralizing impurities and toxins.

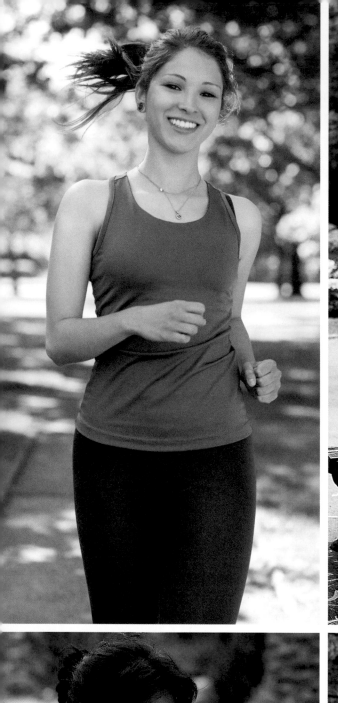

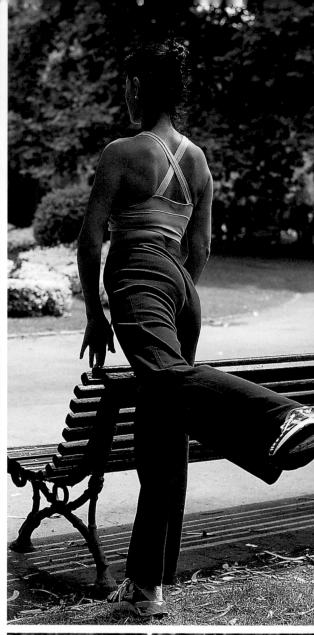

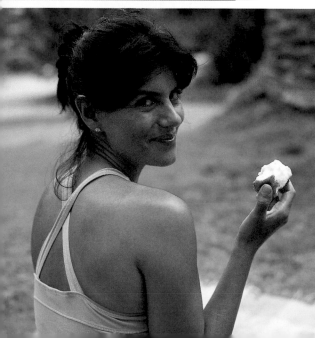

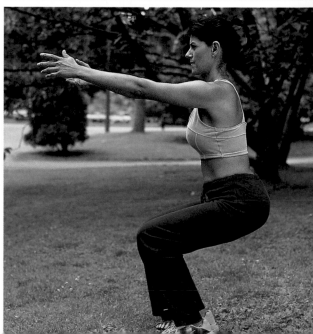

- **Reduce your salt intake.** Sodium is important to the body. In partnership with other minerals (mainly potassium), it carries out important physiological functions, including the regulation of arterial blood pressure, maintenance of the body's water content and powering of the active transport mechanism in cells. Salt attracts and holds water, but too much of it causes cells to absorb more than they need, making them bloated.

- **Eat less animal fat and drink more water.** By consuming foods that are full of vitamins and minerals and healthy plant-based fats, you keep your immune defenses strong. By drinking your daily quota of water, you help flush out toxins.

Exercise and Physical Activity

Exercise stimulates the lymphatic and circulatory systems, and strengthens connective tissues. It also activates cell metabolism, helps nutrients reach cells and tissues more effectively, stimulates combustion in the cells and boosts blood circulation. Physical activity of any kind keeps the lymphatic system pumping, allowing it to carry away and dispose of metabolic by-products deposited in the intercellular spaces.

All types of exercise are excellent at building your general health and well-being. Swimming is especially good for banishing cellulite. There are also specific stretching and toning exercises you can try (see box, page 268) that are highly effective and easy to do daily at home.

Medicinal Plant Treatments

There is a group of plants that are extremely beneficial for treating cellulite, thanks to their stimulating and purifying powers. You can use them in two different forms:

- **Infusions.** Nettle, dandelion and horsetail teas are ideal for preventing fluid retention in connective tissues. They activate your body's immune defenses and eliminate impurities. To prepare them, place 1 to 2 tsp (5 to 10 mL) of the dried herb in a tea strainer in a teacup. Pour 1 cup (250 mL) boiling water over top. Cover and let stand for 5 minutes. Remove strainer and enjoy the tea. Drink one or two cups per day.

- **External applications.** Medicinal plant treatments, made from anti-cellulite superstars (see box, page 270), can also be administered in the form of baths, poultices and masks. The active substances of the plants are either absorbed through the skin or inhaled through the mucous membranes and transported throughout the body. Ivy leaves and seaweed are two other ancient remedies that purify, tone and revitalize cellulite-prone skin.

Targeted Anti-Cellulite Exercises

These exercises are specially designed to stimulate areas of the body that are commonly bothered by cellulite. Choose the area you want to target and do 5 to 10 repetitions of the exercises twice a day to improve the appearance of cellulite:

- **Abs, thighs and glutes.** Lie down on your stomach on a mat or towel. Bend your knees at a right angle. Then, reach back and grasp your left ankle with your left hand and your right ankle with your right hand. Slowly raise your upper body off the floor without pressing down too hard on the ground. Hold this position for a few seconds as you inhale and exhale deeply. Lower back down to the starting position.

- **Abs and legs.** Sit on a mat or towel with your legs together and stretched out flat on the floor in front of you. Raise your arms straight out in front of you, palms facing each other. Lean your upper body back, lifting both legs off the floor and balancing on your buttocks. Hold this position for a few seconds as you inhale slowly and deeply. Slowly lower back down to the starting position.

- **Hips, glutes and thighs #1.** Lie on your side on a mat or towel. Push your upper body up off the floor, supporting it with your arm at a right angle on the floor. Slowly raise your leg as high as you can. Hold for a second and slowly lower it back to the starting position. Repeat on the same side. Then, switch sides.

- **Hips, glutes and thighs #2.** Stand with your back slightly away from a wall, feet slightly apart and toes pointing forward. Rise up on your toes, lean back against the wall as you sink down and bend your knees to a 90-degree angle. Keep your back as straight as possible and your knees in line with your toes. Hold this position for a few seconds. Slowly straighten your knees and push back upward to the starting position.

Dry Brushing

A vigorous daily dry brushing of areas affected by cellulite stimulates the lymphatic system and improves circulation, and is an excellent way to remove toxins. Use a firm natural bristle brush with a long handle. Massage dry skin with the brush, making small circular movements over areas affected by cellulite. After you finish, take a hot shower followed by a cold-water rinse.

Anti-Cellulite Massage

Despite their claims, massage creams and lotions do not dissolve fat that accumulates in specific areas of the body. They do, however, help improve circulation and reduce the appearance of cellulite, especially if you

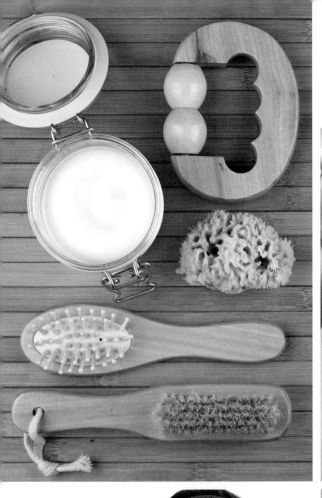
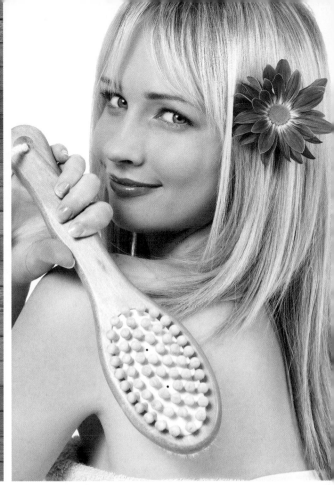
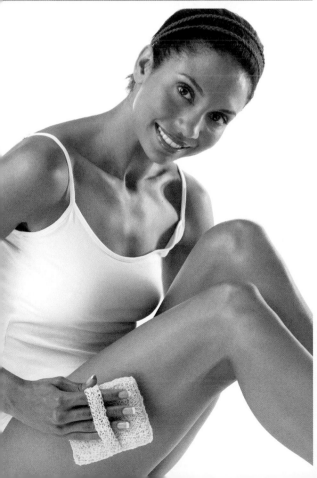
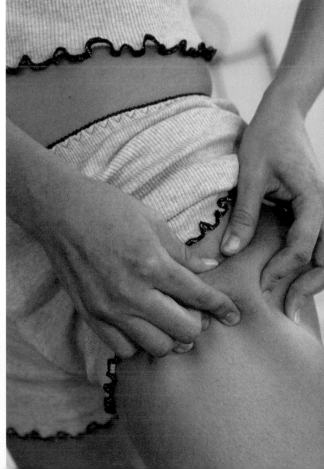

Anti-Cellulite Superstars

- **Marine silt.** This ocean mud comes in paste form. It nourishes the skin, providing magnesium and other minerals and trace elements it desperately needs. The rich iodine content of marine silt also activates the body's natural cell-restructuring system and drains accumulated toxins. Apply it directly to the area to be treated, and let it stand on the skin for 15 to 20 minutes before rinsing off with warm water.

- **Yellow sweet clover.** A poultice made from this herb has a purifying effect, stimulates circulation and activates cell metabolism. Fill a cotton drawstring bag with 3½ oz (100 g) of yellow sweet clover, including the seeds and flowers. Place the bag in a medium saucepan of boiling water; cover and let stand for 15 minutes. Remove the bag from the water and let it cool enough to handle. Gently squeeze the bag to remove excess moisture, discarding the liquid. Apply the damp bag to the affected area when the bag is as hot as your skin will tolerate without burning. Cover with a towel and let stand on the skin for 1 hour.

regularly do lymphatic drainage (see below) with essential oils or seaweed extracts. Seaweed extracts have a diuretic effect and help prevent fluid retention. They are high in vitamins and minerals, and contain amino acids, which strengthen the skin.

Lymphatic Drainage

Lymphatic drainage is a therapy that encourages lymph fluid to flow away from tissues in which it has accumulated. One method involves the fingers massaging the lymphatic vessels in the direction of the lymph nodes. Using strong, consistent pressure, the fingers stimulate the movement of lymphatic fluid and help push it in the correct direction. Lymphatic drainage can correct edema (fluid retention) and reduce the size of swollen fat cells. You can receive a lymphatic drainage treatment from a qualified massage therapist.

You can do a version of this technique at home. For example, on the upper legs, place your hand on one thigh so that your thumb is on the inside and your fingers are on the outside. Massage the tissue in circles, working upward toward the groin. Always follow the direction of lymph flow; on the thighs, lymph moves from the knee to the groin; on the glutes, it moves from the base of the spine toward the hips; and on the abdomen, it moves from the navel toward the groin.

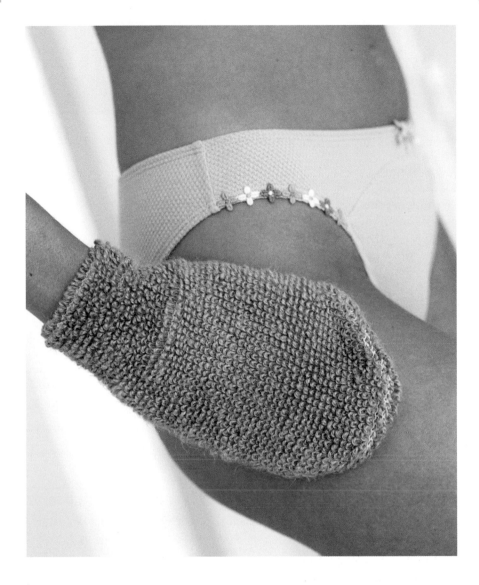

Natural Fiber Exfoliating Gloves

A daily dry massage is another great way to remove dead cells from the surface of the skin and stimulate circulation. Natural fiber exfoliating gloves and natural sponges are ideal tools, because they won't scratch the skin but are not so soft that they merely caress it. Start with your feet and work upward, massaging the insides of your legs, then moving to the outsides. Then, massage your abdomen, buttocks and back. Then, move on to your neck, shoulders, chest and breasts, circling around your nipples but not brushing across them. Finish by brushing your arms from fingertips to shoulders.

Witch Hazel and Clay Anti-Cellulite Bath

This soak is full of astringent herbs and clay, which help tighten skin and nourish it, reducing the appearance of cellulite.

Best for: Areas prone to cellulite

Tips: You can buy dried witch hazel leaves (*Hamamelis virginiana*) and horsetail (*Equisetum arvense*) at many online herb stores.

Large-flake kosher sea salt is easy to find and a good ingredient for this recipe.

Note: Always measure accurately when you're making homemade beauty products. See page 53 for tips.

- Fine-mesh sieve

2 cups	water	500 mL
1¾ oz	dried witch hazel leaves (see tips, at left)	50 g
1¾ oz	dried horsetail	50 g
1¾ oz	dried rosemary	50 g
1 lb	kaolin clay (see tips, page 239)	500 g
⅓ cup	sea salt (see tips, at left)	75 mL

1. In a medium saucepan, combine water, witch hazel leaves, horsetail and rosemary. Bring to a boil. Reduce heat, cover and simmer for 2 minutes. Remove from heat. Let stand for 10 minutes.

2. Place fine-mesh sieve over a medium heatproof bowl. Strain infusion into bowl, discarding solids.

3. Stir infusion, clay and salt into warm bathwater. Soak in bath for 15 to 20 minutes.

Essential Oils That Fight Cellulite

The ideal essential oils to use during anti-cellulite massages are lemon, juniper, orange, cypress, rosemary, bergamot, cedar and sandalwood. These aromatherapy oils are produced by distilling or pressing flowers, herbs, leaves or fruits, thereby concentrating their active substances. Inhalation or application of these scents on the skin causes changes to and healing effects on the body. Mix a few drops with a gentle carrier oil, such as wheat germ or hazelnut, before applying them to the skin.

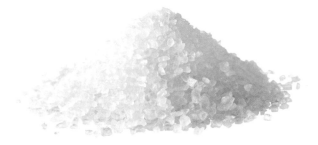

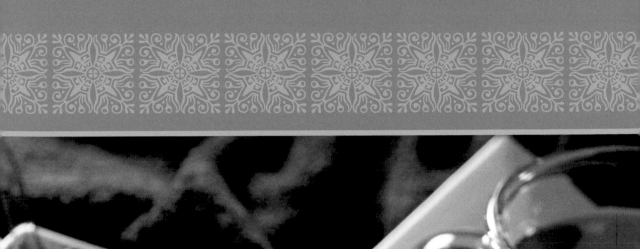

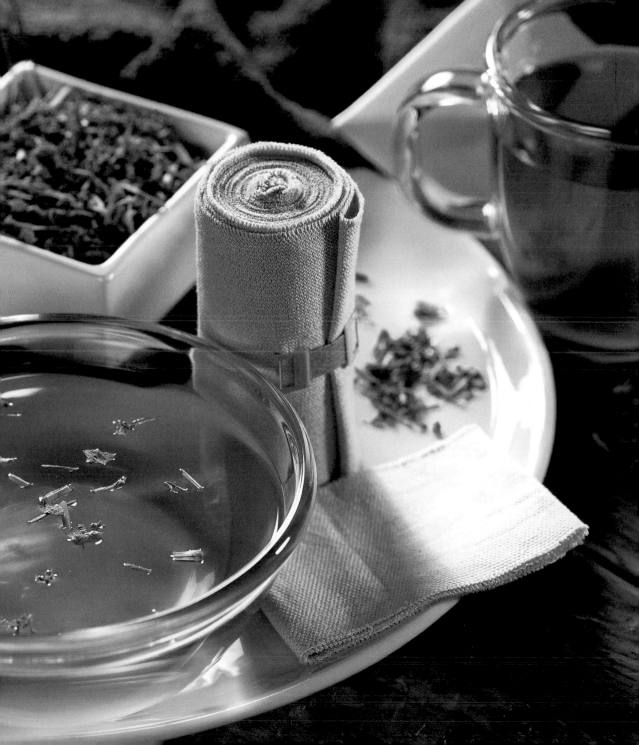

Bran Mask

In this mask, wheat bran works with vinegar to nourish and tone areas that are bothered by cellulite.

Best for: Areas prone to cellulite

Tip: Buy organic wheat bran to make this treatment. It is free of pesticide and fungicide residues, two types of toxins you definitely don't want to put on your skin.

3½ oz	wheat bran (see tip, at left)	100 g
1 cup	cider vinegar	250 mL
5	drops cypress essential oil	5

1. In a small bowl, stir wheat bran with cider vinegar until well combined and moistened. Stir in cypress essential oil until thick and creamy.

2. Spread bran mixture over areas most affected by cellulite. Let stand on skin for 20 minutes.

3. Rinse off mixture with warm water. Gently pat skin dry with a towel.

Banana Mask

This mask moisturizes skin, making it more attractive and resilient, and reduces the unsightly appearance of cellulite.

Best for: Areas prone to cellulite

Tips: Ripe bananas are the most fragrant and easiest to mash. A banana is soft and very ripe when it's yellow all over with a smattering of small brown freckles.

Cold-pressed extra-virgin oils are the purest and most unadulterated type you can buy for making homemade beauty treatments. They are worth the higher price tag.

Note: Always measure accurately when you're making homemade beauty products. See page 53 for tips.

1	ripe banana (see tips, at left)	1
2 tbsp	sweet almond oil	30 mL
1 tsp	soybean oil (see tips, at left)	5 mL
1 tsp	sunflower seed oil	5 mL
5	drops rosemary essential oil	5

1. In a small bowl and using a fork, mash banana. Stir in sweet almond oil, soybean oil, sunflower seed oil and rosemary essential oil until a pasty mixture forms.

2. Spread banana mixture over areas most affected by cellulite. Let stand on skin for 20 minutes.

3. Rinse off mixture with warm water. Gently pat skin dry with a towel.

Revitalizing Masks for Cellulite

Masks are ideal for restoring the vitality of your skin. Start with a hot shower to open your pores. Then, apply the mask. In addition to the recipes on this page, try masks made with seaweed, clay, ginseng, honey, collagen or rose essential oil. Experiment with different ingredients to find the ones you like best.

Q&A: Anti-Cellulite Products

Marie Carrasquedo Lebourgeois, a specialist in natural cosmetics, has her own natural body products laboratory, so she knows the best formulas for authentic natural beauty. She answered the following common questions on this topic. Just remember: when it comes to cellulite, don't expect miraculous results, even from the most natural, balanced, safe products.

Q: How effective are anti-cellulite products?

A: These products alone cannot completely eliminate cellulite or take off excess weight. There is no miracle cream that will do that. They can, however, help activate peripheral and lymphatic circulation; decongest, drain and flush away accumulations of water and fat; and gently and progressively reduce cellulite. They can be useful in activating circulation, as they can enhance the effects of lymphatic drainage.

Q: What are the best ingredients for cellulite treatments?

A: The natural active substances most used in anti-cellulite products are caffeine; English ivy (Hedera helix) and ginkgo biloba extracts; various seaweeds; silver birch leaves; horse chestnuts; and lemon, cedar, orange and rosemary essential oils.

Q: What textures do these products most commonly have?

A: Commercial anti-cellulite products in the natural cosmetics market are increasingly trending toward gel textures, with silicone as an ingredient. These creams are often made with effective aromatic essential oils, but they do not always contain the most suitable carrier oils.

Q: Why do you have to worry about carrier oils?

A: Essential oils are complex substances obtained from aromatic plants. They are very effective in reducing accumulated metabolic waste products, but lose much of their beneficial action when mixed with mineral oils or carrier oils that contain saturated fats. This is why consumers have to pay close attention to the composition of the product, including the carrier oil.

Q: So what are the most effective anti-cellulite formulas?

A: The most effective formulas have a carrier oil that is beneficial to the skin, such as wheat germ or hazelnut oil, which are very rich in essential fatty acids that aid in balancing the skin. What's more, these ingredients are the most compatible with essential oils.

Q: What are the least effective formulas?

A: The least effective carrier oils contain petrochemical fats, such as petroleum jelly, paraffin and silicone. These fats work against the skin's natural elimination and breathing functions, so they are best avoided.

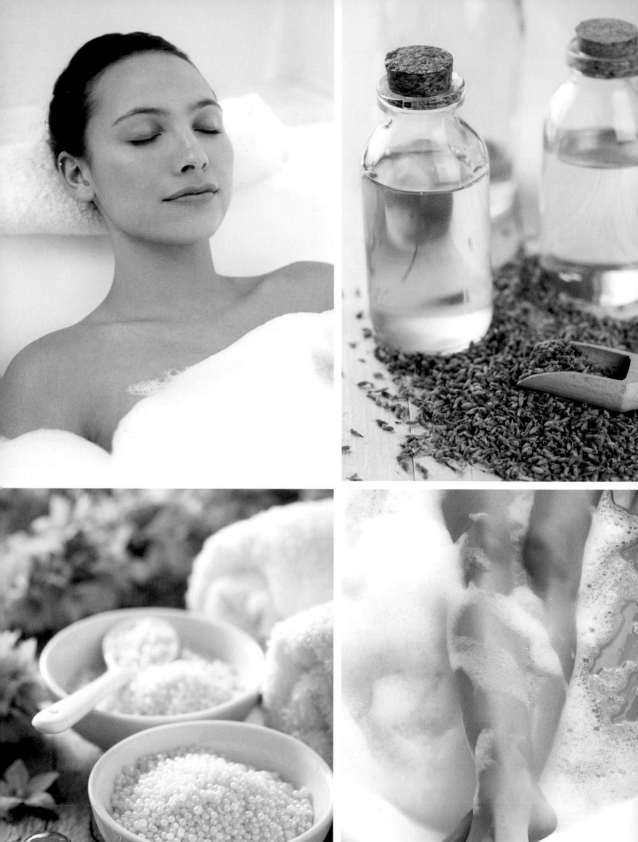

Bath Products and Treatments

Nature provides a nearly inexhaustible list of ingredients you can use to make homemade beauty products. In this chapter, you'll find all the formulas you need to create your favorite herbal baths, bath oils, after-bath body lotions and oils, soaps and soap-free cleansers. Their effects are healing, relaxing, stimulating, purifying and refreshing — and every formula is good for your skin.

Restorative Baths

Enjoying a soothing, aromatic, restorative bath at the end of a long day will relax you and create the ideal atmosphere for putting your thoughts in order. You'll be able to cleanse your body, your mind and your spirit at the same time.

Creating a great bath product starts with the best natural ingredients. Homemade cleansers and moisturizers do not have the big drawback that commercial, chemical-based ones do; namely, homemade formulas won't dry out your skin by removing too much of its natural oils. The medicinal plants and essential oils in these formulations nourish

Bathing: A Fragrant History

In ancient civilizations, bathing had social, religious and even medical purposes and meanings. In Ancient Egypt, the wealthier classes had slaves whose only job was to bathe their masters. For centuries, baths were perfumed with natural ingredients, such as myrrh, saffron and cinnamon. In Ancient Greece, it was customary to receive guests with a bath of tuberose, rose and almond. Later, the Romans built their impressive public baths, where they used susinum, an ancient ointment made from aromatic lilies, honey, cinnamon, saffron and myrrh.

While the ancients loved this custom, bathing fell out of fashion in later centuries. In the court of King Louis XV of France, doctors advised against bathing because they thought it was harmful to the king's health. Fortunately, the late 19th century brought a new interest in cleanliness, and bathing became fashionable again.

the skin, transmitting each of their active ingredients directly to tissues. For example, the essential oils in rose petals penetrate the skin, protecting it from infections and helping renew it. Many medicinal plants also have beneficial aromatherapeutic powers. When you add them to warm bathwater, their fragrant essences travel via your nose and lungs into your circulatory system and brain, where they have a positive effect.

Bath Oils and After-Bath Lotions

Oils contain a high proportion of fatty elements, which mitigate the drying effects of soap and water. Indulging in a bath laced with rich bath oil is especially good for people with dry skin. After rinsing, a thin film of oil stays on the skin, which helps keep it moisturized.

Depending on the ingredients, after-bath body lotions and oils may be softening, skin lightening, nourishing or healing. Choose the one that's right for your skin's needs. If you regularly use lotions and oils that are well suited to your skin, it will look healthier, softer and more vibrant.

Homemade Soaps

Making homemade soaps sounds daunting, but it can be quite simple and the ingredients you need are easy to find. The traditional process for making soap involves mixing caustic soda, or lye, with fat; combining these two elements results in a phenomenon called saponification, which creates a stable, safe mixture that lathers and cleans dirt and contaminants off the surface of the skin.

The recipes in this chapter skip this time-consuming and slightly dangerous process by employing a shortcut. They call for a glycerin soap base or grated ready-made soap bars, which are available anywhere soap-making supplies are sold. By using these, you can make soaps that give the same results as handmade bars without having to handle corrosive caustic soda. This shortcut creates soaps that are excellent for your skin-care needs.

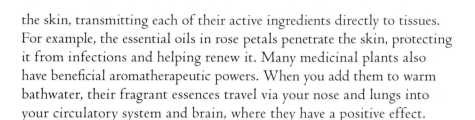

Flower, Herb and Fruit Bath

This highly perfumed combination of flowers, herbs and citrus fruits will drain away the tension and relax you after a hard day at work. It will also soothe skin irritations.

Best for: Sensitive skin

Tips: Gourmet tea shops often sell small cotton drawstring bags for steeping teas. If you don't have one (or yours is too small to accommodate the mixture), place the ingredients on a double-thickness square of cheesecloth and tie with cotton string to make a bundle.

Seville oranges are bitter and usually used to make marmalade. They can be hard to find in North America, so substitute navel or other orange peel if you like.

Note: Always measure accurately when you're making homemade beauty products. See page 53 for tips.

- Cotton drawstring bag (see tips, at left)

3½ oz	dried lavender flowers (see tip, page 281)	100 g
1¾ oz	Seville orange peel (see tips, at left)	50 g
1 tbsp	dried thyme leaves	15 mL
1 tbsp	dried wild rose leaves	15 mL
1 tbsp	dried white willow bark	15 mL
1 tbsp	dried borage	15 mL
1 tbsp	dried spearmint leaves	15 mL
1 tbsp	dried marjoram leaves	15 mL
1 tbsp	dried rosemary leaves	15 mL
2	whole cloves, crushed	2
2 to 5	drops lemon juice	2 to 5
5	drops rose essential oil (see tip, page 281)	5

1. In a large bowl, stir together lavender flowers, orange peel, thyme leaves, wild rose leaves, white willow bark, borage, spearmint leaves, marjoram leaves, rosemary leaves, cloves, lemon juice and rose essential oil.

2. Spoon mixture into bag. Tie tightly. Hang bag ties over tap and let bag float in warm bathwater. Soak in bath for 15 to 20 minutes.

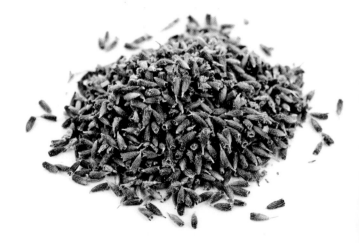

Stress Relief Bath

This calming mix of lavender, ginger, mint and orange relieves headaches caused by exhaustion and stress. It also relaxes tired, aching muscles.

Best for: Reducing stress and soothing aches and pains

Tips: If you like, you can substitute fresh ginger for the dried in this recipe. Peel and slice a 1-inch (2.5 cm) chunk of fresh ginger and add it to the lavender mixture.

Orange blossom essential oil, also known as neroli essential oil, is made from the flowers of the orange tree. Orange essential oil is extracted from the zest of the fruit, and petitgrain essential oil is made from the leaves and twigs of the plant.

Note: Always measure accurately when you're making homemade beauty products. See page 53 for tips.

- Fine-mesh sieve

¼ cup	dried lavender flowers (see tip, opposite)	60 mL
2 tbsp	ground ginger (see tips, at left)	30 mL
2 tbsp	fresh mint leaves	30 mL
2 cups	water	500 mL
5	drops orange blossom essential oil (see tips, at left)	5

1. In a medium heatproof bowl, combine lavender flowers, ginger and mint leaves. Set aside.

2. In a medium saucepan, bring water just to a boil; pour over lavender mixture. Cover and let stand for 10 minutes.

3. Place fine-mesh sieve over another medium heatproof bowl. Strain infusion into bowl, discarding solids.

4. Add infusion and orange blossom essential oil to warm bathwater. Soak in bath for 15 to 20 minutes.

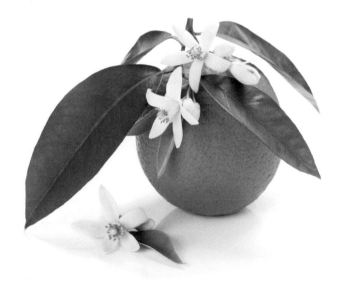

Sleepytime Bath

Valerian root *(Valeriana officinalis)* is a gentle natural sedative that relaxes the body and helps bring on sleepiness. Mixed with lavender, another natural sedative, it's a soothing treatment to help you unwind before bed.

Best for: Reducing stress and inducing sleep

Tip: Look for a reliable source of dried medicinal herbs, such as an herbalist's shop or a reputable online dealer. Make sure it's a business with high turnover, to ensure you're getting the freshest, most effective herbs possible.

- Fine-mesh sieve

3 tbsp	dried lavender flowers (see tip, at left)	45 mL
3 tbsp	dried valerian root	45 mL
2 cups	water	500 mL

1. In a medium heatproof bowl, combine lavender flowers and valerian root. Set aside.

2. In a medium saucepan, bring water just to a boil; pour over lavender mixture. Cover and let stand for 10 minutes.

3. Place fine-mesh sieve over another medium heatproof bowl. Strain infusion into bowl, discarding solids.

4. Add infusion to warm bathwater. Soak in bath for 15 to 20 minutes.

Stimulating Bath

Sometimes you want a bath to give you a pop of energy, rather than relax you into sleep. This one does that with the help of rosemary, roses and lemon.

Best for: Increasing energy

Tip: Buy essential oils sold in dark bottles. Exposure to light can reduce the potency of their medicinal herbal components. Store the bottles in a cool, dark place to keep them fresh.

- Large fine-mesh sieve

4 cups	water	1 L
1¾ oz	dried rosemary leaves (see tip, above)	50 g
1¾ oz	dried rose petals	50 g
5	drops lemon essential oil (see tip, at left)	5

1. In a large saucepan, combine water, rosemary leaves and rose petals. Bring to a boil. Cover, reduce heat and simmer for 10 minutes.

2. Place fine-mesh sieve over a large heatproof bowl. Strain infusion into bowl, discarding solids.

3. Add infusion and lemon essential oil to warm bathwater. Soak in bath for 15 to 20 minutes.

Rose and Poppy Bath

This fragrant flower-infused bath softens and hydrates parched skin. Use your favorite after-bath lotion (see pages 300 and 301) to lock in this added moisture.

Best for: Dry skin

Tips: Marshmallow root (*Althaea officinalis*) contains natural mucilaginous compounds, which make it great for softening skin and soothing irritations. The chopped dried root is available at herbalists' shops and online herb stores.

Use rose and poppy petals from plants that have not been sprayed with herbicides or fungicides.

Note: Always measure accurately when you're making homemade beauty products. See page 53 for tips.

• Large fine-mesh sieve

1¾ oz	marshmallow root (see tips, at left)	50 g
1	handful each fresh rose and poppy petals (see tips, at left)	1
4 cups	boiling water	1 L
5	drops rose essential oil (see tip, page 281)	5

1. Place marshmallow root in a medium saucepan. Pour in enough water to cover by 1 inch (2.5 cm). Bring to a boil. Cover, reduce heat and simmer for 10 minutes. Remove from heat. Let stand for 10 minutes.

2. Meanwhile, in a large heatproof bowl, combine rose and poppy petals. Pour boiling water over top. Cover and let stand for 10 minutes.

3. Place fine-mesh sieve over another large heatproof bowl. Strain marshmallow infusion and rose and poppy infusion into bowl, discarding solids. Stir in rose essential oil.

4. Add infusion mixture to warm bathwater. Soak in bath for 15 to 20 minutes.

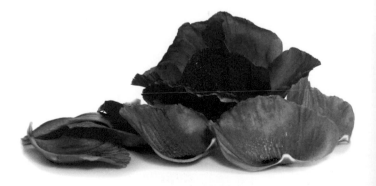

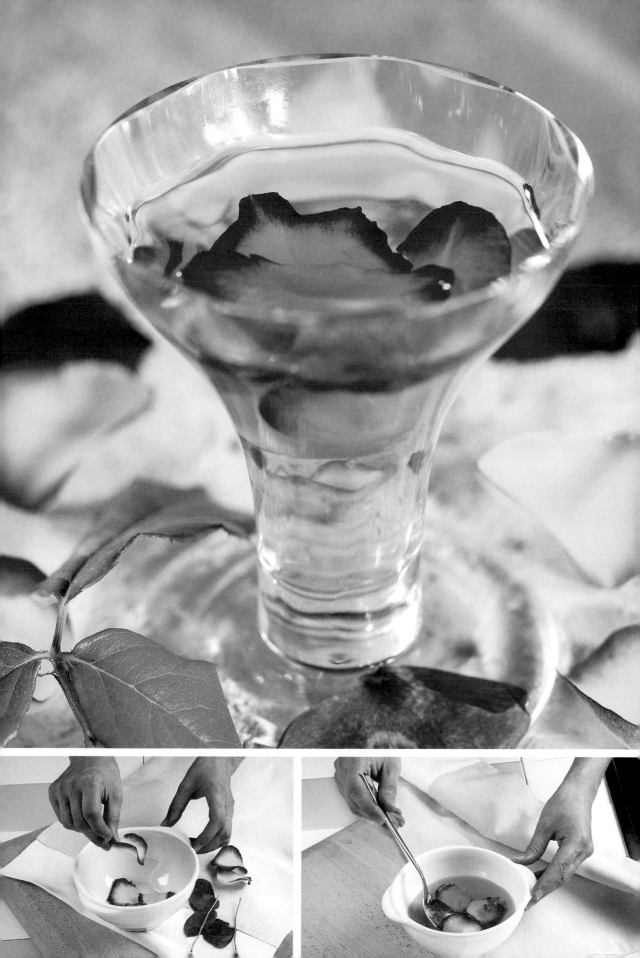

Herbs for Healing Baths

These are some of the most helpful medicinal plants you can enjoy in your bath. Here is a list of the healing properties they offer when they are used in warm bathwater:

- **Calendula.** The leaves of this plant are well known for their skin-healing properties and are found in many medicinal creams. The leaves can be used in warm baths to improve wound healing and help fade scars. They're also good for treating varicose veins and improving circulation.

- **Chamomile.** This herb is one of the most effective and common ingredients in personal-care and beauty products. It is excellent in hair rinses, eye rubs and face cleansers, and it softens skin. Both the dried flowers and the leaves can be used in baths.

- **Dandelion.** The fresh leaves are very rich in vitamin A and have cleansing properties that are ideal for enhancing your bath.

- **Linden.** Linden leaves, also known as tilia or lime leaves, contain vitamins and essential oils that moisturize the skin and improve its appearance. Linden flowers help heal the itchiness and broken skin associated with eczema.

- **Poppy.** This flower's soothing, relaxing properties make it ideal for relieving circulatory problems. The medicinal components in poppies are also helpful for smoothing out wrinkles.

- **Sempervivum.** The leaves of this succulent are considered invaluable for reducing skin inflammation, so they are a soothing and nourishing addition to baths.

- **Spearmint.** The leaves of this plant are antibacterial and refreshing. Used in the bath, they can heal minor skin rashes.

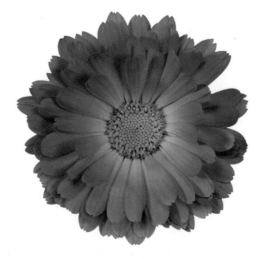

Skin-Softening Milk Bath

Milk baths are an ancient beauty treatment that make skin silky and youthful looking. The softening effect of this bath is very soothing for sensitive or inflamed skin.

Best for: Dry, sensitive or irritated skin

Tips: Powdered milk (also called dry milk) is commonly found in the baking aisle at the supermarket. You can store it in a tightly sealed airtight container in a cool, dark place for up to a year. If you keep it in the freezer, it will last even longer.

Buy organic wheat bran to make this infusion. It is free of pesticide and fungicide residues, two types of toxins you definitely don't want to put on your skin.

- Cotton drawstring bag (see tips, page 290)

3½ oz	powdered milk (see tips, at left)	100 g
4 cups	warm water	1 L
3	drops rose essential oil (see tip, page 281)	3
1¾ oz	wheat bran (see tips, at left)	50 g

1. In a large bowl, combine powdered milk and warm water. Stir until milk is dissolved.

2. Add milk mixture and rose essential oil to warm bathwater. Place bran in bag. Tie tightly and add to bathwater. Soak in bath for 15 to 20 minutes, squeezing bag from time to time under water.

Bath for Oily Skin

Natural astringents are the key to gently keeping oily skin in check. This mélange of herbs, fruit peels, flowers and barks is a natural alternative to overly drying commercial products.

Best for: Oily skin

Tips: Use a sharp vegetable peeler to cut the zest off a lemon quickly and easily.

Peppermint is a natural antibacterial agent. It acts as an astringent as well, tightening and firming up skin.

Note: Always measure accurately when you're making homemade beauty products. See page 53 for tips.

- Large fine-mesh sieve

¾ oz	dried witch hazel bark (see tips, page 272)	25 g
¾ oz	lemon zest (see tips, at left)	25 g
¾ oz	dried white oak bark	25 g
¾ oz	dried peppermint leaves (see tips, at left)	25 g
¾ oz	dried orange blossoms	25 g
4 cups	water	1 L

1. In a large heatproof bowl, combine witch hazel bark, lemon zest, white oak bark, peppermint leaves and orange blossoms. Set aside.

2. In a large saucepan, bring water just to a boil; pour over witch hazel mixture. Cover and let stand for 20 minutes.

3. Place fine-mesh sieve over another large heatproof bowl. Strain infusion into bowl, discarding solids.

4. Add infusion to warm bathwater. Soak in bath for 15 to 20 minutes.

Bath for Dry Skin

Dry skin can be so itchy and uncomfortable. This easy herbal bath helps restore moisture to the skin.

Best for: Dry skin

Tip: The comfrey plant contains allantoin, which is very effective for treating skin inflammation, wounds and premature wrinkles. Comfrey is a perennial herb, which means you can plant it once and it will come up every year. If you don't have it in your garden, you can buy dried comfrey leaves and roots at an herbalist's shop or online.

Note: Always measure accurately when you're making homemade beauty products. See page 53 for tips.

- Large fine-mesh sieve

¾ oz	dried comfrey leaves (see tip, at left)	25 g
¾ oz	dried comfrey root	25 g
¾ oz	dried chamomile flowers (see tips, page 260)	25 g
¾ oz	dried rose petals	25 g
¾ oz	dried rosemary leaves (see tip, page 281)	25 g
4 cups	water	1 L

1. In a large heatproof bowl, combine comfrey leaves, comfrey root, chamomile flowers, rose petals and rosemary leaves. Set aside.

2. In a large saucepan, bring water just to a boil; pour over comfrey mixture. Cover and let steep for 10 minutes.

3. Place fine-mesh sieve over another large heatproof bowl. Strain infusion into bowl, discarding solids.

4. Add infusion to warm bathwater. Soak in bath for 15 to 20 minutes.

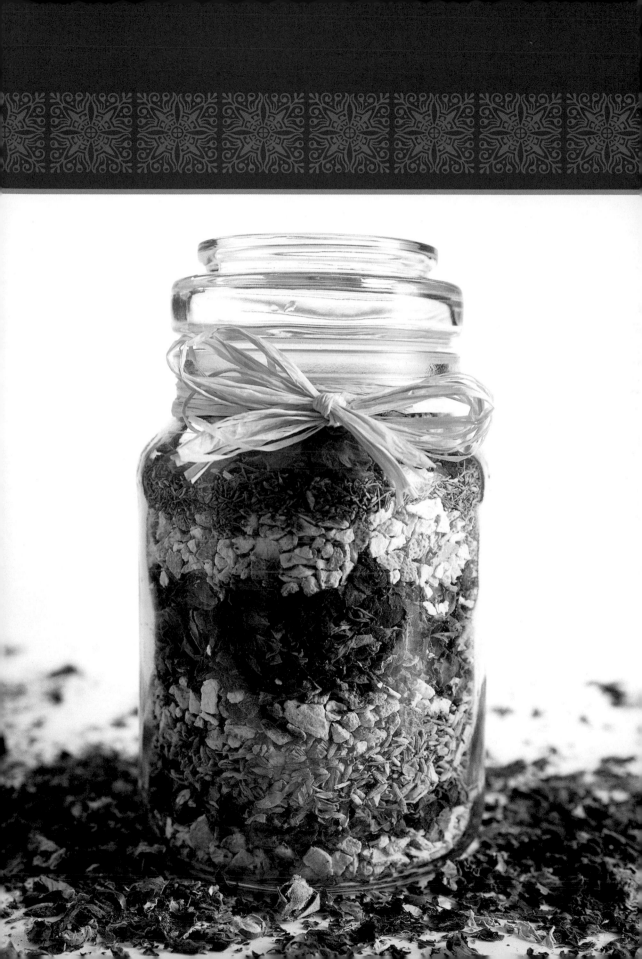

Cold- and Flu-Fighting Bath

This soothing bath will help strengthen your immune system in the winter months, protecting you from colds and the flu. It's also great if you already feel sick; it will help decongest your nose and respiratory tract and make breathing easier.

Best for: Colds and flu

Tip: If you like, you can substitute fresh ginger for the dried in this recipe. Peel and slice a 1-inch (2.5 cm) chunk of fresh ginger and add it to the lavender mixture.

Note: Always measure accurately when you're making homemade beauty products. See page 53 for tips.

• Large fine-mesh sieve

4 cups	water	1 L
¼ cup	dried lavender flowers (see tip, page 302)	60 mL
¼ cup	dried rosemary leaves	60 mL
2 tbsp	dried eucalyptus leaves	30 mL
2 tbsp	ground ginger (see tip, at left)	30 mL

1. In a large saucepan, combine water, lavender flowers, rosemary leaves, eucalyptus leaves and ginger. Bring just to a boil; remove from heat. Cover and let stand for 10 minutes.

2. Place fine-mesh sieve over a large heatproof bowl. Strain infusion into bowl, discarding solids.

3. Add infusion to warm bathwater. Soak in bath for 15 to 20 minutes.

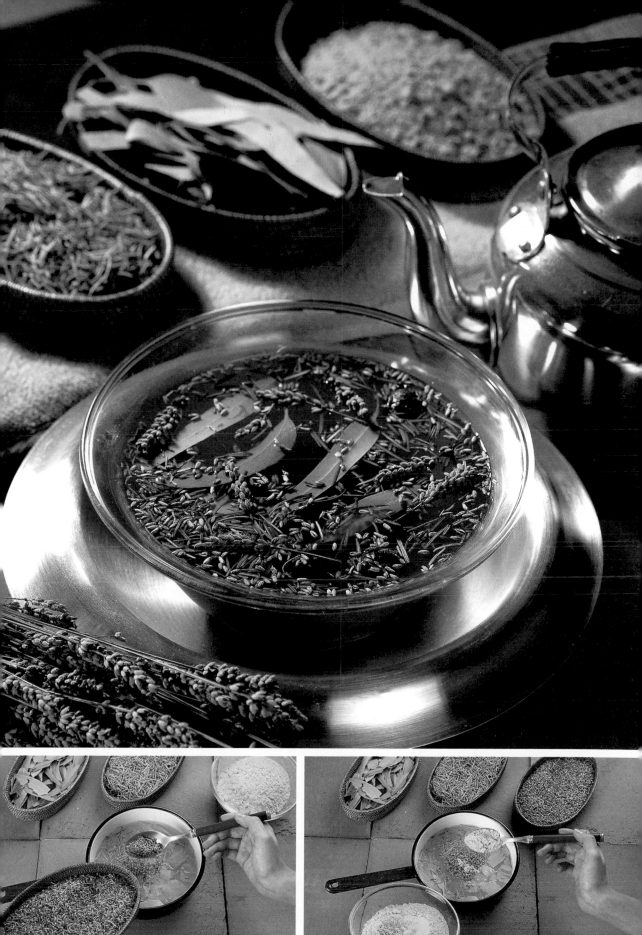

Eczema-Soothing Bath

Linden, also known as tilia or lime (but not the same as limes in the citrus family), is an effective skin soother. It is also a calming agent, so it reduces stress.

Best for: Eczema

Tips: Gourmet tea shops often sell small cotton drawstring bags for steeping teas. If you don't have one (or yours is too small to accommodate the flowers), place the ingredients on a double-thickness square of cheesecloth and tie with cotton string to make a bundle.

Make sure your bathwater is not too hot for this soak. Overly hot water can strip the natural oils from your skin, making eczema worse.

- Cotton drawstring bag (see tips, at left)

1¾ oz	dried linden flowers (see tips, page 292)	50 g

1. Place linden flowers in bag. Tie tightly.
2. Add to warm bathwater (see tips, at left). Soak in bath for 15 minutes.

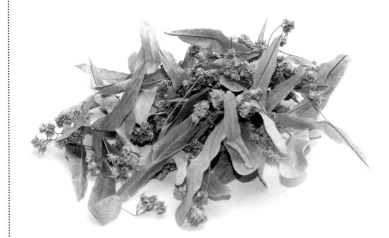

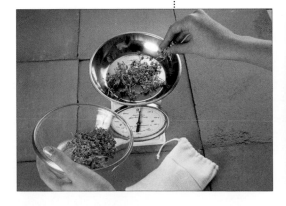

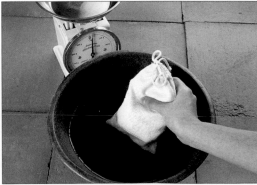

Mint and Lemon Bath Oil

This excellent all-purpose bath oil purifies and tones skin, stimulates circulation and clears out congestion in the respiratory system.

Best for: All skin types

Tip: Jojoba oil is a wonderful addition to bath oils because it is moisturizing. Choose cold-pressed 100% jojoba oil, which contains the largest quantity of bioactive substances.

Note: Always measure accurately when you're making homemade beauty products. See page 53 for tips.

½ cup	jojoba oil (see tip, at left)	125 mL
10	drops spearmint essential oil (see tip, page 294)	10
10	drops peppermint essential oil	10
10	drops lemon essential oil	10

1. In a small bowl, stir together jojoba oil, spearmint essential oil, peppermint essential oil and lemon essential oil.

2. Add to warm bathwater. Soak in bath for 15 to 20 minutes.

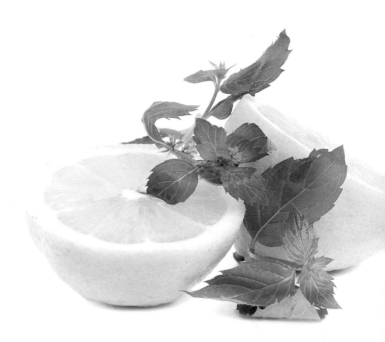

Rejuvenating Bath

Patchouli and sandalwood have warm, rich scents that rev you up. Combined with sage, thyme and eucalyptus, they create a fragrant bath that will make you feel revitalized.

Best for: Soothing tired skin and increasing energy

Tips: Look for a reliable source of dried medicinal herbs, such as an herbalist's shop or a reputable online dealer. Make sure it's a business with high turnover, to ensure you're getting the freshest, most effective herbs possible.

This bath is also pleasant if you have a cold. The menthol scent of the eucalyptus can help make your sore, stuffy nose feel a bit better.

Note: Always measure accurately when you're making homemade beauty products. See page 53 for tips.

- Large fine-mesh sieve

4 cups	water	1 L
¾ oz	dried sage leaves (see tips, at left)	25 g
¾ oz	dried thyme leaves	25 g
¾ oz	dried eucalyptus leaves	25 g
3	drops patchouli essential oil (see tip, page 294)	3
3	drops sandalwood essential oil	3

1. In a large saucepan, combine water, sage leaves, thyme leaves and eucalyptus leaves. Bring just to a boil; remove from heat. Cover and let stand for 20 minutes.

2. Place fine-mesh sieve over a large heatproof bowl. Strain infusion into bowl, discarding solids.

3. Add infusion, patchouli essential oil and sandalwood essential oil to warm bathwater. Soak in bath for 15 to 20 minutes.

Tips for Preparing Baths

- Make your bath a soothing ritual: create a warm, calming atmosphere in the bathroom with relaxing music and soft lighting.

- Soak for 15 to 20 minutes only. Longer baths can be bad for the heart and circulatory system, and may cause the skin to swell excessively and damage its protective acidic coating.

- Make sure that the bathwater temperature does not exceed 96.8°F (36°C), or just below normal human body temperature. When the water is too hot, the bath loses its power to relax you and can make your heart race.

- Always dilute herbal infusions and essential oils by adding them to bathwater. Don't apply them directly to your skin.

- Limit the number of baths you take to two or three per week. Shower the rest of the time.

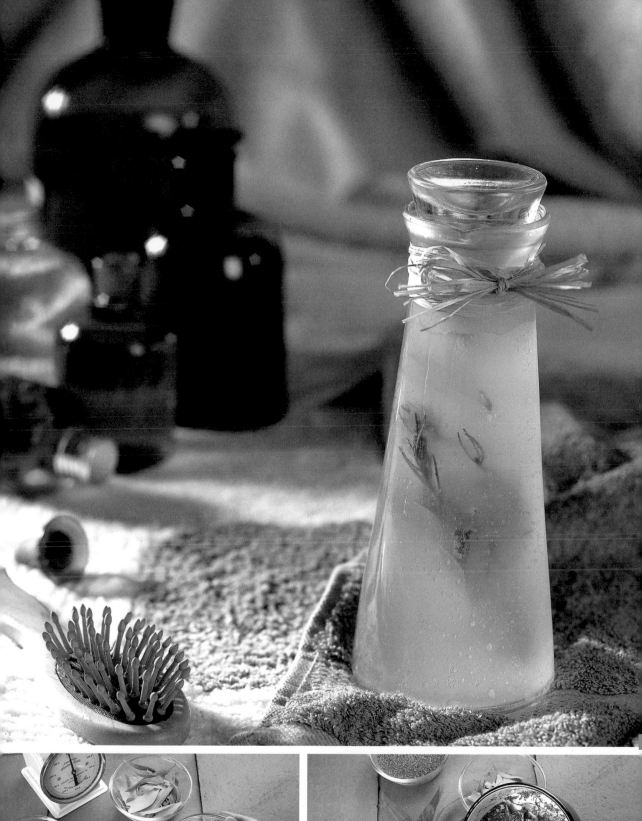
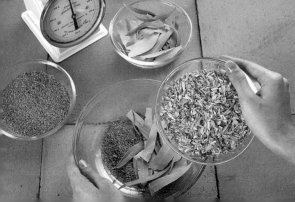
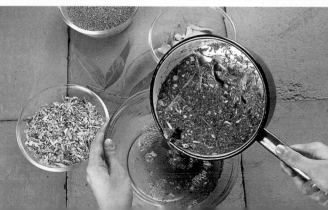

Sleep-Inducing Bath Oil

This is a good bath to take just before bedtime, since it drains away tension and eases you into sleep mode for the night.

Best for: Relaxing and inducing sleep

Tip: Buy essential oils sold in dark bottles. Exposure to light can reduce the potency of their medicinal herbal components. Store the bottles in a cool, dark place to keep them fresh.

Note: Always measure accurately when you're making homemade beauty products. See page 53 for tips.

½ cup	olive oil (see tips, page 296)	125 mL
4	drops chamomile essential oil (see tip, at left)	4
2	drops lavender essential oil	2
2	drops marjoram essential oil	2
2	drops sandalwood essential oil	2

1. In a small bowl, stir together olive oil, chamomile essential oil, lavender essential oil, marjoram essential oil and sandalwood essential oil.

2. Add to warm bathwater. Soak in bath for 15 to 20 minutes.

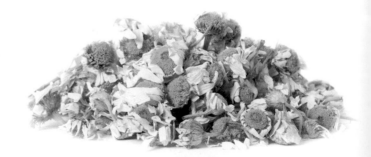

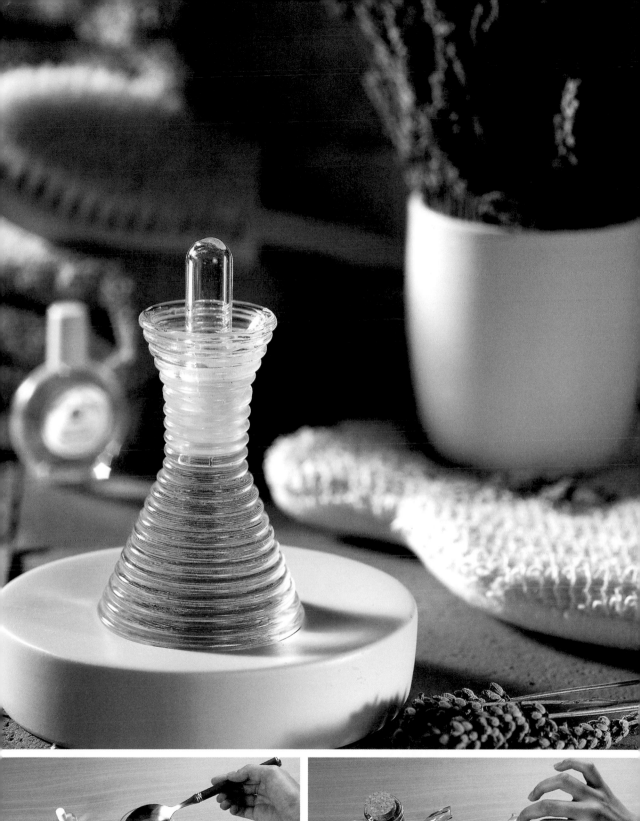
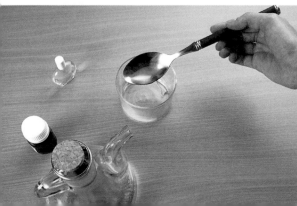
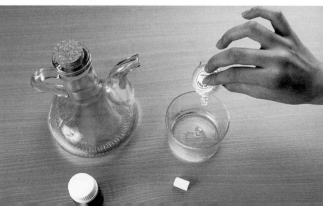

Almond, Rose and Orange Bath Oil

This oil is a delightful softener that smooths dry, damaged skin. It is especially rich and nourishing in the winter, when cold, wind and indoor heating all take their toll.

Best for: Dry, damaged skin

Tips: Sweet almond oil, like other nut oils, can perish quickly if stored in a warm place or exposed to direct sunlight. Keep the bottle in a dark, cool cupboard and use it up within a couple of months of opening.

Rose water is commonly used in Middle Eastern, Mediterranean, Indian and North African cuisine, so look for bottles of this fragrant essence at specialty grocery stores.

- Small dark glass bottle with lid

6 tbsp	sweet almond oil (see tips, at left)	90 mL
2 tbsp	rose water (see tips, at left)	30 mL
3	drops orange essential oil (see tip, page 294)	3

1. In a small bowl, stir together sweet almond oil, rose water and orange essential oil.
2. Pour into bottle. Add a few drops of oil mixture to warm bathwater. Soak in bath for 15 to 20 minutes.
3. Store bottle in a cool, dark place for up to 2 months. Shake before each use to recombine.

Mediterranean Bath Oil

Olive oil is so nutritious, whether you eat it or apply it to your skin. It is one of the best Mediterranean beauty secrets.

Best for: All skin types

Tips: Cold-pressed extra-virgin oils are the purest and most unadulterated type you can buy for making homemade beauty treatments. They are worth the higher price tag.

Wheat germ oil is a good source of vitamin E, but it can go rancid quickly if stored at room temperature. Keep it in the fridge to extend the shelf life.

- Dark glass bottle with lid

1/2 cup	olive oil (see tips, at left)	125 mL
1/2 cup	sunflower seed oil	125 mL
1/2 cup	wheat germ oil (see tips, at left)	125 mL
1 tbsp	lavender essential oil (see tip, page 294)	15 mL
1 tbsp	basil essential oil	15 mL

1. In a medium bowl, stir together olive oil, sunflower seed oil, wheat germ oil, lavender essential oil and basil essential oil.
2. Pour into bottle. Add a few drops of oil mixture to warm bathwater. Soak in bath for 15 to 20 minutes.
3. Store bottle in a cool, dark place for up to 2 months. Shake before each use to recombine.

Macadamia Moisturizing Bath Oil

Macadamia nuts are good for you (and delicious). So is their oil, which is especially wonderful for hydrating the skin.

Best for: Dry skin

Tip: Macadamia nut oil contains a large number of antioxidants, so it will keep well at room temperature for a year or more. It doesn't require refrigeration like some other nut oils.

Note: Always measure accurately when you're making homemade beauty products. See page 53 for tips.

½ cup	macadamia nut oil (see tip, at left)	125 mL
2	drops chamomile essential oil (see tip, page 294)	2
2	drops lavender essential oil	2
2	drops carrot seed essential oil	2
2	drops geranium essential oil	2

1. In a small bowl, stir together macadamia nut oil, chamomile essential oil, lavender essential oil, carrot seed essential oil and geranium essential oil.

2. Add to warm bathwater. Soak in bath for 15 to 20 minutes.

Rose Hip Seed Bath Oil

Rose hip seeds contain a huge amount of fatty acids that are good for the skin. The seeds are considered one of the best natural antiaging ingredients.

Best for: Dry skin

Tip: Rose hip seed oil is very rich, so it's not recommended for use on oily skin or for people who have acne.

- Dark glass bottle with lid

½ cup	sunflower seed oil (see tips, opposite)	125 mL
½ cup	sesame oil	125 mL
½ cup	apricot kernel oil	125 mL
1 tbsp	rose hip seed oil (see tip, at left)	15 mL

1. In a medium bowl, stir together sunflower seed oil, sesame oil, apricot kernel oil and rose hip seed oil.

2. Pour into bottle. Add a few drops of oil mixture to warm bathwater. Soak in bath for 15 to 20 minutes.

3. Store bottle in a cool, dark place for up to 2 months. Shake before each use to recombine.

Basil Body Oil

You may not think of basil when you think of beauty products, but it has a lovely, slightly spicy scent. This oil will retain its fresh fragrance for months.

Best for: Normal or dry skin

Tips: Basil flowers are abundant at the height of summer, and removing them actually helps the plant become fuller and bear more leaves.

When you strain the finished oil, make sure to remove every last fragment of the flowers. Left in the oil, they will rot and spoil the product. The cheesecloth in the sieve should help capture all the tiny pieces.

Note: Always measure accurately when you're making homemade beauty products. See page 53 for tips.

- Two 4-cup (1 L) canning jars with lids
- Fine-mesh sieve lined with cheesecloth

2	handfuls fresh basil flowers (see tips, at left)	2
2 cups	sweet almond oil (see tips, page 296)	500 mL

1. Place basil flowers in one of the jars. Pour in sweet almond oil, turning jar to ensure flowers are completely submerged. Seal tightly and let stand in a cool, dark place for 1 month.

2. Place fine-mesh sieve over a medium bowl; strain oil into bowl, discarding solids.

3. Pour into clean jar. Rub a small amount of oil over skin after bathing. Store jar in a cool, dark place for up to 3 months.

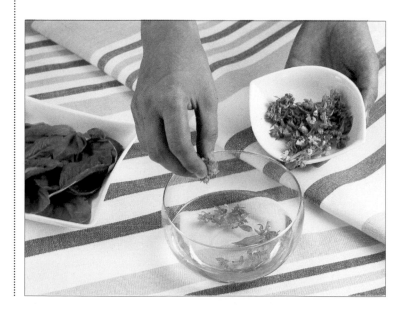

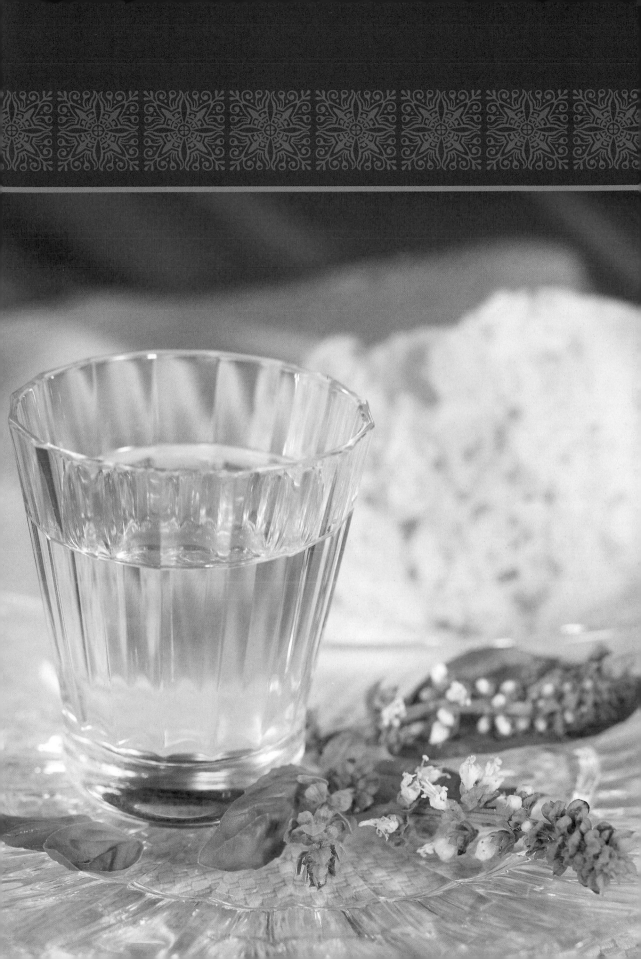

Rose, Honey and Almond Body Lotion

The seeds in fresh quinces are very high in pectin, which creates a gel when cooked with liquid. It gives this lotion a thicker, more viscous texture than other after-bath lotions.

Best for: All skin types

Tip: To make quince gel, you need about 25 seeds from a ripe quince. (If you can't find the ripe fruit, Middle Eastern markets often carry packets of the dried seeds, which can be substituted.) In a small saucepan, combine the seeds with ½ cup (125 mL) distilled water and bring to a boil, stirring constantly. Remove the pan from the heat and stir for a minute or two or until the liquid forms a gel.

- Small glass jar with lid

1 tbsp	quince gel (see tip, at left)	15 mL
1½ tsp	sweet almond oil (see tips, page 296)	7 mL
1 tsp	strong brewed chamomile tea	5 mL
¼ tsp	liquid honey (see tips, page 258)	1 mL
1	drop rose water (see tips, page 296)	1

1. In a small bowl, stir together quince gel, sweet almond oil, chamomile tea, honey and rose water until well combined.

2. Spoon into jar. Rub a small amount of lotion over skin after bathing. Store jar in a cool, dark place for up to 2 months.

Poppy After-Bath Body Lotion

Poppies are great wrinkle fighters and sunburn soothers. Here, they team up with sweet almond oil to make a potent emollient lotion.

Best for: Normal or dry skin

Tip: Poppies are pretty to grow in the garden, and the plants self-seed, meaning you don't need to plant new ones every year. They are useful additions to a medicinal plant garden.

Note: Always measure accurately when you're making homemade beauty products. See page 53 for tips.

- Two 6-cup (1.5 L) canning jars with lids
- Large fine-mesh sieve lined with cheesecloth

1¾ oz	fresh poppy petals (see tip, at left)	50 g
4 cups	sweet almond oil (see tips, page 296)	1 L

1. Place poppy petals in one of the jars. Pour in sweet almond oil, turning jar to ensure petals are completely submerged. Seal tightly and let stand in a cool, dark place for 2 weeks.

2. Place fine-mesh sieve over a large bowl; strain oil into bowl, discarding solids.

3. Pour into clean jar. Rub a small amount of oil over skin after bathing. Store jar in a cool, dark place for up to 2 months.

Almond Body Milk

Almonds are rich in oil and nutrients that soften and nourish skin well. They also lighten and brighten the skin, making it look radiant.

Best for: All skin types

Tips: Blanched almonds have been boiled briefly in water to remove their papery brown skins. Look for them where baking ingredients are sold.

Distilled water has been purified through the process of distillation; in other words, the water is boiled, and the condensation (which is free of impurities) is collected in a clean vessel. Bottles of it are readily available in supermarkets.

- Food processor or mortar and pestle
- Fine-mesh sieve lined with cheesecloth
- Large glass jar with lid

1 oz	blanched almonds (see tips, at left)	30 g
2 cups	distilled water (see tips, at left)	500 mL

1. In food processor, purée almonds until they form a fine paste. (Or in mortar with pestle, grind almonds until they form a fine paste.) Transfer to a medium bowl.
2. Stir distilled water into almond paste until smooth and well combined.
3. Place fine-mesh sieve over another medium bowl; strain almond mixture into bowl, discarding solids.
4. Pour into jar. Rub body milk over skin after bathing. Store jar in a cool, dark place for up to 1 month.

Rose Body Milk

This hydrating combination smells so pretty you won't need any perfume.

Best for: All skin types

Tips: To make the rosemary infusion, pour 1/2 cup (125 mL) of boiling water over 1 1/2 tsp (7 mL) of fresh rosemary leaves. Cover and let stand for 10 minutes. Strain through a fine-mesh sieve and let cool before adding to the recipe.

Benzoin is a reddish-brown resin extracted from a tree that grows in southeast Asia. Soaking the resin in alcohol creates a tincture that smells a bit like vanilla.

- Large dark glass bottle with lid

3 1/4 cups	rose water	810 mL
1/2 cup	rosemary infusion (see tips, at left)	125 mL
2 tbsp	tincture of benzoin (see tips, at left)	30 mL
1 tbsp	rose essential oil (see tip, page 294)	15 mL

1. In a large bowl, stir rose water with rosemary infusion.
2. Stirring constantly, gradually add tincture of benzoin, then rose essential oil. Stir until well combined.
3. Pour into bottle. Rub a small amount of body milk over skin after bathing. Store bottle in a cool, dark place for up to 2 months.

Rosemary and Vinegar Rubbing Lotion

This cool rub is refreshing on clean skin and is excellent for a massage after a relaxing bath.

Best for: All skin types

Tips: Look for a reliable source of dried medicinal herbs, such as an herbalist's shop or a reputable online dealer. Make sure it's a business with high turnover, to ensure you're getting the freshest, most effective herbs possible.

A pinching massage is good for stimulating circulation. Gently pinch and pull the skin upward as you massage the lotion into the skin on your legs, arms and torso.

Note: Always measure accurately when you're making homemade beauty products. See page 53 for tips.

- Fine-mesh sieve
- Large glass bottle with lid

2	sprigs fresh rosemary (or 1 tsp/5 mL dried rosemary leaves), see tips, at left	2
1 cup	boiling water	250 mL
	Cider vinegar	

1. Place rosemary in a small heatproof bowl. Pour boiling water over top; cover and let stand for 5 minutes.

2. Place fine-mesh sieve over a glass measuring cup; strain infusion into measuring cup, discarding solids. Let cool.

3. Check measurement of liquid in cup; add an equal amount of cider vinegar.

4. Pour into bottle. Rub a small amount of lotion all over body after bathing. Store bottle in a cool, dark place for up to 2 months.

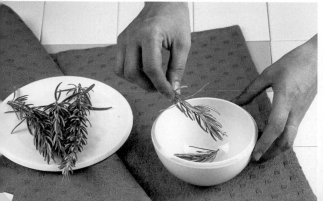
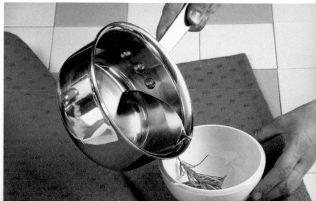

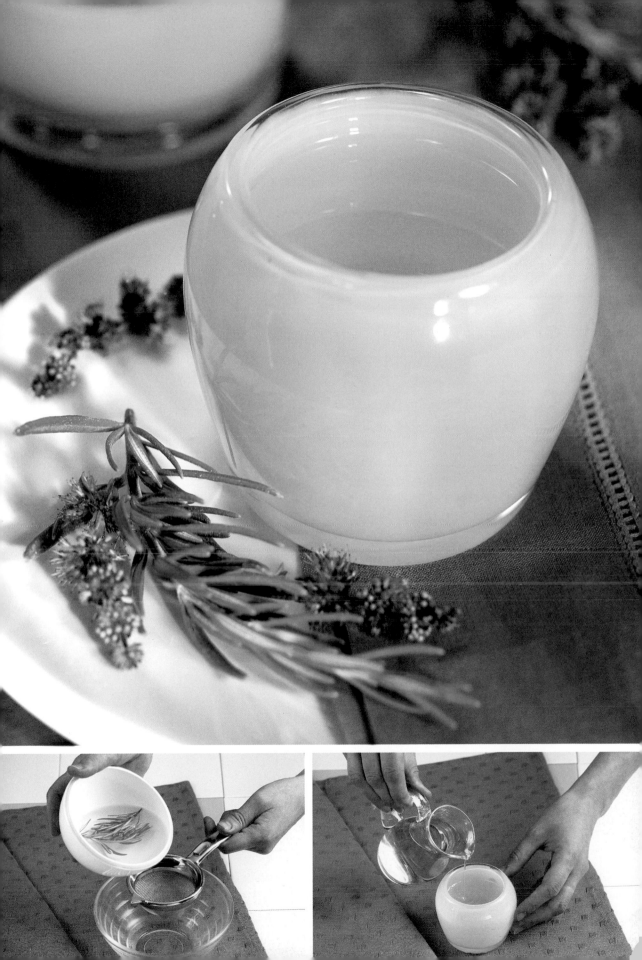

Calendula Body Oil

This is a delicate oil that can be used both as a massage oil for dry skin, especially for children, and as a flavoring in cooking.

Best for: Normal or dry skin

Tips: Calendulas, or marigolds, are versatile medicinal plants that have many healing properties, especially for the skin. They are really easy to grow in the garden or in pots, and they love just about any location, from sunny to shady.

Make sure the calendula flowers you use are in full bloom. They will give your body oil the most active compounds.

Note: Always measure accurately when you're making homemade beauty products. See page 53 for tips.

- Fine-mesh sieve lined with cheesecloth
- Glass jar with lid

2	handfuls fresh calendula flowers (see tips, at left)	2
2 cups	olive oil (see tips, page 296)	500 mL

1. Place calendula flowers in a medium bowl. Pour in olive oil, stirring to ensure flowers are completely submerged. Cover and let stand in a warm, sunny place for 1 month.

2. Place fine-mesh sieve over another medium bowl; strain oil into bowl, discarding solids.

3. Pour into glass jar. Rub a small amount of oil over skin after bathing. Store jar in a cool, dark place for up to 2 months.

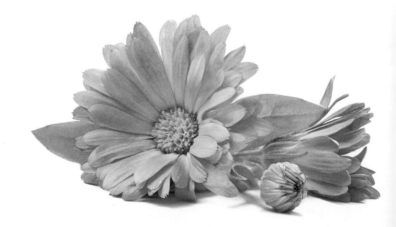

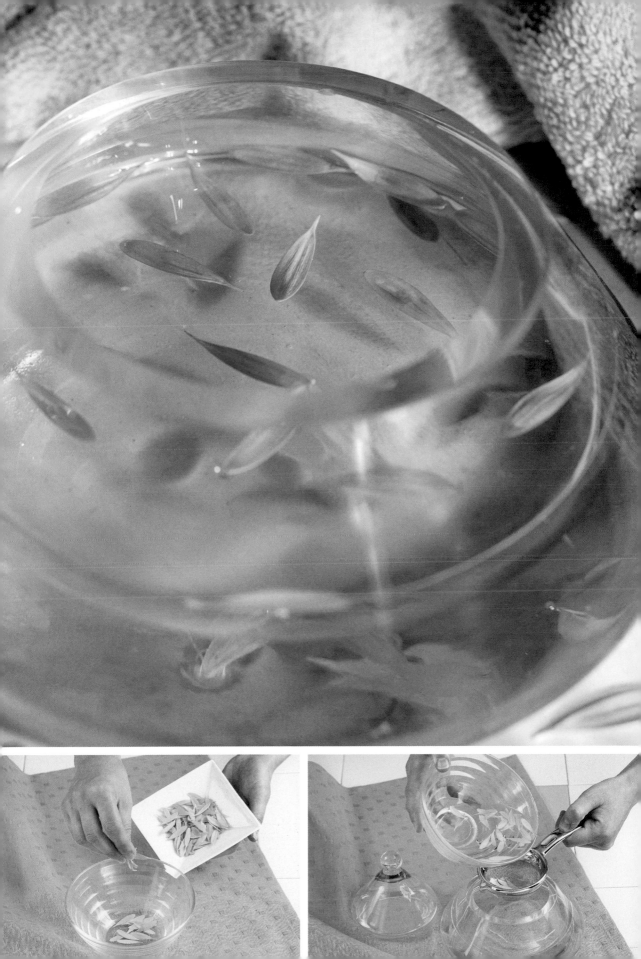

Chamomile Body Oil

Grassy, fresh-smelling chamomile is definitely a plant you want in a medicinal herb garden. Here, it works with cider vinegar and sweet almond oil to smooth skin after a bath.

Best for: All skin types

Tip: You can dry chamomile flowers very easily if you grow the plants at home. Gather a bunch of the flowers and tie string tightly around the stems, about 2 inches (5 cm) up from the bottom of the bunch. (It's important to tie it tightly because the bunch will loosen as it dries.) Hang the bunch upside down in a cool, dry place for a week or two until the flowers are completely dehydrated and crisp to the touch. Gently remove the flowers from the stems and store in an airtight container in a cool, dry place.

Note: Always measure accurately when you're making homemade beauty products. See page 53 for tips.

- Mortar and pestle
- Two glass jars with lids
- Fine-mesh sieve

¼ cup	fresh or dried chamomile flowers (see tip, at left)	60 mL
2 tbsp	cider vinegar	30 mL
	Sweet almond oil (see tips, page 296)	

1. In mortar with pestle, mash chamomile flowers with vinegar until moistened. Spoon chamomile mixture into one of the jars.

2. Pour in enough sweet almond oil to cover chamomile mixture. Seal tightly and let stand in a warm place for 3 weeks, shaking jar once every day.

3. Place fine-mesh sieve over a small bowl; strain oil into bowl, discarding solids.

4. Pour into clean jar. Rub a small amount of oil over skin after bathing. Store jar in a cool, dark place for up to 2 months.

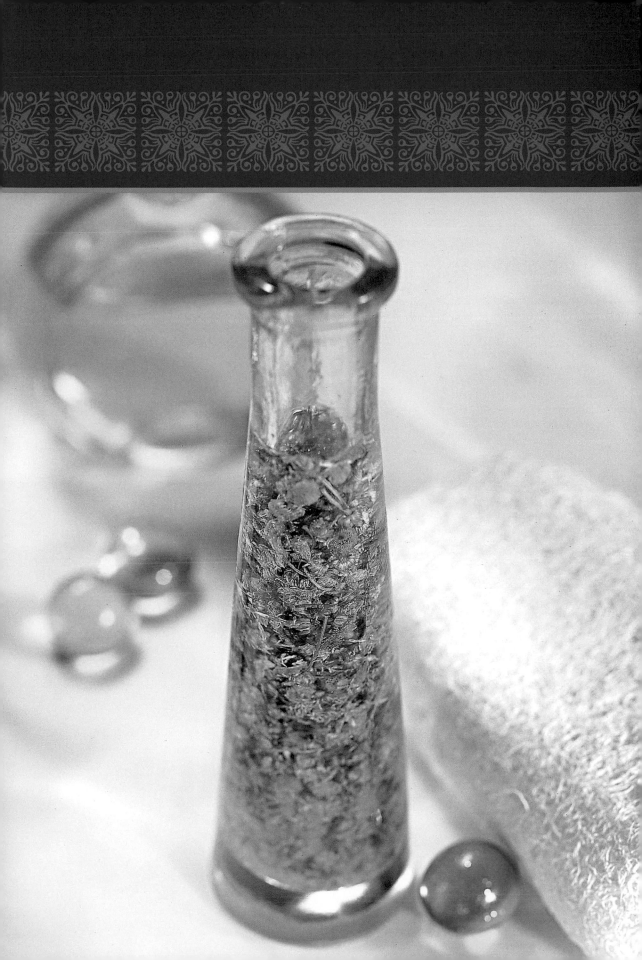

Baby Powder

This is a delicate, talc-free powder that soothes babies' irritated skin. The myrrh gives it a gentle scent; avoid the temptation to add more aromatic essential oils or perfumes.

Best for: Skin irritated by diaper rash

Tips: The bark of the slippery elm tree (*Ulmus rubra*) contains slick, mucilaginous compounds that help wounded skin heal. It makes a soothing addition to this diaper rash formula.

Myrrh is a perfume that was prized in Ancient Egypt. It is a tree resin that has a warm, earthy, smoky aroma. This recipe uses the powdered, ground resin so that it can be mixed with the other ingredients and dusted on the skin.

- Glass jar with lid

½ cup	kaolin clay (see tips, page 323)	125 mL
½ cup	slippery elm bark powder (see tips, at left)	125 mL
¼ cup	myrrh powder (see tips, at left)	60 mL

1. In a medium bowl, whisk together clay, slippery elm bark powder and myrrh powder.
2. Spoon into jar. Dust over irritated skin after cleansing. Store jar in a cool, dry place for up to 2 months.

After-Bath Dusting Powder

This old-fashioned dusting powder keeps skin nice and dry after a leisurely bath. Orris root gives it a gentle violet-like scent that's clean and pleasant. If you want a little more perfume in your powder, you can dress it up with a few drops of your favorite essential oil.

Best for: All skin types

Tip: Orris root powder and rose powder are available online at shops that specialize in medicinal herbs. If you can't find them, you can buy the dried root or petals and grind them yourself using a small food processor or blender (just make sure it's one you plan to use only for homemade beauty products, not for preparing food).

- Glass jar with lid

3½ oz	kaolin clay (see tips, page 323)	100 g
¾ oz	orris root powder (see tip, at left)	25 g
¾ oz	finely ground oat flour	25 g
¾ oz	rose powder	25 g

1. In a medium bowl, stir together clay, orris root powder, oat flour and rose powder. Let stand for about 1 hour, breaking up any lumps that form.
2. Pour into jar. Dust a small amount of powder over towel-dried skin after bathing. Store jar in a cool, dry place for up to 3 months.

Stained Glass Soap

Two different colored soap mixtures come together to make one pretty multihued bar. This technique is fun and surprisingly straightforward.

Best for: All skin types

Tips: Soap molds come in a wide variety of shapes and sizes. Use whatever shape you like; just make sure you have enough molds to use up the entire batch of soap mixture. Don't have any fancy molds? Try silicone baking pans or ice cube trays in interesting shapes.

You can use all sorts of ingredients as natural colorants in soap. You can buy ready-made colorants at soap-making or cosmetic-supply stores, or experiment with spices, teas, vegetables and fruits. Add a little at a time until you get your desired hue without diluting the soap mixture too much.

Note: Always measure accurately when you're making homemade beauty products. See page 53 for tips.

- Soap molds (see tips, at left)
- Cutting board and sharp chef's knife

1 lb	glycerin soap base (see tips, page 310), coarsely chopped	500 g
2	contrasting natural colorants (see tips, at left)	2
1 tbsp	essential oil of your choice (see tips, page 323)	15 mL

1. Place half of the glycerin soap base in a medium heatproof bowl. Set aside. Pour enough water into a medium saucepan to come about 2 inches (5 cm) up the side; bring to a simmer.

2. Set bowl on saucepan so that bottom of bowl is not touching simmering water; stir until soap base is melted and smooth. Remove bowl from heat. Stir in 1 of the natural colorants and half of the essential oil until well combined. Stir well and pour mixture into soap molds.

3. Let molds stand at room temperature for 30 minutes. Refrigerate for 30 minutes. Let molds stand at room temperature for 10 minutes. Unmold soaps onto cutting board. Using chef's knife, cut into thin strips or chunks. Set aside.

4. Place remaining glycerin soap base in a medium heatproof bowl. Set aside. Pour enough water into a medium saucepan to come about 2 inches (5 cm) up the side; bring to a simmer.

5. Set bowl on saucepan so that bottom of bowl is not touching simmering water; stir until soap base is melted and smooth. Remove bowl from heat. Stir in remaining natural colorant and essential oil until well combined.

6. Stir well and pour mixture into soap molds until about half full. Add reserved soap strips or chunks and top with remaining soap mixture. Tap molds on counter to remove any air bubbles.

7. Let molds stand at room temperature for 30 minutes. Refrigerate for 30 minutes. Let molds stand at room temperature for 10 minutes. Unmold soaps.

Layered Oatmeal Soap

Oatmeal is a gentle exfoliant. It makes an attractive addition to this two-layer bar.

Best for: All skin types

Tips: Soap-making supply stores sell a number of different soap bases. They are often sold under the name melt-and-pour soap because you simply melt them and pour them into molds.

To make rose-scented soap, substitute 6½ oz (200 g) of dried rose petals for the rolled oats. For a lavender version, substitute 4 oz (125 g) of dried lavender flowers for the rolled oats.

Note: Always measure accurately when you're making homemade beauty products. See page 53 for tips.

- Soap molds (see tips, page 309)

1 lb	glycerin soap base (see tips, at left), coarsely chopped	500 g
1	natural colorant (see tips, page 309)	1
1 tbsp	essential oil of your choice (see tips, page 323)	15 mL
4 oz	rolled oats	125 g

1. Place glycerin soap base in a medium heatproof bowl. Set aside.

2. Pour enough water into a medium saucepan to come about 2 inches (5 cm) up the side; bring to a simmer.

3. Set bowl on saucepan so that bottom of bowl is not touching simmering water; stir until soap base is melted and smooth. Remove bowl from heat. Stir in colorant and essential oil until well combined. Stir well and pour about three-quarters of the soap mixture into soap molds until three-quarters full, leaving about one-quarter of the soap mixture in bowl. Set molds aside.

4. Return bowl to saucepan over simmering water. Heat, stirring often, for 5 minutes. Stir in rolled oats. Pour over soap in molds until full.

5. Let molds stand at room temperature for 30 minutes. Refrigerate for 30 minutes.

6. Remove molds from refrigerator and let stand at room temperature for 10 minutes. Unmold soaps.

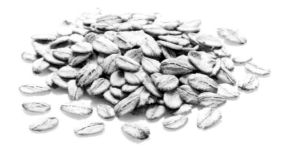

Comfrey Soap

Another simple way to make homemade soap is to grate ready-made bars, melt them and dress them up with the scents and additives you like. Here, a healing comfrey infusion is added to soften and pamper skin.

Best for: Dry, sensitive or irritated skin

Tips: The comfrey plant contains allantoin, which is very effective for treating skin inflammation, wounds and premature wrinkles. Comfrey is a perennial herb, which means you can plant it once and it will come up every year. If you don't have it in your garden, you can buy dried comfrey leaves and roots at an herbalist's shop or online.

This comfrey infusion is also used to make Almond Soap (page 312). Make the entire batch of infusion, and measure out the amount called for in this recipe. Save any leftovers to make a batch or two of Almond Soap.

- Large fine-mesh sieve
- Soap molds (see tips, page 309)

1 cup	grated neutral soap (see tip, page 312)	250 mL

Comfrey Infusion

6 cups	water	1.5 L
2 oz	dried comfrey root (see tips, at left)	60 g
1 oz	dried comfrey leaves	30 g

1. **Comfrey Infusion:** In a large saucepan, combine water, comfrey root and comfrey leaves. Bring to a boil. Cover, reduce heat and simmer for 20 minutes. Remove from heat and let stand for 10 minutes. Place fine-mesh sieve over a large heatproof bowl; strain infusion into bowl, discarding solids.

2. In another large saucepan, combine 3 cups of Comfrey Infusion with soap (save remaining infusion for another use; see tips, at left). Bring soap mixture to a simmer over medium heat, stirring well until soap is melted and smooth. Remove from heat. Let cool slightly.

3. Pour soap mixture into molds. Let cool at room temperature until hardened. Unmold soaps.

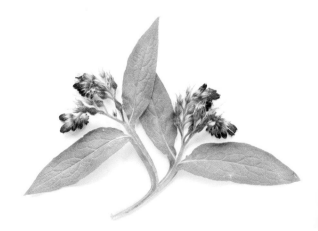

Almond Soap

Ground almonds give this soap exfoliating powers in addition to its fabulous cleansing abilities. By removing dead cells on the surface, it makes skin looks lighter and brighter.

Best for: All skin types

Tip: Neutral soap is pH balanced, so it is neither too acidic nor too alkaline, which complements the slightly acidic natural pH of the skin. Many commercial soaps are highly alkaline, which can strip too much oil from the skin.

Note: Always measure accurately when you're making homemade beauty products. See page 53 for tips.

- Soap molds (see tips, page 309)

1 lb	neutral soap (see tip, at left), cubed	500 g
1 cup	Comfrey Infusion (page 311)	250 mL
8 oz	finely ground almonds	250 g

1. In a medium heatproof bowl, combine soap and Comfrey Infusion (see box, page 82). Set aside.

2. Pour enough water into a medium saucepan to come about 2 inches (5 cm) up the side; bring to a simmer.

3. Set bowl on saucepan so that bottom of bowl is not touching simmering water; stir until soap is melted and smooth. Remove bowl from heat. Stir in ground almonds until well combined. Let cool slightly.

4. Pour soap mixture into molds. Let cool at room temperature until hardened. Unmold soaps.

Storing Homemade Soap

After your soap has hardened and dried, wrap it in waxed paper, fabric or plastic wrap to store it. Never wrap it in foil. No matter how pH balanced your soap is, it will always be a little bit on the alkaline side and will react with foil. Wrapping the bars in paper, fabric or plastic will help maintain their appearance and their perfume.

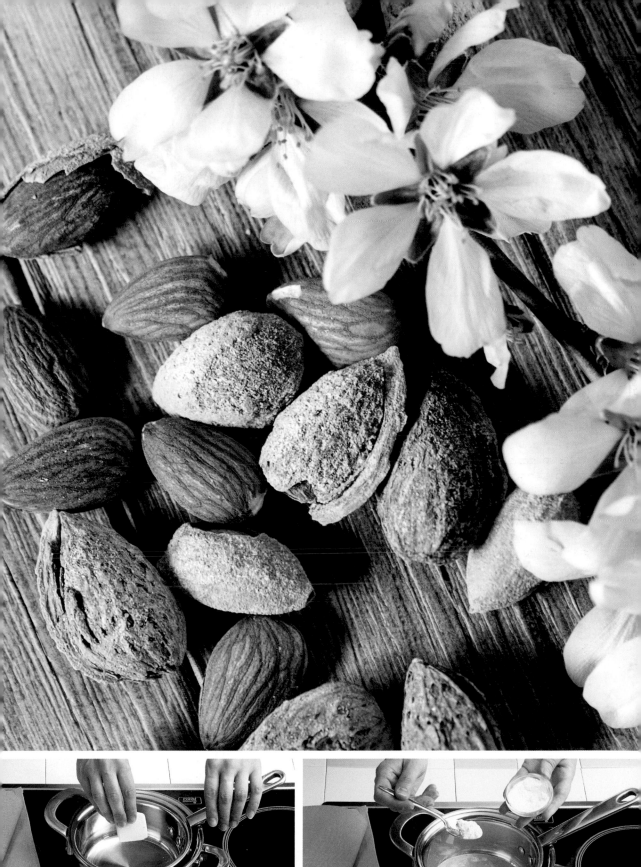

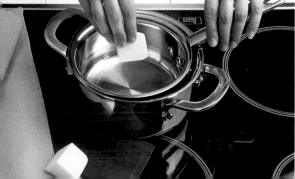

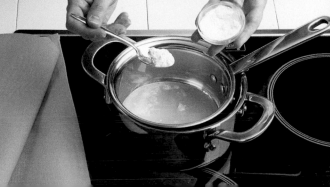

Chamomile Soap

This soap has a delicate herbal scent. If you like a stronger aroma, make a stronger chamomile infusion by adding a larger quantity of the dried flowers.

Best for: All skin types

Tip: Dried chamomile is easy to find at stores that sell medicinal herbs. It's also a very undemanding plant to grow in your garden, so you can grow, harvest and dry your own organic flowers with a minimal amount of effort.

Note: Always measure accurately when you're making homemade beauty products. See page 53 for tips.

- Fine-mesh sieve
- Soap molds (see tips, page 309)

| 1 cup | grated neutral soap (see tip, page 312) | 250 mL |

Chamomile Infusion

| 3 cups | water | 750 mL |
| ⅓ cup | fresh or dried chamomile flowers (see tip, at left) | 75 mL |

1. **Chamomile Infusion:** In a large saucepan, combine water and chamomile flowers. Bring to a boil. Cover, reduce heat and simmer for 10 minutes. Remove from heat and let stand for 10 minutes. Place fine-mesh sieve over a large heatproof bowl; strain infusion into bowl, discarding solids.

2. In another large saucepan, combine Chamomile Infusion with soap. Bring soap mixture to a simmer over medium heat, stirring until soap is melted and smooth. Simmer for 2 minutes, stirring constantly. Remove from heat. Let cool slightly.

3. Pour soap mixture into molds. Let cool at room temperature until hardened. Unmold soaps.

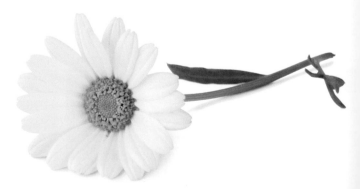

Herbal Soap

This recipe is so easy, and you can customize it with your favorite herbs. If you like, try a combination for a more complex aroma.

Best for: All skin types

Tip: Almost any herb will work in this soap. Strongly aromatic herbs, such as rosemary, spearmint and peppermint, are especially nice. Make an infusion using a heaping spoonful or two of the herbs, and add more if you want a more pronounced scent.

- Soap molds (see tips, page 309)

| ½ cup | herbal infusion (see tip, at left) | 125 mL |
| 1 | bar neutral soap (see tip, page 312), grated | 1 |

1. In a medium heatproof bowl, combine herbal infusion and soap. Set aside.

2. Pour enough water into a medium saucepan to come about 2 inches (5 cm) up the side; bring to a simmer.

3. Set bowl on saucepan so that bottom of bowl is not touching simmering water; stir until soap is melted and smooth. Remove bowl from heat. Let cool slightly.

4. Pour soap mixture into molds. Let cool at room temperature until hardened. Unmold soaps.

Tips for Perfuming Ready-Made Soap

You can customize bars of soap by melting them, adding the essential oil of your choice and remolding the mixture. However, adding scents can be tricky and a little disappointing. The warm soap mixture's alkalinity neutralizes fragrances and can leave you with bars that have only very faint aromas. Even if you add strong essential oils at the last moment, the aroma can be weaker than expected in the finished soap.

One technique that improves the result is to partially cure the mixture to stop the chemical reaction before adding your scent. As the temperature falls, the alkalinity disappears and the aroma of the essential oils remains.

To do this, grate the soap finely. Place it in a heatproof bowl with one-quarter of its volume of water. Melt it over a saucepan of simmering water, stirring until smooth. Remove the bowl from the heat. When the temperature of the mixture drops to 104°F (40°C), add the essential oils, using up to 3% of the total volume of the mixture. Stir well to combine. Then, pour the scented mixture into soap molds.

Strawberry Soap

Juicy and ripe, strawberries make this soap smell almost good enough to eat!

Best for: All skin types

Tip: A potato masher is a useful tool to have on hand for making homemade beauty products. It efficiently mashes fruits and vegetables and gives them a smooth texture so they blend well into mixtures.

Note: Always measure accurately when you're making homemade beauty products. See page 53 for tips.

- Potato masher (see tip, at left)
- Fine-mesh sieve
- Soap molds (see tips, page 309)

4 oz	fresh strawberries, hulled	125 g
1 cup	water	250 mL
4 oz	neutral soap (see tip, page 312), grated	125 g

1. In a small heatproof bowl, combine strawberries and water. Let stand for 5 minutes.

2. Pour enough water into a small saucepan to come about 2 inches (5 cm) up the side; bring to a simmer.

3. Set bowl on saucepan so that bottom of bowl is not touching simmering water; cook strawberry mixture, mashing frequently with potato masher, for 10 minutes or until bubbling and smooth. Remove bowl from heat. Let cool.

4. Place fine-mesh sieve over a medium heatproof bowl; strain strawberries into bowl, pressing with spatula to extract all liquid. Discard solids. Add soap and set aside.

5. Pour enough water into a medium saucepan to come about 2 inches (5 cm) up the side; bring to a simmer.

6. Set bowl on saucepan so that bottom of bowl is not touching simmering water; stir until soap mixture is melted and smooth. Remove bowl from heat. Let mixture cool slightly.

7. Pour soap mixture into molds. Let cool at room temperature until hardened. Unmold soaps.

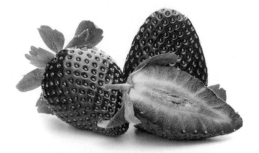

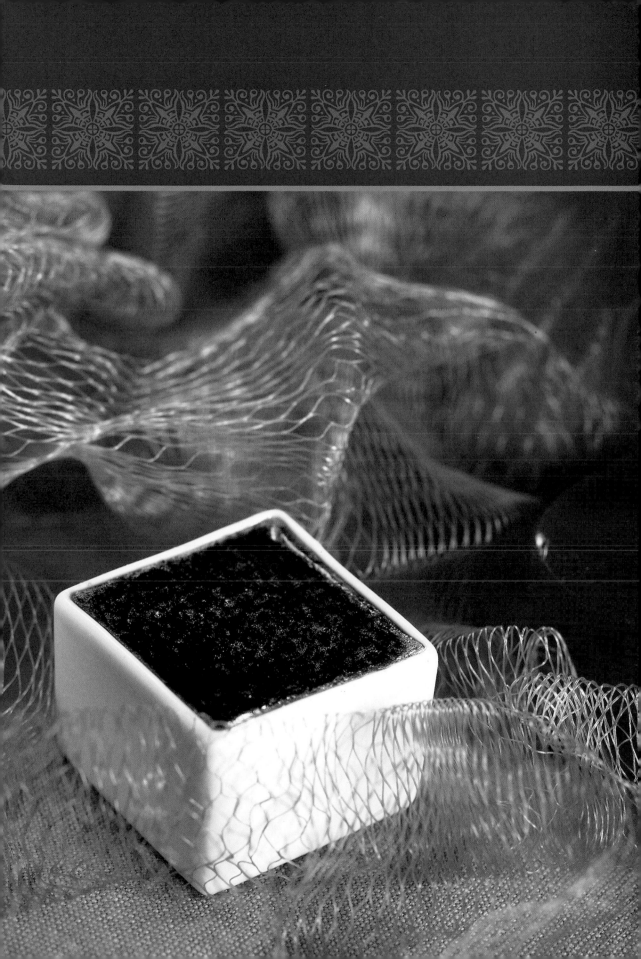

Cornmeal Soap

This is an excellent soap to use after exercising, because the rough cornmeal acts as an exfoliant, stimulating circulation and toning the skin.

Best for: All skin types

Tip: Choose medium or coarsely ground cornmeal for this recipe. Finely ground cornmeal is too powdery to serve as an exfoliant.

Note: Always measure accurately when you're making homemade beauty products. See page 53 for tips.

● Soap molds (see tips, page 309)

1 lb	neutral soap (see tip, page 312), grated	500 g
1 cup	water	250 mL
8 oz	cornmeal (see tip, at left)	250 g

1. In a medium heatproof bowl, combine soap and water. Set aside.

2. Pour enough water into a medium saucepan to come about 2 inches (5 cm) up the side; bring to a simmer.

3. Set bowl on saucepan so that bottom of bowl is not touching simmering water; stir until soap is melted and smooth. Remove bowl from heat. Stir in cornmeal until well combined. Let cool slightly.

4. Pour soap mixture into molds. Let cool at room temperature until hardened. Unmold soaps.

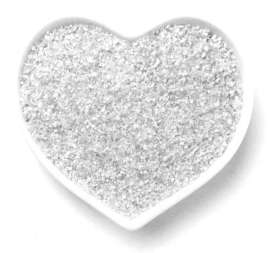

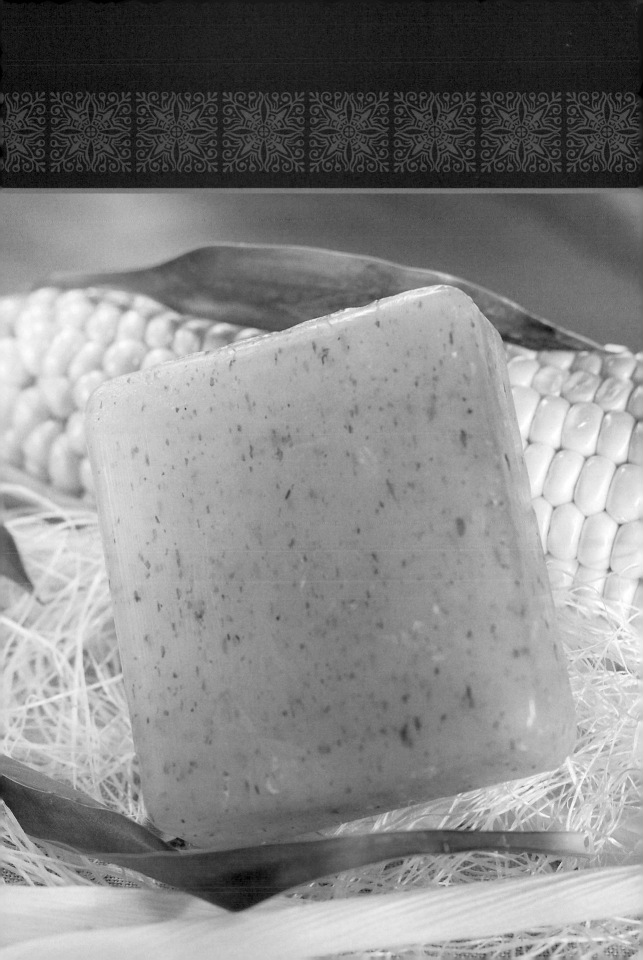

Lavender Soap

Lavender essential oil is known for its health-enhancing, relaxing properties. It relieves anxiety, irritability, stress, headaches and skin problems.

Best for: All skin types

Tips: Brandy can be expensive. Don't splurge on the high-end stuff for this recipe. It requires just a neutral alcohol to draw out the scent of the lavender flowers.

Castile soap is a traditional, simple soap made with olive oil. Some modern versions contain other fats. Look for unscented bars, which will allow the lavender aroma to be the focus.

This recipe makes a big batch of soap. Make sure you have plenty of molds before you start.

Note: Always measure accurately when you're making homemade beauty products. See page 53 for tips.

- Blender
- 6-cup (1.5 L) canning jar with lid
- Large fine-mesh sieve lined with cheesecloth
- Soap molds (see tips, page 309)

8 oz	fresh lavender flowers and leaves, finely chopped	250 g
4 cups	brandy (see tips, at left)	1 L
2 lbs	unscented castile soap bars (see tips, at left), grated	1 kg
1 tbsp	lavender essential oil (see tips, page 323)	15 mL

1. In blender, combine lavender flowers and leaves and brandy. Purée at high speed for 2 minutes.

2. Pour lavender mixture into jar. Seal tightly and let stand at room temperature for 24 hours.

3. Place fine-mesh sieve over a large heatproof bowl; strain liquid into bowl, discarding solids. Add soap to bowl. Set aside.

4. Pour enough water into a large saucepan to come about 2 inches (5 cm) up the side; bring to a simmer.

5. Set bowl on saucepan so that bottom of bowl is not touching simmering water; heat, stirring occasionally, until soap mixture is melted and smooth. Remove bowl from heat. Stir in lavender essential oil until well combined. Let cool slightly.

6. Pour soap mixture into molds. Let cool at room temperature until hardened. Unmold soaps. Let stand in a cool, dry, well-ventilated place for 4 to 6 weeks before using.

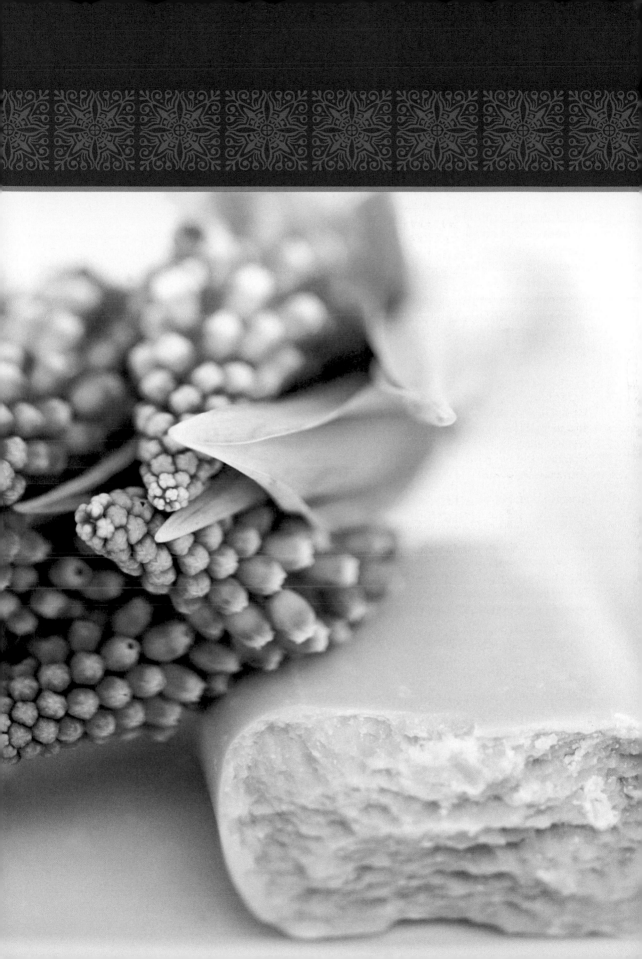

Orris Root Exfoliating Cleanser

This formula contains no soap, but it still gets rid of dulling dead cells and dirt, leaving skin soft and luminous. This gentle cleanser can be used on both the body and the face.

Best for: All skin types

Tips: Orris roots are the rhizomes, or fleshy underground parts, of a beautiful and medically useful variety of iris (*Iris germanica*). Look for chopped dried orris root at herbalists' shops or online herb stores.

Oat milk is a nondairy beverage made by soaking oats until they are soft, then blending them with water, salt and a bit of sugar. There are many easy recipes for oat milk online, or you can buy ready-made packages of it in the health food section of the supermarket.

Note: Always measure accurately when you're making homemade beauty products. See page 53 for tips.

- Fine-mesh sieve
- Glass jar with lid

1¾ oz	dried orris root (see tips, at left)	50 g
1 cup	water	250 mL
½ oz	kaolin clay (see tips, opposite)	15 g
	Oat milk (see tips, at left)	

1. In a small saucepan, combine orris root and water. Bring to a boil. Cover, reduce heat and simmer for 10 minutes.

2. Place a fine-mesh sieve over a small heatproof bowl; strain infusion into bowl, discarding solids. Let cool.

3. Stir clay into infusion, adding a little more water if very dry. Spoon into jar.

4. In a small bowl, mix 2 tbsp (30 mL) of cleanser with enough oat milk to create a creamy consistency. Using fingers and making circular motions, massage cleanser over skin, moistening the mixture with a little more oat milk if it becomes too dry.

5. Rinse off cleanser with warm water. Pat skin dry with a towel. Store jar in a cool, dry place for up to 2 weeks.

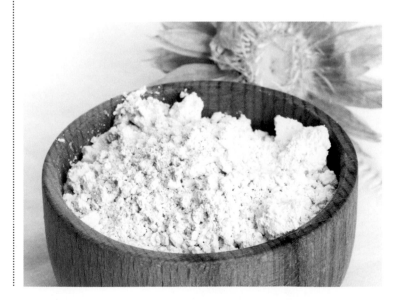

Almond Flour Soap Substitute

This is another simple, hydrating soap-free cleanser. You can form this one into a convenient bar.

Best for: All skin types

Tips: Almond flour is just very finely ground oats. Look for bags of it in the natural food aisle, near the baking ingredients.

There are many different types of clay available for making homemade beauty products. Kaolin, a pure white type of clay, is one of the most common and easy to use. French green clay is also popular for its oil-absorbing powers.

Buy essential oils sold in dark bottles. Exposure to light can reduce the potency of their medicinal herbal components. Store the bottles in a cool, dark place to keep them fresh.

- Soap mold (see tips, page 309)

2 tbsp	almond flour (see tips, at left)	30 mL
2 tbsp	kaolin clay (see tips, at left)	30 mL
2 tsp	sweet almond oil (see tips, page 296)	10 mL
1 or 2	drops essential oil of your choice (see tips, at left)	1 or 2

1. In a small bowl, stir together almond flour, clay, sweet almond oil and essential oil until well combined.

2. Spoon almond flour mixture into soap mold. Let stand at room temperature until hardened. Unmold soap.

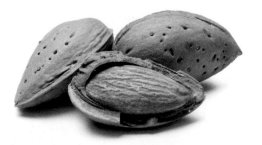

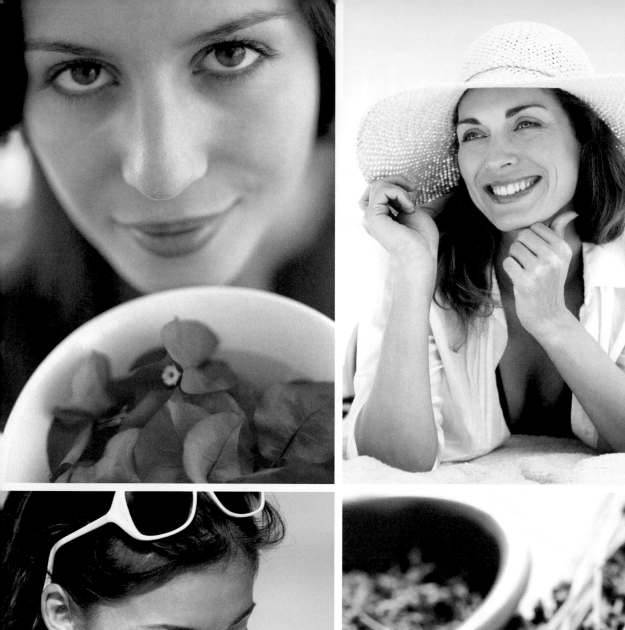
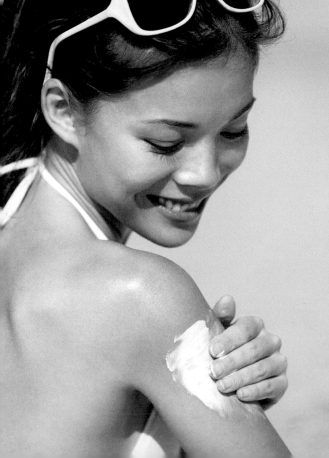
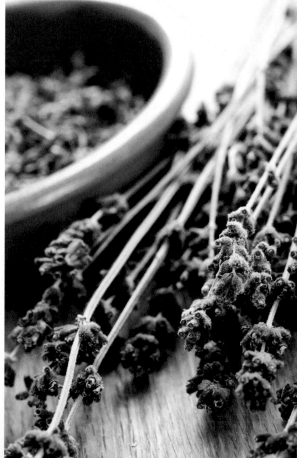

Scents and Sun-Care Products

Homemade beauty products aren't limited to face creams and shampoos. There's a whole world of freshly picked flowers and leaves you can transform into lightly fragrant colognes, intensely sensual perfumes (for both men and women), potpourris and even sunscreens. The possible combinations of plants and flowers are virtually endless.

Perfumes have a wonderful magic. They can awaken feelings, evoke memories, lift your spirits, transport you to a pleasant state of relaxation and dreaming, and energize you. When you make them with pure essential oils, they can even heal you.

Likewise, the sun's healing rays can be a strong ally in building good health. Sunshine stimulates circulation and increases the body's defenses. But the sun can also be a fickle friend. If you don't protect your skin properly and you get too much sun, the consequences can be unfortunate, both in the short and the long term. You can buy a huge number of industrially made, chemical sunscreens, but you don't have to. In this chapter, you will learn how to be sun conscious and discover recipes for a range of homemade sunscreens based on pure, natural oils. Your skin will thank you for this loving care.

A Short History of Scents

The art of perfumery was known in ancient civilizations. In the beginning, perfumes were used for religious purposes; in China, Egypt and Persia, myrrh and frankincense were burned on altars. In the age of the Greek writer Homer, perfumes were part of funeral rites. The sacred uses of perfumes evolved into more secular functions, thanks to the influence of Asian cultures, in which people anointed their bodies with scented balms for reasons other than worship. This was the beginning of the sensual appreciation of perfumes.

The sale and use of perfumes reached a peak in Ancient Rome. But with the fall of the Roman Empire, their appeal faded in Western society. The Crusades reignited a taste for perfumes from the East, and the people of France especially embraced them.

In the 14th century, perfumes were used to mask foul odors that were prevalent as a result of poor hygiene. Bathing was discouraged for health reasons, and intense fragrances, such as musk, amber and civet, were favored. In the 15th century, the first scented water made its appearance: the famous Hungary Water was invented in the country of the same name. This was the forerunner of cologne, created later by Jean-Marie Farina. With the conquest of the New World, Europe was enriched with many new aromatic raw materials, from which a new perfume industry grew. In the court of King Louis XV, perfumes were used as a weapon of seduction.

During the 19th century, flower growing for the perfume industry expanded enormously, especially in southeastern France. The region between Grasse and Nice was said to be a vast garden of roses, tuberoses, jasmine, acacia, violets, lavender and rosemary, all used to create beautiful scents for people to enjoy.

What Are Essential Oils?

Essential oils are volatile components contained in plants. They can be distilled from a variety of plant parts, including leaves (such as eucalyptus), flowers (such as roses or orange blossoms), woods (such as sandalwood), resins (such as benzoin), roots (such as vetiver) or seeds (such as carrot seeds). Different aromas have different powers. Some increase productivity and concentration while others are relaxing (see box, page 336). Medical studies have verified the physical powers of some scents; for example, spearmint has been proven to increase energy and encourage a positive attitude.

Sun Exposure: The Benefits

The sun plays a necessary role in human health. Ultraviolet (UV) rays transform provitamin D in the skin tissue into vitamin D, which plays a part in calcium absorption and therefore bone health. Vitamin D deficiency causes rickets, a bone-weakening condition that was quite common in previous centuries among children who did not get enough sunlight.

The sun's energy is also good for the blood and circulatory system. Exposure to sunlight speeds up blood circulation, increases the heartbeat slightly and increases respiratory frequency and depth, which results in better oxygenation of the blood and better carbon dioxide elimination. When the skin enjoys good circulation, toxic substances are removed more readily, and the body's defenses against infection are heightened by the increased production of white blood cells.

Research has also shown the effect of the sun's energy on the body's hormonal system. When light enters a person's eyes, a signal reaches the hypothalamus, which stimulates the pituitary gland, which directs the functions of all the glands in the body. As a result, the thyroid gland steps up its functioning and raises the metabolism; this helps in weight loss, for example. Sunlight exposure also increases sex hormone secretion by the ovaries and testes, which enhances sexual health.

The sun also affects hair growth because increased circulation means a better supply of nutrients to the roots. This can stimulate hair to grow at a rate of almost ¾ inch (1.8 cm) per month. In addition, moderate sunbathing strengthens the nervous system, helping nerve cells rest and recover; sadly, too much sun exposure can have the opposite effect, causing overexcitement. The sun can also act as a bactericide on skin, because a specific wavelength in the sun's rays destroys germs before they can become hazardous to health.

Natural Sun Protection

While cosmetic and drug companies manufacture a wide range of sunscreens that are easy to use, it is also possible to make homemade sunscreens using plant-based ingredients. Many contain natural oils that are water-resistant on the skin. In addition to protecting your skin from the outside and monitoring your time in the sun, make sure you eat plenty of fruits and vegetables, especially fresh green salads, which are rich in the antioxidants needed to neutralize the negative effects of solar radiation.

How to Distill Essential Oils at Home

You can find all the essential oils used to make perfume in cosmetic-supply stores, but if you are up to it, you can try creating them yourself. Here's how:

1. Place the aromatic plant or herb you want to distill in a pot filled with water. Cover it and bring to a boil. Uncover, reduce heat and simmer.

2. Into the pot, above the boiling mixture, insert a special plastic tube that runs through a container filled with ice. (You can buy this special equipment online.) Place the other end of the tube in a glass receiving container. The purpose of the tube is to carry the steam from the pot to the glass container. As it passes through the tube, the steam comes into contact with the ice, condenses and becomes liquid again. The liquid runs down into the glass receiving container.

3. Let the liquid in the receiving container stand. The essential oil will float on top of the condensed water and can easily be skimmed off.

Orange Blossom Cologne

In the spring in southern Spain, the air is perfumed with the sweet smell of orange blossoms from the trees that line the streets. This perfume evokes that season.

Best for: All skin types

Tip: Fresh orange blossoms can be hard to come by if you don't live in a warm climate. While you can buy dried blossoms, they don't smell as heavenly as the fresh ones.

Note: Always measure accurately when you're making homemade beauty products. See page 53 for tips.

- Large fine-mesh sieve
- Large glass bottle with lid

1½ cups	fresh orange blossoms (see tip, at left)	375 mL
6 cups	boiling water	1.5 L
2 tbsp	ethyl alcohol (see tip, page 332)	30 mL

1. Place orange blossoms in a large heatproof bowl; pour boiling water over top. Cover and let stand at room temperature for 1 day. Transfer to the refrigerator and refrigerate for 2 days.

2. Place fine-mesh sieve over another large bowl; strain liquid into bowl, discarding solids. Stir in alcohol.

3. Pour into bottle. Store bottle in the refrigerator for up to 2 months.

Scents and the Sun

Be careful about using perfumes and colognes if you plan to go out in the sun. Some, particularly those that contain bergamot or musk, can make the skin more susceptible to sun damage.

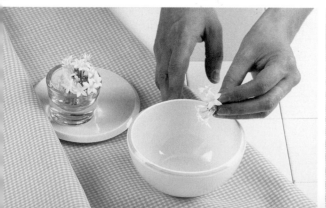
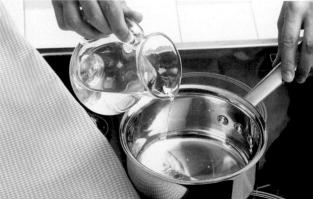

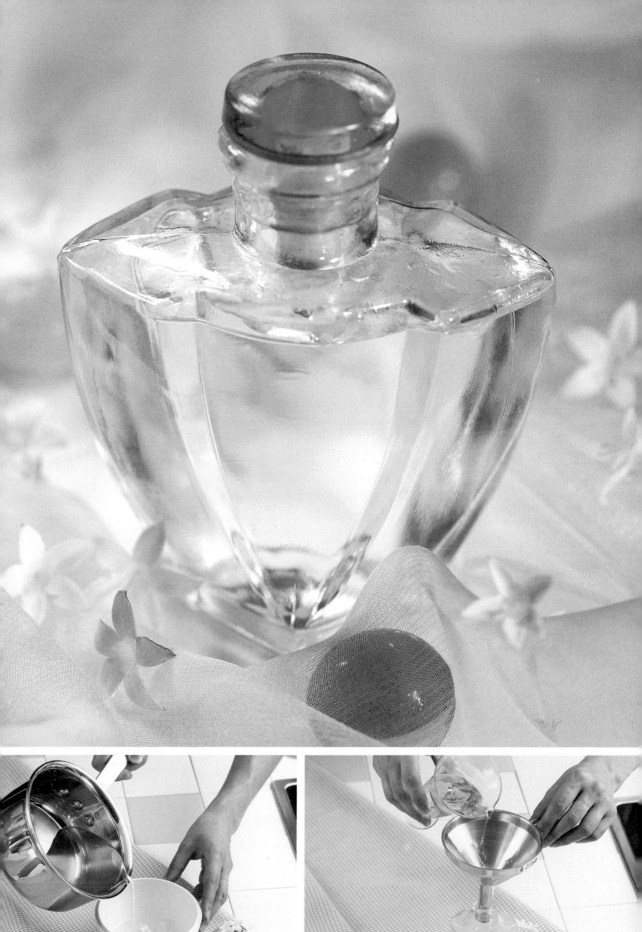

Bay Rum Cologne

A traditional West Indies staple, this cologne makes a nice aftershave for men. It has a slightly spicy fragrance that's neither too masculine nor too feminine.

Best for: All skin types

Tips: Distilled water has been purified through the process of distillation; in other words, the water is boiled, and the condensation (which is free of impurities) is collected in a clean vessel. Bottles of it are readily available in supermarkets.

Buy essential oils sold in dark bottles. Exposure to light can reduce the potency of their medicinal herbal components. Store the bottles in a cool, dark place to keep them fresh.

Note: Always measure accurately when you're making homemade beauty products. See page 53 for tips.

- Small glass bottle with lid

2½ tbsp	ethyl alcohol (see tip, page 332)	37 mL
1½ tbsp	distilled water (see tips, at left)	22 mL
1 tsp	amber rum	5 mL
2 to 5	drops bay laurel essential oil (see tips, at left)	2 to 5

1. In a small bowl, stir together alcohol, distilled water, rum and bay laurel essential oil. Cover and let stand for 2 days in a cool, dark place.

2. Pour into bottle. Store in a cool, dark place for up to 2 months.

Essential Oils Aren't New

The art of aromatherapy is not a modern trend. The use of essential oils can be traced back more than 3,000 years. Aromatic oils were enjoyed in Ancient China, India and Egypt, societies that had highly developed perfume trades. In fact, perfumes were once a form of currency. Essential oils were used in religious ceremonies and even appear in the Bible, where their therapeutic properties are mentioned.

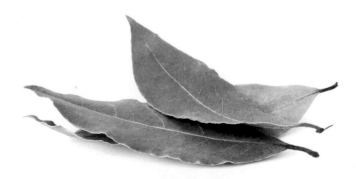

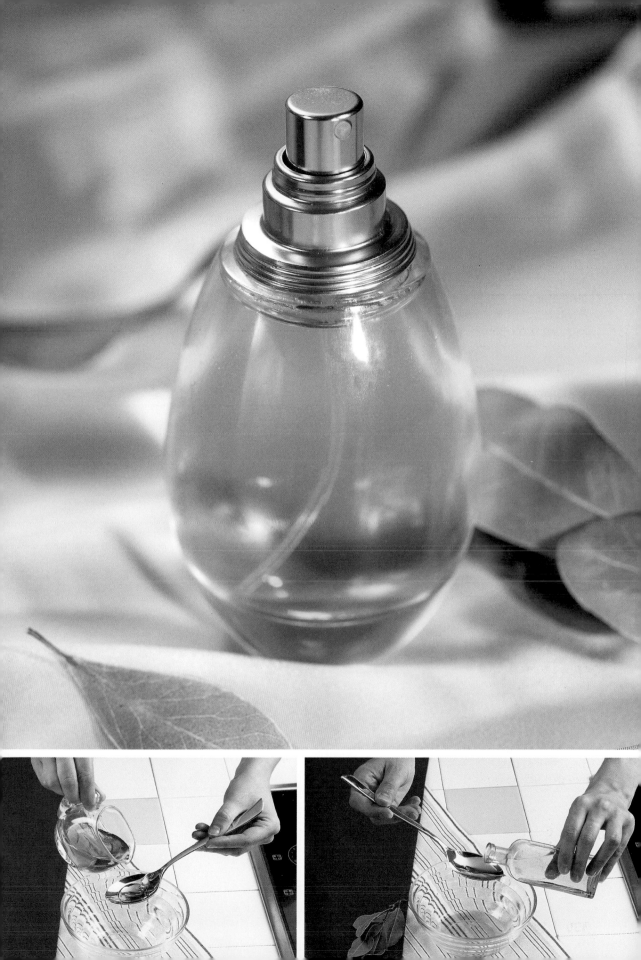

Jasmine Cologne

Jasmine has a pretty floral fragrance that evokes tropical climates and lush gardens. This perfume could not be simpler to make, and it doesn't require fresh flowers.

Best for: All skin types

Tip: Ethyl alcohol is the type of alcohol in spirits and other alcoholic beverages. It is not the same as isopropyl alcohol, the type you find at the drugstore for disinfecting wounds. You can get high-proof grain alcohol from the liquor store (look for the brand name Everclear). In a pinch, substitute unflavored vodka or brandy.

Note: Always measure accurately when you're making homemade beauty products. See page 53 for tips.

• Small glass bottle with lid

3½ tbsp	ethyl alcohol (see tip, at left)	52 mL
5	drops jasmine essential oil (see tips, page 330)	5

1. In a small bowl, stir alcohol with jasmine essential oil.
2. Pour into bottle. Seal tightly. Let stand at room temperature for 2 weeks before using. Store bottle in a cool, dark place for up to 2 months.

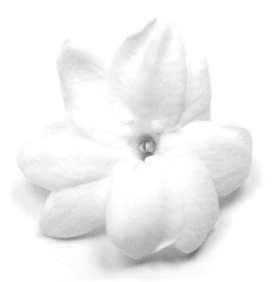

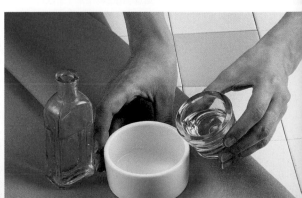

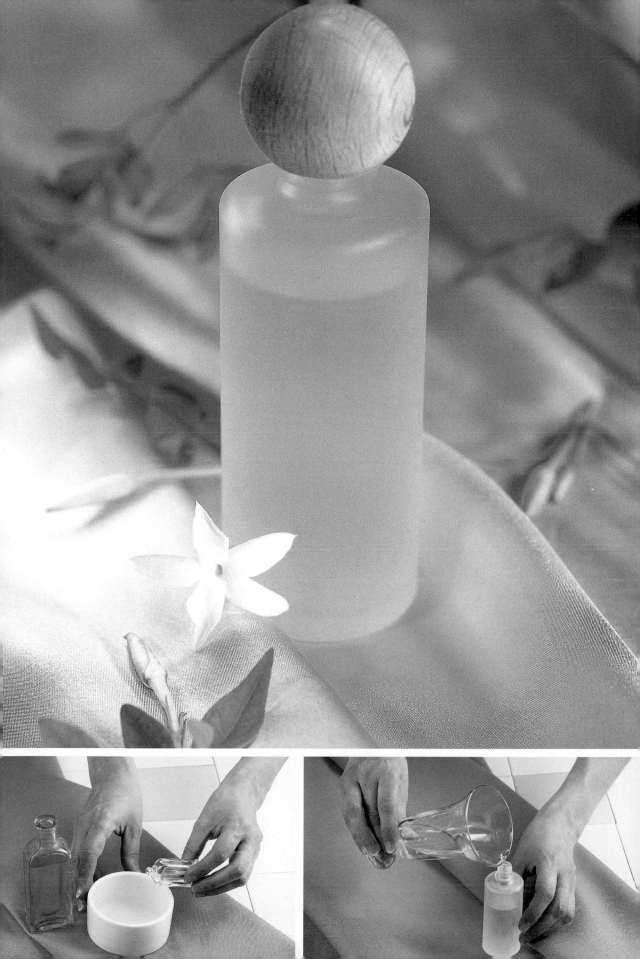

Rose Petal Cologne

Natural perfumes like this keep best in the refrigerator. They are cool and refreshing to apply, especially on a hot day.

Best for: All skin types

Tip: Roses are easy to find in flower shops and supermarkets, but they have often been treated with pesticides and fungicides. Avoid them and use organic, unsprayed petals for any homemade beauty products.

- Fine-mesh sieve
- Large glass bottle with lid

2 cups	fresh rose petals (see tip, at left)	500 mL
	Boiling water	
2 tbsp	ethyl alcohol (see tip, page 332)	30 mL

1. Place rose petals in a large heatproof bowl; pour in enough boiling water to cover petals. Cover and let stand at room temperature for 1 day. Transfer to the refrigerator and refrigerate for 2 days.

2. Place fine-mesh sieve over another large bowl; strain liquid into bowl, discarding solids. Stir in alcohol.

3. Pour into bottle. Store bottle in the refrigerator for up to 2 months.

Violet Flower Cologne

Violets were a favorite in the Victorian era. They have a delicate, old-fashioned aroma that's clean and light.

Best for: All skin types

Tip: There are many different violet cultivars. To make perfume, you need a highly scented variety, such as sweet violet (*Viola odorata*).

Note: Always measure accurately when you're making homemade beauty products. See page 53 for tips.

- Fine-mesh sieve
- Large glass bottle with lid

2 cups	fresh violet petals (see tip, at left)	500 mL
	Boiling water	
2 tbsp	ethyl alcohol (see tip, page 332)	30 mL

1. Place violet petals in a large heatproof bowl; pour in enough boiling water to cover petals. Cover and let stand at room temperature for 1 day. Transfer to the refrigerator and refrigerate for 2 days.

2. Place fine-mesh sieve over another large bowl; strain liquid into bowl, discarding solids. Stir in alcohol.

3. Pour into bottle. Store bottle in the refrigerator for up to 2 months.

Hungary Water

Also called Queen of Hungary Water, this is the first and most famous alcohol-based perfume. It is said to have been invented in the 14th century for Queen Elisabeth of Hungary, and there are many different but aromatic recipes for it.

Best for: All skin types

Tips: Rose water is commonly used in Middle Eastern, Mediterranean, Indian and North African cuisine, so look for bottles of this fragrant essence at specialty grocery stores.

Spearmint is wonderful not only in cooking but also in homemade beauty treatments. It can run wild in the garden, so plant a pot of it instead. That way, you'll always have fresh leaves ready to go into whatever you're making.

Note: Always measure accurately when you're making homemade beauty products. See page 53 for tips.

- Fine-mesh sieve
- Glass bottle with lid

½ cup	rose water (see tips, at left)	125 mL
1 tbsp	fresh spearmint leaves (see tips, at left)	15 mL
1 tbsp	fresh rosemary leaves	15 mL
	Zest of 1 lemon and 1 orange	
¼ cup	ethyl alcohol (see tip, page 332)	60 mL

1. In a small bowl, combine rose water, spearmint leaves and rosemary leaves. Stir in lemon zest and orange zest. Stir in alcohol. Cover and let stand at room temperature for 2 weeks.

2. Place fine-mesh sieve over another small bowl; strain liquid into bowl, discarding solids.

3. Pour into bottle. Store in a cool, dark place for up to 2 months.

Keeping Essential Oils Pure

Bottles of essential oil with eyedropper tops are convenient but not always available. If you have bottles without them, you can use a separate eyedropper to pick up and drop the oils into recipes. To prevent cross-contamination between different oils, you can do one of two things: clean the eyedropper with alcohol after it's been in one oil and before dipping it into a different one, or use a separate eyedropper for each oil. In either case, clean the eyedropper with alcohol after use and before storing it.

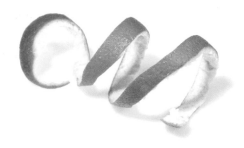

Create Your Signature Scent

You can make perfume with any essential oils you choose. Experimenting with different favorite aromas and combinations will allow you to find the ideal blend for your personality and needs.

To make a perfume with an alcohol base, pour 1 tbsp (15 mL) of ethyl alcohol (see tip, page 332) into a small dark glass bottle. Using an eyedropper (see box, page 335), add the essential oils you have chosen and gently swirl the mixture to dissolve the oils in the alcohol. Add 10 drops of distilled water, one by one, shaking the bottle after adding each drop.

To make a perfume with an oil base, pour 1 tbsp (15 mL) of jojoba oil or coconut oil into a small dark glass bottle. Using an eyedropper, add the essential oils you have chosen and gently swirl the mixture to combine.

For either base, let the perfume stand in a cool place for 2 to 4 weeks to mature and allow the fragrance to develop fully. Shake the bottle once a day to recombine.

Find Your Favorite Aroma

Before you begin making perfumes with essential oils, it is helpful to know their fragrance notes and evocative powers. Below are a number of popular essential oils and their characteristics or the feelings they evoke. Keep in mind that the aroma of the oil in the bottle will not be exactly the same as when it is exposed to the air.

- **Basil:** refreshing, herbal, inspiring
- **Bay laurel:** spicy
- **Benzoin:** pleasant, warm, soothing, similar to vanilla
- **Bergamot:** sweet, fresh, citrusy
- **Black pepper:** spicy, very warm
- **Cardamom:** sweet, warm, slightly musky
- **Cedar:** warm, woody
- **Chamomile:** refreshing, pleasant, lightly grassy
- **Cloves:** pungent, spicy, warm
- **Eucalyptus:** clean, refreshing
- **Frankincense:** sweet, spicy
- **Geranium:** sweet, refreshing, relaxing
- **Ginger:** very warm, spicy

- **Jasmine:** exotic, sensual, relaxing
- **Lavender:** fresh, clean, floral
- **Lemon balm:** clean, gentle, lemony
- **Lime:** refreshing, acidic, bright
- **Marjoram:** pungent, warm, herbal
- **Orange:** sweet, refreshing, citrusy
- **Patchouli:** damp, earthy, pungent
- **Rose:** sensual, sweet, intensely floral
- **Sage:** sweet, floral, green
- **Sandalwood:** woody, spicy
- **Spearmint:** refreshing, penetrating, clean
- **Vanilla:** sweet, warm, similar to caramel
- **Vetiver:** earthy, pungent

Spring Perfume

Floral and fresh, this perfume begs to be dabbed on when gardens start to bloom.

Best for: All skin types

Tip: To make this or any of the perfumes on this page and page 338 with an oil base instead of an alcohol base, substitute 1 tbsp (15 mL) of jojoba oil or coconut oil for the alcohol. Omit distilled water. Gently swirl to combine oils, pour into a bottle and let stand as directed.

- Small dark glass bottle with lid
- Eyedropper (see box, page 335)

1 tbsp	ethyl alcohol (see tip, at left)	15 mL
6	drops sage essential oil	6
6	drops lavender essential oil	6
3	drops jasmine essential oil	3
10	drops distilled water (see tips, page 330)	10

1. Pour alcohol into bottle. Using eyedropper, add sage essential oil, lavender essential oil and jasmine essential oil. Gently swirl mixture to dissolve oils in alcohol.

2. Using eyedropper, add distilled water, 1 drop at a time, swirling mixture after each addition to combine.

3. Seal bottle. Let stand in a cool place for 2 to 4 weeks, shaking once a day. Store bottle in a cool place for up to 6 months.

Summer Perfume

This mix of citrusy, floral and grassy scents is light enough to enjoy in the warm weather.

Best for: All skin types

Note: Always measure accurately when you're making homemade beauty products. See page 53 for tips.

- Small dark glass bottle with lid
- Eyedropper (see box, page 335)

1 tbsp	ethyl alcohol (see tip, above)	15 mL
8	drops lemon essential oil	8
8	drops lavender essential oil	8
5	drops chamomile essential oil	5
5	drops eucalyptus essential oil	5
10	drops distilled water (see tips, page 330)	10

1. Pour alcohol into bottle. Using eyedropper, add lemon essential oil, lavender essential oil, chamomile essential oil and eucalyptus essential oil. Gently swirl mixture to dissolve oils in alcohol.

2. Using eyedropper, add distilled water, 1 drop at a time, swirling mixture after each addition to combine.

3. Seal bottle. Let stand in a cool place for 2 to 4 weeks, shaking once a day. Store bottle in a cool place for up to 6 months.

Autumn Perfume

Warm, woody and spicy notes are complemented by a light spritz of citrusy bergamot.

Best for: All skin types

- Small dark glass bottle with lid
- Eyedropper (see box, page 335)

1 tbsp	ethyl alcohol (see tip, page 337)	15 mL
6	drops sandalwood essential oil	6
6	drops bergamot essential oil	6
3	drops vetiver essential oil	3
3	drops clove essential oil	3
2	drops patchouli essential oil	2
10	drops distilled water (see tips, page 330)	10

1. Pour alcohol into bottle. Using eyedropper, add sandalwood essential oil, bergamot essential oil, vetiver essential oil, clove essential oil and patchouli essential oil. Gently swirl mixture.

2. Using eyedropper, add distilled water, 1 drop at a time, swirling mixture after each addition to combine.

3. Seal bottle. Let stand in a cool place for 2 to 4 weeks, shaking once a day. Store bottle in a cool place for up to 6 months.

Winter Perfume

Holiday aromas of spices, vanilla, incense and citrus mingle in this warm scent.

Best for: All skin types

- Small dark glass bottle with lid
- Eyedropper (see box, page 335)

1 tbsp	ethyl alcohol (see tip, page 337)	15 mL
8	drops cinnamon essential oil	8
5	drops lime essential oil	5
5	drops vanilla essential oil	5
5	drops clove essential oil	5
3	drops bergamot essential oil	3
2	drops frankincense essential oil	2
10	drops distilled water (see tips, page 330)	10

1. Pour alcohol into bottle. Using eyedropper, add cinnamon essential oil, lime essential oil, vanilla essential oil, clove essential oil, bergamot essential oil and frankincense essential oil. Gently swirl mixture to dissolve oils in alcohol.

2. Using eyedropper, add distilled water, 1 drop at a time, swirling mixture after each addition to combine.

3. Seal bottle. Let stand in a cool place for 2 to 4 weeks, shaking once a day. Store bottle in a cool place for up to 6 months.

Herbal Deodorant Powder

This mix of powdered herbs, ground seeds and essential oils is refreshing and helps keep your skin dry and comfortable.

Best for: All skin types

Tips: Arrowroot powder is also called arrowroot starch or arrowroot flour. It's made by grinding the starchy rhizomes of the arrowroot plant. It's a fairly common cooking ingredient, used in baked goods and as a thickener. You can find it in the baking or natural food aisle of the supermarket.

A spice grinder or a clean coffee grinder is a useful tool for grinding spices. If you don't have either, use a mortar and pestle.

Note: Always measure accurately when you're making homemade beauty products. See page 53 for tips.

- Small glass jar with lid

2 tbsp	unscented talcum powder (see tips, page 344)	30 mL
2 tbsp	arrowroot powder (see tips, at left)	30 mL
1 tbsp	coriander seeds, ground (see tips, at left)	15 mL
1 tbsp	ground dried sage leaves (see tips, page 344)	15 mL
1 tbsp	ground dried lavender leaves	15 mL
1 tbsp	ground dried spearmint leaves	15 mL
1½ tsp	whole cloves, ground	7 mL
20	drops lavender essential oil (see tips, page 344)	20
20	drops spearmint essential oil	20
10	drops patchouli essential oil	10

1. In a small deep bowl, whisk together talcum powder, arrowroot powder, coriander seeds, sage leaves, lavender leaves, spearmint leaves and cloves until well combined.

2. Add lavender essential oil, spearmint essential oil and patchouli essential oil to spice mixture. Whisk until well combined.

3. Pour into jar. Dust a small amount of powder on underarms. Store jar in a cool, dry place for up to 6 months.

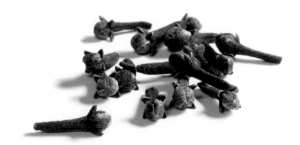

Citrus Deodorant Powder

Dust a little of this light, citrusy powder on your underarms to keep the skin smelling fresh and clean.

Best for: All skin types

Tip: Orris root powder, powdered citrus peels and licorice root powder are available online at shops that specialize in medicinal herbs. If you can't find them, you can buy the dried root or peel and grind them yourself using a small food processor or blender (just make sure it's one you plan to use only for homemade beauty products, not for preparing food).

Note: Always measure accurately when you're making homemade beauty products. See page 53 for tips.

- Fine-mesh sieve
- Glass jar with lid

1¾ oz	powdered dried orange peel	50 g
1¾ oz	powdered dried lemon peel	50 g
1¾ oz	orris root powder (see tip, at left)	50 g
pinch	licorice root powder	pinch

1. In a small bowl, stir together powdered orange peel, powdered lemon peel, orris root powder and licorice root powder until well combined.

2. Place fine-mesh sieve over another small bowl; sift mixture into bowl several times to break up any lumps.

3. Pour into jar. Dust a small amount of powder on underarms. Store jar in a cool, dark, dry place for up to 2 months.

Natural Deodorants

Deodorants work by forming a barrier against perspiration. They contain disinfectant ingredients that prevent bacteria from reproducing, which postpones the decomposition of sweat and the creation of unpleasant body odor.

However, commercial deodorants often cause itching and produce irritation and/or numbness, especially when applied over damp skin that has not been thoroughly dried. Sometimes, irritation is the result of a reaction to alcohol in deodorants, which dries out the skin. People with sensitive skin have it worse, because this drying can cause uncomfortable inflammation. Skin may also be allergic to the antibacterial ingredients in commercial deodorants.

A smarter alternative is to use deodorants that contain natural active ingredients and little alcohol. Herbs and essential oils give these deodorants their powers, prevent bacteria growth and suppress the sweat glands. An even better idea is to try the safe, effective, natural deodorant options on pages 339 to 344.

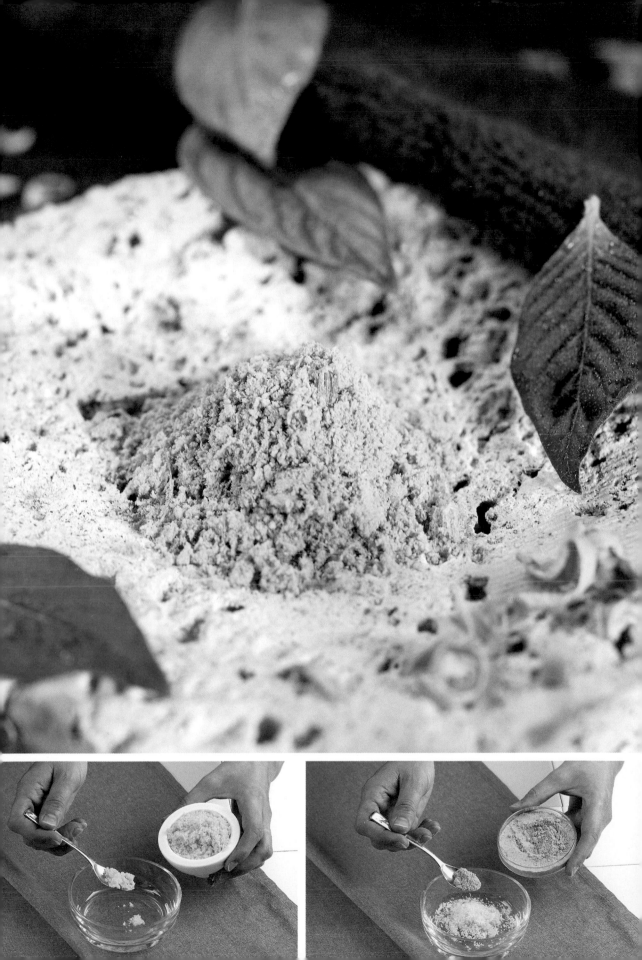

Sage Deodorant

Sage is a powerful odor fighter and astringent, so it is wonderful for keeping perspiration in check. This liquid formulation is convenient to spray on after a shower.

Best for: All skin types

Tips: Look for small spray bottles in the travel section of the drugstore or at stores that specialize in travel accessories. Some cosmetic-supply stores sell small dark glass bottles with spritzer tops, which are ideal.

Ethyl alcohol is the type of alcohol in spirits and other alcoholic beverages. It is not the same as isopropyl alcohol, the type you find at the drugstore for disinfecting wounds. You can get high-proof grain alcohol from the liquor store (look for the brand name Everclear). In a pinch, substitute unflavored vodka or brandy.

Note: Always measure accurately when you're making homemade beauty products. See page 53 for tips.

- Fine-mesh sieve
- Small spray bottle (see tips, at left) or glass bottle with lid

⅓ cup	water	75 mL
2 tsp	fresh sage leaves	10 mL
2 tsp	fresh rosemary leaves	10 mL
2 tbsp	ethyl alcohol (see tips, at left)	30 mL
5	drops sage essential oil (see tips, page 344)	5
2	drops lemon essential oil	2

1. In a small saucepan, combine water, sage leaves and rosemary leaves. Bring just to a boil; remove from heat. Cover and let stand for 10 minutes.

2. Place fine-mesh sieve over a small heatproof bowl; strain infusion into bowl, discarding solids. Let cool.

3. Stir alcohol into infusion. Add sage essential oil and lemon essential oil, stirring until well combined.

4. Pour into bottle. Spritz or dab on underarms. Store bottle in a cool, dark place for up to 2 weeks.

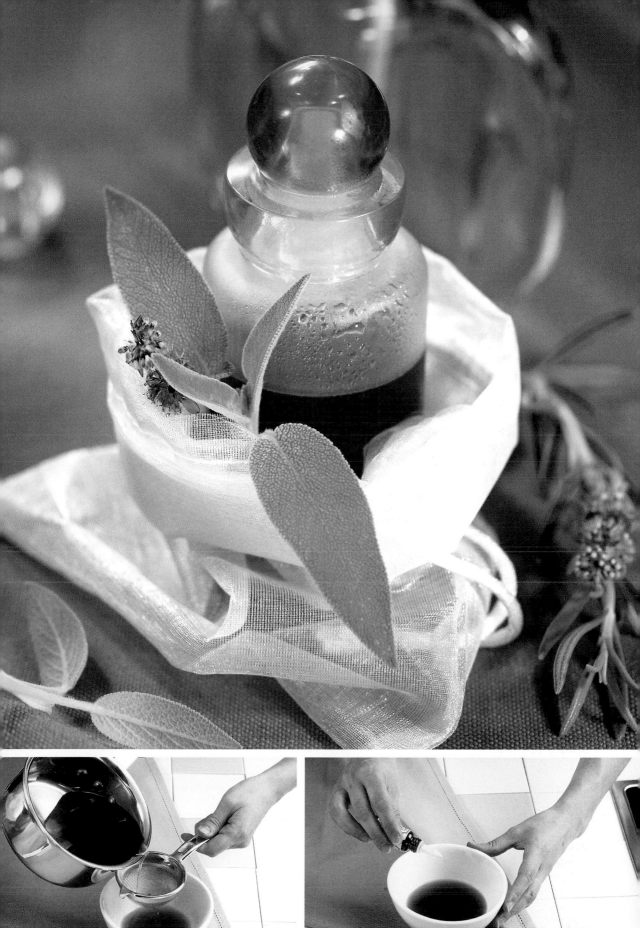

Body Powder for Men

Sandalwood has a woody, earthy, masculine scent. It also has antiseptic properties, so it's good for keeping bacteria on the skin at bay.

Best for: All skin types

Tips: Look for a reliable source of dried medicinal herbs, such as an herbalist's shop or a reputable online dealer. Make sure it's a business with high turnover, to ensure you're getting the freshest, most effective herbs possible.

Most talcum powder you'll find in drugstores is scented. Online cosmetic-supply stores are a good source for the unscented variety, to which you can add the fragrance of your choice.

- Mortar and pestle
- Fine-mesh sieve
- Small glass jar with lid

1 oz	each dried hollyhock and vetiver root (see tips, at left)	30 g
1¾ oz	unscented talcum powder (see tips, at left)	50 g
1 oz	powdered sandalwood	30 g

1. In mortar with pestle, grind hollyhock and vetiver until powdery. Pour into a small bowl.

2. Whisk talcum powder and powdered sandalwood into hollyhock mixture until well combined.

3. Place fine-mesh sieve over another small bowl; sift mixture into bowl several times to break up any lumps.

4. Pour into jar. Dust powder over skin. Store jar in a cool, dark, dry place for up to 6 months.

Deodorant Lotion

Antiperspirants are full of chemicals that block pores and prevent normal perspiration. This natural lotion kills body odor and has no harmful side effects.

Best for: All skin types

Tips: Glycerin is an effective moisturizer that is often added to beauty treatments and cosmetics. Here, it's a softening agent that protects delicate underarm skin from drying out. Look for bottles of it at cosmetic-supply stores or online.

Buy essential oils sold in dark bottles. Exposure to light can reduce the potency of their medicinal herbal components. Store the bottles in a cool, dark place to keep them fresh.

- Glass bottle with lid

1 cup	hazelnut milk	250 mL
1 tsp	liquid glycerin (see tips, at left)	5 mL
30	drops sage essential oil (see tips, at left)	30
10	drops lavender essential oil	10
10	drops thyme essential oil	10
10	drops patchouli essential oil	10
5	drops sandalwood essential oil	5

1. In a small bowl, stir together hazelnut milk, glycerin, sage essential oil, lavender essential oil, thyme essential oil, patchouli essential oil and sandalwood essential oil.

2. Pour into bottle. Seal tightly and shake well to combine. Let stand for 4 days in a cool place before using.

3. Rub a small amount of deodorant lotion on underarms. Shake bottle to recombine before each use.

Scents to Perfume Your Home

Potpourris are perennially popular. The custom of using these mixtures to scent the home is thought to have originated centuries ago in Britain and Scandinavia, where mixtures of herbs were used to counteract unpleasant odors in the home and prevent disease. The term *potpourri* comes from French and literally means "rotten pot."

Making a potpourri couldn't be easier. You simply mix together a selection of flowers, herbs, fruits and/or spices that act as odor fighters. Potpourris can be dry or wet, and there are endless blends and recipes. You can create a heavily scented mixture or one that blends into the background.

Spices are ideal ingredients in potpourris. Cinnamon, cloves, allspice, nutmeg and coriander are common additions. Scented leaves, such as geranium, bay laurel or marjoram, also add lovely aromas. If you want to integrate more sensual, exotic scents, you can add a fruity note by including pieces of dried tropical fruits such as mangos, papayas or passion fruit.

Adding a few drops of essential oil, such as violet or sandalwood, intensifies the aroma of a potpourri and makes it last longer. Just add essential oils sparingly. You can set the fragrance using fixatives such as orris root powder, ground benzoin gum or powdered sandalwood.

There are so many different ways to use and display potpourris. You can hang cloth bags filled with potpourri in your closet or slip them into drawers to scent your clothes. You can place them in wooden, ceramic or glass jars and leave them around the house as a decorative element; try setting large seashells filled with potpourri in the bathroom for a pretty, fragrant accent. Displaying potpourris in multiple rooms of your house will make the overall environment pleasant and welcoming.

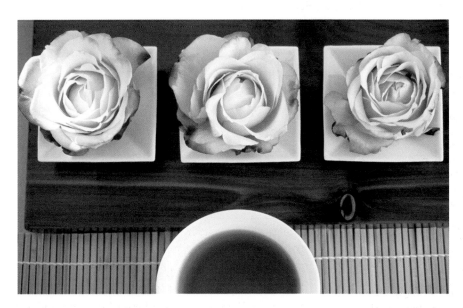

Sandalwood Potpourri

Woody, earthy sandalwood is the aromatic base for this mixture of flowers, citrus fruits and spices. The long curing time helps fix and develop the scent.

Best for: Scenting the home

Tips: Large-flake kosher sea salt is easy to find and a good ingredient for this recipe.

Cinnamon is most pungent when it's freshly grated. A palm-size metal nutmeg grater or the nubbly side of a box grater is tough enough to take on hard sticks of cinnamon.

Note: Always measure accurately when you're making homemade beauty products. See page 53 for tips.

● Cloth bags or decorative containers

1 lb	dried fragrant rose petals (see tips, opposite)	500 g
8 oz	dried peony petals	250 g
8 oz	dried orange blossoms	250 g
	Coarse salt (see tips, at left)	
½ oz	powdered sandalwood	15 g
2½ tbsp	dried thyme leaves	37 mL
2 tbsp	orris root powder (see tip, page 340)	30 mL
1 tbsp	dried bergamot orange peel	15 mL
1 tbsp	dried rosemary leaves	15 mL
1 tbsp	crushed bay leaves	15 mL
	Ground dried peel of 1 orange	
1 tbsp	freshly grated cinnamon (see tips, at left)	15 mL
1 tbsp	whole allspice	15 mL

1. In a large bowl, stir together rose petals, peony petals and orange blossoms. Cover with an equal amount of coarse salt. Cover tightly and let stand in a cool, dark, well-ventilated place for 2 to 3 weeks.

2. If mixture has solidified, using a wooden spoon, break up any chunks gently. Stir in powdered sandalwood, thyme leaves, orris root powder, bergamot peel, rosemary leaves, bay leaves, orange peel, cinnamon and allspice. Cover tightly and let stand in a cool, dark, well-ventilated place for 5 weeks.

3. Place potpourri in cloth bags to hang in closets or in decorative containers for display.

Rose Potpourri

This floral mixture makes a wonderful gift to share with a friend. Pack it in a pretty glass jar and tie with a ribbon to give for a housewarming or other occasion.

Best for: Scenting the home

Tips: Use rose petals from plants that have not been sprayed with herbicides or fungicides. Choose a fragrant variety.

Borax, or sodium borate, is a natural mineral compound that is used as a laundry detergent and brightener. It is also great for drying flowers because it draws out their moisture quickly and efficiently, leaving the petals looking and smelling lovely. Look for boxes of borax alongside the laundry detergent at the supermarket. It is toxic when consumed, so make sure you use separate tools that will never touch food when you make this recipe. Also, wash your hands well after touching borax.

- Large fine-mesh sieve
- Large glass jar with lid
- Cloth bags or decorative containers

1 lb	fresh fragrant rose petals (see tips, at left)	500 g
3½ oz	fresh rose geranium leaves	100 g
3½ oz	fresh lavender flowers, chopped Borax powder (see tips, at left)	100 g
3½ oz	dried jasmine flowers, chopped	100 g
1 tsp	dried thyme leaves	5 mL
1 tsp	orris root powder (see tip, page 340)	5 mL
1 tsp	whole cloves	5 mL
1 tsp	chopped dried lemon peel	5 mL
½ tsp	chopped dried orange peel	2 mL
5	drops rose essential oil (see tips, page 344)	5
2	drops jasmine essential oil	2

1. Pat rose petals, rose geranium leaves and lavender flowers dry if they are moist. Sprinkle borax in a large shallow pan; arrange rose petal mixture over borax. Gently sprinkle more borax over petals until covered. Let stand in a warm, dry place for 10 to 14 days or until flower mixture is crisp and dry.

2. Place fine-mesh sieve over a large bowl; strain rose petal mixture, gently shaking and/or brushing off borax into the bowl. Discard borax. Transfer rose petal mixture to another large bowl.

3. Using your hands, mix jasmine flowers, thyme leaves, orris root powder, cloves, lemon peel and orange peel into rose petal mixture. Add rose essential oil and jasmine essential oil to flower mixture, 1 drop at a time, using a spoon to mix well after each addition.

4. Pour into jar. Seal tightly and let stand in a cool, dark, dry place for 6 weeks, stirring occasionally.

5. Place potpourri in cloth bags to hang in closets or in decorative containers for display.

Q&A: Sun Safety in Depth

It feels so good to sunbathe, and there certainly are benefits to doing it. But there are a few questions to consider before you step out of the shade. Dr. José Castells, a dermatologist with extensive experience in sun-related skin issues, answers some common questions about sunbathing.

Q: What factors should determine my optimal level of sun exposure?

A: There are five different factors. First, phototype, which is your skin type according to pigmentation. There are six phototypes, from people who have virtually no skin pigment (such as people with albinism) and are highly susceptible to the sun's rays, to people with very high pigmentation and whose skin is more resistant to the sun. Second, latitude. The sunshine is much weaker at the poles than it is at the equator. Third, time of year. The sun's rays are direct and vertical during the summer. Fourth, time of day. In the summer, solar radiation is at its strongest and most harmful level between 11 a.m. and 2 p.m.; sun exposure is not recommended at this time. Fifth, amount of sun exposure. You want to sunbathe and get the sun's therapeutic benefits without the risks associated with overexposure.

Q: How destructive can sunshine be to the skin?

A: The sun is an important source of radiation. It is the source of life of course. But its enormous destructive power can also make it a fearsome enemy. The sun generates different types of rays. Ultraviolet C is gamma radiation, which is highly destructive but doesn't reach the earth's surface, because it is blocked by the ozone layer. Ultraviolet A and B rays do reach us, and both are destructive.

Q: What are the short- and long-term harmful effects of sun exposure?

A: The sun has an immediate effect. A few hours of sun exposure triggers inflammatory mechanisms that can vary in severity. We know this phenomenon as sunburn, which fades in 24 to 48 hours and turns into increased pigmentation and peeling.

The effects of sunburn are cumulative. The sun attacks the dermis layer and eventually leads to wrinkles and spots. As a result, skin ages not only from the passage of time but also from the effects of the sun. This process of premature aging is called photoaging, and it may occur in people as young as 30. The next phase is loss of control over the skin's pigmentation system. This shows up as brown spots that appear in the areas that have received the most sun exposure. If the process continues, it alters the synthesis of all the components of the dermis, leading to a thickening of the skin or the fracturing of the elastic fibers. This condition is called solar elastosis. If it continues, reddish lesions that may be precancerous begin to appear and can develop into skin cancer.

Q: What is melanin?

A: Melanin is skin pigment produced by melanocytes, specialized cells located in the epidermis layer of the skin. Melanin is created as a result of exposure to ultraviolet light, and its effect is tanning of the skin. Melanin is the most important protective element shielding the body from the damaging effects of ultraviolet radiation.

Q: Is it true that the sun also powers a photosynthesis process in mammals?

A: Yes, it does. In addition to providing heat, the sun is involved in photosynthesizing vitamin D_3 and helping the body to assimilate it. But don't be overzealous; merely exposing a piece of skin the size of your hand to the sun for five minutes once a week will cover your vitamin D_3 needs. Keep in mind that we also obtain this vitamin from food.

Q: How should a person choose the best sunscreen?

A: Choose one that's right for your skin type. For anyone who has a fair amount of pigmentation, a good bet is a sunscreen with a sun protection factor (SPF) of 15. But that is nowhere near enough for people who have fair skin, because they need a complete physical sunscreen as well as a chemical one. Your sunscreen should totally block the sun. In addition to SPF, the consistency of sunscreen is important. For oily skin, for example, a gel is better than a cream.

Q: Why do people tan despite the risks?

A: Tans are associated with good health and hence higher social status. A pale person is seen as someone who is sickly, or who is less fortunate and cannot afford to ski or to go to the beach. A similar phenomenon happened in reverse in the 19th century: farm workers were tanned, while people in the upper classes were proud of their pale complexions because it showed that they did not have to work.

Q: Are we finally moving from a culture of tanning to a culture of protection?

A: We're getting there. Some people still sun themselves indiscriminately, because it feels good. They want to change only when it is too late. When they find they have spots and wrinkles, they become concerned and seek medical attention. But by then, the damage is done because they have been putting their skin at risk for many years. We should be more conscious that too much sun always takes a toll on the skin.

Walnut Oil Sunscreen

The oils in this formula all contain natural sunscreens and no chemical additives. Still, the best protection is to watch the clock and stay in the shade when the sun is at its peak in the late morning and early afternoon.

Best for: All skin types

Tip: Cold-pressed extra-virgin oils are the purest and most unadulterated type you can buy for making homemade beauty treatments. They are worth the higher price tag.

Note: Always measure accurately when you're making homemade beauty products. See page 53 for tips.

- Small glass bottle with lid

1 tbsp	walnut oil (see tip, at left)	15 mL
1 tbsp	avocado oil	15 mL
1 tbsp	soybean oil	15 mL
1 tbsp	carrot seed essential oil (see tip, page 356)	15 mL
	Water	
	Lemon juice	

1. In a small glass measuring cup, stir together walnut oil, avocado oil and soybean oil until well combined. Add carrot seed essential oil and stir mixture for 1 minute.

2. Pour into bottle. Pour a few drops of sunscreen into palm of hand. Mix in a few drops each of water and lemon juice; massage gently onto skin before sun exposure. Store bottle in a cool, dark place for up to 2 months.

UVA Isn't Safer

Experts used to believe that tanning lamps that emitted ultraviolet A (UVA) rays were a safer option for tanning than exposing yourself to the sun, which also emits skin-damaging ultraviolet B (UVB) rays. In recent years, however, it has been discovered that UVA rays penetrate deeper into the skin's layers and have a greater aging effect than previously understood, so lamps that use them are not safe at all. The bottom line: be sun safe and avoid tanning beds, which will irreversibly age your skin.

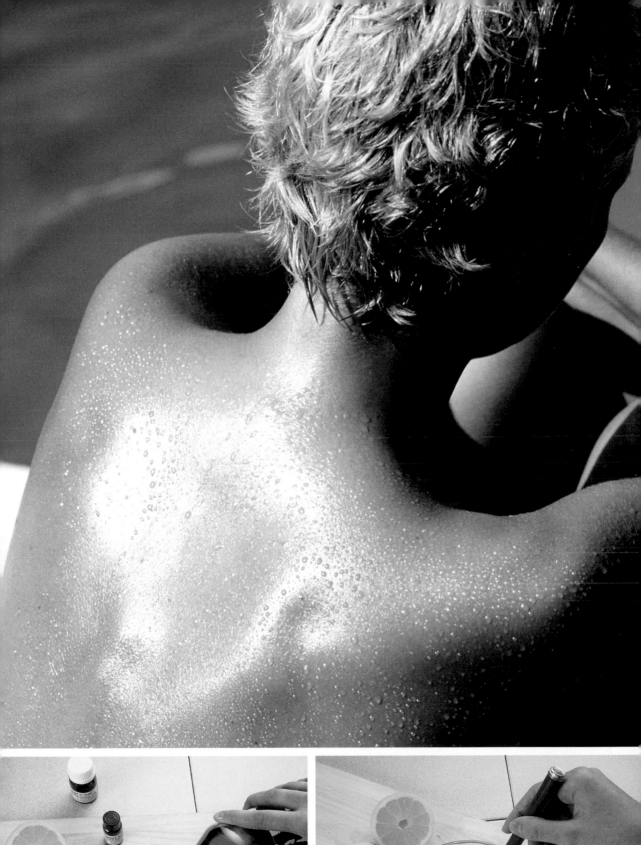
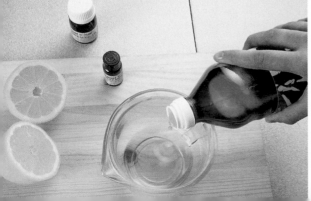
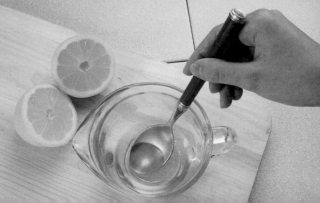

Alfalfa Sunscreen Oil

The tincture obtained by filtering this alfalfa and brandy mixture contains chlorophyll, a green plant pigment, which stimulates melanin production in the skin. The liquid also contains flavones, or substances that plants naturally produce to protect themselves from UV rays.

Best for: All skin types

Tips: Amber glass bottles protect the liquids inside them from exposure to sunlight. Large ones like the ones you need for this recipe are often sold at specialty container stores online. Stores that specialize in chemistry and beer-brewing supplies may also be sources for this type of bottle.

Brandy can be expensive. Don't splurge on the high-end stuff for this recipe. It requires just a neutral alcohol to draw out the chlorophyll and flavones in the sprouts.

Note: Always measure accurately when you're making homemade beauty products. See page 53 for tips.

- 6-cup (1.5 L) amber-colored glass bottle with lid (see tips, at left)
- Large fine-mesh sieve
- Eyedropper
- Small glass jar with lid
- 4-cup (1 L) amber-colored glass bottle with lid

½ oz	alfalfa sprouts	15 g
4 cups	brandy (see tips, at left)	1 L
3½ oz	coconut oil, melted and cooled slightly	100 g
2 tsp	avocado oil or sesame oil (see tip, page 354)	10 mL

1. Place alfalfa sprouts in larger bottle; pour brandy over top and turn bottle to ensure sprouts are immersed. Seal tightly and let stand in a cool, dark place for 28 days.

2. Place fine-mesh sieve over a large bowl; strain liquid into bowl, discarding solids.

3. In a small glass measuring cup, stir coconut oil with avocado oil. Using eyedropper, add 15 drops of alfalfa tincture to coconut oil mixture. Stir until well combined. Pour coconut oil mixture into jar. Pour remaining alfalfa tincture into smaller bottle and save to make more batches of sunscreen; store in a cool, dark place for up to 2 months.

4. Gently massage oil over skin before sun exposure. Store jar in a cool, dark place for up to 2 months.

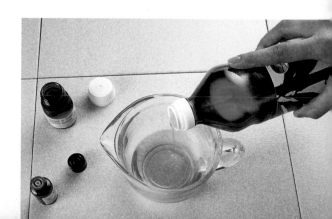

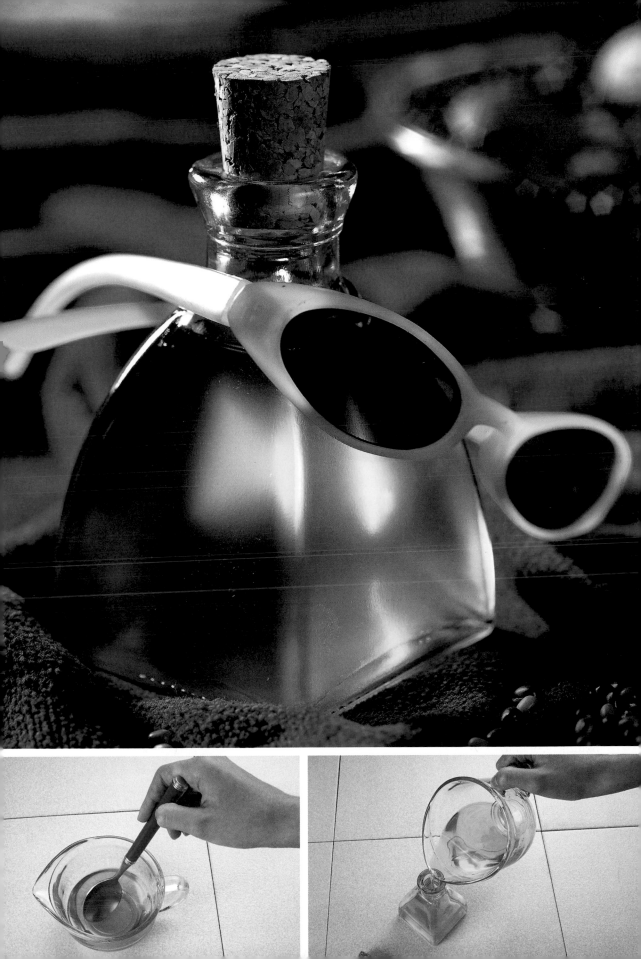

Water-Resistant Sunscreen Oil

Oily sunscreen formulations aren't easily washed off by water, so they are good for time spent at the beach or by the pool.

Best for: All skin types

Tip: Cold-pressed extra-virgin oils are the purest and most unadulterated type you can buy for making homemade beauty treatments. They are worth the higher price tag.

Note: Always measure accurately when you're making homemade beauty products.
See page 53 for tips.

• Small glass bottle with lid

3 tbsp	soybean oil (see tip, at left)	45 mL
2 tbsp	avocado oil	30 mL
1 tbsp	walnut oil	15 mL

1. In a small bowl, stir together soybean oil, avocado oil and walnut oil. Pour into bottle.

2. Massage oil all over skin before sun exposure. Store bottle in a cool, dark place for up to 2 months.

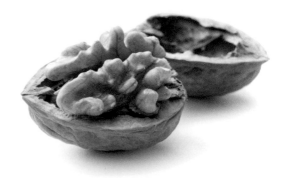

Chamomile and Aloe Sunburn Lotion

For days when you get a little too much of the sun's rays, this lotion will help cool the burn and make you more comfortable.

Best for: Minor sunburns

Tips: Aloe vera oil is a combination of the juicy, burn-soothing pulp of the aloe vera plant and a neutral oil, such as canola or coconut. If you prefer, you can substitute pure aloe vera gel to make a thicker lotion.

Glycerin is an effective moisturizer that is often added to beauty treatments and cosmetics. Look for bottles of it at cosmetic-supply stores or online.

- Small glass jar with lid

1 tbsp	witch hazel	15 mL
1 tbsp	aloe vera oil (see tips, at left)	15 mL
1 tbsp	liquid glycerin (see tips, at left)	15 mL
3	drops chamomile essential oil (see tip, page 356)	3

1. In a small bowl, stir together witch hazel, aloe vera oil, glycerin and chamomile essential oil. Pour into jar.

2. Smooth lotion generously over sunburned skin, reapplying several times a day until discomfort disappears. Store jar in a cool, dark place for up to 1 month.

Sunburn Symptoms

Mild to moderate sunburn appears in the form of redness, itching and peeling of the skin. Severe burns cause blisters, which should never be popped or broken open; doing so exposes the skin to harmful bacteria and can result in infections. Unfortunately, by the time you see these signs, your skin is already damaged and there is nothing you can do but treat, protect and nourish skin as it recovers with the remedies on this page and page 356.

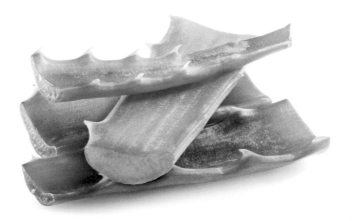

Spearmint and Aloe Sunburn Lotion

Spearmint essential oil is antibacterial, so it's a helpful addition to this lotion. It fights bacteria that can cause infections in tender, burned skin.

Best for: Moderate to severe sunburns

Tip: Buy essential oils sold in dark bottles. Exposure to light can reduce the potency of their medicinal herbal components. Store the bottles in a cool, dark place to keep them fresh.

Note: Always measure accurately when you're making homemade beauty products. See page 53 for tips.

- Small glass jar with lid

2 tbsp	aloe vera oil (see tips, page 355)	30 mL
2 tbsp	liquid glycerin (see tips, page 355)	30 mL
4	drops spearmint essential oil (see tip, at left)	4

1. In a small bowl, stir aloe vera oil with glycerin until well combined. Stir in spearmint essential oil. Pour into jar.

2. Smooth lotion generously over sunburned skin, reapplying several times a day until discomfort disappears. Store jar in a cool, dark place for up to 1 month.

More Home Remedies for Sunburns

There are several natural, simple home treatments that can ease the pain of sunburns and speed up healing. One traditional recipe is to boil equal parts red wine and olive oil together for 15 minutes. Let the mixture cool, and pat onto sunburned skin with a cotton ball. You can also apply the following to red, painful skin:

- Aloe vera gel
- Equal parts cider vinegar and olive oil
- Equal parts cider vinegar and water
- Grated raw potato
- Puréed cucumber
- Stinging nettle or sage infusion
- Strong brewed tea that has cooled

Safe Sun Exposure

Exposing your skin to the sun's rays releases free radicals, which cause aging. But that doesn't mean you have to give up on the sun entirely. You can still enjoy soaking up some rays if you follow these key pieces of advice:

- Protect your skin from overexposure by wearing light-colored clothing, a hat, sunscreen and sunglasses.
- Avoid exposure when UV rays are strongest. Stay out of the sun between 11 a.m. and 2 p.m. in summer, when the sun's radiation is most intense.
- Expose your skin gradually. Limit sun time after a long period of being indoors (such as at the beginning of summer), and let your skin get used to exposure a little at a time.
- Don't trust a cloudy sky to protect you from the sun. UV rays penetrate clouds and can still burn your skin.
- When you're buying or making a sunscreen, make sure you choose one that has the appropriate level of SPF for your skin. Paler skin needs much shorter exposure times and much stronger SPF to prevent burns. Consult a dermatologist if you are not sure what to choose.
- Never expose babies or children under five years of age to the sun during peak hours, even if they are wearing sunscreen.
- In addition to protecting children's delicate skin from burns, be sure to protect them from sunstroke and dehydration caused by excessive sun and heat.
- Drink plenty of water to compensate for the dehydrating effect of sunbathing. Aim for at least 8 cups (2 L) per day.

Protection for Tan Lovers

Even though they understand the risks of overexposure, some people still love to get a deep tan. If you're one of those people, you need extra protection. Externally, you need to apply a good-quality sunscreen and avoid peak hours of solar radiation. Internally, you need to consume foods or supplements that provide plenty of antioxidants, such as vitamin E, to help boost your epithelial cells' defenses. Make sure you also get extra vitamin C and the trace element selenium.

Vitamin A is a crucial skin-protecting micronutrient. Your body synthesizes this from a variety of carotenes (such as beta-carotene) consumed in foods. A specialized protein binds and transports vitamin A through the bloodstream into the cells of the dermal and epidermal layers of the skin, where it is transformed into a series of fat-soluble substances that penetrate all layers of the skin. If skin that has been exposed to a great deal of sun does not receive enough vitamin A, it becomes keratinized, which makes it tough, leathery and much darker than its natural color.

If you tan responsibly, you can make your glow last longer. Increase your consumption of vegetables (such as carrots, squash, zucchini and tomatoes) and fruits (such as melons, apricots and peaches). After a sunbathing session, be sure to help your skin cells regenerate by consuming foods that are high in vitamin C, including red peppers, broccoli, cabbage, oranges, tangerines, lemons, kiwifruit and strawberries.

After-Sun Cream

Skin can get dry when exposed to the sun, and a hydrating after-sun cream is a terrific solution. This one contains a number of natural emollients that protect the skin.

Best for: All skin types

Tips: Choose 100% natural cocoa butter for homemade creams like this. You can buy chunks of this creamy, yellowish substance made from cocoa beans at cosmetic-supply stores and online. It is also sold in uniform-size wafers. Either form will work fine in this recipe.

Stearic acid crystals are commonly added to mixtures that contain beeswax, to help boost the wax's emulsifying powers. Look for them at cosmetic-supply stores or online.

Note: Always measure accurately when you're making homemade beauty products. See page 53 for tips.

- Fine-mesh sieve
- Hand mixer
- Small glass jar with lid

1 tsp	dried horsetail (see tips, page 272)	5 mL
2 tbsp	boiling water	30 mL
¼ oz	raw beeswax, grated (see tip, page 158)	7 g
¼ oz	cocoa butter (see tips, at left)	7 g
⅛ oz	stearic acid (see tips, at left)	4 g
1 tbsp	avocado oil	15 mL
2 tsp	walnut oil	10 mL
3	drops orange essential oil (see tip, page 356)	3

1. Place horsetail in a small heatproof bowl; pour boiling water over top. Cover and let stand for 5 minutes.

2. Place fine-mesh sieve over a small glass measuring cup; strain infusion into cup, discarding solids. Let cool to room temperature.

3. In another small heatproof bowl, combine beeswax, cocoa butter, stearic acid, avocado oil and walnut oil. Set aside.

4. Pour enough water into a small saucepan to come about 2 inches (5 cm) up the side; bring to a simmer.

5. Set bowl with beeswax mixture on saucepan so that bottom of bowl is not touching simmering water; stir until beeswax mixture is melted and smooth. Remove bowl from heat.

6. Add horsetail infusion to beeswax mixture. Using hand mixer, beat for 2 minutes or until beeswax mixture has a milky consistency.

7. Add orange essential oil and beat for 2 minutes or until mixture is thickened and cooled.

8. Pour into jar. Gently massage cream over skin after sun exposure. Store jar in a cool, dark place for up to 1 month.

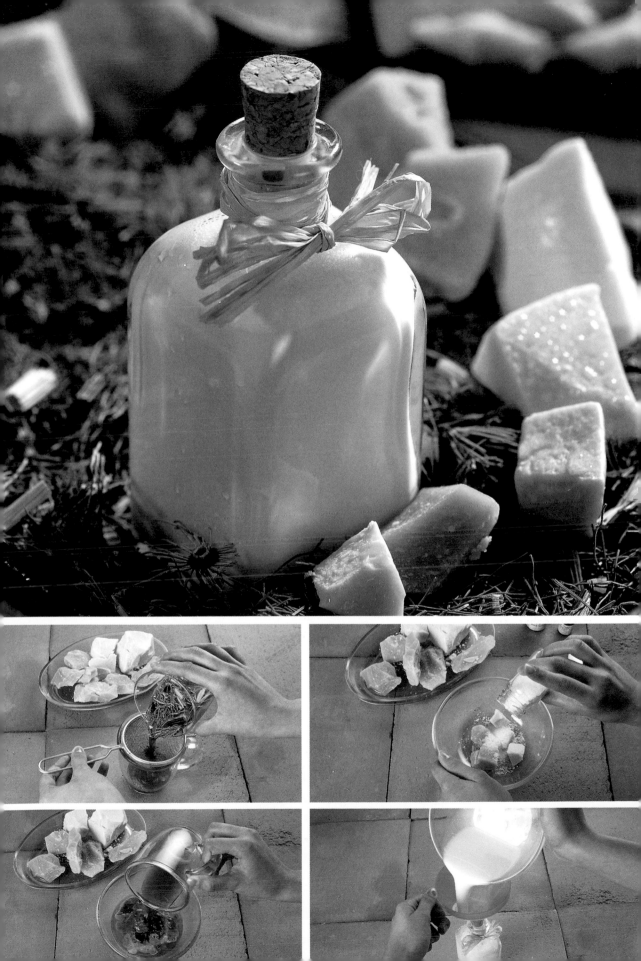

Resources

Associations

Handcrafted Soap & Cosmetic Guild

178 Elm St.
Saratoga Springs, NY 12866, U.S.A.
www.soapguild.org

International nonprofit trade association promoting the benefits of handcrafted soap and cosmetics.

Canadian Guild of Soapmakers, Chandlers & Cosmetic Crafters

www.canadianprofessionalsoapmakers.com

Association of professional craftspeople specializing in artisanal soaps and other personal-care products.

The European Directory of Soap and Cosmetic Makers

146 Glasgow Rd.
Longcroft, Stirlingshire
FK4 1QL, U.K.
www.soapmakers.eu

Europe's largest directory of artisans specializing in handmade soaps, candles, cosmetics and personal-care products.

Information

Cosmetic Ingredient Review

1620 L St. N.W.
Suite 1200
Washington, DC 20036, U.S.A.
www.cir-safety.org

Supported by the Personal Care Products Council, the U.S. Food and Drug Administration, and the Consumer Federation of America, a panel of experts and policy makers publish safety reviews of ingredients used to make cosmetics.

EWG's Skin Deep Cosmetics Database

1436 U St. N.W.
Suite 100
Washington, DC 20009, U.S.A.
www.ewg.org/skindeep

The Environmental Working Group (EWG) is a nonprofit, nonpartisan organization that funds research, education and advocacy for consumer protection from environmental pollutants and toxins. Their database and mobile app contains detailed data on the safety of more than 64,000 ingredients used in consumer beauty and body-care products.

Supplies

Aussie Soap Supplies

P.O. Box 165
Palmyra, WA 6957, Australia
www.aussiesoapsupplies.com.au

Carrier and essential oils, cocoa and shea butters, glycerin, flower waters, witch hazel, beeswax, clays and soap bases.

Bramble Berry Soap Making Supplies

2138 Humboldt St.
Bellingham, WA 98225, U.S.A.
www.brambleberry.com

Carrier and essential oils, cocoa and shea butters, powdered additives, beeswax, soap bases, natural colorants, soap molds and exfoliants.

Canwax Candle & Soap Making Supplies

114 Lindgren Rd. W.
Huntsville, ON P1H 1Y2, Canada
www.canwax.com

Carrier and essential oils, flower waters, witch hazel, zinc oxide powder, cocoa and shea butters, and clays.

From Nature With Love

341 Christian St.
Oxford, CT 06478, U.S.A.
www.fromnaturewithlove.com

Carrier and essential oils, flower waters, cocoa and shea butters, beeswax, clays, stearic acid and soap bases.

Gracefruit Limited
146 Glasgow Rd.
Longcroft, Stirlingshire
FK4 1QL, U.K.
www.gracefruit.com
Carrier and essential oils, butters, beeswax, glycerin, exfoliants, clays and jars.

Healing Spirits Herb Farm
61247 Route 415
Avoca, NY 14809, U.S.A.
www.healingspiritsherbfarm.com
Medicinal herbs, essential oils and extracts.

Horizon Herbs
P.O. Box 69
William, OR 97544, U.S.A.
www.horizonherbs.com
Medicinal herbs, extracts, seeds and plants.

MakingCosmetics
35318 S.E. Center St.
Snoqualmie, WA 98065, U.S.A.
www.makingcosmetics.com
Carrier oils, cocoa and shea butters, glycerin, beeswax and powdered additives.

Mountain Rose Herbs
P.O. Box 50220
Eugene, OR 97405, U.S.A.
www.mountainroseherbs.com
Carrier and essential oils, medicinal herbs, cocoa and shea butters, beeswax, clays, teas, powdered additives, bottles and jars.

New Directions Aromatics
6781 Columbus Rd.
Mississauga, ON L5T 2G9, Canada
www.newdirectionsaromatics.ca
Carrier and essential oils, flower waters, cocoa and shea butters, beeswax, soap bases, soap molds, bottles and jars.

Oregon Trail Soapers Supply
522 E. Main #1456
Rogue River, OR 97537, U.S.A.
www.oregontrailsoaps.com
Carrier and essential oils, cocoa and shea butters, beeswax, clays, soap bases, natural colorants and soap molds.

Richters
357 Hwy 47
Goodwood, ON L0C 1A0, Canada
www.richters.com
Medicinal herbs, essential oils, seeds and plants.

Saffire Blue Inc.
1444 Bell Mill Sideroad
Tillsonburg, ON N4G 4G9, Canada
www.saffireblue.ca
Carrier and essential oils, cocoa and shea butters, beeswax, glycerin, powdered additives, bottles and jars.

Soap Basics
23 Southbrook Rd.
Melksham, Wiltshire SN12 8DS, U.K.
www.soapbasics.com
Carrier and essential oils, cocoa and shea butters, beeswax, clays and soap bases.

The Soap Kitchen
Unit 8, Caddsdown Industrial Park
Clovelly Rd.
Bideford, Devon EX39 3DX, U.K.
www.thesoapkitchen.co.uk
Carrier oils, cocoa and shea butters, beeswax, soap bases, soap molds, bottles and jars.

Soapmakers Store
Unit 3, Quatro Park
Blakelands Industrial Estate
Tanners Drive
Milton Keynes MK14 5FJ, U.K.
http://soapmakers-store.com
Carrier and essential oils, cocoa and shea butters, beeswax, soap bases, soap molds, natural colorants, bottles and jars.

Voyageur Soap & Candle Co.
#14-19257 Enterprise Way
Surrey, BC V3S 6J8, Canada
www.voyageursoapandcandle.com
Carrier and essential oils, cocoa and shea butters, beeswax, soap bases, soap molds, bottles and jars.

Index

Library and Archives Canada Cataloguing in Publication

Ruiz, Amelia
[Belleza y cosmética natural. English]
    The complete guide to natural homemade beauty products & treatments : 175 recipes from scrubs & masks to moisturizers & shampoos / Amelia Ruiz.

Includes index.
Translation of: Belleza y cosmética natural.
ISBN 978-0-7788-0530-4 (paperback)

    1. Beauty, Personal. 2. Herbal cosmetics. 3. Cosmetics. 4. Hair—Care and hygiene. 5. Skin—Care and hygiene.
I. Title. II. Title: Belleza y cosmética natural. English.

RA776.98.R8513 2016   646.7'2   C2015-908241-2

REBELS
ON
EIGHTH
STREET

REBELS ON EIGHTH STREET

JULIANA FORCE
❦ *AND THE* ❦
WHITNEY MUSEUM
❦ *OF* ❦
AMERICAN ART

AVIS BERMAN

ATHENEUM
NEW YORK ❦ 1990

Atheneum
Macmillan Publishing Company
866 Third Avenue, New York, NY 10022
Collier Macmillan Canada, Inc.

Library of Congress Cataloging-in-Publication Data

Berman, Avis.
  Rebels on Eighth Street : Juliana Force and the Whitney Museum of American Art / Avis Berman.
    p.   cm.
  Bibliography: p.
  Includes index.
  ISBN 0-689-12086-9
  1. Force, Juliana, 1876–1948.   2. Art museum directors—United States—Biography.   3. Art patrons—United States—Biography.
4. Whitney Museum of American Art.   I. Title.
N618.B47   1990
709.73'092—dc20
[B]   89-14968
                                                                  CIP

Macmillan books are available at special discounts for bulk purchases for sales promotions, premiums, fund raising, or educational use. For details, contact:

Special Sales Director
Macmillan Publishing Company
866 Third Avenue
New York, NY 10022

10 9 8 7 6 5 4 3 2 1

Designed by Jack Meserole

PRINTED IN THE UNITED STATES OF AMERICA

Permissions and acknowledgments appear on page 573.

For CARL *and* HELEN

CONTENTS

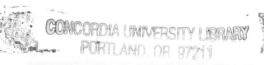

ILLUSTRATIONS

ABBREVIATIONS

AAA   Archives of American Art, Smithsonian Institution
Col. I, AAA   Photographs of Artists, Collection I, Archives of American Art,
        Smithsonian Institution
GVWP   Gertrude Vanderbilt Whitney Papers
RFC   Rieser Family Collection
WMAA   Collection of the Whitney Museum of American Art,
        New York, N.Y.
WMAA, Archives   Collection of the Whitney Museum of American Art Archives

ACKNOWLEDGMENTS

It is a pleasure to thank the many persons who have helped me to prepare and complete this book.

My greatest debt is owed to the members of Juliana Force's family whom I have been privileged to know. No one could have been more tolerant, more intelligent, or more understanding than Carl and Allan Rieser, Juliana Force's nephews. They turned over letters and photographs without caveat, and as the years went by, they spent hundreds of hours answering questions, some of them unpleasant, with candor and grace. Their loyalty and reassurance were unfailing. I am also deeply obligated to Juliana Force's nieces, Marjorie Rieser and Beverly Rieser Smock, both now deceased, for their frank observations and painstaking genealogical research. I cannot thank the Rieser family enough for letting me explore their aunt's rich and varied life and follow the trails wherever they led. Deborah Rieser and Theodore Smock, Juliana Force's niece and nephew by marriage, also displayed extraordinary goodwill in dealing with incessant familial queries. John and Elizabeth Gerald, two of Juliana Force's staunchest friends, said of her, "We miss her more than anyone else who went out of our lives," and I feel the same void now that the biography is done. But if I became enriched from knowing Juliana Force, I continue to be rewarded by my acquaintance with her family.

The cardinal fact of Juliana Force's life was her alliance with Gertrude Vanderbilt Whitney, and a cardinal fact of this biography has been the unstinting cooperation of the Whitney family. To my great benefit, Gertrude Whitney was a hoarder of documents and memorabilia, and I am extremely grateful to Gertrude Whitney's daughter, the late Flora Whitney Miller, and her granddaughter, Flora Miller Biddle, for their part in propelling this book along. Without their trust and their generosity in allowing me to read through Gertrude Whitney's voluminous archives, this book could not have come into being. Among other members of the Whitney family, I am happy to thank Gerta and Macauley Conner for their many kindnesses during the early stages of this project.

Several people made such fundamental contributions to my work that I can only begin to express my full appreciation in print. First, I am honored to acknowledge the advice, guidance, and friendship of the late Lloyd Goodrich. We had many pointed and delightful conversations about his days on Eighth Street, Juliana Force, and the art world he knew and helped to shape. I am extremely proud that both Lloyd Goodrich and his wife, Edith Havens Goodrich,

read the first part of the manuscript and pronounced it accurate and readable. I am equally proud to acknowledge the enormous interest Brendan Gill, Ira and Nancy Glackens, Katharine Kuh, and Helen Farr Sloan took in my progress. They have been acute critics and the most steadfast of friends, so much so, that only they know how much I owe them.

I am most grateful to Thomas N. Armstrong III, the director of the Whitney Museum, for his total cooperation in permitting me to examine his institution's archives. He placed no constraints on the available material, nor did he seek to influence the contents of the manuscript. On the museum's curatorial staff, Barbara Haskell and Patterson Sims graciously shared information and traded insights and speculations over the years. May Castleberry, the Whitney's librarian, welcomed me whenever I turned up and fulfilled my requests with cheerfulness and dispatch. Most of all, I would like to pay tribute to Anita Duquette, the manager of rights and reproductions, for coming to my rescue countless times over the years. Her comprehensive knowledge of Whitney collections past and present, her commitment to pursuing inquiries, and her ready identifications of photographs and works of art have taken on heroic dimensions.

When a memorial exhibition in Juliana Force's honor was organized by the Whitney in 1949, her colleagues Hermon More and Lloyd Goodrich wrote, "The history of her career and the successive organizations that she and Mrs. Whitney built has never been written and must always remain incomplete, for the two protagonists never thought of themselves as historic figures, and left only fragmentary records." Since the time those words were written, much new primary documentation on American art has become accessible, but the paucity of records about the Whitney Studio and Studio Club was an obstacle that had to be surmounted. Although Juliana Force was not one to save papers, many artists who were regular exhibitors at the Whitney did. More often than not, their papers and oral histories were assiduously collected and preserved by the Archives of American Art. Without the invaluable collections of the Archives and the expertise and enthusiasm of its staff, I could not have attempted a biography of Juliana Force. I am especially indebted to William McNaught, William Woolfenden, Garnett McCoy, Jemison Hammond, Arleen Pancza, Robert Brown, Marina Pacini, Paul Karlstrom, and Catherine Keen for their many favors and dispensations.

Other librarians and archivists who assisted me were Van B. Afes, New York University Dental Center; Paula Baxter, Janis Ekdahl, Daniel Pearl, and Daniel Starr, the Museum of Modern Art; Donald Gallup and David Schoonover, Beinecke Rare Book and Manuscript Library, Yale University; Eugene R. Gaddis, Wadsworth Atheneum; Abigail Gerdts, National Academy of Design; Jeanie M. James, Metropolitan Museum of Art; Michael Kelly and Al Minnick, Buffalo Bill Historical Center; Aletha Kowitz, American Dental Association; Terry A. McNealy, Bucks County Historical Society; Terry Miller, Encyclopaedia Britannica; Bruce Brooks Pfeiffer and Indira Berndtson, Frank Lloyd Wright Memorial Foundation; Judith Schiff, Sterling Memorial Library, Yale University; Mike Spangler, National Society of the Daughters of the American Revolution; Catherine Stover, Art Institute of Chicago; Joel K. Thiele, Malden

Public Library; Patricia Tugwell, Pentagon Library; and Deborah Wythe, the Brooklyn Museum. For furnishing me with materials from their institutions, I am also indebted to Michael Culver, Ogunquit Museum of Art; Linda Dost, Nelson-Atkins Museum of Art; Mark L. Drucker, National Park Service; Diana Edkins, Condé Nast; Richard Kuehne, West Point Museum; William Morrow, Northfield Mount Hermon School; and Sealy Hathaway Rodger, Sotheby's.

My understanding of the subject has been enlarged by conversations and correspondence with a number of writers, art historians, and scholars in other fields. Dan Burne Jones, Janis Conner, Rowland and Betty Elzea, Betsy Fahlman, William M. Murphy, Francis V. O'Connor, Bennard Perlman, Pierce Rice, Joel Rosenkranz, Irving Sandler, Frances Weitzenhoffer, James Yarnall, and Marilyn J. Ziffrin have consistently gone out of their way to provide aid and comfort. I also thank William Agee, Mary Black, Susanne Brendel-Pandich, Carol Clark, Wanda M. Corn, Alvord Eiseman, Emily Farnham, John Gable, Emily Goldstein, Christopher Gray, Randolph C. Henning, Douglas Hyland, Sue Davidson Lowe, Stanley E. Marcus, Clark Marlor, Eugene Metcalf, Ann Lee Morgan, Michael Richman, and Carol Troyen for their knowledgeable assistance, from which I have profited greatly.

As a girl, Juliana Force copied out a quotation into her daybook that appealed to her: "How hard and colorless is life without an atmosphere!" This was an aphorism she took to heart, and her feeling for atmosphere was reflected in the *gemütlich* environment she created for herself and the artists in her circle. Whenever possible, I strove to re-create the atmosphere and milieu in which Juliana Force moved—to live over events and phases of her life, as it were—through the testimony of those who remembered her. For reminiscences and time freely given, I am indebted to the following friends, acquaintances, and colleagues of Juliana Force: Faith Andrews, Marie Appleton, Edmund Archer, Peggy Bacon, Eleanor Lambert Berkson, Theresa Bernstein, Isabel Bishop, Lucile Blanch, Aaron Bohrod, Edith Bry, Jeanne Bultmann, Stanton Catlin, Patra Cogan, Gertrude Henry Conner, Horace Day, Joseph Delaney, Elsie Driggs, Maria Ealand, Mary Earley, David Eisendrath, Emlen Etting, Col. Robert Evans, Barbara Fite, Dennis Flanagan, James Thomas Flexner, Karl Fortess, John Frear, R. Buckminster Fuller, Sidney Geist, John and Elizabeth Bart Gerald, Eugenie Gershoy, Ira Glackens, C. Adolph Glassgold, Maurice Glickman, Lloyd Lózes Goff, Harry Gottlieb, Helen Gray, Dorothea Greenbaum, Chaim Gross, Berte and A. Edward Grudin, Ruth Grudin, Karl Gruppe, Albert and Frances Goodrich Hackett, Raoul Hague, Hananiah Harari, David and Katie Harris, Rosella Hartman, John Davis Hatch, Axel Horn, Edward and Anne Powis Jones, Jacob Kainen, Dora Koch, Antoinette Kraushaar, Viette Kroll, Richard Kuehne, Brenda Kuhn, Marchal Landgren, William Lane, Edward Laning, John Laurent, Julian Levi, Florence Lewison, Edith and Milton Lowenthal, Molly Luce, Luigi Lucioni, Eugene Ludins, Betty Bartlett Madden, Peppino Mangravite, Nan Mason, Bena Frank Mayer, Grace Mayer, Eleanor Scarlc McCollum, Yvonne Pène du Bois McKenney, Janet Meder, Flora Whitney Miller, Herbert Morgan, Maud Morgan, Donn Mosenfelder, Reuben Nakian, Elizabeth Navas, Isamu Noguchi, Edith Nolder, William Pachner, Betty

Parsons, Simmons Persons, Eugenie Prendergast, Ethel Renthal, John Rewald, William Robb, Andrée Ruellan, Allen Saalburg, Charles Sawyer, Katherine Schmidt, Bernarda Bryson Shahn, Anne and Margaret Sharkey, Millard Sheets, Irvine Shubert, Helen Farr Sloan, Hannah Small, Isaac Soyer, Raphael Soyer, Harry Sternberg, Henry Strater, Jane Bouché Strong, Allene Talmey, John W. Taylor, W. Lester Trauch, Dorothy Varian, Maynard Walker, Jane Wasey, Gordon Washburn, Monroe Wheeler, Timothy Whitehead, and Edwin Zittell.

For letters, photographs, and other documentary information, I thank Ivan Albright, Elena Barnet, Margaret Scolari Barr, Cecil Beaton, James Benton, Edward L. Bernays, Alexander Brook, Jr., Nathaniel Burt, Ned Cameron, Rodrigo de Zayas, Elizabeth Dos Passos, Sylvia Winsor Dudley, Lois B. Force, Jared and Margaret French, Elizabeth Geissbuhler, Martha Gellhorn, Rosamund Gilder, Malcolm Goldstein, David and Patricia Goodrich, Stephen Greene, Chaim Gross, Alexandre Hogue, John Houseman, Thomas Carr Howe, George Karfiol, Caroline Keck, H. W. Keil, Sara Kuniyoshi, James Lechay, Janet LeClair, John and Norma Marin, William Maxwell, A. Hyatt Mayor, William Ashby McCloy, James A. Michener, Don F. Mills, Sheridan Morley, Paul Nakian, Roy Neuberger, Gerald Nordland, Elizabeth Olds, Audrey Buller Parsons, Carole Pesner, Jan Pirzio-Biroli, Donald Pizer, Edna Reindel, Nicholas Rieser, Genevieve Rindner, Lillian Rixey, William Roerich, Lincoln Rothschild, Daniel and Eleanore Saidenberg, Helen Sawyer, William Schack, J. Nevin Schroeder, Jr., Antoinette Schulte, Ernest Small, Eloise Spacth, Edward John Stevens, Lowell Thomas, Donald Torchiana, H. E. Vinyard, Rebecca West, Cornelius Vanderbilt Whitney, and Alice Winchester.

For sharing unpublished correspondence, diaries, interviews, and memoirs, I thank Benjamin Bernstein, Aileen Cramer, Earl Davis, Emlen Etting, and John Graves.

At Atheneum, I must thank my editor, Carrie Chase, for her patience, hard work, and humor. Ann Finlayson copyedited the manuscript with great care, Karla Knight compiled an expert index, and Benita Korn provided special editorial assistance.

As an independent writer, I could not have borne the entire cost of financing this biography alone. There is no gift like financial independence not only for research and travel, but for the substantial periods of time that sustained thinking and writing require. In the course of working on this book, I was fortunate enough to receive financial assistance three times. The National Endowment for the Humanities awarded me a Fellowship for Independent Study and Research, which gave me an uninterrupted year to spend on Juliana Force. Before and after the NEH fellowship, I received grants from the John Sloan Memorial Foundation that fortified me in completing and revising the first portion of the manuscript. I could not have accepted the Sloan grants without the agency of the Archives of American Art, which administered them for me. I hope that the finished product has justified these organizations' faith in me.

Finally, I wish to thank my family, my friends, and my agent, Helen Merrill, for their support and encouragement.

REBELS
ON
EIGHTH
STREET

FIRE, INTRIGUE, AND LARGESSE

T HERE IS a photograph in existence of Juliana Force, tiny and uncertain, standing near the fireplace in the library of her apartment on Eighth Street, just west of Fifth Avenue. In front of her stretch broadly flowered Brussels carpets, invisibly sewn together. Above her hang four enormous lamps, their globes grasped in the talons of gilded eagles, raised and lowered by silken cords. A profusion of chairs, urns, alabaster ornaments, statuary, bibelots, and paintings threatens to overwhelm her, a collector by her things collected. It is one of the rare occasions when she was dwarfed by her surroundings instead of dominating them.

The opulent setting reflected the owner's reputation as a vivid personality and someone with an eye that ranged far beyond the boundaries of regulation taste. The suite of rooms, which no visitor ever forgot, took up the top two floors of the Whitney Museum of American Art, the center of her career and affections. The apartment was strewn with plump, tufted loveseats, petticoated hassocks, marble-topped tables, carved blackamoors, and velvets, satins, and fringes that were dear to the hearts of the 1870s but eyesores to their grandchildren. The walls were hung with pictures by itinerant nineteenth-century folk artists (another pioneering enthusiasm) and by more contemporary names, such as Charles Sheeler, Joseph Stella, Preston Dickinson, Niles Spencer, Abraham Walkowitz, Guy Pène du Bois, Philip Evergood, and Glenn O. Coleman. At the time, these young Americans were deemed nearly as uncouth as the self-taught limners. More often than not, this blend of art, antiques, and curios was photographed for its sovereign eccentricity rather than as an interior to imitate. Like the woman who assembled it, the decor challenged convention too vehemently to appeal to people who needed the assurance of rules and certainties.

In a far more characteristic portrait, taken at about the same time, Juliana

1

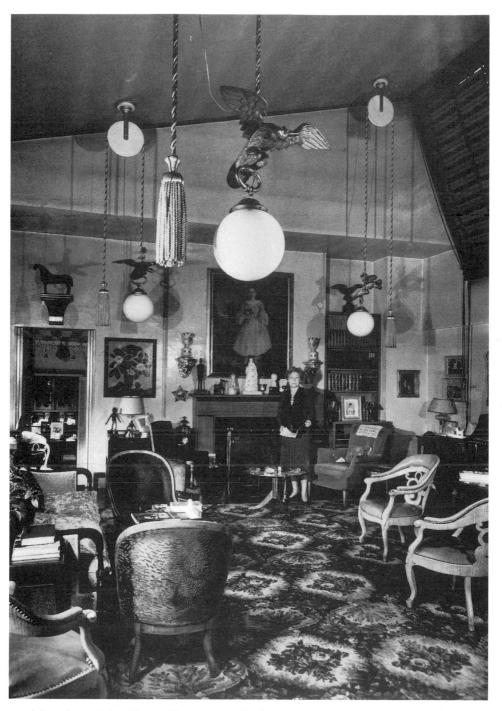

Juliana Force in her library. The chairs are Biedermeier and the carpet, also nineteenth century, has red roses splashed on a white background.

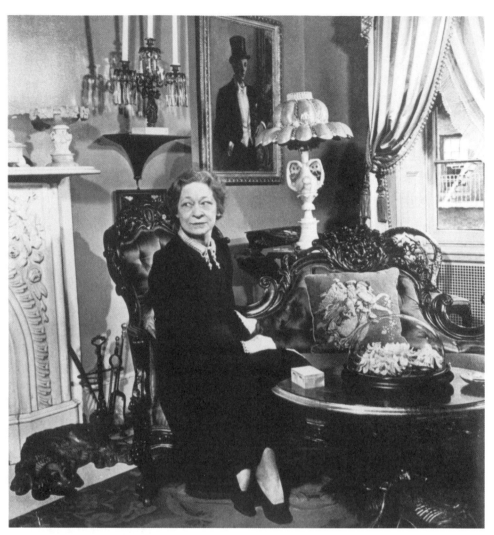

Juliana earning her nickname: Mrs. Fierce. The portrait in the background is by Henry Schnakenberg.

Force roosts regally on a rosewood sofa. She wears a finely tailored wool dress, and the pearl collar knotted around her neck is a pretty echo of the pearls edging the blue satin draperies at the window. The homely, mobile features hint at both kindness and malice. With her unbending posture and hooded green eyes challenging the camera with their piercing gaze, she seems, as indeed she was, one of the more formidable figures in the art world of her day.

The day was late in 1939. The portrait and other photographs were shot to accompany a profile of Mrs. Force, as everyone invariably called her, that appeared in *Vogue* on February 1, 1940. The author was Allene Talmey, then

a feature writer and editor for the magazine. Her assignment was to write a series of stories on New Yorkers in the public eye. The patrician Juliana Force—first director of the Whitney Museum, art patron and impresario, agent and representative of Gertrude Vanderbilt Whitney—was a natural choice to inaugurate the series. "Juliana Force was the most powerful woman I ever knew," Allene Talmey said many years later. "She had made a place for herself, and New York moved over to make room for her. She could make or break an artist. Despite the enormous disparity in size, prestige, and years of operation between the two museums, Mrs. Force had as much influence as the director of the Metropolitan Museum of Art."

Impulsive, arbitrary, innovative, and autocratic by turns, but always striving to gain artists an audience for their work, Juliana Force was a doer and a scrapper who triumphed at a man's job in a man's world. She was a standout even in a profession that cultivated mavericks and applauded originals. By the time *Vogue* presented her to its readers as the model of an executive woman, Juliana's verve—and trenchant tongue—had assumed celebrated proportions, since she was no stranger to controversy and gossip. Peggy Bacon, who had drawn a biting caricature of Juliana in 1931 and secretly subtitled the portrait *The Ugly Duchess*, described her to a T: "Handsome, auburn *chevelure*, cream-colored skin and small menacing eyes that miss nothing. Nose of a Cyrano de Bergerac, mouth like a circumflex accent. Figure erect, trim, magnetic, packed with audacity and challenge. As full of fire, intrigue, poison and largesse as the Italian Renaissance."

When Allene Talmey arrived, notebook in hand, at the salmon-pink building in Greenwich Village that housed the museum, awareness of an entity called American art was already instilled, at least in the better museums and commercial galleries. Enlightened minds granted that painters, sculptors, and graphic artists active in 1935 could be as important as those of a hundred years earlier. As Allene Talmey noted, "Before the Whitney-Force tactics, the status of American painting and sculpture was deplorable. Most of the dealers, collectors, museums had little knowledge or desire to know about American artists, with the exception of a carefully culled few."

Progress had been slow and arduous. It took the small band of trailblazers a good thirty years to prevail, for turn-of-the-century America was narrow, provincial, and smugly ignorant when it came to culture and creative expression. In the main, the citizenry pigeonholed art and artists as useless, lazy, effeminate, decadent, *European*. (Before the early 1930s, when the College Art Association began sending out traveling exhibitions and the New Deal art projects put painters to work designing murals for public buildings, the majority of the population had never seen an original oil painting by a professional artist.) New York City, the magnet for the socially, intellectually, and materially ambitious, was emerging as the nation's cultural capital. As such, it offered the best of universally depressing possibilities. Serious artists were converging on Manhattan by the hundreds, but they were apt to be ignored or scorned. Anyone whose work departed from the reigning requirements of sentimentality, picturesqueness, idealization, or laboriously recorded detail stood little chance of attracting sales

or encouragement. As John Sloan said of that grim period, "We always regarded contemporary success as artistic failure."

The Metropolitan Museum of Art, the preeminent art museum in town, was firmly expatriate in outlook, devoted to accumulating the masterworks of Europe and Asia. The small number of examples by Americans that trickled in typically were gifts of their own work from the conservative artists sitting on the Metropolitan's board of trustees. The prevailing attitude toward local talent was summed up in 1909 by John Cadwalader, one of the trustees. He asked the museum's president, "What do you mean by American art? Do you mean English or French or what? There is nothing American worth notice."

Dealers generally felt the same way. Fewer than six commercial galleries sold or showed living American artists, and only two of them were willing to gamble on anything out of the ordinary. The sole remedy for this stifling state of affairs was the occasional show initiated and paid for by the excluded artists themselves. However, lack of funding or a permanent exhibition space kept these "outlaw salons" sporadic occurrences; hence their effectiveness was limited. Despite the ground swell of independent art shows held during the first years of the twentieth century, culminating in the epochal Armory Show of 1913, most fine arts institutions and authorities regarded the native talent as vulgar and insignificant. Until the body blow delivered by the Armory Show, one organization had an apparent stranglehold on large, prestigious exhibitions in New York. The National Academy of Design was a citadel of conservatism whose acceptance could mean the difference between survival and failure for a young artist. Originally the Academy had served a useful function as an artist-run coalition for teaching and exhibiting, but over the years it had ossified into a reactionary body that excused the submissions of its members from the scrutiny of a jury and rejected or "skyed" above eye level the canvases of almost everyone else. Change would require a strong-willed person who could rally the dissidents, a dynamo to power the democratization of art.

At first, Juliana's status and largesse derived from Gertrude Whitney, the vastly wealthy sculptor and socialite who put her name and fortune at her associate's disposal. Their partnership lasted more than three decades, until Gertrude's death in 1942. From the early teens until her own death in 1948, Juliana made the Whitney Museum and the clubby artists' galleries that were its predecessors the greatest sponsors of living American artists in the nation. Ignoring names and rules, Juliana backed her judgments decisively by purchasing works by artists she liked and believed in. She was impulsive, she had favorites, she stirred up trouble, and she did things she shouldn't have, but she was pivotal to a transformation of taste that took root in the 1920s and is still very much in evidence today. Through her increasingly influential position, Juliana opened the eyes of Americans to their visual heritage, to the vitality and worth of native themes, styles, and traditions. Her dedicated, doughty championship of American painting took many forms. She scouted and subsidized artists, bought what they created, supported scholarship in the field of art history, lobbied for protective legislation, and presided over a full schedule of exhibitions. Gertrude Whitney paid the bills, but Juliana Force ran the show.

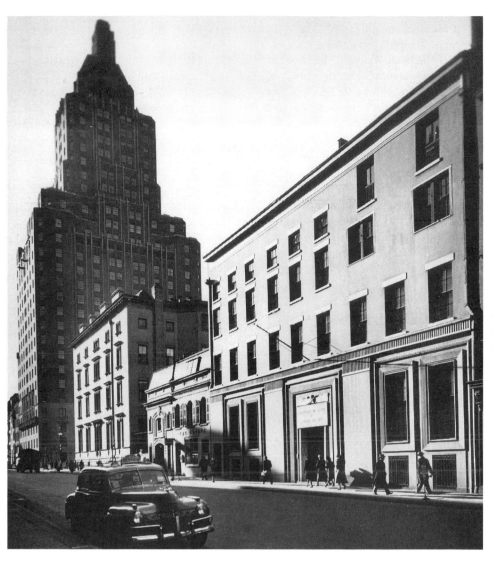

The Whitney Museum of American Art as it looked in 1942. The building incorporated the town houses at 8, 10, 12, and 14 West Eighth Street. The view looks east toward Fifth Avenue.

Juliana became a cynosure of respect and influence in her own right through her most singular achievement, one that was an extension of her own robust temperament. Indeed, her talismanic name, with its intimations of a royal command, fit Juliana so perfectly that it is difficult to write about her without punning on it. Force, tempered by an almost lunatic generosity, was her outstanding characteristic. The sculptor Gutzon Borglum told her, "What with my guts and your force, we could conquer the world."

Juliana changed the received notion of how a museum should look and what

a museum should entail. The conventional function of a museum was to be a repository of the past; its halls were swathed in dark draperies, and the atmosphere was thick with gloom. The existence of the working artist was acknowledged only reluctantly, if at all. Juliana's special and courageous insight—commonplace enough now, but an innovation then—was a wholehearted repudiation of this tenuous, impersonal tie between artists and museums. Aloofness, indifference, and inhospitable premises were anathema to her. First and foremost, she stood for living artists, for guarding their rights and ensuring their future. Juliana valued friendship, loyalty, and intimate involvement, and she demonstrated this to the fullest in her stewardship of the Whitney art enterprises.

Juliana felt as much responsibility toward artists as to the objects they created. Accordingly, the Whitney frequently was less interested in collecting unimpeachable masterpieces than in the more slippery pleasure of nurturing and stimulating artistic creativity. As Juliana explained to one artist, "Our desire [is] to establish a sympathetic relationship between the museum and American artists and to be intelligently informed of what the artists are doing." Put more succinctly, she believed that buying art was good for artists. Juliana once interrupted a roomful of museum directors guilty of proposing abstruse theories on the most proper means of encouraging Art with, "If you love a woman, marry her. If you like a painting, buy it."

She rejoiced in seeing for the simple pleasure of seeing. She urged people to trust their intuitive emotional responses to a work of art and teased them out of worrying about names, fashionable reputations, or established market prices. Her brisk credo, entitled "Think for Yourself" and articulated in a speech given in 1932, caused other museum administrators to quail behind their desks, but it endeared her to the adventurous. The dealer Betty Parsons had this passage from the lecture taped to a wall in her gallery:

> Do not read too much criticism on art. At the beginning it is apt to paralyze thought. . . . Go directly to the work of art and face it alone. Do not remember anything anybody has said about it. . . .
>
> And when you look at a picture be sure you do not search too hard for that little name, or that big name, in the corner of the canvas. Some collectors are made in this very dull, joyless way. It may be good on the day of the auction, but to me it is like looking at happiness through another man's eyes.
>
> . . . Buy pictures, not names. The last thing to interest you in a work of art is the name of an artist. Pictures should be seen, not heard!

No matter how imperious or overbearing she grew, Juliana did not use her position for personal aggrandizement. She enjoyed power, no doubt, but she never lost her sense of obligation. Her power was an instrument for artistic freedom. "Juliana Force used power the way you or I would use a hundred-dollar bill," Allene Talmey explained. "Just use it to do whatever you wanted —simply, directly, without any fuss." If she fought, she almost always had some object other than herself in mind. This is why, regardless of the impact Juliana had on the social history of the visual arts in America and the sturdy hand she gave to hundreds of artists who had nowhere else to turn, her name is virtually unknown except to her own friends and to students of early twentieth-century

American art. There is no physical monument to her in the Whitney Museum at its "new" (since 1966) location on 75th Street and Madison Avenue. Nor would she have wanted one.

Juliana was a mercurial compound of brains, frivolity, rebelliousness, luck, and—as perhaps is inevitable with those who fulfill themselves through the achievements of others—impermanence. Her renown was bound up with the critical fortunes of the young men and women she promoted. Some of the Whitney stalwarts, for the most part exponents of solidly representational painting and sculpture, went into eclipse during the heyday of the New York School; others did not live up to their early promise. That Juliana's record should be mixed was not only fated, but to her credit. If the Whitney helped many artists whose names are best forgotten, it also befriended or crucially aided Edward Hopper, Stuart Davis, John Sloan, Robert Henri, William Glackens, George Luks, Jo Davidson, Gaston Lachaise, Charles Sheeler, Charles Demuth, Charles Burchfield, Peggy Bacon, Joseph Stella, Rockwell Kent, Guy Pène du Bois, Reginald Marsh, Oscar Bluemner, Buckminster Fuller, Edward Steichen, Reuben Nakian, Isamu Noguchi, Raphael Soyer, John Dos Passos, Thomas Hart Benton, John Steuart Curry, Carl Ruggles, and Edgard Varèse. In each case, Juliana gambled on her instinctive sympathy with the person instead of taking the wiser—and utterly uncharacteristic—course of waiting for history to bless him.

But such verdicts were for the future. When Allene Talmey met Juliana, she saw before her the embodiment of money and privilege: a chic, urbane woman who mingled with Whitneys and Rockefellers. She was dressed by Mainbocher and photographed by Cecil Beaton. She owned houses in New York State, Pennsylvania, Connecticut, and England. And she knew an extraordinary range of people. Along with a roll call spanning two generations of American artists, her story was connected, at different times, to personalities as diverse as Noël Coward, Theodore Roosevelt, John Butler Yeats, Emma Goldman, William Randolph Hearst, Christopher Morley, George S. Kaufman, Leopold Stokowski, and Rebecca West.

Allene Talmey appraised Juliana as "[d]ependably indiscreet, brutally witty, she talks effectively, constantly, sparing no feelings, letting people know exactly where they stand." This tart summary was wrong in one important respect. Juliana *was* abrasively candid and dependably indiscreet, except when the conversation turned to two sensitive subjects: Gertrude Whitney or her own origins and background. She remained silent about the first out of love and loyalty; she offered fables about the second out of pride and misguided shame. She believed she had a great deal to hide.

Her deception went beyond the usual feminine fibs about age, although Juliana habitually gouged five to twenty years off that. Relating how Gertrude Whitney enlisted Juliana's services in 1908,* Talmey reported, "Up to that moment, Mrs. Force had had no experience, no training, no Fogg Museum

---

*Evidence points to the date being 1907. See Chapter 3.

coaching . . . to prepare her for gallery running. She was just a pleasant girl who had been born some twenty years previously in Bucks County, Pennsylvania. Most of her childhood had been spent with . . . books; about the only art, in the formal sense, was her father's collection of steel engravings. Instead of going off to Wellesley College, as she planned at eighteen or so, she taught English at a small New England private school, and finally became secretary to Mrs. Whitney." This account implies that Juliana was a frail adolescent creature of genteel antecedents born in 1888. She was supposedly a lady with an independent income whose social position was just a shade less exalted than that of her employer, a Vanderbilt married to a Whitney. No mention was made of her maiden name, her large crop of brothers and sisters, or that she was a twin. In truth, Juliana Rieser Force was a first-generation American born in 1876, the daughter of a poor tradesman. Although born in Doylestown, Pennsylvania, she had grown up unhappy and discontented in Hoboken, New Jersey. Earning a living was a necessity, not an option. Hers was a far more classic—and interesting—American success story than any magazine editor suspected.

There was no question that Juliana misled inquisitive journalists on purpose. "The story was based on an interview with Mrs. Force," Allene Talmey recalled. "I was young then, and we didn't question things as much in those days. If the head of the Whitney Museum told me a damned good lie, I would believe it and not investigate." In a similar vein, for her entry in Who's Who in America, Juliana falsely stated that she had been "educated in private schools and abroad."

A grand, unwitting by-product, and one of the most artful fabrications to issue from Gertrude and Juliana's dashing social service for raw and untried talent, was the highly finished persona of Juliana Force. From her early youth, Juliana was determined to acquire the manner and means of an aristocrat. It was a role she relished, and throughout her life she got away with playing it. Behind the worldly incarnation of confidence and glamour that was Mrs. Force lay the prosaic apparition of Miss Rieser. In burying the evidence of how Miss Rieser metamorphosed into Mrs. Force, Juliana exercised much cleverness and skill. Although she loved the limelight, she feared the glowing coals of memory and acted accordingly. She discarded letters, gave away memorabilia, suppressed details, and refused to reminisce. Even when filling out applications for passports under oath, she never recalled the facts of her life with any accuracy.

She was so firmly possessed by the need to disguise her past that the embroideries became indistinguishable from actual remembrance. By the early 1920s, surface and inner being were united and inseparable. To Alexander Brook, a prominent young painter who worked for Juliana between 1923 and 1927, she seemed a sort of Coriolanus: She was author of herself and knew no other kin. "It seemed incredible," he wrote in 1949. "Juliana Force introduced me early in our friendship to a small, quiet, conservatively dressed man who proved to be her brother. Somehow . . . it did not seem right for her to have a brother or any other relative—even parents, for that matter. I cannot recall that she, at any time, had ever mentioned them in my presence or anything about her childhood or early life. No one I knew could say when she was born, though her birthday was always celebrated with a party on December 25th. To this day

I have met no one who knew her before artists and their work began entirely to absorb her life, and as far as I know, aside from the fun and tragedy of the day, she was never consistently interested in anything else." One of Juliana's nephews confirmed Brook's impression. "We were all gathered together and Aunt Clara and Aunt Mary [Juliana's sisters] were telling a story about the family," Allan Rieser remembered. "Aunt Julia listened to the whole tale, only to say, 'Now that's where you girls go wrong,' and proceeded to turn the entire story around to our benefit. I remember thinking what a beautiful lesson it was in the worldly presentation of yourself."

Juliana fought hard for her seigneury, overcoming poverty and an unpromising physical appearance. She armed herself with everything self-devised: a near-British accent, dramatic gestures, a temper matching her red hair, a wit that devastated the unwary, and a vaguely insinuated pedigree. These weapons intimidated the boors, snobs, and philistines, and entertained everyone else. The patrician forgetfulness that she assumed accounted for many of the ambiguities and contradictions of her career. Impetuous generosity and extravagance were her hallmarks, but a certain arbitrariness and irrationality occasionally crept into her dealings as well. Overearnest or conspicuously educated intellectuals might find themselves targets of her deadliest retorts, and the hostility was more deeply ingrained than a reasonable impatience with pedantry.

"She was one of the great unsung actresses of the age," stated an artist Juliana fired from a curatorial job at the Whitney. His comment was meant derisively, but it has the ring of a compliment, too. Her mental and histrionic gifts were all the dowry Juliana had, and for her they were sufficient even in an era when the majority of her sex could hope to prevail only through the resources of a wealthy and tolerant male relative. For decades Juliana coasted from triumph to triumph. Only in her final years would anything threaten to mar them.

CHAPTER ONE

DOYLESTOWN
AND
HOBOKEN

❦ *(1876–1906)* ❦

T HE YEAR 1876 was a resonant one in American history. The nation celebrated its centennial with pomp, solemnity, and joy. Public meetings, devotional exercises, processions, bonfires, and the ringing of bells around the country all culminated in the huge Centennial Exhibition in Philadelphia, acclaimed as the supreme Centennial city. President Grant, accompanied by the Emperor and Empress of Brazil, opened the ceremonies on May 10, 1876, and in the ensuing months more than 8 million people passed through the turnstile to view the latest refinements in art, science, industry, and agriculture. In the West, Colorado became a state, and Custer was vanquished at the Little Bighorn. *The Adventures of Tom Sawyer* appeared, and Central Park was completed. Thomas Eakins submitted *The Gross Clinic*, the masterpiece of his early manhood, for display in the art pavilion at the Centennial Exhibition, only to have it rejected by the jury, who pronounced its bloodily accurate portrayal of a surgical demonstration too indelicate for the eyes of women and children. Chosen instead were pictures of military heroics, gatherings around the hearth, and Theban maidens singing hymns to the gods. In contrast to these Centennial glories, the presidential election of 1876 saw Samuel Tilden, Democrat of New York, run against the Ohio governor Rutherford B. Hayes. Tilden won the popular vote by a small margin, but Hayes received one more vote in the electoral college, and the election remained in dispute for months. The world did not learn the identity of the nineteenth president of the United States until March of the following year.

The citizens of Doylestown, Pennsylvania, a village twenty-five miles north of Philadelphia, finished out 1876 by recovering from an outbreak of smallpox and debating the outcome of the election. For the family of Max Rieser in

11

particular, the year had not been an auspicious one. Socially and economically, they slipped downward a notch as another two children made their appearance. On December 23, 1876, Juliana and Maximilian Rieser were added to the family's overflowing nursery. The twins, named after their parents, were the eighth and ninth offspring of a woman who would bear a total of fourteen children.

As a girl, Juliana Rieser learned to prize her roots in Bucks County. Her people had carved out a place for themselves in the German community there, and they enjoyed some standing among its members. They prided themselves on their self-sufficiency, military valor, love of liberty, and freedom of conscience, and they were devoted to their new homeland.

Juliana's maternal grandparents, Hermann and Elisabetha Schuler Schmutz, emigrated from the Grand Duchy of Baden in the aftermath of the Revolution of 1848. Hermann Schmutz, the son of a cavalry officer who served in the Napoleonic wars, was also raised to be a soldier. Although social and political conditions in his native Engen forced him to spend some time as a tailor, he nevertheless attained the rank of major. Photographs of him record a tall, square-jawed, stern-looking man who stood at attention with the upright bearing demanded by his profession. In 1848 Hermann was made a delegate from Engen to the rebel congress. He went on to serve under the Baden insurgent Franz Sigel, who later became an American general in the Civil War. At the close of the rebellion, Hermann, Elisabetha, and their five daughters fled to America and settled in New Britain, Pennsylvania, a rural township in Bucks County outside of Doylestown. The area had a large German population, for the Schmutzes' countrymen had been emigrating to Pennsylvania ever since William Penn founded the Commonwealth.

The Schmutzes bought a small farm in New Britain, raised dairy cattle, and harvested oats, wheat, and hay. Hermann owned less than twenty acres—which would yield no more than subsistence homesteading—but in the barter and exchange economy of the region, diligent husbandry as well as actual capital could make for a simple yet comfortable life.

Although merely one of many struggling farmers in his adopted land, Hermann Schmutz became a prominent citizen. He involved himself in civic affairs, was one of the founders of the local German aid society, and stayed loyal to his soldierly past and political tenets. Because of the severe political oppression in the old country, the passion for liberty was a common and ingrained characteristic of German-Americans, who looked upon their participation in elections and government as a serious and God-given duty. Hermann connected voting with the military defense of freedom and the protection of sacred rights. On election days he would arrive at the polling place clad in a top hat and dress coat, a gesture that signified his respect for the democratic process but was also calculated to be noticed. Keeping to his lofty standards in other matters of conscience as well, Hermann abandoned his Catholic religion when the parish priests in Pennsylvania failed to satisfy him intellectually. For the source of Juliana's burning individualism, her impulse toward the theatrical, and her refusal to be

impressed or browbeaten by authority, one need look no further than her up-standing grandfather.

Julia Schmutz (1844–1920), Juliana's mother,* had inherited her father's penchant for dramatic statement and his streak of South German romanticism, as well as his erect carriage and a strong sense of being someone special. She was neither rich nor beautiful—her long nose and conspicuous ears deprived her of any claims to conventional comeliness—but she caught one of Doyles-town's more popular bachelors. In December of 1865, Julia married the town's deputy sheriff, Julius Kuster. Striving and energetic, Kuster was a model new American. He was born in Prussia in 1836 and arrived in Philadelphia in the late 1840s. After several years working as a printer's devil and newspaper editor, Kuster joined the *Doylestown Democrat*, one of the town's two main journals. When Fort Sumter was fired upon, he was one of the first to volunteer for duty. He served in the army for a year, and his commander later wrote that Kuster "spent all his means in endeavoring to raise a company for a three years regiment. He went to Harrisburg with a portion of a company, but failing to obtain a commission, he returned home, paying the expenses of the men who declined entering any other company."

When Julia wed Julius Kuster, he was not only a law officer, but a clerk of the court and an editor of his paper. He was considered a person of substance, and social notices chronicling the couple's comings and goings began turning up in the *Democrat* with cozy regularity. Given his patriotism, military record, and German origins, Julius must have been an ideal son-in-law for the Schmutzes. Whether in acquiescence to Hermann's disdain for the local brand of Catholicism or because Julius's faith made it impossible for a priest to perform the ceremony, the couple were married in the bride's house by a pastor from the Reformed church.

The Kusters set up housekeeping in Doylestown, and on October 15, 1866, twin sons, Herman and John, were born. Within months of their birth, Julius's health began to deteriorate. Medical records suggest that his disease was tuber-culosis. In May of 1867, he set out on an extended, therapeutic tour of the West. He mailed lively dispatches to the *Democrat*, describing his adventures from Harrisburg through Pittsburgh, West Virginia, Ohio, and Kentucky to St. Louis and Kansas. Then, one month into his trip, Julius realized that his con-dition was hopeless. Wanting to die amid family and friends, he started east. He reached Philadelphia on June 20, 1867, and collapsed with a fatal hemorrhage of the lungs. Julius died unaware that the previous week his son John, not yet eight months old, had been carried off by scrofula.

Julia, unaccustomed to owning property or handling large sums of money,

---

*Juliana Force's mother was christened Juliana, but she was called Julia. To avoid confusion in discussing mother and daughter, I use the shortened name to refer to the older woman. When Juliana Force became an aunt, her nieces and nephews called her "Aunt Julia," "Aunt Jule," or, most affectionately, "Aunt J." However no one outside the family circle used any first name other than "Juliana."

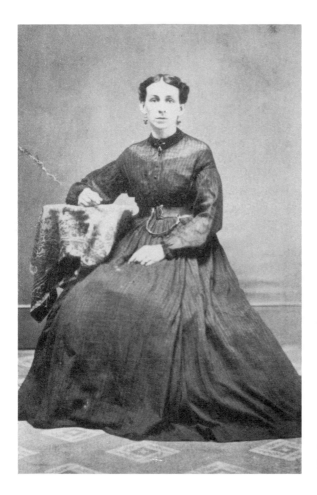

Julia Schmutz Kuster Rieser, Juliana's mother, probably in the 1870s.

was suddenly the head of a household. At a time of great sorrow, she had to begin administering Julius's estate. She had to buy a funeral plot for husband and baby and endure their near-simultaneous burials. Julius died intestate, and his widow had to inventory all of their belongings and find a suitable guardian for her surviving child, who would receive his inheritance in trust. She shouldered these duties with efficiency, as local records and deed books show. And all the while, she had to keep up with the sunup to sundown job that was rural housekeeping. Julia's settlement was $700 in cash and $300 worth of possessions of her choice. She was further aided by the German benevolent society, which donated $125 toward funeral expenses.

Julia was better prepared to cope with her losses and adjust to a diminished situation than her upper middle-class contemporary might have been. The intensely practical Pennsylvania Germans valued industry and resilience in a woman more than ornamental grace, and all members of the family unit were expected to work hard and contribute to its prosperity. German-American wives and mothers had a reputation for strong-mindedness and were respected for their

productivity. This would have been Julia's experience. The feminine flutterings so admired in more cosmopolitan settings would have been scorned as spinelessness or malingering in these hardy communities. The farm household's goal of near self-sufficiency would have schooled her to do what was necessary and face up to realities.

Julia could manage the legal and administrative burdens of widowhood with some degree of skill. What she could not accept so easily were her shrinking prospects and lowered social status. Since she was no longer sharing an interesting future as the wife of a trusted citizen bound for advancement, her prime means of glory had evaporated. To add to her troubles, Hermann Schmutz died in June of 1869, and his farm and equipment were sold at auction. After her father's debts were paid, Julia received almost $1,200, but she had become a completely unprotected woman. Her combined legacies, although a bulwark against immediate insolvency, were not going to last very long. As a dowry, however, the money was a significant sum. The solution to the uncertainties before her was marriage.

Julia's choice was Maximilian Rieser (1843–1917), a distant cousin. According to family legend, Max and Julia first met on board the ship taking them to America. Since Julia was about five and Max about six years old at the time of their journey, the story—whether true or not—was not so romantic as their descendants fancied. More significantly, Max's father, Mathias Rieser, had lived in Engen and married Maria Schmutz, a relation of Hermann's, so all four of Juliana's grandparents had been acquainted in Germany and held similar political views. Mathias Rieser entertained his children, who would subsequently entertain their children, with tales of how he escaped from Germany by a ruse. Mathias received word from a cousin in the government that the authorities were apprised of his revolutionary sympathies. He was warned to leave Baden before he was put in jail and his property confiscated. Having first sent Maria and their children, Max and Matilda, to Paris on a "vacation," Mathias got into the habit of sitting on his front steps in his slippers. In the evenings he would smoke his long pipe, take a short stroll, and then retire. After establishing this pattern, Mathias varied it by casually walking into the Black Forest. His enemies did not guess he would travel far in his bedroom slippers, and Mathias padded nonchalantly along until he was out of sight. He was met in the woods by a friend who gave him a change of clothes and, sturdily shod, Mathias joined his family in France. The four of them landed in New York City with $25 in their pockets.

The Riesers rented rooms on the Lower East Side of Manhattan. In this heavily German district, rapid assimilation was not essential to being employed or understood. Although Max Rieser came to America at an early enough age to speak English like a native, he retained a guttural accent. Julia, however, shed hers.

Outside his small country village, Mathias was without an occupation. A new one presented itself through a charming accident. Shortly after their arrival,

the Riesers were exploring the neighborhood near their apartment. They chanced upon a man puffing on the same long pipe that Mathias preferred. The two started talking. The man made hats by the piece and offered to teach Mathias his craft. Hat making became Mathias's livelihood and eventually Max joined him at it, dropping out of school in his early teens.

Eighteen years after landing in New York, the Riesers had saved enough money to leave the gritty Lower East Side for 153 East 52nd Street, a less crowded residential neighborhood uptown that was a mecca for better-off Germans in the city. About this time a correspondence ensued between Max and Julia, and Julia visited the Riesers in Manhattan. Max and Julia were married on August 19, 1869, in St. Peter's Lutheran Church.

The couple planned to live in Doylestown. Julia was already set up and lived on her own; Max did not. Julia was known in her town; Max was not. Julia had money to invest or spend as she wished; Max did not. Despite the incalculabilities of the millinery trade in Doylestown, Max wouldn't have deliberated long in forsaking the metropolis for the clean air and pastoral beauty of Bucks County, enhanced by a wife with the means to establish him in business.

Max was taciturn and easygoing, and quite early in the marriage he assumed a secondary position in the household. Julia, accustomed to managing, continued to run things as she had when she was alone. Engulfed by the robustness of his many children and effaced by the domination of his wife, Max plays a minor role in Rieser family memories. In contrast to their acrid but colorful accounts of Julia's exploits, Max Rieser's grandchildren speak of him as a remote, nearly ghostly figure, a sweet-tempered soul who kept to himself. Like Mr. Bennet in *Pride and Prejudice*, he loved to read and buried himself in his books, a protective measure that allowed him to blot out reality and remain oblivious to much of what went on in his large, clamorous family. Thus for parental models, the Riesers grew up with a mother who was powerful and active yet often capricious and overwrought and a father who, for all his amiability, was weak and yielding.

Every indication pointed toward a stable life for the Riesers in Doylestown. The Civil War had stimulated a land rush in the area. Money was plentiful, or so it seemed. The number of residents (all of whom presumably wore hats), rose from 1,601 in 1870 to 2,070 in 1880. (The Riesers themselves would contribute mightily to the local population boomlet.) A referendum to introduce running water to the borough, defeated for lack of enthusiasm in 1852, was carried in 1869. Gas lamps, another recent invention, were also installed. In 1870 Julia bought a small brick house in the north end of town, known as the "Germany" or "German hill" section. Max, bankrolled by Julia, opened a shop specializing in fur hats, collars, and gloves, although all types of caps, scarves, and mittens could be found on the shelves. As an old engraving shows, Max's store was in the grandest building in town.

This prosperous start could not be maintained. Business reverses and the exploding size of the Rieser family made the struggle to survive respectably an

intractable problem. Max's work as an independent hatter and furrier yielded a steady income, but not a rising one. The carriage trade most likely to buy fur accessories took its custom to Philadelphia, and the craft of hat making was being rendered obsolete by industrialization. Mass-produced hats, plentiful and cheap, would usurp the rest of Max's customers. Add to this the propensity of the little Riesers to arrive in sets of two—Juliana and Max were but one of four pairs of twins—and financial embarrassment was all but inevitable. Joseph Rieser was born in 1870, followed by Mary in 1871, George and Clara in 1873, Francis (Frank) in 1874, Max and Juliana in 1876, Robert in 1881,* Louis and a stillborn baby in 1881, and Charles Frederick in 1883.

In 1874 the Riesers sold their house. Perhaps it was too small a space for the burgeoning tribe, but since they did not buy another place to live, it is likely that they could not meet the mortgage payments on top of day-to-day expenses. Doylestown property rolls indicate that the Riesers' taxable assets declined every year after 1874. In a town where house-proud residential property owners far outnumbered tenants, renting rooms meant a slippage that was visible to everyone. The Riesers' social ignominy (by Doylestown standards) was compounded in the early 1880s when Max was forced to close his shop and accept a job working for his competitor.

Julia suffered the most from this dip in the Rieser fortunes, not solely because her money was lost, but because of the damage to her precious sense of superiority and self-esteem. During her years as Miss Schmutz and Mrs. Kuster, Julia had been upwardly mobile. Her father and husband had been men of enterprise and universally popular. They provided well and accumulated savings. Formerly Julia had the satisfaction of reading complimentary squibs about Hermann Schmutz and Julius Kuster printed in the flag-waving *Democrat*, which missed few opportunities to praise patriotic joiners and excoriate shirkers. All Max ever rated from the *Democrat* were infrequent recommendations to the townspeople to visit his shop for the latest in headgear. More often than not, his name was spelled "Reiser." He was labeled the "mad" or "happy" hatter who purveyed "nobby neckties" and the like. The undertone was one of benign contempt. The Rieser family, already insular, was encouraged by Julia to become more close-knit than ever. The children were taught to play only with each other and to see themselves as better than those who had slighted them. One of Juliana's brothers said that their mother, "in one of her angry moods," called him a "ruffian" and whipped him with a rattan switch until the welts on his back showed scarlet because he wanted to play football with a bunch of ragtag boys instead of staying at home.

The condescension and snubs were not entirely of Julia's imagining, for Doylestown was a town inordinately pleased with itself. Its old guard maintained elaborate snobberies and upheld a caste system complex enough to convince a Hindu that his social divisions were crude and oversimplified. Bucks County was one of the three principal counties settled by William Penn, and its com-

---

* Probably 1880, although 1881 is the date entered in the family Bible. However, the handwriting is Robert Rieser's, and he later lied about his age.

mingled German, English, Welsh, Scotch, and Dutch families, tracing themselves back to 1682, constituted the homegrown aristocracy. Their ancestors fought in the American Revolution, preserved the house where Washington slept, and they let no one forget it. In 1880, when Doylestown was just over a hundred years old, local buffs and antiquarians founded a county historical society. The group added considerably to the preservation and understanding of the past, but it also served to remind newcomers of their place. As the county seat, Doylestown was home to doctors, lawyers, judges, and gentlemen of leisure, all of whom contributed to its stuffy and complacent atmosphere. Doylestown had the reputation for being the most snobbish and clannish town in Bucks County. The same people headed all the committees, ran for office, organized dances, gave teas, played bridge, and rented pews at the Episcopal Church.

For a village, Doylestown was teeming with private schools. Public schools were not deemed suitable for boys and girls from good homes, and any parents who could afford it sent their children to one of the many lyceums, seminaries, or academies. The young Riesers went to public school, yet another mark of their poverty. Well into the twentieth century, a wealthy resident of Doylestown who remembered little Juliana Rieser with approbation, nonetheless betrayed some entrenched condescension about her background. "She was such a brilliant little girl, the smartest one and the brightest one in the family," the woman said. "But, my, my, who would have ever expected her to do as well for herself? Where she came from was so poor. She didn't even go to private school."

Social sensitivity was not a virtue practiced to excess by Doylestowners. One of the principal good works of the town's elite was the Doylestown Relief Society, organized to aid the deserving poor. In December of 1880, the *Bucks County Intelligencer*, whose editors were on the society's board, printed this announcement for public consumption:

> Though no action was taken [by the committee] and no particular course was agreed upon, it was decided not to call the committee together, or to contribute money or provisions at present. The past season has been a prosperous one, those who wanted work have generally been able to obtain it and to provide it for themselves, provisions are cheap, and there should be little suffering this winter, certainly none at this early time. One or two applications were made for assistance as soon as the first fall of snow came, but the committee concluded not to respond to them.

Shortly after this less than charitable pronouncement, the society singled out the Rieser family as being among the truly needy by awarding them a check for $25. When Max informed his benefactors that the money "was not needed," they were mystified as to why the gift was returned.

Doylestowners categorized the Riesers as poor but a little too proud. The incident of the refused check apparently deepened the rift between the family and the more solvent citizens of the community. Their mortification must surely have been intensified by the generally held view that poverty was a moral defect, a condition resulting from the victim's own lethargy. Still, for the Rieser children, Doylestown was a peaceful, joyful place in which to grow up, and throughout their lives they considered it their true and rightful home. Their village was picturesque, situated on a rise overlooking low hills, orchards, and plowed fields.

The main avenues were fronted with large frame or brick houses that were quaintly interpreted versions of Queen Anne and High Victorian architecture. The buildings were shaded by oak trees older than the town. The side streets, little more than crooked lanes, led to farmhouses dating back to colonial times. Doylestown was a popular summer spa for Philadelphians seeking relief from the urban heat, and to complement the advantages bestowed by nature the villagers constructed an inviting promenade and made the town a center for concerts, strawberry festivals, dances, fairs, and parades.

It was this kernel of sweet impressions—of swimming in the Neshaminy Creek, of sleds and picnics and pastures—and not the less happy ones that the Riesers would retain when their thoughts traveled back to Doylestown. Although the children had been hurt there (or at least Julia told them they were), in their imaginations their sojourn in rural Pennsylvania became a golden interval, a garden from which they had been unfairly exiled. As adults all the Riesers felt a strong attachment to Bucks County, but only Juliana managed to return them to their birthplace, and in a style that was a revenge on her beginnings.

In January of 1885, the haberdashery where Max worked was absorbed by a department store, and he was out of a job. After looking unsuccessfully for employment in town, he left home in early spring to find work in New York. He rented a room in Jersey City and promised to send for his family once he had a job. A few weeks of silence elapsed, and Julia, rustling impatiently around Doylestown, decided to investigate why she'd had no news. Without advance notice to her husband, she gathered the younger children together and instructed them to select a favorite toy for a long journey. The party, which must have numbered at least six, headed for Jersey City and arrived in the late afternoon. Their destination was 215 Ogden Avenue, where Max was boarding. Julia and her brood rode a trolley that stopped at the upper portion of Ogden Avenue. Unaware that the thoroughfare ran for several miles, the Riesers trudged down the street; the children became hungry and cranky and began to cry. Somewhere short of their goal, a neighborly woman leaning over the front fence asked Julia what the trouble was. After hearing their story, the woman invited them in. She fed the children milk and buttered bread, after which they all dropped off to sleep. The hostess then had little choice but to ask the Riesers to stay the night, and Julia accepted without a qualm. The next morning they set off for No. 215, a short block or two away.

After surveying Max's lodgings, even Julia agreed that he was not ready for the family, and she and the children returned to Doylestown. But the May 12, 1885, issue of the *Democrat* was able to announce, "Our former townsman, Max Reiser [*sic*], has a situation in the grocery house of Park and Tilford, Broadway, New York." Three days later Doylestown said farewell to the Riesers, as Herman Kuster, Julia's son by her first marriage, collected Julia, the children, and their belongings and removed them to New Jersey.

After a brief stay in Jersey City, where Charles Allan, the last Rieser baby, was born in 1886 (Charles Frederick died in 1884), the Riesers relocated to

Hoboken, a port city on the Hudson that was undergoing rapid industrialization. Although Max and Julia were attracted by its proximity to Manhattan, the low rents, and vigorous German community, Hoboken, compared to Doylestown, seemed paltry and blighted. The town was eminently more habitable than it would be in the period of decay between the wars, when graft and a tentacular political machine transformed it into a haven for gangsters and a personal fiefdom of the ruling political dynasty, but for the average resident Hoboken was not an idyllic place.

Hoboken, which juts into New York Harbor, was a hub of shipping, trade, and industry. Only a mile square, it was dense with people—48,026 resided there in 1890. Nearly three hundred plants turning out paint, varnish, leather, rubber goods, silk, and iron and steel blackened the air. Within the factory walls and on the docks and piers servicing six transatlantic steamship lines and the trans-Hudson commuter ferries labored thousands of badly paid, unskilled workers. Most of them were Irish immigrants, and they were wedged into flimsy wooden tenements in the flat marshy acres behind the factories and waterfront. The "uplands," a strip of high ground with a river view, was reserved for the first families of Hoboken.

But even if Hoboken had been a place of great charm, it would have appeared unlovely to Julia, who was convinced that her life had been ruined by the move from Bucks County. To her, New Jersey represented social and economic disinheritance. Moving frequently to escape the spread of encroaching saloons, the Riesers lived in a succession of dignified but prosaic town houses in the city's

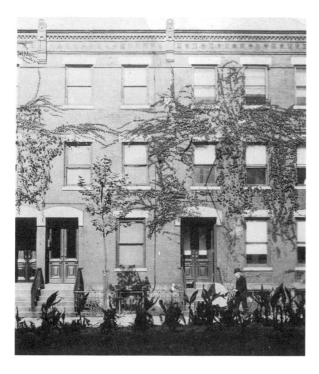

The Riesers' final address in Hoboken, at 208 Eleventh Street.

middle section, ending up at 208 Eleventh Street. Their neighbors were professionals, skilled workers, and tradesmen.

The clubs and parties sponsored by the cultivated German community had little impact on the Riesers. Their lives, centered around home and church, assumed a steady routine. Max remained with the grocery store until he retired. Julia filled their home with massive, unremarkable pieces of furniture upholstered in black horsehair. (Juliana's originality in interior decoration had no roots in her early surroundings.) The children responded to "good music," and they learned to play instruments and sing. As the boys grew older, they took part-time jobs to help out at home. At dinner the family convened around a long mahogany table, where the squeal of voices signaled the collision of egos and childish rivalries asserting themselves. The evening meal over, Max would tell stories or the children would take turns reading aloud, exuberantly acting out the narratives. The atmosphere was one of happy, boisterous disputation. The older boys needled the younger ones, and everyone fought to be heard. Juliana, the veteran of a house full of unruly brothers, was accustomed to thriving on tension and conflict as well as jovial banter, and she learned to give back what she got. Sibling squabbles, both minor and serious, plus her own combativeness, prepared her for the long, controversial struggle that distinguished her later life.

Resilience and ebullience were qualities indispensable to any child under Julia Rieser's roof. Worn out by twenty years of childbearing and domestic drudgery, and in reaction to her involuntary displacement from her beloved Pennsylvania, Julia took out her frustration and anger on Max and the children. In middle age Julia's rancor would not be curbed. The old independence and self-reliance, poisoned by resentment, degenerated into an unpredictable tyranny and vindictiveness. No one was safe from Julia's spleen or spite. One way she kept her sons and daughters in line was to terrify them with chilling anecdotes of babies choking to death. Her children, unable to say a good thing about her, testified that Julia berated Max for his inadequacies as a wage earner. Charles Rieser wrote that his mother "left her easy-going husband without a shred of respect in the eyes of his children." Julia instilled in her children a gripping fear of poverty and a wild desire to spend money as an act of defiance. And she continued to drill into them the sense that they were superior to everyone else. As a result, Charles Rieser said, the Riesers were "cursed with over-nice tastes in the art of living and an income almost too scant for the bare essentials."

Julia herself was the victim of her impulses and her malaise; she could not refrain from disrupting any semblance of domestic tranquility the household sometimes attained. Visiting friends or relatives, she would present herself unannounced at mealtimes and expect to be served the choicest morsels. Her peremptory royal progressions were notorious within the family. While she wailed about the dire circumstances in which she scraped along, Julia would buy herself strawberries in December or any other expensive delicacy she craved. "I needed them," she said, and that was the only explanation she offered.

To all of this, Max raised no objections. He took refuge in his major after-work project: to read the entire *Encyclopaedia Britannica* from first volume to last. Julia thus learned that if her behavior was outrageous enough, she would

get away with it because her audience would be too stunned to stop her. This lesson Juliana absorbed and would perfect in later life. Julia's neuroses and the myth she perpetuated of Max's failure unquestionably contaminated her children, but her extreme self-absorption may also have worked to Juliana's good. Neither mother nor daughter wasted any energy on self-blame. Whereas the average girl was taught coy wheedling and other means of indirection at her mother's knee, Juliana had the rare example of an unsubordinate female parent who got what she wanted by assertiveness rather than stoicism, submission, or pathos.

In Hoboken Julia divested herself of housewifery by conscripting her two eldest daughters. When Mary and Clara reached the age of twelve or fourteen, their mother permanently removed them from school. They were instructed in cooking, sewing, and cleaning and became the unpaid servants of the family, functioning as seamstresses, laundresses, chefs, and bakers—even nursemaids, for Julia handed over the care of little Charles to them. Mary and Clara spent most of their days at home, which left Julia free to shop, visit, and rest. The sisters were prematurely consigned to a life of spinsterhood and dependence upon others.

Louis Rieser told this story to illustrate how his mother disciplined his sisters and controlled the rest of the family as well. "The whole family once sat down at the dinner table for dinner and immediately ran out of bread. Mary and Clara hadn't baked enough, so one of the boys said he would hop down to the store and get some. Julia said, 'No!' and walked out herself. Everyone thought she had gone to fetch the bread, but they were wrong. They didn't see her for three days. She went to stay with friends and never let a soul know, which was typical of her. She always found excuses to disappear."

When Juliana reached adolescence, her mother made plans to withdraw her from school. But a teacher interceded, persuading Julia that this child was too gifted to lose. (It is likely that Juliana, alarmed by the prospect of impending domestic servitude, alerted school officials to her predicament before it was too late.) She was allowed to continue her studies. Whether or not Juliana was ever taught to keep house is unclear; in later years she made great show of her inability to do so much as boil an egg. She loved Mary and Clara deeply, but she took care not to identify with them or the foreshortened feminine horizons they represented. After Max and Julia's deaths, Juliana supported her maiden sisters, who could not earn a reasonable income on their own. She bought them a house in Chatham, New Jersey, and provided a monthly allowance for running it. Juliana often said that she had been set free by her sisters, and her generosity acknowledged that Mary and Clara had been sacrificed to the rest of the family's comfort.

Julia frightened her children into obeying her, and her despotism was effective with all but Juliana. In mother and this daughter two fierce wills were pitted against one another. Julia unwittingly raised Juliana in her own image, and the two could not abide each other. In general, Julia preferred her sons, who were

more amused than appalled by her antics. (Daughters-in-law came in for automatic disapproval.) Only Juliana contested her bizarre behavior. Her stubbornness, independence, and earthquake temper equaled her mother's, and their relationship was one of open warfare. At some point the two women no longer bothered to conceal their mutual animosity. Juliana on one occasion was rebuked by her mother for not showing sufficient respect. Juliana replied, "You haven't earned my respect." Julia was no less brutal. After Juliana became engaged to Willard Force, the two sets of parents gathered to meet each other. While the prospective in-laws were sitting around and digesting each other, Juliana stepped out of the room. Seconds later Julia started ticking off her daughter's faults. Juliana's later sensitivity to any hint of criticism can be traced to the wear and tear of this long, destructive conflict. The lack of warm, shielding parental affection moved her to take disagreements and challenges much too personally, and so to suffer much unwarranted—and unintended—pain.

The friction between mother and daughter also had its comic element. As a young working woman, Juliana began wearing modish clothes and buying herself little luxuries. In response Julia appropriated her daughter's things when-

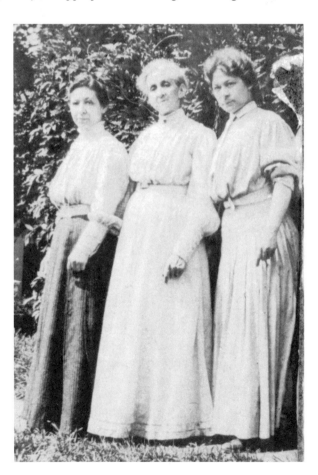

From left, Mary, Julia, and Juliana Rieser—a powerful but tiny trio. Even when leaning forward Juliana is the tallest of the group, and she was only five feet one.

ever she could. Marjorie Rieser, one of Julia's grandchildren, recalled, "Grand-mother Rieser had her cotton-picking fingers into everything. I remember one day at her house, before they had electricity, that Aunt Jule was going out somewhere and was going to wear a beautiful black tulle hat, a big dress hat on a wire frame. The only way to keep this prize out of Grandmother Rieser's clutches was to put it where she couldn't reach it, so Aunt Jule hid it behind the gas jet. Well, Grandmother Rieser came in, she was tired, she automatically struck a match, and there went the hat. When it was time for Aunt Jule to leave for wherever she was going to wear this gorgeous creation, she reached up and nothing was left but the wire frame. All hell broke loose between the two of them. And Grandmother Rieser said so innocently, 'I wondered why all of those little black specks kept falling down.' "

Despite her contempt for her mother, Juliana identified with Julia's drive and her methods of handling emotional crises and trampling opposition to her wishes. Charles Rieser said of his mother, "Her temper swung on a quick pendulum—from over affection [for her sons] to petulant anger. With the tem-perament (and probably the aspirations) of Sarah Bernhardt, she not infrequently dramatized her troubles before a trembling captive audience." Julia would reg-ularly take to her bed and groan that she was dying, temporarily engaging her children's sympathy and attention with descriptions of her latest mortal ailment. Juliana never stooped to hypochondria, but she did deal with frustration through fits of temper and hysterical scenes. Moreover, she not only endorsed the emo-tionally labile myths created by her mother, but evolved into their most dedicated exponent within the family. She too agreed that the Riesers had been cruelly ejected from Doylestown to languish in Hoboken. Class distinctions mattered to her. Louis Rieser often talked of his sister Juliana's tantrums. As a girl, she would stamp her feet and shout, "I won't be poor! I hate being poor! I won't be poor!" Her cries expressed the thwarted dreams of Julia Rieser. Outwardly Juliana adopted her mother's decisiveness, histrionics, arbitrariness, and brass. The quieter, less visible side of her nature—the side that read omnivorously, and responded with sensitivity to the Lake Poets, to the serenity of the Shakers, to long stretches of country life, to the pleas of young artists—was the more intro-verted legacy of Max Rieser.

Julia's influence usually prevailed: It was a riskier way to live, but the potential gains were greater. Emulating her mother's patterns, Juliana later ordered her brothers and sisters around. Although not the eldest, she became the undisputed head of the Rieser clan by making the best marriage, ascending the highest professionally and socially, and having sheer strength of character. It was she who took over the custodianship of Julia's cemetery plot, chose where Clara and Mary would pass their old age, and decided the extent of her nephews' education. She didn't think much of her brothers as providers and told them so. In other words, Juliana held a position of authority that families normally reserve for men. Her brothers resented her interfering, but from her point of view, she was merely trying to embellish and improve lives she perceived as being starved for texture and color. The roles of arbiter and good angel that Juliana had assumed

in her professional career she extended to her blood relatives, resolving her private and public concerns in a similar manner.

In the Riesers' big family, with births spread over decades, the children were closer to some of their siblings than to others. The ones of most importance to Juliana were Mary, Clara, Max, Robert, and Charles.

Mary (1871–1943) and Clara (1873–1952) were five and three years older than Juliana, respectively, but they gradually subordinated themselves to her. These gentler personalities, cowed by their mother and unending household responsibilities, were awed by their sister's intelligence and bravado. Juliana was grateful to her sisters for accepting their burdens, and her bond with them was protective and tender. She felt keenly that they had missed out on life's favors in order to let the younger Riesers fulfill themselves. Mary and Clara were welcome companions and guests in her many establishments, and she spent time at the house she had bought them in Chatham. At the same time, they were cautionary role models. Their domesticity, cloistered existence, and choking virtues of faith and renunciation held little attraction for her.

Max (1876–1954) and Juliana were volatile opposites, and in their relationship they seemed to reenact the enmities and defense mechanisms of the parents whose names they bore. Although twins, they professed mutually incompatible philosophies of life and reacted to their environment in opposite ways. Whereas Juliana responded to the family's financial discomforts and her parents' separate retreats into petty tyranny and introversion with explosions of feeling, impulsive extravagance, and a determination to fight free of Hoboken, Max deflected these same tensions with rigid routines, fixed habits, and inertia. He insulated himself from anxiety by obtaining one job and holding onto it all his working life. From 1908 until his retirement in 1945, Max was a clerk in the Hoboken post office. He kept to himself and lived frugally, first with his parents and then with Mary and Clara in Chatham. A resolute bachelor, he accepted his sisters' slavish attentions. (Mary and Clara doted on all their brothers and enjoyed living vicariously through their adventures.) Grouchy and skeptical, Max confessed to three passions: books, opera, and socialism. His political views never went farther than the armchair, and perhaps he advocated them chiefly to pique the rest of the Riesers. He made no secret of his disapproval of the circles in which Juliana traveled once she was working in Manhattan. He railed against the Whitneys and Vanderbilts as ruthless capitalists and wrote off their philanthropies as decadent. "Under socialism," he would admonish Juliana magisterially, "all of this will change." Certainly Max, her twin, was the family member least respectful of Juliana's stellar career, but he chose not to notice the irony of denouncing her multimillionaire employers while living in a house that was financed entirely by the income she earned happily in service of the oppressors. Max was not known to have contributed anything himself to the mortgage or upkeep of the Chatham house, and he was nothing if not lordly in his refusal to help with chores and repairs. If a sidewalk needed shoveling or a gutter had to be replaced, Max would sit aloof and immovable with his book while Mary or Clara telephoned brother Rob in Hoboken for assistance.

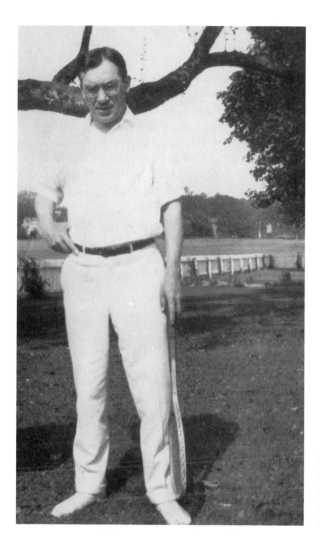

Max Rieser, Juliana's twin brother, in an uncharacteristically athletic moment at the Forces' farm in Pennsylvania.

Juliana had little use for Max's passive-aggressive egoism and lack of ambition. Rob Rieser (1881–1950), her junior by five years, was a different sort altogether, a flamboyant model of her own creative energies and emotionalism gone awry. In Rob, Juliana's dynamism and fun-loving whimsy were foolishly distorted, as if her most memorable attributes were being grotesquely reflected in a funhouse mirror. After Juliana, Rob showed the most potential for achieving, but he frittered away his time and talents instead of channeling them productively. Nor was he one for deliberating very judiciously on the consequences of his actions, and he was always embroiled in causes, right or wrong. As Marjorie Rieser put it, "Rob was a busybody, a self-appointed curator of anything that went on. . . . He liked to swagger around town and make a pest of himself."

Charles Rieser (1886–1976), the baby of the bunch, was also the handsomest of the boys. He was Juliana's favorite and his mother's darling. Julia would not

let him go to school until well after his eighth birthday, and he enjoyed being spoiled and cosseted by his sisters. Playful and good-natured as a boy, he grew into a bright, dapper man who relished parties and good company.

Juliana and Charles had many things in common: Both were fastidious and wore clothes well, both spoke vividly and were drawn to the literary life, and both were extroverts who loved socializing, staying up late, and drinking. Charles's first job was with a New Jersey newspaper, but he was quickly hired as a city reporter by the *New York Sun*. On the side he wrote hair-raising adventure stories for the pulp magazines. From Juliana's standpoint, he was her most charismatic and presentable sibling. Charles *was* cherished on his own merits, but it would be unrealistic to deny that some part of Juliana's special fondness for him was tied to the fact that he was the only Rieser besides herself capable of appreciating and participating in the social and intellectual milieu she was resolved to enter. Even in parceling out her early affections, Juliana distanced herself from the peripheral existence of her sisters and the mundane vocations of her other brothers.

Julia Rieser came into the world a Catholic and was married by Dutch Reformed and Lutheran ministers. Her four eldest children were baptized Catholics, but all the babies born thereafter were christened in Doylestown's Pres-

Charles Rieser, Juliana's favorite brother.

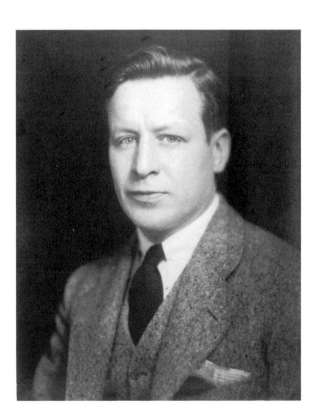

byterian church. Yet there is no record of the Riesers' membership in either institution. Presumably religion, or at least religious observance and theological consistency, was not of great moment to husband or wife during the Pennsylvania years. After the Riesers settled in New Jersey, however, a change came over Julia. She joined a Presbyterian church in Jersey City, and once in Hoboken, she started attending the First Presbyterian Church, located a block from her house. Religion became the anchor she clung to in an unfamiliar community, though the solace it provided clearly was not great enough to calm her inner turmoil. Julia, Mary, and Clara received certificates of membership in the First Presbyterian Church in 1888. The elder girls joined the Christian Endeavor, a social club for young people, and signed up as Sunday school teachers. The rest of the Riesers were enrolled in Sunday school classes. As they got older, Frank, Joe, Max Jr., Robert, and Charles professed their faith and became members of the church in their own right. Frank emerged as the most pious in the family, and in 1896 he was elected a trustee and made a secretary of the church board. Under his influence, the Riesers' involvement with the First Presbyterian grew positively fervid. Even the perennially skeptical Max, who in his later years looked upon organized religion as counterrevolutionary babble, rented a pew and taught Sunday school.

Throughout this flurry of prayer and good works, three in the family abstained from churchgoing: Max Sr., Louis, and Juliana. (Herman and George were out of the house by this time.) After Sunday school, the next step for a child was to join the Christian Endeavor, profess the faith, and apply for a single membership. Juliana did none of these. Her own faith was in individualism—she was unwilling to surrender any portion of her autonomy, even to God—and her mounting rebelliousness made the notion of conforming to any form of orthodoxy insupportable. One can only marvel at the power of her youthful resistance, her mettle in withstanding what must have been grinding pressure to reverse her stance. In Juliana's eyes, rules were for other people, and the preordained paths other young girls took didn't apply to her.

Paradoxically, it was through the Riesers' church connections that Juliana was able to make the initial break from Hoboken and win a chance at a richer life. One of the elders of the First Presbyterian was a leading citizen of Hoboken named Palmer Campbell. As vice-president of the Hoboken Trust Company, chairman of the parks commission, and president of the Hudson Land and Improvement Corporation (which controlled all the important parcels of real estate in town, including the Riesers' own block), Campbell was consulted on most business, civic, and religious affairs in his city. He also believed in direct and unostentatious charity, and he became Juliana's first benefactor.

Campbell was tolerant enough to overlook Juliana's lack of enthusiasm for religion and to see her as an exceptional mind in danger of being thwarted. She was enrolled in the classical curriculum, and her average was 94. She had finished two years at Hoboken High School when her education was interrupted by a serious deterioration of her eyesight. She needed to leave school to be cured. Juliana had wanted to be a poet and hoped to go to Wellesley. "I want to be a writer," she ventured at the age of nineteen, "and I believe I mean, not startling

the world, or revolutionizing it, but earnestly and honestly learn that 'life's the soul's song' and then to sing it sweetly for the echo's sake."

Campbell proposed that Juliana apply for admission to Northfield Seminary for Young Ladies in Northfield, Massachusetts, a village near the Vermont border. He helped her procure letters of recommendation, agreed to lend her the tuition fee of $100 per year, and presumably joined in the efforts to convince the reluctant Riesers that a child of theirs should be sent to boarding school as preparation for a thoroughly impractical career.

Today Northfield Mount Hermon School is a nonsectarian coeducational preparatory school catering to the children of the affluent. But in its first years its conditions and commitments were very different. Northfield Seminary was founded in 1879 by the evangelist leader Dwight L. Moody as a boarding school designed for poverty-stricken girls. It provided "opportunity education" and trained its students in "Christian living." "The central book in the curriculum was the Bible," wrote Burnham Carter, the school's historian. "The education was to be above all, 'earnestly Christian.' " Students had to raise $100 for room, board, and tuition, approximately half of what expenses actually were. To supplement this fee, each girl was expected to do manual labor every day. Northfield was not free, because Moody felt that his charges would be more thankful for their training if they earned it.

Northfield's emphasis on evangelical Christianity was not to Juliana's taste, but the school was modeled on Mount Holyoke and Wellesley and considered a stepping-stone to either college. It is obvious why Campbell would recommend sending Juliana there. More intriguing is her continued rejection of religion. Even when beholden to the pillars of the First Presbyterian, she offered no profession of faith out of gratitude or opportunism.

The entrance application Juliana filled out for Northfield is a revealing testament to her forthrightness. She stated that she had been raised a Presbyterian and that her mother was a member of a local congregation. She admitted that she had not been received into the church herself, and to the question, "If not a member of the Church, has [the candidate] shown any interest in religion?" she replied, "Practically, shown by good works, no; selfishly, for my own good, yes."

Apparently Juliana's sponsors were concerned about the sketchiness of her belief, for they remark upon it in correspondence with Northfield and cite it and her stormy home life as especially compelling reasons for exposing her to a sustained dose of Dwight Moody. They were at least as interested in cleansing her soul as in nurturing her intelligence. For example, William Willcox, a minister recruited by Campbell as a character reference, composed a letter of recommendation that dwelled more upon salvation than scholarship. He wrote to Moody:

> She is a young lady of more than usual thoughtfulness & ability, but her inner life greatly lacks the repose & strength that comes from intelligent faith & christian discipline. I fear her home surroundings have not been favorable to her best development, but I think she has in her such material as may make her an influential

and useful woman. I propose to send her through Wellesley* if she shows herself worthy, & I hope you will cooperate with me as far as you can, by opening to her the opportunities of your school. Can you do so?

The principal of Hoboken High School confined himself to a report on his student's mental powers and general demeanor. "Miss . . . Rieser . . . is an independent thinker rather than one who blindly follows others," he wrote. ". . . If her mind were properly trained, we believe she would make a brilliant woman."

The most unblinking appraisal of the candidate's character issued from the candidate herself. Requested to enumerate her outstanding traits, Juliana wrote, "Love of beauty is the only decided good one; for the rest, I have to fight hardest against a tendency to dictate . . . temper, uncharitableness, selfishness, pride, pessimism . . . and a sharp tongue." This extreme breast-beating may well have been exaggeration for the sake of winning Northfield over, but it is uncanny how many of those faults dogged her through life. At nineteen she knew herself well.

Two other curious items are recorded on Juliana's application. She listed as her guardians her mother and Palmer Campbell. As if to affirm his irrelevance, Max Rieser is not mentioned. And in answer to the question asking for her father's occupation and income, she skipped the first part and replied, "Father is a workingman who became too poor late in life ever to be even comfortable." In Juliana's presentation of herself, Max was a figure who could be done without.

Juliana was eager to attend Northfield, and she was accepted in the winter of 1896. Her letters to Evelyn Hall, the principal of Northfield, about her arrangements at the school portray not the stubborn and romantic young woman she was, but still a person to be reckoned with. She is seen angling for the academic credits and domestic amenities she thought she deserved. On January 11, 1896, Juliana told Miss Hall of her intention to enter Wellesley in September of 1897. She had missed at least a year of secondary school and lacked French, a requirement for matriculation. Yet she assured her adviser that she could catch up—doing otherwise would be a waste of her time and money. "I am sure I can do it: perfect health and love of study for study's sake help wonderfully, is it not so?" the aspirant wrote. She was not as persuasive as she had hoped. Evelyn Hall informed her that a minimum of three years' preparation would be necessary before she was ready for Wellesley. In her reply, Juliana tried to whittle the period down to two years, adding on a less confident note, "And would you write to me if you think I shall be too old? Nineteen is not old age, I know, but most girls enter college at eighteen."

Thwarted in her campaign to shorten her time at Northfield, Juliana next concentrated on bettering the conditions of her stay. Privacy was not a feature of the narrow town house the Riesers were piled into, and Juliana wanted a room of her own. She pleaded her health, intimating odd, vaporous habits and implying how disastrously her presence would affect an unsuspecting roommate.

---

*Willcox was a trustee of Wellesley, and his daughter, Mary A. Willcox, taught zoology there.

Miss Hall took offense at the letter. The new applicant was upbraided for her lack of humility, and her reply, tinged with enforced meekness, also discloses the financial arrangements for her schooling. On July 20, 1896, Juliana wrote:

> I was surprised to find by your letter that my request was a presuming one; believe me, I never meant to ask too much. Your suggestion that I board outside was a temptation, but it is my guardian who pays my expenses, and as I have accepted it as wholly & only a loan, you see I dare not increase the obligation one whit for my comfort's sake. Therefore I am ready to room with a dozen others, if it is my place.

Two weeks later, she registered at Northfield.

With its maples and birches blazing forth in crimsons and golds, its white clapboard buildings, and its 500-acre campus close by the Connecticut River, Northfield was far removed from the streets of Hoboken, and the earnest poet-in-waiting who knew her Emerson and Thoreau must have savored the New England landscape before her. Five dormitories, two "recitation halls," a library, an auditorium, and a gymnasium stood ready to receive the 300 or so girls who were accepted as pupils that autumn.

Juliana's desire for privacy went unsatisfied, for the average day at Northfield was essentially spent in the company of others. The girls, housed in double rooms opening onto long corridors, arose at 6:15, and ate breakfast at 7:00. The first class began at 8:15 and the last ended at 4:30. Lessons were broken up by a midday meal and compulsory attendance at chapel. Supper was at 6:00, followed by a prayer meeting. Students prepared and served their meals and were in charge of all the cleaning and laundry for their residences. Upon completion of their tasks, the girls were permitted a study period. Then came "silent time," when each girl was given twenty minutes alone in her room for meditation and prayer. These brief moments of reflection constituted the only solitude allotted to Northfield students. They went to bed immediately afterward, at 9:30.

The academic courses at Northfield were varied, but typical of their time. Instruction was given in algebra, literature, Latin, history, spelling, grammar, composition, basic arithmetic, the sciences, music, art, homemaking, and Bible study. The most exceptional offering was an offshoot of Evelyn Hall's conviction that her girls should be fortified in both mind and body. She initiated a vigorous program of sports and exercises, and Juliana, like her schoolmates, played tennis, field hockey, and basketball. Miss Hall was strict in her insistence that Northfield girls attain faultless posture. She made gymnastics mandatory and declared war on the slouch. In later life, Juliana was a walking advertisement for her principal's ideas. More than one eyewitness commented upon her rigorous carriage, which contributed to the overall aura of mastery she radiated.

Life was sober and straitlaced at Northfield, but there were diversions. The girls had parties among themselves, and sometimes students at Mount Hermon Boys' School, the seminary's affiliate for young men, were invited for suppers, dances, or taffy pulls. Befitting the respectable character of the institutions, "contacts between Mount Hermon and Northfield were few, decorous, and

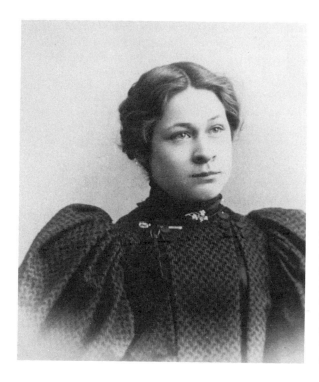

Juliana had to submit a photograph with her application to Northfield, and it is the earliest surviving likeness of her. She wrote about the picture, "It is thought to be good, except that I tried to look pleasant, which is wholly foreign to me."

heavily chaperoned," but they gave the students something to look forward to during the isolation and harshness of a Massachusetts winter.

No amount of compensation would have made Northfield congenial to Juliana. She lasted there only three semesters, forfeiting the dream of Wellesley, and she did not talk about her school days afterward. Louis and Charles, on the other hand, had fun recounting their experiences at Mount Hermon. On long weekends and holidays when the Riesers gathered as a clan, a favorite amusement was outlandish storytelling, in which brothers and sisters would try to top each other. That Juliana did not regale them with Northfield anecdotes is an indication of how distasteful those eighteen months were to her.

The religious commitment that was solicited and the clear linkage of North-field with penury rankled Juliana to the bone. Dwight Moody wanted pupils to leave his schools with a solid intellectual grounding, but his first educational priority was to ensure that those under his roof led "lives that count[ed] for the cause of Christ." The Sabbath was kept inviolate, of course, and Bible study and daily attendance at religious services were mandatory. Students actively leading persons to God were praised more lavishly and ranked as more important than those who merely earned high marks. Indeed, both boys and girls had to promise in writing to convert at least one soul to Christian belief every year. It was Northfield custom to post these signed pledges in the girls' rooms.

It was the designation of poverty that Juliana would have detested even more than the religious coercion. No pupil at Northfield could come from a rich family, and the faculty checked incomes carefully. As Evelyn Hall explained,

"In order that mistakes may not be made and girls be accepted who could afford to go elsewhere, we ask now for the name of some business man who can speak of the financial standing of the family. We write him a very specific letter, inquiring whether the candidate is able to pay more than $100." Palmer Campbell was the businessman asked to give an account of the Riesers' financial status. Northfield was evidence of her parents' failure and the world's knowledge of it, and Juliana's ruling thought was to erase all that.

Juliana dropped out of Northfield and was repatriated to Hoboken in January of 1898. An eighteen-month immersion in Dwight Moody's doctrines had not changed her mind about professing her Christianity. She stayed away from the First Presbyterian and did not worship formally. As Juliana grew older, she equated organized religion with cant, hypocrisy, parsimony, repression, and middle-class dullness, as did so many other American bohemians intent on breaking away from the constraints of a nineteenth-century upbringing. Her later scorn of conventional piety was another repudiation of her past.

Northfield did furnish Juliana with the training to become a teacher, one of the few careers then open to a woman of her class. She got a job at Eagan's Business School, a busy commercial academy located near the Hoboken railroad terminal, teaching English composition, grammar, practical correspondence, and stenography to men and women not much younger than herself. A student of hers (circa 1905) "remembered her vividly; trim, erect, and proud, she brought a sense of excitement to her classes." But once she was in the art world, Juliana no longer wished to be connected with a Hoboken institution. When questioned by Allene Talmey, she conflated Northfield and Eagan's. *Vogue* reported that "she taught English at a small New England private school."

Eagan's Business School did not take all of Juliana's time or energy. Her goal was still to become a writer, and she apprenticed in three ways. She signed up for literature courses at Barnard College. She sent poems and stories to *Harper's, Scribner's, The Atlantic Monthly*, and other prestigious magazines of the day, using a male pen name in order to avoid being stereotyped as a lady scribbler. In conversations she later had with artists, Juliana said that her submissions were rejected. As nothing of it survives, she must have destroyed her work. Lastly, Juliana was keeping a daybook of quotations collected from her reading.

The daybook, which has come down nearly intact and dates from Juliana's return to Hoboken, was an exercise in learning how to develop a distinctive voice. There she recorded sixty-three pages of phrases, thoughts, and rhythms that startled and tickled her. Some of the lines she inscribed became verbal signatures or were incorporated into the prose style of her maturity. "Details are melancholy," from Emerson, was, for example, the motto she invoked whenever the petty exigencies of administrative work overwhelmed her.* She also employed

---

* Not entered in the daybook, but utterly Juliana, was Emerson's famous passage from "Self-Reliance": "A foolish consistency is the hobgoblin of little minds. . . . With consistency a great soul has simply nothing to do. He may as well concern himself with his shadow on the wall. Speak what you think now in hard words, and tomorrow speak what tomorrow thinks in hard words again, though it contradict every thing you said today."

it to wave away certain telling lapses in memory. Juliana did not record any of her own observations directly, but from what she chose to copy it is possible to discern her primary values, her reigning fancies, and her perception of her niche in life. She drew sustenance from all sorts of authors: Plutarch, Epictetus, Shakespeare, Jonson, Prior, Johnson, Burns, Coleridge, Shelley, Arnold, the Brownings, Ruskin, Kipling, George Eliot, Tennyson, Scott, Swinburne, Stevenson, Whittier, Emerson, Thoreau, Eugene Field, and Kate Douglas Wiggin. The entries, ranging from drinking songs and doggerel verses to aphorisms and familiar essays, show her inclination toward the worldly point of view, the witty turn of phrase, and the sharp revelation of human foibles. Many excerpts exalt grand flourishes of emotion, the transcendentalist belief in the impact of a radiant individuality, and the triumph over the tribulations of existence by living every minute joyously and intensely. Juliana favored sayings and verses with a cheerful or picturesque twist, and she also liked wistful discourses on loneliness and on friendship. Her choices were natural for a romantic twenty-two-year-old whose hankering after a larger and more elegant world separated her from her more earthbound contemporaries in Hoboken. For example, the authors Juliana quoted most frequently were George Eliot, the literary idol of a generation of sentient, heroically minded women, Thoreau, the apostle of disobedience, and Kipling, the spit-and-polish instructor in making the best of things in adversity.

The habit of writing down interesting or affecting quotations stayed with Juliana as she grew older. Her mature letters are highly allusive, sprinkled with snippets of unattributed prose and poetry. After her death, the curators cleaning out her office at the Whitney Museum found the desk crammed with slips of paper, each with a handwritten quotation from classical or popular literature.

Juliana stopped making serious attempts at writing by 1906 or 1907, about the same time she resigned from Eagan's Business School. It is impossible to know if she would have succeeded as a writer, but she could count among her natural endowments a racing mind, a quicksilver temperament, a robust sense of humor, and a far-flung curiosity. These gifts, along with an instinctive grasp of prose rhythms (her rich contralto voice enthralled listeners when she read aloud), a passion for reading, and an alertness to piquant phrasings and eccentric diction ("a pudding is a prejudice," "acclamations hyperbolical," "fine inspirations of prudence," and "do the misanthropical" were jotted down in the daybook), combined to produce an imaginative woman responsive to style and sentiment.

So commanding was Juliana's verbal acuteness that she was a whiz at wordplay, persiflage, and naming and nicknaming. In the early days of the New Deal art projects that were putting artists to work painting walls of public buildings, Edith Halpert, the director of the Downtown Gallery, marched into Juliana's office and declared, "I think we should all be more mural-minded!"

"Oh," Juliana queried, "do you mean wall-eyed?"

When Guy Pène du Bois, who specialized in acrid portrayals of sleekly cloched flappers out on the town with their leering sugar daddies, needed titles

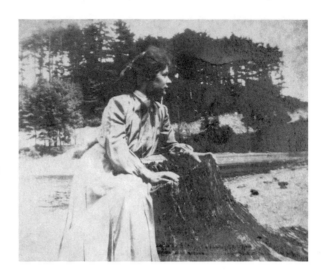

The young poet-in-waiting. One of the many quotations from Thoreau that Juliana copied into her daybook was, "The universe is wider than our views of it. Thank Heaven, here is not all the world."

for some of his most barbed paintings, he turned to Juliana. She suggested "A Window in the Union Club," "Pouter Pigeon," "Chanticleer," and "Mr. and Mrs. Middle Class," all of which he used. Not long afterward, a young Englishman having trouble thinking of a name for his new play arrived at West Eighth Street. "My aunt told me quite matter-of-factly about a tall, thin, chain-smoking, nervous young man who came to see her for help," Allan Rieser said. "It was Noël Coward."

But other elements of Juliana's personality were incompatible with a literary career. She was too fully extroverted, and power was too much to her liking, for her to remain immured with pen and paper for protracted amounts of time. She preferred formulating and participating to observing, ruminating, and interpreting. But given Juliana's limited experience at the time, and the general narrowness of employment options for women, professional writing would have seemed a likely path to creative, productive labor and more exciting surroundings.

As it turned out, the traits that led Juliana away from the typewriter were her real capital. Gregariousness, energy, lightning judgments, and an inexhaustible capacity for activism were what carried her throughout the years. Her supreme achievements, her unshakable belief in the new and vital, and "her courage and skill in fighting for it," were manifestations of her driving, aggressive personality. Juliana's genius was for picking up ideas before they could be abandoned and then swiftly distilling and translating them into workable, successful realities. "She had an extraordinary sense of quality, and she made up her mind about things more quickly and unerringly than anyone I ever knew," said Lloyd Goodrich, who met Juliana about 1924. "I can still see her wheeling around a gallery and pointing her finger at all the best pictures—'that one and that one and that one'—just like that." Her instincts were just as sure on substantive issues: "She might know nothing about a project in detail or by logical analysis,"

Goodrich observed, "but she never failed to recognize its importance and the necessity of carrying it out; and before one knew it, it was being done." Her magnetism heightened the most insignificant event. Juliana, said the art critic Forbes Watson, flashed with "such a gusto for life that wherever she was there was always something doing. It might be a morning meeting, a business lunch, an evening celebration or just a plain row. It was never mere quietude."

For Juliana Rieser, feeding her mind on the Romantic poets, the Victorian sages, the transcendentalists, and the down-to-earth electricity of Walt Whitman, Eagan's classrooms seemed a little too much like quietude. Hoboken had become intolerable for a variety of reasons, and a change of scene was imperative. Writing might not have been the perfect career for her, but then neither was anything else. The position she would shine in—"to personify," as one grateful painter put it, "the spirit of genuine appreciation, sympathetic understanding, and encouragement"—had not yet been invented.

CHAPTER TWO

THE GREAT HEIRESS

🌸 *(1875–1905)* 🌸

WAS THERE reason to suppose that Gertrude Vanderbilt Whitney, daughter of one millionaire and wife of another, would make distinctive use of herself? Shy, self-involved, romantic, fretful, and often silly, she was an heiress whose life revolved around cotillions and dinner parties. Her destiny was to dress expensively, entertain splendidly, and do very little else. All the ingredients for insignificance and triviality were there, and she might easily have metamorphosed into a placid, solemn dowager so like the numerous cousins and family friends she never quite dispatched from her life.

But Gertrude Whitney did not collapse into the future that stood every chance of claiming her. She tired of her endless leisure and slowly sought a focus for her existence. From being a sedulous, secret diarist, she emerged as a persistent writer, a serious sculptor, and one of the most important patrons in the history of American art.

Such things were not expected from a woman of her social position. One of seven children of Alice Gwynne and Cornelius Vanderbilt II, Gertrude Vanderbilt was born on January 9, 1875. Her great-grandfather was "Commodore" Cornelius Vanderbilt, who started as a ferryman on Staten Island and ended his days in control of all the shipping and railroad lines in New York. Between 1829, the year he went into the steamboat business, and 1877, the year of his death, he had amassed a fortune of $100 million and was famous for the ruthlessness with which he crushed his competition. The Commodore's millions were doubled by his son and principal heir, William H. Vanderbilt. In 1885 Cornelius Vanderbilt II, Gertrude's father and the Commodore's favorite grandson, inherited the major portion of the family's money, lands, and trusts. He was reported to be the richest man in America.

Money on such a scale, at a time when a miner earned about $400 a year and a schoolteacher about $250, meant identity as much as leverage. The greater one's wealth, the more well-defined and secure was one's sense of individual authority and happiness. The new rich not only lived but acted like sultans. By virtue of their influence, complained one writer, the multimillionaires' "slightest doings were chronicled, and their flimsiest sayings were construed oracularly as those of public opinion." He might have been referring to the view expressed by *Collier's Once a Week* in 1889, which was widespread: "The Vanderbilts have come nobly forward and shown the world how millionaires ought to live." Gertrude herself noted at a very early age that "everything my parents did and said was more right than what anyone else's parents did or said." This high prestige extended to the Vanderbilt children. Society reporters in all regions of the country churned out columns of unctuous prose about Gertrude, cooing over her appearance, ancestry, and marital and financial prospects.

In Manhattan Gertrude and her family lived in a house spread over a square city block and dominating the southeastern (and most fashionable) entrance to Central Park at Fifth Avenue. The address was 1 West 57th Street, a site now occupied by Bergdorf Goodman. The mansion, a caricature of a French Renaissance chateau, contained 137 rooms under a roof erupting with turrets, balconies, towers, and dormers. This urban palace could only be maintained by a battalion of servants who scrubbed and polished every inch of it between 6:00 and 9:00 in the morning, and then vanished from sight before their masters came downstairs. The staff was on a similar schedule in Newport, Rhode Island, where the family summered. There they were in residence at The Breakers, the famous seventy-room summer "cottage" designed by Richard Morris Hunt and modeled on a sixteenth-century Genoese palazzo.

Whether in New York, Rhode Island, or elsewhere, Gertrude spent much of her girlhood being instructed in what she could and could not do. A lady walked a tightrope, even a Vanderbilt; one tiny misstep could plunge her into the abyss of social disgrace. She could not show anger, she could not complain aloud, she could not go out alone. Unless she was driving out of town, she would see nothing of New York City unless it lay in the narrow rectangle of Manhattan bounded on the north and south by Fifty-ninth Street and Washington Square and to the east and west by Park and Sixth Avenues, although exceptions were made for Central Park, the Metropolitan Museum of Art, and one or two other northern outposts. It is doubtful that Gertrude ever rode a bus or, before she was married, even went into a restaurant by herself. She passed many hours being tutored in the accomplishments of dancing, drawing, French, and sewing, and she showed some flair for watercolor. Within the limits permitted by her mother, she went to parties; she arranged tableaux; she swam and sailed; she took drives; she played tennis; she made calls; she dreamed of dashing men. She lived a life of complete luxury, privilege, and pleasure. But somehow something was wrong.

To the adolescent Gertrude, who was sensitive and guilt-ridden about being different, the limitations that riches and social prominence placed upon her were the central problem of her life. Until she grew easy using status as the

Open Sesame it was, the Vanderbilt name was a source of deep distress to her and accounted for the disconnectedness she often felt. As a child, it had kept her isolated: Tightly supervised by her mother and obedient governesses, she was not allowed to speak, play, or form close friendships with other children unrelated by blood or marriage. Caring about anyone too much was discouraged, and knowing the wrong people, she was warned, would be dangerous.

By the time she reached the age of eleven, Gertrude no longer trusted in the sincerity of anyone's affections. Her private writings of these years reveal her suffering and entrenched suspicions. In an unsent letter to a favorite teacher, she wrote, "If I thought that because I am Gertrude Vanderbilt it made any difference to you in the way you treated me, I would be more unhappy than if I never saw you again. For then I could keep the memory of one whom I consider noble and in the other case I would never believe in human nature again." An autobiographical sketch of 1893 prophesied, "I look into the future and imagine I see myself, grown up and out. I meet a man. I love him. He is attentive to me for my money. He proposes, makes me believe he loves me. I accept, since I love him. We are married. Now, since money is secure, he shows me that he does not love me. I love him still and am wretchedly unhappy." Even traveling abroad could lead to embarrassment. " 'A Vanderbilt, and oh a Miss Vanderbilt—this will bring to light all the fortune hunters,' the people I suppose say . . . oh I hate it so I can't go on," she wrote. At this stage, although she understood the power of money to manipulate human relationships, it had no meaning for her in the ordinary sense. One year, for example, she was given $5,000 to spend on clothes and had some trouble staying within that budget.

Gertrude expressed her doubts about the life laid out for her only to herself. Raised in a regimented atmosphere of servants, governesses, and nurses, in which enthusiastic outbursts of affection were thought to be grossly undignified and speaking one's mind a ghastly breach of decorum, Gertrude learned, in the way that shy people customarily do, to present a frozen face to the world. Externally she was aloof and undemonstrative, an expert at hiding her feelings, but inside she was a molten personality capable of sliding from the lushest romantic melancholy into mordant cynicism. By her tenth birthday, Gertrude was recording her rebellious thoughts in journals and diaries. The pages abound in descriptions of table settings, corsages, yachts, and frocks; besides the relishing of things, she was trying to impart significance or make sense of an environment in which she was not always comfortable. The ceaseless diarizing compensated for her lack of confidantes and the Vanderbilts' own failure to communicate with each other when difficult truths needed to be said. Among Gertrude's masses of personal papers are quantities of unsent letters, many of them addressed to her closest relations. She could not speak bluntly and openly about her inner life for no other reason than that it might disturb someone. Therefore, she did not.

Gertrude's accounts of her own life and feelings were intermingled with poems and tales of changelings, Gypsies, lingering illness, stilettos, scoundrels, and unappreciated (often suicidal) maidens. These fervid efforts at fiction document more than passionate longings or the hidden world for which her stormiest impulses were reserved. They speak of situations she did not yet know how to

escape. In the Vanderbilt dining room or reception hall, she was the demure, dutiful daughter who "had to be nice to everyone"; upstairs at her desk, in her boudoir curtained in white lace and carpeted in white velvet, she confessed her wayward urges. Gertrude's characters showed a freewheeling tendency to laugh in each other's faces, make coarse remarks, and kill themselves or one another when events took an unexpected turn. Nor is it a great surprise to find a quantity of murders and other humiliations visited upon brothers, sisters, parents, and potential suitors—all representatives of the stultifying conventions and attitudes to which a Miss Vanderbilt was tied. Ever a fantasist, her journalizing was her means of contending with a family situation in which her mother read her letters, selected her reading matter, and told her what to think. Her brothers (one of whom, the Vanderbilts agreed, had "all the brains of the family") were being prepared for the future in ways she ached to experience. Gladys, her lovely baby sister, usually stole the show. "G. V.," she convinced herself, "is *dull*."

Gertrude's sensitivity, her penchant for dramatizing, and her fondness for thinking of herself as misunderstood by those around her were signs of creativity, but Cornelius and Alice Vanderbilt ignored or were immune to those messages. And had they perceived that Gertrude was imaginative, they would not have been overjoyed about it. As long as they were in charge, no daughter of theirs would attempt any vocation outside society. Before even the part-time assumption of an artistic "hobby" was allowable, Gertrude was obligated to make her debut, become engaged, be married to an approved young man, and produce children. These events were considered stimulation enough for a woman of her age and class. Gertrude herself would have been quick to agree with those fixed beliefs, although early on she sensed the thinness of her existence. She, who had met more grandees and visited more exotic places by her eighteenth birthday than most other Americans could hope to do in a dozen lifetimes, wrote disconsolately, "My childhood passed almost completely without incident." Her statement echoes that moment in *The Importance of Being Earnest* when Lady Bracknell is confronted with evidence of Cecily Cardew's "birth, baptism, whooping cough . . . vaccination, confirmation, and measles." She comments, "Ah! A life crowded with incident, I see; though perhaps somewhat exciting for a young girl."

Learning to think for herself, let alone to act on the results of what she concluded, would be Gertrude's first true insurrection. Someone who asked questions—even a girl whose thoughts went no further than her diaries—was bound to emerge in some degree as a rebel and a misfit. No one in the immediate Vanderbilt circle was blessed with much intellectual curiosity. And unlike European society, which welcomed writers, politicians, musicians, and artists, the best New York families closed their drawing rooms to all but the well-born and the profusely rich. When one society hostess planned a "bohemian" party, she needed a "bohemian" and invited Edith Wharton. "The Four Hundred," noted one of its members, "would have fled in a body from a poet, a painter, a musician, or a clever Frenchman."

Gertrude watched the Vanderbilt energies, as embodied in her great-grandfather, grandfather, uncle, and father, deployed in cutting bold and bruising swaths through the annals of transportation, commerce, finance, and government, giving shape and tone to the era. In a contrast that couldn't have been other than blatant to Gertrude, her female kin spent their potential in distinguishing themselves in the history of social excess. Locked out of the marketplace, the wives and daughters of the rich took over the management of society and elaborated its hierarchies into a simulacrum of court life. They exhausted themselves giving dinners and balls and making calls; they vied to outdo each other in the extravagance of their gowns, jewels, carriages, flower arrangements, receptions, and residences. Gertrude's aunt, Alva Smith Vanderbilt, was so successful in this sphere that her name has become synonymous with unquenchable—and remarkable—social athleticism.

In the 1870s the Vanderbilts were still outsiders, downright parvenus in the small, closed world of knickerbocker New York. As the foremost examples of the breed nicknamed The Suddenly Rich, they were disdained by Mrs. Caroline Schermerhorn Astor, the city's indisputable social leader by virtue of the seniority of her wealth. The Vanderbilts would continue to be snubbed until the tobacco-spitting, fanny-pinching old Commodore was safely dead, buried, and forever removed from the possibility of doing something unspeakable at grand soirees.* The Commodore expired on January 4, 1877, and shortly afterward Alva (Mrs. W. K. Vanderbilt) went into action. First, she commissioned the de rigueur François I chateau on Fifth Avenue to be built as a fitting domain and backdrop for her activities. In the meantime, she went in for glamorous, expensive dances and dinners to which the city's first families were persistently invited. Since the old guard gave duller and less lavish parties, its younger members were eager to attend Alva's splendid entertainments, with their hired orchestras, banks of hot-house flowers, and out-of-season foods. As the completion of her new castle drew near, Alva set about organizing the most glittering costume ball of the 1883 spring season. She was said to have spent $155,000 on costumes, $65,000 on food and drink, and $11,000 on roses and orchids. The ostensible reason for the party was to inaugurate her new town residence. The true one was to kick open the door to the Four Hundred.

One of the main entertainments Alva devised was the dancing of a series of quadrilles by the young people in attendance. Prominent on the list of prospective dancers was Carrie Astor, Mrs. Astor's youngest daughter. Everyone was invited to practice under Alva's supervision. Through the agency of a mutual friend, Carrie was informed that it would be impossible for her to attend the ball. Mrs. Vanderbilt, the hostess, had never been properly introduced to Mrs. Astor. Carrie left off rehearsing to rush home and tell her mother the terrible news. What had happened convulsed New York hostesses. Mrs. Astor was maneuvered into

---

* To add to their difficulties, the Vanderbilts' newly acquired money came from shipping, which was too much like trade for established society. Astor wealth, originally obtained by exploiting Indians in the fur trade, by that time was derived from real estate, much of it from rents on slum properties.

reappraising Alva's qualifications—and by extension, the whole Vanderbilt clan—for society. "I think the time has come for the Vanderbilts," Mrs. Astor announced, and went to call upon the enterprising striver. Carrie received the last invitation to Alva's ball, and the Vanderbilts were awarded a permanent victory in the "supreme court of social appeals." The rest of Fifth Avenue and Washington Square fell into line, and when the first edition of the *Social Register* appeared in 1887, the Vanderbilts were in it.

For Alva, Mrs. Astor's concession was just the beginning. She invented a coat of arms for the Vanderbilts and plastered the crest over the walls and gates of her town and country houses. Feeling the need of less freshly minted heraldry, in 1895 she coerced her daughter Consuelo into a loveless match with the ninth Duke of Marlborough. The misalliance was so blatant and Consuelo so wretchedly unhappy that several newspapers ran editorials criticizing Alva's conduct. Alice Vanderbilt, Gertrude's ultradignified mother, also approved of coronet hunting among the European houses (Gertrude's little sister Gladys wed a Hungarian count in 1908), but she played the game more sedately and avoided notoriety. Alice made such a fetish of privacy (or, more accurately put, exclusivity) that she refused to enter a shop; any goods she wished to consider for purchase were sent to 1 West 57th Street for inspection.

At Alva's dazzling party symbolizing the Astor capitulation to Vanderbilt ambition, Alice created her one and only public stir. Costumed in white satin and diamonds, she made a grand entrance as Electric Light. She was photographed on that occasion, but otherwise her aversion to reporters and cameramen was unrelenting. If she spied a photographer snapping her picture, she would instruct her chauffeur to take the man's camera and smash it to bits. This was the future held out to Gertrude: the granting and withholding of social recognition, an existence based on the administering of snubs. Like Edith Wharton's Mrs. Welland, what she would have to show for her years on earth would be a lifetime of authority over trifles.

For all her material advantages, Gertrude did not grow up in a visual environment shaped by imaginative taste. Alice and Cornelius Vanderbilt were not people of discernment, but they were shrewd enough to understand that in matters of art and architecture they should bow to the herd instinct. Unlike the entrenched knickerbocker families who lived soberly behind brownstone fronts, the recently arrived tycoons, having much more money to spend, paraded their wealth in front of each other. Building a house that imitated past architecture was the most conspicuous way to do this, and the new nabobs seemed unopposed to any style as long as it looked expensive and wore the aspect of power. Thus the Vanderbilts were not alone in preferring awesome size to fitting proportions and competitive display to restraint. Their redbrick palace, rising five stories high on 57th Street, was elephantine. Built in 1879 and enlarged in 1893, it was a gaudy union of Henry IV and Queen Victoria. The architect, George B. Post, had orders to engineer the biggest house in town, and he succeeded. In Henry James's words, the house was "bristling with friezes and pinnacles, but

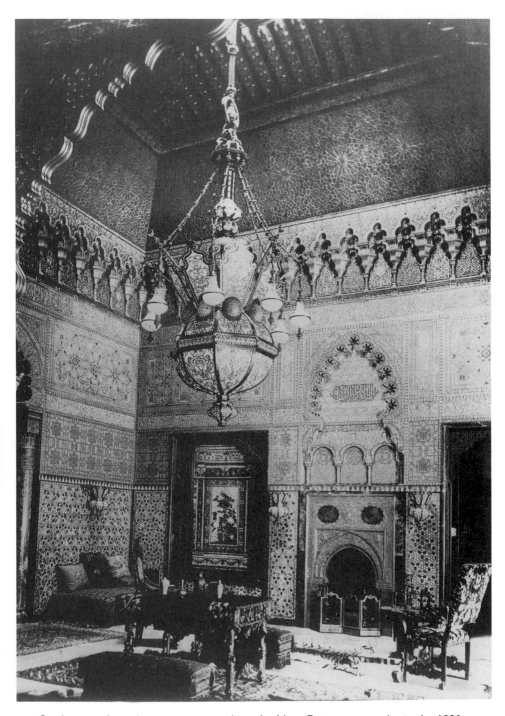

Smoking nooks and cozy corners evoking the Near East were popular in the 1880s, and the Vanderbilts followed the fashion. The stained-glass window was designed by John La Farge.

discernibly deficient in reasons." The first floor alone contained a 40- by 50-foot reception hall, a ballroom, a library, a Persian room (a nook atmospherically decked with striped awnings, satin pillows on which no one ever reclined, spears, and scimitars), a watercolor room, a breakfast room, large and small salons, and a dining room that could seat 200. (To complement the gilded chairs, the Vanderbilts ordered a solid gold service for 200 dinner guests.) The top floor held a bowling alley and a printing room—the latter presumably to handle the volume of engraved invitations and menus Vanderbilt entertaining required.

The effect was one of sumptuous incoherence. No area of the house was related to any other, either structurally or decoratively. Each room had its own geographic theme, making the place a smorgasbord of interior design. Connected by cavernous halls pillared in marble, the ersatz French, Italian, Colonial American, and Moorish rooms were stuffed with tapestries, potted palms, carved furniture swaddled in velvet and tassels, and various trophies torn from European castles. Just as a married woman could never have—or wear—too many jewels, her home could never have too many tables, too many draperies, too many bibelots, or too much silver. The art critic Charles Caffin, writing in 1903, summed up the Vanderbilt style of furnishing when he lamented that the American rich "prefer a room in which every detail is dryly imitated from a dead period to one animated by the art spirit of to-day. So they take their morning coffee *à la Louis Quinze*; their luncheon in a Dutch kitchen; drop into an affectation of Japan for a cup of afternoon tea; dine in the splendour of the *Grand Monarque*; sip their liqueurs in Pompeii, and rest at length from this jumble of inert impressions in a chamber *à l'Empire*. Small wonder if their appreciation of art should be a pose and their actual encouragement of it nearly null!" Although John La Farge and Augustus Saint-Gaudens had contributed elegant decorations to the entrance hall, dining room, and watercolor room, less delicate tastes ruled overall. One guest at the Vanderbilt mansion remembered that "gilt panels of birds and fruits were everywhere, along with ponderous red velvet hangings and paintings—family portraits and badly painted cows and unnatural trees." The staggeringly ornate Breakers, although majestically designed, was first and foremost an assertion of how much it cost. Gertrude, it seems, took the grandeur of her childhood dwellings for granted. In the millions of words she logged about herself and her emotional circumstances, there is not a line about the architectural behemoths she called home.

Gertrude's parents were keenly aware that earning social approval depended in part on hanging the correct paintings on their walls. To the Vanderbilts and their peers, the right brands were the historicizing and sermonizing specialties of the French *pompiers* and, if possible, canvases by certain Old Masters. Within their immediate family, Alice and Cornelius had witnessed the outcome of misguided versus educated picture buying. W. H. Vanderbilt (Cornelius's father and Gertrude's grandfather) had a brief and enthusiastic fling as a patron of American artists. From the mid-1850s until the late 1870s he was a regular supporter of New York painters. He paid frequent visits to 51 West Tenth Street, the supreme artists' domicile for over half a century, where everyone from Winslow Homer, Frederic Edwin Church, and Albert Bierstadt to La Farge and

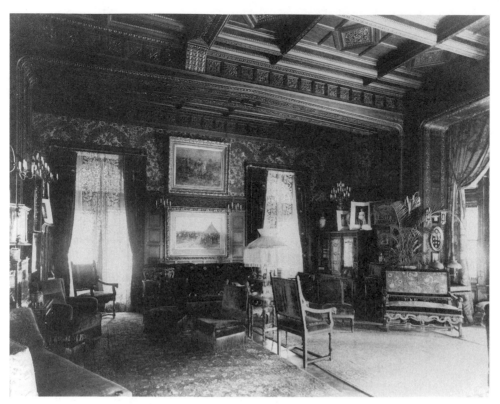

A first-floor sitting room in the Vanderbilt house at 1 West 57th Street. The two paintings depict Orientalist subjects and might well be French.

William Merritt Chase maintained a studio at one time or another. Sociable painters living there stood a good chance of retaining his custom. W. H. favored cheerful genre scenes and romantic landscapes. His favorites were Seymour J. Guy, whose anecdotal paintings bore titles like *Stolen Sweets* and *The Lost Treasure*, and J. G. Brown, nicknamed the Bootblack Raphael for his saccharine pictures of shoeshine boys, newspaper hawkers, and ragged street urchins capering happily in sunlit poverty. But along with these mediocrities, W. H. was gradually making his way toward better paintings by Jasper Cropsey, Sanford Gifford, and Eastman Johnson.

But because of an affront to his pride, W. H. cut back on his acquisitions of American landscapes and conversation pieces after 1874. That spring Guy borrowed a group portrait he had painted of the Vanderbilt family* to hang in a big exhibition at the National Academy of Design. After the show opened, critics ridiculed the picture for the sitters' and owner's folly in supporting home-

---

* *The William Henry Vanderbilt Family*, now in the collection of Biltmore House.

grown talent. Worried about social rebuffs (Alva's conquest of Mrs. Astor was still nine years in the future) and angered by the jeering at his family, W. H. caved in to the art critics. He resolved thereafter to acquire art beyond reproach.

W. H. retained as an adviser the well-positioned New York art dealer Samuel P. Avery, who steered him toward the most acclaimed official art in Europe—paintings by Meissonier, Gérôme, Bouguereau, Lefebvre, Couture, Landseer, and Alma-Tadema. These set pieces, laden with academic honors, were best-sellers with prices to match, but W. H. could afford to indulge himself. With the death of the Commodore in January of 1877, over $90 million was placed directly in W. H.'s hands. As Avery later intoned to a group of reporters, his client "did not continue to make a collection of American pictures after he came into the possession of his fortune, since he was able to buy the best and most costly in the world. He decided, at the outset, to procure nothing that was not important."

Consuelo Vanderbilt once wrote that everyone she knew on Fifth Avenue prized an object far more for its price than for any originality, grace, or imaginative power. Correspondingly, the new Croesuses, who were more at home with possession than appreciation, reasoned that the bigger a painting, the more valuable it was bound to be. The owner of an agglomeration of art for which he paid more than $1.5 million, W. H. believed he had scaled a new pinnacle of connoisseurship.

The times being what they were, W. H.'s collection was ratified by the local cognoscenti. In 1880 the Metropolitan Museum of Art borrowed ten paintings from him for an exhibition of "modern" European art. Two years later, following the fashion set by other wealthy collectors, W. H. opened the doors of his private gallery to the curious public on certain afternoons. Gawkers jammed the premises, stealing flowers and pushing their way into the private rooms, and the viewings were discontinued. W. H.'s greatest source of pride was the publication in 1884 of an oversized four-volume catalog of the contents of his house and collection. It was bound in thick leather, printed in an edition of 500 copies, and distributed to those Vanderbilt hoped to impress. Of the hundreds of works of art shown in the book, there is not a single American painting to be found.

None of this was lost on Alice and Cornelius, who stood by during W. H.'s humiliation, repudiation, and reward. Careful to avoid similar mistakes of their own, they prudently affirmed the superiority of European culture. In 1880 the Metropolitan elected Cornelius to its board of trustees. He expressed his gratitude by giving the museum a group of nearly 700 drawings that the art critic James Jackson Jarves said contained many Michelangelos, Raphaels, Titians, Tintorettos, Rembrandts, and Leonardos. Unfortunately, not one of these optimistic attributions was correct. Every sheet proved to be a copy or from the hand of a student. (Seven years later Cornelius was to do better with his presentation of Rosa Bonheur's *The Horse Fair* to the museum.)

Gertrude's aesthetic orientation was, not surprisingly, sharply angled toward Europe. From the time she was five, she was making several transatlantic crossings a year and notching the customary sights and monuments in her travel albums. As she grew older, she was expected to acquire a familiarity with the

fine arts, and between visits to the dressmaker and the races she sandwiched walks through the Luxembourg and the Louvre. (Society women went to Paris at least twice a year for clothes and spent most of their time in shops and fitting rooms.) In London Gertrude made perfunctory notes about works she saw by Reynolds, Romney, Rubens, Bouguereau, and Sargent. Mired in the prejudices and prerogatives of her class, she categorized the pictures as "ideal," "disgusting," or "expensive." Making the rounds of the galleries would prepare a Miss Vanderbilt to embrace the shopping-bazaar mentality of the new rich and their impresarios, who assumed that all and any treasures of Europe could be borne away for a price. The 1880s marked the beginning of a great American buying spree. Industrial magnates, hungry for sophistication and social grace and abetted by the cupidity of Europeans with a patrimony to sell, were persuaded that not only importing works of art but transporting whole environments to their mansions back home would turn them into men of polish welcome in the best drawing rooms and clubs.

New York's most prominent artists were no different from the plutocrats. They drew upon the artistic vocabulary of the academies in Paris and Rome, which in turn were perpetuating a debased interpretation of classicism, and vitiated it further by espousing an extreme gentility in subject and treatment. Polite thoughts and noble images were presented with prettiness or finicky decorum. Artists who did not conform ran the risk of becoming nonpersons in the eyes of the ruling critics. Eakins and Ryder were the victims of misunderstanding, and Cassatt and Whistler voluntarily exiled themselves rather than work in such an atmosphere.

In October of 1889, after years of being educated at home, Gertrude was admitted to the Brearley School, a private girls' academy then on West 44th Street that took exception to the rule that young ladies should not be exposed to too much learning. Convention decreed that a woman of breeding should know enough about the arts and sciences to adorn her husband's table with grace, but should not become tiresome about her discoveries. Brearley instructors, however, despised the ideal of ignorance. They insisted that a girl could think and reason without coming to harm, and they drilled their students in English, French, German, mathematics, history, civics, science, and Latin. The historian Nathalie Dana, who attended Brearley at the same time as Gertrude, remembered the stimulating effect of the curriculum on sequestered schoolgirls. "Fresh from a parochial atmosphere where women were expected to stay at home except for shopping, associating with their friends, or engaging in church work," she reminisced, "education at the Brearley was breath-taking to a girl who even dimly felt its implications. The first intellectual experience had a novelty and an excitement that is almost impossible for a person born in the twentieth century to understand. It was thought that intellectual activity took the bloom from ladies, and it was insulting to call one a 'bluestocking.' Life was incredibly dull."

Despite her frequent absences (the Vanderbilts showed little concern about

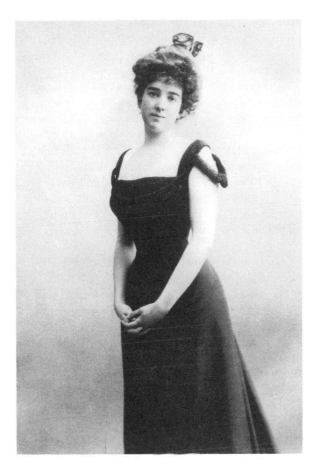

Gertrude as a young woman.

interrupting their daughter's schooling for seasonal peregrinations to Newport, Palm Beach, Paris, and London), Gertrude performed very well scholastically and was considered academically advanced for her age. Classes at Brearley were the high point of her adolescence. Within the pages of her diary, Gertrude deluded herself into thinking that she could abandon "conventionalities," that she might pursue her education. But her parents would not allow her to go to college; she was to get on with the business of coming out. Graduating in the Class of 1894, Gertrude understood, as she had to, that the formal education Brearley offered was no more than an interlude leading up to her being presented in the season of 1894–1895.

During that season, Gertrude was nineteen, young enough and product enough of her upbringing that the vivid round of parties and flirtations filling a debutante's hours seemed ample recompense for college. She was "crazy about going out," and had become an accomplished list maker of topics for sprightly conversation. Conversation, as Gertrude was trained to practice it, consisted of

the speakers handing out subjects to each other. There were beaux and a marriage proposal or two. Gertrude was not especially pretty, but she did possess several attractive features: dark, wavy hair, fair skin, almond-shaped eyes, and long, thin hands. She was tall and lithe, and at her best she could be an effective-looking woman. The fashions, restrictive as they were, enhanced Gertrude's appeal: high-necked lace blouses drawn tight at the waist, skirts that swept the ground, cartwheel hats anchored by long steel pins. Now that she was of marriageable age, all sorts of new amusements were hers for the trying. The novelty of the entertainment blinded Gertrude. It was not yet in her power to realize that the same set of companions and diversions was supposed to occupy her for a lifetime.

The old fears and frustrations of being a Vanderbilt oppressed her still, but Gertrude had grown up an exceedingly sheltered girl who remained in many ways a naive woman wedded to wildly romantic fantasies. This went beyond her versifying about "spooning bliss" and rosebuds; her innocence was evident in her attitudes toward men, most notably in the pseudo-wise generalizations she loved to fabricate (and once fabricated, unquestioningly believed) about the men who courted her. To these twenty-year-olds she ascribed well-formed characters and rich experiences. "Interesting, intensely fascinating, clever, entertaining, deep and passionate. . . ." Gertrude wrote about one caller. "A man of the world who has seen life and profited by what he has seen. . . ." Later she added, "You have had disappointments, but they have not soured you. You are capable of the deepest and most intense feelings. . . . You love life, yet have deep fits of the blues." In describing this young man, Gertrude was also writing about herself. The confluence of romantic distortion, optimism, artistic leanings, and diminished sense of self that accounted for the odd, tortured blend of Gertrude's nature influenced her selection of a husband. She chose her next-door neighbor, Harry Payne Whitney.

Three years older than Gertrude, Harry Whitney had been a part of the Vanderbilts' circle since childhood. His parents—Flora Payne, whose family fortune came from Standard Oil, and William Collins Whitney, a lawyer turned stock manipulator—were part of that tiny group able to keep pace with the Vanderbilts in piling up wealth. William C. Whitney had enjoyed a reputation as a decent lawyer and politician, becoming Secretary of the Navy under Grover Cleveland, until his obsession with joining the $50,000,000 Club got the better of him. Fifty-million dollars was the sum current opinion deemed necessary for a man to live minimally well on Fifth Avenue. Whitney made $40 million in ten years for his part (stock watering) in obtaining a monopoly on Manhattan's street railway lines. He then retired, accumulating the remaining $10 million through loans and investments. Whitney had houses in Newport, Old Westbury, Long Island, Aiken, South Carolina, and Bar Harbor, Maine, as well as a 110,000-acre "camp" in the Adirondacks and an 8,000-acre tract in Lenox, Massachusetts. In the New York house, he was known for maintaining a staff that could serve a meal to 100 diners at an hour's notice.

Harry did not inherit his father's drive. He was a lackadaisical playboy and an avid sportsman, with few intellectual or political interests. Although he was educated at Yale, his letters are barely literate. Harry's assets were good looks,

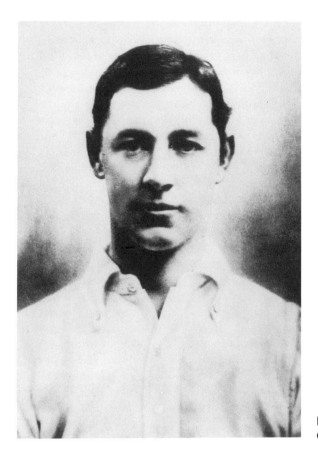

Harry Payne Whitney, whom Gertrude wed in 1896.

common sense, natural athleticism, a zest for sports and society, an old family name buttressed by plenty of hard cash, and a willingness to preserve and manage capital. This very conventionality—the epitome of the sterling young scion— made him a perfect choice for a Miss Vanderbilt. It is not difficult to see how Harry's levelheadedness betokened strength and seriousness to Gertrude, while his charm and good manners hid his laziness, hypochondria, shallowness, and rigid snobbery. Seeing Harry on formal and well-chaperoned occasions, she mistook his obtuseness for self-assurance.

But Harry didn't pretend to imagination, wisdom, or humor in order to win Gertrude. By her own account, she fell in love with him because once, off-handedly, he had spoken with a directness unusual in her universe. One August night in 1894, Gertrude was seated next to Harry at a dinner in Newport. "I'm having such a good time," she said. "You will always have a good time because even when your looks give out, you will still be a great heiress," he replied. With this one remark Harry stunned Gertrude. She was smitten enough to pepper her diary with analyses, reading all sorts of virtues into Harry's bit of frankness. "No one else would have said it—I was delighted." She found "perfect

trust and confidence" in him, "so strong and true . . . He cannot act what he does not feel." She even composed an imaginary note to Harry that focused on the great question of her life—the brute insistence of money. "What I want to know is this—do you think it possible for anyone to love me for myself entirely? That the money would—no, could—make no difference? That anyone in all the world would not care for the money would care as much as his life for me?" Such was Gertrude's innocence that she was able to accept one bald remark as the solution to all her doubts. Candor and openness, worth more than money because they were independent of money, drew her to Harry, and would, in the future, bond her to Juliana. (Artists said that Juliana had the reputation of being the one person who consistently told Gertrude the truth.)

Harry liked clubs, polo, and shooting, and Gertrude liked poetry, novels, and solitude, but somehow his indifference to every activity save sports was an obstacle she was sure she could surmount. More astute observers disagreed. Upon learning of their engagement, one of Gertrude's acquaintances said to him, "Why I thought you were engaged to sport." Sincerity was so rare in Gertrude's circumstances—for her, it existed only within the pages of her journals—that she equated Harry's outspokenness with moral fiber. She even imagined that Harry's habit of plain speaking would extend to winning for them a modest, informal life in a small house—a modern pastoral for an urban heiress. Not the least of the joys of wedlock was its promise of liberation from her mother's supervision and the weight of the vast Vanderbilt household.

With such inordinately inflated expectations in the air, Harry Payne Whitney, even had he been a larger person, was bound to disappoint his wife. His stolid nature did not complement or protect her creative energies or her capacity for romantic fantasy, and nothing in the rest of his character gave him the imagination to understand his wife's ambitions. Disillusionment came, as it had to, in a brief span of years, when Harry withdrew to his clubs and chronic promiscuity. He knew his defection to be a standard marital practice among members of his set, whereas Gertrude, who was not supposed to take notice of such infidelities, would view the situation as an unheard-of betrayal.

On August 25, 1896, in the Gold Room of The Breakers, Gertrude became Mrs. Harry Payne Whitney. She brought a dowry of $10 million to the marriage.

The newlyweds honeymooned in the Berkshires before going on to Japan. The bride exulted in being off on a lark with a man, but soon enough the two were being trailed by unsolicited advice from both families. Alice sent Gertrude a check covering her quarterly allowance and a note suggesting she should send her laundry to Newport. Having chosen to build a new house for himself on Fifth Avenue, William Whitney cabled an offer of his house at 2 West 57th Street to the married pair. Before they received the wire, the senior Vanderbilts and Whitneys had already discussed the matter among themselves. Alice dispatched a strong letter of approval, adding that everything was all arranged— Cornelius was standing ready to furnish the entire house. If the new Mrs. Whitney were unaware that she had wed a man who wanted to be no different

from his father and his father's generation, she certainly learned it during their honeymoon. The dream of a small, cozy establishment was over; Harry was overjoyed about taking over his father's house. The jubilant young husband saw this as the right moment to secure their resort cottage as well, and he bought a waterfront property in Newport close by The Breakers.

Gertrude was in the startling predicament of having exchanged one set of strictures for another. She had not metamorphosed into the someone else she hoped marriage would make her, but she was pregnant. Her closest neighbors were her parents, her in-laws, and the gaggle of cousins who lived up and down Fifth Avenue. When Harry and Gertrude returned from Japan, all was in order, including their destinies. Nothing was left to be sorted out, or so everyone assumed. In an autobiographical fragment written about 1912, Gertrude looked back on her homecoming with sorrow.

> The house I stepped into after my marriage was furnished complete & full. Beautiful Renaissance tapestries, Louis XV and Louis XVI furniture, old French & Italian pictures. The very same atmosphere in which I had been brought up surrounded me again. Just as physically I had moved some fifty feet from my father's into my husband's house, so I had moved some fifty feet in feeling & period of environment. No more than that. . . .

During the first two or three years of her marriage, Gertrude did her best to submerge herself in the routines of wealthy young couples. Shuttling from the town house on West 57th Street to the country retreat in Old Westbury and the shore estate at Newport, Gertrude devoted herself to the demands of society. Her first child, Flora, was born on July 29, 1897, and a son, Cornelius Vanderbilt ("Sonny") Whitney, followed on February 20, 1899. Her old vision of a great love that would fulfill her completely had fled, and there were worse discouragements to face as Harry became more blasé about their marriage. Gertrude, in turn, tried to disguise her impatience with Harry's failure to be attracted to any vocation but play. For years she was ready to adapt, even as she watched with disgust while his token curiosity about law and politics waned (aside from the amount of work involved, he would not associate with men who were unacceptable "for social reasons"), and he lost himself in golf, polo, and racing. Gertrude chafed at the cosmic unfairness of it all. She, who wanted to leave her mark, was relegated to a minor sphere, whereas he, who had been brought up to lead, only wanted to play games.*

An indifferent husband and two dependent children exacerbated the emptiness Gertrude felt. She had done everything that was wanted of her. Why then was she not content? Her diaries of the late 1890s register some general, unfo-

---

*This division of interests along lines of gender exemplified a growing tendency for upper-middle and upper-class women, as dabblers in the arts and displayers of polite accomplishments, to pursue culture while their husbands, brothers, and fathers knew only business and money. The schism led Henry Adams to observe that "the American woman of the nineteenth century was much better company than the American man."

cused strivings, a hunger for emotional satisfaction (but without strategies for attaining it), and the simple human need to be of use. Initially Gertrude saw the barren climate she dwelled in as one of her own making, and she subjected herself to intense examination. "The more I tried to forget myself in life the less I succeeded in doing so," she wrote. "I found myself analysing with minute care . . . looking into a future that held neither pleasure nor satisfaction." Self-scrutiny was the first stage in shaking off the palace-bred helplessness of her background, but the habit of passivity did not die easily. This was, after all, a woman whose clothes were so elaborate and who changed in and out of them so often that she could not even dress without help. "If one has been surrounded all one's life by a great high fence . . ." Gertrude wrote in discouragement, "then when . . . one is liberated from prison one's wings are so inconceivably weak that though one longs to fly one has abrupt falls which are painful. . . . My wings have neither grown nor have they spread."

One exception to the blandness of Gertrude's days occurred during the winter of 1898, when she and Harry began to refurbish 2 West 57th Street. Seeking guidance, they visited the studio of John La Farge, one of the most cosmopolitan American artists of the time. The introduction was arranged by Harry's father. William C. Whitney, whose perceptions seemed largely governed by his pocket-book, regarded La Farge as "a sort of protégé" because he had hired him to design woodwork, embroideries, and stained-glass windows for his house.

Penetrating the sanctum of a painter's studio thrilled Gertrude. Artists made up a "Secret Society" that not even her social position allowed her to enter as an equal. The physical facts of La Farge's rooms alone must have been a revelation. Coming from a world in which no surface was left unembellished, she would have been stunned by his painstakingly plain studio, the consequence of a profound knowledge of the Orient. He did not redo the young Whitneys' premises, but Gertrude went on to buy one of his watercolors at a local show. She later wrote of the "privilege of meeting so great a man. . . . I began to realize the opportunity I had of acquiring." Gertrude did not really begin acquiring art for another three or four years, but La Farge was also intriguing proof of a thought slowly obtruding itself on Gertrude: that talent, unlike yachts or stables, was one of the few things that could not be bought. From the evidence of her 1912 autobiography, the visit took on the aura of a sacred moment as the years went by; in retrospect, it was the only event of 1898 she cared to mention.

By late 1899 Flora and Sonny could be handed over to the care of servants. Harry was taking fewer pains to conceal his mistresses or his lack of interest in understanding his wife. For Gertrude, his rejection was the classical kind of crisis that unleashes and sublimates energies. The sad impetus of Gertrude's drive to improve herself and help others was her husband's unbearable behavior. In more ways than anyone can guess, American art is indebted to the philandering of Harry Payne Whitney.

In the first flush of determination, Gertrude contemplated becoming a writer, the obvious advance on her journalizing. She produced short stories and began,

but did not finish, several novels. Some of her fiction continues the old, retaliatory themes of her adolescence. The writing also served as a vehicle through which she could recognize and explore her sexual nature, a part of herself neglected during the past few unhappy years. Because she had been denied affection and starved for emotional attachments, her novels and short stories overdo infatuation and passion. Because it did only harm to speak of emotional or physical need, Gertrude claimed that she "would rather die than show my real feelings." She was coming to see herself as ruled by impulses and longings a married woman was not supposed to have. If she did, she would do better to suppress them.

Writing, Gertrude's first mode of achieving selfhood, was not a vocation she could pursue on the scale she required. One night she dreamed of working in a cellar and modeling the figure of a man. From that incident she fastened onto the idea of becoming a professional sculptor. Her extrapolation was extraordinary. In the absence of any outright skill or manifest talent, Gertrude radically reinvented herself in the form of an artist. Doing so was a triumph of will and application over nature, and as much a sign of desperation as authority. She wanted something to happen to her, and the world of art and artists was essentially unmapped territory.

Writing dazzled Gertrude, and she could never leave it alone. It was through the authorship of a novella in 1911 that she was to cement her association with Juliana. But there were irreducible reasons why Gertrude, who had a history of being "encouraged" in her literary aspirations by her teachers and childhood friends, chose—and chose permanently—to be a sculptor instead of a writer. Her station and her thin skin ruled out a career in journalism. What was possible for her then was the realm of autobiographical fiction; for a woman as much in the public eye as she was, any resentments or grievances, however subtly transmuted, could not have seen print without bringing down an avalanche of press coverage, gossip, and familial recriminations. For Gertrude herself, writing was associated with her loneliest moments and the urge to retreat into the adolescent fancy that distorted her judgments and intensified her reserve. To be reminded of the topics of Gertrude's juvenile essays—betrayal, entrapment, weakness, boredom, loss of love, and dashed hopes—is to comprehend what she was battling in herself and within her class. She could keep these demons at arm's length in her private musings, but unlike Edith Wharton, her fellow fugitive from the vacuities of New York society, she was not tough enough to expose them to public evaluation.

Whereas the life of an author was a perilous one for Gertrude, the fine arts (and sculpture in particular) would offer the fullest participation in life. No sculptor worth his Beaux-Arts certificate (Paris training was the great and sought-after goal of just about every American art student then) expected to make a living or win acclaim by making small, individual pieces for a client's parlor pedestal or garden fountain. He strove instead for profitable, prestigious public commissions: to ennoble a town square or national exposition with a figure signifying War, Peace, Commerce, Beauty, or Justice.

Monumental public sculpture was an extroverted enterprise that would carry

Gertrude into a community of teachers, pupils, studios, artists, artisans, foundries, and models because it was utterly collective in execution. The atelier and apprentice system was flourishing when Gertrude first dreamed of modeling clay, and its dependability as a source of sympathetic companions kept her from being buried alive. The sculptors she met were a clubbable bunch devoted to dignifying the human figure, and they did not blanch when they saw it naked. Their unprudish attitude and the manual labor involved in shaping plaster and clay represented for Gertrude an explosive defiance of the entirely ladylike existence she had known. A Vanderbilt would be muddying her hands and building up her physical strength.

Perhaps Gertrude thought she would begin so humbly, but she had little time (and no financial provocation, of course) to start at the bottom as an apprentice to an established artist. Instead she took intermittent courses of private tutoring, and within a year of instruction she was engaged in making a monumental figure of her own. Despite her seriousness about her new profession, Gertrude never really studied long and effortfully enough in those early stages to master the plastic understanding necessary to achieve the highest technical proficiency. Gertrude did have imagination, but her powers of invention were weak. This deficiency, coupled with her inability to be single-minded and remove herself sufficiently from the social obligations of being Mrs. Harry Payne Whitney, severely limited the quality of her work. She accepted clichéd symbolism too easily, and her compositions had a predictable sameness to them. Her early sculptures, by and large, were clumsy, idealized rearrangements of Rodin; many reflected the archaisms of Bourdelle, in her hands a manner more assimilated than felt. Eventually Gertrude fell into the practice of hiring (and occasionally forming a liaison with) a respected journeyman sculptor to help her with her commissions. Just what kind and degree of assistance she received over the years became a subject of some rumor in less friendly corners of the art world.

Routine love affairs and suspect collaborations were reserved for the future. But even in 1900, whether or not she confronted it consciously, the excitement of hiring muscular young men to pose nude was undeniable. Gertrude had suffered much sexual frustration from her husband's neglect. She was now a lonely woman aware of a pronounced streak of eroticism, however firmly it was controlled. Paradoxically, traditional figurative sculpture destined for public places was tailor-made for Gertrude's dissociated nature—both the sensual awakening she craved and the discretion she had to maintain. She was exhilarated by the physicality of the work and the necessity for intimate knowledge of the human body. Yet the purposes of late-nineteenth-century sculpture itself, so entwined with architectural or landscape decoration and intended for the public gaze, left little latitude for searching expression or private obsessions. Only sculptors of the highest imagination—say, a Rodin in France or a Saint-Gaudens in America—had the personality to dominate their commissions and attain some autonomy. The rest, regardless of their talent, labored under an insuperable handicap. The destiny of their work dictated its appearance and the range of subject matter was restricted. The allegorical and symbolical trappings that often cloaked and thus legitimized the typical nude statuary of the period almost parody

Gertrude Whitney's own conflicts as the romantic believer in passion and ad-ulation and the icily insecure, emotionally prudent daughter of the upper class. It was the *act* of sculpting and the surprises it would bring into her life that constituted this woman's daring. The lack of emancipation in the art she pro-duced was ultimately secondary to the fact that she had taken the initiative of producing it at all.

The times themselves were receptive to a young woman, even one of means, eager for an artistic career. Never before had belief in the possibility of elevating oneself through the arts been as popular—or as easy to test—as it was in the United States during the Centennial epoch. With the West largely settled and the continent linked by railroads, the nation, entrepreneurial and mobile, was stable enough to invest in universities, museums, public parks, and monuments. Much of what passed for civic pride was in fact self-aggrandizement, and cul-tivation was sometimes inseparable from affectation, but some genuine achieve-ments did result from the fashion for having taste. In 1870 the Metropolitan Museum of Art was incorporated, as were the Boston Museum of Fine Arts and the Corcoran Gallery of Art in Washington, D.C. And in New York, competing with Boston and Philadelphia for the right to be recognized as the country's social capital, the arts and their allied institutions were booming. Between 1875 and 1892, the Art Students League of New York, the Architectural League of New York, and the Municipal Art Society came into being.

The vogue for aesthetic discernment also created a need for more art dealers, auction houses, purveyors of antiquities, and consultants. The publishing in-dustry responded with specialized art journals and popular weekly and monthly magazines that all did their share by running many articles on the importance of aesthetic cultivation. Throughout 1895 and 1896, *Godey's Magazine*, that bible of fastidious womanhood, recognized the growth of art appreciation and the new margin of freedom allowed to women in a series of reports on visits to artists in their studios. Successful painters, sculptors, and architects of both sexes were interviewed and accorded equal critical treatment. In one essay, the writer pointed out the scarcity of women practicing sculpture and recommended that more of them join the artistic community.

Sculpture, despite its potentially subversive effects on the socialite mind, was almost compatible with high society because of its association with lofty purpose. "No art," observed the art historian Daniel Robbins, "was so identified with spiritual values . . . as sculpture in post-Civil War America." The outcome of the war and such huge public convocations as the 1876 Centennial celebration and the 1893 World's Columbian Exposition were greeted as triumphs of the Republic. As such, they generated a further clamor for the enshrinement of heroes in imperishable materials. No library, railroad station, courthouse, or cemetery could be without its bronze or marble statue to the illustrious local military hero, statesman, or poet. Sculpture thus became synonymous with

dignified subjects and inspiring ideals, and its maker an instrument of morality and civic virtue.

This appropriation of national significance—the chest thumping of commemorative sculpture as compared to the breast-beating of confessional fiction —was an unequivocal boon to Gertrude. She was steadily fighting her way toward using her money productively, but she was conscientious about remaining considerate of Whitney and Vanderbilt proprieties. (At times when she wasn't, her mother tartly called attention to her deviations.) Her decision to have a career, no matter how bold a step for her, had to be kept within certain limits for Harry's sake. Patronizing the arts was one thing, but practicing them was another. Nathalie Dana, who had hoped to become a concert pianist at about the same time Gertrude was transforming herself into a sculptor, explained the prevailing attitude.

> [A]lthough we were criticized for our peculiar desire for hard work, our enthusiasm for the arts was accepted. It was better to work in the arts where we were unlikely to earn money; for a girl who earned money insulted her father, who took pride in providing for his family. It was also considered wrong for a girl to compete with poor women who needed money.

Afraid that signing her own name would invite unfair judgments, Gertrude exhibited her sculpture pseudonymously until 1910. Her primary reason was, as she said, to avoid the condescension and skepticism inevitable when a socialite attempted something creative. But the assumed name would also help guard against censorious scenes at home and accusations about the vulgarity of pushing oneself forward. What might be considered an insult in the more modest Dana household would have been a supreme mortification in Harry's.

To return to the winter of 1899, Harry's multiplying infidelities increased the pressure on Gertrude to make a separate, purposeful life for herself. She had no professional connections and little idea how to make advances to people outside her own circle. However, the Vanderbilt and Whitney influence was powerful, and she was beginning to want to capitalize on it. Gertrude asked her mother to arrange a meeting with Saint-Gaudens, which did not come about, and the architect Stanford White to write on her behalf to Daniel Chester French, sculptor of *The Minute Man* and the seated Lincoln of the Lincoln Memorial, who did not accept pupils. She then turned to Howard Cushing, a fellow member of Newport society who had succeeded in becoming a painter. Cushing, six years her senior, became Gertrude's artistic mentor, and he recommended her first instructor, Hendrik Christian Andersen, a Norwegian-American sculptor who specialized in gargantuan nudes.

Andersen, whose work ranges from the dull to the frightful, is best known today as the flaxen-haired young man who infatuated Henry James. James met the sculptor in Rome during the summer of 1899 and was helplessly attracted to him. For his part, Andersen kept a vigilant eye on the main chance and saw no reason why James should not be enlisted to promote his work. Andersen's

association with Gertrude evolved in a similar manner, typical of the way clever, manipulative personalities were able to use her until she found a trustworthy assistant in Juliana, who protected her from the bloodsuckers and parasites.

Andersen did possess real teaching ability, but his primary qualification was social acceptability. He and his family, living in genteel poverty in Newport, were on the fringe of the Whitney set. They inched closer to the center when Hendrik's brother Andreas became engaged to Olivia Cushing, Howard's sister. Had Hendrik not been known to Newport society, it is doubtful that he would have been asked to give lessons to Gertrude.

After a stay at Lamb House with James, Hendrik arrived in New York in the fall of 1899, eager to earn money to finance his colossal statues. He reported on his progress to the Master, who seconded him in his determination to perform any labor, no matter how tedious, in order to return to Europe and himself. "So, most assuredly, boil the pot by sorry art and every cunning you can contrive or cultivate," James urged. "Gird your strong loins, nurse your brave visions, bear with your stupid sitters, gouge in your master-thumb. . . ."

The pot that would boil most rapidly was the job of teaching Gertrude Whitney. On January 27, 1900, Hendrik informed his mother that he was going to teach Gertrude how to sculpt. As she was the daughter of Mr. Vanderbilt, he noted, giving lessons was bound to be remunerative. A month later, Hendrik was making headway. He had constructed a temporary studio for Gertrude at 2 West 57th Street and nailed down a monthly allowance for himself. But he could not resist confiding that Andreas's socially prominent friends were a witless lot. In letters to his mother, Hendrik effusively declared his great liking for Gertrude and what fast friends they had become. To Andreas, with whom he could afford to be candid, he wrote, "I am not over anxious about anything, at least I make her *think* so! For I want to make her excited. *Not myself!* And although she is *very foolish* I will put the *world* in a *new* light for her! and make her say only nice things and I see how she can be of use to us in a hundred ways! so I play a slow game, and have my sleeves full of trumps!"

Although he was not above telling Gertrude that Henry James empathized with her and sent his good wishes, Hendrik *did* keep his part of the bargain. He put the world in a new light for Gertrude merely by being himself. He fulfilled an important function if only because in his impassioned devotion to art and the people he chose to befriend, he was such a devastating counterpoint to the jaded philistines she knew. Within a month of meeting Gertrude, he introduced her to Ellen Terry. The threesome visited a group of Andersen's sculptures on view at the Metropolitan and made the rounds of the art galleries, brazenly breaking the Four Hundred's taboo on well-born women mixing with actresses. * Hendrik impressed upon Gertrude the importance of having a studio physically separate from her living quarters and designed one to be erected that spring on the cliffs of her estate in Newport.

---

* All women in the theater were thought to be disreputable, but Ellen Terry was especially scandalous because she was known to have borne "unfathered" children.

When not working on *Aspiration*, a life-size male nude Gertrude had begun under his tutelage, Hendrik would read aloud from Ibsen. On her own, he expected her to draw and study anatomy, to ground herself in the fundamentals of technique. Too subtle to fawn on his rich pupil, Andersen dignified her by criticizing her strictly, which often sent Gertrude scurrying from the studio in tears but also imbued her with "faith in my own capacity." Hendrik was wise enough to advise her to see even failure as a kind of coming into one's own. "It makes little difference who you study with, as long as your instructor is not too *artistic* or sentimental. . . ." he counseled. "Use your own judgment about the modifications [for the statue] and ask *the advice of no one!* as the figure must stand alone, and since it is your first work, let those things that others consider faults be *your faults!* and not subjected to a lot of *assimilated* hysterical and well intended suggestions." Hendrik's solicitude and appeals to Gertrude's nascent sense of independence, regardless of the cynical motivations behind them, outweighed the value of whatever money she had paid him.

By the summer of 1900 Hendrik had been so slow and canny in drawing his trump that both he and Andreas were installed in Newport as Gertrude's teachers. Andreas, instructing her in drawing, was less predatory than Hendrik and more sweetly disposed toward her because of his intimate involvement with the Cushings and their friends. He tried to dissuade Hendrik from his maneuvers. "About Mrs. Whitney, she's all right and likes you," Andreas wrote to his brother. "She, poor thing, wears a mask, because her situation demands one. Society is a masked ball, and by way of hint, some of the dancers are weary; so if you go to Mrs. Whitney frankly and honestly, you won't need a disguise and you'll really get things surprisingly quick." Gertrude commissioned a painting from Andreas, and Hendrik sold her a double portrait bust of her and Harry as well as another portrait head. He had indeed "gouged in his master-thumb" with a profit beyond anything he could have imagined when he landed in New York. A year after his arrival in America, Andersen had saved enough money to embark for Lamb House and eventually Rome.

Gertrude did not see him again until the summer of 1902, when Hendrik visited Newport and helped her finish a figure she was modeling. But while he was abroad, he continued to write her rousing letters that buoyed her confidence and kept her apprised of his own plans and parlous financial state. They were reunited in New York in June 1905, and in Newport that July he gave Gertrude pointers "in expression of sentiments in relation to sculpture," namely, "despair, agony, joy etc." The lessons were followed by more purchases. Within a year or two, however, Andersen faded from Gertrude's life as his requests for subsidies grew too exorbitant even for her to consider. Always in love with the grandiose (James sighed over his friend's "mania for the colossal, the swelling or the huge, the monotonously and repeatedly huge"), he conceived a notion of a World City of Peace, a new metropolis to be designed by a team of eminent architects. The demand for sculpture in this public-spirited place would be enormous and, conveniently enough, it was all to be filled by Hendrik Andersen. Once he latched onto this idea, he poured every spare cent he had into its realization,

and no one else was exempt from his demands for money, either. Gertrude received a begging letter from him as late as 1920. Nevertheless, she would remember Hendrik with fondness and remain grateful for his tutoring.

After Hendrik left for Europe, Gertrude began searching for another teacher. She was also storing up the strength to challenge family opposition to her sculpting. Originally, when her dissatisfaction with home and society seemed to be a passing oddity, the objections were cunningly low-key. Later, after the uncompliant Gertrude gave no quarter in shutting out Harry and returning to her studio, antagonism was swift and extremely sharp.

Fussy, belligerent Alice Vanderbilt was the first to question her daughter's propriety in modeling a nude figure from life. Throughout September and October of 1900, in response to seeing a photograph of *Aspiration*, she composed notes to Gertrude that were little darts of blame. "I hope you do not apply yourself too closely to [your work]. . . . Do give him a scarf. [A]nd don't let little Flora be shocked. . . . The fig leaf is so little! . . . What becomes of him when you leave your Studio—and how does Harry like him?" "I hope your baby is well—do not let him get ill like last year. Keep him warm & leave the Statue—what is anything compared with the health of those we love!" When matched with Alice's skill as an emotional saboteur, Harry ranked in the amateur class. He declined to notice the importance of sculpting in his wife's schedule, or he would assert that she would really get more fun out of hunting and riding.

Gertrude needed a vacation from these reproofs. She persuaded Harry to take her to Europe, which she had not toured since 1895. Sailing in the winter of 1901, they stayed for five months and for diversion brought along another couple and three bachelors, one being the indispensable (to Gertrude) Howard Cushing. The trip was another expansion of her freedom. She flirted with the unattached men, reveling in her "mood of deviltry." Visiting museums and artists' studios with Howard, Gertrude was painfully reminded of Harry's apathy toward the life of the mind. He could not "see beyond the boundaries of nondescript ideas," whereas traveling abroad left her "irretrievably changed," "in a tumult," and no longer able "to fight the temptations in my life."

Back in the Newport studio, Gertrude sent *Aspiration* to the 1901 Pan-American Exposition in Buffalo, a fair now primarily remembered as the scene of McKinley's assassination. With a year's worth of sculpting behind her, Gertrude entered one of the most caustic passages to be found in her journals. The object of her contempt was Harry, but in the process of flaying him she was denouncing her own former ways with the zeal of a recent convert.

I pity, I pity above all that class of people who have no necessity to work. They have fallen from the world of action and feeling into a state of immobility and unrest. They have become inert, both mentally and bodily, also from an emotional standpoint, and they are not even spared the ignorance of their condition. . . . They can scarcely be called weary of life for they have never tasted it. . . . The great and grand unemployed—the dregs of humanity.

Gertrude backed up her words with actions. She located a place to work on West 33rd Street in New York, knowing that the Newport studio was too near Alice Vanderbilt and too far away from everyone else.

Next Gertrude began studying with James Earle Fraser, a sculptor recommended by Daniel Chester French. Nearly two years younger than she, Fraser knew his calling early in life and was already a figure of some note when Gertrude met him. In 1894, as a result of witnessing the Indians being herded farther and farther into the West, the seventeen-year-old Fraser made and showed *The End of the Trail*, in which an exhausted brave on a worn-out pony plods ever onward. Merely by being reproduced in photographs, the maquette had become one of the nation's most popular statues. (Fraser became just as famous again one generation later for designing the Buffalo and Indian Head nickel, issued in 1913, and today New Yorkers know his equestrian statue of Theodore Roosevelt at the main entrance of the American Museum of Natural History.)

Gertrude absorbed some of Fraser's gift for spontaneous-looking movement, but their breezy camaraderie and the sculptor's personality seemed to matter just as much. Fraser was a kindhearted man whose generosity toward other artists must have impressed Gertrude, as did his studio picturesquely located in Greenwich Village, a part of Manhattan she had little cause to visit in those days. Here, in a row of converted stables and carriage houses lining a dead-end street called MacDougal Alley, labored a dozen other painters and sculptors. Fraser introduced Gertrude to this charming neighborhood, which would one day be her own.

By mid-1902 Gertrude's struggle to bridge the distance between socialite and artist appeared doomed, although the preceding months had passed constructively enough. The lessons with Fraser continued while she attempted to write a travel book that would sort out the upheavals of her European vacation. She corresponded with Howard Cushing and Hendrik Andersen, and their benign prodding fueled her intention to work. But Gertrude became pregnant for the third time—most inconveniently, and not much to her liking, one suspects.

And Harry, she learned, was carrying on a heated affair with a distant cousin by marriage, someone of their own social stratum whom she would be obliged to see and entertain. Reeling from this cruelly timed infidelity, Gertrude stopped doing much of anything but living through those months. She did manage to sponsor art classes at a settlement house on the Lower East Side, but the depression did not lift. On the contrary, she hoped she would die. Gertrude addressed a long letter to Harry, to be opened in the event of her death. Her mental state had so deteriorated that she could only condemn herself as a person of no consequence. "If I could not hold you I had only myself to blame . . ." Gertrude wrote. "Could I have gone on without that for which I pine for the most. I doubt it & been a good woman. I love love and I need it as we all do & perhaps I would have taken it even if I could not give it, rather than starve forever. . . . As for Sonny be good to him. He seemed at times really to like me. I think we could have been very close."

The extent to which Harry understood how much he had injured his wife is impossible to guess, but something chilled and hardened in Gertrude during that bleak winter of 1903. She recovered physically, had a daughter, and rehearsed, as she never had before, compartmentalizing and sealing off sections of her life. She mustered a distrustful self-sufficiency and self-centeredness, derived of bitterness but positive in their ends, an adamant determination to find gaiety, sympathy, and freedom as an artist and a woman of affairs. The artist's mantle would cloak her with welcome detachment and self-definition; the amorous secrets would help avenge the scars she had sustained. She would battle for respect and take love rather than starve for it.

Not only did Gertrude now loathe the existence—"the arranging of life to fit surroundings"—she had chosen for herself in 1896, but her family was set more obstinately than ever against the effrontery of her ambitions. In the autobiography of 1912, which was originally slated for public consumption while all parties involved were still alive but which never did see print, Gertrude presented a whitewashed version of her relatives' opposition to her work during the years between 1900 and 1904. Gertrude stated that it had "positively no effect on me." "On the whole," she concluded, "they might have been much more disagreeable and I never had a real struggle, only a rather scornful attitude to combat."

That was the tactful version, written to prevent hurt feelings. The truth was more tempestuous, as this 1905 diary entry attests:

> You have known always that whatever you did in the line of art would be a fight. It is a fight, it always has been one & will go on till doomsday to be one. Now you have won a point—the point being that you can get out of the . . . trip* to do your work, do not expect to have any sympathy for having gotten out of it. . . . Never expect Harry to take the work seriously & that because you have promised to do a thing you must do it if possible. To the other kind of person in the world (the non-artist) no struggle is considered serious . . . but you have won battles already and will win more. Think of the great advantages that this trip (now that you do not have to go) will give you. Two weeks of absolute freedom . . . three weeks. . . . No one to wear you out, no one to discourage you, and no one to keep up for. . . . Are you going to be discouraged & forlorn simply because Harry fails to see your viewpoint. It has never made any difference to him that I feel as I do about art and it never will (except as a source of annoyance) so there—I realize *that* when I stop and think about it, and it is only in moments of discouragement that I expect other things. . . . I undertook this thing really to convince him I was serious & the result is—nothing at all.

As can be seen, Gertrude now accepted herself as an artist. Perhaps the ultimate casualty of the couple's alienation and Gertrude's fight to be taken seriously was Barbara, the child born on March 21, 1903. She was an eternal reminder of a period of unremitting misery, and her mother had comparatively little to do with her. From the evidence of Gertrude's journals and date books, Barbara received far less maternal warmth and attention than Flora or Sonny.

The end of 1903 found Gertrude toiling under Fraser and another sculptor

---

*A voyage abroad that Harry wanted to make.

and designing bas-relief panels for a house some cousins were building. When Fraser signed on to teach at the Art Students League, the largest art school in the city, Gertrude joined his classes a few months later. Meanwhile, events again conspired to overpower her. William C. Whitney died suddenly on February 2, 1904, of peritonitis. The despondent Harry, who had idolized his father, attempted to comfort himself by usurping Gertrude's love again. Howard Cushing, whom Gertrude considered her own, married, and then a childhood friend also died unexpectedly. This time Gertrude did not founder into a depression. Calloused from her experiences, she was capable of beginning again. Her knowledge of her real preferences and dislikes led her to admit with increasing frequency the startling disproportion between the lavishness of her family's and friends' physical world and the threadbare quality of their mental and emotional furnishings. Most of the people she was "thrown in with" and most of the things she did were "not congenial" to her.

Gertrude couldn't defy the social ethic, but she could bend it to her purposes, as resourceful persons had always done. She stopped looking at her wealth and position chiefly as barriers to artistic people. Her advantages, now that she was ready to wield them, were shortcuts that would let her do whatever she wished. In the form of patronage and enlightened philanthropy, money and influence were passports out of a suffocating milieu. Gertrude matter-of-factly vanquished

Gertrude with her younger daughter, Barbara, a few months after her birth in 1903.

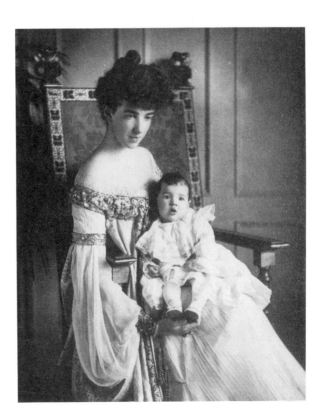

her insecurities, writing in her journal of 1904—and how these sentiments would have shocked the young Miss Vanderbilt, so longing to be like everyone else—

> your real power . . . is your money and position. . . . Why do what is fitting for Jane Smith when you are not Jane Smith? . . . . This road through life is the only one for you. Do not sink into a nonentity when the path for other things is open to you. And it is open. Go to your friends, to people who know you well & make them tell you what your good points are . . . so that you may make something of them. Why should you waste these talents anymore than your money and position which are also talents. . . . Do not let this burst of enthusiasm pass.

She made a list of useful persons and cited the assets of each one. Several cousins had "business knowledge" or "financial value"; her brothers Alfred and Reginald also had a "name"; others possessed an open mind, and some were even aware of art and artists.

From Fraser, from the young people she observed at the Art Students League, from the apprentices in the large ateliers she'd visited, Gertrude saw firsthand how exhausting the contest to maintain oneself as an artist was for men and women who could not afford extensive schooling or travel abroad, who had to make do in parochial, provincial surroundings. Here was an area in which Gertrude could offer sorely needed help, and where she could put the weight of her name to advantage. She felt renewed and confident as she set down her ideas in a new notebook.

> To see artists and find out [their] wants would be a good start. . . . To found a Beaux-Arts—with painting & modeling in connection. Tuition low. Scholarships. Exhibition rooms in connection. How much demand is there for Architecture in N.Y.? . . . S[tanford] White. [Charles] McKim. Painting? J[ohn White] Alexander. . . Modeling? [Daniel Chester] French. Raise money for building. $1,000,000 at 5% interest. $50,000 for me to pay. . . Best teachers. Lectures from prominent artists . . .

Gertrude knew what she was doing when she hit on this plan. All of her grief, self-consciousness, and frustration could not be poured into her art alone. Helping other artists would provide her with great merriment and contain the melancholy. Her aims would bore Harry and anger Alice. Within this form of advocacy, Gertrude's own struggle for recognition and fulfillment could be played out. No charity, even if it is a refuge from despair, is untainted by egotism, and the execution of her project would be an outlet for the love and admiration missing from her personal life. But she would achieve a larger rather than selfish purpose and effect great change.

In trying out her schemes for an art school and accompanying exhibition space, Gertrude was poised to refashion her life in a manner impervious to interference. She was thirty. Her childbearing was behind her. She had a cause. She had every social and monetary means at her disposal. She intended to make use of them all, and she did. And that change—the choice of the mature, seasoned manipulation of her public identity to serve her rebellious spirit over the passive, forlorn, rueful sulking that characterized her earlier years—was the real victory of the great heiress.

CHAPTER THREE

GETTING TO NEW YORK

❦ (1906–1912) ❦

> Of all the ambitions of the great un-
> published, the one that is strongest,
> the most abiding, is the ambition to
> get to New York.
>
> —FRANK NORRIS, *Blix*

ON THE EVENING OF MAY 2, 1906, John Sloan attended a preview of an exhibition held by the American Water Color Society. The members had requested ten of his latest etchings delineating New York City life for the show, and he was eager to see them on display. But between the time Sloan dropped off the prints and the opening that night, the society's hanging committee pronounced four of them "too vulgar" and banned them from the public gaze. The committee's embarrassment lay in portrayals of families asleep on a tenement roof on a hot summer night, a couple embracing with obvious relish while their child looks on, a slatternly woman scanning the fashion page of the newspaper, and another woman putting out the light as her companion waits for her to join him in the darkness. Three out of the four scenes took place in a bedroom and the other was set in an improvised sleeping area. Such backdrops were too suggestive—they sullied the good name of art.

Sloan was incensed by the society's action and demanded that the other six etchings be returned to him at once. The society, after all, had *invited* the works of art that now offended them. He also averred that the prints were honest transcriptions of incidents he had actually observed from his own windows, which overlooked the tenements, fire escapes, and rooftops of Chelsea. "I know these plates are not vulgar—not indecent," he declared in his diary. At the same time, Sloan wasn't inordinately surprised at the society's rejection. By now he was

almost resigned to the various cold-shoulderings he'd received, for he had long ceased to conform to official expectations of good taste. He was thirty-four years old and had not sold a single painting. Nor would he find an interested buyer for another seven years. Although Sloan was already well embarked on his pictures of the metropolitan milieu, he could find little support for his art outside a loyal group of friends. The critics were certain that Sloan's sooty intimacies defiled the fair rose of art. As one reviewer thundered, "Is it fine art to exhibit our sores?"

Sloan lived with his wife, Dolly, in a fifth-floor apartment at the top of 165 West 23rd Street. Since their move to New York from Philadelphia two years before, their life together was one tinged by hardship. Sloan earned some money as a free-lance magazine illustrator, but his only steady income came from designing a weekly puzzle for the *Philadelphia Press*, an assignment he first received in 1899 and had hung onto ever since. Their rent was a stiff $50 a month, and the Sloans had to live carefully to meet it. The New York they knew was indeed the city seen in the artist's paintings and prints—hearty, lively, extravagant, flamboyant, rich in contrasts, and frankly sordid. The millionaires' palaces were strung along Fifth Avenue in ever greater numbers, but three quarters of the population were crowded into tenements. (The Sloans themselves resided close by the Tenderloin, a wide-open zone running between West 14th and West 34th Streets. Beer gardens, gambling dens, policy shops, dance halls, and worse flourished there. The streets swarmed with confidence men and prostitutes, abetted by the connivance of the police.) The sporting set consumed lavish dinners at Sherry's and Delmonico's, and their idea of fine entertainment was an evening with the Floradora Sextette or a dozen naked girls bursting out of an enormous Jack Horner pie. Yet none of this—nor the existence of ordinary wage earners—could be acknowledged in aesthetic works with claims to cultural legitimacy. The libertine and the puritan alike wanted his art sugarcoated.

Sloan was not an isolated target of prudery. This was the heyday of Anthony Comstock, the founder of the New York Society for the Suppression of Vice and a one-man censorship squad ready to collar any person, practice, or expression he judged to be obscene. What Carry Nation was to alcohol, Comstock was to images of the unclothed human body. In February of 1905, the art dealer William Macbeth hung in the window of his Fifth Avenue gallery a picture by Bryson Burroughs of naked children playing together in a pool. Burroughs was a follower of Puvis de Chavannes, and his paintings were nothing if not chaste in appearance. Comstock nevertheless was disgusted by what he saw, and insisted that the wicked thing be removed from view.

On August 2, 1906, the vice hunter struck again, this time at the Art Students League. The school put out its usual fall catalog for prospective students, and Comstock heard rumors about the horrors inside its covers. Accompanied by two policemen, he raided the League and confiscated the publication because reproductions of nudes could be discovered therein. Acting in his capacity as a special agent for the U.S. Post Office, Comstock placed the bookkeeper under arrest for distributing obscene materials through the mails. One sculptor then proposed that Comstock organize raids on any store selling *Gray's Anatomy*.

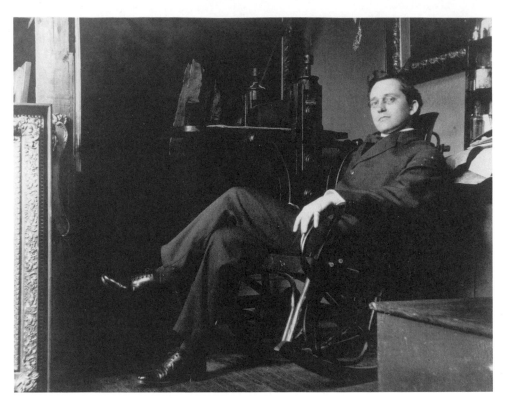

John Sloan in his studio at 165 West 23rd Street, about 1906.

In the provincial environment that was turn-of-the-century New York, art was expected to be arty: pretty, ennobling, and, most of all, reassuring. The aestheticism and refinement of the nineties had daintily laced mainstream creative expression into a straitjacket of gentility. In the name of idealism and hallowed tradition, portrayals of day-to-day existence, especially when that existence recognized the facts of an imperfect world, were disparaged for their crudity. Artists were expected to be the handmaidens of society rather than its critics, and they earned the most praise when, in William Dean Howells's words, they lingered exclusively on "the more smiling aspects of life." Not only unpleasant social or moral truths were to be suppressed, but actual observations from nature. The most popular painters and sculptors (those who carried off the big prizes at local exhibitions) practiced a very commercialized art. Their stock-in-trade ran to pastiches: synthetic pastoral scenes, simpering nudes draped in the requisite classical allusions, ethereal women with cherubic tots seen in a gracious interior or a fresh meadow, and falsely scintillating portraits. These productions were typically executed in a cloudy froth or with an accretion of lugubrious detail that Sloan characterized as "an obnoxious kind of clever photographic painting."

The last modern movement in art to have been completely accepted on

American shores was Impressionism, but the native variant was often tame, having been much traduced by slick or unadventurous imitators. Formulas prevailed, and there was a general ebbing away of character and vigor. Fauvism and Cubism were fermenting in Paris, but most American artists were still oblivious even to Post-Impressionism, whose leaders had died by 1906. The painter Leon Kroll, who studied at the National Academy of Design in 1906 and 1907, later said that during his Academy days he "had never heard Cézanne's and Van Gogh's names mentioned."

Because acclaim went to the painters and sculptors who paid homage to values society held high, most artists were not adversarial, and next to no galleries handled American art. Those that did represented the salable names. Everett Shinn remembered those early picture salons as "funeral parlors wherein the cadavers were displayed in sumptuous coffins." Hence anyone without an established reputation wishing to reach an audience was at the mercy of the various exhibition societies (such as the American Water Color Society) that regularly organized shows throughout the year. Memberships in these groups, the most powerful of which was the National Academy of Design, interlocked. Predictably, the governing officers within the larger bodies were narrow and intolerant. Fiercely conservative and bound to the ideal of the antique, they were preoccupied with guarding civilization and defending authority. Convention took precedence over invention. Unfortunately, the classicizing tradition the establishment upheld was no longer nourished by life, and thus had become increasingly irrelevant to it. Wallace Stevens, after attending one of the Academy's annual shows, noted in his journal that "the pictures, taken one by one, were hardly worth the trouble. . . . The artists must be growing as stupid as the poets."

As is inevitable with the institutionalizing of taste, the academicians wanted to protect their raison d'être by perpetuating their own creed and influence. The Academy censored opposition most effectively through the selection process for exhibitions. Shows were nominally open to all comers, but nonmembers' offerings had to undergo a trial by a jury of academicians and were subject to being blackballed, whereas members' submissions were *hors concours*. As one newspaper reviewer put it, "Inanities by the older academicians . . . have the divine right of wall space." The Academy's hegemony made for the virtual disenfranchisement of most liberal or independent artists. In this respect, the politics of art mimicked big business practices of the time. Benefits and profits were distributed among a very few, who monopolized sales, exhibition space, awards, and commissions. In arranging for the consolidation of power in its own hands, the National Academy of Design seemed as unreasonable—and invincible—as any trust.

But a bankrupt authority can serve as a whetstone on which the opposition can sharpen itself. Aesthetic revolutions take place only when "feeling drops out of the work and it must fight to get back in again," testified Robert Henri, a veteran of many such skirmishes. The very artificiality of the art being laureled offered a ready-made focus of discontent, but there were larger forces also accounting for the creative turmoil. Immigration, which was restructuring the demographic, political, and social makeup of New York, would affect the arts

as well. Furthermore, the influx of population was not restricted to the foreign-born. All kinds of people who felt they didn't fit in anywhere else in the country poured into New York, intent on bending the leviathan to their will. William Dean Howells, Stephen Crane, Upton Sinclair, Theodore Dreiser, Lillian Wald, Edward Arlington Robinson, Margaret Sanger, Lewis Hine, Isadora Duncan, O. Henry, D. W. Griffith, Willa Cather, Wallace Stevens, and Lincoln Steffens not only laid claim to the city, but revealed new possibilities for it. They rejected outdated attitudes and art with a surface like a retouched photograph or a manicured green. Responding with the outsider's fresh—and often outraged—perspective, they studied the rawness, squalor, and tumult of the industrial metropolis, the very facets of urban living ignored by polite society and the housebroken artists it rewarded. Even if the newcomers did not interpret or recast their environment directly, they drew strength from New York's plenitude and, in turn, they reinvigorated the city with their fresh opinions.

Out of the several hundred artists who called New York home, two breakaway groups emerged as major forces ready to attack the Academy, organizationally and aesthetically. Both were formed around a charismatic leader, both took the vibrations of the city as crucial to their aims, and both refused to court official recognition. The artists of each group were iconoclasts in conflict with the establishment; they left their audiences behind them and risked rejection, ridicule, and oblivion.

One circle was constituted of the painters and photographers clustering around Alfred Stieglitz and 291, his tiny gallery on lower Fifth Avenue. Originally named the Little Galleries of the Photo-Secession, Stieglitz's temple began as an exhibition center for photography. Stieglitz had already won international acclaim as a photographer, and his gallery was founded to persuade scoffers that photography was a valid art form. Taking up the cudgels for photography was at the time an act of great courage in itself, but Stieglitz went a step further in 1907 when he expanded the scope of the gallery to include painting and graphic work of the most advanced sort. To the accompaniment of jeers and insults, he introduced Cézanne, Matisse, and Picasso to America. Consequently, the New York artists (Marsden Hartley, Arthur Dove, John Marin, Abraham Walkowitz, Max Weber) who hovered around 291 could monitor the European avant-garde. They were part of a handful of people in the entire country who could comprehend modernism and were equipped to interpret Fauvism, Expressionism, and Cubism.

The other group was a band of painters marshaled by Robert Henri. In 1906 Henri was not only an established painter, but a gregarious teacher and firebrand. The nucleus of his coterie consisted of Sloan, William Glackens, George Luks, and Everett Shinn. Henri met these four men in Philadelphia fourteen years before, when he was returning from Paris and they were artist-reporters for the local newspapers. Henri urged his friends to set their sights beyond illustration and toward easel painting. "Henri could make anyone want to be an artist," said Sloan, who often stated that until then he had had no ambition to be a painter.

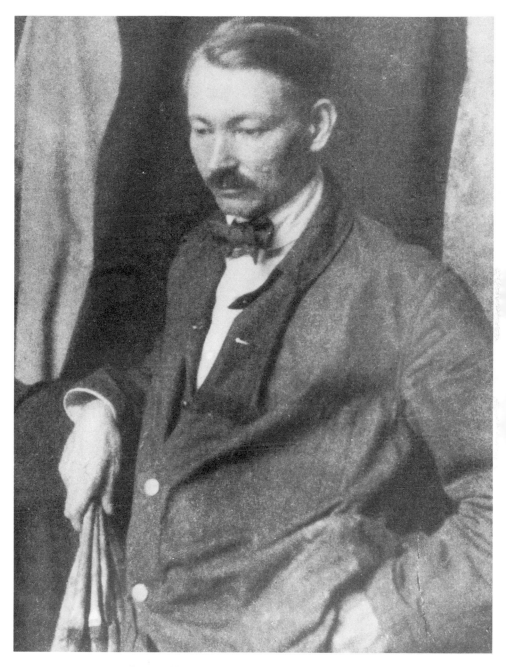

Robert Henri—painter, teacher, and firebrand.

The same transformation later occurred with George Bellows. Yet Henri was careful that his disciples retain their impulse toward the sharply observed, on-the-spot impression, their preference for noting what went on around them. Their brushes recorded contemporary costumes and attitudes that the academicians, yearning for the perfections of chitons and garlands, categorized as ugly. "Be willing to paint a picture that does not look like a picture," said Henri.

The painters in the Stieglitz circle focused on formal innovations, drawing on Post-Impressionism, Fauvism, and Cubism, whereas the Henri coterie, which stopped stylistically with Manet and Forain, was more involved with expanding the realm of subject matter fit for art. Yet both groups seized on authentic, firsthand experience instead of invoking older formulas for what the world was supposed to look like. They had a common indebtedness to the crowds, rhythms, shadows, and spaces of New York, another affinity that made them all modern in outlook. The concept of the city as a living, highly influential entity was fundamental to the work they produced. The difference lay in how the raw materials of the urban environment were processed into art. Early American modernists such as Marin and Walkowitz saw the city as a cacophony of imploding forms and dynamic movements lending itself to a semiabstract treatment. The Henri school was more traditional in that its members saw the city as an inexhaustible source of incidents that, observed realistically, would allow them to express a democratic humanism. Sloan explained it this way: "We found beauty in commonplace things and people. With a rather limited palette and through quick and direct work, we made pictures which have design and form because the intention was graphic and honest."

Henri and his protégés had adopted the Impressionists' approach to motif—that of finding one's subject matter anywhere—but they shied away from their dissolving forms and pure, spectral colors. The Americans turned back to Velázquez, Hals, Goya, Daumier, and especially Manet. They emulated these masters' broad, summary brushwork and dramatic use of blacks. As the epitome of the vanguard artist scorned during his lifetime but ultimately vindicated, Manet gave them license to take an "interest in the wrong side of things." Henri identified with Manet because he "did not do the expected. He was a pioneer. . . . Told the public what he wanted it to know, not the time-worn things the public already knew and thought it wanted to hear again." Considered in relation to what was happening in Europe in 1906—the Fauves and Expressionists had already made their debuts, and Picasso was moving toward Cubism—the American Realists were provincial, and their rebellion was moderate. But given the somnolence of the great majority of American artists, the Henri group's credo of art-for-life's sake provided a brave and much-needed opposition.

Among their American forebears, the Henri circle's hero was Thomas Eakins. Still a commanding and intransigent presence in the stuffy Philadelphia the five men had deserted, he was the deity around whom their moral and artistic convictions had coalesced. Eakins's resolve was to "peer deeper into the heart of American life." In sticking to his native environment and finding beauty in it, he demonstrated the value of recognizing one's heritage and discovering what

was usable in the past. Eakins, of course, was unable to harmonize his painting with popular opinion. He made few sales and received fewer commissions; many of his sitters refused to accept their portraits. In 1886 he lost his teaching job at the Pennsylvania Academy of the Fine Arts—where Henri, Sloan, and Glackens would later study—because during a lecture before a class of men and women, he became so impatient at having to explain the structure of the male pelvis without pointing to it that he removed the model's loincloth. This was taboo in a mixed class, and Eakins was asked to resign. In his uncompromising enforcement of standards, he was again a model to the younger men, who could have easily uttered, as Eakins did, "Respectability in art is appalling." (Eakins's choice of subject matter and intense personal courage were paramount to the Henri group. They had neither the training nor the inclination to pursue his technique.)

To the core group made up of Henri, Glackens, Sloan, Luks, and Shinn, who came to be known collectively as the New York Realists, were added three other artists interested in achieving more lyrical effects with paint. They were the brilliant watercolorist Maurice Prendergast, the landscapist Ernest Lawson, and Arthur B. Davies, the last a romantic symbolist, a behind-the-scenes activist, and a whiz at charming money out of wealthy women for good causes. These painters were to show together only once—in February of 1908, as The Eight, in the historic exhibition that became the opening wedge in the struggle to democratize the process by which American artists put their work before the public. Associated from the beginning with the Henri coterie, the push for independent exhibitions, and the espousal of unidealized contemporaneity were the painters Jerome Myers, Randall Davey, and Walt Kuhn, as well as some of Henri's best-known students, including Edward Hopper, Stuart Davis, George Bellows, Glenn O. Coleman, Guy Pène du Bois, and Rockwell Kent.

Gertrude Whitney gravitated to the men around Henri rather than the group led by Stieglitz. She was not ready for the advanced art Stieglitz defended, the intellectually intimidating atmosphere of his gallery, or his daunting behavior. Inseparable from Stieglitz's prescient vision and his willingness to nurture deserving artists was his sizable ego. That ego was an invaluable asset to the modernist cause, but its preenings did offend people. For many, including Gertrude, Stieglitz's shortcomings would overshadow his knowledge, ardor, and discernment.

Because his gallery was so often condemned and vilified, Stieglitz, fighting for the new against heavy odds, often adopted a siege mentality toward strangers. Whoever was not with him was an enemy. That applied not only to unsuspecting gallery goers off the street, but even to other artists. The young William Zorach, for example, was made to feel quite uncomfortable whenever he dropped in. Sometimes Stieglitz showed endless patience; at other times, he would hector visitors or talk to them in parables. As Van Wyck Brooks put it, Stieglitz had "an element of the mystagogue in him," and his premises were difficult for the uninitiated to penetrate. Stieglitz measured his visitors as strictly as if they were entering a ministry, and in a sense they were. The ambiance was churchlike, with only one true prophet. Although a penetrating comment would be rewarded

by Stieglitz's own passionate response, an obtuse one would be met with silence or an annihilating stare.

In inveighing against a commercialism and philistinism that he abhorred, Stieglitz often careered to the other extreme—a corrosive elitism. To this deterrent might be added two other factors that would have militated against Gertrude's being a part of 291. First of all, Stieglitz was a Jew, as were several of the artists in his gallery. Mixing with Jews as friends or colleagues would have been repugnant to Gertrude at that stage of her life. She was still too socially rigid to accept Jews in any sort of personal relationship. Second, Gertrude had grown up hating the Vanderbilts' stringent drawing of barriers between her and other people. She now wanted to broaden her sphere and slip away from small cliques closed to lesser mortals. The intellectual and aesthetic exclusivity of the Stieglitz group, although sharply different from the money-minded snobberies of the Vanderbilts and their peers, might have struck Gertrude as but a variant of the oppressiveness she was trying to escape.

Finally, the main reason Gertrude was not drawn into the Stieglitz orbit is that the modernist art he advocated was not compatible with her still-unfolding sympathies. She was committed to the cause of realism in American painting. By 1906 she was aware of Eakins, saving a newspaper clipping about him and the reception of his paintings. Gertrude felt that realism was a modern American style, and she was not wrong, either.

Her preference for realism was by no means timid or *retardataire* in the America of 1906 and 1907. Whether as an antidote to the formality and high-flown diction of Victorian poetry or the fastidiousness of academic painting, realism was then equated with modernism in the United States. The allegiance to facing facts, making direct statements, sinking art deeply into the visible world in order to transform it, united not only ground-breaking painters who went outside the studio for inspiration but writers as diverse in outlook and technique as naturalistic novelists and Imagist poets. Crane, Norris, and Dreiser made the squalor, smoke, and surging energy of the metropolis integral to their work; so, too, did Henri, Sloan, and Luks, followed a few years later by William Carlos Williams and Marianne Moore. Just how antithetical these views were to the majority belief at the time of Gertrude's awakening was illustrated by Samuel Isham in his *History of American Painting*, published in 1905.

> The American man finds enough of prose in the day's work . . . when he turns from it he demands that art shall do its duty in furnishing delight and that uncomplicated by too much subtlety. He dislikes problem plays that finish badly and realistic novels that simply give again the life he knows, and he wants his pictures beautiful or at least pretty.

Henri, Sloan, and Glackens were friendly with Hartley and Dove, but they stayed away from Stieglitz, who did not like their work. Henri's good humor and openness, which contrasted with the standoffishness of 291, was no small attraction for Gertrude, who was more entranced by the world that art could bring her than by art itself. The Henri crowd gathered at Shanley's (an all-night

restaurant), the Café Francis, and Mouquin's, the artists' and writers' hangout captured so memorably by Glackens's brush in 1905.* They welcomed editors, reporters, cartoonists, illustrators, actors, and musicians to their table for evenings of genial, bibulous argument. The painters were so at home at the Café Francis that they would exchange pictures for meals. Ernest Lawson estimated that he had "eaten up" seven of his paintings there. James B. Moore, who owned the Francis and appeared there nearly every night with a voluptuous young woman he would introduce as one of his "daughters," had a town house at 450 West 23rd Street that he named The Secret Lair Beyond the Moat. In the Lair's cellar, artists who partook of his hospitality painted antic scenes on the walls. While they were decorating the basement, Edward Arlington Robinson, another beneficiary of Moore's largesse, lived rent-free in the attic.

Perhaps as important to Gertrude as the conviviality of his group was the considerable personal impact of Henri himself. In mid-March of 1906, six weeks before Sloan's etchings perturbed the American Water Color Society, Henri left for a working vacation in Aiken, South Carolina. He had been commissioned to paint a group portrait of the three children of Mrs. George Sheffield. While staying at the Sheffield estate, he met Gertrude, who was at the Whitney farm nearby. He noted it in a diary entry of March 30, 1906. "Today Mrs. Harry Payne Whitney is come to see [the portrait]. . . . I believe she is the one who is interesting herself in sculpture and decoration. . . ." The substance of the encounter was not recorded by either party, but there is no question that the dark and dashing artist made an impression, especially on a woman who spent so much time sizing up men. Henri was forty-one, a tall man with slanting eyes and high cheekbones that gave his face a Eurasian cast. That exoticism was enriched by a gift for mesmerizing talk: He ranged tirelessly over art, music, politics, dance, literature, and baseball, always arguing the place of art in everything we do and the necessity of leading a creative life.

Henri also had the distinction of being the most politically emancipated artist Gertrude had met to date. The artist, Henri liked to say, "disturbs, upsets, enlightens," and he was a prime example of productive agitation. He was newly a member of the National Academy of Design, but he did not close ranks with the rest for his personal advantage. Instead, he jeopardized his place within the organization by lobbying for fairer exhibition procedures that would allow more artists to participate. Guy Pène du Bois said that Henri reminded him of "a rock dashed, ripping and tearing, through bolts of patiently prepared lace."

More than a foil to the artists Gertrude already knew (who were more or less content with the system as it was), Henri was squarely a product and reflection of the progressive era. As the leader of the movement to be free of tightly controlled exhibitions, Henri was the Teddy Roosevelt of American art, the trustbuster who wrested power from the entrenched combines of juries and academies. Shortly after the trip to Aiken, Gertrude began clipping articles about Henri's disagreements with the Academy and pasting them into her scrapbook. She was introduced to Arthur B. Davies, Henri's fellow artist-dissident. As the

*Chez Mouquin, now in the collection of the Art Institute of Chicago.

battle lines for independence were being drawn, Gertrude hoped to be pulled into the fray. Unlike the director of the Metropolitan Museum of Art, who was soon to declare, "There is a state of unrest all over the world in art as in all other things; and I dislike unrest," Gertrude's mind was not bolted against the new. She was looking forward to her share of excitement.

The young woman whom Henri met at Aiken was herself a figure of some assurance, although she had not yet reshaped her circumstances to suit her purposes. Gertrude was beginning to make efforts, but she had carried nothing through to completion. Her blueprint for a Beaux-Arts had been abandoned. Harry wouldn't listen to her proposals, and she was not yet autonomous enough to muster support for such a large undertaking on her own. Nonetheless, she was managing very well, especially in the matter of self-definition. She was buying works of art, and, more tellingly, she had effectively segregated her life into several discrete existences. One portion, given over to being an obedient wife, mother, and socialite, revolved around Fifth Avenue and the estates in the Adirondacks, Old Westbury, Aiken, and Newport. Gertrude spent less time in those places than she had in the first days of her marriage, but when she was there, she did her duty. Her escape hatch in Manhattan was a studio overlooking Bryant Park. There she sculpted, read, wrote, made appointments, and saw the people she wanted to see. Gertrude's activities in the United States were supplemented with travel to Europe, at a frenetic pace she would sustain for decades. She had reached an accommodation with Harry, who allowed her to live abroad three to six months a year as long as she did not attract gossip.

Gertrude's base in Europe was Paris, a city she had loved since childhood and the only spot where she felt she could truly live and breathe. She leased a studio and began befriending other Americans studying art abroad. Membership in her entourage grew or diminished with the seasons and transatlantic crossings, but in the main it consisted of Arthur Lee, Herbert Haseltine, Mahonri Young, Alfred Maurer, John Gregory, Andrew O'Connor, Edgar McAdams, Morgan Russell, Andrew Dasburg, and Jo Davidson. Most of these men received monthly allowances from Gertrude, and she purchased work from Maurer, Gregory, and Davidson. In Paris a rich artist was not automatically regarded with contempt; rather, she was looked on as someone who had had some luck and was sport enough to share the bonanza with everyone else.

The privacy and tolerance of Paris intoxicated Gertrude, and she wanted to duplicate the magic in New York. That was proving to be impossible in the midtown studio, because she could no longer be sure of remaining undisturbed. The location was too convenient to fashionable shops and restaurants, and her society acquaintances had gotten into the habit of dropping in. James Earle Fraser asked Gertrude to move near him in Greenwich Village, and in early 1907, one of Fraser's best friends, the painter Blendon Campbell, located a vacant stable at 19 MacDougal Alley, just north of Washington Square. He suggested that Gertrude rent the stable, which had once served a mansion on the square, and remodel it. (Converting stables into residences and studios as a step in the assumption of the artistic life came into smashing vogue in 1881, after Stanford White renovated one on East 15th Street for the magazine editor

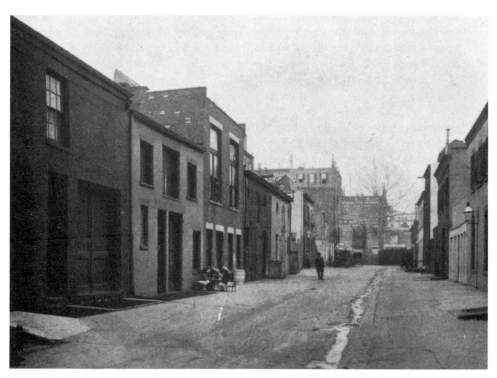

MacDougal Alley as it looked when Gertrude moved in. The children of her neighbor, the artist Edward Deming, are having tea in front of the building that became her studio.

Richard Watson Gilder. The boom accelerated with the advent of the auto and the subsequent ruin of many liveries.) Gertrude leased the property and ordered construction to begin.

Over the spring and summer of 1907, Gertrude moved piecemeal into 19 MacDougal Alley. Once she was settled in, she found herself promptly at home. Around the corner from West Eighth Street, accessible only through MacDougal Street and closed off to the east by Fifth Avenue, MacDougal Alley was soothingly secluded. The Alley is today, as it was in 1907, a quiet and charming street of exquisite, ivy-covered houses where the twentieth century scarcely intrudes. And within the block, No. 19 was the perfect hideaway for Gertrude. She left the work area a large, plain, open space, raising the ceilings and keeping the planked wooden floors of the original stable. She installed modern lighting and an arsenal of equipment. The sculptor Malvina Hoffman, who was an apprentice in another Alley studio at the time, remembered a great "array of modeling tools and glistening saws and chisels that hung over the workbenches, turntables that really turned, stands that did not wobble." The sitting rooms were hung and upholstered in red velvet. The furniture was dark and ornately carved, but the pieces were kept to a minimum and the effect was modest compared to the sweeping modes of studio embellishment—spinning wheels, fishnets spangled with bits of glass,

and other picturesque accessories—favored by successful artists of the day. The rooms were threadbare if compared to the palatial trappings of Gertrude's new uptown residence. She and Harry would soon move from 2 West 57th Street to 871 Fifth Avenue, the fifty-four-room town house formerly owned by William C. Whitney. It was decorated, as one would expect, with French and Flemish tapestries, Renaissance and Baroque furniture, and hundreds of paintings in heavy, gilded frames.

When Gertrude was downtown and wanted some companionship or shoptalk, her neighbors were artists who could supply either. For the most part they were traditional and not very original sculptors filling commissions for portrait busts, monuments, and architectural decorations. Along with the steadfast Fraser in No. 3, there was Gertrude's old acquaintance Daniel Chester French, the most sought-after American sculptor of his time. He owned an entire house: Its stable at No. 7 MacDougal Alley he had transformed into a studio, and the rest of the dwelling, fronting on 12 West Eighth Street, was rented to other artists and their friends. Andrew O'Connor, a sculptor who had assisted Sargent, Saint-Gaudens, and French, worked in the Alley when he was not at his atelier in Paris; he would become Gertrude's mentor. Philip Martiny specialized in ornamental reliefs, and Alexander Phimister Proctor was a gifted *animalier* in the tradition of Barye. Edward Deming painted and sculpted images of American Indians. The street was also home to the portraitist Charles Hawthorne and to Ernest Lawson of The Eight. These artists were all quite chummy with each other, but they were united in their suspicions of Henry Hudson Kitson, a later renter in the Alley. Kitson, in their opinion, was not an artist at all but a clever fraud who scooped up commissions, farmed out the work to his technicians, and put his name on the results.

Gertrude was never entirely accepted by her peers. Her position was not as unfortunate as that of the despised Kitson, for she did not exploit other artists financially, and her enthusiasm and generosity won her friends. But the general feeling among other sculptors was that she was an unqualified amateur who depended on influence and had not paid her dues.

Part of the problem was Gertrude's early decision to exhibit work under an assumed name. This created the impression that the sum of her achievements was what she had attempted as a student of Hendrik Andersen and Fraser. Sloan's first significant diary entry about Gertrude, dated February 20, 1908, refers to her as "Mrs. Harry Payne Whitney, the rich sculptor—at least she has a fine studio for the purpose." Sloan had no way of knowing that she was sincere, and his astringency was justified by a controversy that had erupted in the press three weeks before. On February 1, 1908, the *New York Herald* reported the outcome of a contest sponsored by the Architectural League of New York for the best design for a swimming pool and pavilion. Gertrude collaborated on a design with Hugo Ballin, a mural painter, and Grosvenor Atterbury, a socially prominent architect who was squiring Harry's younger sister, Dorothy Whitney. Gertrude's contribution was a fountain from which sprouted a statue of Pan. Their entry was awarded first prize, but Atterbury was the chairman of the committee appointed to choose the winner. When the other contestants complained that

the chairman was ineligible to enter the competition, Atterbury did not help things much by stating that he compensated for his presence as both judge and entrant by voting on the others' designs but not his own. Besides, he noted, he had entered the contest for the sake of Gertrude and Ballin, who had no architect and needed someone to frame their work in a winning setting.

Most of the newspapers were blandly circumspect about Gertrude's part in the contest, but the scurrilous *Town Topics*, the gossip sheet of the Four Hundred, had no intention of being so respectful. On February 6, 1908, The Guyer spoke of a "Mrs. Aitch Pea Doubleyou," whom he described as advancing "with the simple self-importance of any unmillioned prizewinner and the air of 'I won but did not take the money.' " The Guyer appended several verses chronicling the affair, including this stanza directed at Gertrude:

> But a studio is the proper thing,
> And I'm primed chock full with bids;
> My praises all the journals sing,
> I'm great on caryatids;
> I love the appreciative stare
> Of critic friends and lauders,
> 'Tis facile for a millionaire
> To be assured of orders.

Gertrude did gain in Sloan's estimation by 1910. He, Henri, Kuhn, and Davies were the prime movers that year behind the Exhibition of Independent Artists, the first large-scale invitational show of unallied and liberal artists of its kind, and The Eight's next assault on the Academy. The exposition, in which 103 artists participated free of juries and prizes, was a landmark in American art, and the organizers knew it. All of The Eight except Luks entered pictures. So did Hopper, Davis, Bellows, Coleman, du Bois, Myers, Kuhn, Kent, Morton Schamberg, and Arnold Friedman. Only seven sculptors were in the show, and Gertrude was one of them. She submitted a study of a head and contributed $200 toward the rent of the hall. The backers would not have asked her to be a patron if they were in doubt of her professional integrity.

Yet Gertrude was extremely insecure about her status as a sculptor. When that status was threatened, she had no sense of humor or perspective. Her imperiousness prevailed over her better instincts, as an incident that took place during this period attests. The Independents' exhibition, which ran from April 1 to 27, 1910, was scheduled to coincide with and tease the Academy's spring annual. Meanwhile, Gertrude had a piece accepted by the Academy. The sculpture, called *Paganisme Immortel*, after some lines from Sainte-Beuve, consisted of two figures: a girlish nude sitting on a rock and a man lying beside her hip. The female figure's arms were stretched out toward her feet. At the time, the Academy was located in the American Fine Arts Society Building at 215 West 57th Street, and it was sharing quarters with the Art Students League. (The AFAS Building is still the home of the League, and the galleries originally belonging to the Academy were a gift of George Vanderbilt, Gertrude's uncle.) To raise money for scholarships and let the students exercise some cleverness in the bargain, the League threw a party every year for enrollees, billed as the

annual meeting of The American Fakirs Society. The fund-raising efforts culminated in a séance, an auction, and the bestowing of prizes—in oil, watercolor, and sculpture—for the best student fake or caricature of a work on view in the Academy galleries. *Paganisme Immortel* reeked with self-consciousness, and to one young man the placement of the woman's arms was too silly not to parody. Karl Gruppe, a Fraser pupil at the League, perpetrated a statue of a woman wielding an enormous scissors and cutting her toenails. *Manicure Artistic* took second prize in the contest.

Gertrude was furious at Gruppe's burlesque and demanded its removal from the League's galleries. When this was refused, she offered to buy the piece so she might take it away before the public could see it. That too was denied, and Gruppe's fake was singled out by the *New York Times*. On April 11, 1910, the secondary headline over the story read, "Mrs. H. P. Whitney A Victim"; on April 17, *Manicure Artistic* was reproduced in the paper's Sunday magazine section.

But Gertrude took her revenge. A month after the Fakirs' festivity, she initiated a competition for young sculptors in which $800 was to be distributed for the best public drinking fountains, wall decorations, single figures for gardens, and andirons. Karl Gruppe wanted to enter the contest, but he was barred from doing so on Gertrude's orders.

The community of sculptors had more serious objections to Gertrude than her display of petulance. They alleged, again and again, that other artists—specifically, her neighbor and teacher, Andrew O'Connor—helped her beyond legitimate bounds with the fine points of design, shape, and detail that Gertrude was unable to resolve. Some of these claims can be discounted as sniping or anger over Gertrude's promotion of artists who rebelled against the Academy and hence the sculpture establishment, but their frequency and persistence, voiced by both conservatives and liberals, point toward dissimulations that can't be ignored. For example, both Gruppe, who had cause for rancor, and the muralist Edward Laning, who enjoyed excellent relations with Juliana and the Whitney, stated in interviews that O'Connor did considerable work on Gertrude's public monuments. Juliana once admitted to a nephew an episode in which O'Connor was summoned in great haste late at night to fix a model that had gone wrong and that had to be ready for a committee's inspection the next day.

The question of assistance versus actual creative labor in gigantic sculpture destined for marble or bronze is a perilously murky one to analyze, especially when separated from its practices and ethics by eight decades. The sculptor thought of the original conception and made small clay and plaster models of it. Letting technicians prepare the armature, rough out surfaces, enlarge proportions with a pointing machine, cast the model into bronze, and do some preliminary carving was normal and acceptable. (Gertrude was solely a modeler, so it is very likely that she did no carving at all.) And the two areas of responsibility were apt to overlap.

O'Connor and some other technicians apparently did repair awkward passages and correct mistaken proportions. One instance was obliquely given credence by Daniel Chester French, who was in a position to appraise the styles and

capacities of O'Connor and Gertrude better than anyone else. Ever discreet, French would not commit such an accusation directly to paper, but he hinted at what he thought was the truth and hoped that his former apprentice would confide in him. "I was very interested the other day in Mrs. Whitney's fountain of three male figures [her Arlington Fountain of 1913, executed in Paris] which has been exhibited at Knoedler's," he wrote to O'Connor in France. "The figures are certainly very handsome. I have heard it rumored that you helped her with it, which accounts for a good deal." O'Connor did not reply to this letter, but in his subsequent correspondence with French he neither affirmed nor denied his collaborative role.

Another indicative letter was written by the sculptor John Gregory in 1919. He was supervising the enlarging and pointing up of a few pieces of Gertrude's sculpture, and both he and the artisans were permitted to improve them. Gregory was more experienced than Gertrude at enlarging statuary; presumably he would be more sharp-eyed than she in spotting weaknesses. That Gregory was more of a collaborator than an assistant is apparent in his report to her.

> I went to Horton's today and found that the group is going well.
>
> He has greatly improved the blind head [referring to the figure of a soldier blinded in World War I] following your suggestions and the other head has come out splendidly.
>
> I told him not to touch it until you saw it.
>
> On the blind figure the right arm is finished smooth and the front pointed except the right foot and left leg. The left arm is not yet finished and I told him to leave it as I think you will want to push back at the elbow to make it longer, it is a good deal shorter than the other.
>
> On the stooping figure . . . there is some uncertainty about the arrangement of the clasped hands. The gun also is a problem and is awaiting your return.

Karl Gruppe, who was long an active member of the National Sculpture Society, said that Gertrude never attained full membership in the organization and remained at the associate level because the majority were convinced that O'Connor was doing the work that counted. In arguments, they cited the case of Gertrude's equestrian statue, *Buffalo Bill* (1922–1924). O'Connor, they contended, was in charge of the large plaster model that was entered in the Paris Salon of 1924 and that won Gertrude a medal of honor. Gruppe believed that her election as an associate member of the National Academy of Design was delayed until 1940 for similar reasons, but by then her efforts had figured so decisively in draining away the power of the Academy that straightforward resentment would have guaranteed Gertrude a blackball.

By taking a studio on MacDougal Alley, Gertrude was thrown in with people of whom she had only been vaguely aware. Her territory now extended to the precincts of Greenwich Village, an older neighborhood into which artists had drifted. In 1907 the Village was not yet the community of free spirits that backward-glancing writers would celebrate with nostalgia and wistfulness. It had,

nevertheless, over the past decade bloomed as a corner of New York seemingly given over to authors, artists, reformers, educators, and real and parlor radicals. The area had an air of informality and individuality that set it apart from the middle-class culture above 14th Street. The Village stood for ambitions other than organizing one's life around great amounts of money. For this reason alone, society considered it a bit queer for Gertrude to be there.

She, of course, preferred it that way. Establishing herself downtown was a key passage in her general declaration of independence. The Village had a peaceful, isolated quality. Seventh Avenue stopped at Eleventh Street then and traffic could not barrel through the main thoroughfares. The lesser streets, which had names, not numbers, were homey and cloistral. Laid out on diagonals to the north-south axis of Washington Square, the downtown streets crossed and recrossed each other or zigzagged into cul-de-sacs, unlike the proper gridiron governing the rest of Manhattan, and Villagers adopted the analogy as an apt one for their own conduct. There was a strong belief that a change in address would bring about a change in identity.

Living in Greenwich Village signaled a like of exoticism and a craving for experience. The Italian immigrant populace, the dominant ethnic group in the West Village, implanted Mediterranean customs on Manhattan soil. They opened up cafés, spaghetti restaurants, and coffeehouses, and when the weather was mild, they lived in the open air. Their casualness helped give the Village its sense of a small town within the great city. Added to that, rents were cheap. A few dollars a month bought a room with high ceilings and a fireplace in a redbrick Greek Revival town house or an Italianate mansion wreathed in curlicued wrought iron. A little more money secured an entire floor of a brownstone. People could and did survive marginally, pursuing their whims or convictions while holding a part-time job on the side. The labor movement, feminism, socialism, modern art, free love, birth control, progressive education, and psychoanalysis were topics on everyone's lips.

Gertrude's most licentiously bohemian acquaintance did not live in a garret in the Village, but in a big house on East 19th Street. He was a painter and libertine named Robert Winthrop Chanler, whom Gertrude met in 1905 and took to immediately. Chanler painted exotic jungle fantasies of parrots, monkeys, trees, and flowers, in lacquered black, gold, red, and iridescent green—a sort of Douanier Rousseau in chinoiserie. A descendant of Winthrops and Stuyvesants and an heir to part of the Astor fortune, Chanler led a riotous life. As errant as Gertrude in not fitting in—he was a millionaire who befriended Emma Goldman—his stratagem for overturning a stuffy life was to revel in dissipation. "Peace," said his friend Guy Pène du Bois, "wasn't one of the qualities Chanler sought."

When Gertrude first set eyes on Bob Chanler, he was only thirty-three, but he looked a good deal older. He was a huge and noisy imp, and the painter Louis Bouché remembered him as standing "about six feet four or five.* He was heavy with a fairly protruding belly which he fondly called his 'Josephine.'

---

* Histories of the Chanler family give his height as 6 feet 3 inches.

His enormous head fitted his frame and was capped by a crown of bushy curls, not unlike Alexandre Dumas. His features were large as well, his neck enormous, his voice booming." Du Bois saw Chanler as "a Gargantua arrived too late, a Gulliver forced to step with more care than he could easily muster in a tidy Lilliputian world. . . . Like his person, his energy was colossal."

To Gertrude, the ribald, profane Chanler represented an uproar of life. He overflowed with the sensuality she had learned to suppress. Gertrude wrote in her diary that Chanler "says live—live—get all you can out of life and he wishes the best of all things. 'I would like to see you go to the Devil' were his words and instead of being shocked or reproving him I merely smile & I suppose my puritan ancestors would turn in their graves were they to hear our conversations."

Chanler was doing his best to go to the devil and having a wonderful time in the process. He was just surfacing from a secret divorce and a tipsily fought campaign for the post of sheriff of Dutchess County, New York, home of the Chanler country seat. He spent $20,000 on being elected. That insured him the office temporarily and the nickname Sheriff Bob forever. Sheriff Bob now gamboled around Manhattan in a chamois shirt and leather chaps. On more subdued days he encased himself in a white smock or overalls, topped by a flowing black silk tie. The effect was reminiscent of a beached white whale.

Gertrude and Chanler were particularly close in 1907, as they were working almost in tandem. They were each awarded a commission—his for a mural and hers for a fountain—for the very chic Colony Club, which was about to open a new building at 30th Street and Madison Avenue. The Colony Club was one of the first private women's clubs in America, and Gertrude was a charter member. It was founded to provide women of leisure as well as eminent professional women a place to go that would rival the various male sanctuaries in town. Besides offering comfort, convenience, and luxurious facilities, the Colony Club was making a statement about a woman's place in the world—she had the right to the same gratifications as a man. Within the club's rooms women could smoke cigarettes and order wine and cocktails—these were clandestine or impermissible pleasures elsewhere. Many of the members were staunch suffragists, and leaders of the women's rights movement lectured there to receptive audiences.

An event of some moment to New York society, the opening of the Colony Club building took place on March 12, 1907. Gertrude, who was serving on the club's art committee, was asked to select and install an exhibition of arts and crafts to augment the inaugural parties. The show was scheduled to open on April 9, and her choices of art reflected an intersection of the disparate worlds she inhabited. Society was appeased with a selection of laces from the cabinets of club members, as well as portraits from such well-known brushes as Whistler and Sargent. Several conservative younger painters (Paul Dougherty, Jonas Lie, and Barry Faulkner) were invited, and MacDougal Alley was represented by Fraser, Campbell, and Deming. Gertrude's interest in the Henri contingent was advertised by her inclusion of Davies, Lawson, and Jerome Myers. She also solicited works by the underappreciated John Twachtman and the extremely popular Maxfield Parrish.

In demonstrating her approval of the partisans Davies, Myers, and Lawson, Gertrude made a gesture toward insurgency at a crucial moment. Art circles had just been shown indisputable proof that the Academy's dictatorial policies had worsened and that self-interest was the ruling principle. (The National Academy of Design, Sloan once quipped, was "no more a National agency than the National Biscuit Company.") During the first week of March 1907, in preparation for the spring annual, the Academy's jury convened. Henri, who was one of the judges, tried to get pictures by Glackens, Luks, Shinn, Sloan, Rockwell Kent, and Carl Sprinchorn into the exhibition. Every canvas but one—*The Picnic Grounds,** by Sloan—was rejected, first by the jurors or subsequently by the hanging committee. In protest, Henri withdrew two of his three entries.

The outcome was too controversial to be kept within studios and galleries, and journalists rushed to cover it. Meanwhile, Sloan and Glackens met to discuss what would turn out to be the genesis of The Eight show. Sloan recorded in his diary on March 11, 1907, that they talked over "the advisability of a split exhibition from the National Academy of Design because they seem to be more and more impossible." The space they wanted was in the Macbeth Gallery at 450 Fifth Avenue, which had already taken paintings by Davies, Luks, Henri, Lawson, and Prendergast. Apart from 291, it was the only gallery in New York that consented to show living American artists of a nonacademic persuasion.

Gertrude's ties to the rebels were recognized on the spot. On April 10, 1907, the day after the Colony Club show opened, Davies moved quickly to reinforce her allegiance with a congratulatory letter: "Mr. Fraser has spoken to me of your desire to insist on a vital movement in those American artistic qualities as yet not sufficiently perceived elsewhere. There is so much to commend the variety of interest and attraction about your present Art Exhibition." Davies then hammered home his main theme: "Believe me I hope you may be a turning point in this movement, a means of attainment for an art of style and true beauty." As Davies wrote those flowery words, he, Lawson, Myers, and thirty-three other nominees were being blackballed from Academy membership.

Once the results of the mass veto became known, the call to strip the Academy of its power gained momentum. Henri swung into action with a long, ardent interview in the *Times,* declaring that the Academy "shows that it is going to stick to its old rut." In the same article, Sloan called the Academy's stance "honest stupidity." Gertrude clipped subsequent stories on the schism. From the *Evening Sun* of April 11, 1907, she saved "Academy Bars Noted Artists," in which Henri was quoted as saying, "The action of last night shows that the academy is hopelessly against what is real and vital in American art. What the outsiders must do now is to hold small or large group exhibitions so that the public may see what the artists who have something important to say are doing." Henri selected the "outsiders" for such a group show and went to the press with their names: Davies, Glackens, Lawson, Luks, Prendergast, Shinn, Sloan, and himself. The group, sharing no artistic creed but a kindred belief in indepen-

* Now in the collection of the Whitney Museum.

dence, was named The Eight by the critic James Huneker. The title harkened back to The Ten, a group of American Impressionists who had been denied exhibitions in the 1890s and then formed their own group in response. (Hostile critics branded Henri's new coalition "the revolutionary black gang" and "the apostles of ugliness.") Gertrude kept a follow-up story on the backlash against the rebels that ran in the May 4, 1907 *Evening Post*. The headline read, "Academy Artists Oppose the Eight." That same month, Gertrude bought a Lawson painting from James Moore of the Café Francis, who was in a financial scrape. Secession was an activity that aroused Gertrude's sympathies.

Watching and listening to Gertrude throughout all this, slipping in and out of the Colony Club and MacDougal Alley, was a new addition to her employ. The administrative chores engendered by the club's exhibition were too burdensome for Gertrude to handle by herself, especially because she also had to cope with the ongoing renovations of her new studio at No. 19. But she knew just the person to assist her. To supervise the assembling and running of the Colony Club show when she could not be present, Gertrude borrowed her sister-in-law's secretary. The woman she tapped was Juliana Rieser.

In 1906, after leaving her job at the business school in Hoboken, Juliana had set herself up as a free-lance typist and stenographer in Manhattan. Occasionally she worked for a secretarial agency that served society women, and she filled in for Whitney and Harriman secretaries when they were on vacation or indisposed. Presumably this is how she came to be hired as a social secretary by Helen Hay Whitney, the wife of Harry's brother, Payne, and the author of two books. Besides fulfilling the clerical duties of the position, Juliana may have helped Helen with compiling a volume of poems. *Gypsy Verses*, Helen Hay Whitney's third book, appeared in 1907. Helen was an officer of the Colony Club, and aiding Gertrude with a club-sponsored project would have been a natural transition for Juliana to make. By the time she went to work for Gertrude, she knew the *Social Register* from cover to cover and was acutely attuned to the etiquette and habits of the moneyed elite. Gertrude was so taken with Juliana that after the exhibition closed, one painter recalled, she wouldn't let her go.

Juliana rented an office at 185 Madison Avenue (at 34th Street, four blocks north of the Colony Club) in 1907. Even at that early point in her association with Gertrude, she was no mere runner of errands. Had she been, she would have bored her new boss. Juliana was erudite and deferential, but not obsequious. She could make suggestions, hold her own in conversation, and take initiative. And though she knew next to nothing about art and artists, she was eager to learn and soaked up information like a sponge. Furthermore, she understood many things intuitively. From the beginning the artists around Gertrude recognized Juliana as "an amazing creature" and "so jolly and nice." She was able to fit in at once because she had the wit to perceive that success lay in being striking rather than sedate.

Vividness attracted Gertrude, who was always on the lookout for "big personalities." Possessed of an operatic temperament, Juliana could dare opinions

that Gertrude might have had but could not bring herself to express. Gertrude's calm—the product of someone who had been trained not to show passion—was stretched tautly over the surface of her life. Juliana was the opposite—blazing with emotion, she would attack the world head on. Correspondingly, she was adept at turning any little happening into a drama with a splendid ending, even a thank-you note acknowledging the receipt of some flowers. In contrast to the icy, undemonstrative Vanderbilts, Juliana was emotionally affluent.

185 Madison Avenue

Dear Mrs. Whitney,

Of course, you didn't know, you couldn't, but the grimness of life and all *is* getting on my nerves and you have done a most beautiful thing. I hardly knew until the roses came that I was so hungry! And the "thickest cloud earth ever stretched" has lost its terror for a whole day long. If there be joy in the world, the echo of the happy thank you my heart sings must bring you some of it.

Very gratefully yours
Juliana Rieser

She was also the embodiment of a type fantasized about, half-envied, and heretofore observed from afar by Gertrude—the self-made, self-possessed professional woman who had marched beyond the boundaries of servant or governess to stake out a satisfying new role for herself. Gertrude, who lived in several worlds for propriety's sake and was constantly resorting to subterfuges, was fascinated by the bold New Woman who openly defied convention and asserted her own power directly. This was a woman who had not had things handed to her, a woman who had learned how to compete. Gertrude longed to merge into that life, or at least a fantasy version of it. In an autobiographical story of 1911, she wrote of "[t]he little restaurants on Sixth Avenue" and the thrill of "mingling [there] with the working girls and being taken for one," which made her "feel the immensity of life as no extensive trip abroad or book of wisdom could." And among Gertrude's unpublished nonfiction writings is an incomplete essay begun in the 1920s. Recalling her past and her quest to fulfill herself, she compared her own predicament and the conditions against which she had struggled with the position of a young woman such as Juliana Rieser in 1907.

The general economic situation of the girl who must work takes care of itself. She comes into competition with all the other girls similarly situated. She sticks to the job of first learning the job, next being better than the next fellow & finally keeping her job because of necessity. The girl . . . who for financial reasons does not have to work has . . . no conception of what arriving at a competitive satisfaction means . . . with no necessity facing her [she] stumbles at the first ditch & having no jockey to push her [over] . . . the next fence, flounders and never faces it.

Gertrude continued with the steeplechase metaphor, the analogy's connection with land and wealth unconsciously emphasizing the chasm separating the two experiences she juxtaposed. She further lamented the fate of young women like her former self, those who "never have to face the second jump, who would

not even have to face the first, only that they have a desire to jump." Failure, she concluded, was unavoidable, especially when these sheltered souls had to challenge "girls who have faced supporting themselves." When Juliana entered Gertrude's life, she had been out in the world and providing for herself for at least six years. That was a track record Gertrude would have respected.

Gertrude's worldliness was of a different sort. To a degree beyond the usual restraints binding an employee, her associates had to maintain absolute discretion because Gertrude had advanced beyond flirtations into a steady succession of love affairs, consummated in the Paris and MacDougal Alley studios. She proceeded in the blithe and largely correct assumption that, since she was rich, she could do exactly as she wished. If something went wrong, she could simply pretend it hadn't happened. Gertrude's lovers typically fell into two distinct categories: artists and models she met through her work or men about town she had known from adolescence. What each set of men had in common was the ease with which they lent themselves to being manipulated. "Take what you can," Gertrude wrote in her journal, "you need not think men cannot take care of themselves." Her calculatedness extended to her love letters: She made many drafts of each one, revised them to her satisfaction, and kept copies for herself for later review.

Gertrude used her money, sophistication, and sexuality as provocative weapons. In the case of the artists, such as John Gregory and Andrew O'Connor (and perhaps Morgan Russell), she would buy their work or ask for criticism of her own. She might then offer a monthly allowance for travel or living expenses. A friendship would develop, and then intimacy. At this juncture in the affair, the man would attempt to deal with Gertrude as an equal or reestablish what he viewed as a position of rightful male dominance.

When a Wall Street man or Newport regular became intimate with Gertrude, the financial lever became irrelevant. She dazzled these men by the novelty of her vocation and the whiff of dangerous glamour she exuded. Compared to most other society women, Gertrude was an exotic creature shining within their own midst. As the Gypsy from the *Social Register*, Gertrude and her allure were thrilling yet impeccable. But whether her partner was an artist or a stockbroker, Gertrude entered into what became a predictable pattern of coquetting, testing, teasing, discarding, and freezing out the current amour.

Gertrude's detachment during her romances was another consequence of her segmented life because she would not divorce Harry. Most of the time she commuted with great composure among the various parts of her psyche, but not always. Keeping up appearances and functioning creditably across a variety of pastimes made for intense strain. She was subject to mood swings and hypersensitivity. In her travels, her attitude toward her lovers, and her reactions to people in general, Gertrude was like a nervous racehorse bolting out of the gate.

Perhaps the key to Juliana's immediate triumph and ultimate staying power with Gertrude was the irregularity of her own private life. Her conduct was so atypical for someone of her background and milieu as to be classified as un-

thinkable. Juliana had done something analogous to Gertrude in severing herself from her own family and the values of Hoboken. Even in 1907 there was reason for Juliana to dissemble; in 1904, her interest in her future husband, Willard Burdette Force, was shocking by the mores of the time.

Juliana was twenty-seven when she met "Doctor," as she and the rest of the Riesers always called him. She was on the threshold of unalterable spinsterhood by conventional wisdom. No one knows why she had not married, but a good guess would be that she was far too independent to subdue her intellect or opinions during courtship. Lack of beauty or style does not seem to have hampered her, for Juliana's appearance was much improved since the Northfield days. Her hair, a mass of long, thick, wavy red-gold tresses, hung halfway down her back, and it was an arresting complement to her creamy complexion. When she smiled—a quick, broad flash—her lips parted slightly to reveal two rows of tiny, babylike teeth, slightly separated. Juliana's figure was slim and well-formed, and her curves were attractively set off by clothes handmade by her sisters. Her nose, which was her poorest feature, protruded well past the promontory of her face. It overshadowed her eyes and mouth and sometimes lent her face a harsh expression. But that was redeemed by her vivacity, enjoyment of life, and "a personal magnetism that struck one instantly on meeting her, like a physical sensation." Juliana's charm lay in an instinctive understanding of the person at hand, and a gleeful delight in the human comedy.

Doctor was 5 feet 10 inches tall (to Juliana's petite 5 feet 1 inch), square-jawed and broad-shouldered. A stylish dresser who was partial to the boaters, tailored suits, and bow ties favored by dandies of the day, he had blue eyes and parted his brown hair in the middle. He wore gold-rimmed glasses and resembled the young Franklin Roosevelt. Normally, he would have been considered quite a catch. The problem was that Doctor was a married man and the father of a baby girl.

Willard Force was born on November 13, 1870, in Whitehouse, New Jersey, one of four children of David and Sarah L. Force. He spent his adolescence in Plainfield, New Jersey, where his father worked as a carpenter. Of Huguenot extraction, the Forces were a long-established family in the central part of the state, their ancestors having settled there in the late seventeenth century. Among the descendants of those first progenitors were Peter Force, who became an important collector of books and a mayor of Washington, D.C., and Mary Heaton Vorse, the author.

In Plainfield, David Force and his family attended the First Methodist Church. Their minister, the Reverend Charles Barnes, made his house a gathering place for young people. The Barneses had three daughters, and one of them, named Mary Grace and called Grace for short, caught Doctor's eye. He began paying attention to her while he was in high school; she was three years older and at home. In 1897 the Barneses moved to Jersey City. Doctor, meanwhile, was accepted as a student at New York College of Dentistry, the predecessor of New York University's College of Dentistry. He matriculated in the 1897–1898 school year and boarded with the Barneses at their new residence, which was just across the river from Manhattan. Doctor and Grace naturally saw each other nearly

every day, and it was not long before they became engaged. The Reverend Mr. Barnes married them on January 2, 1900. The newlyweds continued to live in Jersey City, sometimes by themselves and sometimes with Grace's parents, until their daughter was born on February 5, 1904. After Grace recovered from childbirth, the Forces moved to Hoboken, taking an expensive flat in the best part of town. Doctor kept up a dual practice, working by day in New York and at night treating patients in the neighborhood.

The Forces' marriage was deteriorating by the time they moved to Hoboken. The two were no longer in agreement about what they wanted, and Juliana's introduction into Doctor's life that year happened to tip the balance. Grace preferred a simple, home-centered existence, whereas Doctor was interested in living well and being seen in the right places. During the summers, he transplanted his practice to Stockbridge, Massachusetts, where he could enjoy the cooler weather and minister to the wealthy summer people. Grace didn't care about fashionable seasons and stopped accompanying her husband to Stockbridge.

Juliana, however, was not content with living in Hoboken, and she would have applauded Doctor's desire to win a life beyond its purlieus. The two of them wanted to make something of themselves and on terms that Hoboken could not match. Indeed, Juliana's distaste for acknowledging her New Jersey antecedents meshed with Doctor's own snobbery. The Force clan held enormous family reunions every year, but according to Lois Force, Doctor's grandniece, Willard Force never attended any of them, even in the 1920s, when the shock of his divorce had receded. She suspected that he kept his distance because he felt he had climbed above his relatives socially. By the 1920s, he owned a big house, had been to Paris, and knew many members of the smart set in the arts—accomplishments undreamed of by the rest of the family. Her observations are corroborated in some letters preserved by a professional genealogist hired to compile a history of the Forces in America. The genealogist repeatedly wrote to Doctor requesting information. Doctor would not only not answer his queries, but balked at admitting his kinship to the other Forces.

Juliana appreciated Doctor's panache, his presentation of himself as what was once popularly called a man's man. He liked good cigars, detective stories, poker games, big dogs, and the outdoors. He was never without an automobile and drove a big, black, shiny Packard. Just as Doctor's style appealed to Juliana, so did his attitude toward money. Both felt that money was to be spent—freely, bountifully, without hesitation or regret—and neither of them had any head for managing it. Juliana despised closefistedness and even necessary thrift. Any kind of putting by carried with it the negative association of Julia Rieser's harping on the privations she and the family suffered from Max's failure as a wage earner. Divesting herself of money, often cavalierly, was Juliana's aristocratic retort to those bleak memories. In dealing with the world, Doctor was genial and trusting, often too much so for his own good. He would listen to anyone with a "business proposition," and his financial gullibility was bottomless. He was a plunger and a soft touch, forever sinking money into worthless properties and dubious inventions. Doctor was conned, for instance, into buying a eucalyptus plantation

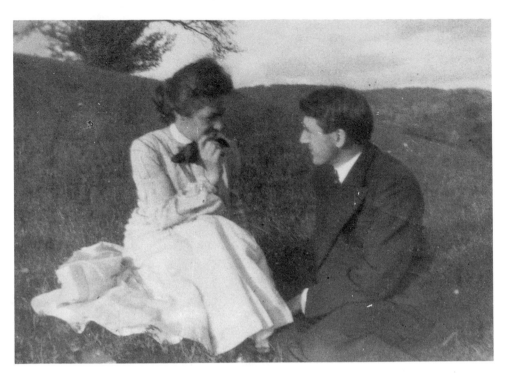

Juliana with Willard Force during the early days of their courtship.

in California; the land he purchased didn't have a tree on it. Carl Rieser remembered growing up with huge stockpiles of Vanessa Toothpowder, a product
Doctor marketed in expectation of making a killing. He also recalled his uncle
investing in a faulty prototype for experimental tires.

How well the lovers hid their romance is impossible to gauge, but Hoboken
was a small town. The Force and Rieser residences and the school where Juliana
worked were all within fifteen short blocks of each other. Encounters would
have been noticed and remarked upon. Doctor made his first attempt to separate
from Grace in late 1904, so she knew that something was amiss by then, if not
before. The Riesers were aware of the affair, and it rocked the household.
Respectable women, and certainly not unmarried ones, did not persist in such
scandalous connections. An illicit attachment could jeopardize the career of a
professional like a dentist in middle-class environs; it would ruin the future of
a female schoolteacher.

One can imagine the reaction at the First Presbyterian Church to such "social
deviance," as adultery was called then. The girl who had been packed off by
anxious relatives to be molded by Dwight Moody and returned without an ounce
of newfound piety remained insubordinate. Juliana was supposed to tread the
path of altruism and Christian morality and renounce Doctor, but she did not.
In Mary and Clara, Juliana had seen enough of self-sacrifice and its consequences, and she would not allow herself to be boxed into a similar prison.
Julia's was the precedent that she followed, but with a difference. The mother

put her needs first within the family; the daughter extended her wants beyond it.

On the morning of October 10, 1906, Doctor dressed himself for the office, wished Grace good-bye, and said he would be back that afternoon. Instead, he sent a letter confessing that he was leaving her and establishing a domicile in Manhattan. Thus he furnished her with evidence for divorcing him on the grounds of "willful, continued and obstinate" desertion across state lines. Doctor gave Grace most of the furnishings and promised her an allowance for child support, but not before advising her to move to a cheaper flat and dismiss the maid.

Juliana was already working in New York when Doctor decamped. A base there offered her anonymity. If she were seen in Hoboken less, tongues might wag less, and she could meet Doctor more conveniently. His New York address, on West 38th Street between Fifth and Sixth Avenues, was just six blocks away from her own office at 185 Madison Avenue. Juliana continued to live in her parents' house in Hoboken, and she would do so until her wedding day. This meant that five or six days a week she journeyed to Manhattan via the ferry from the Hoboken pier to the terminal at West 23rd Street. Every morning she crossed the Hudson, seeing the tugboats bobbing on the waves and the jagged skyline of the Battery coming into focus. The downtown towers, those shrines to commerce glittering white and gold in the eastern sky, symbolized hope and promise to Juliana, in bitter contrast to the indignities to be endured during the ride. She would have been subjected to comment by knowledgeable passengers—she was, in their eyes, the home wrecker who had come between husband, wife, and baby. With what relief must she have stepped off the boat each day and turned toward the unsanctimonious precincts of Greenwich Village and the Colony Club! There Juliana could melt into a world in which traditional moral and social values were challenged or flouted. To partake of the camaraderie of artists, to hear about the courage of a Henri or the audacity of a Chanler, to see women who smoked, drank, and relished their pleasures—such occurrences must have been as fortifying to Juliana as they were inspiriting to her employer.

Living at home with her parents was not pleasant for Juliana. The fights between mother and daughter were devastating, yet Juliana maintained her authority within the family. Whatever disgrace the Riesers felt Juliana brought on them by her affair with a married man, she was not ejected from the house. On the contrary, she was free to move back and forth between Hoboken and New York City. Attempts to stop her, if any, she defied or ignored. As Marjorie Rieser, who remembered the family's horrified reaction to Juliana's "running around" with Doctor, put it, "Whatever most girls did had nothing to do with Aunt Jule. She was a law unto herself."

Having been subject to much gossip herself, Juliana was discretion personified with respect to Gertrude. The silence she preserved ranged from small matters to the greater secrets of Gertrude's love life and the degree to which hers was the sole hand behind the design and execution of her public monuments. Of the more than 120 artists, dealers, curators, relatives, and friends of Juliana Force interviewed for this book, not one could recollect a single instance of her

discussing Gertrude Whitney with them. Carl and Allan Rieser, who were closer to their aunt than anyone else, cannot remember Juliana making more than four or five remarks about the woman she served for thirty-five years.

By a rewarding coincidence, the Colony Club's art exhibitions that Juliana assisted with were scheduled at dates when American art history was being made. Gertrude's first show lent support to Henri as he and his stalwarts defied the Academy and banded together as The Eight; the second one she was asked to organize opened in early February of 1908, just days after the debut of The Eight themselves on the third of that month at the Macbeth Galleries. Juliana had a chance to witness events that would put Gertrude on the map as a daring collector and propel them both to the center stage of American art.

Much of what transpired in art circles did so in the face of public indifference, but the reaction to The Eight's showing was vociferous. The instigators, who wanted to broaden exhibition opportunities for all artists as well as deflate the Academy, were out to create a sensation. Sloan, the secretary-treasurer, was indefatigable in compiling the mailing list and getting a catalog printed. As half of the exhibitors had once worked for the press, they knew how to attract publicity and had well-placed friends in the newspaper world. Charles FitzGerald of the *Evening Sun*, for example, was Glackens's brother-in-law and a champion of The Eight. Guy Pène du Bois, who wrote for the *New York American*, was a painter and a Henri disciple. James Huneker and James Gregg, who worked for the *New York Sun* and the *Evening Sun*, respectively, were regulars at Mouquin's. The show ran for two weeks, and an article appeared in print nearly every day of it.

The critics were divided fairly evenly between praise and brickbats. The *Town Topics*, however, reveled in the chance to do its worst. In the same issue that ran the doggerel maligning Gertrude as a sculptor, The Gilder, the paper's purported art critic, vesuviated with invective. The Eight were purveyors of "unadulterated artistic slop," their combined output "create[d] a distinct feeling of nausea." But the cumulative effect of the show, explained William Innes Homer in 1969, was to validate The Eight "as significant artists who honestly spoke the language of their own time and place. . . . The exhibition at Macbeth's was a rallying point for those, particularly the young, who wished to see a realistic treatment of contemporary themes win out as the modern idiom; and the show's success gave courage, again to the young, to carry on the fight against the Academy by organizing larger and more radical exhibitions of contemporary American art."

The public flocked to see the show. Over 300 spectators per hour filed into Macbeth's two rooms to see the sixty-three works on view. By the end of the first week, more than 3,000 people had seen the paintings. Sloan did not attend the preview or the public opening. He thought his old clothes would be poor advertising. Because of his absence, he missed meeting Gertrude, who walked into the gallery on February 2, 1908, and reached for her checkbook. Of the seven pictures sold from the show, she bought four of them for $2,225. Gertrude

chose Henri's *Laughing Child*, an animated portrait of a blond Dutch girl; *Revue*, by Shinn, a vignette of a musical comedy star, bathed in blue-black light, bowing to her audience; *Winter on the River*, a scene of the open country above West 125th Street, by Lawson; and Luks's *Woman with Goose*, an unidealized study of a battered-looking old woman.* A month after these purchases, Gertrude bought five more works by Shinn—four red-chalk drawings and a monotype.

Within the context of Gertrude's own growth and self-realization, the new acquisitions represented not only a major gesture of support, but a far-reaching assertion. As Sloan said many years later, "At that time, to buy such unfashionable pictures was almost as revolutionary as painting them." Before these four paintings, the works of art Gertrude bought were either slight or acquired almost as a souvenir of a visit with a personality who had impressed her. The paintings and sculpture she had gotten from John La Farge, Daniel Chester French, Howard Cushing, Hendrik Andersen, and James Earle Fraser fit one or both of these categories.

Gertrude did know Henri and Lawson, but perhaps not Shinn and Luks except by reputation. She bought their paintings because she liked what she saw and for political reasons: She wanted to defend art that was not yet accredited, and she wanted to boost art that was concerned with the condition of being American. Buying those canvases—especially the one by Luks, which was small and dark and uningratiating—was, consciously or unconsciously, a statement of class rebellion. Gertrude understood that these were the paintings of democrats, and collecting them was an act of engagement. The more stylish art preferred by most of Gertrude's peers celebrated the world of appearances— which counted for everything—and recognized no world outside its own fantasies of sweetness and prosperity. The Eight, however, attempted to embrace a totality of life, and much of their work was flavored with social commentary. Henri and Sloan were politically radical, and the group as a whole stood for youth, forthrightness, pungency, and experiment. Resistance buoyed these artists along, because generosity, not alienation, prompted them to defy the system. Their advocacy of spontaneity and art for life's sake and the struggle they waged against the Academy's despotism were equivalent to Gertrude's own determination to break out of a repressive environment and find a meaningful identity.

The purchases from Macbeth's marked Gertrude's first foray into buying art that would be unappetizing to her friends and relations. That Henri, Lawson, Luks, and Shinn's paintings were meant for MacDougal Alley, not Fifth Avenue, was a foregone conclusion. Contrary to the custom of American millionaires, Gertrude chose against or indifferently to fashion and investment. She did it without advice, and she risked making a mistake. She was not the sort of buyer who, in Henri's words, "sits like a pack rat on a pile of collected art of the past," but someone who elected to be in on the beginnings of things. Forbes Watson, in surveying the pattern of Whitney collecting, wrote in 1949 that Gertrude's initial

---

*All are now in the collection of the Whitney Museum.

collection was an incident of her generosity. It was not made with a museum in view. She could easily have had one of the outstanding collections of the world with all the correct names from Cézanne to Picasso. She could also have had her Goyas and El Grecos. She could have been a collector most utterly correct. She could have made the dealers of New York and Paris dance with joy and sing her praises to the heavens. Instead she bought hundreds of works by young artists who at that time didn't have dealers, artists unknown to the type of correct collector which she herself might have been had she less human interest in the artist.

Laughing Child, Revue, Winter on the River, and *Woman with Goose* and their makers assumed a significance beyond their place in Gertrude's personal advancement. They became anchors and reference points for much of the art Gertrude and Juliana later chose to sponsor. The Whitney Studio Club and the museum that came after it were nothing if not catholic in intent—they embraced multitudes and contradictions with gusto. Yet certain tendencies, loyalties, and ways of doing things went back to the bedrock of The Eight and those epochal acquisitions of 1908. Lively humanism, especially as it manifested itself in depictions of the American scene, was a staple. The orientation was progressive and liberal, but not avant-garde. Works of art were bought quietly and unostentatiously, without fussing about publicity or waiting for a critic's sanction. Henri and his friends emerged as trusted advisers to the two women; paintings by these artists and their students were consistently invited to be in Whitney shows.

No records survive to recount Juliana and Gertrude's association between 1908 and 1910. The first extant letters date from 1911, when Gertrude once again turned to writing. Under the pen name Phyllis Lane, she completed a novella called "White Voices," and Juliana was to be her reader and literary agent for the manuscript.

The assignment was ideal for her. She was an avid reader who kept up with books and magazines, and her own experience as an aspiring author had familiarized her with editors and reviewers and helped her to meet people in the publishing world. And as the recipient of many rejection slips, she was sensitive to the fragility of an author's hopes and the importance of cushioning disappointments with sympathy and care. An index of the confidence Gertrude had in Juliana was the amount of money she paid her—Juliana received $300 a month for wages and basic expenses. This was a prodigious sum for a woman to earn in 1911.

In July of that year, while Gertrude was relaxing at the Whitney camp in the Adirondacks, Juliana was making the rounds of New York publishing offices with "White Voices." She sent Gertrude several progress reports, which are interesting both as documents of the growing bond between the two women and as windows into the personality of the writer. The letters are written by hand, a sign of some informality between employer and employee. The most curious and fascinating aspect of Juliana's handwriting is that it had evolved to become nearly indistinguishable from the penmanship of Helen Hay Whitney. Juliana

may have begun imitating it when she worked for Helen, and it is the first indication of her aptitude for picking up the mannerisms, habits, and flourishes of a class well beyond her.

"White Voices" was a difficult property to sell—the author and her pseudonym were unknown and the story was narrated in a singsong tone. Juliana's letters to Gertrude, however, betray no doubts about the manuscript's probable fate. They are compounds of encouragement and criticism, grounded in real warmth and sympathy, yet also cunningly devised to parade the writer's idiosyncratic charm and cleverness. Juliana told Gertrude the truth, but she rounded its sharp corners with entertaining metaphors and digressions. Poking fun at the proprieties enabled Juliana to persuade Gertrude of her loyalty in a lighthearted way. Humor also helped to deflect the blow of rejection, as can be seen in this letter of August 2, 1911.

185 Madison Avenue

Dear Mrs. Whitney:

Your copy came to me yesterday, thank you. It is now in the hands of a man whose opinion I value, but who is not a "professional" critic.* He has promised to read it today and let me know his opinion tomorrow.

[The rest of the letter was written after Juliana received the man's appraisal of the manuscript.]

I was tremendously upset over the word "disreputable,"† because, unless one decides it has been used by a most commonplace person, it is unjust. I met my brother at dinner and casually inquired what sort of a man Mr. Metcalfe was. "Very nice fellow" I was assured, and then the most enlightening afterthought—"a sort of proper little man." Don't you know all about him now? I quite forgive him. Wasn't it the Fireside Companion, or The Household Friend, where none of their contributory geniuses were allowed to have a man marry his wife's cousin, nor a horse to trot any faster than just so fast? It was really nice of him, too, not to forget to say that it wasn't badly written. . . . Have you seen the article on The *Corrupting* Influence of Walter Pater? That dear indifferent man who warned us not "to sleep before evening!"

Another bitter disappointment awaited me—My interview with Mr. Gilman [the editor of *Harper's Weekly*] wasn't an interview! He slipped into his coat—before he received me minus—and insisted upon shaking hands with me. My heart sank, but I was determined then to make the most of the situation, which is—the story is too long for a weekly, in fact the size of a novel. Mr. G. had that morning sent it downstairs to Mr. Fair, the book reviewer, to whom I was introduced in turn, and who said he was snowed under and would read it "some time soon." After a little while his eyes, way back under bushy white brows, smiled at something said, and the humanity of him encouraged me to beg for an early perusal. I am to see him tomorrow at eleven. He warned me "we don't give literary advice; ours is a purely commercial interest, you know." I said that I was sure it would not be inconsistent

---

*Possibly Charles Rieser, at that time working for the *New York Sun* and successfully moonlighting as a writer of pulp fiction, or an acquaintance of Charles's named Metcalfe.

†"Disreputable" was evidently the word used to describe "White Voices" by the man Juliana enlisted to criticize the work. She refers to a reader's report he gave her, but it has not survived.

with the commercial interest to say whether or not it was worth while in any way, and he laughed again and said "We shall see."

Mr. Gilman had read it, I am sure, because he looked like he had. His eyes are extremely clever, and he would make an ideal witness in a murder case. I think he considers it too good to condemn, and does not want to risk his opinion. Otherwise, there is the very usual and most effective "returned with thanks."

I know you will be disappointed; but please believe that I am too, and that I did all I could with any dignity do to get his honest expression. Are you really satisfied with what I am doing?

This "man-stifled" town was just a little too much for me yesterday so that I could not write sooner.

Very briefly yours,
Juliana Rieser

The efforts to place "White Voices" came to naught, but the story did accomplish something in that "man-stifled" summer of 1911. It seems to have been the vehicle for bringing Gertrude and Juliana together as a permanent team. Juliana, with her thoroughness and ability to amuse, had proved that there was room in Gertrude's life for a creative woman who would support her and take her seriously, yet not compete with her artistically. In spite of their differences in temperament, Juliana and Gertrude shared important qualities— aesthetic sensitivity, nonconformity, and an appetite for experience. Their dissatisfaction with orthodoxy and the obstacles they had faced because they were different enabled the two women to understand each other across the gulf separating them in wealth, position, upbringing, and education. They were both members of the small company of women who chose to break the mold before the mold broke them. One woman, impetuous and ebullient, wishes to forget a difficult home life and the constrictions of a small town. She meets another woman, secretive and shy, but as full of dreams as herself, struggling against empty routines and the narcissism that comes from being trained as an ornament. One woman with a flair for doing impresses a woman who wants to get so much done and can pay any price to realize her desires, but who is immobilized by her need for privacy. Separately the pair's progress would have been erratic; together they could achieve almost anything.

If anyone could help broaden the perimeters of Gertrude's patronage, it would be Juliana, even if she were inexperienced in art matters. Practical considerations dictated that Juliana be chosen as Gertrude's manager, secretary, and confidante, but what really drew Gertrude to her new associate was Juliana's absolute and unswerving grasp of what it meant to live. In an impromptu talk Juliana gave years later, she spoke ringingly of her belief in receptivity and vitality as the governing poles of her being. Her speech was as close as she ever came to articulating a personal philosophy. She spoke of the distinction between living and existing and of the importance of heeding the claims of the imagination. This was the message Gertrude must have heard:

In New York there are only two kinds of people—the quick and the dead. . . . There are only two peoples anywhere—the quick and the dead, if we use "quick" in the old Anglo-Saxon sense, to quicken, to be sensitive, to be alive. You call it energy,

intelligence, responsiveness—but it is really being alive. . . . One must go on or go back, and we are only important . . . in so far as we are able to go on. There are two kinds of people, the people who go on and the people who shrink back; . . . I have really felt it . . . this feeling that we have got to progress, to be alive, to be quick.

Together Gertrude and Juliana could go on. Juliana, who shrank from nothing, was able to actualize Gertrude's plans, and she emerged as Gertrude's intermediary and buffer for her downtown activities. Besides watching over the private art exhibitions in the MacDougal Alley studio, Juliana screened Gertrude's callers and took care of the clerical work involved in submitting sketches, budgets, and the like for commissions for public monuments that Gertrude hoped to win. Her position was that of executive secretary, but her easygoing relationship with her employer as it matured was one of two confederates in bohemia, learning as they went. Juliana was a firecracker lobbed into Gertrude's life; sparks ignited in her wake. Gertrude in turn held out a lifeline to Juliana by which she might swim into a fluid new pool of New York culture.

While "White Voices" was circulating, Juliana received another piece of news. On November 13, 1911, Doctor's forty-first birthday, his divorce from Grace became final. But after seven years of waiting, Juliana wondered if she should marry him after all. According to Carl Rieser, Juliana discussed the matter with Gertrude after the latter's return from Europe. Juliana did not confide the reason for her hesitancy to her nephew, but only that Gertrude, apparently counseling her with the voice of worldly wisdom, advised her to go through with it. In this case, she may have believed it was best to observe the rules. That Juliana even considered breaking with Doctor is astonishing, particularly if it is assumed that the two were lovers before they were married. New York offered them a privacy unobtainable in Hoboken, and seven years was a long time for either party to remain celibate. Moreover, both Juliana and Doctor were gregarious, highly sensual persons who enjoyed drinking, parties, comfortable surroundings, and Rabelaisian stories. Yet it seems too much to expect that Juliana, a product of a moralistic upbringing (no matter how hated it was) and the general strictures of the era, could have been so sexually free as to forgo legitimizing her relationship.

Any doubts that lingered in Juliana's mind were dispelled or repressed. Her wedding took place on June 20, 1912. A church ceremony in view of gawking Hoboken was inappropriate, so the bridal couple was united in Julia and Max's parlor on Eleventh Street. The Reverend Henry Beatty, the Riesers' faithful pastor even for the family black sheep, performed the ceremony. Doctor was forty-one. Juliana was thirty-five, but she gave her age as thirty on the marriage certificate, and her statement was accepted.

The couple would live in Manhattan. Juliana moved out of her parents' house, returning only for the occasional visit. Miss Rieser of Hoboken was now Mrs. W. B. Force of New York City. As far as Juliana was concerned, the world was not to know she had ever been anyone else.

CHAPTER FOUR

FRIENDS OF YOUNG ARTISTS

❧ *(1912–1917)* ❧

A S GERTRUDE'S DOWNTOWN SECRETARY, Juliana found herself in a kind of waking dream. She almost had to pinch herself for reassurance that it was real. Gertrude was the fairy godmother who had whisked her into this wonderland, and now she was granting her permanent admission. Juliana was enthralled by Gertrude's glamour and the magical ease with which she got whatever she wanted.

In 1912, Gertrude's good works were at the point where they either had to stop or expand. If she wanted to sculpt, a lieutenant was required for her other activities. So what counted in a partner were certain qualities of mind and temperament: elasticity, adventurousness, vitality, wit, grit, and a positive outlook. Most of all, the job called for a fighter—the conservatives were heavily entrenched in the art world, and without a champion, artists outside the citadel, persevering though they were, didn't stand much of a chance. John Sloan put it well when he said, "Artists, in a frontier society like ours, are like cockroaches in kitchens—not wanted, not encouraged but nevertheless they remain."

Juliana recognized that her main deficiency—she was starting from scratch in art matters—could be neutralized, or even converted into somewhat of an asset by virtue of her energy. The classic strength of an amateur is the determination to tackle large, new, and often intractable projects. Whereas the more knowing might shake their heads dubiously, Juliana, not being familiar with the pitfalls, could and would push forward unafraid.

Nevertheless she was not so foolish as to rely on innocence and personal chemistry to see her through. Her job was multilayered, her employer quixotic, and there was much to learn. If Juliana were to master the art world, she would have to move quickly to cover the great stretches of her inexperience. A good

portion of her instruction was basic—she was familiarizing herself with the museums and galleries and paying attention to what Gertrude said. But her true education, which would spice her own life, further her understanding, and establish important lines of communication, lay in the forming of friendships with artists. In their company, good times and tutorials were one. Juliana relished it all, and she was gifted at winning their confidences. Her training was never scholastic or didactic—later she would say of this early education, "I didn't learn anything, but I just grew more and more astonished." She focused on the solving of artists' problems, and that was what she learned to do best.

In those first years with Gertrude, Juliana was also the doorkeeper at 19 MacDougal Alley, and she built up many an acquaintance in her capacity as a greeter. She conferred with Gertrude about who should be invited to exhibit, made sure the submissions were delivered to MacDougal Alley on time, planned the layouts, reported on difficulties the artists were having, and served tea in the late afternoons. During the run of any show, she kept attendance and dispensed catalogs. She piloted interested spectators around the shows, looking out for important guests and newspaper reviewers. She sold pictures and made sure their new owners received them. To Gertrude's position as gallery director, Juliana was, in these first few years, a combination of salesman, policeman, and curator. Visitors to the Whitney Studio remarked on her enthusiastic boosting of art and artists, and they were struck by her unabashed desire to improve the artists' well-being.

Before long, Juliana's solicitude—in tandem with her discovery that artists were rare and wonderful beings—overflowed into her home life. She and Doctor lived briefly on East 58th and 49th Streets before moving into a pleasant three-room apartment at 138 East 36th Street. According to Forbes Watson, who remembered the rooms in East 36th Street, the establishment "contained a single borrowed picture. And since her love of interior decorators had not yet blossomed, it was a simple, homey, and cosy little place, untouched by early American and Victorian highlights." The Forces were at home to artists on Sunday mornings, supplementing with their own hospitality the Whitney bounty Juliana administered. The Sunday morning breakfasts began late and lasted long enough to slide affably into cocktails and lunch. Over Scotch and gin and bourbon, hostess and guests talked nonstop about painters and paintings, galleries and shows, studios and art schools. Juliana heard shoptalk, gossip, admirations, enmities, and philosophizing. In this agreeable fashion, she gained much working knowledge for her purposes, and it was the way she preferred to operate throughout her career. Juliana was consistently more partial to knowledge absorbed from direct experience than knowledge acquired by study.

Blendon Campbell remembered that Juliana was indispensable to Gertrude's first benefit shows at the Whitney Studio because "she could sell practically anything to anybody." Her flair for salesmanship was a surprise only to those who did not know her. After all, she had taught at a business school and afterward she kept afloat her own stenography business, small though it was. Despite the

failure of "White Voices" to interest a publisher, Gertrude did not attribute its rejection to Juliana's shortcomings. Instead she was sufficiently impressed by her assistant's diligence to hazard switching her from literary to artistic agentry. Gertrude was now being regularly encouraged to submit bids for monuments and large sculptural decorations. Winning a commission for a work of art destined for the public view was (and is) not merely a matter of conceiving a competent design. Applications must be written, budgets drawn up, fund raisers and judges met and charmed.

Juliana demonstrated that she was a shrewd negotiator of contracts for Gertrude and a graceful minister to the selection committees of architects and civic officials responsible for awarding commissions. These skills were essential to the business side of Gertrude's sculpture. In 1912 the New Arlington Hotel in Washington, D.C., hired Gertrude to design a fountain; in 1913 the Pan-American Building (also in the capital) requested a frieze and fountain based on the legend of El Dorado. At the end of 1912, she was sounded out about the possibility of creating a statue commemorating the victims of the *Titanic*. Negotiations began in 1913, and on January 6, 1914, she learned she had won the job. The *Titanic* memorial, which was also to be erected in Washington, D.C., appears to be the first sculpture commission for which Juliana represented Gertrude. But certainly from 1914 onward, she was in charge of the welter of social, aesthetic, and technical details inherent in winning commissions and bargaining in the artist's interest.

Juliana's specialty was her adroit courting of the various delegations of pooh-bahs bent on dictating their artistic conceptions. She came into her own in this after World War I, when Gertrude competed successfully for several war memorials. Juliana, as several witnesses recalled, would invite the military brass to luncheon. She chatted with them and took them on excursions. She could laugh them into seeing Gertrude's point of view, and they would all feel mightily entertained. As her agent for sculpture, Juliana obtained an immutable power base within Gertrude's entourage. Quite as usefully, the experience prepared her for directing the bigger and more complex enterprises of the Whitney Studio Club, the Whitney Studio Galleries, and the Whitney Museum.

Gertrude's growing renown as a professional artist meant even greater celebrity. By 1912 Gertrude was, as a pendant to her fame as an heiress, famous as an art patron and an active sculptor. She seemed especially open to appeals because her giving was far-flung and eclectic. In 1910, for instance, she gave money to both the liberal Independent show and the hidebound American Academy in Rome. In late 1911, another stronghold of mossbacks, the National Academy of Design, benefited from a donation. Shortly afterward she expressed interest in supporting the Association of American Painters and Sculptors, the group behind the epochal Armory Show.

"Besieged" was the word to describe Gertrude's state from morning until night. Letters from poets, musicians, decorators, painters, sculptors, seamstresses, artists' models, art dealers, and cranks deluged her two Manhattan addresses and the Westbury house. They poured in every day from all over the United States and two or three European countries. The correspondents wanted

appointments, testimonials, photographs, and certified checks. Young people offered to be her secretary, her maid, her pupil, her studio aide. And these appeals were separate and distinct from the hundreds of solicitations received from charities traditionally underwritten by socialites. The situation had deteriorated to the point that not even MacDougal Alley was safe from predators. Artists waylaid her as she walked from the street into her studio, and small boys in the neighborhood offered to guide sightseers there for a fee.

A more elaborate city refuge was necessary, a fact further underscored by the completion of a studio at Old Westbury in the summer of 1912. Two years before, Gertrude had hired the architect William Adams Delano to make her a studio as "splendid as a temple" on Long Island to replace the converted barn she was using. He responded with an exquisite Italianate marble pavilion surrounded by formal gardens and woodlands. MacDougal Alley could not hope to match the serenity of a neoclassical villa or its parklike acreage, nor was it supposed to. Yet it could be made less assailable. Gertrude instructed Thomas Regan, the Whitneys' business manager, to buy her the lease to the town house (the property was not a freehold) fronting on 8 West Eighth Street. This was the dwelling attached to the stable that became her studio in 1907, and she planned to build a passage between the structures. Gertrude could then enter her studio via Eighth Street, a busy crosstown thoroughfare, and elude any person waiting for her around the corner. Some of the rooms in the town house could be turned into galleries. She could show more art, and she would no longer have to let strangers into her actual place of work. Regan made the down payment on November 4, 1912. Two months later Gertrude sailed for Paris.

Securing 8 West Eighth Street, which would be the official address of Gertrude's studio for the remainder of her working days, was of substantial consequence to her life. By rights another such pivotal event should have occurred three months later, on February 17, 1913. On that day the most important art event ever held in America—the International Exhibition of Modern Art, swiftly abbreviated to the Armory Show on account of its location in the Sixty-Ninth Regiment Armory at 25th Street and Lexington Avenue—opened its doors to a public eager to be shocked. It could hardly have been otherwise. Ben Hecht accurately characterized the state of things when he wrote, "In 1913 Americans thought that Art was men who wore long hair and talked like sissies; naked women in a garret; something J.P. Morgan was interested in; a Chinese kimono thrown over a chair in the vestibule; something they had in Europe; any statue in a public park."

Because of its huge scope—nearly 1,300 works of art, with every progressive tendency in Europe and America on view—and implications—the inevitability of revolution, the legitimate claim of the avant-garde to a great tradition, the demonstration that American artists were roughly twenty-five years behind their European counterparts—the Armory Show and its aftermath forever transformed the course of art in America. (That would lead Hecht to issue a progress report: "In 1923 Americans think Art is something that doesn't look like a photograph;

marrying a negro in the South Seas; anything a Russian does; turning colored lights on the orchestra in the movie palace; a rape scene in a moving picture.") The contents of the Armory Show called into question the age-old faith that mimetic representation of nature was the ultimate goal of a creative artist. Consequently, every serious American artist—many of whom had never laid eyes on a Cézanne or Van Gogh, let alone a Picasso, a Picabia, a Brancusi, or a Duchamp—had to reexamine his aesthetic. The sweep of the show, an organizational feat *extraordinaire*, toppled the totem of Academy omnipotence conclusively. As Milton Brown wrote in his history of the Armory Show, "The most vital artists in the United States . . . had done what the National Academy of Design always maintained was impossible without public support . . . that is, put on an exciting exhibition of monster proportions. . . . The Academy never again played any significant role on the American artistic stage." Modern European art entered the marketplace, and devotees gamely opened galleries showing it by itself or in conjunction with the more radical Americans. The Armory Show was imperative to the prescient collections made by John Quinn, Lillie P. Bliss, Walter Arensberg, Stephen C. Clark, and Arthur Jerome Eddy. If the germ of the Whitney Museum can be traced to the coming together of The Eight, then the Armory Show was the seedbed of the Museum of Modern Art.

Gertrude and Juliana's attitudes about the Armory Show were dichotomous. Broadly speaking, they approved the ferocity of commitment and maverick style by which the artists brought off an electrifying phenomenon and trounced the nay-sayers, but their immediate reaction to the more experimental art was negative. Judging by the art Gertrude and Juliana exhibited during the first two years of the Whitney Studio, they were not only not persuaded by modernism, but determined to ignore it. Not until 1916 did the women gradually accept the School of Paris and its American adherents. Wholehearted support came a few years later. Although Gertrude was involved in the initial planning of the Armory Show, her dealings with it are ultimately somewhat puzzling—and startling.

In December of 1911 Gertrude met with Walt Kuhn, Elmer MacRae, Jerome Myers, and Henry Fitch Taylor at the Madison Gallery, an establishment run by Clara S. Davidge, a decorator and antiques dealer. These men were tossing around the idea of a confederation for exhibiting worthy artists neglected by the New York galleries. Any such venture would require financial backing, and Gertrude was an obvious patron to enlist. Their proposal was compatible with her own broad-minded inclinations, and familiar, reassuring names, such as Henri, Davies, Glackens, Lawson, Luks, Fraser, and J. Alden Weir, were elected charter members. A few weeks into the Association's incorporation in 1912, Davies took over its presidency. To Gertrude, the Armory Show initially must have appeared, as indeed it was ideologically, an outgrowth of The Eight and the 1910 Independent shows. More than forty Americans whom Gertrude knew personally, had exhibited in the Independent show, or had been supported by her stipends or purchases of art were going to take part. But she was kept in ignorance of the plans Davies, Kuhn, and MacRae—who were emerging as kingpins of the undertaking—had for including the giants of European modernism.

When did it dawn on Gertrude that she would not be invited to be in a show she was supposed to help guarantee? For much of 1912 she must have thought that she would be in the thick of it. She agreed to lend a screen she owned by Chanler. Alfred Maurer and Jo Davidson, one a protégé and the other a close confidante, introduced Davies and Kuhn to Ambroise Vollard, who made important loans to them. Moreover, Gertrude saw herself as a rebel, as a bohemian well-versed in the arts. Her tastes, which had advanced as far as Manet, the Impressionists, and American Realism, lagged behind Stieglitz, Davies, and John Quinn, but she was miles ahead of most of her countrymen. Gertrude had seized upon the democratic humanism, the "antiartistic" subject matter bodied forth by Henri and his followers, as a gratifying form of insurgency and a liberating corollary to her own search for self-realization. She was typically American in that she could conceive of radicalism in the context of politics, but not in the cause of formal revolution. The Cubist attack on the object and the possibilities suggested by the Fauvist freedom of color did not, in Gertrude's mind, relate to her interests or her life. Because she attached so much importance to subject matter, in 1913 the new art was too unnerving for her to absorb or internalize.

Milton Brown has described the masterly diplomacy required of Davies and Kuhn to prevent the marmorean "nightmare of sculptured rhetoric" produced in the New York ateliers of the academic sculptors from encroaching on the uncompromisingly advanced character of the Armory Show. *Retardataire* Beaux-Arts sculptors were incessantly being suggested for inclusion by Gutzon Borglum, the Association's vice-president (and future carver of Mount Rushmore). He complained that too much space was given over to paintings and sought to correct the imbalance by packing the sculpture section with soothingly respectable carvers and modelers. After Davies vetoed Daniel Chester French, Borglum saw the wisdom of withdrawing from the Association. If establishment figures such as these were left out of the show, then Gertrude could rationalize her own omission. Yet Fraser, Robert Aitken, Chester Beach, and George Grey Barnard—senior academicians all—*were* invited to submit work, as were several conservative women sculptors with careers comparable to Gertrude's. Presumably Gertrude was handled with extreme delicacy, because she retained an admiration for Davies, and he, Kuhn, MacRae, and Taylor were asked to exhibit their work at her studio in 1914.

Exclusion from the approved list of sculptors may very well have precipitated Gertrude's decision to miss the Armory Show altogether. Her diaries and letters show that she left for Paris by January 9, 1913, and did not return to New York until the middle of May. The Armory Show opened on February 17 and closed on March 15. It rocked Chicago from March 24 to April 16, and Boston got an abbreviated version from April 28 to May 19. Gertrude did not see the big production at all.

Her absence explains why she never bought anything from the Armory Show. But it does not explain why she underwrote the decorations for the exhibition, a fact reverently cited in histories of the event. According to ledgers kept by MacRae and corroborated by other accounts, a check for $1,000 is listed as coming from Mrs. Harry Payne Whitney on January 24, 1913, but by then she

was no longer in the country. The money was collected during a personal visit by Clara Davidge, who was canvassing wealthy women she and Davies knew to see if they would make up the Association's rising deficit. The one person Davidge could have seen with the authority to release money for art in Gertrude's absence was Juliana.

The original impulse to give, as well as the enabling power to do so, might have emanated from Gertrude. She could have been prepared for the eventuality of subsidizing the show and told Juliana about it. However, the span of time between the meeting at the Madison Gallery in 1911 and the actual assemblage of the art, plus the fact that Gertrude was brought back into financial discussions at the last minute—a bare three weeks before the exhibition was scheduled to open—militates against this reconstruction of events. Two other possibilities suggest themselves. Juliana, when approached by Clara Davidge, recognized that Gertrude would want to be affiliated with the show and cabled Paris for approval. Or, Juliana took her chances—she agreed to help, pledged $1,000 in Gertrude's name, and broke the news to her afterward. If the second or third explanation is true, American art owes much to the alacrity of Juliana's judgment. And it is to Gertrude's credit that she did not permit personal disappointment to prevail over her general interest in bettering the lot of other artists.

More engrossing than Gertrude's eschewal of the Armory Show was her reaction to its shockwaves. She was tolerant of the new art's partisans, but European or American modernism didn't overtly excite her, either as an artist or a patron. She concentrated, perhaps unconsciously, on remaining in isolation, even though her intimates were strongly aware of the School of Paris. Morgan Russell was writing her copious letters filled with talk of Matisse, Picasso, and the Steins, and he dedicated a key Synchromist painting to her that was exhibited in October of 1913. Bob Chanler, whose painted screens turned out to be one of the surprise hits of the Armory Show, bought Redon etchings and a bust of *Mlle. Pogany* from the exhibition. Bernard Karfiol, who was close to Gertrude in the early teens, recalled trying to talk to her about Cézanne, "but she admired Zuloaga and Sorolla* and . . . [I] was never able to win her over to . . . [my] side."

A good number of American painters who were instrumental in putting over the Armory Show (most vocally, Henri, George Bellows, and Myers) resented its outcome. Whereas they believed that the exhibition was formulated to bolster native artists, it had, in their opinion, only worsened the situation. Not only had the Europeans run away with the publicity and sales, once more preempting buyers and newspaper columns, but the hosting Americans were shown up as provincial. The Realists' sense of being betrayed and ill-used reached Gertrude's ears. She took their side wholeheartedly, as the one surviving record of her response to the Armory Show attests. The fragment of an unpublished speech, it is a surprising document, uncharacteristic of the writer.

* Ignacio de Zuloaga and Joáquin Sorolla y Bastida, two Spanish painters then having a vogue in New York.

I was very glad to find that I agreed with anyone as distinguished as Mr. Royal Cortissoz* in my opinion of Post-Impressionism and Cubism.

He finds fault with people for taking them so seriously. For instance in speaking of Matisse he says: "These things are not works of art; they are feeble impertinences."

Referring to Cubism: "Are we to be at great pains to explain that a chunk of marble is not a statue?"

Later he remarks: "I cannot too often repeat the statement that there is nothing grand, gloomy and peculiar about these freak pictures."

These schools had their origin in France, they had big followings in other foreign countries. It is easy to observe their growth in the history of art and it has seemed to me that there is one point, interesting and true, which I deem to be to the credit of America. We have never gone to the same extremes to which the French, Germans, Italians and Russians have gone in this regard. Even those . . . exponents of the Independent schools preserved some semblance of sanity in their madness. The longing for something new, which unfortunately has often found its answer in something freakish lacks construction, and as a contrast we revert to that old formula from which a true inspiration may arise.

During the winter of 1913 we were able for the first time in this country to compare at close range the works of foreign artists with those of our own artists. I would not presume to rely on my own judgment in this matter. Much has been written about the Armory Exhibition, and many connoisseurs and critics both American and foreign were of the opinion that America held its own & more than held its own in this interesting and unusual Exhibition. Not only this, but that America is now showing an individuality, a progress from the source of its inspiration which is a very impressive & to many people a surprising thing.

Both Alden Weir and Childe Hassam, in using a given method, developed a personal and distinguishing creative power. Davies, a visionary painter who is still a realist, and Albert P. Ryder who though like Puvis is utterly different, were here seen in the best of company and inspired only a feeling of hope in the minds of those most deeply interested in the art of this country.

The result which comes after the passing influence of a great painter, if it is a real result is not that of imitation, it is rather that of a big principle discovered, and it is this fertilization which we with our strongly marked American personalities have, I truly believe, carried forward. I would like to lay stress on this particular phase of our development. We have always had individuality in all that we have endeavored to do. Our heroes stand out not quite like the heroes of other countries. They have particular traits, potent points, weak or strong as the case may be, but still just a little different, just our own, and as they are our own we must of necessity express those points in our art.

The draft is undated, but it was written in 1914 or early 1915. In 1916 Gertrude edged toward a reappraisal of Post-Impressionism. After World War I she arranged to export a comprehensive show of modern French and American paintings overseas and then lobbied the Metropolitan Museum to mount a big survey of Post-Impressionism. Another argument for dating the speech as 1914

---

*Royal Cortissoz, the art critic of the New York Tribune, wrote two articles adverse to the Armory Show. The first appeared in the Tribune on February 13, 1913, and the second in the April 1913 issue of The Century. The passages quoted by Gertrude are from the newspaper review.

or 1915 is that the writer assumes that Cortissoz's statements are still fresh enough in the audience's memory to have wide currency.

What is especially remarkable about Gertrude's opening commentary is its know-nothingism. She was not a philistine, and one of her admirable traits was a resolve to learn and decide things for herself instead of relying on secondhand verdicts. In this case, instead of investigating personally, she took someone else's word on a controversial subject and based her condemnation on it.

The sixth paragraph is even less forthright. Gertrude pretends that she attended the Armory Show. (By now to admit that she, an artist and collector of liberal sympathies, had skipped a momentous and sensational event that 70,000 other people had seen, an event which artists did not so much visit but live in, would have been a grave embarrassment.) Beyond hiding behind Cortissoz, she damns with the paired adjectives "interesting and unusual," which are so bland in this context that any compliment bestowed is negated by the triteness of the application. Gertrude further pecks away at the impact of the exhibition by incorrectly reporting that informed critical opinion pronounced it a triumph for the Americans.

In the last paragraph of her speech Gertrude advances toward a valid point: The need for American artists to cultivate their individuality as Americans and refrain from borrowing just for the sake of novelty. However, her wish for an organic evolution and synthesis is rendered suspect by the chauvinism and defensiveness of the preceding passages, and by the refusal to accept that Post-Impressionism and Cubism had as trustworthy an artistic pedigree as Eakins, Whistler, or Ryder.

The foundations on which Gertrude had erected her own art were shaken by the ascendancy of modernism. Her repetition of Cortissoz's "Are we to be at great pains to explain that a chunk of marble is not a statue?" indicates that she understood Brancusi and Archipenko to be repudiating sculptural notions of truth and beauty as she perceived them. Her attempts to wrestle with this affront to Beaux-Arts assumptions can be seen in a few figures Gertrude completed after the Armory Show. She modified her style in an embrace of archaism. Abandoning the Rodinesque muscularity of her previous figures, she modeled smoother torsos and masklike faces closer to Oriental statuary and the pre-Phidian Greeks.

We do not have Juliana's reactions to the Armory Show, but in 1913 her aesthetic preferences didn't diverge from Gertrude's. As she did not try to introduce any vanguard art into the early exhibitions she orchestrated, there is scarce reason for thinking that the Armory Show affected her any differently than it did her employer. It would have left Juliana unprepared, skeptical, and jolted, but glad that she had a hand in subsidizing it.

The final touches on the studio in Old Westbury were completed in 1913, and Gertrude spent much of the summer working there. On July 1, Regan wrote that he had closed the deal on 8 West Eighth Street; the lease was hers for $15,000. In August, Grosvenor Atterbury (Gertrude's partner in the disputed

Architectural League award) remodeled the building to her specifications. After receiving the architect's estimate for alterations—about $7,000—she left once more for Paris.

The changes were simple and functional, taking into account that the building, although three stories high, was just 25 feet wide. The outside was painted a tawny pink, and its bright face was accented by a dark green door and casements. The ground floor was divided into two exhibiting rooms plus a small back hall where Juliana sometimes sat during visiting hours. A public staircase led to another gallery room taking up the front half of the second floor. The rear half of the second story became Juliana's office, and the third floor was set up as a workroom for artists. Juliana's office contained the entrance to a private "umbilical staircase" connecting it with Gertrude's studio. Only the two women, Gertrude's children, and her good friends had access to this flight of steps, which was invisible from the galleries and reception areas. In the coming years the hidden staircase would take on symbolic overtones. To Stuart Davis it stood for "Mrs. Whitney . . . very quietly but very efficiently behind the scenes doing a lot to help young American artists long before she founded the museum in 1930."

While construction proceeded at 8 West Eighth, Juliana was doing some house hunting. She and Doctor were looking for a weekend and summer house in the country. In January of 1914 they realized their dream by buying property in the Pennsylvania village of Holicong, just a few miles from Doylestown. Their new estate, named Barley Sheaf Farm, consisted of an eighteenth-century fieldstone farmhouse, an icehouse, a clapboard barn, an underground spring, and sixty acres of arable land. They paid $7,000.

Juliana and Doctor wanted to make Barley Sheaf Farm a showplace as a manor house and a working farm, and they were responsible for extensive alterations. Doctor stocked the place with animals and oversaw the landscaping. Juliana took to renovating with an almost alarming vigor. She transformed dark, cramped rooms by demolishing interior walls, raising the ceilings and the roof, enlarging doors and windows, and installing bathrooms and closets. She also added a huge screened-in porch. When Juliana tore out the old kitchen walls, she had them redone five times, according to the neighbors' recollections, before she was satisfied. The formerly humble "Georgian farmhouse was transformed into a French chateauette," with a mansard roof and wrought-iron railings and balconies, although some of the better architectural features—such as the wide-planked flooring and the carved and molded mantelpieces—were spared. The icehouse became a guest house. Doctor put in a board fence around the boundaries of the property and planted bushes and trees along the entry drive. Because the main house was set well back from the public road, the landscaping ensured that the top of the new mansard roof was the only sight visible to outsiders.

Barley Sheaf Farm marked Juliana's first thorough experience in obliterating and reshaping her physical environment, but she started as she meant to go on. She had a passion for making over. In subsequent apartments and houses, a hallmark of her decorating was not the slight addition or minor repair, but a top-to-bottom, full-scale redesign of the premises, usually accompanied by new

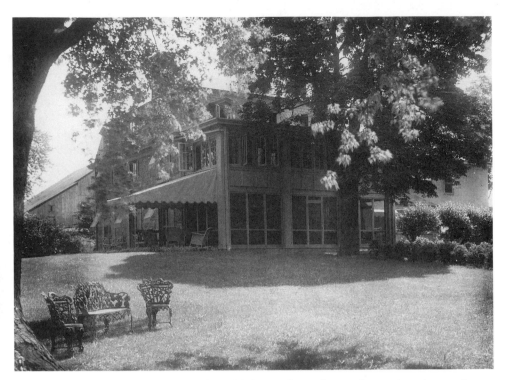

The main house of Barley Sheaf Farm, Holicong, Pennsylvania, after undergoing much remodeling at Juliana's hands.

plumbing, wiring, and the latest appliances or conveniences. Juliana's views on the inviolability or permanence of architecture were notably casual. Irrespective of the native appearance of any house she owned, it inevitably took on a sprightly aspect and imposing breadth that was pure Juliana.

Transforming her surroundings found its parallel in redefining lives in accordance with her own prescription. Juliana saw Barley Sheaf Farm as a symbol of the rightful restoration of Rieser status and a long-awaited redressing of old inequities. It was a recovery of the world she and her siblings had been born into, but improved by her embellishment. With the farm, what Juliana had invented came true.

The acquisition of the Holicong property meshed with Juliana's complete victory within her family. She became its head, in acknowledgment as well as in fact. As a natural consequence of marriages, births, and the depredations of age, the weight of the Rieser family configuration shifted. Juliana's parents were fading out of her life. Julia's health began to fail, and she was too weak to engage in combat. Her hold on the family slipped, and the ineffectual Max could not abdicate what had never been his in the first place. He died in 1917 and Julia in 1920. In 1913 Charles Rieser married Irene Grosel, an attractive young woman whom Juliana liked. They produced two boys—Allan, born in 1914, and Carl,

born two years later. The childless Juliana doted on her nephews, and they were her favorites among her brothers' children. Her affection for Allan and Carl, absolutely genuine and open-hearted, often was maternally possessive. In addition, Juliana started assuming more responsibility for Mary and Clara. Adopting her whole family en masse, she attempted to situate herself as mother and father to both her own siblings and their children. Accordingly, she insisted that they share in her good fortune.

As part of re-creating the family, Juliana tried to repair old disruptions by transferring the family seat to a more promising setting. The new center of Rieserdom was to be Barley Sheaf Farm. Its enlargement and modernization made it ample for family gatherings on holidays and weekends.

Juliana and her siblings remembered Bucks County with sentimental fondness, and they still felt its strong pull. The presence of Julia's relations living in the area and the maintenance of the Rieser burial plot in the Doylestown cemetery reinforced this attachment. Pennsylvania was their first home and the site of their earliest memories. Now in a position to set right—that is, revise—the past, Juliana exerted herself in avenging it. Returning to her birthplace as the chatelaine of a splendid country house was merely the beginning. She felt compelled to lift the rest of her family up to this new level of affluence and influence.

Juliana no longer admitted that the Riesers had been middle class. Instead, she recast them as aristocrats who had suffered unfair reverses. Her nephews and nieces were indoctrinated with a heightened social sense. "Aunt Jule had a very strong feeling for the way the family should look and behave," said Beverly Rieser Smock. "If she didn't like the coat you were wearing, she would march you down to the store, take you in hand, and get you what she thought you should have." Marjorie Rieser recalled, "We learned, We are the Riesers. We have nothing to do with other people."

Juliana was ambivalent about her hometown, and it disapproved of her. After settling into the farm, she snubbed the Doylestown gentry and teased them with her behavior. Remembering the Bucks County stuffiness, she stayed pointedly away from their flower shows and club meetings, and did her best to keep the young Riesers from playing with the local children. "We were told never to talk to the other children," Beverly Rieser Smock said. "I would get invited to places and then want to have the kids back to go swimming with me. Aunt Jule, giving the orders and seconded by Aunt Clara and Aunt Mary, didn't like it." Even worse in the eyes of Doylestowners were Juliana's own appearance and demeanor. Her hair was bobbed. She wore knickers and smoked in public. Guests at Barley Sheaf Farm were suspected of being freethinkers and Jews.

There was not much for Juliana to do for Gertrude during most of 1914, save for the executive duties surrounding the *Titanic* memorial. Gertrude went abroad from January until late March to work on the monument, her spring was spent in Old Westbury, and in the summer she was stricken with a crippling attack of colitis. Her galleries on West Eighth Street were completed but empty.

Giving the *Titanic* memorial commission to Gertrude created some controversy. Other sculptors groused about her getting ahead too easily, and once more she was accused of benefiting from a biased jury. There were three judges, one of whom was Helen Hay Whitney, who did not disqualify herself from voting. The sculpture, of an idealized youth—meaning an androgynous male figure discreetly wrapped in drapery—with his arms limply outstretched, was an obvious allusion to the crucifixion and resurrection. (The cruciform figure would become Gertrude's standard design solution, and it was used in several of her memorials.) Unnoticed by any of Gertrude's contemporaries was that the rendering of the youth's face was heavily indebted to Andrew O'Connor, who helped Gertrude with the statue when she worked on it in France during the spring of 1914. In a journal entry from then, she wrote about him, "You said if I would work hard you would make me the greatest woman sculptor. . . ." O'Connorisms also show up in Gertrude's *Head of a Spanish Peasant*, a portrait bust she started in 1911, and the fountains she made for the New Arlington Hotel and the Pan-American Building.

Gertrude was passing through a phase of ardent self-involvement, extreme even for her. Winning the three big commissions in Washington, D.C., especially the *Titanic* memorial—which was the basis of her reputation—hyper-inflated her ego. Believing perhaps that O'Connor would indeed make her the greatest woman sculptor, Gertrude pandered to her most romantic schoolgirlish fancies. "[I]n the face of the *Titanic* Memorial," she exhaled, "will be seen the love, the agony, the joy of my soul. I love what I have written now, for it is the truth." Among her writings of this period is a half-finished essay on the virtues of selfishness, in which she played with voguish Nietzschean ruminations and identified with Napoleon, Wagner, and Alexander the Great. In her diaries she occasionally spoke of herself as a "genius." Previously she had been readier to concede the slenderness of her sculptural gift.

Another literary project Gertrude undertook was her autobiography (never finished), which presupposed that the author had profound sensations to communicate. Of course there was a splendid social story to be told had she been prepared to reveal it. Gertrude, however, presented her life as a series of unruffled transitions culminating in her easy emergence as an artist of stature. That her eye was on posterity is suggested again by the number of portraits—several of which were by ultrafashionable artists—she posed for between 1912 and 1914. Gertrude sat for Emanuele de Rosales, John Singer Sargent, the Princes Paul and Pierre Troubetzkoy, Count Francesco de Guardabassi (a current flirtation), Baron de Meyer, and O'Connor. Her belief in her power to inspire, which empurpled the 1911 "White Voices," was given more intense expression three years later. She wrote to O'Connor about his portrayal of her: "I do not wish you to sculpt me for the world to admire and my pride to be satisfied. I want you to do it so that your ideal through me may give to the world a work of art such as no man has yet produced!"

The excesses of Gertrude's fascination with herself were swept away with the outbreak of World War I. The war emancipated her from petty obligations and caused her to rethink her priorities. In 1914, on account of the impact of the

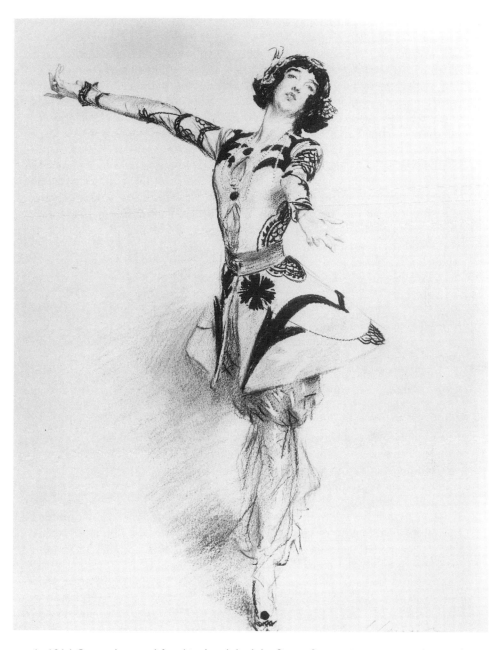

In 1914 Gertrude posed for this sketch by John Singer Sargent in a costume designed for her by Leon Bakst.

Great War, Gertrude regained whatever ground she may have lost to the doldrums of vanity and never surrendered it again. A fierce Francophile, she was afraid for France in particular, and generally overcome "by the fact that people were tearing themselves to pieces. I could not bear the idea that civilization could stand for it." Her dormant sense of responsibility was roused and she acknowledged that sacrifice had a place. The human suffering reported brought out the best in her—her capacity for disinterested generosity and the desire to be of use.

The first thing she did was one of the most selfless—and consistently overlooked—actions of her career. She offered $200,000 of her own money (Harry was against her involvement, but she defied him) to the French government as an initial payment toward opening a field hospital in France. By the time the war ended, Gertrude had contributed more than $1 million to her hospital, plus a separate fleet of thirteen ambulances. Photographs sent to her from the front in 1915 provided blunt proof that when automobile transport was lacking, the wounded were taken to medical facilities on stretchers yoked across the backs of mules.

But sending an enormous sum of money was not enough for Gertrude. She understood at once that the war was the central crucible of experience of her time, and she would not stay on the sidelines. The climate of glory and sacrifice stirred her craving for adventure as much as the spectacle of a world blowing itself apart outraged her sense of decency.

Overlooking the derisive protests of Harry, Gertrude crossed the Atlantic on the Lusitania on November 4, 1914. With her were eight doctors, twenty-five nurses, twenty ambulances, and as many blankets, linens, warm clothes, drugs, and surgical instruments as she could collect. Gertrude's party, aided by French and American officials, set up a hospital in Juilly, a town northeast of Paris near the front. Gertrude was escorted to Red Cross stations behind the Allied lines, where she saw thousands of casualties and stacks of corpses awaiting burial. She wrote in her diary on December 18:

> I know that when Harry realizes that I have made up my mind to come back [to Juilly] he will try and say a great many disagreeable things and ridicule the idea of my being of any use. If this experience has done nothing else . . . it has made me see more clearly the line of usefulness in life and cast behind me more ruthlessly these people who will acknowledge no duties or responsibilities.

Gertrude's war effort was waged on two fronts—Juilly and New York. To be effective in France alone was not good enough. She knew she could use her influence to raise money at home and sway her fellow citizens. Those activities had to go forward as soon as possible. However, she was to be abroad from November until Christmas, and then sail again in early January of 1915. How to do it? The answer was both simple and momentous: Sponsor an art exhibition for the benefit of war relief in her own new galleries in the Village and let Juliana run it. Thus it was World War I that launched Mrs. H. P. Whitney's

Studio, as the galleries were first called, and crystallized Juliana's position as an art impresario.

Bringing off a profitable art show in the Whitney Studio was a challenging assignment. Not one but two fund-raising affairs were planned. The first one, which ran from December 3 to 10, 1914, was a benefit exhibition in which the works on view were donated by well-known artists and sold on behalf of a charity aiding European civilians made destitute by the war. This show was followed by a "50-50" Christmas sale and exhibition. Because artists could not be expected to contribute their work outright for a second time, 50 percent of the proceeds would go to the American Ambulance Hospital in Paris and 50 percent to the participants. To compensate for Gertrude's absence, society women were asked to lend their names as patronesses and nominal managers. Their names on the invitations increased the exhibitions' attractiveness to potential buyers and guaranteed that the newspapers would print something about the shows.

Throughout November Juliana busied herself with coordinating lists of American painters and sculptors to be invited. Working with the patronesses and the dealer William Macbeth, who rounded up pieces from his artists for both shows, she assembled a mixed combination apparently drawn from the following categories: artists Gertrude knew and trusted, artists who would donate work, artists whose work would sell well, artists who would place reasonable prices on their offerings, and younger artists whose pictures she liked. (In this last category, she seems to have been guided by recommendations from Macbeth, Henri, and Davies.) Solid reputations were favored over experiment, yet a sprinkling of more adventurous talents leavened the brew.

The first show, with seven sculptures and nine paintings, was genteel in content and presentation. The Studio was open in the afternoons from 2:00 to 6:00, and tea was served. All the bronzes were conservative: a standing figure of Lincoln by French; a seated representation of John Ruskin by Borglum; Janet Scudder's *Lady of the Sea* (described in one review as a "full-length nude wringing water from her tresses of seaweed"); a dancing girl by Malvina Hoffman; another dancer, this time an English countess writhing away with scarcely a stitch on, by Paul Troubetzkoy; a bust of a young girl by James Earle Fraser; and Gertrude's *Head of a Spanish Peasant*. The painters sent offerings just as characteristic. John White Alexander and Cecilia Beaux donated portraits, Howard Cushing a still life, Blendon Campbell a view of MacDougal Alley, Ernest Lawson a landscape, Sorolla a beach scene, J. Alden Weir a view of a country church, and Henri a full-length portrait of a Spanish woman in a showy costume. Juliana earned her selling spurs here—$8,000 was raised in relief money, and she or Helen Hay Whitney, who was one of the patronesses, probably bought French's statue of Lincoln for Gertrude from the show.

The Christmas sale and show were much bigger. More than 200 items were exhibited by at least fifty artists. This time Juliana asked for smaller and less expensive pieces. The invitations advertised "pictures and small bronzes in the exhibition room" and "fancy articles for Christmas gifts upstairs." A price list compiled for Juliana by Macbeth, who was storing the objects at his gallery until the art from the first show had been cleared out of the Studio, indicates the

effort made to keep prices modest. For instance, drawings by Davies went for $60, $65, $70, and $80. Macbeth was extremely helpful to Juliana, and he persuaded his artists to take less money for the good of the cause.

Eight veterans of the first Whitney exhibition—Fraser, Lawson, Troubetz-koy, Scudder, Weir, Chanler, Hoffman, and Beaux—sent work again. Included for the first time were Glackens, Paul Manship, and John Twachtman. Also among the new invitees was a group of younger painters, several of whom would become fixtures of the Whitney Studio and Studio Club in the next few years. They were George Bellows, Eugene Speicher, Allen Tucker, Randall Davey, Guy Pène du Bois, Walt Kuhn, and William Zorach. All were disciples of Henri or Davies. There was even room for photography. Clarence White, one of the founding members of the Photo-Secession but who had broken with Stieglitz, was represented by some prints. A definite attempt was being made to branch beyond fixed points of reference, to curb an idolatrous attitude toward reputation, although one artist could not restrain his ego. Zorach, recently back from Paris in 1914 and not overwhelmed by offers to exhibit, would reminisce, "I was very happy to be invited but when I went to the opening I found my painting hanging behind the door! I was indignant and took it down and took it home.

"Mrs. Force . . . was insulted. I think she said, 'Never darken my door again.'

"I didn't but when I had my first show at Kraushaar's, Mrs. Force bought two pieces of mine, a wood carving called Pegasus* and a small panel relief. After that we were friends and comfortable with one another again."

The variety and low prices of the Christmas show made it a great success. The newspapers quoted Juliana as announcing that $10,000 was raised for the American Ambulance Hospital,† which meant that she sold $20,000 worth of art in a week—at 1914 dollars.

After this, Juliana also took on the correspondence for another nascent enterprise. Gertrude and four other wealthy and public-spirited New Yorkers banded together with the architect Thomas Hastings (of Carrère & Hastings, the firm that built the New York Public Library), the muralist Edwin Blashfield, and the sculptor C. S. Pietro to form a philanthropic society they named The Friends of the Young Artists. With a war on, the financial predicament of young, unknown American artists was worsening. Retrenchment among collectors and dealers was severe, and destitute foreign artists were arriving every day, desperate for any job. To relieve this distress, the Friends would create opportunities for young artists to show their work and receive cash prizes. These competitions would alert the public to their existence. Pietro and Gertrude emerged as the leading spirits of the committee, and most of the Friends' exhibitions were held in Gertrude's galleries under Juliana's supervision. As such, they became un-witting dry runs for future Whitney-Force practices and procedures. Any entry

---

*Pegasus, which Juliana later gave to the Whitney Museum, is dated 1925. However, Zorach's first show at Kraushaar's was in 1924.

†This figure seems overoptimistic, given the prices of most of the works. It is more probable that the $10,000 was the *total* amount of money raised. In that case, $5,000 went to the hospital.

could be submitted, regardless of aesthetic tendency, as long as it was sincere; the raw, the untried, the unready would get a chance.

The Friends moved sedately. Knowledgeable but not exciting older artists to whom Gertrude and Juliana turned as if by rote were chosen to be the first contest's jurors. The impending competition was publicized in November and December of 1914, with notices sent to the local art schools, newspapers, and the Metropolitan. Five sets of prizes were offered, and the winning designs in painting, sculpture, and architecture would be shown at West Eighth Street from January 16 to 24, 1915. Admission was to be charged for the benefit of families of French artists.

The categories of entries were strictly dictated by the Friends. The sculpture had to be allegorical. Apprentice sculptors were to submit plaster casts of up to three figures depicting "The Struggle"; art students were asked for a single figure of "Youth." Painters had to come with a decorative picture of "Philosophy" for a lecture hall. Architects collaborating with sculptors had to design a model of a mantelpiece for an actors' clubhouse. Those working with painters had to devise a dining room.

The combination of narrowly designated subject matter and a prospectus that did not spell out practical or formal specifications led to dire confusion. Juliana was bombarded with inquiries from artists requesting entry blanks and better directions. "Is the figure of Youth *necessarily* a *standing* one?" one Philadelphia student wanted to know. "Is there any objection to two students using the same model? We feel we can hardly afford a model many hours except this way. *Must* it be a nude figure?" Hugh Ferriss, who competed in the architecture division, asked for detailed instructions about proportions and elevations that revealed his knowledgeability and the sponsors' lack of it. Nevertheless, figures got modeled, sketches drawn, and fifty finalists were culled from 200 contestants. Saul Baizerman took one of the student prizes, and 800 visitors passed through. Because nothing was for sale, only $142 was raised for war relief. But that first competition was judged to be good exposure for the participants and worth repeating.

Along with aiding war victims, Gertrude and Juliana were interested in inaugurating a varied agenda of exhibitions in the Whitney Studio. From February 2 to 16, 1915, they borrowed a significant portion of a private collection. The lender was thirty-four-year-old Albert Eugene Gallatin, a patrician New Yorker (he was the great-grandson and namesake of the second Secretary of the Treasury) who had already made a mark as an art writer and connoisseur. In the 1920s he would champion Picasso, Léger, Braque, Neo-Plasticism, and Constructivism, but in 1915 his tastes coincided with Gertrude's. They both admired The Eight, American and French Impressionism, Whistler, and Tonalism, although Gallatin's eye was already astuter and more historically conditioned.

Gallatin was devoting much of his energy to war relief, and when Gertrude proposed a loan show of eighty of his paintings, drawings, and etchings for the benefit of the Fraternité des Artistes Fund, he consented. He chose the show, hanging "intimate documents" that would illuminate the artists' working pro-

cesses. Internationalism was a subordinate theme because artists from ten different countries were selected, although the bulk of the exhibition was American and French. With works by Cassatt, Hassam, Steichen, Shinn, Glackens, Lawson, Luks, Daumier, Degas, Forain, Manet, Fantin-Latour, Rodin, and Puvis, the caliber of the Gallatin holdings was admirable, and the general opinion was that of the *American Art News*: "It is one of the most agreeable exhibitions yet held for foreign artists, suffering from the war's effects. The owner, whose unusual taste and knowledge are well known, has collected his treasures con amore. There is an 'intime' and delightful atmosphere to the display, that well repays a visit."

This estimable show was followed, alas, by one that sank to the level of calendar art. The first one-man show at the Whitney Studio went to Warren Davis, a painter and pastelist whose forte was "neo-classical designs of auburn-haired nymphs dancing in draperies against backgrounds of russet, black or gold." Davis was much admired for his "refined" nudes, meaning that their bodies were hairless and nearly breastless. Juliana hung the pastels in the front galleries, against red velvet hangings, and the oils upstairs. Davis, who went on to produce many versions of nudes wafting here and there for the covers of *Vanity Fair*, has since slipped from view.

Gertrude returned from Paris in mid-March of 1915. Two months later she went into deep mourning and seclusion. Her younger brother Alfred Vanderbilt was on the *Lusitania* when it was fatally torpedoed by a German submarine on May 7, 1915. He drowned after giving his life preserver to an old woman who had none. In late July Gertrude underwent an appendectomy, subsequently complicated by phlebitis. Accordingly, from May through September of 1915, Juliana assumed the brunt of the administrative and curatorial tasks demanded by two contests held under the aegis of the Friends of the Young Artists and seen at the Whitney Studio. These shows were educational experiences, with attendant ups and downs.

The May 1915 competition stipulated that entries should depict "War," an idea proposed by Daniel Chester French. Gertrude pointed out that vivid portrayals of a horrible reality did not stand much of a chance of selling. She hoped that the next competition, one for painters, would yield attractive pictures suitable for home decoration. In this she was disappointed, as the next theme was not one to inspire the Friends with jubilant visions of sales. The young artists were to execute pictures of "Labor."

Out of approximately 200 submissions, fourteen prizewinners were picked. It was reported that "the youngest competitor was a school girl of thirteen and the oldest a man of sixty who claimed the right to compete as he had only studied art for a year." Most of the offerings were descriptive scenes of men and women at a fixed task; the reviewers spoke of the "discouraging quality" of what they saw. Perhaps a discouraging assignment contributed to dreary results. Third prize of $100 was won by Eugene Higgins, who depicted a team of horses struggling to pull a loaded cart up a hill. Theresa Bernstein won one of ten

honorable mentions of $25 with a factory scene, and Louis Bouché took another with a canvas of dockworkers straining against a gigantic ship. Along with the distribution of some money to young painters, another benefit of the show was an acquaintance with Higgins and Bouché. Higgins was then married to the satirist Mabel Dwight, and she eventually worked as a receptionist for Juliana. Bouché, a tall, mustachioed dandy who liked sauntering up Fifth Avenue in his best English suit, bowler hat, and matching pearl-gray kid gloves and spats, became a charter member of the Whitney Studio Club and a favorite guest at Juliana's parties.

The Friends' commendable intentions of uncovering and spurring on budding talent were being defeated by their own rules for exhibition schemes, and some revamping was in order. The form of the enterprise could not do justice to its guiding idea. Forbes Watson, writing in the *Post*, spotted the problems in May of 1915, after he attended just two shows. Taking care to acknowledge the generosity of the founders in stirring an unresponsive public into taking an interest in fledgling artists and granting that a great many bad artists were needed to bring forth one good one, he still wondered if "the wholesale encouragement of every young person who thinks it would be nice to be an artist [is] merely adding to the bitter struggle of the rare new talent by intensifying the competition." Watson criticized the rule of preordained content more severely. "[N]o doubt many of these young artists would have been shown to greater advantage if they had been permitted to express an idea of their own, rather than to be tied down to the prescribed subject." Ranking contestants and handing out awards, he continued inexorably, "tends to encourage superficiality, exhibitionism, prize-hunting, and the quest of publicity, which are four of the deadliest enemies to lasting achievement."

For the time being, Watson's disapproval was ignored. Even with the Friends' flaws, Gertrude was satisfied with the organization's usefulness. The society had started as a service to alleviate economic suffering—indeed, throughout 1914 and 1915 *all* exhibitions held at the Whitney Studio were hatched with a charitable, patriotic, or educational motive in mind—and a service it would remain. Kindliness took precedence over connoisseurship. The Friends also took the democratic and very commonsensical view that no one could tell if someone who shone at twenty would retain his glow at thirty or forty or fifty. Besides, by limiting eligibility to beginners, they recognized that what they showed would, by definition, be immature. Last, Gertrude and the rest of the advisers were assured of the competitions' popularity among the constituency they aimed to help. Students and assistants entered each show by the hundreds. Looking back fifty years after he won an honorable mention in the first easel contest, Louis Bouché wrote proudly about it as his first artistic recognition. He had saved every clipping and piece of memorabilia connected with the occasion.

Overzealous nationalism was a primary incentive behind the Whitney Studio's next artistic function. In July of 1915 Gertrude was approached by Frances Kellor, a prominent reformer and social investigator in the city. Kellor was

heading the Society for the Americanization of Immigrants in America, an assimilationist body worried about the immigrants' adjustment (or lack of it) to the New World. The society desired an art show that would attract attention to the 13 million unnaturalized—and in consequence, unregenerately ethnic—foreign-born residents of the United States. The exhibition would celebrate America as the alembic in which alien traditions were tested and transformed, an idea popularized by *The Melting Pot*, Israel Zangwill's play of 1908, and still au courant seven years later. With luck, the Whitney show would inspire new arrivals to apply for citizenship and shed their greenhorn manners. Young artists, preferably foreign-born, would create paintings, drawings, sculptures, and posters on "the meaning of America to the Immigrant and the Immigrant to America." Visualizations of the passage through the Golden Door, with its ample quotient of moral uplift, were no more or less deadly than the themes of previous shows, but the personal alliances that would be forged from the endeavor changed Juliana's life and redirected the course of the Whitney Studio.

Gertrude agreed to host The Immigrant in America, split the expenses with the Americanization Society, donate prize money, and assemble a jury. She solicited not only Henri, but his friends and cobelievers Bellows, Tucker, and Sloan to judge the entries. This was the first time Sloan was associated with Whitney-Force activities, and the Henri contingent added some freshness to the proceedings. Of greater importance was that Sloan, Bellows, and Tucker were quickly accepted by the two women as confreres and as regulars on the Whitney exhibition roster.

Gertrude's illness and convalescence overruled a second trip to Juilly that had been scheduled for September of 1915. She stayed on Long Island, and Juliana oversaw the preliminaries to the immigration show. They met in early October to compare notes. Later in the month Juliana wrote for more guidance, but she was rebuffed. The letter was not written or signed by Gertrude herself, but Irene Givenwilson, a woman originally hired as a governess for Flora and Barbara Whitney. Of late she was doubling as a social secretary at Fifth Avenue and Old Westbury. Miss Givenwilson revered Gertrude as fervently as Juliana did, and it was not long before the two of them were engaged in a polite, low-key but nonetheless intensely felt tug-of-war for ascendancy in Gertrude's good opinion.

Irene was the uptown adversary who had a claim on Gertrude's other existence, and Juliana wanted to dethrone her. Nothing overt could be dared, for Irene was an infinitely better secretary. She was consistent and punctilious where Juliana could be erratic and forgetful. Unlike Juliana, who had grown somewhat careless in looking after minutiae once she shouldered greater responsibilities, Irene never mislaid papers or let the melancholy details escape her. She typed and saved copies of her transactions, and her correspondence files often furnish the only surviving documentation of the workings of the infant Whitney Studio. By contrast, Juliana wrote to artists and to Gertrude by hand; she was not rigorous about making copies. Those that she did make were thrown away after she no longer had a perceived need for them, and she cleaned out her files every few months. Juliana appeared to be distancing herself from the ironclad rules of the

bookkeeper and the stenographer, their vestiges a petty and disagreeable reminder of a past she was sloughing off. Concomitantly, she had a great deal invested in the view that too much practicality destroys art, instinct, and poetry.

Irene was as indispensable to Gertrude in teaching and chaperoning Flora and Barbara as Juliana was essential in securing sculpture commissions and arranging exhibitions. Each had a function in making Gertrude's life easier. On the surface they had to remain friendly. Irene herself was too intelligent for open warfare; she merely chided Juliana for oversights and mix-ups in managing the Whitney Studio. Sometimes Irene caught her rival in a messy mistake. Then she could suggest to the parties involved that they deal only with her in the future. Juliana responded by ignoring the trivial admonitions, countermanding the more intrusive proposals, and growling acerbically about Irene to her own artist-allies. She reported to them that Irene was trying to drive a wedge between herself and Gertrude. As a true daughter of the contentious Julia, she was not blameless in inciting frictions. Issues divided themselves naturally into factions and opponents for Juliana, because she took criticisms, major and minor, so personally.

Neither woman was effective in eliminating the other. The end was in a sense predetermined, and not even a close match, if Juliana could have seen the situation in a cooler light. For all her virtues, Irene had no imagination, no artistic discernment, no sense of humor, no poetry, no *dash*. Gertrude hated being bored, and being exposed to Irene for long stretches was boring. Juliana, however, lived by the self-imposed maxim "Never bore the boss." One of her missions was to make the studio hours as entertaining as any of the other compartments of Gertrude's life. But in late 1915 Irene and her encroachments seemed undetachable.

In between being vexed by Irene's perfections, Juliana was exploring exurban amenities. Barley Sheaf Farm, idyllic as it was, was then a five-hour drive from New York on roads that iced over in winter. Weekend trips were impractical, so the Forces scouted for a place closer to the city. They rented a big brick and stone house in Montclair, New Jersey, a prosperous residential town in easy commuting distance of Manhattan. With its three floors, three fireplaces, and chestnut paneling, the house fit the image of a busy dentist and his cultivated wife. Doctor and Juliana kept the apartment on East 36th Street, and they shuttled between both places.

The Immigrant in America opened on November 15, 1915. The next day Gertrude left for San Francisco to attend the Panama-Pacific Exposition, a vast fair that had a sizable group of her own sculptures on display. Juliana was entrusted once more with holding the fort. She recorded attendance figures and made sure the press knew that on weekends the show drew 250 persons daily. She was rewarded on December 2, 1915, when Frances Kellor, who had been a top committeewoman in the Progressive party, brought her chief by. Wearing a big black campaign hat and aspirating through glistening teeth, Theodore Roosevelt was paying a visit to the show.

Besides the thrill of having the ex-President of the United States as a guest, a nod from T. R. was the equivalent of a papal benison in the arts. As Roosevelt

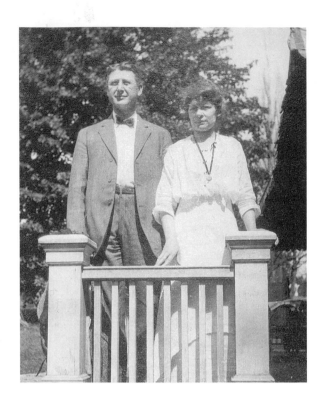

Juliana and Doctor at their house in Montclair, New Jersey, 1916. Juliana has on the same dress that she wore when Sloan painted her.

was one of the very few presidents who was well-informed about the fine arts or took them seriously,* his visits to controversial cultural ventures gave them instant credibility. He had inspected the Armory Show and attended the touring Abbey Theatre's opening performance of *The Playboy of the Western World*, which hostile Irish-Americans denounced as immoral. T. R. was ebullient about both events and his positive commentary was quoted extensively in the press.

T. R. announced to Juliana and the cadre of reporters stalking him, "My friend Royal Cortissoz said long before there was a party of that name that I had the taste of a bull moose." With that as prologue, Roosevelt, escorted by Juliana, made a brisk circuit of the galleries, emitting rapid bursts of impromptu art criticism as he went. Most of his broadsides were directed against the verdicts of the jurors. If he had his way, he said, the palm would have been awarded differently. A prize should have gone to contestant Winifred Ward for her plaster figure, *The Brow of Egypt*—a stately, columnar statue standing for, one supposes, American immigration in the Ptolemaic period. "By Jove, that Winifred Ward's a wonder!" T. R. boomed.

The party marched on. Once more T. R.'s gaze swept over the rooms and lighted on a mildly Cubist sculptural group. "If I had not seen it here," he told Juliana and the feverishly writing press corps, "I should have said those were devils."

* He was surpassed only by Thomas Jefferson.

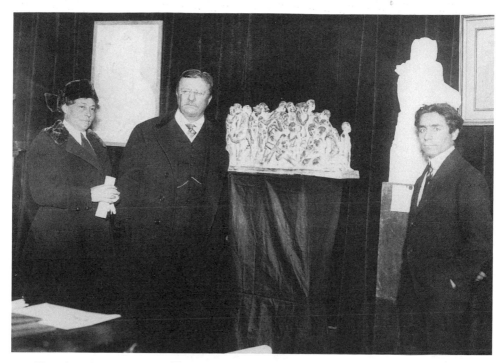

Theodore Roosevelt visiting the Immigrant in America show at the Whitney Studio. With him are Frances Kellor and Beniamino Bufano. Bufano's sculpture (center) won first prize, but T.R. preferred the statue on the right.

The finale was a photography session. T. R. refused to have his picture taken unless *The Brow of Egypt* was included. The statue was moved from its corner into position and narrowly escaped toppling off the pedestal into disaster. Roosevelt posed jovially and exited, but not before telling everyone assembled that he'd had a bully time. The newspapers, not unexpectedly, emphasized the bull-moose details of the visit. "Colonel's Big Stick Batters Cubist Art," ran the *Times* headline.

With a presidential endorsement, The Immigrant in America was an un-qualified triumph in terms of numbers of visitors, attention focused on unnat-uralized residents, and publicity for the Whitney Studio. From 1916 on, art activities emanating from West Eighth Street were covered in greater depth and detail in the popular press and the art journals.

The Immigrant in America closed on December 15, 1915, and Juliana reacted by inaugurating the tradition of a big Christmas party at West Eighth Street for artists, friends, and families in the neighborhood. Sylvia Dudley, who was born in 1909, grew up in Gramercy Park and started going to those Whitney open houses when she was a small girl. Her father was Louis Sherwin, the drama critic for the *New York World,* and both he and his wife, Ann, were Juliana's friends. Mrs. Dudley has written, "Juliana Force was a delightful and honoured

personality. She was always invited to my family's parties, but came rather to tea and small dinners, seldom to large affairs. I remember her quick trot, tailored dresses rather than suits, straying strands of hair wisping around her face. She was an elegant-looking, trim lady, even to my childish eyes. Masses of children were going to that Christmas party. My mother for her own reasons thought it better not for me to go, but Juliana Force came round herself and with a brisk, 'Nonsense, Ann,' whisked me off."

Juliana and Doctor also celebrated the holidays in Montclair with a party for the Riesers. Their house had a wide front window and Juliana set a huge tree in its bay. She trimmed it with dozens of glass icicles and white candles, which when lighted transformed the tree into a twinkling pyramid of fire and ice. Her little nieces and nephews were enthralled by the welcoming blaze and could not leave off staring at it, according to Marjorie Rieser, who remembered the sight some sixty years later.

Gertrude returned from the Panama-Pacific Exposition in early December of 1915. Apparently she was inspired by what she saw there, because she immediately began to plan a group show of "modern" paintings by American and European artists, to run from January 5 to 18, 1916. This was the first exhibition in the Whitney Studio not directly triggered by charity or proposed by an external agency. As the Studio's first independent gathering of art for art's sake, it says much about the evolution of Gertrude's tastes and her approach to the contemporary scene in 1916.

Besides relying on her own information, Gertrude called on William Macbeth and Roland Knoedler, art dealers with extensive knowledge of the whereabouts of American and European canvases. She sought the names of collectors who owned good examples of Jacques-Emile Blanche, Sorolla, Zuloaga, Zorn, Boldini, Carolus-Duran, Frederick Carl Frieseke, Charles Hawthorne, Luks, Lawson—and Cézanne and Matisse. Three years after the Armory Show, Gertrude changed her mind about the wisdom of dismissing these last two painters as "feeble impertinences." Along with providing the information Gertrude requested, Macbeth went on to recommend collectors with Redons, Van Goghs, and Gauguins, whom she did not have on her list. Arthur B. Davies, the dealer reported in another unsolicited aside, possessed excellent examples of Redon, Derain, Villon, Picasso, and "three fine marbles" by Brancusi.

The extent of the assistance Gertrude wanted from Macbeth consisted of names and addresses of owners. Matisse and Cézanne were dropped from the roster of foreign artists, and Derain, Redon, Villon, and Picasso—and even Carolus-Duran—were edged out by Besnard, Mancini, Boldini, Brangwyn, Lavery, Edmund Dulac, William Orpen, Gaston La Touche, Gennaro Favai, Lucien Simon, Sorolla, Zuloaga, and Zorn.

These choices denote an attraction toward clever, superficial, self-important painting, as well as a baggy definition of modernism. Even then the word was reserved for artists swimming in the wake of the School of Paris. Writing about the show, Forbes Watson commented that "modern" in this assemblage of talents

was used merely as a synonym for art done within "our own time, for the exhibition is practically untainted by that insistent and troublesome spirit of modernity which . . . is continually challenging the cherished tradition that a picture 'should look like something.' "

In selecting Americans whose pictures looked like something, Gertrude was more sure-footed. She was good at judging native realism, especially when it was salted with the strong local flavor of New York. The Luks she borrowed was the superb *Spielers*. Glackens with *Cafe Lafayette*, Henri with *Laughing Child* and *Herself*, Lawson with *Winter on the River*, and Bellows with *Floating Ice**were ably represented, too. Rounding out the selection was *Before Her Appearance*, a large picture of a woman at her mirror, by Frieseke, the expatriate American Impressionist, portraits by Sargent, Beaux, Hawthorne, and Cushing, fantasies by Chanler and Maxfield Parrish, nudes by the treacly Warren Davis, and watercolors by John La Farge.

Modern Paintings by American and Foreign Artists marked Gertrude's first sizable public display of her art collection, for she owned approximately half of what was in the show. Shortly after it opened, Gertrude bought *Nude with Parrot* by Bellows, *Portrait of a Man by Benjamin Kopman, and Mahonri Young's bronze, Man with Wheelbarrow.*† Her Frieseke, along with several other purchases, came from the Panama-Pacific Exposition. Notwithstanding the uneven quality of the art to be seen, New Yorkers were crowding into the Studio. Modern Paintings by American and Foreign Artists drew 1,800 people during its two-week run.

The only major Realist who had not yet shown at the Whitney Studio was John Sloan. As of January 1916, he had sold only one painting, to the Philadelphia collector Albert Barnes, and that was in 1913. (A brewer and his wife had commissioned portraits from him, but he did not consider that equivalent to a buyer of a picture freely composed.) In 1915 Sloan went so far as to send notices to 1,600 individuals and institutions offering a set of thirteen of his city etchings for $35. Two sets were sold. He had exhibited steadily and gained the respect of the more enlightened critics, but no collectors were forthcoming. Sloan was forty-four years old, and he still had not had a one-man show.

In the summer of 1915, Sloan and Dolly moved to Washington Place West, close to MacDougal Alley. Gertrude wanted him represented in the American and European paintings show, but the invitation was mailed to the old address and failed to reach him until after the opening. Sloan was chagrined by the missed chance, but he worked up his courage and wrote to Gertrude.

The Spielers is now in the collection of the Addison Gallery of American Art; *Laughing Child* is now in the collection of the Whitney Museum; *Herself* is now in the collection of the Art Institute of Chicago; *Winter on the River* and *Floating Ice* are now in the collection of the Whitney Museum.

†*Portrait of a Man* and *Man with Wheelbarrow* are now in the collection of the Whitney Museum.

May I take the opportunity of asking you to consider giving me a "one man show" in your galleries? The dealers in the city are not inclined to show more than one or two of my pictures at any one time—most of them not at all—and I feel that a collection shown together would be, at least, an artistic success, and might attract considerable public notice.

Should you care to talk of the matter or see my work I will be greatly favored.

The proposal appealed to Gertrude, though in her reply to Sloan she hedged that his show would have to take place late in the season. On January 11, 1916, Sloan called on her. His conversation must have swayed her to hold the show as soon as possible—she magnanimously moved the date of the first New York showing of her own sculpture, which had been set to follow the painting show, to late February. Sloan's work was to be shown from January 26 through February 16. Within three weeks of asking, the artist was preparing for his first one-man show.

Historically, the Sloan retrospective—for it turned out to be a thorough survey of his time in New York, thanks to the unrestricted hand he was given in selecting what he wanted seen—was the most important exhibition sponsored by the Whitney Studio in its fledgling years. Gertrude's old ties to The Eight were reinvigorated; the future spirit and orientation of Juliana's exhibition policies were announced. Sloan's show was the most provocative seen at the Whitney Studio since the Gallatin collection a year before. And with twenty-one paintings, sixteen etchings, three lithographs, four monotypes, and forty drawings, the exhibition was as comprehensive as it was worthy. The oils gave an extensive account of the painter's free and easy grasp of his milieu and his acuity in evoking character and atmosphere. They ranged from scenes painted the summer before in Gloucester, Massachusetts, where Sloan had experimented with plein air painting and Post-Impressionist brushwork, to the dark, trenchant genre pictures that have become emblems of the roundness and savor of old New York life.*

As the art press knew, Sloan was in a different league from Warren Davis, the sole other recipient of a one-man show to date, and the event was covered as it deserved. The *Herald*, the *Sun*, the *Brooklyn Eagle*, and the monthly *Arts and Decoration* filed reviews of unalloyed praise. While Forbes Watson in the *Post* had reservations about the oils, he had nothing but congratulations for Sloan's etchings: "He is in another world from the dealer's etcher who works up architectural landmarks from photographs. As first-hand observation and humorous comment on the life of the streets and tenements Mr. Sloan's etchings have a place all their own in American art." The *Globe*, however, regretted that Sloan "presents too often the squalor and sordid aspects of life," yet allowed that "his sincerity of purpose justifies the ugliness of his themes."

Sloan's art had been put before the public, but nothing sold from his show. Yet lack of sales didn't disappoint Sloan, for his visibility at the Whitney Studio

---

*Some of the canvases shown, now in public collections, were *The Haymarket* (Brooklyn Museum), *Three A.M.* (Philadelphia Museum of Art), *Isadora Duncan* (Milwaukee Art Museum), *Carmine Theater* (Hirshhorn Museum and Sculpture Garden), and *Six O'Clock, Winter* (Phillips Collection).

brought him long-term benefits of much value. He wrote to Gertrude, "For it is quite due to the prestige which my exhibition at 8 W. 8 established that I have passed through the most successful winter of my career and I have many reasons to hope that next season may pass it in results—Mr. Kraushaar is to handle my etchings and paintings as well—his attention was quite surely attracted to my works by my 'Whitney Show.' " Kraushaar Galleries went on to represent Sloan for the rest of his life, and the firm still handles his artistic estate.

Having Sloan noticed by a dealer was the ideal result, as envisioned by Gertrude and Juliana. An artist was to be given a boost, which, with any luck or justice, would flow into a commission, a berth in a gallery, or a perceptive write-up by a critic. Soon enough the two women had reason to be as grateful to Sloan as he was to them. Without him, their progress would have been somewhat less direct and much less fun. Gertrude had been the first to clear away a new road to freedom, and Juliana had widened and fortified it, yet in 1916 the women were stumbling toward a dead end. But Sloan providentially came along with his talent and his wit and his fighting spirit, to steer them straight into the exuberance of the highway.

Through assembling and hanging the works in his exhibition, Sloan and Juliana became friends. "Sloan was a salient figure from the early days of the Whitney-Force activities," wrote Watson. He said Juliana and Sloan got along like a house afire because both had in abundance a "happy combination of wit and scrappiness," which made being in their company "so gay." Juliana derived great pleasure and came by much education from listening to Sloan. He was short on tact, long on rapid, puncturing argument, and erupting with novel ideas about art and life. His self-described "tabasco tongue" was a match for her own.

That Sloan reciprocated with equal warmth can be seen in the portrait of Juliana* that he began painting not long after his Whitney show. Wearing a soft white dress and seated next to a vase sparsely filled with sprigs of spring blossoms, she radiates compassion and thoughtful sympathy. The likeness is unique for the sweetness of her gaze. Later on, painters emphasized the fierce and commanding facets of her character that had crept into her face; in 1916, however, Juliana had an unmarked, almost girlish aspect about her, despite the fact that she had just turned thirty-nine. Watson, who got to know Juliana in 1917, stated that his first impression of her was of "a romantic little girl."

One touch of humor in the picture, a private joke in compositional guise, may lie in the old-fashioned straw hat trimmed with flowers that rests on Juliana's lap. It seems to have migrated intact from Glackens's *Nude with Apple*† of 1910. Such a colorful hat would have been a useful studio prop and perhaps Sloan borrowed it from his friend Glackens for a foil to the pale dress Juliana wore.

The portrait was lightly undertaken. As Sloan had invited Juliana to sit for him, he was under no obligation to complete the picture. The portrait was only sketchily laid in when he gave it up because he was having trouble with the

* Now in the Whitney Museum.
† Now in the collection of the Brooklyn Museum.

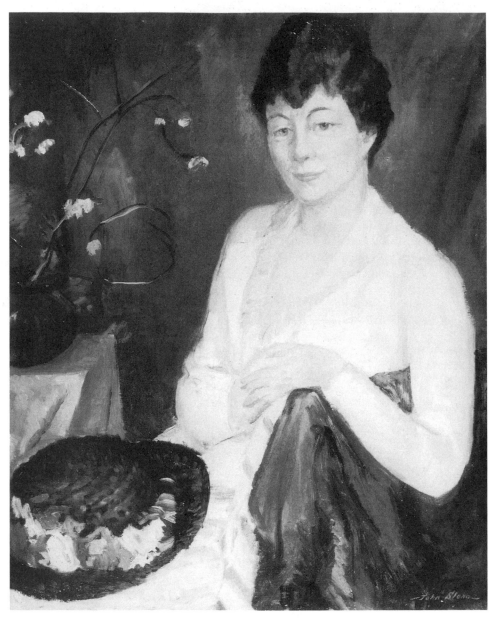

Sloan began this portrait of Juliana in 1916 after his one-man show at the Whitney Studio, but didn't complete it until 1949.

perspective. Sloan's studio on Washington Place was so small that he could not move far enough away from the sitter to judge the proportions correctly. Juliana's unfinished portrait stayed as it was in the artist's studio until after her death. Then, in 1949, he was moved to repair the distortions.

The look of empathy and concern rendered in paint mirrored Juliana's impressions as she sat for her sessions at the Sloans'. If she had not realized the painter's problems before, she became painfully attuned to them now, with prolonged occasions for observing the household. Dolly Sloan was an incorrigible alcoholic, prone to scenes, blackouts, delirium tremens, and disappearances. Her drinking caused or was brought on by a manic-depressive disorder that a physician who examined her said was "too deep-seated to be cured." Two drinks changed her personality. She would metamorphose from a loving, loyal helper into a terrifying and unreasoning stranger, or she would vanish for long stretches of time. Sloan was under constant stress, as he never knew what the next day would bring. Juliana felt protective of the artist and his wife. She was not alienated or embarrassed by Dolly's illnesses. In Dolly's good moments Juliana was very fond of her, and she pretended not to notice the bad spells. She did notice, of course, and those memories would stay with her.

Juliana was also initiated into the happier side of the Sloans' world. They had all kinds of diversified friendships with people in art, literature, and politics. One of the most captivating acquaintances she made through the Sloans was that of John Butler Yeats, the charming, impecunious painter and father of all the Yeatses. The elder Yeats arrived in New York at the close of 1907, his announced intention to indulge in a holiday of a few weeks. But in Manhattan he found himself free to read, write letters, sketch, take long walks, drink wine, smoke cigars, and philosophize, unfettered by the debts and family responsibilities that dogged him in Dublin. Sloan said that Yeats preferred the "hopeful penury" he enjoyed in the United States to the "hopeless penury" he endured in Ireland. Within two or three months of his New York debut, he was a sought-after dinner guest and had transcended his Dublin status of superannuated father to famous sons. Yeats then slipped into his long, artfully guileless, and ultimately victorious maneuver of perpetually deferring his return to Ireland. As Henri said, "Yeats was an old man who ran away from home and succeeded."

Nominally Yeats affected to live by his pencil sketches and portrait commissions, as well as an infamous self-portrait commissioned by John Quinn, the country's leading collector of modern art and his principal patron. This last work of art was, in Helen Vendler's words, "his Penelope's web." The picture was never finished, but always begun, scraped out, and begun again. Its main utility, as the disarming old man discovered, was its magnificence as an excuse for doing or not doing whatever he pleased. His expenses were surreptitiously paid by William Butler Yeats and Quinn, the latter fruitlessly attempting to export his charge to Ireland. These two furnished Yeats with financial support; for emotional solace he depended on the Sloans, who nursed and coddled him in a hundred ways.

The Sloans liked to take Yeats for airings outside New York. On April 21, 1916, Yeats wrote to Quinn, "I am off this afternoon to Montclair with the

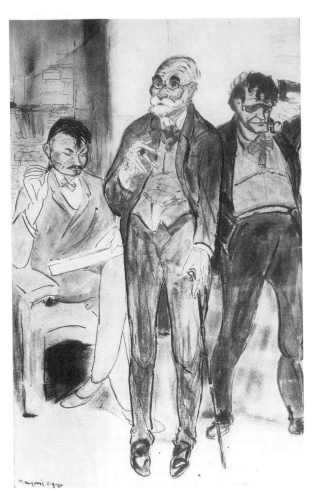

Before she married Henri in 1908, Marjorie Organ had been a cartoonist for the *Journal* and the *World*. Here she caricatures her husband, seen with John Butler Yeats and Sloan.

Sloans, to stay till Monday. I don't know the names of the people, but I am told they are delightful." Unbeknownst to him, the couple he was describing were the Forces. After Yeats returned, he was fizzing with good reports about the weekend, writing two letters to Quinn about it during the course of one day. Of his hosts Yeats said, "There could not be nicer people."

While in New Jersey Yeats had sketched Juliana and made a slight pen-and-ink copy of it for Quinn's benefit at the top of his second dispatch. Below the portrait he wrote, "I had one 'success' at Montclair—our hostess is not suitable for photography except as its victim, yet really a woman charming to look upon and I made a successful sketch." Regrettably, the original pencil portrait has disappeared, so we cannot judge the artist's success for ourselves, but Yeats's perception of Juliana's homeliness being vanquished by her personal spark was the first of many such reactions. His impression tallies closely with that of Margaret McKellar, a former registrar of the Whitney Museum, who began her

career there as a secretary in 1940. The first time she laid eyes on Juliana she thought she was the ugliest woman she had ever seen in her life. Within two days at the Whitney, McKellar was so awed by Juliana's manners, actions, and way of dressing and carrying herself that she asked for a photograph of her to adorn the top of her desk. She now considered Juliana one of the handsomest women she knew.

The Forces, once the initial introduction was made, began going to hear Yeats talk at Petitpas', the boardinghouse and restaurant at 317 West 29th Street where he lived and held court. Juliana and Doctor responded heartily to this picturesque figure, and they became regulars at the Yeats table. Besides the Sloans, their fellow diners were the Henris, the Glackenses, and Bellows, as well as Van Wyck Brooks, the art critic Mary Fanton Roberts, her husband William Carman Roberts, who was editor of *The Literary Digest*, and Heywood Broun, the newspaperman. That Yeats was a painter seemed secondary to Juliana. She enjoyed him as a sage, but one devoid of pomposity because of his optimism, his accent on the young, and his unbroken spirit. "Don't daunten youth," Juliana liked to caution audiences, proud to identify the source of the saying as her old friend John Butler Yeats.

Sloan's gregariousness pulled Juliana into other circles. He had long been an active socialist, even running as a party candidate for state assemblyman in 1910 and 1915. Although he quit the party in the spring of 1916, he remained sympathetic to its objectives and to political radicalism in general. Sloan shared his enthusiasms with his friends, which occasionally led to some pretty unusual get-togethers. In his book about The Eight, Ira Glackens told this story:

> Sloan was a friend, though not a follower, of Emma Goldman, the anarchist. Art makes strange bedfellows, for there occurred a dinner at which Miss Goldman, Sloan, Mrs. Harry Payne Whitney and Juliana Force were all present. As soon as she was served, Emma Goldman started to eat. Then she noticed that everyone else was waiting until all were served. She said, "Excuse me, I learned my manners in jail."

The incongruity of this encounter—the direct descendant of Cornelius Vanderbilt breaking bread with the notorious anarchist whose lover once tried to assassinate Henry Clay Frick—illuminates a vital facet of Juliana's relationship to Gertrude and what Forbes Watson called "the serious subject of boredom." Particularly in the year of 1916, Gertrude's ennui and frustration were becoming dangerously high. Because the war ruled out another trip to France, she was trapped in America until the fighting was unequivocally over. In New York she had to face the verdict on her sculpture retrospective, which opened on February 18 to reviews implying that she was little more than a banal technician. The impact of these brickbats may have been softened by a letter from Daniel Chester French, who, among other things, was the chairman of the Metropolitan's sculpture committee. In this capacity he asked if he might buy a bronze of *Head of a Spanish Peasant* from the Whitney Studio show. A cast entered the permanent collection of the Metropolitan in May 1916.

From May to December of 1916, the Whitney Studio was dormant. During those intervening months and subsequent fallow periods, no small part of Juliana's job lay in the delicate art of human relations. Much of her time centered on making Gertrude's studio more absorbing than the life away from it and acting as a counterweight to the social influences undermining Gertrude's concentration on artistic pursuits. This task was not easy, but neither was it dull. Juliana was unflaggingly interested in what she was accomplishing, and she believed in Gertrude. At one level, Juliana was to develop the market for Gertrude's commissions, improve and expand her art collection, and prompt the creativity of young painters and sculptors. At another, she was to create an interest for Gertrude that society was incapable of supplying and which she couldn't obtain by herself on account of her position and disposition.

Juliana did not go about her business unopposed. Irene Givenwilson's quiet but insistent pressure was bothersome, but nothing compared to the leverage of the uptown crowd of Whitney friends and relatives. Their opinions, conveyed to Gertrude without hesitation, fell into two camps. Some thought the Whitney Studio futile, a waste of time and money. It was still very much a testing ground in 1916, often directionless and error-prone, and Gertrude and her manager were criticized for not unveiling sensational short-term results. Nothing seemed to be paying off. Others saw the Studio as a sweet display case for their own favorites. Society artists, often with titles, arrived bearing letters of introduction from the fashionable on both sides of the Atlantic, and they were infiltrating the Eighth Street galleries.

The most intricate conflicts for Juliana, and those on which a duller person would have foundered, were the ones generated by Gertrude's own warring nature. Juliana had to keep in mind how swiftly bored her employer was, how easily she could shift to other diversions that would remove her physically and psychologically from sculpture and the art life. If the dimensions of the Whitney Studio—and Juliana's creative needs—were to be fulfilled, Gertrude "was not to be bored except when constructively necessary." Even so, the quest for her attention was intimidating because Gertrude was in incessant demand in social circles and could sample any entertainment the world had to offer. Fifth Avenue, Newport, Long Island, the Adirondacks, and Palm Beach were all at her disposal, and sometimes she was lost to them.

Moreover, Gertrude's makeup contained elements that Juliana could not amend, particularly her refusal to accept for herself the principle that art was not a profession she could pick up and drop at will, but a completely encompassing and self-defining existence. Gertrude did not put in the day-to-day hard thought and labor that art exacts. She believed she could leave her sculpture behind her when she commuted to and from her various spheres; she believed that her art would not suffer much from her desertions. However, Gertrude was not impervious to the requirements of competent sculpture, and she would go into fits of depression over her shortcomings. Such times, when Gertrude's continuing struggle to sustain a career caused a great strain, were dark ones for Juliana and the Studio. So much of Gertrude's courage was absorbed by the effort to live differently from the rest of the Vanderbilts and Whitneys, who

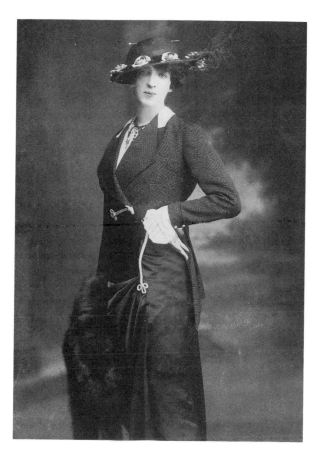

Gertrude in Paris in 1914,
living the life she desired.

never believed she would stick to what she was doing. Perhaps this was why so little intensity or risk was left over for her art. At these moments, Juliana needed all her finesse to reassure. "I should not, perhaps, be doing the work I am today," Gertrude was to say, "if it were not for the battle I've had to fight to show that I'm not merely amusing myself."

Gertrude's wealth was also an adversity, as it still occasionally created a powerful undertow of frustration and lack of purpose. Rubbing shoulders with people her parents would never have dreamed of entertaining helped ward off boredom. But Juliana preferred to introduce new faces through the widening and diversifying of aid to artists. Gertrude's generosity was seconded and expanded by Juliana, who loved performing benevolent acts. As she sifted deserving from fraudulent claims, she was on the watch for promising young people in need. Money went to Frederick G. R. Roth, a sculptor of animals who had exhibited in the Panama-Pacific Exhibition and wrote to Gertrude about his financial plight. For the first time, women received some assistance, too: Helen Farnsworth Mears, a former pupil of Saint-Gaudens who was near starvation; Laura McLane,

another sculptor; and Winifred Ward, whose statue Teddy Roosevelt had singled out while visiting the Immigrant in America show.

The bounty was a godsend to the four who received it, but it did not quite satisfy Juliana. Buying a work of art, even when a masterpiece was not involved, was better than handing out money for nothing received. (The women still had no thought of a museum; art was acquired not so much to establish a collection, as to help those who were trying to maintain themselves as artists.) Yet why stop at buying or giving? Juliana reasoned. Her growing intimacy with artists in straitened circumstances developed insights into means of providing assistance, dignified means that she would foster and build upon in years to come. Securing advances for artists from Gertrude and other wealthy persons she had come to know, getting them teaching jobs, framing their pictures or casting their sculptures for an exhibition, selling their works elsewhere—these were some of Juliana's ingenious emendations to conventional patronage.

Juliana's parties, which were unfolding beyond those long Sunday mornings into dinners and suppers and late-afternoon get-togethers as she befriended more and more artists, also did much to lift both women's spirits. The guests were men whom Gertrude knew first—Henri, Chanler, Campbell, and Gifford Beal. Or, they were painters Juliana met through their inclusion in Studio shows. The Sloans fit this latter category, as did William and Edith Glackens, a pair she adored. Another regular was Bellows, with his wide-eyed and often strident excitement about all things native. (Bellows, Watson once quipped, "was American as donuts, and not much more subtle.") Two of Bellows's friends were in and out of Juliana's apartment, too—Eugene Speicher, a handsome, athletic man who was on the brink of a lucrative career as a portraitist, and Randall Davey, a particularly snappy member of the group. Davey had done some vaudeville on Broadway, and Juliana, who delighted in theatrical people, was taken with his singing, jokes, and mimicry. Another instant favorite was Guy Pène du Bois. Gertrude and Juliana were fond of this painter's hard-boiled social satires of New York nobs and strivers. Du Bois was also an excellent writer, and from 1913 to 1915 and 1918 to 1921 he edited *Arts and Decoration*, a freewheeling monthly that had been the first journal to support the Armory Show. He was an affable, raffish sort who didn't mind loafing, especially when cocktails and gossip were in the offing, and he basked in Juliana's welcome. Quieter foils to these extroverts were Allen Tucker, a landscape painter with an ear for music and poetry, and Henry Schnakenberg, who entered Juliana's life when one of his canvases was accepted for The Immigrant in America. (Everyone except Sloan and Schnakenberg had shown in one or both benefit exhibitions of 1914.) This close-knit circle of artists, nearly all of them associates or ex-students of Henri, constituted the second (and last) wave of artists who knew Gertrude at all. (The earlier group, which she met between 1900 and 1916, consisted of elder statesmen of the art world, her teachers and mentors, the Beaux-Arts sculptors of the heroic and the ideal, the Paris expatriates, and her MacDougal Alley neighbors.) The majority of the artists, most notably the younger ones coming into the Whitney fold from 1917 onward, did not mingle with Gertrude.

They glimpsed her at openings and big receptions, but their firsthand dealings were with Juliana.

The Whitney Studio's location was Juliana's confederate in diversion, for the Village had heated up in the teens. More artists, poets, novelists, musicians, actors, composers, and dramatists moved there, hoping to make the area an American equivalent of the Left Bank and the Latin Quarter.

Rebelliousness, shallow and serious, was in full simmer downtown. In 1916 George Cram Cook established on MacDougal Street the Provincetown Players, the first theater group to stage the plays of Eugene O'Neill. *The Masses* (with illustrations contributed by Sloan, Henri, Glackens, Bellows, Stuart Davis, Glenn O. Coleman, Boardman Robinson, and Art Young) had its headquarters in the Village, as did several less consequential periodicals. In 1917 *The Little Review* was transplanted from Chicago to 27 West Eighth Street, above the Washington Square Bookshop (a cozy haunt for writers) and diagonally across from the Whitney Studio.

Villagers relaxed in clubs, cafés, coffeehouses, bookstores, and saloons. The Liberal Club, a MacDougal Street hot spot, featured earnest free-for-all discussions, advanced art on the walls, and the presence of women with short-cropped hair and rolled stockings. The queen of eating establishments was the dining room of the Brevoort Hotel, at Eighth Street and Fifth Avenue. This was where Gertrude and Juliana customarily lunched. The cuisine, service, and atmosphere were pungently French. Louise Varèse called it "Paris in New York" and remembered the café and lounge as swarming "with the usual American artist habitués, that is, all the drinking intelligentsia of New York."

The feeling of bravado was given affectionate graphic expression by Sloan in his etching *Arch Conspirators* (1917), which commemorates a legendary episode in Village history. One January night in 1917, an art student named Gertrude Drick led Sloan, Marcel Duchamp (temporarily, another Eighth Street resident), and several actors from the Provincetown Players company to a door she had discovered at the base of the Washington Square Arch. (Drick, in good bohemian style, chose to be known as "Woe" so she could introduce herself as "Woe is me.") Provisioned with candles, balloons, Chinese lanterns, hot drinks, sandwiches, and hot water bottles to sit on, the revelers climbed to the top of the arch for a nocturnal picnic. "A document," Sloan said, "was drawn up to establish the secession of Greenwich Village from the United States and claiming protection of President Wilson as one of the small nations." Then, looking northward up Fifth Avenue, he declared the Village a free republic, independent of uptown.

Interactions among Village artists were fluid and densely overlapping, enhancing the collegial ambiance of the neighborhood. Bellows, for instance, had once roomed with O'Neill, and Charles Demuth and William Zorach were charter members of the Provincetown Players. O'Neill often drank at the Golden Swan saloon, a Sixth Avenue dive nicknamed the Hell Hole, and O'Neill at the Hell Hole was a subject illustrated by Demuth and Sloan. The Hell Hole also found its way into *The Iceman Cometh*, as Harry Hope's saloon. Theodore Dreiser, who moved to West Tenth Street in 1914, collected background in-

formation for his novel *The "Genius"* (1915), by visiting the nearby studios of Sloan and Everett Shinn.

Juliana spent the summer of 1916 away from Village enticements. Gertrude asked her to work in Newport for July, August, and part of September because of a busy schedule. Flora Whitney was coming out, and that special occasion demanded superhuman hospitality from Gertrude and Harry: parties, receptions, dances, teas, breakfasts, luncheons, and dinners. B. H. Friedman estimated that the Whitneys entertained between 700 and 1,000 people over the month of August alone. To accommodate their guests, Gertrude had a ballroom added to the house.

Gertrude also had consented to furnish the Newport Art Association (now the Newport Art Museum) with an exhibition for the high season that would open on August 29. What she sent to Newport was essentially a reprise of the two surveys held at the Studio in the beginning of 1916—the "modern" American and European paintings show was supplemented with her own retrospective. As she had done before, Juliana was to install the art and make sure the show ran smoothly. Diagrams written in her hand indicate that the floor plans went through multiple drafts before she and Gertrude were satisfied. The galleries were spread over two floors, and in the hall downstairs, Juliana intermingled paintings and small sculptures. (The large models for Gertrude's memorials and fountains were placed on the lawn.) Upstairs, etchings and watercolors had a room to themselves, and Gertrude's statues were in another, "arranged with candles against a green background."

Juliana must have liked observing Newport at close range. At Gertrude's invitation, she stayed at the Whitney cottage on Bellevue Avenue, the millionaires' promenade. Though her participation in social affairs would be limited, the beach, the cliffs, and the sea stretched before her. Doctor did not accompany her, but some of the isolation was mitigated by the fact that although Juliana was with Gertrude, Irene was not. She had been sent to France as Gertrude's emissary to straighten out problems that had arisen at the field hospital. Assigning Irene to Juilly meant not only removing her from the art sphere, but thrusting her into a whole different set of urgencies. If any event signaled the beginning of Irene's withdrawal from the field as Juliana's professional rival, it was this one. Irene would return to Fifth Avenue and her typewriter. She would perform her duties impeccably, but she did not recover her former standing.

At the end of 1916 the Forces gave up the lease on the Montclair house and made their Manhattan apartment their primary residence again. By then Juliana had renewed her friendship with the Sloans, as a print in the Whitney's collection indicates. The museum's etching of *Girl and Beggar* (1910) is inscribed to Juliana by Sloan. He and Dolly brought the signed print—and John Butler Yeats—to a party the Forces gave on December 23. That was the actual date of Juliana's birth, but she preferred to observe the day on December 25. (Within a few years,

Christmas Day was the only date she would admit as her birthday. She would celebrate the day by combining it with the Christmas party at the Whitney—an open house that started about 11 A.M. with a champagne breakfast, was sustained by an excellent punch, and didn't break up until 2:00 or 3:00 the next morning.)

Juliana's fortieth birthday party—not that she disclosed that secret—began festively enough, but the atmosphere grew tense after Sloan, a pacifist, brought up politics and war. His incendiary views—would it matter so much to the workingman if Germany won the war?—upset everyone present, according to Yeats, who complained to his daughter Lily:

> Sloan started holding forth on war and on Germans and his object seemed to be to insult and humiliate everyone. His wife sat in indignant silence. I overheard the hostess asking her if she was enjoying herself and she replied, "No, I am not." "Ah, why?" "Because of Sloan.". . . he must have seen how bored we all were.

Any ill feelings Juliana harbored blew over, and she and Sloan were soon friends again. He had blundered into a sensitive area, but she realized that his rhetoric sprang from passionate convictions that could not be contained. Gertrude and Juliana supported the Allies unconditionally—that was common knowledge. Yet Sloan was unlikely to know of Juliana's uneasiness about her German ancestry or her antipathy to her brother Max's hectoring socialism.

Temperamentally and politically, Juliana found socialism abhorrent. She was too much the idiosyncratic, intuitive individualist to believe in systems, especially those based on collectivism. She was too much the self-reliant Emersonian to approve of social engineering of any sort. But in general, Juliana was as indifferent to politics and political movements as Sloan was consumed by them. She was content to adopt many of Gertrude's views as her own. A staunch Republican who admired Theodore Roosevelt, Juliana would later dismiss his cousin Franklin as "that man in the White House." The sole political cause outside the arena of art and artists she is known to have advocated and demonstrated for was women's suffrage. According to Rieser family stories, in the early teens Juliana marched in the great suffrage parades up Fifth Avenue and carried a banner.

Juliana was not a thoroughgoing feminist. Her habit of mind was to reach out to individuals expressly affected by trouble or injustice rather than theorize about larger systems of oppression. But she believed unshakably in the equality of women, especially in the workplace and in the struggle for creative recognition. Carl Rieser said of his aunt, "She believed in applying the same standards to men and women alike. She would never use the once-familiar 'aviatrix' any more than she would say 'painteress.' Years later, as a museum director, she refused to hold special exhibits for women artists on the grounds that this was condescending to women." Little need existed for having such exhibitions at the Whitney because women were significantly represented (between 30 and 35 percent) in group shows, one-artist shows, and the permanent collection.

When it came to art insurgency, Sloan and Juliana agreed entirely, and here she was prepared to listen receptively. The cardinal principle on which they

were united was independence: Artists should be free to choose their own way of working. Sloan, Henri, du Bois, Schnakenberg, and Tucker—the artists who had Gertrude and Juliana's ears—were also united in their hatred of the prize system. Awarding prizes to artists, they argued, as Watson had in 1915, aroused a false sense of competition and perpetuated the self-congratulatory trappings of academic hierarchies. In their view, it was a spurious, gaudy trick to catch the public interest, and one which lofted the "victorious" works into a fictitious notoriety. Most perniciously, jockeying for prizes forced artists to please the judges before they pleased themselves.

In late 1916 Henri and Sloan exerted their influence to reform the procedure of shows sponsored by the Friends of the Young Artists. Instead of handing out prizes and then sending the contenders home with their works of art, they suggested that the only dignified way to reward artists was to *buy* what they made. A purchase was the more sincere and the longer-lasting gesture of faith in someone's talent; it would also build up and generate collections.

The war cry of "no juries, no prizes," although dear to the hearts of Henri and Sloan, was not their brainchild. The premise originated in 1884 with the French Société des Artistes Indépendants, an artist-run exhibition cooperative *independent* of selection committees that became a haven for painters too radical for the Paris Salon. Seurat, Signac, Redon, Van Gogh, and Henri Rousseau— all Salon rejectees—took their canvases to the Independents' annual shows.

Independence also happened to be in the air in 1916 because the art critic Walter Pach was spearheading a movement to start an American version of the French group. Pach worked on organizing it throughout 1916, with advice from Glackens, Maurice Prendergast, Morton Schamberg, and several French artists living in New York on account of the war—Marcel Duchamp, his brother Jacques Villon, Francis Picabia, and Albert Gleizes. The Society of Independent Artists came into being in late 1916, with Glackens selected as the first president and John Quinn as legal adviser. Gertrude put up $1,500 to defray expenses for the inaugural exhibition, to open in April of 1917, and she entered a cast of her figure for the *Titanic* memorial.

The society and its first show, which contained 2,125 entries, leapt into art and social history through the serious whimsy of Duchamp. To test the much-vaunted guarantee that any object submitted by a member (someone who had paid $5.00 in annual dues and an initiation fee of $1.00) was automatically accepted for public display, he anonymously submitted an upside-down urinal. It was titled *Fountain* and signed "R. Mutt." The directors were in an angry quandary about what to do with this controversial article, and arguments about artistic freedom raged. They eventually rejected the piece, which was then spirited away to Stieglitz's gallery for safekeeping.* After *Fountain*'s removal, the harmony between the directors was shattered, and Glackens stepped down from the presidency. The office was assumed by Sloan, who remained in it until 1944, when the society ceased to exhibit. The Independents survived *Fountain* and earned a reputation as a legitimate addition to the spring art season in New

---

* *Fountain* has since disappeared.

York. Their annuals, which consistently offered new discoveries, were backed by forward-looking critics like Watson and Henry McBride of the *Sun*.

Because it evolved out of a concern for the betterment of American art and was headed by men they liked and trusted, the Society of Independent Artists became a regular beneficiary of the spreading net of Whitney-Force philanthropies. Between 1921 and 1930 Gertrude was the most generous contributor to the society, which was perennially in debt. Sloan would tell Juliana how much money he needed, Juliana would report to Gertrude, and Gertrude would erase the deficit. Sloan illustrated their arrangement in a cartoon he sent Juliana one spring. In it the artist-president, of grimacing mien, rescues a squalling baby representing the independent artists from a huge pail of red ink. He writes below—"Dear Mrs. Force:—In it again! Help! Help! Details enclosed." Gertrude's annual payments ranged from $784.90 to $2,000. Juliana also contributed to the Independents' treasury with money of her own in 1919, 1920, and 1939–1942.

The Independents' example fed into the reshaping of the Friends. Sloan modestly guessed that "[p]erhaps it was through the influence of the Independents that she [Gertrude] and Mrs. Force made a change in the policy of the Friends of the Young Artists." Unfortunately, that change was not as rapid as Gertrude and Juliana wished. The other board members were loath to change the format because the prize money for the next show, in February of 1917, was already

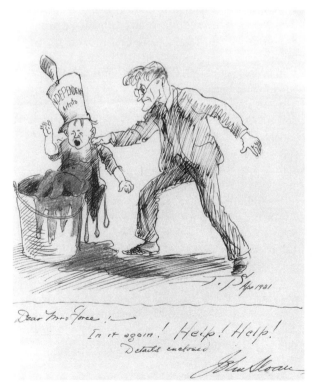

In Sloan's sketch, dated April 1931, he is determinedly pulling the Independents out of a pail of red ink.

collected. However, they agreed that the new policy could go into effect afterward.

Determined to rehabilitate the Friends, Gertrude used the occasion of its latest opening, on February 19, 1917, to distribute a manifesto. She spelled out the predicament young artists faced, declared the new policy of no juries and no prizes, and characterized the customary method of rewarding artistic ability as demeaning.

> The annual exhibitions of the various established societies are already overcrowded, and the private galleries seldom accept the works of unknown men, so that by organizing such exhibitions, as we have done, . . . we bring before the public work which they otherwise would have no opportunity of seeing and estimating. . . .
>
> After this competition we intend to adopt a new scheme in regard to our exhibitions. There will be no prizes. But the money which has been offered as prizes will be spent by the prizegivers themselves in purchasing any work of art sent in for the exhibition which appeals to them for its beauty or its merit.
>
> The object of this new scheme can be readily understood. First, the general public will not be influenced in its judgment by the verdict of a jury; second, the young artist will be encouraged by the fact that some one actually wants to possess his work, instead of being encouraged merely by a jury whose opinion he perhaps does not value, or by a society that sends him a check and returns his picture; third, the young artist cannot complain that he has not been given a fair chance to show his capacities and make his work known. . . .
>
> We hope that American art will become what it promises to be, a fresh and vital expression of a new great art.

This important statement contained, in embryo, the credo of all future Whitney organizations. It recognized the reality of artists needing to *sell* as well as show their works, a reality overlooked before. From 1917 onward, Juliana would buy at least one work for herself or Gertrude out of nearly every show held in their galleries. Future exhibitions were liberated from ill-conceived restrictions, and the deadly philanthropic climate of the past charity- and other service-related shows was dispelled. Gertrude's announcement endorsed American artists and sided confidently with the destiny of American art.

The Friends appeared to be saved from themselves, but the concurrent shows at the Whitney Studio were also ripe for rescue. Gertrude and Juliana came up with the idea of three consecutive group exhibitions, each exploring the theme To Whom Should I Go for My Portrait? The motive behind them was to prod the public into commissioning likenesses, and Juliana had charge of the series from first to last, from inviting artists and fixing prices to alerting journalists and art students and arranging sittings for interested spectators.

The first selection, running from December 4 to 18, 1916, and encompassing oils, sculptures, and drawings, was dominated by the familiar. The stars were the tried-and-true, such as Henri, Glackens, Bellows, Luks, Beaux, Davidson, and French, and now-forgotten society favorites were represented too amply with foolish statues and pictures. The gamut of talent was summed up by the reviewer

from *Arts and Decoration*, who wrote that the portraits "extend from the work of George Luks to the work of Walter D. Goldbeck [known for his idealized countenances and lavish attention to accessories and costume] and that is to say that they extend from an insistent determination to give an evidence of truth telling to an insistent determination to flatter the truth."

The second assemblage of portraits (on view from January 8 to 22, 1917) was larger, more diverse, and in some aspects more distinguished than the first, but it was heir to the same weaknesses. Juliana made sure that she included Sloan, a sign that all was well between them after her uncomfortable birthday party. (She then bought his *Signorina Cherubino* in January of 1917. The first Sloan to enter the Whitney collection,* the painting cost $600.) Another exhibitor was John Butler Yeats. Since his perpetual self-portrait was in no condition to be seen, Juliana borrowed a painting of George Moore† owned by Quinn. Quinn was generous about lending, and he was especially well-disposed toward anyone who watched over his elderly charge. In contrast to this excellent grouping there appeared, once again, an egregious set of commercial portraitists to the undiscerning rich.

The show's most interesting section was photography, although Juliana didn't seem to know much about it. In the catalog she credited two portraits by Edward Steichen—his famous image of J. Pierpont Morgan, plus a print of Bernard Shaw—to Alfred Stieglitz, who had merely lent them from his collection. But ignorant or not, she did manage to find outstanding photographers for the show—Stieglitz (with a print of Abraham Walkowitz), Baron de Meyer, Clarence White, Gertrude Kasebier, and Arnold Genthe. Jean de Strelecki, who had made portraits of Gertrude and Juliana, was also invited.

During the second week of the show's run, Juliana was working in her office when she chanced to observe a short, dark-haired man hovering around the table of photographs reserved for the critics. He picked up some reproductions and attempted to shove them into an envelope. As the man turned to leave, Juliana trotted up to him and said, "Are you from the press?" Reluctantly, he said yes. She asked the visitor his name. More reluctantly he gave it. The man she had surprised was Forbes Watson.

Watson of course had been watching the Whitney Studio for years, but until that day in January of 1917 he and Juliana had not met formally. At the time, his policy—and that of his paper, the *Post*—was to avoid disclosing his identity as he made his rounds. He had eluded her before, all the while attacking the Whitney Studio and the Friends of the Young Artists as well-meaning but inept. Now the inevitable was about to happen. Juliana buttonholed Watson and asked, "What do you think of the exhibition?"

"I think it's terrible," he answered.

"Why?" she demanded.

Watson did not flinch. The Studio had no direction or sense of continuity. It tilted one way and then another. One heterogeneous exhibition followed the

---

*Now in the collection of the Delaware Art Museum.

†Now in the collection of the National Gallery of Ireland.

next, without apparent connection or pattern. He once thought that a defining stand had been taken in giving Sloan a one-man show, but nothing matching it in quality or initiative had been offered since. (Watson was unaware that it was the artist himself who had proposed this highlight in Whitney history.) The effect of the good work displayed, as in the portrait shows, was diluted by the flood of flimsy, inferior products from the society hacks. The shoddy commercialists had to be eliminated from the invitation list altogether, and the preferences of socialites with false pretensions to discrimination had to be ignored. Furthermore, the same artists, most of them far removed from the cutting edge of art, were appearing at the Studio again and again. Juliana was presenting well-rehearsed, well-worn anthologies of the predictable. Surely that was not what she and Mrs. Whitney intended? They could not forever be forgiven their failings or their amateur status. To foster talent and give art shows was not so simple a job as it might seem. It had to be done suitably and intentionally, not nebulously.

Reeling from Watson's criticisms, Juliana nevertheless saw their justness. She recovered enough to concede that he was right. She implored him to become their art consultant and admitted that Guy Pène du Bois had already recommended that she enlist him. Watson remained uncommitted, but their meeting had ramifications beyond the Whitney Studio's immediate predicament. His knowledge and candor won Juliana's respect. No matter how grievously stung she was by Forbes Watson's condemnations, she wanted him on her side.

The critics judged the third and final installment of To Whom Should I Go for My Portrait? (January 29 to February 12, 1917) as the best in the series. The exhibition was commended for its catholicity of taste. McBride, heretofore not very excited about the Studio and its doings, heartily applauded the show in the *Sun*, singling out for praise the contributions by Sargent, Zorn, Charles Grafly, and Weir. Besides these men, twenty-one other artists participated in the show, including Alexander Stirling Calder, who submitted *Sandy*, a finely modeled figure of his son Alexander. Among the younger artists, the two to note were du Bois and a painter who may have been hurriedly added to the roster. Her specialty was flowers, but she painted portraits, too. Her name was Nan Watson, and she happened to be married to Forbes.

The final portrait exhibition drew 1,200 (a substantial figure for a midwinter event lasting only two weeks), but suddenly that kind of show seemed hopelessly old hat to Juliana. The next project she was managing was one compatible with Watson's liberal leanings. Four struggling artists in their twenties—Claude Buck, Abraham Harriton, Benjamin Kopman, and Jennings Tofel—asked permission to use the Whitney Studio for a group show in late spring. They called themselves the Introspectives, because they felt an artistic kinship with the introspective, subjective, romantic tradition of Inness, Ryder, and Davies. (A suggestion was made to invite the latter two venerables to exhibit with the younger men, but that provocative possibility did not materialize.) The Introspectives had banded together in "protest against superficial surface art, however excellent in craftsmanship, and as a plea for the art which expresses insight, feeling [and] imag-

ination." None of them had gotten any exposure to speak of, and none of them were society pets. Their promise was being recognized, but not patronized. The Introspectives' show established the precedent of artists choosing artists: The original Introspectives were asked to extend the Studio's hospitality to four other artists. They invited Van Dearing Perrine (an older painter, but one whose work they felt was in harmony with their theories), Jacques Chesno, Felix Russman, and the early modernist sculptor Robert Laurent. The caliber of the show was respectable, and it fulfilled the purposes for which Gertrude intended her galleries to be used. The exhibition was sent to Chicago, where it scored a big success.

The Introspectives came to Gertrude and Juliana's attention through the Friends of the Young Artists because they presented their petition at its office in C. S. Pietro's studio. At long last, owing to Gertrude's prodding, the society had freed itself from the gropings of the formative years and was emerging as a mature sponsor. But then its affairs took an improbably disastrous turn.

Winifred Ward, late of *The Brow of Egypt* and recipient of a stipend from Gertrude, was a shrewd young woman adept at playing on other's sympathies. In 1917 her subsidy from Gertrude was over, and she was not above dropping sorrowful hints about having to give up her studio and nascent sculpture career to return home to Philadelphia. Ward seemed capable and efficient, so Gertrude gave her a job as corresponding secretary for the Friends. The organization was slated to hold its first unjuried show in April of 1917.

Ward's position was strictly clerical, but she used it to promote herself within the sculpture establishment and insinuate herself into society. Capability and efficiency metamorphosed into officiousness and unadulterated cheek. Immediately transgressing her authority, she overruled her benefactress behind her back (Gertrude was in Florida for most of March) by *reinstating* the very prize system Gertrude fought to dislodge. As the one in charge of assembling a jury, Ward could make valuable contacts who would otherwise have been unavailable to her. She further trivialized the Friends by arranging to have *little children* choose the prizewinners for the April exhibition. On her own initiative Ward brought several boys and girls to the Whitney Studio to judge an exhibition already in progress. She wrote airily to Gertrude, "It was a very amusing experiment and they [the children] re-awarded the prizes very cleverly. It seems to me, that well managed, this will make an opportunity for an amusing, and successful afternoon affair."

Ward's subsequent actions were even more presumptuous. She took it upon herself to enlarge the size of the Friends from the original eight to at least twenty-five members. She sought to load the advisory board with influential artists, rich collectors, and socialites. Her list was heavy with precisely the mix of persons an ambitious sculptor without connections would find extraordinarily handy to know. Each patron—for Ward had reinstalled that dubious concept—would select his or her pet young artist and finance the protégé's entry into the show. In short, Ward was twisting the Friends' apparatus and whole raison d'être into something more regressive than it had been in its most benighted hours. Ward's final grotesque proposal was to have the judges award the prizes in front of the contestants, which showed an astonishing insensitivity to the losers. Having lined

up everything, she reported to Irene Givenwilson on March 14, 1917, that Knoedler Gallery had donated its space for the first two weeks in April. (The Introspectives were on view at the Studio during that time; perhaps Ward did not want to wait until that exhibition closed for fear that the changes she had pushed through would be revoked by Gertrude, who would be back in New York by then.)

Upon learning that the Friends was being sabotaged, Gertrude clamped down on Ward to the extent she could. But she heard of the scheme too late to undo it. The odious reversion to prizes was vetoed in time, but the democratic admissions procedure was beyond resurrection. Ward had already mailed invitations to the men and women she wanted as patrons, and many had accepted. The exhibition, which ran from April 2 to 16, featured thirty painters. So as not to embarrass the donors or Knoedler's, Gertrude maintained a furious silence. As soon as the canvases were out of the gallery, she fired Ward and told her that all ties between her, the Friends, and the Whitney Studio were permanently severed.

The damage inflicted by Ward in her three months on the society's payroll was irreparable. She had quarreled with Pietro, and her high-handedness drove away everyone else who was formerly involved. The Friends broke up, never to be re-created. Ironically, the Friends' "no juries, no prizes" rule, once adopted, was never applied to any of their exhibitions.

April of 1917 was a chaotic month for Gertrude and Juliana. Aside from the Ward fiasco, life was in ferment all around them. On the sixth, the United States formally declared war on Germany, and New York, like the rest of the country, began to mobilize. At 291, Stieglitz was devoting his gallery to the paintings of a young woman named Georgia O'Keeffe; concurrently, the Society of Independent Artists was in the news for its first exhibition and the tempest brought on by Duchamp and his urinal. There was zip in the Village, there was zip in the art scene. But the Friends of the Young Artists lay in ruins, and the Whitney Studio was in limbo. The question, one which fell to Juliana to answer, was this: How could she and Gertrude put some of that zip into shows of their own?

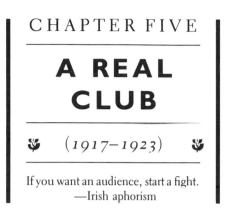

CHAPTER FIVE

A REAL CLUB

❧ (*1917–1923*) ❧

If you want an audience, start a fight.
—Irish aphorism

I N APRIL OF 1917, despite the haziness of the Whitney Studio's future, one thing *was* firmly established: Juliana had absolute hold of its reins. Gertrude, of course, remained vitally interested in the art center she was sponsoring, but war relief, travel, and sculpture commissions made greater claims on her attention. And after the debacle of Winifred Ward and the Friends of the Young Artists, she was wary of entering into art entanglements unless they were overseen by someone to whom she could entrust complete authority. The home front was Juliana's, and she asserted herself.

Her way unencumbered (and reinforced by a salary raised to $500 a month), she took to power smoothly. It was noticed. Juliana's enhanced status was made clear to the art community in print by Jerome Myers, who in the guise of a "young lady artist," was writing a column of gossip and news for *Arts and Decoration*. In the June 1917 issue, he reported, "We formed a party at the Brevoort the other night with Mrs. Force, who directs art destinies." However, to wear the crown of authority for no other reason than to set off her own triumph was not Juliana's object. On the contrary, she happened to be extremely discontented.

Forbes Watson's dressing-down and the contrast between the premature stodginess of the Whitney galleries and the exuberance of the Independents made a strong impression. These events thrust into sharp relief the long, slow, and often retrograde apprenticeship of the Studio under her management. It had not made sufficient progress, and save for a few comforting exceptions, it had not had a profound effect. The Studio had been merely a sideshow, never a main

event, and the time for reshaping its form and character was overdue. Fortunately, it was not too late to start afresh.

Juliana's instincts were good. First she turned to Watson, her most persistent critic, for advice. His judgment would have been invaluable, but after war was declared, he volunteered as an ambulance driver and left for what would be a two-year stay in Europe. She then consulted artists, and she was wise enough to pick several who knew what it was like to be at the mercy of worldly circumstances. Henri and Sloan were solicited for their opinions, as were du Bois, Speicher, Tucker, and Schnakenberg. These men were open-minded, and they believed in fighting for others besides themselves.

From these discussions emerged more flexible and challenging methods of encouraging talent. The competitions, with their prescribed subject matter, were abolished, as Gertrude wished. Adopting the Independents' rallying cry, the Whitney Studio would uphold the principle of "no juries, no prizes." Instead of issuing mass calls to exhibitions, Juliana would invite individual artists to show, and they could submit whatever work they wished. No one would be instructed to execute a specific representation of anything. Juliana would buy works out of the shows for Gertrude or herself, and she hoped that the public would follow her example. Concomitantly, the nominal patrons and patronesses disappeared. Those who painted with drawing-room smartness in mind were to be eased off the exhibition roster and serious artists added to it. The Whitney Studio was prepared to embolden itself at last.

By 1917 a few painters in the Henri group had surmounted the barriers of the National Academy of Design and other salons, and they were in possession of reputations. But many younger artists were now coming along who found themselves in the same harsh predicament as that of Sloan twenty years before. Juliana and Gertrude would have to prove their courage by showing artists who did not have dealers and were not accepted by officialdom. The value of this work would not become apparent for years; in the meantime they would be rewarded by public apathy or disdain.

The direction Juliana chose to pursue was not one solely devoted to the up-and-coming and unheralded generation, although younger artists would receive the most prominence in the future. In a sense, concentrating on the young alone would have been easier than what she did, because her course would have appeared to be more consistent. Instead, she chose to encourage the independent artist, known and unknown. She thought it foolish to bar good artists from her galleries because, after a long struggle, they had earned a mark or two of recognition. The notion was also foreign, perhaps even distasteful, to her emotionally—it tried her loyalty and her belief in friendship too severely.

Another policy deriving from the Henri circle and the Independents was that of inclusivity. As artists with histories of being denied access to large audiences, they could not overstate the value of extending broad sympathies to all varieties of aesthetic impulses. Camaraderie was infinitely superior to competition. They were cool to the single-mindedness of exclusive societies, be it embodied in the gross protectionism of the Academy or even the prescient discernment of a

Stieglitz, who confined himself to helping a handful of people. The pitfall of such democratic practices was that in attempting to do well by everyone, the promoter could end up doing well for no one. To be eclectic was to risk being only miscellaneous, for to be generous to talent also meant being gentle to mediocrity. But being raw and fallible was preferable to being conservative and secondhand. "We have always maintained the open door," Juliana would say, "with larger exhibits and more artists exhibiting."

Juliana, it should be understood, never pretended to perfection or clairvoyance in the artists whose pictures she chose to buy or show. The photographer David Eisendrath was once on assignment at the Whitney Museum, taking pictures of several works of art. One of them was a painting that had achieved a near-classic status and was bought early by the institution, and Eisendrath said to Juliana, "It's wonderful that you had such foresight." In response she rolled her eyes and said, "Yes, but the storeroom is full of things that can never realize that appreciation." She never expected more than a small percentage of the art she bought over the years to have staying power.

If West Eighth Street was to attract exciting artists to its midst and radiate youth and high spirits, a more distinctive attitude would have to be communicated. The Academy remained a useful center of reaction: Its fort, although crumbling, still stood. The organization no longer retained the prestige of the pre–Armory Show days, but acceptance into its big shows practically guaranteed a sale. Academy members controlled the purse strings of the Metropolitan Museum in the field of contemporary art, and Academy officers continued to advertise the organization as a national and disinterested institution, instead of what it was: a private body working for the benefit of its members. Accordingly, taking issue with the Academy's so-called official standing and its support of official honors was still valid and necessary in any campaign to support maverick artists and educate the public. Juliana's renewed opposition to the Academy's inequities on behalf of an independent American art gave the Studio a focus and confirmed her as a champion of progressive artists without prospects. Slowly but confidently, the Whitney galleries joined the small number of places sympathetic to living artists. Now Juliana was exactly where she wanted to be—critical of the status quo and allied with youth, rebellion, invention, and optimism.

These changes were instituted in the fall of 1917. Before then Juliana had other pressing business. Once again Gertrude arranged to furnish the Newport Art Association with summer art exhibitions, and Juliana had to be on hand to organize them. This time a series of one-man shows, with all expenses assumed by Gertrude, was organized for Paul Manship, Ernest Lawson, George Bellows, Jo Davidson, Arthur B. Davies, James Earle Fraser, William Glackens, and John Gregory. (For Newport these artists were strong fare.) In New York Juliana was working on a charity event called the Alley Festa, conceived for the benefit of the Italian Red Cross. From June 6 to 9, 1917, MacDougal Alley was transformed into an Italian street fair. Juliana was attached to the executive committee,

whose key members besides Gertrude were Manship, the architect Paul Chalfin, Malvina Hoffman, *Vanity Fair* editor Frank Crowninshield, and Elsa Maxwell. A massive coordination of material and personnel was required, and everyone's abilities were tested. Chalfin, for example, was to "Italianate" the plain faces of the Alley's stables and town houses with Potemkin facades. Before long the cul-de-sac bristled with ersatz bell towers, parapets, balconies, and flying buttresses. Juliana distributed tickets, persuaded artists who worked in the Alley to open their studios to the public, and searched for magicians, ventriloquists, guitarists, flower girls, singers, and puppeteers to populate the street concessions. The Alley Festa grossed more than $70,000 and sold over $540,000 in Liberty Bonds in its four days. After the war, both Gertrude and Juliana were decorated by the Italian Red Cross in recognition of their efforts.

In between engagements Juliana retreated to Barley Sheaf Farm, if any dwelling being remodeled can be called a retreat. A tennis court and huge swimming pool were in the offing, and she was embarking on what would prove to be an enduring love affair—the seeking out and collecting of American folk art. Portraits by self-taught limners, theorem paintings on velvet copied by school-girls, fanciful etchings of historical incidents, vernacular furniture fashioned by a local artisan or whittled by a tramp who happened to be passing through, quilts, whirligigs, cigar-store Indians, hand-carved toys, the odd article of homely whimsy—Juliana had an eye for them all. Such things were all around her in the antique shops and secondhand stores of rural Pennsylvania, and because no one else prized such castoffs, they were cheap and plentiful. In Bucks County Juliana piloted an old station wagon, and she rarely returned from a ramble in the country without a chair or a footstool or a picture in the back seat. She interspersed these almost seditious articles of Americana with squat, self-impor-tant Victorian settees, formal Brussels carpets, and English china animals. The effect was so insouciant that marveling guests sometimes wondered if the whole assemblage wasn't a stunt. However, in her domestic surroundings as in art entrepreneurship, Juliana felt that play was a part of wisdom, and there was no condescension toward the folk idiom in her decor. Describing her collecting, Robert Bishop, director of the Museum of American Folk Art, wrote that "she did not view folk art as a minor expression of American art, but an extension of craft traditions into the realm of fine art." For the times, this opinion was radically imaginative.

Juliana became one of the earliest and most authoritative collectors of folk art in this country: Items she owned are now in the Abby Aldrich Rockefeller Folk Art Center in Williamsburg, Virginia, and the New-York Historical Society, and they were exhibited in several ground-breaking shows in the 1920s and 1930s. Her collecting was important not only on account of the quality of the objects,* but because of the influence it had. Visitors to her apartment and

---

*For example, such landmark portraits as *The Brown Family, Picking Berries,* and *Child in Blue Dress*; the romantic *Runaway Horse*; an ingenious genre engraving of Perry's victory at Lake Erie (now in the collection of the New-York Historical Society); *Indians, Salmon Falls, New Hampshire* by Samuel Seymour; an exquisitely modeled wooden horse; and early Shaker tables, dressers, chests, and desks.

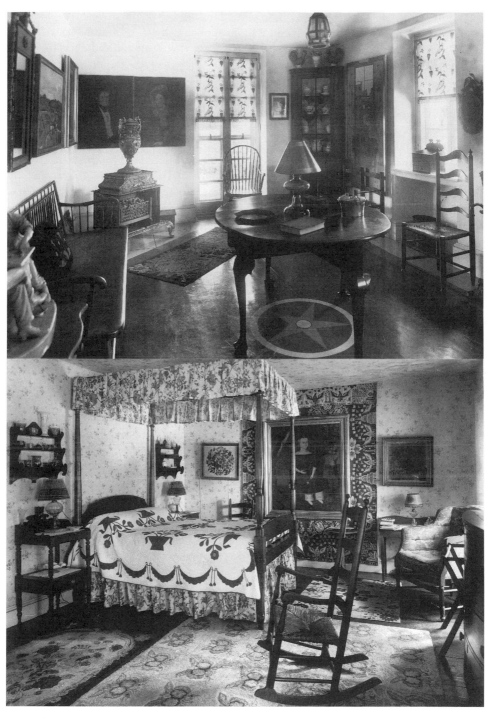

Juliana's long-standing interest in Shaker furniture and American folk art was expressed in the decoration of the entrance hall and bedroom at Barley Sheaf Farm.

various houses over the years, and readers who later saw the interiors featured in magazine layouts, were struck by what they saw. In emulation, they began buying similar objects and furnishings.

In forming such an adventurous collection, Juliana took inspiration from her milieu and from artists, although vernacular art itself was destined to attract her. She spent the first decade of her life in Bucks County, a rich source for Pennsylvania-German artifacts, and an undeniable part of the appeal of folk art was symbolic. Its items were tangible ties to the lost (yet now recaptured) Bucks County heritage.

The folk idiom also intrigued Juliana because it was a vigorous yet essentially undiscovered manifestation of the indigenous American culture she and Gertrude were working so assiduously to legitimatize. It spoke to her, as it did to contemporary artists, in the charm of its self-sufficiency, gravity, directness, humor, and lack of pomposity. So-called American primitive art had great personal flavor, and it was unconventional to like it—these two characteristics alone would have captivated Juliana. What most people overlooked, she took care to scrutinize. With folk art Juliana was also commenting on the stultifying nature of the academicians and their closed exhibits. Henry Schnakenberg said that he and his fellow artists embraced folk art because of its rebellious contrast to the artifice-laden products of the National Academy of Design. It was the "freshness of the primitives" that appealed to them. The folk artists offered a historical alternative to academic training; the Whitney galleries, where young and emerging artists could exhibit, provided a contemporary alternative to the Academy. Several painters whom Juliana knew had been collecting folk art since the early teens, but how early she was aware of their shared interest is unknown. She seems to have come to the collecting of indigenous Pennsylvania furniture and handicrafts independently, and pure luck may have prodded her to begin as she did: After the Forces bought their farm, Juliana, in going through the contents of the barn, found a filthy canvas that she felt to be of some value. She had it cleaned and knew her instincts were correct. The picture was later identified as one of several versions of *Nature's Bounty*, a still life painted by Severin Roesen. *

By 1920 Juliana certainly knew that artists in her circle were scouring New England, New York State, and Pennsylvania for paintings, carvings, weather vanes, and furniture. About that time she became friendly with Charles Sheeler, who was already immersed in the art and culture of the Shakers and, according to Forbes Watson, it was he who first steered her toward forming a collection of their crafts. (However, a photograph of the living room at Barley Sheaf Farm in 1920 shows some Shaker furnishings.) Juliana did not consider the Shaker artisans to be untutored, and she separated them from folk painters. Always citing the "elegance" of everything they made, she saw the Shakers as a bastion of American individualism and a creative culture that had not been given its due. In 1932 Juliana met the pioneering husband-and-wife team of Shaker scholarship, Faith and Edward Deming Andrews. By then she had already accumulated

---

* Roesen was not a naive or untutored artist, but because he worked mainly in Pennsylvania, he was one of many painters Juliana collected under the loose rubric of folk and provincial art.

a sizable collection of Shaker furniture, but through their scouting, she added many other outstanding pieces.

Barley Sheaf Farm was more than a storehouse for burgeoning art holdings. The Riesers—Juliana's sisters and brothers, and their young offspring—were now repairing to it with the sense of paradise regained that its chatelaine had hoped for. Mary and Clara moved in for the summer, and their nephews and nieces came for weeks at a time. And when Juliana was there, doing her best to entertain her small charges, the children felt that she diffused "an air of lovely things about to happen." Allan Rieser wrote of his vacations in Holicong:

> [I]n the foreground of my memory will always be the early years—the years of my boyhood when Aunt J. was in her early middle age—before Dr. Force died . . . when the family was in full force and most of them spent some part of their summers on the Farm. There were the large family dinners, with two long tables set— uproarious with laughter from beginning to end—drives through the . . . countryside . . . picnics. Gargantuan shopping sprees in back-country antiques warehouses— swimming parties—tennis parties—a party in a canal barge hired for the day— charades (serving mainly as an excuse to rummage for costumes in the attic)—family readings and card-games—comedy croquet-games in the apple orchard—walking trips around the farm, which included mass hay-jumping in the barn and bullfighting with a young but crafty ram—visits in force to the local fair . . . flower-gathering and fruit-gathering—epidemics of furniture-shifting (Aunt J. could never stay in a room for long without re-arranging it)—burglar-hunting at night (a regular feature) —a constant turmoil and a constant wave of laughter from day-beginning to day-end—and of course all presided over, led, directed, urged on, and controlled by Aunt J.

The likelihood of these adventures becoming harrowing multiplied if Juliana got behind the wheel. She was a demon driver, or rather, steerer. Like Gertrude Stein, she could not or would not learn to park or reverse. She went forward and that was all. It did not endear her to the shopkeepers of Doylestown when she rocketed up to their front doors and planted the car horizontally or diagonally across the entrance, taking all the parking spaces allotted. Not surprisingly, Doctor forbade her his shiny, immaculate Packard; hence the assignment of a brigade of sturdy station wagons able to withstand assault and battery as the world made way for her. Allan Rieser summarized motoring, Juliana-style: "Aunt J. drove . . . fearlessly and dreadfully—always, it seemed, in a brilliantly inappropriate costume. Once she overturned [her station wagon] in a ditch. Another time she started on a trip to Philadelphia, changed her mind, asked a passing stranger to turn the car around for her, and headed back. Just as well for Philadelphia."

An exhibition of contemporary landscapes, which belatedly opened the Whitney Studio's 1917 season in December, made it plain that changes had taken place. The caliber of the artists participating rose significantly: Maurice Prendergast made his long overdue debut in the galleries, and Charles Demuth and the twenty-five-year-old Stuart Davis (the latter recommended to Juliana by

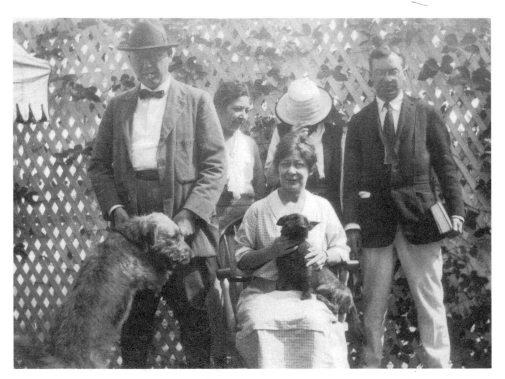

Doctor, Mary, Clara, and Max Rieser, and Juliana relaxing at the farm with several members of the Force menagerie.

Sloan) were invited to show. Other noteworthy first-time exhibitors were Max Kuehne, Augustus Vincent Tack, Paul Burlin, and Glenn O. Coleman. In response to the new regime, the *Brooklyn Daily Eagle* wrote appreciatively, "The exhibition at the Whitney Studios seems to have shaken itself free from the oppressive spirit of patronage which was the keynote of the exhibitions held there last year. This exhibition consists of works of our proudest and most independent young painters. It is the most vigorous, sincere group that has been shown this year."

Sloan and Juliana were consulting each other on matters other than new artists for the Studio. In 1917 Dolly's alcoholism and its attendant problems had worsened, and Sloan was devoting immense time and energy to rescuing her from wherever her drinking led her. Dolly could not always account for her actions, and she got into trouble with the police. When Juliana learned of this, she immediately offered to arrange an appointment for Dolly with one of the foremost neurologists in New York. The Sloans went to him, and the physician said that although he could guarantee no cure, long-term institutionalization was the only answer. Juliana offered to pay for it. Sloan said that he would consider a sanitarium, but upon reflection he refused it. He thought that if Dolly were separated from him involuntarily, "it would break her heart." He feared she would kill herself.

Juliana was touched by Sloan's unselfishness, and after the conference with him about getting medical help for Dolly, and over the years, she aided him in ways he could accept. Sloan was an artist she believed should be fully represented in the Whitney collection, and Juliana bought his work steadily for its merit, but if she heard he was ill or short of money she often purchased for that reason or tried to sell something to sympathetic collectors.

Sloan never forgot Juliana's offer of psychiatric care for Dolly, and he saw that quick, voluntary effusion of generosity repeated over the years on behalf of other artists and their families who were sick or homeless or hungry. He sent many to Juliana himself. They were helped, but Juliana, out of respect for their privacy and "possibly because of a certain arbitrariness in her personality," kept no written account of these transactions. Sloan conjectured that decorum and sensitivity lay behind the piecemeal records and hiding of good deeds in his remarks about Juliana in 1949. Perhaps the memory of his own sorrow led him to write with veiled allusion:

> No one will ever know the extent of the private benefactions Mrs. Whitney performed through Mrs. Force. The records have been destroyed, probably at Mrs. Whitney's request. But of my own knowledge I know of innumerable artists whose studio rent was paid, or pictures purchased just at the right time to keep the wolf from the door, or hospital expenses covered, or a trip to Europe made possible. Mrs. Force's office was always open to such pleas, even when she had a secretary, even when you had to surmount two secretaries to reach her.

The modest success of the 1917 landscape show was soon topped by an affair that not only afforded much amusement to all who devised and participated in it, but assumed a great symbolic importance in Whitney annals. The event was called the Indigenous Exhibition, and it was, in essence, a painting bee.

In late January of 1918, twenty painters were bidden to West Eighth Street to draw lots; they were asked to reappear at the Studio early on February 1. As the painters trickled in that morning, awaiting them in the galleries were twenty virginal canvases of different sizes and shapes. Each was stretched, primed, framed, mounted on a wall, and ready to be swabbed with paint. Stacked on a table in the center of the room were brushes of all varieties, palettes, tubes of paint, and turpentine ordered from one of the city's best dealers in art materials. Another table held sandwiches, cigarettes, cigars, and bottles of whiskey. Juliana handed out crisp gingham smocks and escorted the arrivals to the canvases representing the numbers they had drawn. They had to paint pictures on the spot, she told them, from memory and without models or sitters. Hence the formerly mysterious title "Indigenous Paintings." All the pictures had to be completed within three days, and participants were allowed to adjourn only for lunch, dinner, and a night's sleep. Except for that, there were no rules but to have fun.

The novelty of an impromptu painting tournament took most of the artists by gleeful surprise. "Most," because after they were apprised of the working conditions, Henri and then Bellows "raised the question of sanctity with only a

minor sense of proportion and no sense of humor." They turned up their noses at the party and left. Of the artists who remained, quite a few were perplexed about a subject and spent much time thinking one up. The craftier ones, who had guessed or heard about what an Indigenous Exhibition might actually mean, took care to smuggle in some preparatory work. Stuart Davis brought in a sheaf of sketches of Gloucester, Massachusetts, and as he drew a large canvas, was able to incorporate them into a composite panorama called *Multiple Views*. The painting, although by no means a mature work, contained the seeds of several ideas Davis was to explore with increasing power in the years to come. Gifford Beal, who preferred to use models, was the first to hit upon the idea of reproducing what was going on around him. His was a small, charming picture documenting a moment of the marathon.* Gertrude, in street clothes, has stopped by to visit. She is inspecting everyone's progress. Around her stand George Luks, Guy Pène du Bois, Paul Dougherty, Jo Davidson (a sculptor, but, smelling a party, he had infiltrated the premises), and the gingham-clad Bob Chanler. In the background other artists are at work, coaxing their pictures into indigenating on the walls. Although captured at a quiescent moment by Beal, Luks was anything but static. His energies were not channeled into painting. Uninhibited under any circumstances, he abandoned what little restraint did govern him at the prospect of an all-day audience and limitless drink. His opening gambit was the pixilated performance of a musical revue, with music and lyrics by Luks, all parts played by Luks, and scenery impersonated by Luks. After that he lurched through wild renditions of Russian dances.

The party got rowdier as the refreshments exerted their effect. Luks, occasionally making swipes at his picture, was stationed next to Davis. From time to time Luks waltzed over to his neighbor and said, "That's pretty good, kid." Then he returned to his own canvas. Armed with six-inch house-painter's brushes, he would show off all the effects he coaxed from them as he worked on the bottles of Scotch, rye, and bourbon. Swinging his brushes like a conductor, Luks was itching to wipe them across someone else's picture. He approached Davis and wheezed, "You're pretty good, but rather young. You haven't had as much experience as I have. Let me show you how." As an eager arm shot in the direction of the meticulously prepared montage of Gloucester, Davis grabbed Luks and held him off with all his strength. So ended the first day.

Enough of the other participants worked productively in a characteristic vein. Du Bois, with his hard-boiled view of the upper crust, painted "an old rounder seated in bulging dress shirt looking . . . to surprise . . . a lily." Juliana named the picture *A Window in the Union Club* and bought it.† Coleman, who loved the alleys and crisscross streets of Greenwich Village, painted Minetta Lane in winter. He also loaded up on the art supplies. Davis later said that the paint and brushes Coleman picked up during those three days lasted him for years. That was as it should be. One reason Juliana laid out materials in extravagant

---

*In *The Figurative Tradition and the Whitney Museum of American Art*, a catalog published by the museum in 1980, the painting is incorrectly attributed to George Luks.
†Now in the collection of the University of Minnesota, Minneapolis.

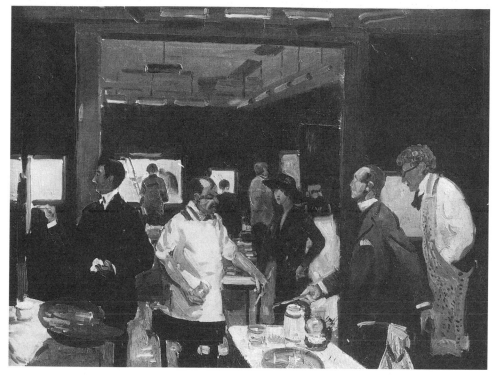

One of the participants in the Indigenous Exhibition, Gifford Beal resourcefully painted everyone else's progress. From left, Guy Pène du Bois painting neatly in suit and tie; George Luks in apron, about to demonstrate some brushwork; Gertrude, Jo Davidson, Paul Dougherty, and, in gingham, Bob Chanler.

quantities was that she wanted the artists to feel free to take them. In 1926 Coleman was given a one-man show at the Whitney Studio Club, where he confessed to Juliana that all of the pictures in the exhibition had been painted with supplies purloined from the Indigenous show. "Oh, that's all right," she replied cheerfully. "I knew it all along."

As the three-day period drew to a close, the remaining stalwarts annexed the blank canvas that had been reserved for Bellows. Each of them worked on it, mixing his strokes into an artifact he hoped would pass for a Futurist composition. For the signature, each one contributed the first two letters of his last name. The result sounded determinedly Russian: "Kudo du Slmodach Bey-Oglhi," from Kuehne, Dougherty, du Bois, Sloan, F. Luis Mora, Davis, Chanler, Beal, Mahonri Young, Glackens, and Eugene Higgins. The canvas seemed, wrote du Bois, "to any casual observer, exceedingly modern. The gentleman critic on the *Herald* celebrated a new though somewhat confusing genius in his columns."

Gertrude gave an evening party to celebrate the steady if bibulous efforts made by all the geniuses involved. Artists and society folk attended. Luks came in, three sheets to the wind. Making a beeline for his hostess, he threw his arms around Gertrude and caroled, "Oh, Mrs. Whitney, I love you." Then he plas-

tered her with sloppy, drunken kisses. But Gertrude did not flinch, bearing his smotherings valiantly until he was pried off her by Blendon Campbell. Luks was ejected from the party, he knew not why. Taking umbrage at the mysterious snub, he reeled back into the building, intent on avenging his injured honor. He stood in the vestibule of the Whitney Studio, micturating in the corner, as men and women in evening clothes passed to and fro. In a letter to Gertrude, Chanler summed up the event: "The Exhibition looks fine, a great deal better than the painters."

The Indigenous experiment imparted an afterglow to the Studio that lasted for weeks. While the exhibition was in progress, Gertrude went out of town, and Juliana wrote effervescently of her activities. She bought a full-length portrait of a dancer by Mora, confessing, "It costs $1500 & I'm paralyzed with fear that you won't have money to come home." She was preparing for an exhibition of Chinese paintings and winding up the business affairs of a one-man show given to Andrew O'Connor, which realized a mere $237. Juliana was concerned and suggested to Gertrude that the blow be softened. "Shall I send . . . a cheque . . . for $250," she asked, "and a note for you explaining that the very cold and cruel winter had a lot to do with the bad showing?" The most savory morsels were saved for last:

> Mr. Cortissoz came in yesterday & had a lot of fun with the Indigents & wished you God-speed! He is terribly nice & boyish—on warm days; otherwise rheumatism. What shall I do with the paintings—remember they have never seen the light of day! . . . Mr. Beal took me to lunch today & we buried Mr. Henri.* It is great fun to joke with an engineer-painter. I didn't mean to but we ate 5 dollars of your cheque to him.

Things were working out so well that the women decided a second Indigenous Exhibition should be held for sculptors. It would await Gertrude's return in March, so that she could participate. As before, Juliana mixed the old and the young, the established and the obscure, and over thirty sculptors were invited. The most outstanding participants were two émigré artists whose points of view and choice of subject matter were earning them reactions ranging from blank incomprehension to disgust: Gaston Lachaise and Elie Nadelman. As in the first show, the indigators finished their work by collaborating. They molded a caricature of Gertrude perched on a pedestal. At her feet are a host of clamoring artists attempting to reach her exalted position. The inscription on the base of the statue read, "Erected in admiration of the woman and sculptress who can cage twenty sculptors without bloodshed resulting therefrom." Jo Davidson was elated by the event. "[T]he Exhibition looks perfectly splendid, surprisingly so," he wrote. "It was a great experiment, and a revelation—in many ways. It helped me dot my I's—and cross the T's. Greg [John Gregory] is fine—Manship timid. Nadelman—altogether impossible—[Hunt] Diederich not so wild, slightly mad . . . Fraser: Dull—[Mahonri] Young nice but dull. [Chester] Beach clear—but uninteresting—[Arthur] Lee, consistent etc., etc. Yet taken altogether, quite

---

*Perhaps because of Henri's refusal to be in the Indigenous Exhibition. And according to Sloan, both Henri and Bellows thought it beneath their dignity to join the Whitney Studio Club and "high-hatted" it.

representative of the world we live in—here and there a spark of something quite intangible which helps sculpture a good deal."

Davidson spoke perceptively about the overall results. For all their horseplay, the painting and sculpting bees transcended their frivolity by exposing artists of various outlooks and stages of accomplishment to each other in congenial surroundings. Reporting on the gracefulness of the Whitney galleries as a backdrop for fine art, *The Touchstone* seconded Davidson's words. "Not only are the rooms . . . delightful in their high-ceilinged proportions, in their . . . arrangement," its critic applauded, "but there is, under the management of Mrs. Force, an air of friendliness, good comradeship, appreciation of art, and, what is even rarer, an enthusiasm for the artist, that creates a flavor of interest and joy that is seldom brought together in any art exhibition in New York. . . . After you have seen the pictures you have a cup of tea with the painters or a critic or Mrs. Force, if she has a minute, and sometimes Mrs. Whitney is there to receive the artist. Altogether it is one of the places in New York where art has a choice and where artists are respected."

The receptivity to younger and more startling talents can be gauged by comparing the second Indigenous Exhibition to a survey of "contemporary" American sculpture Daniel Chester French assembled for the Metropolitan. Like the Whitney show, it opened in March 1918, but there the similarity ended. The setting was gloomy—Henry McBride was one among many alienated by the "chilly, jaillike salon d'honneur of American art in the Metropolitan Museum." Within these icy caverns, French's choices were supremely backward-looking. Everyone invited was connected with the National Academy of Design or the National Sculpture Society, for French believed that few sculptors of ability could be found outside those groups. The boldest work on view was *Man with a Pick* by Mahonri Young, a finely crafted work of art, but it stood as the sole example of the whole spectrum of newer sculpture. There was no room for the independent point of view, let alone the uncompromisingly modernist. Lachaise, fresh from an important show at the Bourgeois Gallery, asked French to include him, but Young and Manship (Lachaise's employer) were as far as French's conservative tastes could be pushed. Once Juliana and Gertrude were aware of Lachaise and his need for money, they chipped in with stipends, purchases, and commissions.* They were able to reconcile tradition with innovation—or at least give innovation a fair chance.

That impulse, combined with the pleasure of providing a warm place for artists to mix and mingle regularly, had immense appeal for Juliana and Gertrude. They pondered how such laudable esprit could be kept permanently and vibrantly alive. Out of their talks came the proposal that a club be formed for the care, feeding, propagation, and entertainment of that precariously surviving species,

---

*Lincoln Kirstein, one of Lachaise's most effective champions, would write, "Gertrude Vanderbilt Whitney[,] with unquestioning generosity, purchased important pieces at the first price asked, not in charity, but as a sculptor's recognition of distinguished sculpture." Between 1924 and Lachaise's death in 1935, Juliana bought four of his sculptures and two drawings. One of the sculptor's unfinished commissions was a portrait bust of Juliana, which was given to the museum in 1953.

the young and uncredentialed American artist. Outlining the genesis of the club, Gertrude later wrote, "I have often asked artists and students where they went when they were not working, what they did in the evenings and what library they used. The answers opened up a vista of dreariness which appalled me, revealing a terrible lack in our city's capacities." This new enterprise, which was devoted to abolishing dreariness, was christened the Whitney Studio Club, and from then on, the prospects of hundreds of painters and sculptors were forever changed. The tenets of the Club were for the moment vague, except for two items: The headquarters would be physically separate from the Whitney Studio and the director could be no one but Juliana.

The Whitney-Force combine sped into action with a celerity that artists were learning to recognize as customary. Three blocks south of the Whitney Studio, they found a four-story brownstone at 147 West Fourth Street, off Washington Square. Gertrude took over the lease in February of 1918. The *Greenwich Village Spectator,* a local newsletter and the only journal covering the event, reported:

> For the present the membership will be confined to the fine arts, either men or women. Applicants will be asked to furnish two references. The membership fee will be small. Those who are accepted will have the use of a reference library, and writing tables, and all of the best art publications will be kept on file. . . . The Whitney Studio Club shall be a meeting-place and consultation room for those who take their work seriously, and have either already accomplished something worth-while, or show an ambition and talent to achieve.

Juliana was in charge of getting West Fourth Street remodeled, decorated, and comfortable. The first and basement floors plus the backyard were altered at once; the second, third, and top floors would wait until the fall. She spent most of March on the job, and the pace she set affected her spirits. A crisis threatened, and Juliana wanted Gertrude, who was in Texas, to come back to New York. She was putting her soul into her work, and she was dependent on Gertrude for reassurance.

> Everybody here seems to have lost heart here. Mr. Chanler has really been down in bed & asked me yesterday to tell you that he has had bad luck ever since you went away & won't you please come home if only for a day! I hate to sound forth all this selfishness, but you do not know how much is real need. We all have reached a point where unless you could step in night will overtake us. I am not fooling. I'm just so sick at heart that I can't be of use to anybody anymore. And the troubles are not the kind to write out, no, nor will you have to listen to them if you come—Just come!

The worries only hinted at in her letter were not the sole cause of Juliana's agitation. Her brother Rob was acting up, and in Hoboken the Riesers suffered from his misdeeds. While the United States was still neutral, Rob hooked up with a German prince who slipped into this country in disguise to avoid the British blockade and got involved with disseminating pro-German propaganda. After America entered the war, Rob switched sides. He joined the American Red Cross, and Juliana helped buy him his own ambulance. While he was abroad, he transferred to the American Field Service, but wound up in the

French Foreign Legion. With this improbable career behind him, Rob resurfaced in New Jersey and fell into some form of busybodying that seemed to have military connotations. Rob was too flamboyant a person to slide by unnoticed, and his information-gathering activities (which, such as they were, were probably futile, given his inability to be surreptitious) placed the other Riesers in an awkward position.

In Hoboken, which became a port of embarkation for thousands of troops and had warehouses and shipping lines of vital strategic importance, fears about security were justified. As the war progressed, prudence escalated into a phobia that eventually destroyed the town's German-American community. German-language newspapers were banned, German dishes were renamed in local restaurants, and meetings at German social clubs were outlawed. In this climate all German-American families were suspected of being sympathetic to the fatherland. Mrs. Jared French, who grew up in Hoboken and met Robert Rieser there, said that her relatives told her that he had been a spy during the war. The statement was more gossip than fact, but it was believed by most Hobokenites. Consequently, the Riesers' place in the community was threatened. Any hint of disloyalty tainted a whole family in those days of intense anti-German feeling, and Clara and Mary Rieser were investigated by government agents. Even as a lieutenant of Gertrude Whitney, who had been identified with the Allied cause since 1914, Juliana was in danger of being accused as well. It was during this time that she began to avoid drawing attention to her Hoboken background and her German heritage. In time this defensive habit hardened into a reflex.

On April 8, 1918, Frank Crowninshield wrote to Gertrude that Juliana had alerted him to the Club and its new premises, so he "hiked down there to look the place over." By April 11, some sort of procedure for keeping track of admissions was instituted, because on that day Juliana was able to write to Carl Zigrosser, a print dealer and scholar she hoped would join:

> Have you heard about the Club? Won't you come and find out or if you know and want to join, fill in the accompanying slip and mail it to me here right away and help to make it a real Club. The place is open every day and evening including Sundays, so do come in and see at least.

Juliana also asked the artists involved in the Indigenous Exhibitions to become charter members. In addition, those invited to be in the shows and presumably to join the Club were Lawson, Maurice Prendergast, Rockwell Kent, Samuel Halpert, Robert Laurent, Leon Dabo, Jonas Lie, Davies, Bryson Burroughs, Walt Kuhn, Jerome and Ethel Myers, Speicher, Bertram Hartman, and William and Marguerite Zorach. But Juliana wanted the Club to reach beyond people she already knew. Accordingly, a major source of new members was to be the Art Students League, then the most interesting art academy in the city. The pupils, who ran the school themselves, were seething with intensity and rebellion, and their presence would infuse the Club with creative turmoil. Sloan taught at the League, and Juliana asked him to announce the Club's existence in his

classes. Dorothy Varian, then studying with Sloan, learned about it from him, and became one of the first to be affiliated with the Whitney Studio Club. Kenneth Hayes Miller, one of the most influential instructors the League has ever seen, also participated in the first Indigenous Exhibition and became a charter member. Many within his large following of students streamed down to West Fourth Street to sign up.

The Indigenous Exhibitions, the concurrent birth of the Whitney Studio Club, and the profusion of newcomers to be welcomed conferred the durable freedom Juliana had been seeking for the art activities sponsored by Gertrude. The galleries were now associated with a sense of crackling intellectual mischief, with a productive sort of *larking*. In other words, from 1918 onward, Juliana, the Whitney Studio, and the Whitney Studio Club derived their character from each other. The individual was inspiration to the organizations, and the organizations were a ratification of the individual. Together their lights flared brightly on the New York art scene. Their personalities—synonymous, inseparable, and identical—were rich in optimism, bravery, energy, generosity, and comic gaiety. The galleries and Juliana could be, and sometimes were, mercurial and perhaps quixotic. But in the long run, they were both fixed on the larger aim of easing the personal and professional problems of American artists by accepting them as their own and, in doing so, nurturing the cause of a native art.

For it to be a real club, West Fourth Street's facilities and its physical setup had to strike the right balance. The Club had to be genial and useful, practical and inviting. First-rate exhibition space was essential, but recreational rooms could not be neglected. The furnishings would be hopeless if they connoted pretension, yet they had to be sufficiently pleasing aesthetically to meet the exacting standards of artists. The first floor, one flight up from the ground, consisted of two closet-sized galleries, plus an anteroom where the secretary-receptionist sat—initially, the satirist Mabel Dwight, the first in a long line of artists who worked for Juliana. In deference to the art on view, the walls, carpets, and occasional settee or upholstered chair were light gray. Downstairs, which had been constructed on the plan of an English basement, was divided into a billiard room, an office, a library filled with new art books (one could also find a Ouija board there), and a writing room. In these downstairs rooms, Juliana demonstrated her flair for creating unconventional interiors. A writer visiting the Club in the spring of 1918 reported that in these rooms "the most pure brilliant colors have been used together with great success. Orange or yellow furniture, with blue cushions and delightful designs in gray, green, vermillion and purple, will delight even the most conservative, so cleverly have they been handled." The curtains in these salons were of royal blue satin, lined with chartreuse-colored silk and tied back with scarlet cords. Guy Pène du Bois sold Juliana on the idea of installing a squash court in the backyard, so Club members could get some exercise. Coincidentally, du Bois happened to be the sole member who liked to play, so he and his partners seemed to be the only ones who ever used it. But Jo Davidson remembered that he and other artists would also stroll over to West Fourth Street in the evenings "to play billiards and exchange ideas."

If the rejuvenation of the Studio and the opening of the Club meant the

apotheosis of Juliana, the shift in character and direction just as surely hastened the withdrawal of Gertrude from the epicenter of activity. Gertrude's friends among the growing coterie who gravitated to West Eighth and West Fourth Streets were of some years' acquaintance. They also were men of the world, like Chanler, Chalfin, O'Connor, Davidson, Henri, and du Bois. Gertrude could never, of course, be at home with the next wave of rising, struggling artists. She was painfully sensitive to the fuss that went with face-to-face thanks. Correspondingly, she was somewhat embarrassed in the presence of emergent painters and sculptors who could barely get along. The disparity between her three studios, her storage facilities, her array of tools, and her unlimited access to models, assistants, and expensive materials and their lack of the basic necessities often caused her to feel uncomfortable in their midst, and some of the artists were similarly ill at ease. Katherine Schmidt, a painter who joined the Club about 1920 and became close to Juliana, said of Gertrude that "she was someone from afar. I used to be trotted up every once in a while to talk to her, but I never knew what to say to her. She was too grand a dame to chatter with. She didn't participate in our way of life or the artists that we were identified with." Gertrude entertained the new crowd of artists, and she put in appearances at the openings and other important social functions at the Studio and the Club. She was gracious as she could be but impenetrable: a tall, elegantly gowned figure standing in the receiving line but unbending no further. She needed Juliana to mediate between herself and the painters and sculptors she was doing so much to help. Juliana knew this and respected the reasons why.

The Club was constituted so rapidly that its functions were a bit nebulous at first, but a primary objective was to have shows. Juliana assembled two for June and July of 1918. One was comprised of camouflage paintings by Abbott H. and Gerald Thayer, showing "protective coloration in nature and its bearing on camouflage in war." The other consisted of works by members, who numbered about sixty by then. The Club was dispensing hospitality, too, and it kept its doors open throughout the perishingly hot summer for any artist unlucky enough to be wilting in New York. Dorothy Varian, stuck in a "wretched little studio" the whole summer, spent a part of every day refreshing herself in the Club. "I had art books to read, the fans were going, and an attendant brought me glasses of ice-cold ginger ale. It was wonderful!"

As fall approached, Juliana faced the job of lofting the Club off the ground. She turned the second and third floors of the West Fourth Street building into apartments. Salvatore Bilotti, a stonecutter who was Gertrude's chief assistant, moved into one floor and Blendon and Alice Campbell into the other. Juliana hired Alice Campbell to help Mabel Dwight as a secretary and keeper of the reading room, and thus built-in caretakers were secured as tenants. The top floor was converted into studio space for what was going to become a Club legend— a sketch class with live models. Twenty cents was the admission price per session—a real boon for young artists who could not afford the hourly rates of professional models. The classes were crowded affairs, and Peggy Bacon and

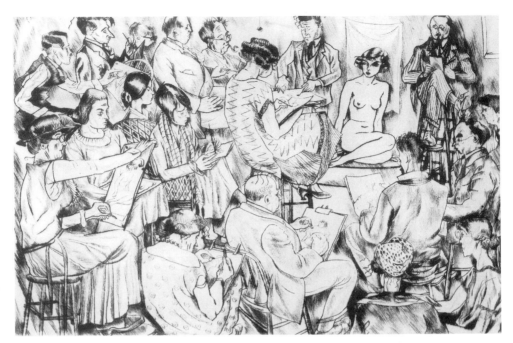

The sketch class at the Whitney Studio Club, here pictured by Peggy Bacon, was one of its most popular activities.

Mabel Dwight saw them as excellent material for humorous prints. Bacon's witty drypoint carries two titles: *The Whitney Studio Club* and *Frenzied Effort*. Edward Hopper, Stuart Davis, Reginald Marsh, Katherine Schmidt, Yasuo Kuniyoshi, Leon Kroll, and George "Pop" Hart were regulars at the sessions. Along with the initiation of a life-drawing class was supposed to come the levying of an annual fee of $5.00. In practice, however, dues were seldom collected. No one ever received a bill, and anyone who attempted to resign on account of not having $5.00 was assured that the money didn't matter. When John Flannagan handed in his resignation because he was too broke to pay his dues, he was told to forget about what he owed. Juliana, who thought Flannagan had a great talent, then said to her assistant, "He can't resign for the reason he gives. Go and tell him we'll give him an exhibition, if he wants one, whenever he's ready." Thanks to her impulse, Flannagan was asked if he had enough sculpture completed for an exhibition. He did, and the artist's early works were shown as a group for the first time anywhere.

In November of 1918 Juliana was again in touch with Carl Zigrosser, brought together by his close friend Rockwell Kent, who had been in the first Indigenous show and had cultivated Juliana ever since. Quick-witted, literate, pugnacious, ebullient, and enterprising, he was a hornet full of hell and ready to sting. Kent's provocative, nonconforming personality mesmerized many who met him, especially women. A man who projected an invincible sense of himself, he excelled

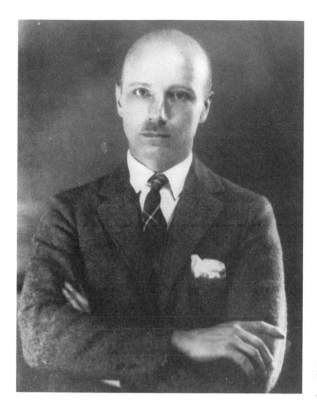

Rockwell Kent had a talent
for art and literature and a
genius for trouble.

at getting useful people in his corner. Juliana, whose primary mission was to
marry the eleemosynary with the aesthetic, was not only useful, but glad to be
of use.

In November of 1918, Kent was paying court to her by letter from his camp
in Seward, Alaska, where he and his son were spending several months. Kent
needed money for various purposes—to paint, to write and illustrate a book, to
finance future trips to Alaska, to buy land in New England, to support his ever-
increasing circle of wives, ex-wives, paramours, and children. One of several
solutions he initiated to ease his money problems was self-incorporation, complete with stockholders and shares. Because of Juliana's access to the Whitney
purse, Kent laid siege to her. On November 22, 1918, he wrote her a long letter.
Shrewdly, it was not cloaked in the usual sincere tones of needy despair. He
gambled instead on ripely flirtatious badinage. He addressed her as Becky Sharp,
and he spoke in the character of Joseph Sedley. With remarkable lightness, Kent
parodied the flow of Thackerayan diction. He even abandoned his own handwriting style for a nineteenth-century script. Its allusiveness inherently flattering
to the knowledgeable recipient, Kent's letter was a master effort, and as such,
deserves lengthy quotation. After saluting Juliana as "My dearest Becky," he
wrote:

I feel that some share of your thoughts and attentions is due to me who hold myself ever in my thoughts so close to you. . . . But, dearest Becky, it is not to voice my own complaints against fortune and your favor that I now address you but to introduce you to and lay before you a project for the welfare of an extraordinarily brilliant and accomplished young friend of mine, Mr. Rockwell Kent. Him the world has unfortunately denied its rewards in proportion to his deserving them; and this is the more pitiable when we know the sweet simplicity and purity of his character, which these respects I liken to my own as it was in those days far, far back in Russell square before you, sweet Becky, came into my life. . . . I will proceed at once to lay before you the plan that I have devised for the mutual benefit of Mr. Kent and of that select portion of the public that shall be fortunate enough to become associated with him in the glorious furtherance of Art, and ask you for your opinion of it.

Mr. Kent has in the last two years earned many thousands of dollars by the sale of his pictures. It has largely been squandered, not in willful dissapation [sic] but because owing to the uncertainty and unexpectedness of the returns he was in no position to profit by them and they ultimately were consumed by the high cost of living in the city where, in the meantime, he had for the better earning of his livelihood, settled. We have figured that Mr. Kent and his family could take up a residence in some remote and rural district and live within the sum of Fifteen hundred dollars per annum. Of this amount Five hundred dollars is already assured him. . . . The remainder, One thousand dollars, remains for us to consider. . . . Altogether Mr. Kent's yearly product, if he can be assured the undivided opportunity to work, is worth at his present prices no less than Five thousand dollars and probably as much as Ten or higher. And for these the ready market is constantly improving. We have then in Mr. Kent's talent and energy and present reputation a decided business asset can it but be made available. And the Thousand Dollars will do this. I propose that he shall *incorporate*—if with the advice of legal minds this is found to be possible —and sell bonds to the total amount of a thousand dollars, payable on a certain date either in cash with added interest or, failing that, in Art work, valuing that at a specified rate considerably less than the market valuation. . . .

I have at last won Mr. Kent over to submitting to my management though you can imagine the difficulty I had in overcoming his repugnance to even the mention of money when I quote his answer to me on my first broaching the subject. "Mr. Sedley, we artists are but the instruments of God and are fed by His hand on heavenly manna."! Mr. Kent has undertaken to write to two influential friends of his to solicit their cooperation in the work of organizing the company. They are Mr. Zigrosser and Mr. Chappell [an architect, and Kent's former employer]. But it is you, Rebecca, from whom I hope for the most useful counsel—although I must beg you not to attempt to interest that well known and kind hearted woman Mrs. Force whose activities in behalf of the struggling artist are already so complete. . . .

I send you a charming [landscape] sketch . . . by the hand of Rockwell Kent himself.

Believe me, dearest Rebecca, ever your most abjectly devoted slave and profound admirer

Jos. Sedley

Rather than trust completely to this extended conceit, Kent followed it with a note in his own voice. After sending Juliana his "best Christmas wishes adorned with real affection," he brought up his previous letter. "Do you know Jos. Sedley?

Becky Sharp's friend?" he queried. "He has a scheme for establishing artists in businesses of their own, and if it can be made businesslike I am the one to do it. He has written to Becky about it—says she's got a great head for such things." In closing Kent asked Juliana, "tell me your [maiden] name—and your favorite traits of your own character, and I'll make you a nice bookplate. I'd have done it long ago but that I needed this data."

Juliana did not respond immediately to Kent's blandishments, perhaps because of sheer busyness. She was running both the Club and the Studio, and between December 1918 and March 1919 she presented a Club members' exhibition (sixty-five works) and seven shows for individual artists, and planned a traveling show called MacDougal Alley Sculpture for the Art Institute of Chicago. Zigrosser was skeptical of Becky Sharp's willingness to underwrite the scheme. He interpreted Juliana's light touch as flightiness. "I do not think Mrs. Force will be of much help; she is too unstable," he wrote to Kent. " 'Out of sight, out of mind', with her you know." However, a week after Zigrosser confided his misgivings to Kent, Juliana prodded him to come see her about the proposal. On February 13, 1919, Zigrosser reported that she was in favor of it. She would confer with George Chappell and let Kent know the results.

Before Zigrosser's positive letter reached the outpost in Alaska, Kent admitted to his friend that Juliana's silence might have a basis in a past altercation. But he played the innocent in his version of events. "She compelled me last spring to offend her in a way that we are told a woman never forgives," he wrote melodramatically. "Maybe it's quite ungallant of me to speak of it but I have tried so hard with her to be decently friendly and helpful and generous as to personal favors that I'm quite out of patience with her. For I've written to her three times as interestingly and amusingly as I could and sent her occasional cards—and all without the slightest acknowledgment from her. Of course there has been some method in my persistence but . . . she has always seemed to me a good sort of woman and certainly an entertaining one."

Kent was either being disingenuous or blind to his own defects. A practiced womanizer, he led on a new acquaintance until she succumbed to his attentions. By comparing Juliana to Becky Sharp, one of the most brilliantly realized coquettes in literature, and styling himself as Joseph Sedley, Becky's supine suitor, Kent more than hints at rekindling whatever it was that had passed between them. That his end was forwarding his career and supporting his dependents— as opposed to the promptings of a trumpeting male ego—made the means no less reprehensible.

Evidently Kent spurned her because she was not beautiful. In his autobiography, the first thing he had to say about Juliana, who aided him substantially for five years, is that she was "a woman utterly lacking in good looks." This comment tells more about the author than the subject, but Kent's seductive behavior and rejection must have left their mark. Juliana had always been insecure about her lack of conventional comeliness. Allan Rieser believes that his aunt "always felt cheated because she was not beautiful. She joked about it herself, saying that one summer Theresa Hellburn had described her as 'the ugliest woman in Venice.' Furthermore, Aunt J. constantly referred to men in

a scathing way, saying that they 'fell for a pretty face.' " Mrs. Lloyd Goodrich never forgot an incident that took place once in a powder room. After she and Juliana fixed their hair and straightened their seams, she watched Juliana, dressed in understatedly elegant clothes and carrying herself with the utmost dignity, survey herself in the mirror. "Oh, that face!" she said disgustedly, shuddering without a trace of moderating facetiousness. Edith Goodrich, who always thought of the fastidiously groomed Juliana as a magnetic woman of arresting style and looks, was astonished at the degree of her dissatisfaction with her appearance.

Juliana could tolerate almost anything in an artist, and in May of 1919 she showed that magnanimity was one of her virtues. She put Kent in the Club's spring exhibition, and to ease his financial predicament, she entered in earnest the proceedings for setting up "Rockwell Kent, Incorporated." She was one of the four shareholders. The others were Kent, the suffrage leader Caroline O'Day, and George Palmer Putnam, the publisher and explorer who would later marry Amelia Earhart. The original estimate of $1,000 was too small; of $4,000 worth of stock issued, Kent owned $2,000 worth; Juliana put in $1,000, and the other two each contributed $500. The stock certificates were hand-drawn and painted with, said Putnam, "a typically Kentian allegory with a naked human figure prone at the base of a tree towards whose rich fruits a serpent winds." A formal employment contract was drawn up, in which Kent promised to pay a 20 percent dividend within a year; if he failed, the shareholders would be allowed to choose "Kent products of market value to balance the account." That never came to pass. Kent as a business venture was a glorious success. His work sold briskly. By January of 1920 he sent the shareholders $1,500, and not long afterward he bought out the three investors. Their largesse enabled Kent to paint, buy a farm in Vermont, and write *Wilderness: A Journal of Quiet Adventure in Alaska* (1920).

The abortive dalliance with Kent in the spring of 1918 adds a concrete, identifying detail to a general and more indistinct state of affairs—the gradual but growing estrangement between Doctor and Juliana. Juliana's life, with its responsibility and travel, now outpaced her husband's. Compared to the imaginative, cosmopolitan, iconoclastic men she was meeting, Doctor, affable though he was, lost his luster. Juliana had always been Doctor's intellectual superior, but his professional status and ambition were equivalent assets. Her ascendancy in Gertrude's service and her development into a creative personality in her own right took her into a scintillating society in which his pleasant but not inspired views and his hobbies of cards and detective fiction began to seem pedestrian. (Forbes Watson, who was not a disinterested party in all this, later called Doctor "the deadliest bore God ever created" and snobbishly added that his grammar was faulty.) Doctor preferred Barley Sheaf Farm and Bucks County to New York, and he spent as much time as he could in Pennsylvania. The Riesers strongly suspected that Doctor had a mistress in Doylestown, but he obeyed the social code and conducted his liaison discreetly. The Forces stayed together in a friendly arrangement in which they politely ignored each other's comings and goings.

Although they maintained a respectful distance from each other, they did appear together on many occasions and continued to enjoy each other's company. Their marriage remained an alliance and a working partnership, but affection-tinged neutrality replaced their original closeness.

One reason Kent's reappearance and epistolary advances may have failed to distress Juliana unduly was that another man was in her thoughts, and she had no time to waste on old perfidies. Forbes Watson was in New York again, this time as the art critic of the *New York World*. He now shared an office with Heywood Broun and Alexander Woollcott, and he was cutting an impressive figure in the New York art world. Upon his return from Europe, he headed directly for 8 West Eighth Street. He inspected the Club and approved of the changes in the Whitney Studio. Forbes and Juliana renewed their acquaintance, on what was to be a much closer basis. Within months of his resettlement in Manhattan, Forbes and Juliana were lovers and neighbors. The Forces now lived in an apartment at 58 West Ninth Street, near Sixth Avenue. In 1920 the Watsons moved into an apartment at 12 West Eighth Street, two doors from the Whitney Studio and two blocks from the Force residence. (This was the building owned by Daniel Chester French.) Forbes and Juliana became fully involved in each other's lives and careers, and their affair lasted twelve years.

Forbes, who immediately began guiding and advising Juliana on art matters, was poles apart from Doctor in background, interest, and manner, and Doctor could only diminish in comparison. Born in 1880 into a proper and peripatetic Boston family, Watson grew up in Cambridge, Florence, and Paris. Of his boyhood, he told Van Wyck Brooks that he "went to school with the Danas and the Jameses" and "played baseball in the Longfellow backyard." In France he

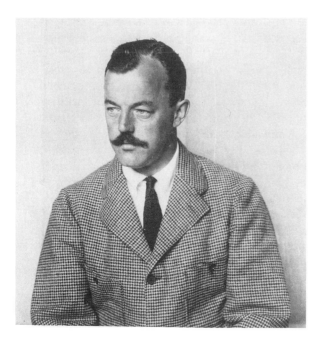

A passport photo of Forbes Watson taken in 1917, before he left to drive an ambulance in France.

met Mary Cassatt, beginning a friendship that lasted until her death. As a young man, Forbes was torn between becoming a writer and becoming an artist. He studied painting with Alfred Collins, a Boston painter to whom he was related. He went to Harvard, where he wrote short stories, some of which were published in the *Advocate*. After receiving his degree in 1904, he enrolled in Columbia Law School. He was admitted to the New York bar, but he never practiced. In 1910 Forbes married Agnes (Nan) Paterson, a painter of portraits and still lifes, who was four years older than he. She encouraged him to write, and the couple moved to Europe for a few years. When the Watsons returned to New York, Forbes went to work for the notorious newspaperman Frank Munsey, but he was fired for "rudeness"—he sat with his feet on the desk in the publisher's presence. These bursts of "rudeness," showing his disrespect for authority, were a constant in his life.

Through a neighbor in his apartment building, Forbes learned that the position of art critic for the *New York Post* would soon be vacant. He took over the job in 1913, and the first article he wrote was a blast at the stupidities of the National Academy of Design. The pattern was set for the rest of his tenure at the *Post*, the *World*, and any other publication that regularly carried his byline. In Forbes Watson the art world was given a born fighter who was at his best scenting the smoke of battle that arose from the blaze of ideas. His weapons—education, knowledge, a lawyerly gusto for argument, a capacity for scathing sarcasm, and a lethal force of expression—made him a fearsome opponent. Forbes would say anything to anybody. In a government report summarizing his tour of federal art projects throughout the country, he wrote, "Omaha is a place to make you feel like a snob and like it."

Watson's grasp of Western art spanned the Greeks and Romans through Cézanne, but he was shaken by the Armory Show. He later wrote, "My first visit to the Armory Show made it clear that the conventional world of art was living in a false and protected security." Instead of lashing out at the unfamiliar things before him, à la Cortissoz, he went every day until he had mastered the epic exhibition and absorbed Picasso, Matisse, Brancusi, and their peers. From then on, he was their partisan. He was also a discerning defender of traditional American art. His real enemies were pomp, pretense, and the brazen pursuit of publicity for its own sake; nothing ignited his pen like a silly fashion or bloviating self-advertisements.

Juliana and Forbes were enormously alike. They reveled in trading ripostes, laughing at life's absurdities, and using their quickness and sharpness to fight other people's battles for them. And just as Juliana was in flight from her background, Forbes had turned away from his old allegiances. His repudiation, however, was predicated differently. Unlike Juliana, whose rebellion against gentility was based on the need to rectify a sense of social inferiority, Forbes, because he was from the upper-middle class, denied nothing about his origins. He could afford to be a permanent adversary of the comically benighted respectability of his hometown and his people. In upholding European modernism and worthy strains of American art, for example, Forbes was shedding his Harvard indoctrination and the famous influence of Charles Eliot Norton, who taught

that America was a cultural void and everything modern smacked of an ugly and degenerate age. But the ineradicable fact remained that Forbes had been to Harvard.

Bostonians would have looked more sternly on another aspect of Watson's makeup. He was an unabashed sensualist. An expansive personality, he had an eye for women, and his job, which took him all over the city, into studios, art galleries, and private homes, demanded flexible hours and accrued its share of glamour. Then too women were attracted to him. In his prime, when Juliana first became intimate with him, Forbes possessed a jaunty, chipper look, much in the style of the young Ernest Hemingway. His dark hair and mustache were well-clipped; his eyes were bright and danced with lively innuendo. Short and trim, he dressed in understated tweeds. While he was involved with Juliana, he saw other women as well.

Forbes held enlightened views about women as individuals who should maintain creative and professional careers. In print he deplored cases of marriages between artists in which the wife's talent was sacrificed to the husband's. At home Forbes did not compel his wife into domestic subservience. Nan Watson had a long career working and exhibiting as an independent painter. She was regarded by her spouse and her peers as a full-time professional artist. Forbes's career was not forged at the expense of hers.

Throughout his infidelities Forbes stayed married to Nan. Nan was aware of her husband's entanglements, but she closed her eyes and held her tongue. She remained silent and benefited professionally from her position as tolerant spouse. Juliana bought several of Nan's floral still lifes for her New York apartment and Barley Sheaf Farm. Moreover, by the time the Whitney Museum opened in 1931, Nan Watson was represented in its permanent collection with eight oil paintings.* For a single artist, this was the institution's fourth-largest holding—as against Sloan, Luks, Davies, Bellows, Kuniyoshi, Reginald Marsh, and Charles Sheeler, represented by three oils each; Thomas Hart Benton, Oscar Bluemner, and Maurice Prendergast, represented by two; and Georgia O'Keeffe, Charles Demuth, Marsden Hartley, Max Weber, and Edward Hopper, who were then represented by one painting apiece. The notion of conflict of interest seems not to have entered any of the principals' heads, perhaps because making money from contemporary American art was yet a phantom in the ludicrous distance.

Good food and drink and their associated bonhomie also meant a great deal to Watson. He delighted in meeting friends for lunch and conversation at the Brevoort, he luxuriated in the sociability and volubility conferred by a bottle of wine. "Forbes was a great one for taking you out to a nice lunch," one of his secretaries said. "He'd have two martinis at least, and chat and chat and chat." In his enjoyment of cocktails and cozy talk, Forbes was joined by Juliana, who loved to drink. Alcohol began to play an important part in her life after she was married and away from Hoboken. Social drinking was not sanctioned by the

---

*After Juliana's death in 1948, many of her purchases were deaccessioned or exchanged for other works. The Nan Watson canvases were reduced from eight to four.

Riesers, and before World War I middle-class women were more likely to dine in tearooms than restaurants serving spirits. But with the liberation of Greenwich Village came the liberation of liquor—and cigarettes—for women in advanced circles. Drinking and smoking in public were signs of urbanity, an emancipated outlook, a willingness to embark on other daring ventures. Juliana's drink was Scotch, which she was able to ingest in huge quantities (especially considering her small size) without visible effect. A woman who had drinks alone with Juliana wrote in her diary that during their encounter "[Mrs. Force] was really very nice and also sober. She has more vitality than any other woman I've ever known and her ability to consume liquor seems to know no bounds." Her impressions echo the observations of others.

Was Juliana an alcoholic? Although the line between a person who enjoys drinking and someone dependent upon alcohol is not easy to draw, especially across the span of years, the answer would have to be yes. In Juliana's case the outward signs of habitual and excessive drinking did not become noticeable until the early 1940s. Then, during the last five or six years of her life, age, illness, and devastating circumstances contributed to a greater consumption of liquor and a lesser ability to conceal that she had been drinking. On the basis of eyewitness accounts, Juliana was a progressive alcoholic who for most of her life was able to control her drinking as much as was socially necessary. She craved excitement, and she often used alcohol to sustain excitement. Her friends and relatives thought she was a heavy drinker, but not an excessive one, because she imbibed "responsibly" and followed the rules of her set. During the Prohibition era, hard drinking, provided it did not lead to obvious antisocial behavior, was accepted as the zest of the times by many Americans. Flouting an ill-advised, unenforceable law was a dimension of being modern. In Juliana's milieu, her own tolerance for drink was considered a part of hospitality. Thus it was viewed as an asset rather than a potential problem or disease.

In 1917 Gertrude had begun renting space at 23 MacDougal Alley for the use of artist-friends who needed a temporary place to work. One of the floors was given to Guy Pène du Bois and the other to Jo Davidson, who was ever in transit between New York and Paris. Their presence in the Alley, plus the addition of Forbes, led to a lively series of luncheons and other parties for visiting celebrities during the 1919–1920 and 1920–1921 seasons. Juliana, Forbes, du Bois, O'Connor, and Gregory had regular berths at these gatherings; other artists, such as Kent and Childe Hassam, rotated. (Du Bois was so involved in MacDougal Alley socializing that in honor of one of the hostesses, his daughter Yvonne named her pet chicken Juliana Force.) One party was in honor of Hugh Walpole, the English novelist. Another featured the opera diva Mary Garden and the monologist Ruth Draper. Although Prohibition was now the law of the land, wines and spirits flowed freely at Studio parties, the Whitney cellars as bottomless as the Whitney coffers.

Guy Pène du Bois made a sketch from memory of an ill-fated experiment that took place about this time. Forgiven his social misdemeanors during the

Indigenous Exhibition, Luks was invited to Gertrude's studio to paint a portrait of her on the spot. Juliana, Forbes, du Bois, and a few other artists were asked to make up the audience. Luks, pirouetting about, set up a full-length canvas and made jokes at the expense of one of the painters watching him. Gertrude stood with her arms akimbo, waiting for the coming pyrotechnics. Luks picked up his palette and a fistful of tubes. Grabbing a tube of vermilion, he yelled, "All my life I've wanted to do this!" and emptied the entire contents onto the palette. As he applied his colors in slapdash gobs, he commented on every stroke he made and solicited the audience's compliments. Eventually Luks came up with something resembling a likeness of Gertrude, but he ruined it by an additional hash of brushstrokes. Luks then strolled blithely away from the mess he made. Du Bois's illustration, *The Three Hour Portrait: A Comedy by George Luks in Six Acts,** shows Gertrude patiently posing on the model's stand. In the foreground stands Luks's canvas, with the broad lines of her figure roughed out. The artist is nowhere to be seen.

These gatherings at MacDougal Alley refreshed Gertrude and catered to her need for diversion. She wanted to be in Paris for more than flying visits, but preparing for a show of her own work in the Whitney Studio detained her in New York. Additionally, MacDougal Alley was serving as a hideaway from her husband. In middle age Harry had become increasingly priggish and mindful of his position. He could no longer dictate his wife's future, but he struck back with petty blows, even intruding on Gertrude's studio, which formerly had been off-limits. Guy Pène du Bois told his daughter that sometimes he was asked to stand outside Gertrude's studio door and warn her if Harry was approaching. She and her friends were taking yoga classes, and they knew he would trample on their latest enthusiasm.

In August of 1919 Harry found some letters to Gertrude from a former lover. Revealing a stunning capacity for ignoring the tenor of their twenty-three years of marriage, Harry wrote to Gertrude, "Now the bottom is knocked out of life. It's all lies. Are you all a lie? Are you all false? Is nothing real?" His own unfaithfulness notwithstanding, she was supposed to have stayed Harry's long-suffering and inviolate property. He went on to demand, "I have got to know how many men. . . . But I don't want to know names. . . ." Gertrude countenanced none of this anymore, but the accusations still seared. At this moment, Juliana, Forbes, du Bois, and Davidson were not only pillars of friendship, but bulwarks of protection, understanding, and jollity for her. Two versions of a limerick Gertrude penned about Juliana's attitude toward the playful conspiracies of MacDougal Alley convey affectionate gratitude for her partner's solidarity and fund of humor. Gertrude wrote:

> Mrs. Force in a new snappy frock
> Didn't tell a lot that could shock
> Encouraged each ass
> Allowed openings to pass
> And was always the last one to knock.

* It was made for Juliana and is now in the Whitney's archives.

And,

> Mrs. Force in a new snappy frock
> Didn't tell a tale that could shock
> Encouraged each one
> Was the heart of the fun
> And always the last one to knock.

Impressions of the War, the body of sculptures Gertrude exhibited in late 1919, was her best to date. World War I brought about an abrupt change in her work. Instead of having to rely on idealized or secondhand versions of experience, she was, through her visits to the front and Juilly Hospital, a direct witness to a reality more grave and solid than any make-believe. To convey a fraction of the conflict's impact on the participants would be task enough. Gertrude's small studies of soldiers and anguished refugees are invested with genuine pathos and sturdiness as well as a documentary accuracy. Finally, if briefly, she had data that served as a point of departure for emotionally engaged, emotionally authentic works of art.

Du Bois wrote the preface to the catalog for Gertrude's exhibition, and in general was acting as Juliana's unofficial adviser. He recommended that one of his best friends be inducted into the Whitney Studio Club. Believing in the man's talent, du Bois told Juliana that he deserved an exhibition to himself. He would arrange everything. And so in January 1920, Edward Hopper was given his first one-man show and "a tea presided over by Mrs Force in an ugly orange hat and a very amiable smile." He was thirty-seven. Sixteen oils were shown— the painter's scenes of Paris, Massachusetts, and Maine. Hopper's famous raking light and his unadorned treatment of his subjects were already evident. That distinctive sensibility did not appeal to potential picture-buyers, and none of the paintings sold.* But a strong connection was made between Hopper and the Whitney Studio Club, and he became a loyal member.

In the adjacent gallery on West Fourth Street, Kenneth Hayes Miller had a show of drawings and etchings. In his wake, a new crop of his ex-pupils joined the Club. Katherine Schmidt, Yasuo Kuniyoshi, Reginald Marsh, Isabel Bishop, Louis Bouché, and Niles Spencer were some of the more prominent young people who began to be seen around West Fourth Street. They flocked to the plentiful teas with their cakes and thick sandwiches and Juliana's "wonderful warmth and appetite for young people." Katherine Schmidt said that the Club became an important part of her circle's social life because she and her friends were rebelling against a middle-class background, and when they needed bolstering, the companionship and encouragement they found at the Club were invaluable to their morale. Schmidt was not represented by a gallery until 1927, so her visibility at the Club helped her to build a reputation. "The Club and Mrs. Force were looking for anyone who had promise," she remembered. "There were not too many of us, so if you had the least promise, you stuck out like a sore thumb. . . . They [Juliana and Gertrude] were really helping, developing

---

*Most of them are now owned by the Whitney.

a side the [National] Academy was overlooking. [We had] a great feeling of animosity toward the Academy."

The Hopper and Miller shows were followed by a collection of photographs of American Indians by Edward L. Curtis, drawings by Old Italian Masters, and a members' exhibition of 161 works, but they were ancillary considered in relation to art activities simultaneously preoccupying Juliana. Gertrude was asked by the directors of the twelfth annual International Art Exhibition in Venice to send a representative sampling of contemporary American paintings to their pavilion to be shown from May to November of 1920. To Gertrude, the timing couldn't have been better. Tired of hearing Americans apologize for the poverty of their culture and certain that if she cured European audiences of their ignorance of American painting they would stop believing that "American artist" were two mutually contradictory words, Gertrude agreed to organize the exhibition at her own expense. She and Juliana chose the artists, and Juliana conferred with them about which pictures to send, arranged the loans, and prepared to go to Venice to install the exhibition.

On the whole, the art (115 pictures) represented two generations of American Realism and Impressionism, although a few young modernists were included. The selections spanned the nineteenth and twentieth centuries, with the connections between active artists and their predecessors clearly delineated. No attempt was made to be comprehensive—on purpose, the living painters were all previous exhibitors at the Whitney Club or Studio; the deceased painters had taught or inspired them. * The common denominator of the nineteenth-century painters was that they were underappreciated. In America their advocates were few; in Europe no one had heard of them. Juliana and Gertrude were eager to present Eakins to Europe. Their show marked the first time his work was seen abroad since the artist, who died in 1916, last sent to the Paris Salon in 1890.

As a trial run for this undertaking, and because of a shortage of storage space for the pictures, Forbes and Juliana organized a show in March 1920 at the Colony Club, the very place she had first assisted Gertrude thirteen years before. Most of the American art on view was destined for Venice, but Forbes added Cassatt and two more contemporary painters whose talents he felt deserved exposure: Max Weber and Charles Sheeler. Sheeler, who shared Juliana's love of Bucks County and American design, would soon be the beneficiary of her assistance. For the Colony Club, the American paintings were augmented by Impressionist and Post-Impressionist works borrowed from the fine collections of Marius de Zayas, Lillie P. Bliss, and Adolph Lewisohn. With a little assistance from Forbes, Juliana and Gertrude demonstrated that they had made their peace with the Armory Show.

---

* The younger contingent consisted of all The Eight except Shinn, plus Bellows, Beal, Burlin, Chanler, Kent, du Bois, Tucker, Hassam, Halpert, Max Kuehne, and Maurice Sterne. At the head of the nineteenth-century group was Eakins, represented by six canvases, including *The Concert Singer*, the early version of *William Rush Carving His Allegorical Figure of the Schuylkill River*, and *Between Rounds*, now all in the collection of the Philadelphia Museum of Art. Shown with him as contemporaries were Ryder, Theodore Robinson, and Twachtman.

In April of 1920 Juliana sailed for Venice. It was her first trip to Europe, and the experience promised a sweetness beyond her wildest dreams. The city was, under any circumstances, one of the most romantic places in the world, but for Juliana the romance was more than historical, as she was not a delegation of one. She needed a co-commissioner to share the work involved, and she got the person she wanted—Forbes.

Yet Forbes and Juliana's time together was not one of unalloyed bliss. As Forbes later reported in several magazine articles, the exhibition became a "terrible official spectacle" with the requisite "official vociferations on art." For decorative presence, it was opened by a member of the Italian royal family, who spent seven and a half minutes eyeing the pavilion and its 115 paintings, and then sped thankfully away in his gondola toward "a well-earned lunch." Among the remaining Italians (artists, art authorities, and civilians alike), the occasion was regarded as sport. Criticism of the living artists was carping. Debate centered on whether their paintings were too French or not French enough. The visiting Americans were especially tried by the spectators who either laughed openly at Eakins or condemned him in whispers everyone could overhear. Even the Italian painters of the day were unable to see any merit in his art. To them he was hopelessly old-fashioned.

Despite the Italian reaction, Gertrude decided to send the show, augmented by a selection of her own war sculpture, to London, Paris, and Sheffield for the summer of 1921. It would do the French and British good, she believed, to become more familiar with recent American art. In December of 1920 Juliana made a brief scouting trip to England and France to find suitable and willing galleries for both exhibitions. This time Doctor would accompany her, making his first and last trip abroad. But Juliana sailed before he did, and she passed her first days in Paris sick and alone in her hotel. Auguste Jaccaci, a learned writer and connoisseur and one of the deans of the American art world then, had gotten to know Juliana and was fond of her. While she was in Paris, he was in the South of France, and Juliana reported on her work setting up the exhibitions. From Vence, Jaccaci replied:

> I am distressed in thinking of you for the first time in Paris, with so much to see that is equally helpful, and of the very few days you can spend there, every one precious, many are blotted. . . . And here it is not like being . . . at home where your friends would come & cheer you up. . . . But my hat is off to you for your courage & cheerfulness at least in your letters to me. . . .
>
> I am so glad you are now entirely satisfied and feel sure about the time for Exhibitions. And that my good friend (and yours) Mr. Jean Guiffrey* is showing his keen interest. Rest assured of what I told you, you can depend upon him. He has the same art ideals you have & is sympathetic to your views which are his. He has the rare advantage of knowing something of America. Moreover his official position—after all the highest in the picture world in France—gives weight to what he says and in what he is interested in. . . .
>
> I should consider this a pleasant day if I was not thinking of you away from all friends alone in a hotel room.

*A curator at the Louvre and formerly the director of the Museum of Fine Arts, Boston.

Doctor arrived, and Juliana was glad of his company. They enjoyed the enchantments of Paris together, and the visit was a happy interlude for them. Doctor and Juliana made the rounds of the galleries, and in one of them Juliana saw a drawing of a couple dancing that she longed to own. It was a study by Renoir for *La Danse à la Campagne*, a painting now in the Musée d'Orsay. The next day the sketch was delivered to her as a gift from Doctor. Many years later Juliana learned that it was a facsimile of such exactitude that it had fooled several experts. But she continued to cherish it as a memento of her husband's burst of sentiment.

In 1921 it was apparent that Juliana and Gertrude were listening to Forbes's advice. The women actively joined him in attacking one of his pet subjects of critical displeasure: the policy of American museums, particularly the mighty Metropolitan Museum of Art, with respect to the acquisition of modern art. Forbes usually directed his ire at the Metropolitan; he boiled over at the museum's refusal to acknowledge that the twentieth century had actually happened. He characterized New York's premier fine arts institution as an extension of the ossified National Academy of Design. Bryson Burroughs, the curator of paintings at the Metropolitan, was open-minded about art and sympathetic to the School of Paris and nonacademic American painting and sculpture, but the purchasing committee controlling his requests was hostile. Back in 1913 Burroughs nearly lost his job for buying a Cézanne from the Armory Show for the museum. Ever since then his was an embattled position. Forbes knew that the Met's failure to add modern art to its collection was not the fault of Burroughs, and he rightly laid the blame at the feet of the "experts" on the purchasing committee. He argued that the committees on Egyptian or Far Eastern or medieval art had specialists in their field, persons who were not only well-versed in their subjects but were passionately interested in them. In the case of twentieth-century art, the museum's committees were made up of men who automatically saw them-selves as authorities because the art was of their own time. Their pronouncements were overwhelmingly negative, and Forbes suggested that instead of trying to force people averse to modern art to try to like it, the Metropolitan should reconstitute their committee with enthusiasts of proven vision. He recommended John Quinn, Albert Barnes, and Arthur B. Davies for the job.

This splendid suggestion was ignored, and the fight to influence the museum's policy was waged on two fronts. In the cause of Post-Impressionism, the president of the Metropolitan received a letter urging him to hold "a special exhibition, illustrative of the best in modern French art," specifying that it should feature Degas, Cézanne, Renoir, Gauguin, Monet, Derain, and others. The letter, dated January 26, 1921, also said that the show should open "if possible, not later than April 15th." It was signed by six of the most respected advocates and collectors of contemporary art in New York: Quinn (the probable instigator of the letter), Lillie Bliss, Davies, Paul Dougherty, Agnes Meyer, and Gertrude. Confronted by this consortium of wealth and influence, the Metropolitan's elders acquiesced. Group pressure was responsible for the important Loan Exhibition

of Impressionist and Post-Impressionist Paintings, the first show of modern art ever held at the museum. Quinn, the major lender, had twenty-nine paintings in the show. Picassos, Derains, Redons, Van Goghs, Dufys, Rouaults, Vlamincks, and Matisses hung on the museum walls for the first time. For Quinn, who tried to get the Metropolitan to buy a Gauguin in 1915 and was flatly turned down, the show was a moment of vindication. It was also, of course, a circus for reactionaries, who parroted the usual objections of unintelligibility and incompetence. Quinn overheard one woman say to another, "Well, I was up there and invariably the awfullest pictures belonged to John Quinn."

Juliana wanted independent artists to be represented in public collections, but saw that the institutions were loath to buy their work. Knowing that few museums would turn down a gift from a Whitney, she entered into an informal but concerted dialogue with museum directors around the country, suggesting that Gertrude purchase the paintings and present them to the galleries. Juliana's half of the bargain was the easier one, for the curators had to argue the pictures' merits before viewers wishing they had never been brought into the room. But their teamwork paid off. In 1921 the Metropolitan accepted four American paintings by artists not previously in the collection: Sloan, Luks, Glackens, and du Bois. Of the four, the painting by du Bois was bought by Gertrude and coaxed into the collection by Burroughs and Juliana. As three out of four of these pictures were painted before 1910, the museum had hardly ventured out on an aesthetic limb in their definition of the contemporary. But for the artists involved, attaining the Metropolitan's portals was cause for great joy, and their euphoria would gratify Juliana as intensely as any larger shattering of precedents. By the end of 1921, Juliana placed six more of Gertrude's gifts into American museums. The most important was *The Haymarket*, by Sloan, which went to the Brooklyn Museum. Another was Rockwell Kent's *Bones of Ships*, donated to the Phillips Collection in Washington, D.C.

In January of 1921 Juliana gave Sloan a show of his etchings at the Club. Another artist she believed in and felt it imperative to sponsor was Stuart Davis, and in April he was invited to assemble a one-man show of his latest paintings and watercolors. Davis's work had taken a pivotal turn, one important to herald. The paint was hardly dry on the canvases when the Club exhibited several of his "tobacco" pictures, including *Bull Durham* and *Lucky Strike*.* These were oils painted to simulate Cubist collages. Besides demonstrating an advanced understanding of juxtaposition and spatial division, the tobacco series set forth with characteristic directness the foundations of Davis's artistic vocabulary: the use of American commercial imagery for its iconographic properties and the incorporation of letters, numbers, and words as independent elements of his design. The toughness and hypnotic dynamism of American production and modern society, epitomized by the throwaway pack of cigarettes and the connotations of cigarettes themselves, possessed Davis while he painted these pictures. He wrote in his journal for April of 1921, "I do not belong to the human

---

* Now in the collections of the Baltimore Museum of Art and the Museum of Modern Art, respectively.

race but am a product made by the American Can Co. and the New York *Evening Journal.*"

Davis was installed in one of the Club's galleries, and in the other were mural sketches and studies of New York and Spain by Joáquin Torres-Garcia, a leading figure in the Barcelona avant-garde who was in New York on an extended visit. Despite good reviews, commercial success eluded Torres-Garcia, so he earned no money for his return passage to Europe. Juliana lent him the fare, with the tacit understanding that the money would not be repaid. Torres-Garcia also had more than 100 paintings that had to go into storage; they were stored gratis until 1933, when the artist asked for them.

Juliana had traveled a long road from Warren Davis to Stuart Davis, from the undistinguished to the remarkable. On that journey she learned, sometimes painfully and sometimes gaily, where she was going. She could not always steer in a straight line, so occasionally it seemed as if she had lost her direction. And sometimes she did—when dealing with the flux and fray of living art, there are no guarantees of error-free choices. But once she had her objective—as Stuart Davis testified, the Whitney Studio Club was the first organization that "encouraged the artist's right to explore and investigate outside the expected norms of picture making"—she could not only realize it in concrete form, but permute it.

That Juliana had identified her direction did not preclude her from spreading the Whitney manna to innovators in other arts. The more she did, the more indefatigable she became in using her gift for getting things done. In the spring of 1921 she heard about the plight and plans of Edgard Varèse, the vanguard composer who was determined to build a following for innovative music in New York. Varèse and Carlos Salzedo, a gifted harpist and teacher, wanted to establish a society for the performance, appreciation, and faithful interpretation of modern music, which in those days meant work ignored by the musical establishment and therefore denied an audience. They called their organization the International Composers' Guild, and as soon as Juliana learned of it, she became an ally. To her it seemed—and the facts bore out her assumption—that Varèse and Salzedo's aims paralleled her own, and she agreed that something must be done at once. She persuaded Gertrude to support the Guild and Varèse, who was then imprisoned in a job as a piano salesman in a department store. In April of 1921 Varèse began receiving an allowance of $200 a month. He quit his "piano nightmare" and returned to organizing concerts and composing.

The International Composers' Guild formally came into being on May 31, 1921. It soon asserted itself as a primary forum for the discussion and performance of modern music. The founders' manifesto and their accompanying grievances were a declaration of independence in complete agreement with the ideas and principles animating all Whitney-Force activities. Varèse and Salzedo proclaimed:

> The composer is the only one of the creators of today who is denied direct contact with the public. When his work is done he is thrust aside, and the interpreter enters, not to try to understand the composition but impertinently to judge it. Not finding

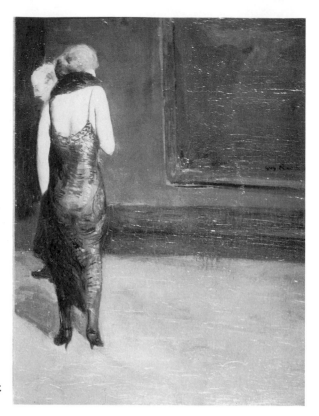

Although du Bois chose to paint Juliana from the back, his portrait of her at the Studio Club is an excellent likeness and catches her in a characteristic act—looking at a picture.

in it any trace of the conventions to which he is accustomed, he banishes it from his programs, denouncing it as incoherent and unintelligible. . . .

The present day composers . . . have realized the necessity of banding together and fighting for the right of each individual to secure "fair and free presentation of his work." It is out of such collective will that the International Composers' Guild was born. . . .

The International Composers' Guild disapproves of all "isms"; denies the existence of schools; recognizes only the individual.

The Club's spring season closed with a members' show, after which Juliana would sail for Europe to superintend the Overseas Exhibition, as the traveling show first assembled for Venice was now called. Before she left, she learned that Guy Pène du Bois was having financial difficulties. She asked Gertrude for $2,000 for him and dreamed up a commission: a series of humorous drawings that together would comprise a pictorial history of the Whitney Studio and an oil portrait of herself. The sketches were slight and not up to du Bois's usual standard of satire, but the portrait was incisiveness itself. Everyone who knew both Juliana and the du Bois portrait (*Juliana Force at the Whitney Studio Club**) said he caught her to the life. This compliment has some meaning

* Now in the collection of the Whitney Museum.

because the artist elected to paint Juliana *from the back*, as she appraises a picture hung on a wall at one of the Club's openings. Juliana is in evening clothes. The heavy coils of red-gold hair are wound loosely back into a chignon, which nestles into a black fur boa. Her dress, a low-cut black gown, clings to a shapely figure. Her arms, shoulders, and legs—all well-proportioned and alluring—are exposed. Allan Rieser thought that du Bois pictured Juliana from the back to avoid painting her face. Alternatively, he may have decided on a presumably anonymous rear view to demonstrate the unmistakability of her person. Juliana does not merely inhabit the space, but through her stance and posture imprints herself on it. And in the protruding curves of her shoulder blades, du Bois introduces an element of erotic promise. There is an aura of sexual provocativeness and confidence in this likeness of her. In suggesting such electricity, du Bois could have been thinking of the exaltation that came from Juliana's relationship with Forbes, or perhaps it was a reflection of the changes in feminine fashion and demeanor the twenties wrought.

At forty-five, Juliana had not lost her looks. Instead she had victoriously gained them. She began to be mistaken for Alla Nazimova, the great tragic actress. The resemblance between the two was undeniable: Both women were simultaneously attractive and homely, with similarly shaped faces, noses, and chins. The eloquent play of their features—particularly the narrow, penetrating eyes—made people forget their lack of conventional prettiness. Most pertinently, both Juliana and Nazimova presented themselves to the world along comparable lines—as central characters in vivid dramas created and directed by themselves. Juliana's theatricality was accented by her hands and manner of speaking. She had long, beautifully articulated fingers, which were unobtrusively but artfully manicured. Her deep contralto voice, which had a whiskey-and-cigarettes worldliness to it, had a range of nuance worthy of a trained actress. That nuance was exercised, for Juliana had a voice for every occasion. "She would answer the telephone with a soft, refined 'Hellooo,' " Charles Rieser said. "Then she would hear me and snap, 'Oh, it's only you, Charles,' and revert to her everyday growl."

Juliana spent July in France, installing and watching over the Overseas Exhibition and Gertrude's retrospective. A few French artists came to pay their respects, including Maillol. After sailing home, she went to Bucks County for August. Charles, Irene, and the boys joined her, and she invited Rockwell Kent to enliven her stay. Kent wouldn't have been Kent if he had not capitalized on a few days in Juliana's company, and he emerged with a commission to decorate the living room doors. In a letter confirming the details, he asked Juliana to lend Carl Zigrosser some money and write on his behalf to a woman friend, who he implied was insecure, that he loved her. Three days later, this bizarre request was repeated. Kent once more insinuated that the woman was caught up in a silly paranoia about nonexistent amorous intrigues. He again asked Juliana to reassure her that such fears were groundless. (They were not—Kent was infatuated with another woman, as Juliana suspected.) Juliana knew better than to furnish dynamite for that explosive situation, and she ignored him. Kent could not understand her reticence and complained to Zigrosser about it.

Kent, however, was capable of disinterested generosity, and through one such act, he expanded the Whitney patronage of modern music. In the fall of 1921 he alerted Juliana to Carl Ruggles, the musician, composer, and associate of Varèse. Ruggles, an exact contemporary of Juliana, was struggling to pay his rent and put food on the table. His output was small, and what music he allowed to be performed was too radically dissonant to become popular. A crusty individualist who served an austere muse, Ruggles was nonetheless a salty, practical man with a booming voice and an earthy sense of humor. Ruggles also painted, and he and Juliana rapidly took to each other. They were fond of trading snatches of poetry and reading verse aloud, a passion that could and did range from Browning and Whitman—Juliana was in her element acting out the monologues and she revered "Out of the Cradle Endlessly Rocking"—to ribald limericks. (Juliana also adored Gertrude Stein, Keats, the hothouse novels of Ronald Firbank, and T. S. Eliot, especially the last's more fleshly passages. She would roar with laughter after a recitation of:

> Grishkin is nice: her Russian eye
> Is underlined for emphasis;
> Uncorseted, her friendly bust
> Gives promise of pneumatic bliss.)

Juliana secured Ruggles an allowance in the autumn of 1921. He received it until November 1925, when another wealthy patron agreed to subsidize him for the rest of his life, and he no longer needed the Whitney largesse.

The world of the Greenwich Village avant-garde was still quite small, and everyone knew each other. Ruggles became a member of the Composers' Guild, and about the time he began to receive Whitney money, Juliana informed a worried Varèse that his allowance also would continue. Varèse celebrated his guarantee of security—which would last for six years—by getting married. Ruggles was also a friend of Henry Schnakenberg, and Varèse of Joseph Stella. All four lived in the Village, close to the Whitney Club and Studio. In November of 1921 Stella and Schnakenberg were given one-man shows at the Club; the Studio received the Overseas Exhibition, to which Juliana added Demuth's illustrations for Zola's *Nana*. (Nevertheless, only 200 people attended the show.)

Juliana bought one of Stella's botanical drawings, and began the negotiations with other museums to place the seven paintings Gertrude bought out of the Overseas show. By now, along with the purchases mentioned, Juliana had bought work out of nearly every Whitney show since 1917. Yet the acquisition of art, beyond a commitment to nonacademic Americans, was not programmatic. It was done mainly as a means of financial assistance or as a testament of belief. Neither Gertrude nor Juliana could live without art around them, but their priorities then lay not in building a collection—otherwise they would have held onto a key painting like *The Haymarket* instead of giving it to the Brooklyn Museum, and they would have waited for artists to reach maturity instead of buying serially out of their own limited exhibitions—but in fostering an artistic

community and seeing to its welfare. The point was not to refine their holdings, but to offer meaningful gestures of faith in the artists' future. After all, they observed, without artists, museums or academies would not exist.

Just as crucial to Juliana was the provision of exhibition opportunities, which also took precedence over conventional collecting. The newly married Doris and Edward L. Bernays took a flat a block away from Eighth Street in 1922 and met Juliana shortly thereafter. The three saw each other quite often, and, wrote Edward Bernays, "The most vivid memory I have of these occasions is her articulate insistence on artists showing their creative work. I think her words, often repeated, were 'Show, show, show.' "

What tells most about the haphazard benignity of these years is that no such entity as the "Collection of the Whitney Studio Club" ever existed. Until 1930 every work bought from a living artist was assigned either to the "Collection of Mrs. H. P. Whitney" or the "Collection of Mrs. W. B. Force." Save for obvious exceptions, such as folk carvings and nineteenth-century provincial paintings, which were the sole enthusiasm of Juliana, and works by personal friends of Gertrude's, such as Chanler, O'Connor, Davidson, and Howard Cushing, it is impossible to decipher or understand the divisions between the collections. Juliana bought roughly 80 percent of the American art in Gertrude's name, and she also bought with her own money.

Paintings, sculptures, and drawings acquired by both women were scattered through Juliana's apartment, Gertrude's studio in MacDougal Alley, her Fifth Avenue and Long Island houses, and the storage areas and walls of the Whitney Club and Studio. Yet location does not always yield clues to possession because art floated around with uncommon casualness. For example, from photographs and an inventory of Juliana's apartment, we know that at some point she displayed the following: several works by Charles Sheeler, which were in her personal collection and remained so throughout her life; a 1919 landscape by Allen Tucker, bought out of his one-man show of that year, with Juliana's home address label on it and now in the museum's collection; still lifes by Leon Hartl—some bought for herself and some bought for Gertrude—from his one-man shows at the Club in 1925 and 1927, which all ended up in the Whitney's permanent collection; and Lawson's *Winter on the River*, one of the four pictures Gertrude purchased from The Eight exhibition in 1908. But the number of cases in which a work of art can be traced from its origin with the painter or sculptor to its entrance into the Studio, Club, or Juliana's premises is maddeningly rare. The odd archival notation, the infrequent newspaper or journal article, or the artist's own ledgers tend to furnish the only traces of the date and circumstances of a sale to the Whitney-Force collections, for Juliana was cavalier about record keeping, and Gertrude didn't object. At the time, the two women had no sense of themselves as making history, no thought of an institution in the future. They neglected to spend the time on establishing a provenance for each object coming into their hands, perhaps because they thought that an emphasis on cataloging would dampen the informality of Club and Studio proceedings. Accordingly, the whens, whys, and hows of most of the art Juliana

acquired from 1916 until the late 1920s are a matter of guesswork and a frustrating enigma.

Compared to the frenetic exhibition schedule of the year before, 1922 was relatively quiet. No shows were held in the Whitney Studio, but the Club sponsored small one-man exhibitions of Glackens, Kuehne, Boardman Robinson, and Hopper (who was still unknown, had no dealer, and was supporting himself as a commercial illustrator). And there was the customary members' show (from 1919 through 1928, a members' annual took place every spring). The two women were busy elsewhere. Gertrude was heavily involved with family obligations: Barbara, her younger daughter, was making her debut, and Sonny had to be extricated from a lurid breach-of-promise and paternity suit filed by an ex-mistress. Juliana was conducting two sets of negotiations for Gertrude's sculpture commissions.

The first commission was a war memorial to the Fourth Infantry Division, to be placed in Arlington National Cemetery. Juliana negotiated with Brig. Gen. Mark L. Hersey, a veteran of the division. Hersey was taken with Juliana and respected her efficiency and her administrative shrewdness, saluting her smartly by calling her "Mrs. Whitney's executive officer." His complimentary estimate was not returned. Hersey, Juliana related to her nephews, was a dreadful bore, and one requiring endless ingratiatory invitations to the farm, but she endured him for Gertrude's sake. "No one will ever know what I went through [to place Gertrude's sculpture]," Juliana confided to Allan Rieser. Hersey was an eager visitor to Bucks County for nine years (1921–1930), throughout the vicissitudes of the negotiations, which became entangled and broke off without the monument ever being realized. However, Hersey staunchly admired Gertrude's sculpture, and he later wrote helpful letters that expedited the progress of subsequent commissions.

A more successful and speedier conclusion was reached in the planning and execution of the second memorial, which was completed in 1924. Gertrude was to make an equestrian statue of Buffalo Bill Cody for the town named after him in Wyoming. Sonny Whitney said that the genesis of the monument took place between 1920 and 1921, when the Whitney family toured the Far West in their private Pullman car. "My mother purchased forty acres of land which she donated to the town of Cody to create a museum complex of Western art,"* C. V. Whitney wrote in his memoir *High Peaks*. "In order to start the project, she agreed to create and sculpt a lifesize statue of Buffalo Bill, who had died in 1917, and erect it on the site where she had chosen." Gertrude's generosity— and the reservoir of wealth behind it that could be tapped if necessary—was certainly a factor in making her the sculptor of choice of Buffalo Bill's niece, and the Wyoming fine arts authorities and townspeople of Cody assented. The press reported that Gertrude got the job because "she was the only woman sculptor

---

* Now the Buffalo Bill Historical Center.

with whom the Colonel was acquainted." (The acquaintance, Gertrude's biographer noted, consisted of her attending a Wild West Show in 1908.) Several of Cody's relatives were given to making exaggerated public statements and promoting their interests at the expense of Gertrude's, and Juliana and Gertrude soon grew wary of them. But unlike the Fourth Division memorial, the solicitors of the Buffalo Bill statue were safely located in Wyoming, well out of reach of New York and Barley Sheaf Farm. Juliana corresponded effectively with the architect and surveyors by telegram and letter and kept hyperactive Codyans at arm's length. She did not go to Wyoming until 1924, on the occasion of inspecting the site.

But there were always diversions from the petty diplomacies and tiresome details of contractual arrangements. The Composers' Guild was thriving, and on February 19, 1922, the first of three concerts scheduled for the spring season took place. Afterward Juliana hosted a party at West Fourth Street and invited the entire audience to it. Presumably in conjunction with the Guild's program, in March and April of 1922 three musical evenings were held at the Studio Club, with Carl Ruggles lecturing on "The Present Situation in American Music," "The Historical Background of Music," and "Technique and Phantasy in the Study of Composition." These were not dry perorations—at one evening six musicians performed his "Men and Angels," and Ruggles himself was a crackerjack speaker. Carl Zigrosser, present at a Ruggles lecture, remembered that while chewing on a cigar the composer "directed a miniature orchestra, and among other things analysed the thematic structure of Beethoven's Eroica Symphony with the aid of considerable profanity."

The third concert of the International Composers' Guild was held in April 1922. The program was devoted to Varèse, who was overjoyed because it was the first time his music had been performed publicly since 1910. His symphony *Amériques* and several songs were on the bill, conducted by Salzedo. Louise Varèse remembered the event as one of the shining moments of her life. "The audience was vociferously enthusiastic and shouts of *encore* brought Salzedo back to conduct it [*La Chanson de Là-haut*] a second time. Mrs. Force gave a reception . . . after the concert and there has never been a happier, gayer party. Varèse's pioneering venture had passed the test of the anxious first season." And Varèse's cause—the understanding and appreciation of modern music in America—was on a surer footing.

Rockwell Kent was still bobbing in the stream of Juliana's social life. His personal life was as tempestuous as ever, and as an escape from commercial pressures and extramarital flings that had gone beyond his control, he decided to go on a painting and adventuring trip to Tierra del Fuego and Cape Horn. (From his journals of his exploits there Kent wrote the very successful *Voyaging: Southward from the Strait of Magellan*, published in 1924.)

Kent peppered Juliana—occasionally addressed as Becky—with shipboard letters over the summer and fall of 1922. She had presented him with a barometer as a going-away gift, and he reported on its perturbations during the storms as his boat was battered by the heavy seas. These were nothing to the disturbances he was causing on land. Kent wrote opaquely of Punta Arenas, Chile, which

he reached in July, as "a wonderful little city . . . full of English and Germans, full of liquor—and good clubs to drink it in, and dice boxes to shake for drinks. That's the national pastime—and the gods, thank Heaven, are on my side." He did not tell Juliana that, within hours of being invited by a British newspaper editor to a club where many Englishmen drank, he was making loud remarks —probably pro-German declarations—that angered a member. Kent, feeling threatened, picked up the man by the neck and pitched him into a nearby dining table.

Even during those rare times when he eluded trouble, Kent made a better friend when an ocean or continent separated him from his well-wishers. He was the exception, as most artists were far less brutal, though they could be rough-hewn. This was true of Reuben Nakian, whom Juliana met in the fall of 1922, while he was sharing a studio with Gaston Lachaise. Nakian was poor, blunt, and in his own words "a young savage who wasn't social at all." Yet he possessed a genuine talent, and other artists who saw his sculpture respected it. He had the good fortune to get a piece of his sculpture (a limestone *Jack Rabbit*) reproduced in the May 1922 issue of the *Dial*, the vanguard magazine of the arts, and Lachaise astutely suggested to Nakian that he show the magazine to Juliana. Nakian saw her, and she made an appointment to visit him a week later. She arrived at the studio with Forbes, and they watched the young man, who was short, burly, and powerfully built, carve in stone. Another week went by, and then Juliana telephoned with the news that she would like to sponsor him. He would shortly be receiving a stipend of $250 a month, enabling him to buy stone and have his own studio.

To Nakian, who needed to separate himself from Lachaise's overpowering presence to establish his artistic independence, the allowance was a godsend. In gratitude he presented Juliana with five graceful chalk drawings* and moved to a studio in Weehawken Heights, New Jersey. The checks started arriving in 1923, and they arrived every month for the next five years. Nakian, nearly half a century after Juliana's help, marveled at the freedom of the arrangement.

> There were no strings attached. The checks came in the mail. I never met Mrs. Whitney. Everything was done through Mrs. Force, who let me alone for years. She trusted me and comprehended what I was—a strange artist who needed my privacy. Without the Whitney it would have been tough—I don't how I would have gotten through. Too bad that I was so goddamn uncivilized. The money stopped [in 1928 when the Whitney Studio Club metamorphosed into the Whitney Studio Galleries], and I was shocked when Mrs. Force dropped me. I was so stupid that I didn't even thank her for the five years and all she did for me. But it didn't matter to her. We became friends again later.

Another contemporaneous "discovery" was John Dos Passos. Dos Passos had already won recognition for his novels, most notably *Three Soldiers* in 1921, but he had also studied art since 1916. He was painting seriously, but he had nowhere to exhibit. His friend Adelaide Lawson, a Whitney Club member, was probably

---

* Now in the collection of the Whitney Museum.

the one to introduce him to Juliana in late 1922. Juliana liked Dos Passos's pictures and would show them as soon as she could.

As 1922 drew to a close, Juliana could be certain that she had done her job with skill and imagination. The Studio was a fresher place and the Club had come into its own. Up-and-coming painters, sculptors, writers, and musicians were congregating at West Fourth Street, as the word circulated of the welcome they would receive. The members' show had been the best ever: Its highlights reflected the capable core of artists the Club was now able to attract. In all, 300 artists had joined the Club, about fifty of them that year. Waving its broad charter of benevolence like a wand, Juliana had given Sloan, Kent, Kuehne, Davis, Torres-Garcia, Hopper, du Bois, Varèse, Ruggles, Lachaise, and Nakian financial and moral support during critical phases of their careers. Growing sturdily and spontaneously, welcoming beginners and ratifying professionals, there was no doubt that it was a real club.

CHAPTER SIX

DEA EX MACHINA

❧ *(1923–1926)* ❧

It seems to be fun to belong to the
Whitney Studio Club.
—HENRY McBRIDE

T HE YEAR 1923 marked the beginning of an inspired period in Juliana's life and Whitney history. It seemed that she could do no
wrong that couldn't be righted, make no mistake that couldn't be
fixed, touch no one without leaving him happier or more self-
confident. Flanked by Forbes, backed by Gertrude, and propelled by her own
vision, serendipity, and qualities of quicksilver and acid, she attacked and wooed,
intrigued and dared, ever managing to skate gracefully over difficulties. There
were tiffs and tears, to be sure, but their effect was minor when weighed against
her dedication to art and her endless encouragement of individual artists. If
Gertrude was universally known as the artists' fairy godmother, then Juliana was
just as widely acknowledged as their dea ex machina, arriving providentially to
intervene in desperate situations. By now she carried around a small black book
wherever she went; when she heard about artists in distress or worthy of attention,
Juliana jotted down their names and followed up on their stories later.

Henry James said that "the great thing in life is to be *saturated* with something," and in 1923 Juliana was happily sharing in the problems of an artist's
life. She did not merely want to make artists productive: She wanted to make
them *joyful*. Within the space of a few months in that year, besides keeping up
her round of exhibitions and purchases, Juliana was responsible for reviving a
moribund magazine, rescuing a young painter who had become too impoverished to take care of his family, and installing other artists in more comfortable
studios. Louise Varèse's experience during the summer of 1923 was typical. She
described Juliana appearing "as a kind of a juggler, with one hand paying the

rent of a painter's apartment so that he and his wife could go to Europe, with the other giving us the key so that we could live free of rent for a few months." Along the same lines, Juliana would write to the painter Ernest Fiene in May, "I am enclosing a check for $1000 for the two pictures. We will talk about the price later, but I thought that at the moment you needed this to go ahead with your plans for the summer."

Yet it was all managed without bother or fuss. There was such ease, for example, in arranging the first exhibition of 1923. The invitation read:

THE WHITNEY STUDIO CLUB
147 West 4th Street
INVITES YOU TO AN EXHIBITION OF
paintings by
JOHN DOS PASSOS
and
ADELAIDE J. LAWSON
and sculpture by
REUBEN NAKIAN
January third to January twenty-fourth
Open daily 11 A.M. to 11 P.M. Sundays 3 to 9 P.M.

Nakian remembered the informality surrounding his first one-man show. He was then working in his Weehawken Heights studio, the establishment made possible by his Whitney stipend. Juliana had evidently directed him to these particular premises (an old garage) because they formerly belonged to a stone-cutter who used to cut marbles for Gertrude. The man had given up the business, leaving the studio filled with tools, pulleys, and turntables. Consequently Nakian had to buy very little equipment himself and could move in immediately. The thought of receiving a show or any further tokens of favor had not occurred to him. "I didn't ask for a show," Nakian recalled. "Mrs. Force just said to me, 'Bring your things to the gallery and we'll have a show.'"

Although the contents were brought together quickly, the exhibition was sizable. Dos Passos was represented by fifty watercolors and gouaches, Lawson by thirty-one paintings, and Nakian by six carvings of animals. The occasion was Dos Passos's first extensive public showing of his work, but perhaps too embarrassed to feel openly proud about it, he spoke slightingly of the Club to his cosmopolitan friends. To Scott and Zelda Fitzgerald, holed up in Great Neck, Long Island, but ready to career into town in their secondhand Rolls-Royce, he addressed a mocking, self-consciously witty note that did nothing to disguise his hope that they would accept his invitation to the opening party. He wrote to Scott on the back of the announcement:

Come and bring a lot of drunks

A desperate tea fight will be held at the Whitney S Club Friday afternoon Jan 5—Contestants are advised to wear masks and raincoats. Lost articles such as happy phrases, critical conundrums et al will be confiscated by the management. Rules: Catch as catch can. Any contestant looking at the pictures or mentioning the syllable art will be declared to have fouled and will be removed from the floor. Consolation

prizes . . . will be administered. Follow the Green line It'll probably be a hellish bore—

Dos

Dos Passos was not as indifferent to the Club as he claimed, for he became a member and exhibited his work there at least five more times between 1923 and 1925. Furthermore, the pictures he showed at the Club—urban scenes of steam and smoke registering the gigantism, wealth, and industrial might of New York City and partaking stylistically of Cubist montage and Futurist serial repetition— appear to have contributed to his literary development. These portraits of the metropolis gave Dos Passos a preliminary mode of probing the themes, imagery, rhythms, and characterizations that were to be represented so successfully in his mature fiction—*Manhattan Transfer*, which was shortly to follow, and the *U.S.A.* trilogy.

January of 1923 also saw the debut of the reconstituted *Arts* magazine, which Juliana had recently salvaged from a premature demise. The magazine, a monthly journal of art news and criticism, was started by the collector and writer Hamilton Easter Field. A wealthy man, he was the magazine's owner, editor, and publisher. But Field died suddenly in April of 1922, and *The Arts* seemed destined to lapse without him. Juliana, however, felt that the publication should not disappear. She told Forbes that if he were willing to take over the editorship of *The Arts*, she would ask Gertrude to subsidize it. According to his unpublished memoirs, he and Juliana had talked in 1921 about the idea of starting a magazine. In an art journal lay the means to proselytize for the enjoyment and love of art in America and elevate the career of Watson, whose critical abilities were not being sufficiently challenged by his newspaper columns. Thus, Forbes recognized this as the prize opportunity of a lifetime—his own forum, kept solvent by dependable infusions of capital whenever necessary, and his chance to defend and illumine the vital art of all places and periods, partic- ularly modernism and nonacademic American art. He accepted, whereupon Gertrude offered to buy the rights to *The Arts* from Field's heir, Robert Laurent, an active member of the Studio Club. As a working sculptor, Laurent had no wish to continue *The Arts* himself, and a speedy conclusion to the negotiations was reached. Juliana got Forbes $8,500 in seed money and a salary of $50 a week. The wage, which was not huge, apparently was envisioned as a supplement to Forbes's regular salary from the *World*; he did not have to quit his job to run the magazine.

Since it was Juliana who initiated the revival of *The Arts*, no one else but Forbes would have been awarded the post of editor, but in this case her choice was justified, for the union of personality and position was unimpeachable. As someone long accustomed to using his writing as a platform for his activism, Forbes was a dynamic and enterprising editor, open to new suggestion, original thought, and provocative differences of opinion. He made *The Arts* into one of the leading art journals published in America during the 1920s. Its tenor was liberal, and its coverage of art ranged from Lascaux and Altamira to El Greco and Piero della Francesca, from Japanese prints and Persian miniatures to Max

Beckmann and John Marin. The magazine emphasized the visual arts, but Forbes also ran many articles on music, dance, poetry, fiction, and film—and treating the last as an art form was hardly common in 1923.

In his first issue, Forbes established the tone and variety of *The Arts* with a remarkable mix of essays. There were several memorial tributes to Hamilton Easter Field, plus Ananda Coomaraswamy on Indian art, Lee Simonson on stage design, Henry McBride on Modigliani, and a conversation with Brancusi that summarized the sculptor's ideas. Forbes contributed two articles. One was on Charles Demuth and the other was the beginning of a two-part report, accompanied by extensive reproductions, that was the first public announcement of the opening of the Barnes Foundation in the Philadelphia suburb of Merion, Pennsylvania.

The Barnes story was an enviable journalistic coup, and one can only marvel at Forbes's powers of tact and persuasion. He was one of the very few art critics of his time to earn the goodwill (although only temporarily) of the magnificently irascible Albert Barnes, the self-made multimillionaire and self-taught art patron who was notorious for refusing entry to his incomparable collection of nineteenth- and twentieth-century art to any person associated with a newspaper, art magazine, museum, or gallery.* Juliana was merely one among many art professionals who were denied permission to visit Barnes's estate, her crime being that she was an art professional.† Barnes had never forgiven the Philadelphia art establishment for making fun of his paintings, and he translated his resentment into a ruling policy. This was a hardship on art lovers, because until the Museum of Modern Art opened in 1929, the Barnes Foundation was the only place on the East Coast where one could see a concentration of work by Cézanne, Renoir, Picasso, Matisse, and Soutine, as well as first-rate examples of Van Gogh, Daumier, Gauguin, Maurice Prendergast, and William Glackens: In essence Barnes held his art hostage from any viewing. With the exception of *The Arts*, he never cooperated with a publication, nor did he allow his collection to be photographed or reproduced. On this occasion, however, Barnes not only opened his door to an editor and a photographer, but he allowed Forbes to print one of his treatises on analyzing art.

In his first editorial, Forbes declared his intentions with his usual brio. The magazine would be "a mouthpiece for neither the radical nor the conservative exclusively, but for art quite regardless of tags." What he said next showed how closely he and Juliana agreed in outlook. Both saw American art as a cause,

---

*Perhaps Forbes's 1921 recommendation that Barnes be one of the three men advising the Metropolitan Museum on modern art accounts for the honeymoon.

†Barnes's first biographer, William Schack, reported that the *refusés* of the Barnes Foundation were so numerous that they constituted an unofficial club. In the words of one member, "almost anyone who was anyone in the art world of the 1920's and 1930's belonged to it." Because he was employed by the Whitney Museum, Lloyd Goodrich was not given an admission card. Alfred Barr was allowed into the collection while he was a student at Princeton, but afterward he was no longer welcome. From then on, he began to make reservations under an assumed name or sneak in with approved tour groups.

both believed in approaching issues from the artist's point of view, and both were all for controversy, letting the sparks fly where they may. Forbes wrote:

> THE ARTS is not afraid to enjoy American work just because it is American. It does not intend to wave the flag, but quite frankly it does intend to stand with the American artist against timidity and snobbery. . . .
>
> Whenever it is possible, articles will be secured by artists. Those who are engaged in creating pictures, sculpture and so forth, are not always, as everybody knows, the most impartial critics. But the most impartial critic is seldom the most stimulating critic, and a special interest and character are often found in the words of a craftsman about his own craft that rarely exist in the writings of those who observe from the outside.

These standards were met, for Forbes knew how to match subject and author, and he tried to feature writers with distinctive points of view. He could coax articles out of artists, even those as chary of making public statements as Picasso or as legendarily laconic as Edward Hopper (who wrote four pieces for *The Arts* between 1925 and 1928). Forbes also had a knack, sharpened by years of critical writing and reading, for seeing the potential in young, unknown writers and scholars. As he did not believe that age had a monopoly on wisdom, he encouraged these tyros to prove themselves in print. Long before any of them had attained eminence as authorities in their fields, *The Arts* published Meyer Schapiro on Greek art, Henry-Russell Hitchcock on architecture, A. Everett Austin on the Fogg Art Museum, Alfred Barr on Delacroix and on Sergei Eisenstein, Alan Burroughs on Eakins, and Lloyd Goodrich on Winslow Homer, on the Hudson River School, and on Edward Hopper (this last assignment inaugurated a sympathetic working relationship between artist and critic that would last forty years).

Forbes's record as an editor has not diminished with the passage of time. A partial list of the essays and authors appearing in the pages of *The Arts* during the first five years of his management was a cross section of international culture then and remains so today: poetry by William Carlos Williams and Dos Passos, Ambroise Vollard on Degas, Waldemar George on Rouault, Leo Stein on Renaissance art and on Renoir, Henry McBride on the discovery of Louis Eilshemius, Walter Pach on Seurat, Alain Locke on Negro art, Mabel Dodge Luhan on Mexican santos, and Virginia Woolf on films. Stravinsky, Varèse, Diego Rivera, Thomas Hart Benton, Archipenko, and Picasso commented on their own work, and verbatim conversations with Maillol, Bourdelle, and Despiau were transcribed and printed. Among the artists who wrote on their peers were Francis Picabia, du Bois, Hopper, Sloan, Andrew Dasburg, William Zorach, Henry Schnakenberg, and George Biddle. For the first two years *The Arts's* chief photographer was Charles Sheeler, whom Forbes and Juliana had taken under their combined wing and wished to help.

The active collaboration between Juliana and Forbes on *The Arts* was made closer by an arrangement of intense physical proximity. The Watsons had been living in Daniel Chester French's building at 12 West Eighth Street until late

1922, when a legal quarrel between Forbes and French caused the Watsons to move next door to 14 West Eighth. Juliana in the meantime rented an apartment *for herself* in No. 12, with a lease beginning on October 1, 1922; it was directly across the hall from the rooms Nan and Forbes were soon to vacate. During these same last months of 1922, Doctor rented an apartment in his name at No. 14, where the Watsons had just migrated. The Forces were maintaining two establishments for what must have been a trial separation, but as husband and wife were living next door to each other, the agreement must have been friendly. It was also temporary. Juliana gave up her lease at No. 12 in June of 1924, on the eve of an extended holiday in Europe. When she returned, she rejoined Doctor (and the Watsons) at No. 14.

Thus Juliana saw to it that she and Forbes had time for many afternoons of enjoying each other's company and plotting projects for the good of art and artists. Their trysts were often preceded by lunches at the local speakeasy of the moment. Besides dispensing liquor, the speakeasies' allure was tied in with their clandestine status, which fed the heady brew of elation and secretiveness that keeps a love affair simmering. As Dos Passos wrote about the Village speakeasies he sampled in the early 1920s, "In some places you whispered your name through a slot in the door. The waiter smiled with sympathetic understanding at your lady friend. From the moment the door clicked to behind you, you had the feeling of being in the Fortunate Islands, where there were no rules and regulations, no yesterday and no tomorrow, no husbands to complain, no private entanglements with other women, only this moment."

Juliana's unflagging hospitality continued, invincible to Prohibition. All of the openings at the Studio and the Club were celebrated with teas that often became cocktail parties or evening parties featuring heaping platters of food and stronger stimulants. Elegant dinners and luncheons honored visiting artists. At the end of January 1923 Juliana threw a party for Katherine Schmidt and two other artists to celebrate the opening of their individual shows at 147 West Fourth. Schmidt was then married to Yasuo Kuniyoshi, and the two of them were at the center of a sociable group of young artists who had known each other since their days together at the Art Students League. Most of the Schmidt-Kuniyoshi set attended the opening, and on that evening Juliana met Peggy Bacon and her husband, Alexander Brook. Apparently Brook was loaded with plenty of Whitney Scotch, and upon being introduced to Juliana—and in his astonishment at his hostess's rapid advance toward him, for she roared up to him "like a fire engine"—he backed into one of the Schmidt paintings with such violence that it fell off the wall. As Brook tried to shake hands and restore the picture to its original position, Juliana growled, "You'll hang for this." In view of later events, neither of them could have guessed how prophetic her remark happened to be.

Although she was approaching her fiftieth birthday, to these twenty-five-year-olds Juliana became the very model of youth and contagious high spirits. They were drawn to her and found her memorable because in her company "you felt braver, happier, and wittier than you were." She was someone who made the very air around her more vivid, more alive: Lloyd Goodrich often said that "the social temperature would go up ten degrees when she entered a room." Katherine

Schmidt said, "There was always a gaiety about Mrs. Force in whatever she did. Even when something was serious an aura of youth and gaiety surrounded it. They [she and the Whitney Club] were gaily breaking new ground." One time while they were together, Schmidt was struck by the beauty of Juliana's tawny hair, burnished and thick, and she exclaimed over its lovely red-gold shade. Juliana thanked her with a little laugh. Looking back on the incident, Schmidt realized that Juliana had been dying her hair for years and that she was amused by her young friend's naiveté about it. But at the time she had no idea of Juliana's age, or more precisely, of the decades that separated them in birth. She did not associate her with an older generation.

The phenomenon Katherine Schmidt described was not so much agelessness as wholeness. By the time she got to know Juliana, surface and inner being were completely united. There was no more discrepancy between desire and actuality. Fate had come to agree with the high value she set upon herself. She now had confidence and security and panache to spare, so much so that she could lavish them—her own bounty, which personalized and ran parallel to Gertrude's material stipends—on the young people she wanted around her. She was wise and free enough to refrain from delivering lectures and making those ponderous comparisons between past and present (always to the detriment of the latter) that mark the old.

Another reason Juliana seemed to have no age is that she treated young people she liked with respect. She endeared herself to rebellious teenagers whose parents she knew by listening to what troubled them and avoiding stale homilies. If they passed inspection, she responded to neophyte collectors or sincere students as equals. One college boy who met Juliana through his parents would ring her on his trips to New York during his school vacations and ask if he could visit. She welcomed him, poured him drinks, questioned him about his plans, showed him around the latest exhibitions, and asked him what he thought. The young man took it all in stride. Only later in his life did the man (who became a serious art collector) understand how extraordinarily accessible Juliana had been.

Besides being inveterately interested, Juliana had another trait immemorially associated with youth rather than middle age. When it came to highlighting her love of the dramatic, she could be reckless. Some of her devil-may-care escapades originated in the temporary momentum of alcohol, but most of them were inseparable from her flair for the spontaneous, and from being the confirmed upper bohemian that she was. In conjunction with Juliana's volatility it also must be kept in mind that while Juliana was long on generosity and tolerance, she was short on temper—a firecracker with a quick-burning fuse. One explosion was set off by a rich woman who was trying to put her artist-husband on the map by giving a round of fancy dinner parties. Juliana was invited to one and accepted. After the hostess greeted her at the door, she suggested to Juliana, whose salary had risen rapidly and could afford to be dressed by Herman Patrick Tappé and Hattie Carnegie, that her appearance would be much improved if she went to her seamstress. As an incentive, the woman sent her an entire bolt of yellow chiffon the next morning. "Juliana boiled with rage all during that dinner party and she boiled with impatience the next morning because there

was no one to tell the story to until I came over," said Katherine Schmidt. Juliana's remedy, characteristically, was to have a party, so she invited a dozen or so artists for that same evening. She wore a beautiful hostess gown in exquisite taste as a further reproof to the dreadful woman who had dared to malign her costume. The artists drifted in and took seats around the fireplace. Reciting the whole tale from start to finish with the requisite embroideries and flourishes, Juliana paused dramatically and brought forth the offending chiffon. A glance told her that she held her audience in the palm of her hand. Without warning or hesitation she finished her story by flinging the entire length of cloth into the fire.

One of the guests at this bonfire was the ceramicist Carl Walters, who planted himself in a pink satin chair next to the fireplace. "Smoke began to fill the room," Katherine Schmidt related, "and we all thought it was the chiffon, which was flimsy and burning up in flames as soon as it hit the fire. I looked over at Carl. He'd become so amazed at the goings-on that he let the bowl of his pipe knock against the side of the pink satin chair and it, too, was now going up in flames. Meanwhile, Juliana continued with feeding bits and pieces of her chiffon into the fireplace as Carl tried to put out this second blaze by beating it with his hands."

Assured as she was that artists were at home at Eighth Street, Juliana was just as certain that the public was unconvinced that art was essential to life. Making an art-buying citizenry feel warmly welcomed to the Studio and the Club still demanded much effort, and *The Arts* was of great use to Juliana as a billboard for benign propaganda. Besides running a calendar of the season's exhibitions in the magazine, she started placing full-page advertisements exhorting readers to support contemporary art. There was nothing subtle about these manifestos: they were the Whitney versions of twenties boosterism. The most hortatory were headed, "I KNOW WHAT I LIKE" and "WHAT IS HOME WITHOUT A MODERN PICTURE?" The first pounded home the message, "Don't be afraid to buy because someone else may not like what you buy. . . . There is no possession with more thrilling possibilities than the work of art that you yourself have selected, uninfluenced by the artist's reputation or by what your friends will think about it." "WHAT IS HOME WITHOUT A MODERN PICTURE?" argued that although painting and sculpture are legitimate branches of contemporary thought, they are the only arts "which, in their contemporary manifestations, people are permitted to overlook while still retaining some sort of claim to cultivation. A person whose bookshelves held nothing later than Thackeray would be a curiosity. . . . Just as you couldn't imagine not having contemporary books in your library, so really you shouldn't be able to imagine living in rooms that are entirely barren of contemporary art." The writers—the prose sounds as if it came from Juliana and was added to by Forbes—then equated a lack of receptivity to art with the denial of the pleasure principle. To be deprived of this inward need was to be only half-alive. "Make up your mind," the copy concluded, "that next season you will buy at least one work of art by a living

artist—not to 'encourage' the artist, but simply for the joy of it—because you want to!"

The tone of the notices did moderate, and sometimes the messages became almost picturesque. One of the lighter ones was headed, "BRING BACK A WORK OF ART FROM YOUR SUMMER TOUR!" and it is a period piece cheering readers on to yet another means of do-it-yourself art collecting. The copy ran, "During the winter season the Whitney Studio Club presents regularly the recent work of vigorous American artists. During the summer, when driving through a village where some artist has his studio, why not alight and make your own discovery? Bring back a work of art from your summer tour!"

The effect of these advertisements was intangible, of course, but they made the Whitney-Force philosophy plain to readers of *The Arts*. Far less overtly missionary, but not without its own influence, was Juliana's invitation to Marius de Zayas to organize exhibitions at the Whitney Studio. A whiplash caricaturist, a dealer of impeccable refinement, and a discerning prober of the new, de Zayas was abreast of all vital currents on both sides of the Atlantic. In 1907, not long after de Zayas moved to New York and became a minor celebrity because of his witty caricatures, an admiring critic described him as "radically Spanish, natally Mexican, residentially American, temperamentally universal."

In 1923, however, de Zayas was not so much a celebrity as a victim of business reverses. His gallery had failed, and in March 1923 he was forced to put much of his collection up for auction. The proceeds of the sale were not high, and de Zayas was in need of income. The Whitney offer not only gave him dignified, suitable work and took some of the curatorial weight off Juliana's shoulders, but set into motion another experiment. This was the expansion of the Whitney Studio into the steady showing of European art, with an emphasis on the French avant-garde. De Zayas was greatly talented at arranging art exhibitions, but he was no salesman. He had failed as a dealer because he could not stand the relentless pressure to sell. He was thus in his element in the noncommercial setting of the Whitney Studio.

De Zayas immediately arranged a show of Picasso's work—twenty paintings done between 1919 and 1923, plus a selection of his graphics—in tandem with African sculpture, which opened in May. None of the canvases had been seen before in America, and the show earned rave reviews from the critics, while artists were grateful for the chance to see the Spanish wizard's latest work. John Quinn stopped by and snapped up a set of lithographs plus a photograph of the artist for forty dollars. Juliana and Gertrude were satisfied with the results—the latter noting, "[t]he Picasso show was a huge success, looked really distinguished + I was really surprised at the interest taken"—and de Zayas was engaged for the 1923–1924 season to arrange six more exhibitions of European art. (Final decisions on exhibitions rested with Juliana, but she obviously respected de Zayas, and after a perfunctory nod from her, he would have worked independently.)

Concurrent with de Zayas's employment, Juliana's collecting habits evolved in conjunction with the new international character of the Whitney shows and the eclectic yet advanced tastes of *The Arts*. When in Paris, Juliana bought fine examples of French art. By the mid-1920s, a bronze *Prometheus* by Brancusi,

a 1914 collage by Picasso (*Pipe, Glass, Bottle of Rum*),* a Degas pastel, two paintings by Henri Rousseau purchased from Vollard, lithographs by Ingres and Daumier, and a portfolio of photographs by Man Ray turn up in her collection. In terms of Juliana's relationship with Forbes, these purchases constituted a challenge as much as an influence. Being so much alike temperamentally and in the same professional milieu, Juliana and Forbes were somewhat competitive with each other, and Forbes liked playing the mentor. He had taught her much and opened her eyes, but Juliana was not one to remain the pupil, submissive and subordinate. In buying the French art, her primary motive, to be sure, was aesthetic pleasure. But she also showed that her judgment had deepened and that she was capable of choosing on her own.

De Zayas's help was especially valuable because Juliana and Gertrude had decided that the physical premises of the Whitney Studio Club were inadequate. The old quarters on West Fourth Street were now too small for the 300 members; during the group shows, the walls were overcrowded. The floor space was diminished by sculptures on pedestals, and the bases caught guests on the shins during openings. The lease to the town house at 10 West Eighth Street, the property adjacent to the Whitney Studio, had become available, and Gertrude took it. The house was a marked improvement on West Fourth Street in both convenience and square footage, and in the spring of 1923 the Club moved out of its old headquarters. The annual members' show, the spring fixture, moved into the galleries at 8 West Eighth with over 180 paintings and sculptures. This huge and inherently heterogeneous mob scene of art won unexpectedly good notices. The *Tribune*, in a review that summarized the views of the other newspapers, approvingly labeled the roundup "a barometer of activity among the young New York independents, though the latter are chaperoned by many well-known men and women." The core group of Club exhibitors—Sloan, Davidson, Jerome Myers, Joseph Stella, du Bois, Kent, Hopper, Glackens, Davis, Laurent, Halpert—were joined by newer members such as Nakian, George Ault, Kuniyoshi, Schmidt, and Agnes Tait.

Juliana spent the early summer supervising the renovations for the new building. No. 10 was painted to match No. 8, so the town houses presented a united facade of salmon-pink stucco and jade-green doors and window casements. The Studio and the Club sponsored separate exhibition programs, but connecting doors were cut through the two lower floors to allow an entire floor to be devoted to one exhibition. Apparently the main public entrance to both buildings was now No. 10, whose galleries were painted pearly white, with the top floor usable for offices and living quarters. No. 8, the original Whitney Studio, retained its galleries on the bottom two floors. Its top floor, however, was given over to Juliana. She now had a luxurious suite of offices and sitting rooms where she and her secretary worked. And of course the house retained its "umbilical staircase" and courtyard garden that led back to Gertrude's studio on MacDougal Alley. Because the door to 8 West Eighth was now essentially a personal entrance for the two women, a butler was engaged to guard the entry

* Now in the collection of the Museum of Modern Art.

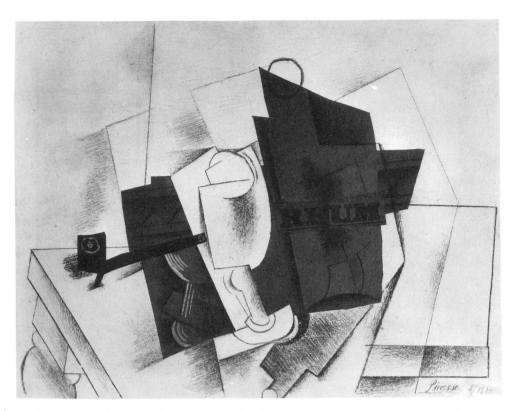

Picasso's 1914 collage *Pipe, Glass, Bottle of Rum* was one of many modernist works Juliana bought in the 1920s under Watson's tutelage.

and announce visitors. To the young painters who dropped by, the man was straight out of an English drawing-room comedy: Tall, somber, and expressionless, impeccably clad in a black cutaway and striped morning trousers, he appeared to see nothing that went on around him.

Toward the end of the summer Juliana took herself to Europe, and may have stopped afterward in southern Vermont, close to Schnakenberg, Kent, and Carl Ruggles. It was during this time that Ruggles, in commemoration of their friendship and her generosity, dedicated the first song of his three-song work "Vox Clamans in Deserto" to Juliana and made her a present of the manuscript. The text of the song is Robert Browning's poem "Parting at Morning," a reminder of their mutual literary admiration.

As for Kent, he was still reaping the benefits of Juliana's favor and retaining it with bantering letters. Earlier that year she bought another of Kent's paintings—*Mount Equinox, Winter* of 1921—for Gertrude, who then donated it to the Art Institute of Chicago. Just after Juliana left Vermont, Kent's wife and two children fell gravely ill, and they all required hospitalization. His pleas

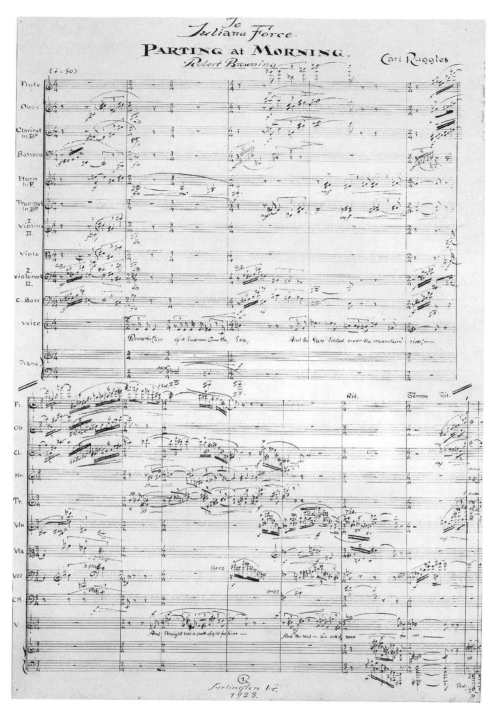

The title page of Carl Ruggles's original manuscript of "Parting at Morning," dedicated to Juliana.

for money went unanswered until he wrote to Juliana, who either bought a painting again or sent a check outright. In expressing his gratitude, Kent wrote in his smoothly honed style of ironic flirtatiousness:

> About the only way to thank you for the enormous kindnesses that you do as if they were nothing at all is just to say "thank you,"—and then hope that some day there'll come the chance to lay down my life for you—and all that sort of thing. But if you were here I know that I would cast aside all the reserve of my nature and sweep aside the chaste scruples of yours, and overwhelm you with my affection. May God spare you that!

In the fall of 1923, Juliana began looking around for a permanent assistant who could be more than a secretary. The Club and the Studio were mounting more ambitious exhibitions, *The Arts*, although Forbes's domain, did take up her time, and Gertrude's sculpture commissions could be negotiated by no one but herself. It was normal to want an assistant; it was Juliana to want no one but an artist for the job.

Her first choice was Katherine Schmidt, who declined because she felt it wasn't the right sort of position for her. Instead, Schmidt agreed to run the Club's evening sketch class. For two years she hired the models and collected the twenty-cent fee from each member, but "if you didn't have any money it didn't make any difference." During that time, Schmidt recalled, "Hopper was my pal in the sketch class. He never missed."

Juliana next turned to Alexander Brook, who had passed the last few months of 1923 in a deep depression. His savings had run out, and his prospects were meager. Forbes was giving him assignments for *The Arts*, but the wages paid for art journalism did not add up to an adequate income. Brook and Peggy Bacon were living in a "sunless chamber" on Patchin Place, innocent of heat or hot water. They were so badly off that Brook's mother-in-law had taken the couple's two children to live with her. As Schnakenberg discovered when he paid a call that fall, Brook was sitting around all day in a funny-looking lavender dressing gown, unable to rouse himself and unable to paint. Schnakenberg silently diagnosed Brook's condition, said little, and vanished. Within an hour the telephone rang. It was Juliana, wanting Brook to stop by her office. "When would you like me to come see you?" he asked. "Now," Juliana replied.

Brook peeled himself out of the purplish bathrobe and headed south to Eighth Street. "Without preliminary remarks or questions," Juliana offered him the job as her assistant. At first it was to be secret—Juliana wanted him to be her underground talent scout and plainclothesman among his contemporaries. Brook was to circulate through various studios, spotting exceptional "and preferably unknown" young talents and reporting to her about them. Finding anywhere from one to six artists a year would be enough, Juliana assured him. The salary was $200 a month, and the hours were from 4:00 to 6:00 P.M., four to six days a week. Since Brook, like many other artists of the period, was a studio painter who depended on natural light, the job took nothing away from his working hours. Being Juliana's gumshoe, Brook wrote later, "was a glorious opportunity

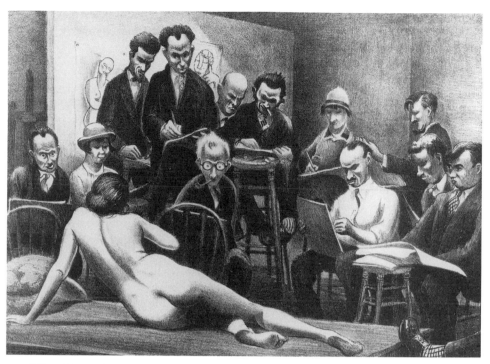

When Mabel Dwight caricatured the Club's life class, she included Edward Hopper (back row, third from right) and Jan Matulka (front row, extreme right).

for steady income with plenty of time to paint, which was the exact combination I had been most wishing for."

Brook's post did not remain quite so light in its duties. He began work in December 1923. A month or two later, one of Juliana's receptionist-guards at the Club quit, and she stretched Brook's job into taking general charge of baby-sitting the exhibitions. He did not select or originate many shows until late 1924, but in his new responsibilities Brook fulfilled what Juliana had prophesied when they met: For four years he hung every show put on by the Club.

Brook was given a little room in 10 West Eighth Street as an office, but there was still leftover space in the new Club building. It did not stay vacant long, however. Juliana offered the space to the International Composers' Guild, which had been practicing in a music room belonging to a wealthy, overbearing woman who expected Varèse to dance attendance on her. As Louise Varèse recounted, her husband "missed the gatherings at Mrs. Force's or at the Whitney Club of the year before. *For us* something had gone out of the Guild—something for which, lacking an English word, I fall back on that precious overworked *Gemütlichkeit*."

To the Varèses' enormous relief, they moved their organization into the Club for the 1923–1924 season and contentedly remained there, unsupervised and

untrammeled, until the Guild disbanded four years later. Varèse, Salzedo, and Ruggles were joined by Henry Cowell, the composer and theorist, and he occasionally gave lectures at the Club. The Guild's officers lost no time in making their appreciation known; on January 13, 1924, "Vox Clamans in Deserto" was given its premiere. However, Ruggles was dissatisfied with the work, and it was not performed again in his lifetime.

Such gratitude, directly displayed, was not exacted or expected—though she would have been inhuman not to savor it—and Juliana unendingly gave artists the benefit of the doubt. But finally, after several preliminary wavers and wobbles, one friendship did founder irrevocably. The artist was Rockwell Kent, and his transgression was so egregious that Juliana could not forgive it.

In his autobiography, Kent wrote evasively—as he had to, given the laws governing libel and invasion of privacy—that he became persona non grata at the Whitney Studio Club because the Club "was human, all too human." Kent accurately observed, "And although it was from the human standards by which in part its inner coterie was chosen that the circle drew its warm conviviality, it was those very standards that I was at last to fail to meet. Yet for a time, for years, the Whitney sun shone bright on me. And I was glad." By "human, all too human," he meant casual sexual dalliance. Throughout much of 1924 Kent, who was then between wives, was notching conquests in a driven manner that suggested he was keeping score. "Seduction followed seduction, affair affair," as David Traxel wrote in his life of Kent. Sadly, one of the objects of Kent's serial seductions was Irene Rieser, Charles Rieser's pretty young wife and Juliana's sister-in-law. Juliana had introduced Kent to Charles and Irene in 1921, and had probably brought them together again in late 1923 or early 1924 at one of her parties. Irene fell under Kent's fascinating spell and the two had a brief affair, but one with destructive consequences. Whereas Kent afterward went on his way unscathed, the Rieser family was devastated. Charles and Irene's life together had not been ideal before Kent's intervention because Charles was in the grip of a serious drinking problem. Irene's infidelity, probably a by-product of her frustration over Charles's weakness and her consequent vulnerability to an attentive man, strained beyond tolerance the already fragile fabric of their relationship. The Riesers began to talk about separating. Eventually Charles and Irene patched up their marriage, but it never regained its previous stability, and the children (Allan and Carl Rieser) suffered.

Juliana's fury at Kent was mixed with anger at herself. Charles was her favorite brother, Allan and Carl her adored nephews. Any harm that came to them was also an assault on the family castle she had constructed. The real bitterness stemmed not so much from all that Juliana had done for Kent over the years, but from guilt. None of this would have come to pass if she, knowing that Kent was a sexual live wire, had kept him from the Riesers. Whereas she could recover from Kent and deal with him on his own terms, Irene lacked her experience or resilience. In her drive to manage their lives, Juliana had only herself to blame for introducing the Riesers into this terribly worldly milieu of persiflage and nonchalant alliances. Kent could devise no more excuses or explanations for his behavior; once the 1924 spring season ended, he no longer exhibited regularly

at the Club. The ingratiating letters stopped, and there were no more flowery allusions to Becky Sharp. But although she would have nothing more to do with him personally, Juliana did relent in matters artistic because in that sphere she was unable to hold a grudge. In 1928 she bought for her personal collection a set of Kent's illustrations. Appropriately, their subject was Casanova.

Offsetting Kent's faithlessness was Juliana's growing friendship with Charles Sheeler, which was deepening just as her association with the former drew to its stormy close. Sheeler, a self-effacing man of some reserve, did not have Kent's like of notoriety, and his friendship did not record itself in flamboyant actions or missives. Sheeler first attracted her attention in 1920 at the Colony Club exhibition she worked on with Forbes but he was not absorbed into the Whitney fold until 1923, apparently through his professional connections with Watson and Marius de Zayas. Forbes thought Sheeler's photography "incomparable" and took care to give him plum assignments for *The Arts*. He also endorsed Sheeler as a painter, which he demonstrated by being the first critic to write a lengthy appraisal of him. (It appeared in the May 1923 issue of *The Arts*.) Sheeler had been de Zayas's gallery assistant, and may have helped de Zayas arrange his exhibitions at the Whitney Studio. Juliana admired Sheeler's immaculately drawn and painted studies of flowers, New York buildings, and the barns of her beloved Bucks County. (Indeed, she had a great liking for Precisionist painting in general. By 1924 Juliana had bought for herself and Gertrude two paintings by Preston Dickinson.* She had been an ardent admirer of Charles Demuth for several years, and sponsored two exhibitions of his work in 1923 and 1924, with purchases quickly following. Niles Spencer's architectural paintings also attracted her, and she bought *Pittsburgh*,† Elsie Driggs's deep, dark, sonorous ode to industry, as soon as she saw it on the walls of the Daniel Gallery.)

Juliana bought some of Sheeler's drawings for herself, and in the summer of 1923 she invited him and his wife, Katherine, to move into the newly completed top-floor flat at 10 West Eighth Street, rent-free. They stayed in the apartment for the next eighteen months, with Sheeler taking an energetic part in Whitney activities. Juliana and the Sheelers and the Watsons were trotting back and forth between each other's apartments. Katherine Sheeler, when she invited the others to dinner, had but one company dish. It was waffles, which she made incessantly. Juliana soon grew heartily sick of those waffles, but chewed on them in silent endurance.

When Juliana went to Barley Sheaf Farm, the Sheelers visited her there. Sheeler, of course, drew inspiration—and many pictures—from the indigenous architecture, arts, and crafts of rural New York, New England, and Pennsylvania, and the Force property had a clapboard and stone barn that appealed to him. His interest became the source of an oft-told anecdote. Sheeler had been visiting her over the weekend, and as she was preparing to go back to New York, he

---

* *Still Life, Flowers* and *Industry*, both now in the collection of the Whitney Museum.
† Now in the collection of the Whitney Museum.

said he would like to paint a picture of her barn. Juliana liked the idea and summoned the head hired man. "Mr. Sheeler is staying over to paint the barn," Juliana announced. To which the man replied, "But we just painted it last year." Unfortunately for the resolution of the story, no Sheeler painting, drawing, or, indeed, photograph of Juliana's barn has been found to date. However, a visual record of his residing at 10 West Eighth Street exists. This is *Stairway to Studio* (1924),* worked in tempera, crayon, and pencil, in which the artist probes his long-time fascination with the enigmatic and forbidding quality of a long, winding staircase.

Publications, purchases, and a rent-free apartment were not all that Sheeler received through Juliana's offices. As Juliana told Edward Bernays, artists should "show, show, show," and for Sheeler she was set on following her own advice. In the middle of 1923 she and de Zayas arranged for the Durand-Ruel Galleries in Paris to hold a group exhibition of seven American painters she felt the French should see; it was the Overseas Exhibition all over again, but on a smaller scale and mostly for younger painters. The show would open in November of 1923, each artist would be represented by several works, and the Whitney Studio would bear all costs. The artists selected were Walt Kuhn, Charles Demuth, Henry Schnakenberg, Allen Tucker, Eugene Speicher, Nan Watson, and Sheeler. The participants must have been pleased about this showcase, for Durand-Ruel stood for the summit of French art. Paul Durand-Ruel was the Impressionists' dealer, and he was one of the few in France who supported Monet, Renoir, and their compatriots in their years of struggle. Furthermore, it was the first time most of these artists had exhibited abroad. In terms of Parisian reaction, the Durand-Ruel group was indeed an echo of the Overseas Exhibition. The French critics were concerned with assigning the painters to their French sources of inspiration and otherwise constructing School of Paris-derived artistic genealogies for what they saw.

In 1924 the Whitney Studio and Studio Club presented a string of vital exhibitions, and Sheeler was at their center, either directly or indirectly. He showed his work in several, selected the artists to be featured in another, and was bound by spiritual affinity to the rest. In January the Durand-Ruel group was presented, and the February snows brought an avalanche of first-rate art, for de Zayas had done his work well. He began with a selection of lithographs and etchings by American and French artists, among them Bellows, Braque, Cézanne, Daumier, Davies, Delacroix, Derain, Hopper, Ingres, Kent, Kuhn, Laurencin, Manet, Matisse, Picasso, Boardman Robinson, and Sheeler. Succeeding this lineup was a remarkable two-man show of terra-cottas and bronzes by Maillol and canvases by Henri Rousseau. Maillol had not been widely exhibited in this country and was definitely underappreciated, but to spotlight Rousseau was an even greater measure of de Zayas's knowledge of a void in the art scene that needed to be filled. A group of Rousseau's canvases had been seen

---

* Now in the collection of the Philadelphia Museum of Art.

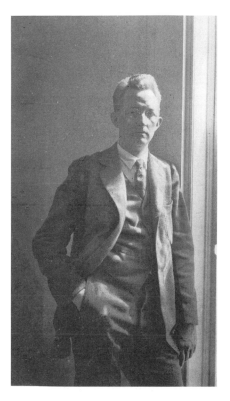

Charles Sheeler was showered with Juliana's help for four years.

in America only once since the Armory Show, and none would be shown again until 1931. At least eight paintings were on view (no catalog survives). One was *Mauvais Surprise,** and two were jungle scenes from Juliana's private collection. It must be acknowledged that no matter how modern, original, and necessary these shows were, they retraced territory pioneered years before by Alfred Stieglitz and 291. But de Zayas and Juliana believed that maintaining and widening an unfamiliar trail, even if it had been first charted by someone else, was worth doing. There was always a younger generation who had not toured New York or Paris, who had not seen the work of the modern masters face-to-face.

Throughout the month of March, Sheeler had a one-man show at the Studio. Twenty-two examples of his work were hung, which made for a full survey of his work over the past two years. Juliana bought *Gloxinia* and *Bucks County Barn*. Going by what is deducible from the vague titles listed in the catalog, other notable works on view were *Timothy†* and the photograph and drawing *New York.‡ Bucks County Barn* has since achieved classic status in twentieth-century American art and is a cornerstone of the museum's extensive Sheeler holdings. *Pertaining to Yachts and Yachting*, another fine drawing by the artist

* Now in the collection of the Barnes Foundation.
† Now in the collection of the Santa Barbara Museum of Art.
‡ The latter is now in the collection of the Art Institute of Chicago.

in this show, had already come into Juliana's hands.* One day on a visit to his studio she saw the drawing and asked him what he was going to do with it. Sheeler made a dismissive motion, as if he were on the verge of throwing it away. Juliana said something on the order of "We'll see about that," and nipped out the door with it.

Of comparable importance were the shows that could be seen next door at the Club that spring season. They were by and large an American counterpart to the internationalism reigning at the Studio. As they were also organized by artists, the contents and concepts behind them were notably fresh. Having recently propagandized in *The Arts* that "the ideal exhibition . . . is an integral part of an artistic plan," Juliana announced that five different artists would be asked to select and hang five separate shows at the Club. The five turned out to be six: Sloan, Schnakenberg, W. E. Hill (a pal of Schnakenberg's and a cartoonist for the *Tribune* who drew a strip called "Among Us Mortals" and inserted wicked distortions of his friends' faces when he felt like it), Brook, Sheeler, and Kuniyoshi. Sloan made thirty-four selections from the Independents' spring annual, and Hill's show, a survey of contemporary paintings and drawings led by entries from Stuart Davis and Peggy Bacon, was competent but not out of the ordinary. The contents of Kuniyoshi's assemblage of portraits and religious works are unknown. Similarly, there is no extant catalog of Brook's provocative-sounding combination of two Mexican artists of disparate sensibilities—José Clemente Orozco,† with watercolors and drawings, and Miguel Covarrubias, with his mock-Cubist caricatures of the fashionable and famous—with oils by E. L. Henry, a nineteenth-century genre painter. But Schnakenberg's and Sheeler's contributions were not only innovative, but better documented and better publicized, and they earned the Club much acclaim.

Schnakenberg, like Juliana, was an early devotee of folk art, and he elected to show examples owned by him and other artists. Early American Art, which opened on February 9, 1924, was the first exhibition of folk art held in America. Naive engravings, paintings on velvet, portraits by untutored artists, a cigar-store Indian, a ship's figurehead, a brass bootjack, and pewter serving bowls were put before the public as authentic works of art and vigorous evidence of a creative impulse in which Americans ought to take pride. The catalog, by virtue of listing many of the lenders' names, recorded a friendly group of early collectors in the know. Most of them were artists who could see art in what others disdained and

---

*These purchases illustrate the difficulties and confusions in sorting out the destination of works of art acquired by Juliana. *Gloxinia* and *Pertaining to Yachts and Yachting* went into her personal collection and stayed in it until 1948, when the latter was bought by the museum. *Bucks County Barn* was in her private collection until the decision to establish a museum was made, and then it was transferred to its holdings. In his catalog on Sheeler (*Charles Sheeler: A Concentration of Works from the Permanent Collection of the Whitney Museum of American Art*, 1980), Patterson Sims mistakenly says that *Pertaining to Yachts and Yachting* was first shown in a group exhibition at the Whitney Studio Club in 1925, instead of at the artist's one-man show in 1924. He also states incorrectly that Sheeler lived at 10 West Eighth Street from 1923 to 1927. The correct dates of occupancy are 1923–1925.

†This was Orozco's first show in this country, not, as reported by Alma Reed, Orozco's biographer, in 1928 at the Marie Sterner Gallery.

who then learned from what they bought. Besides showing some favorites from his personal collection, Schnakenberg borrowed objects from Juliana, Demuth, the decorator Robert Locher, Sheeler, Brook, Bacon, Dorothy Varian, Schmidt, Kuniyoshi, and the poet Elinor Wylie. Whereas the artists had been buying for years, he had much consciousness-raising to do among storekeepers and other owners. "Cigar-store Indians were still to be seen outside tobacconists' stores," Schnakenberg reminisced, "and I finally persuaded one old dealer to lend me his for a few weeks, although he was afraid that the neighborhood children would not know his place when they came to buy candy and found their beloved Indian gone. But he came to the opening and was delighted to see his Indian there shown for the first time as a work of art."

Of real historical importance, the show heralded, as did the opening of the Metropolitan's American Wing later that year, the beginning of a tilt toward—and eventually a craze for—the vernacular. The American Wing, however, concentrated on more polished and mainstream examples of native craft. At that time the Metropolitan looked on folk art as a bit foolish for its marble halls. The *New York Times* also felt that the primitives were a shade too close to junk. In reviewing Schnakenberg's presentation at the Whitney, one of the paper's critics categorized what was seen as "odds and ends of not very early decorative art." Another, diverted by the humor and homely patterns, condescendingly hedged that "[i]t may not be altogether to scoff that one goes to see the early American art at the Whitney Studio Club."

The increased popularity of folk art as the 1920s wore on has been linked to a concommitant Colonial revival that was also gaining momentum, but Schnakenberg surmised that the source was less provincial than that. He stated that he and his friends were inspired by all things primitive, whether American or not, in their quest to express themselves in a direct manner. It had not been accidental that in response to the artists' needs Juliana had shown African sculpture in 1923. And while Early American Art was on view at the Club, the Henri Rousseau exhibition was taking place at the Studio.

The aesthetic of the castoff, so central to folk art, also underlay the show selected by Sheeler and seen at the Club in March of 1924. He proclaimed his own tastes and influences and celebrated Cubism and Dada with works by Picasso, Braque, de Zayas, and Marcel Duchamp, all of whom were masters at valuing the throwaway, at siting the *objet trouvé*. The exhibition, which also included African sculpture, ran concurrently with Sheeler's own one-man show next door. The star was indubitably Duchamp, there in force with five canvases Sheeler borrowed from Walter Arensberg, John Quinn, and several other collectors: *Nude Descending a Staircase, The King and Queen Surrounded by Swift Nudes, Apropos of Little Sister, Chocolate Grinder, No. 2,* and *The King and Queen Traversed by Swift Nudes.** Because these paintings were sequestered in private apartments and Duchamp's output was tiny—by 1924 he professed not to paint anymore—seeing the *succès de scandale* of the Armory Show and its

---

*All are now in the Philadelphia Museum of Art except for *Apropos of Little Sister*, which is in the Solomon R. Guggenheim Museum.

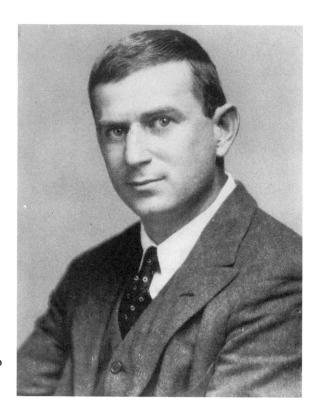

Alexander Brook, the
assistant director of the Club
from December 1923 to
May 1927.

companion pieces once again was a great privilege. Recalling the gallons of ink
once spilt about *Nude Descending a Staircase*, Henry McBride remarked that
the pictures at the Club now had "the air of classics. They are painted in reticent
grays and browns and the whole atmosphere of the room has become thoughtful
and serious."

In his role as gallery concierge, Alexander Brook was chafing at his lack of
influence over the exhibitions presented, as not all of them were to his taste.
Brook was a frequent visitor and a sometime resident of Woodstock, New York,
the headquarters of a highly visible artists' colony much practiced in logrolling.
In early 1924, Konrad Cramer, one of the leaders of Woodstock's modernist
faction, asked Brook for a show at the Club in the near future. Since Juliana,
de Zayas, and the artists in charge of assembling their own exhibitions had
determined the schedule in advance, there was no room for Cramer on the
agenda. Brook wrote to his friend, "Next year, however, more can be done about
such matters. I have not full authority to give people exhibitions, but I have
quite a bit to say." Feeling embarrassed about the admission of his own relative
powerlessness, he closed with a little boasting: "I wish also to inform you that
the standards of the shows, beginning next fall, will rise, at least as I hope."

Perhaps Brook was in just such an ornery frame of mind when he decided
to increase attendance at the Duchamp show by reviving the dependable old

ghost of 1913. He hoped to make capital from those squads of outraged philistines who couldn't wait to storm the portals of West Eighth Street once the horrors on the Club's walls were made known to them. Brimming with the confidence of the initiated, Brook took out an advertisement in a weekly guide to New York happenings on condition that *Nude Descending a Staircase* be reproduced. He thought the bait had been swallowed when he saw two suburban-looking matrons clutching guidebooks and advancing sternly on him. One demanded to know if the *Nude* was indeed installed in the gallery. As Brook recounted it, upon his saying yes:

> The ladies looked and burst into laughter, which, however, was directed not at the "Nude" but disconcertingly at myself. The one who had spoken held up the guide for me to see.
> "Well," said I, now on the defensive, "what's wrong with that?"
> "It's upside down!" the lady said with further merriment, and so it was, turned topsy-turvy by the printer. Those . . . ladies had not seen the "Nude" since the Armory Show, yet their memories and eyes were keen and completely accurate, whereas I with my 20/20 vision had been unforgivably careless. It was a hell of a way to start my gallery-guy career.

By the spring of 1924, Gertrude's equestrian statue of Buffalo Bill Cody was nearly completed and ready to ship to its destination of Cody, Wyoming. The memorial was the best public sculpture Gertrude ever made, and as a work of public art, it still exerts a certain vitality. The specificity of the subject (Cody is portrayed as a scout riding the trail) and its unabashedly American frame of reference anchored the piece in a down-to-earth realism to which Gertrude responded very well. In depicting a characteristic, exciting action—Cody reins in his pony to scan the tracks on the ground—as opposed to an attitude struck, she escaped the inertness and high-flown symbolism that mar her other large works. Andrew O'Connor was rumored to have a share in the execution of *Buffalo Bill*, and in sculpture circles its merit came as some surprise. "[Mrs. Whitney's] statue is better than I had been led to believe," Daniel Chester French wrote to his daughter. "It has a good deal of spirit and gives the picturesqueness of the subject."

From the time Gertrude had accepted the commission two years before, Cody's relatives and some of their followers among the townspeople threw themselves into celebrating their Western heritage. But honest pride and exuberance had turned into glory hunting. The Codyans had become positively messianic: Lately they were intent on launching a national movement for erecting shrines to the pioneers, with Buffalo Bill as their supreme deity. None of these enthusiasts had the money or celebrity for propelling such dreams into reality, but they were sharply aware of who did. The Codyans began exploiting Gertrude's name, and emboldened by her generosity, asked her to underwrite their uncapitalized project. (Gertrude had already paid for the land on which the monument would stand and volunteered to maintain the site, but that only excited them more.) The Cody family and their friends indulged themselves in hyperbole. "The happiest two hours of Mrs. Whitney's life were spent in Cody," Buffalo Bill's niece assured the Wyoming newspapers.

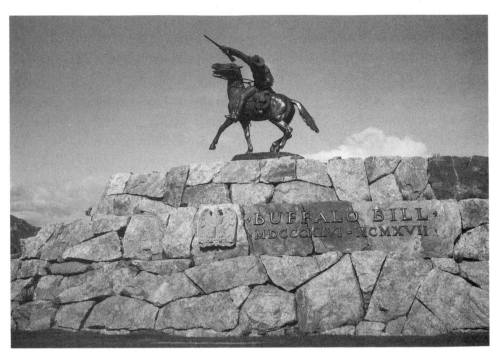

Gertrude's sculpture of Buffalo Bill Cody, now known as *The Scout*, high on a plinth above the Shoshone River.

As their untempered determination grew, the Cody brigade became pests to Gertrude, and the situation got messy. She did not want to set foot in Wyoming until the dedication of the statue, which was scheduled for July 4, 1924, so Juliana boarded a train bound for the Rockies in her stead. Juliana was going primarily to inspect the stone base, confer with its architect, and prepare the political ground for the unveiling, but she also had to make Cody see reason. Money would have to come from local and state fund-raising, and no more liberties were to be taken with the Whitney name.

As a representative of new art, old-line culture, piles of money, and the society page, Juliana was news in Cody. The local dignitaries acted as if she were the biggest thing to hit town since statehood. They rushed her off her feet with sightseeing and engagements. She approved the magnificent site (placed atop a high plinth, rearing above the Shoshone River, Buffalo Bill and his mount would face the eastern entrance of Yellowstone Park and be flanked by the Rattlesnake and Cedar mountains) and made vivacious informal speeches to the leading civic organizations. Her appearances made the front page, and the newspapers printed her every utterance. Because of their coverage, the addresses Juliana delivered in Cody constitute the only extended illustration of her gift for holding an audience, of her warmth and magnetism as a speaker and impresario.

Addressing a women's club, Juliana persuaded her listeners to see Gertrude's sculpture as an interpretation of American life. In her talk she cleverly guided

a group of people with little experience in judging or looking at art toward a way of apprehending it. Using herself as an example to avoid charges of patronizing, she told them to trust to their intuitions and emotional responses:

I have never been further west than Chicago, and yesterday I realized that I did not know anything about geography. All of my education has been with artists, and I have something to substitute for that lack of knowledge. I realize for the first time the grandeur and beauty and the freedom in the midst of which you are living and I think it has had a great effect. I do not see how you could be any different from what you are living as you do in the midst of this. . . . They say in New York that all good Americans when they die go to Paris; but I say good Americans when they live should come to Cody.

In New York there are only two classes of people the quick and the dead. This applies to Cody and every other place. Mrs. Whitney and you and I are appreciated in the world only as much as we show this sensitiveness, quickness, and responsiveness to all that life means. There are only two peoples anywhere—the quick and the dead, if we use "quick" in the old Anglo-Saxon sense, to quicken, to be sensitive, to be alive. You may call it energy, intelligence, responsiveness, anything you want, but it is really being alive. And that is the thing which I think Mrs. Whitney has put into her statue of Buffalo Bill. As has been said, one must either go on or go back, and we are only important, you and I, Mrs. Whitney and Buffalo Bill, only important insofar as we are able to go on. There are two kinds of people, the people who go on and the people who shrink back; and I feel out here the tremendous feeling of going on . . . and I think the monument which Mrs. Whitney is making has that feeling.

I want to say a word about the monument itself. I am not an artist, so I can boast. It is a monument, not so much to Buffalo Bill as a man who wore a certain kind of coat, or who wore a certain kind of boots, or hat, or played cards this or that way— it is the spirit which animated him throughout his life as the artist has tried to interpret it—the spirit of every American whether he was known or not, which contributed . . . to this country's success. . . .

You know there are two ways of making monuments. You make a symbol or you make a figure. I was in the foundry when I went over to see the Buffalo Bill cast a week or so ago, and the man who runs that foundry showed me another monument, and I looked at it—a gigantic portrait of a man represented in all his grandeur— morning coat, braid on it in bronze; waistcoat just right in appearance, watch chain across his waistcoat, all the links in the cuffs just as we would stand there, cuffs just the right length, creases in trousers—all in bronze. The head of the foundry asked: "What do you think of it?" I said, "That is not a monument, that is a pickle." He replied: "That is a funny thing; this monument is a memorial to the head of the 57 Varieties."

The high thing in a work of art is what is technically called "gesture." If that work does not say something to you that makes you go on, that "quickens" you, then that is not a work of art; it is just a historical document. And this monument, when you get it, I am sure you will realize, as I have realized for a long time, is a gesture. Look at it that way. I am so proud of it, and I am so glad to be able to tell you I am proud of it, and so glad in fact that I have met you, and I know you will understand when I say I am proud of this gesture which Mrs. Whitney has made.

Juliana also spoke to the best students at the town high school. Much of what she said was the same, but she varied it with some humorous (and untrue)

reminiscences about herself. No one knew she was taking poetic license for the sake of rhetorical symmetry and euphony, so the wit was what counted. And because Juliana could never bring herself to be straitlaced around young people, her remarks voluptuously reflected her own private enthrallment with art. As a reporter on the scene summarized it:

> Speaking to the honor roll of students (those who had attained at least a grade of 90% for the past semester), Mrs. Force said she scarce had the courage to address so august a body; that she never had such a chance. She had never gone but to one school, a private one [wildly incorrect] and never had but a single teacher. And the only percentage she'd ever received was when someone told her during the war she was 100% American.

After repeating her praise of Cody and her pride in Gertrude's statue, Juliana concluded, "I could tell you a lot of things about art. As my teacher said, 'My dear young lady, Art is like Love; you don't talk it, you make it.' "

No wonder Juliana captivated Cody. But through it all, except for those brief little jokes, she kept the focus on Gertrude and Gertrude alone. Besides extolling the monument and its site, Juliana also explained the particulars of Gertrude's life as they related to her struggle for a career in art. She talked of the gossip and resentment Gertrude faced because of her social position. Meanwhile, Juliana took care to stress, Gertrude was always working for other artists and for the furtherance of American art. About her own part in that campaign, she said nothing. In Cody she introduced herself as Gertrude Whitney's secretary, toned down her personality, and did not elaborate on her responsibilities.

Juliana consistently gave full credit for their joint enterprises to Gertrude. This was a rule which amounted to a statement of principle, for she remained grateful to Gertrude for placing absolute trust in her. Even though Gertrude was no longer directing the course of the Studio or the Club, she had originated the idea of helping artists, and she still bankrolled everything done in her name. And although she remained bound by the world she was born into, Gertrude had succeeded in expressing her individuality to a degree beyond the majority of other women—or men—in similar social spheres. Juliana never forgot that Gertrude had made her possible.

Juliana could only admire Gertrude's perseverance in maintaining an active, continuous involvement with art. Accordingly, she went about educating people as to Gertrude's valor and largesse with a sense of sacred personal duty. Numerous artists have testified to Juliana's reiteration that Gertrude was the best friend they ever had, but the Philadelphia painter Franklin Watkins conveyed it best when he wrote to Juliana:

> Isn't it strange how much she [Mrs. Whitney] has meant to me through you? I wonder how many painters must be thinking this today as they look back to that bleak period of a few years ago when American art was "out"; and then you came along and told us we had a meaning. . . .
>
> In a few brief years your sympathy became one of the reasons why we mustn't fail.

The only aspect of the expedition to Cody that flopped was the attempt to restrain the Cody family. Since Juliana had taken the town by storm on her

trip, she, along with Gertrude, was now a heroine to one contingent of Codyans, who pressed her for further visits years and years after the statue was dedicated. Most of the time Juliana could plead overwork, but the cat-and-mouse game took on a comic dimension one summer when Buffalo Bill's niece arrived in New York with the purpose of bringing Juliana back to Cody. She didn't succeed in that, but she was in the very unusual position of having Juliana on the run. After dodging her for several days—the lady was visiting the galleries and lying in wait at her office—Juliana was reduced to hiding out and sending preposterous telegrams to keep her at bay.

The Club's New York season ended with the now traditional members' roundup. Good, even verging on the indulgent, notices had gradually become a part of that tradition, because the unevenness inherent in presenting artists in all stages of endeavor was now accepted rather than disparaged. Among the unknowns making their Club debut were Isabel Bishop, Reginald Marsh, Ernest Fiene, John Flannagan, William Gropper, Martin Lewis, Wharton Esherick, and William Lescaze. Henry McBride led off his review with, "The Whitney Studio Club of late years has been steadily improving and the present season, now brought to a conclusion with a members' exhibition, has been lively and effective throughout. It is one thing to mean to do good and another to achieve it. The institution provided an excellent gallery and all sorts of enticements to young artists for a number of years before it finally caught on." His colleagues heaped on similar praise.

Juliana and Gertrude girded themselves for returning to Cody for the July 4 dedication ceremonies. But fate in the form of another war monument kindly intervened. Gertrude was awarded a commission for a memorial to the American Expeditionary Forces; it was to be placed in the harbor of Saint-Nazaire, the first French soil the American troops touched when they landed in 1917. Gertrude had to select a site for the monument, and the expediency of sailing in June and skipping the festivities in Wyoming became apparent. But to avoid giving offense to Cody, her departure was kept secret until the last possible moment. Only after she was safely aboard ship did she cable her regrets. Meanwhile, the newspapers printed stories about the special train bringing Gertrude and her party West.

Juliana also wriggled out of going to Cody to join Gertrude at Saint-Nazaire. As she was planning to spend the summer in France, she asked the Varèses, who were already in Paris, to take a villa for her. The composer rented a house on the river near Fontainebleau. Juliana closed the Club to the public and conferred about what should be shown the following fall. Brook loyally plumped for Konrad Cramer, and Juliana accepted his judgment. Brook purred to Cramer, "I asked you in a previous letter for some photographs of your work as Mrs. Force has not seen any for some time and wanted to see what you had done recently. She took my word that it was good, however, so it is unnecessary to send them if you have not done so."

Juliana's holidays were passed exactly as she liked—long drives around the

countryside, plenty of art, and even more socializing with her friends. She saw the Varèses, but not for very long. Varèse, the irreducible urbanite, had trouble sleeping in the country, because he was kept awake by the noises of the birds and frogs. The Davidsons, of course, were guests, and Juliana ordered clothes from Jo's wife, Yvonne, who had become a sought-after couturier with a successful dressmaking establishment. (Gertrude was one of Yvonne's steady clients and over the seasons had bought ensembles for herself and Juliana.) The du Boises and the Glackenses were also in France, and so were the Watsons. Forbes was gathering material for articles to run in *The Arts*, based on his visits to artists' studios in Paris. Inconveniently for Juliana, Forbes was only in pleasure-loving France a few weeks before he was obliged to visit his stuffy Scottish in-laws in the Border counties. In a letter to Gertrude, he retailed his change of scene.

> Since I left Paris I have been to church three times, heard grace at every meal, climbed the Cheviot Hills day after day, slept ten hours a night, read Anthony Trollope's autobiography, made no mention of any sex problem, sworn not once, and heard nothing of the existence of wine, liquor or cigars, had afternoon teas served as regular meals with forty different kinds of scones and oat cakes and a dozen different kinds of jams, discussed Scotch ecclesiastical laws, as well as ballads and legends, and in general been a perfect imitation of a country parson. I feel rested, healthy, full of pep, grateful, and amply ready to depart toward regions where life is not quite so 1860.

Forbes was not the only one sending bouncy letters. Before she left, Juliana had asked Brook to write and fill her in on all the Village gossip she was missing. He covered sheets of paper with animated descriptions of their friends' assignations in juicy prose. No reply came from Juliana, but then Brook didn't expect to hear from her. When she returned in September looking blackly at her employee, he learned the reason why. Her mailing address that summer was the Guaranty Trust in Paris, to which Brook sent his letter, but he had neglected to write her name on it. Meanwhile, Juliana had not been receiving all her mail, and some important correspondence had been due for weeks. The day came when Juliana completely lost her temper over the delay, and blamed it on the bank. As Brook related in his memoirs, she

> went storming into the bank, demanding rather than asking for her mail. The quiet man behind his cage smiled slyly, went to the pigeonholes behind him, and said as he proferred her a letter, "Perhaps this is for you, Mrs. Force. We opened it because there was no name but ours on the envelope."

It was, of course, Brook's salacious letter. The contents had obviously been read by the snickering clerk at the Guaranty Trust; her consternation was total. It was soon Brook's turn to wish that the floor would open wide and swallow him, but Juliana was a connoisseuse of the ridiculous and that ensured his forgiveness. Juliana and Brook were constantly thwarting intrigues, both comical and deadly. One memorable instance of deviousness was tantalizing for not being realized. In 1922, Brook met John Graham, the painter, collector, and theorist who was to figure importantly in the development of the New York School. After Brook became Juliana's assistant, Graham would visit him at the

Club. During their talks, Graham quizzed him closely about the organization and its practices.

These visits, for all their amiability, hinted at a motive Brook could not fathom, because most of the time Graham could "barely contain his scorn" for what was on the Club's walls. To this cosmopolite, born in Kiev and familiar with the School of Paris and the Russian avant-garde, the Club was hopelessly provincial. But he must have seen some potential in Eighth Street, for in 1925 he wrote to Juliana requesting Brook's job. Graham argued that he was better qualified for the work, which, in retrospect, was true, but he did himself no good by informing her that the Club "was a dull and unprogressive institution offering unimaginative, mediocre exhibitions that demonstrated no awareness of changing times." Maligning the basis of Juliana's career was hardly the way to influence her, and Graham was not invited to advise or work for the Club. Had he used better judgment, he might have been tried out in some curatorial capacity, as had happened with Marius de Zayas. The outcome is fascinating to contemplate, for if Graham had imposed his tastes on the Club, the shows and purchases would have been significantly different. Brook and Juliana did not ostracize Graham, and Graham had no qualms about staying on the scene. He exhibited at the Club between 1925, the date Brook assigned to the letter to Juliana, and 1928, the year the Club was disbanded.

But such equanimity was not automatic because the less attractive streak in Juliana's character—the vitriolic irrationality and cruel sarcasms that were the dark side to her pep, impulsiveness, and fondness for whimsy—was a combustible reality ever ready to flare. And flare it did, in insults and rages and mix-ups when she concluded—many times mistakenly—that she was being slighted or criticized. Carl Zigrosser, who had been so friendly with Juliana during the first few years of the Club's existence, began to pull away from her because he was disturbed by what he saw. He could not reconcile the coexistence of so much unkindness with so much sympathetic accord, but he ascribed the contradiction to the pressures of her job:

> The years she spent acting as a buffer between Gertrude Vanderbilt Whitney and a horde of hungry artists began to leave their mark. She became artful and politic, more prone to search for the *arrière pensée*. In her position as the intermediary between wealth and need—or sometimes greed—her only chance for survival was to anticipate every trick of the beggar and sycophant, and manoeuvre to remain in control of the situation. She lived in an artificial world of indirection and deceit— outwardly *toujours la politesse* but inwardly a cutthroat game indeed. Needless to say I saw less and less of her: I would not put myself in a position where my motives might be questioned. . . . Our relations were cordial but infrequent. If she invited me to an opening at the Club, I accepted.

Some years after the museum opened, Juliana and Zigrosser spent an evening together. She confided to him that her position was one of minefields eternally traversed, and as she made her weary confession, their friendship was resumed. For Zigrosser the excesses of Juliana's behavior made sense:

She talked of the venality of the dealers and critics and what helpless adolescents artists were. She cited the vulgarity of one artist who sent Mrs. Whitney twenty-five dollars' worth of orchids, and the impudence of a writer who asked for $10,000 a year for five years to study abroad. These were but samples of . . . stories she told of pettifogging manoeuvres which she had to circumvent.

Yet it was true that Juliana's flair could get out of hand and take very unpleasant forms. The heat from her tongue could barbecue anyone. Raillery was not always distinguished from gratuitous insults nor playful chaffing from brutal taunts, especially after several rounds of cocktails. She had a loud, raucous laugh that could destroy someone—"it sounded like a Mack truck changing gears," one museum director said. Guy Pène du Bois, a scathing satirist himself when he wanted to be, analyzed her mordancy from a kindred point of view. He wrote of Juliana, "Life was her meat. She loved to report on how badly it could behave and stir it out of any angelic pose it might momentarily adopt. It has often seemed to me that she considered silence as an invalid in want of vitamins and that in conversation she preferred the bite, even of calumny if a substitute was wanting, to the toothlessness of a considered and polite statement."

A personality far better prepared than Zigrosser to withstand Juliana, but who nevertheless was humiliated by her, was Rebecca West, who came to New York several times between 1924 and 1926. She knew Juliana slightly, and on one of her American trips she received unpardonable treatment at her hands. Juliana's version of events is not extant, but Dame Rebecca remembered the incident with such horror that she felt "an absurd desire to burst into tears on some sympathetic shoulder" in recounting it a half-century later. In 1978 she wrote:

I had met her [Juliana] once in France, with, I think, M. [Etienne] Bignou of the Bignou Galleries in London and New York, and a Philadelphia family called Ridgway, and I had only a pleasant enough impression of an agreeable, chattering woman up to the night that I was invited to a dinner-party given before the hosts and guests went *en masse* to a reading of poetry by Edna St. Vincent Millay. When I got there I was rather surprised to find she seemed to be the hostess at the dinner, and quite surprised when she almost at once began to make rallying remarks about me, which got stranger and stranger. Finally she said, out of the blue, while someone else was talking to me, "Well, Rebecca, I had always heard of you as brilliant and charming, and when I met you I was so surprised. I knew [at] once I couldn't stand you, and I was right." By this time I had come to the conclusion that she was either drunk or drugged, for she was making faces at me, so I answered amiably.

This made an awkward situation at the dinner-table and I was relieved when we got off to the theater for the reading. There I heard no more of her until Edna St. Vincent Millay read a long poem called "Carnival," which I couldn't quite hear. Mrs. Force asked me, "What did you think of that?" I answered, "I am afraid I did not catch it." She said nothing more. The party then broke up and went on somewhere else, and I refused to go on some pretext and went back to my hotel. . . .

Two or three days later I saw a caricature of myself in a New York newspaper, which was plainly meant for me, and was described as "English visiting lecturer looks bored as she insults her hostess." I rang up . . . a close friend of Flora Tower's

[Gertrude's eldest daughter, Flora Whitney, now married to Roderick Tower] and asked if he could explain this fresh insult (which was drawn by a man who had been at the party, a well-known caricaturist).* He then came to see me and told me that Mrs. Force was under the impression that I had insulted her. He said that according to her I had called her a bitch. This wretched nonsense Mrs. Force told not only . . . [him] but everybody she met for quite a considerable period of time.

I think you will realize that this statement is hardly one that I would have made in answer to an enquiry as to whether I liked a poem.

I met Mrs. Force two or three times after that and each time she gave me a triumphant smile.

Rebecca West was right in claiming that Juliana spread around the "wretched nonsense." Both Allan Rieser and Alexander Brook heard from Juliana that Rebecca West said to her, "There sits the queen of the bitches." Juliana also told them, "Rebecca West called me a bitch, and I don't know why." It is apparent that Juliana heard "I am afraid I did not catch it" in West's rapid, clipped English as "queen of the bitches." Doubtless she was expecting the quick-witted author to return her guying with a retort of her own, which made her receptive to interpreting as a slur whatever assailed her ears. No aspect of this discreditable episode redounds to Juliana's favor, but the worst of it, besides her publishing of the story, is her dead certainty that she had heard slander and her instantaneous and vehement acting upon it. The verdict was irreversible: She did not challenge Rebecca West on what she thought was said, and she did not try to straighten things out or make amends. Hence the story went on unchecked, and ten years later it was still circulating as debased scuttlebutt.

At this stage of her life, apology was not a common word in Juliana's vocabulary, even with friends. As she once said to a curator who, in her view, was exonerating himself too wordily from a charge, "Sir, there are two times when you have to defend yourself: one is in a police court and the other is on Judgment Day." In one notable instance, the unjustly blamed victim of her pique was Stuart Davis, who was twice cursed by inept installations of his paintings at Whitney shows. Juliana's irritation was temporary—even Davis dismissed it as an "occasional difference"—and should be measured against years of financial support and genial relations, but whether out of loyalty to her staff or plain arrogance, she refused to own mistakes. The first time Davis crossed Juliana was over his landmark Eggbeater series. In an interview about his association with Juliana and the Whitney, Davis stated that the paintings "were pretty abstract, but the Whitney was always willing to show experimental work and they invited one of my Eggbeaters† to a group exhibition [the 1928 annual]. The only trouble was that I hadn't marked which was the top and they hung it on its side between two windows. It just fitted that way . . . you couldn't turn it right side up and still get it in the same space. I had what I thought then was a pretty novel idea. I went back to the studio and brought in another picture that would fit right

*This must have been W. E. Hill.

†*Eggbeater, Number 4.* Davis changed the numbering of the Eggbeater series several times, so it is impossible to know if the painting shown in 1928 as *Eggbeater, Number 4* is the painting known today as such.

side up. But Mrs. Force was a strong character. She liked that eggbeater on its side and that's the way it stayed all through the show." The second time Davis's canvas was physically interfered with, and he was indignant. In an exhibition of flower paintings, he contributed a picture with edges bordered in lemon yellow. When he arrived at the opening he was stunned to see his "picture with another frame on it, a frame nailed to the picture through the canvas on the edges from the front—. . . a barbaric thing!—and the yellow border had been painted white. . . . I wrote [Mrs. Force] a letter . . . saying I was sure she didn't know about this vandalism on my painting, and that I hoped she would take notice and find out who was responsible for it." According to Davis, who was a touch prickly himself, Juliana took the letter as a personal assault and wrote to him saying that *he* was the one being outrageous. No such vandalism ever occurred in *her* galleries, and hence he had erred in his charges.

Juliana was prone to mishearing or misinterpreting and then judging too quickly. She liked or hated on sight, and that was that. On the positive side, living her life like a projectile in flight made her superbly responsive to problems; on the negative side, it swept her into catastrophic assumptions and vendettas or clouded the air with confusion. Eleanor Lambert, who worked as a publicist for the Whitney Galleries and Museum before she became a luminary of the fashion world, remembered Juliana rushing pell-mell into a furor when reflection would have been wiser. The scene was an elaborate party Juliana gave featuring Gypsy fortune-tellers. The affair had been uninhibited, and the guests made themselves at home. After the revels were over, Juliana retired to her bedroom. Beginning to undress, she discovered that her jewels were gone and then roused the household. The Club and her apartment were turned upside-down in the search for the missing jewelry. But Juliana refused to call the police. Only artists attended the party, she said, which meant that only an artist could have been the thief, and she could not bring herself to accuse an artist. The atmosphere at the Whitney fluctuated from dismal to poisonous as everyone tried to adjust to the idea that a friend or a colleague was dishonest. Several days elapsed before Juliana remembered a crucial detail. Before the party she had sent her maid to the bank with her jewel case. It had been in the vault all along.

These rampages and careless misunderstandings elicited and were resolved by short spurts of anger. In a whole other category were Juliana's hysterically drawn-out seizures of rage, terrifying not only to those on the receiving end but to anyone in the vicinity. Her disarray signaled that control had slipped away from this customarily strong and poised woman. These frenzies bore a close resemblance to her mother's tantrums, and they were as much a mode of prevailing by intimidation as surrendering to emotion. Allan Rieser, who watched many of these squalls build to a passionate intensity, linked them to a very purposeful working up of feeling. Seeing them as fixtures of Juliana's dramatic kit, as part of the theater she carried around with her, he was more apt to marvel than tremble. He wrote of his aunt:

No portrait would be complete without some mention of her famous rages. They were the most impressive I have ever seen, either in life or on the stage. Her deep

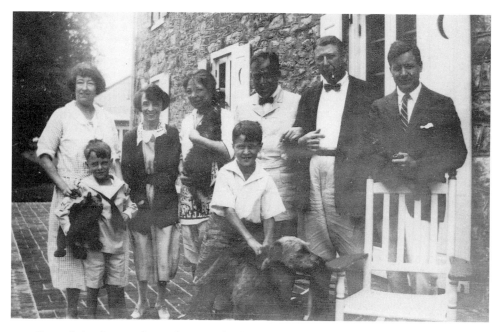

Part of the Rieser clan gathers at the farm: from left, Mungo Park with hands on shoulders of Carl Rieser; unknown woman; Juliana holding either McTaggart or McDuff; unknown man; Allan Rieser; Doctor with his Airedale; Charles Rieser.

voice changed into a roar, straight from the chest; her eyes glared histrionically; she pounded things and flung things. I think Napoleon would have given ground. . . .

I heard that once . . . when she learned that some antique seller had cheated her, she threw an entire set of furniture into the fire. Given her temperament and the size of the fireplaces, it is very believable.

But I don't want to distort the picture. In all honesty, the things I have been mentioning, added all together, amounted to some stormy days in a life which in general was sunny . . . and generous. If she manipulated people, it was the people themselves she had in mind. If she fell into a rage with them, it was because they had disappointed her, and if she laughed at them, it was because she thought that life itself was funny, and she relished oddity.

Thanks to Alexander Brook's lobbying and increased influence, Konrad Cramer had his show at the Club in December of 1924. Other highlights of the 1924–1925 season were the first one-artist shows ever given to Reginald Marsh, Joseph Pollet, Molly Luce, Cecil Howard, and Andrew Dasburg, and the entrance into Juliana's life of a consumingly peculiar person, an Englishwoman named Eirene Mungo-Park.

Mungo, as she was known to everyone, was a direct descendant of the Scottish explorer of Africa, and as Katherine Schmidt said, "She looked odd, she acted odd, and she *was* odd." Mungo had red-brown hair, cropped straight around her head in a Buster Brown bowl, and a redder face. She painted a little, sculpted a little (she entered her pieces in Club annuals), played the piano a little, and

was good at sports and games. Unlike her distinguished ancestor, however, Mungo was incompetent at functioning in the larger world. If England had nurtured her, Greenwich Village protected her, and she existed there marginally but cheerfully as a middle-aged waif.

Someone who felt sorry for Mungo told Juliana about her, and Juliana invited her to her office. Before their interview, Mungo heated a pan of milk on the stove in her flat. On the shelf above the stove was a box of matches and somehow the matches fell into the milk. Mungo did not notice them until she poured the milk into a glass, but she drank it and went off to her appointment without a second thought. By the time she reached the office, her ruddy face had gone white, and she was on the verge of collapse. Juliana took one look at this blanching weirdo and sent for a doctor at once. He examined Mungo and, hearing what had happened, told her that the milk had kept her from getting even sicker. No more concrete demonstration of Mungo's helplessness could have been furnished, and Juliana took her under her protection. Mungo was absorbed into the Force household—she was around when Juliana needed her for errands, she carried bits of gossip to and from Eighth Street, she sometimes looked after the Rieser children, and she evolved into a companion for Doctor now that he and Juliana were under the same roof again. Mungo and Doctor would have dinner together or play checkers, leaving Juliana free to exit with her friends for the evening. About this time Doctor took up sculpting, no doubt due to Mungo's encouragement.

In the country, Mungo was a semipermanent guest at Barley Sheaf Farm. She spent much of the summer there and quite a number of weekends the rest of the year. In town, however, Mungo did not live with the Forces; she stayed in a primitive room nearby. It had no bathtub, but now that she could come and go as she liked at the Club, Mungo started making use of the full bathroom at No. 10 belonging to the Composers' Guild. Brook was not always glad to see Mungo because of her bumbling and her hotline to Juliana, but once in a while she would accidentally do something transcendant.

In January of 1925 Peggy Bacon had a show of drypoints and pencil drawings at the Montross Gallery. The most outstanding work was a large and subtle pencil drawing entitled *The Blessed Damozel*,* which Juliana bought. Some months later, she discovered that she had laid the drawing unwrapped on top of a cupboard in her office. The paper was coated with dirt and dust, and the original image was now invisible. She turned it over to Brook to clean. He took the drawing to the Club and put it in a butler's pantry in one of the back galleries until a solution suggested itself.

While he was attending to other business, Mungo drifted in to take one of her baths in the Whitney tub, which was situated directly above the butler's pantry. When Brook returned, the room was steaming and the ceiling dripping with moisture: Mungo had wandered off somewhere and left the faucets running. Bacon's drawing was now not only grimy, but sopping wet. Not knowing what

* Now in the collection of the Whitney Museum.

else to do, Brook turned off the faucets, laid the drawing flat on a board, and left the premises without hope of restoring the *Damozel* to some vestige "of her former pristine self." But the next day, he unbelievably found

the white paper as bright as ever or brighter, the drawing as delicately gray as it had been with none of it smudged or lost. After surprise had subsided I reasoned, rightly or wrongly, that the ceiling must have been painted with calcimine which had dissolved in the bathwater as it dripped down, removing the drawing's loose dust and no doubt, with the glue that was in it, performing the extra function of fixing the pencil lines. Good old Mungo! She had started out as a potential villainess, but through carelessness and dumb chance had been transformed into a glowing heroine.

All of this, the comedy and the errors, as well as the benisons and the inspirations, kept the Whitney enterprises in their perpetual whirl. For Juliana, an unadulterated personal triumph came on March 1, 1925. Edgard Varèse had dedicated *Intégrales*—his most rhythmically complex and innovative symphony—to Juliana, and it was to have its premiere that night. The first public performance of *Intégrales* took place at the Aeolian Hall, and it was conducted by Leopold Stokowski. In his study of Varèse, Fernand Ouellette observed that *Intégrales* was important not only in the Varèse canon "but in the whole history of music. It was in reference to this work that the expression 'spatial music' was to be formulated for the first time." Varèse and his ideas had been ridiculed by some reviewers on the daily papers, and friends and enemies of the composer looked forward to the performance with excitement. *Intégrales* was enthusiastically received: At its final notes, the cheering audience clamored for Stokowski to repeat the entire symphony. From this memorable event, Juliana and Stokowski got to know each other quite well, and the conductor spent many weekends at the farm. (When *Intégrales* premiered, Gertrude's niece Gloria Vanderbilt, who would marry Stokowski in 1945, was one year old.)

The members' annual, which opened on May 18, 1925, provided proof (if any more were needed) of the Club's popularity among artists and its indispensability as a showcase for their work to be seen. The exhibition was so big —over 350 items, with Thomas Hart Benton (who submitted panels from his first mural project) and Bradley Walker Tomlin making debuts as promising newcomers—that it had to be given uptown. The Anderson Galleries at 59th and Park Avenue were rented for sufficient space. With an indifference to chronological accuracy that was already second nature to Whitney-Force institutions, the Club (established in 1918, but assuming the founding date of the ill-fated Friends of the Young Artists) proclaimed the annual its tenth anniversary show. The "anniversary" was duly celebrated by critical plaudits, and Juliana capped the season with an enormous party in honor of Katherine Schmidt and Yasuo Kuniyoshi. From her job running the sketch class and his sales (in addition, Kuniyoshi may have worked as a photographer for the Club), the couple had saved enough money—$1,200—for a trip to Europe. Before they set sail, Juliana sent them off with a supper party at her apartment and a dance at the Club that lasted until dawn.

About the same time as the advent of Mungo and the departure of Kuniyoshi

and Schmidt, Juliana invented a commission for Charles Sheeler, who had moved out of the top floor of 10 West Eighth and into rooms across the street. The results are interesting chiefly as a pendant to Juliana's relationship with her mother and her past. Julia Rieser died in 1920, and none of her descendants recalled her passing as being extensively mourned. Yet five years later Juliana asked Sheeler to paint a full-length likeness of Julia, to be copied from a daguerreotype of her mother in widow's weeds, taken in between her marriages to Julius Kuster and Max Rieser. Sheeler was not the ideal candidate for this, but perhaps she assumed that his interests in photography, American culture, and folk art would make the job palatable. (Julia was posed against a crudely painted background typical of those in photographers' studios of the period.) However, the portrait of Juliana's mother turned out to be an uninspired picture.* The drawing is poor, the color is dull, and the overall execution lacks conviction. The most illuminating aspect of the painting is its title, which Juliana created. She called it *Lady of the 'Sixties: Portrait of Mrs. Custer.* The title not only neglects to indicate that the subject was Juliana's mother, but the German "Kuster" has been Anglicized to "Custer." It also seems significant that Juliana selected a photograph of her mother that showed her while she was living in Doylestown and before her social descent as Mrs. Max Rieser. Now that her mother was safely out of her life, Juliana could stand a memento of her, but in a once-removed form that wasn't necessarily identifiable. In how Juliana hung the portrait, there was a tinge of heartlessness, not commemoration. She trivialized her mother by putting her into the decor as a piece of Victorian melancholy.

Juliana spent the summer of 1925 at the farm. Sojourns in Bucks County now diverged along two different but basic lines, depending on the guests. If the Riesers were down, the children were the center of attention, with Doctor, Mungo, and the aunts as playmates and Juliana as mistress of the revels. Doctor enjoyed his nieces and nephews, and Beverly Rieser Smock remembered playing many games of hide-and-seek with him. He was such a strappingly built man that Beverly would hide from him under a bed because his arms were too big to reach for her there. Another entertainment was the séances held in a darkened room. The table rocked back and forth at a dangerous angle, loud rapping came out of nowhere, disembodied voices spoke from the astral, and the little Riesers emerged ecstatically terrified by what they had been through. Years later the children realized that Mungo customarily disappeared before the séances began, and it was she, of course, who tipped the table so thrillingly and hallooed messages from the dead.

Juliana had been thoroughly successful in making the farm a stronghold of family stability and influence. Beverly Rieser Smock cherished the orchard where she and her cousins played croquet and had tea brought to them by a butler. In its meadow they also went for "rides" on a big wooden horse Juliana bought for them. Carl Rieser wrote to his aunt about the centrality of the farm to his

* Now in the collection of the Museum of Fine Arts, Boston. When Carl Rieser owned the painting, William Lane, a Sheeler collector, advised him to burn it.

life. "[In New Jersey] I used to close my eyes and pretend that I was down here," he said. "I could always recall the way the locusts sang down here, the way a gate closed, the sound people's footsteps made on certain floors. 'The Farm' has become almost a symbol to me. I think that it has had a great effect aesthetically on me, too. Its beauty has cut more deeply than that of any other place." What mattered most to him was the togetherness the farm fostered: "There is Allan writing; Uncle Max going off on his solitary walks; the whole family collecting at supper time at a pleasantly set table with the amber setting sun streaming warmly through the windows; my birthday parties, always so gay; the family sitting around after supper reading."

An equally strong and recurring theme at Barley Sheaf Farm was Juliana's taking everyone else in hand and announcing how he or she should behave. Beverly Rieser Smock said that she and her family sometimes felt caught in the vise of Juliana's imperial largesse. "If Aunt Jule didn't like your dress or your hairdo," she said, "she would change it. In 1930 we drove up to the farm in our 1924 car. Aunt Jule was so horrified by our old car that she gave us one of the late-model Fords in her garage. It was generosity, but you had to do it her way."

Doctor tried to make a go of the farm, but neither he nor Juliana were cut out for making it pay. Juliana didn't keep track of expenditures, and Doctor, who was extremely soft-hearted, was often cheated in the most obvious fashion by the local people. Charles Rieser told his sons about being at the farm after the Forces' truck was stolen by a workman. He and Doctor went over to confront the thief and found him standing next to the truck. When he saw them coming, the man swung his foot over the license plate and kept it planted there while he talked. Doctor couldn't bring himself to accuse the man, and he and Charles went away without the vehicle.

The Riesers also spent hours following the latest fad or craze Juliana would import from her most recent trip to Europe. "She thought you could discover doctors the way you could discover artists," her nephews said, and every year there was a new genius who had to be obeyed. The Riesers, captive guinea pigs, would religiously comply with the new regimen for a few weeks and then forget it. One year the guru was Emile Coué, the popularizer of autosuggestion—that summer, everyone on the farm went around mumbling, "Every day in every way I'm getting better and better." Another season brought the gospel according to the Abbé Dimnet. The lessons of his book, *The Art of Thinking*, were presented to the younger Riesers as an ideal system for acquiring poise. While the Abbé reigned, Allan Rieser said that Juliana "told us how we had to be prepared mentally for everything. Before we walked into a room we had to decide how we would enter, how we would look, what we would think, and what we would say." Coming from a woman who was ruled by instinct and impulse, such advice must have struck even children as outlandish.

But all the mental exercises in self-improvement were easier to take than the quack nostrums Juliana imposed as cure-alls on her relatives. Worried about evacuation, she attempted to institute a daily enema; another time a high colonic was universally recommended. It was Fletcherism, the practice of chewing every

morsel that passed one's lips at least twenty-eight times, that embedded itself in the younger Riesers' collective consciousness as the quintessential health fad temporarily but furiously promoted by their aunt. Under Juliana's direction, Fletcherizing was mandatory even when drinking liquids. "I was made to do it for some time," Allan Rieser said, "and I became hypnotized by it. I lived in fear of not chewing my food enough, though several times I came fairly near to strangling myself while Fletcherizing a glass of milk."

When artists were guests at the farm, the social elixir was stronger than masticated milk. Doctor played a less prominent part during those weekends. He was amused by his wife's friends, but he didn't join in their more exuberant activities. Everyone was free to fan out and tour the grounds, swim in the pool—the men were handed laugh-engendering two-piece bathing suits if they hadn't brought their own—or play tennis. Cocktails were served on the screened-in porch, on the garden patio, or by the pool. If she was in good emoting form, Juliana would read aloud, her choices ranging from *The Pickwick Papers* to *The Eternal Moment*. For Dorothy Varian, who accompanied the Brooks to Holicong one time, the indelibly etched incident of the weekend was definitely not literary. "A group of us were . . . having cocktails on the second-floor terrace with Juliana. The butler came up about three times to announce dinner and we never budged. We just went on drinking. We did have dinner sooner or later, and about midnight somebody suggested going for a swim. All of us except Dr. Force went for a swim in the river. Alex was driving like a madman, and I never came closer to being killed in my life. We went swimming, and on the way back Juliana was holding her wet underwear in her lap. She must have gone in wearing it. Everyone was keyed up, and on the spur of the moment Juliana suddenly tossed her underwear out of the car window. The next morning she came downstairs with a long face. 'You know,' she said, 'all my underwear is monogrammed.' "

To Alexander Brook must go the credit for many of the livelier exhibitions, astute talent spottings, and general good works effected during the Whitney Studio Club's 1925–1926 season. Promoted from gallery assistant to assistant director, he was organizing and hanging shows, borrowing and selling works of art, and searching for new faces. To keep the Club going full tilt, Brook was spending more time than the promised two hours a day on the job; in his memoirs, he estimated that in his heyday he was responsible for suggesting 60 percent of the exhibitions to Juliana.

Although Juliana did not dictate to the artists she subsidized, she did monitor their progress lightly with sporadic visits and calls. After a couple of trips to New Jersey, she saw that Reuben Nakian was not producing much work in the studio she had located for him. She sent Brook to investigate; he reported that Nakian was demoralized because he was stuck in Weehawken and advised that a studio be found for him in a livelier and more sympathetic environment—namely Manhattan and, more pointedly, Greenwich Village. Juliana, who was never content assisting one artist if she could help two in the same stroke, asked Brook

to find a studio large enough for two people to share. Then Brook could use it in the mornings and Nakian in the afternoons while he was at the Club. Nakian liked the idea, the deal was on, and the two moved into a walk-up on Christopher Street in 1925. For a while the arrangement worked well, so well that Brook's best friend, Louis Bouché, sometimes came over and shared a model with him. Brook initially had reservations about the communal studio, but they were dissipated by the flexible schedule. However, he had not counted on the unbidden appearance of Eros in the now-crowded room on Christopher Street.

In his role as gumshoe, Brook made a habit of visiting most of the art schools in the city. One of the places he cased was the Master Institute of United Arts, an affiliate of the Roerich Museum at 107th Street and Riverside Drive. Robert Laurent taught a sculpture class there, and in the fall of 1925, Brook dropped in to watch. He observed two students he thought had more than ordinary ability: Concetta Scaravaglione and Duncan Ferguson. Brook asked to see some of their finished pieces, and made appointments with them at the Club. Although neither student was a mature artist, Brook and Juliana had enough faith in them to start putting them into exhibitions. Scaravaglione went on to sustain a long career; Ferguson did not live up to his promise and disappeared into obscurity.

In the course of launching Scaravaglione, Brook introduced her to Nakian, and the two became inseparable. Nakian brought his new love and photographs of her work to Forbes, who reproduced some examples in *The Arts*. Juliana helped out again by recommending Scaravaglione to the Tiffany Foundation for a fellowship. The only loser in this litany of lucky breaks was Brook. Nakian was no longer very willing to have Brook and Bouché as studio mates. He naturally wanted to reserve the space on Christopher Street for himself and Scaravaglione. The undesirability of his presence became plain to Brook, and he was back to having no studio.

The Club was peripatetic, too. Needing even more room for exhibitions and storage for what was now a bulging collection culled from several dozen shows, Gertrude took over 14 West Eighth Street and the Club moved there in October of 1925. (The Club and the Studio were now spread over 8, 10, and 14 West Eighth Street; No. 12, the building of artists' studios owned by Daniel Chester French, lay in between Gertrude's properties.) This expansion caused the Watsons to move uptown and the Forces to move into the top floor of No. 10. For Juliana it was the beginning of the ornate setting with which she would be identified. The connecting wall between No. 10 and No. 8 was knocked out and the space was remodeled into a suite of rooms running the width of both houses. Collaborating with the decorator Robert Locher, who helped her create this first version of her ever-elaborating Victorian world, Juliana installed carved marble fireplaces, floral carpets, and satin curtains that spilled prodigally onto the floor. The drawing room, a library, a dining room, and a bedroom were filled with pieces of Belter and Biedermeier furniture, which were then roundly castigated as the disgraces, excesses, and foibles of an ugly age. As a foil to what one Italian artist called the "humoristic" decor in the other portions of the apartment, the dressing room and bar were done in a smart Art Deco. Living directly above the Whitney Studio Club represented the convivial intersection

of Juliana's work life and personal life, her public and private enjoyment of art and artists. Upstairs at Eighth Street would be home to Juliana for the next two decades; when she vacated its premises, neither she nor the Whitney Museum would be the same again.

Brook next came to the aid of John Flannagan, the gifted and tormented sculptor whose alcoholic self-destructiveness would end in suicide. Brook had known Flannagan for several years, because they were neighbors on Patchin Place, and Flannagan used to display his finished pieces in the cul-de-sac formed by the street's warren of little buildings. Brook brought Flannagan into the Club, and Alice Campbell introduced him to Juliana. She recognized that he was troubled as well as out of the ordinary, and she was very kind to him over the years. As Robert J. Forsyth wrote about the sculptor's affiliation with the Whitney, Flannagan became one of those artists singled out for Juliana's "special attention, a life-long association in which Mrs. Force and the Whitney promoted Flannagan and his work whenever they possibly could within their working policies." The Whitney Museum was the first public collection to purchase his sculpture. When Flannagan applied for a Guggenheim Fellowship in 1932, Juliana was instrumental in securing him the award, and she consistently invited his work to the museum's annuals. As previously noted, when Flannagan tried to resign because he couldn't raise the five-dollar membership dues, Brook told Juliana, who countered by offering a show in December of 1925. Twenty-one pieces were exhibited, with prices between $150 and $500. Brook sold enough of them to ease Flannagan's financial problems temporarily. After his exposure at the Club, Flannagan met Carl Zigrosser, who was then running the Weyhe Gallery, and he began handling Flannagan's work.

Hung in a room next to Flannagan's sculpture that December were oils by Leon Hartl, a painter of lyrical landscapes and still lifes. Hartl had to work full-time to support himself, so his art was confined to Sunday painting and exhibiting from time to time at the Independents' spring annual. Juliana was delighted by the modesty and quietude of his work. She especially liked the delicately executed flower paintings and bought two of them. She then offered him a one-man show in the new galleries. Hartl assembled twenty-five canvases, priced from $15 to $50, and the exhibition was a minisensation: glowing reviews applauding the Whitney's discovery, including an essay in *The Arts* by Lloyd Goodrich, plus sixteen pictures sold. Juliana bought one for Gertrude and many of the rest were purchased by artists. This set a pattern—Hartl's most devoted following was among other painters. Hartl was collected by artists ranging from Arthur B. Davies to Fairfield Porter, and he was appreciated by many other practitioners of the intimist mode. His Whitney show gave him the confidence to pursue a career as an artist.

Juliana did not neglect Alexander Brook's well-being, and she came up with another proposition for funneling more income in his direction. If he would agree to find an apartment spacious enough to accommodate an extra boarder of her choice, she would raise his salary $50 a month. Brook could use the money, and Juliana told him to save the spare room for Mungo. Even someone as freewheeling as Brook could not consider Mungo as other than a walking

hazard, but he gritted his teeth and thought of the extra cash. He found an apartment on West Tenth Street with a room for Mungo that was separated by a long hall from the rest of the flat. This was as good a setup as could be managed, and Brook braced himself for Mungo to make her appearance. Meanwhile, time passed, and the room stayed empty. Mungo had gone to live somewhere else and forgotten to tell him about it. But no matter—Brook was now free to rent to whomever he pleased. He let it be known that he had a spare room, and an appointment to see it was made by Mrs. Alexander Stirling Calder, who arrived with her son Alexander, then a painter. Mrs. Calder looked the place over and said it would do for her "bear cub," as she called her good-natured and shambling son. The Brooks, both senior and junior, took to the playful Sandy, who fashioned ingenious toys from wire and wood and made up all manner of wonderful games. Brook and Bacon introduced him to all their friends and took him to rowdy artists' gatherings, including a famous party for the visiting Brancusi, which Calder re-created in paint.* It was not long before Sandy, with the blessings of Brook, was inducted into the Club.

The Whitney Studio Club, with over 300 artists on the rolls, had in its membership a perfect grab bag of personalities, styles, creeds, attitudes, and degrees of experience. There were the old friends and supporters from the earliest days, like Sloan, Chanler, du Bois, William and Edith Glackens, Ethel and Jerome Myers, Lawson, Gifford Beal, Jo Davidson, Mahonri Young, and Paul Manship. There were the novices, like Concetta Scaravaglione and Elsie Driggs, and Pamela Bianco, a child prodigy. There were the younger Realists, like Edward Hopper, Reginald Marsh, Katherine Schmidt, Glenn O. Coleman, and Isabel Bishop. There were the experimenters, who explored abstraction and representation in their attempts to come to terms with modernism in a language of their own, like Andrew Dasburg, Konrad Cramer, Jan Matulka, Stuart Davis, David Burliuk, John Graham, Charles Sheeler, Charles Demuth, Bradley Walker Tomlin, Niles Spencer, Walt Kuhn, Samuel Halpert, and Ben Benn. There were socially conscious artists, like Boardman Robinson, Harry Gottlieb, and William Gropper, sophisticated primitives, like Kuniyoshi, and those still in the throes of developing a style, like Alexander Calder and Thomas Hart Benton. There were academicians-in-the-making, like Eugene Speicher and Leon Kroll. There were conservative sculptors, like Gertrude, and lively ones, like Gaston Lachaise, John Flannagan, Reuben Nakian, Wharton Esherick, and Robert Laurent. There were graphic artists, like Peggy Bacon, Louis Lozowick, and Martin Lewis, and cartoonists, like Otto Soglow, W. E. Hill, Rudy Dirks, and John Held, Jr. There were those temporarily passing through the art world who would distinguish themselves in other professions, like John Dos Passos and William Lescaze, and there was room for resident foreigners, like Jules Pascin. And mingled with these more or less well-known names were many hardworking

---

*Now in the collection of the Whitney, and given to the museum as a gift by the artist.

but not outstanding artists who are now forgotten or who never attained fame at all, and, as was unavoidable, a percentage of Village dilettantes, would-be bohemians, escapees, and hangers-on like Mungo, who enjoyed the Whitney ambiance. Although Juliana's personal tastes ran to naive art, decorative still lifes, romantic landscapes, and the crisp refinement of Precisionism, as far as the Club and the Whitney Studio were concerned, she wanted all kinds of artists involved, from conservative to radical, as long as they were outside the rule- and prize-mongering crowd.

The Club tried to be nonpartisan, but it couldn't escape being biased toward the Ashcan and Fourteenth Street schools of urban realism, a preference that went back to Gertrude's purchases from The Eight exhibition and which was sustained through enduring friendships with the Henri group. However, Juliana was open to most trends, and as a rule, the Club was an accurate reflection of an American art still very much in the process of defining itself. It registered the foolish and ephemeral along with the classic and enduring, and exhibited its fair share of dross in the course of seeking the genuine article.

Despite Juliana's stated aim to be all-embracing, she let stand a gaping and conspicuous omission: the artists represented by Alfred Stieglitz. When after eight years of comparative inactivity, Stieglitz opened the Intimate Gallery in 1925, the core of his stable consisted of Arthur Dove, John Marin, Marsden Hartley, Georgia O'Keeffe, Paul Strand, and himself. Other artists, such as Demuth and Lachaise, made guest appearances in his galleries, and they, as has been seen, were assisted by Juliana. But the inner circle, which was made up of the first six, did not participate at all in the Club or Studio.

Between Juliana and the Whitney enterprises and Stieglitz and his galleries existed a state of polite but many-stranded antagonism. Because it was polite, much of the friction must be pieced together by inference, but a convincing picture of hostilities can be delineated. Because of the absence of the Stieglitz group from the Club's galleries, critics have often branded the Club as anti-modernist. It was not antimodernist (if it had been, many of the best shows of 1923, 1924, and 1925 would never have occurred and Marius de Zayas would not have been hired), but anti-Stieglitz. There is a distinction, although most keepers of the Stieglitz flame do not concede it.

The quarrel between Juliana and Stieglitz was first and foremost determined by their fundamental disagreement as to how American art might best be served and encouraged. Juliana and Gertrude, deriving their policies from Henri, Sloan, and the Independents, believed in helping as many as possible, in tolerating the chaff to obtain the precious grain of wheat, and leaving it to history to sort things out. Henri himself volunteered his blessing for what the two women had achieved over the last decade. He wrote in his diary on January 25, 1926, "Met Mrs. Force [at a reception], told her that while I did not meet them very much I had a great love for her and her boss (Mrs. Whitney) for all the splendid things they did for the younger artists, and I might have added for the way they do it—for much is done without anyone knowing that it is being done." To use a metaphor from Virginia Woolf, Juliana viewed the Club and Studio exhibitions not as

finished compositions, but as preliminary studies and notebooks preparing the ground for the future. "Time," wrote Woolf about the business of judging contemporaries, "like a good schoolmaster, will take them in his hands, point to their blots and erasions, and tear them across; but he will not throw them into the waste-paper basket. He will keep them because other students will find them very useful." Stieglitz, however, took a more limited and elitist line. He chose six or seven individuals he believed (correctly, for time has borne him out) had staying power, presented them and talked about them as Old Masters comparable to the greatest artists, and promoted them to the exclusion of everyone else. A fastidious artist himself and blessed with a remarkable eye, Stieglitz could sustain an intensity of focus and develop one idea in all its permutations no matter where it led or how long it took (as in his suite of photographs of Georgia O'Keeffe), whereas Juliana was best at seeing broadly and quickly rather than searchingly.

Juliana showed a wide variety of art and made no bones about it. The Whitney was capable of being avant-garde at one exhibition, traditional at the next, and unclassifiable the time after. There was no special drive to be consistently among the vanguard: The aim was to be pro-artist, regardless of styles or schools. Stieglitz was adamantly modernist, concerned only with Americans who had absorbed the implications of revolutionary European painting. The Whitney *presented* points of view; Stieglitz *advocated* them. And Stieglitz despised such heterogeneity: His artists had to share his ideology. In his *Alfred Stieglitz Talking*, the photographer's acolyte Herbert Seligmann recorded that Stieglitz "had been told during the day [February 13, 1927] that the Whitney Studio Club was finally admitting that he had accomplished great things for America and for the world. 'They used to complain because I focussed on one or two individuals. Do they think I could have done what I've done by concentrating on a hundred and ten million Americans?' " (In the reams of his letters and remarks attributed to him, Stieglitz, who could not share attention, allowed no parallel comment, not even a grudging or qualified admission, that perhaps Gertrude Whitney had done something worthy after all.)

Financial need was another criterion to which Juliana responded; Stieglitz generously supported his artists with gifts and loans, but sentimental considerations like need weren't primary if he took on an artist. Juliana would have been loath to sponsor Stieglitz's artists precisely because they had a prestigious gallery and an industrious dealer. The Club was supposed to act as a stepping-stone for artists trying to gain recognition from critics and dealers, and the one-man shows were principally reserved for those who did not have other outlets for their work. In the 1920s Marin and O'Keeffe had already become well-known through Stieglitz's efforts and comfortably off from the high prices he got for their pictures.

Along with the basic contrasts in how they chose to operate, the personal element figured strongly in keeping Juliana apart from Stieglitz and his artists. Juliana liked to meet and get to know the artists she helped. As Forbes observed, "The life of the artist and the production of the artist were not separate entities to [her] any more than they were to me." Commonly, Juliana would hear about

an artist's problem and invite him to come see her, or an artist would be recommended or make a friendly overture to the Club. The personal contact somehow had to be made, and those who remained uncommunicative or aloof were generally not smiled upon.

Emotional and geographic distance effectively prohibited most of the Stieglitz stable from being shown at the Club: Marin divided his time between New Jersey and Maine, Hartley was traveling abroad or in the Southwest during most of the 1920s, Dove was living in eastern Long Island, and O'Keeffe was not only Stieglitz's wife but temperamentally indisposed to want to join another coterie. The one she was in tried her patience and independence too often. (Stieglitz and Strand were photographers, and since the Club wasn't interested in photography, they were automatically disqualified as exhibitors.) Juliana did get to know Sheeler, Demuth, and Lachaise, which led to Whitney patronage, but it was precisely their openness to other acquaintances that barred those artists from Stieglitz's ultimate favor.

It seemed that if an artist "belonged" to Stieglitz, he could not be too friendly with Juliana. De Zayas, for example, did not work for Juliana until after he and Stieglitz were estranged, and the Whitney did not aid Hartley until after he drifted away from Stieglitz's suzerainty. The only one who managed to oscillate between them without calamity was Demuth, probably because Juliana was already an established client and confidante of Robert Locher, his lover.

Juliana was autocratic herself and could act like a queen at her court, but she drew the line at circumscribing an artist's network of useful friendships. Her possessiveness never extended to controlling a career. Stieglitz demanded that he be the omnipresent and exclusive intermediary in his artists' lives, and he worked to keep them isolated from competing influences. At his most egregious, his manipulations prevented Dove from meeting Duncan Phillips, his unswerving patron and founder of the Phillips Collection, more than once. If Stieglitz did not scruple—and he did not—to call Dove's rescuer, the eminently decent and sensitive Phillips, an "enemy" in order to maintain his hold, then one can begin to imagine what he said about Juliana, Gertrude, and the Whitney Studio Club to keep his artists from casting a curious eye in that direction.

A key player in this drama of enmities and egos was Forbes, who no doubt reinforced Juliana's inclination to dislike Stieglitz and contributed to Stieglitz's belligerent perception of Juliana. Watson had known Stieglitz since his early days as an art critic, when he worked for the *Post* and reviewed shows at 291. These visits became a trial, because whenever Stieglitz spotted Forbes, he would nab him and pour forth long-winded testimony about the art on view. The orations threatened to drive Forbes from the gallery until he hit on the idea of checking with the elevator boy to find out if Stieglitz had gone to lunch. If the answer was yes, Forbes went into the show and made up his mind in peace. Stieglitz was unaware of this ruse for several years, and it was, characteristically, the pugnacious critic himself who revealed it. The two happened to meet in the studio of Paul Burlin. Wrote Forbes, "Stieglitz immediately asked me why I wrote longer reviews about Marin when his work was exhibited by the Daniel

Gallery [in 1917–1918] . . . than I did when it was exhibited in his galleries. I told him without a noticeable degree of politeness that Mr. Daniel did not talk about his exhibitions. That remark closed our conversation."

Forbes often went out of his way to fight with someone, and Stieglitz was an irresistible opponent because of his insistent sermonizing and exquisite sense of personal grievance. Relations between the two soured once and for all after Forbes became art critic for the *World* and took some potshots at him. One such aside ran, "He does not sit modestly aside and allow the works of the artists whom he has sponsored to speak quietly to the beholder. An accompaniment of words is always to be heard, with the final result that long ago Mr. Stieglitz became such an accomplished impresario that all of his particular pets in the art world are now well known, even disproportionately well known." Stieglitz was quick to lash other people with his pen, but he did not like feeling the sting himself. Furthermore, he was dissatisfied with anything less than a rapturous review. Once Forbes, who felt that Marin had a pure talent but not a grand one, did not acclaim him ardently enough. Because his appreciation was qualified, he heard about it from Stieglitz. For Stieglitz to be happy, Forbes learned, "One must place Marin with the great. He must become the best of all watercolor painters, the most imaginative of artists." Then there was the matter of O'Keeffe, whom Stieglitz would praise maunderingly to Watson when he appeared at the gallery. O'Keeffe became so embarrassed by these adulatory monologues that she told Forbes "that her family had nicknamed Stieglitz 'Caw Caw' because he crowed so much."

To Stieglitz, anyone who associated with Forbes became tainted and risked ostracism from his clique. In 1922 Charles Sheeler was close to Stieglitz and Strand; in 1923 he was no longer intimate with them, and letters between Stieglitz, Sheeler, and Paul and Rebecca Strand suggest that Sheeler's growing friendship with Forbes—considered tantamount to betrayal—helped cause the breach. Sheeler, who first transgressed by working for the now-shunned de Zayas but evidently had been forgiven, then dared to work for Watson and *The Arts* as a photographer and writer. Sheeler's first article was about Stieglitz's photography, and although the essay was full of praise, he did venture a reservation about the master's continued use of platinum prints. This was too much for Stieglitz—Sheeler had lapsed again, and there was no choice but to cast him out as a heretic. Perhaps an underlying reason why Juliana welcomed Sheeler so effusively into the Whitney fold was to show Stieglitz what she thought of his schoolboy expulsions.

Stieglitz's hostility to Forbes and his coworkers remained constant throughout the 1920s. Inslee Hopper, who was hired by Watson at the end of the decade, remembered, "I went to a show at Stieglitz's, and introduced myself as covering the show for *The Arts*, for Forbes Watson. I got a reception which would have chilled a polar bear. I went back to Forbes and said, 'What is this? He doesn't seem to be too friendly toward us.' Forbes said, 'It's not you. He and I are not exactly pals. We don't see eye to eye about a lot of things.' " Lloyd Goodrich, who worked for *The Arts* and Forbes before going on to the Whitney and Juliana, inherited a double legacy of Stieglitz testiness that dogged him in his encounters

with the man. His visits to the gallery were dominated by cranky harangues, and when he brought in his sister, the playwright and screenwriter Frances Hackett, to buy a Marin, Stieglitz refused to sell her one because she was unworthy of it.

It was this high-handedness that really drove Forbes mad. Stieglitz protested that he wasn't an art dealer or businessman of any kind, as if selling art were on a par with committing a crime or incubating a deadly disease. Whereas Juliana believed that, in the pantheon of art, there were many beings worthy of worship, Stieglitz took the position, said Forbes, "that he is the one and only Pope in the religion of art. He has given a lifetime to this work of establishing an uncommercial status in a purely commercial venture."

For someone who inveighed loudly against wealth, rich people, and commerce, Stieglitz's own statements and correspondence harp incessantly on money and business matters. This financial acumen was shrewdly couched in lofty rhetoric, which Forbes, Juliana, and Duncan Phillips saw through and relished puncturing. Others, like Herbert Seligmann, swallowed uncritically whatever Stieglitz said and published it. This vignette from Seligmann is typical of the Intimate Gallery's brand of idealism. "The first days of February [1927] recorded a victory for Stieglitz. A flower painting by O'Keeffe sold for three thousand dollars and another painting for six thousand. It was not the money, as Stieglitz wrote in a letter, but the togetherness of creative spirits, the taking root of something he had been working for, for 37 years."

Another evil Stieglitz was vociferously on record against was publicity—unless he desired it, originated it, or controlled it. He wrote to Dove in 1925 about an exhibition, "I must see to it that the press gets to see nothing—that is the professional press—the Henry McBrides and the Luther Careys* and all the rest of that unspeakable crowd." Yet to the unspeakable McBride, an avid supporter of 291 and the Intimate Gallery, Stieglitz was heartiness itself. As a result, whenever he wished to establish public credit for something he had done, he need only write to McBride and his letter would be published in the *Sun*.

If he wanted to broadcast his own propaganda and price levels, Stieglitz could be as shameless as the merchants he snubbed so contemptuously, thrusting aside privacy and discretion for publicity and money while employing McBride as a conduit. In March 1927, against the wishes of Duncan Phillips, Stieglitz leaked the sensational (and distorted) news that Phillips bought a Marin for $6,000, which was then published in *The Dial* and *The New Yorker*. Phillips, who had grounds to ask, "Who's commercial now?" wrote angrily to Forbes:

> Field Marshal Stieglitz maneuvered negotiations so that I paid his record price for the Marin I liked best, receiving as compensation two others of the very finest of Marin's 1925 vintage *as gifts*. Thus I secured for $6000 three of the best Marins in existence at an average of $2000 each. No doubt the misleading statement that I bought a single Marin for $6000 helped the cause of modern art in general and Marin in particular. I must say however that I would have been unable to consider any one Marin this year, no matter how wonderful, for such a price, and it was only

* Elisabeth Luther Cary, conservative critic of the *Times*.

the opportunity to get three A-1 watercolors by this great artist at a price below their value which tempted me. . . . And I can assure you that I buy Marins not because of Stieglitz but in spite of him, though it is probable that people are saying he has exercised on me his hypnotic powers. . . .

Four months before, Stieglitz had written to Phillips, "I am a bit amused that you class me among the dealers! I have to bear it—I often wish I could be a dealer—but dealing in human souls is just a bit beyond—or short—of my make up."

What Juliana and Forbes found most abhorrent about Stieglitz's protestations of having nothing to do with the marketplace or materialism was his game playing in regard to prices and selling. He liked creating an artificial scarcity, and sometimes it was done at the artist's expense. Stieglitz's habit of refusing to sell if he decided the buyer was ignoble meant that the artist went without. To Juliana, who would go to any lengths to relieve an artist's suffering, this practice was outrageous. Stieglitz, who was never without a private income, wrote scornfully to Dove, "Hartley wants admiration—and cash!" At that time Hartley was deeply depressed and anxious about how he would support himself.

As far as Juliana was concerned, Stieglitz and his artists were more trouble than they were worth. She was not going to court Stieglitz, and Stieglitz was not going to approach her, so each ignored the other. This was perfectly easy to do, as Stieglitz restricted himself to seven Americans and Juliana to the other "hundred and ten million." Time has proved Stieglitz right in his choice, but it has also validated Juliana's. After all, in the mid-1920s the Museum of Modern Art had not been born, the Metropolitan Museum of Art was a closed brotherhood, the National Academy of Design was full of fussbudgets and reactionaries, and the government gave no help to living artists. For the young and unpedigreed, Juliana and the Whitney were their faint gleam of hope, and Juliana and the Whitney were what counted. As Reuben Nakian said of his support from Gertrude and Juliana, "It was way before . . . anything else. They sparked art."

Juliana's failing in passing over the art Stieglitz stood for lay in her inability to set aside personalities for aesthetic judgments. Doing so would have been tremendously galling, of course, and utterly foreign to her makeup. As long as the Club and the Studio were private agencies, Juliana could elect to avoid Stieglitz. But once the Whitney was to become a museum with a public agenda and public accountability, Juliana was not so free. She had to bow to the imperative of getting Hartley, Marin, and O'Keeffe represented in the collection. It became necessary to deal with Stieglitz on his terms. Stieglitz knew this and would make her pay.

The question of personal sympathies versus aesthetic judgments was one that shadowed the Club and would later haunt the museum. Sentiment was their pride and their albatross. A major purpose of the Club was to solve artists' problems, and in writing about Juliana's leadership, Sloan recalled that she

"once said that she did not judge pictures, she judged people; for just this reason she was the right person for her job at that time." For good and for bad, the Whitney and Juliana were known for their human touch. Certainly the artists were grateful, whether or not they were direct beneficiaries, because they were moved by the beauty of the gesture. Aesthetic judgments tended to be suspended when Juliana could not contain her concern about an artist in trouble. Sometimes the destitute or discouraged person was of the caliber of a Flannagan or a Varèse, and sometimes he was not. Once her heart went out to an off-and-on painter who was so despondent about his progress that he said he was pulling out of the Club's upcoming show of his work. Brook and one of the artist's coexhibitors went round to his studio to persuade him otherwise, but the man was immovable. Brook met with Juliana, and they hashed and rehashed the problem from all possible angles. They were about to give up, Brook wrote,

> when Mrs. Force suddenly said, "Try him again, Alex; make him show. I'd rather him sorry he had an exhibition than sorry he hadn't. He may never have another chance. If he paints better in the future it will have been worthwhile; if he gets worse he will, at least, have shown at his peak. See to it that he is supplied with frames if he needs them. Give him whatever help is necessary; do whatever you can."
>
> Whether it was Mrs. Force's power behind my persuasion or the reluctant artist's weakened resistance I do not know, but exhibit he did and I am sorry to say his only reward was a few small, gentle words of kindness from the critics to brighten his life. What course was right would be hard to tell, but I like to think that Mrs. Force's decision, aside from the charitable impulse, was sensible and just.

These discrete demonstrations of caring were not ill-advised, and few would be so hard-hearted as to wish that Juliana had curtailed her bounty. But when personal sympathy and companionability swelled into a favoritism and privileged status that began to dominate exhibitions and alter the balance of the Club, then Juliana's attachments were open to question and challenge. The omission of the Stieglitz circle was compounded by overfriendliness to another group. Starting in the mid-1920s, the Whitney Studio Club became excessively involved with, indeed mired in, the art colony at Woodstock.

Woodstock, New York, a small town in the Catskills and an easy drive from New York City, began its life as an artists' retreat in 1902, when two idealists founded a community for painters and artisans who would attempt to live by the social and aesthetic ideas propounded by Ruskin and Morris. The colony was given a great boost four years later, when the Art Students League opened a summer school there. Because of its rural setting and cheapness—the founders built primitive cottages for artists, who were allowed to live there free or for a nominal sum—the area began attracting a number of vigorous artists, including Dasburg and Cramer. Woodstock made a giant leap forward in terms of reputation and visibility when George Bellows and Eugene Speicher, then kingpins on the exhibitions circuit, bought summer houses in the late teens. Henri taught at the League during the summer of 1921, and the place was made. There were now enough artists in residence to split into factions and have raging arguments about their heroes. Dasburg, Henry Lee McFee, and their friends would sit up

all night parsing Cézanne, and Arnold Blanch once punched Carl Walters in the jaw over significant form.

By then Woodstock had also developed a distinct reputation for unconventionality, and it was one that many bohemian types did their best to nurse. Playing the free spirit and looking flamboyant were good for business. The men wore subversive Russian blouses, and the women often traipsed around in long, flowing dresses. Tourists and locals were easily titillated by the sight of rusticating artists.

With this atmosphere and the presence of people like Speicher, who was looked up to as the great master painter and one of the most important artists of his time, Woodstock thought of itself as a nationally significant school of landscape painting. Mythmaking was already rampant, and in 1923 a local writer actually said, "To the map where we find Sèvres, Barbizon, Bayreuth and Kelmscott [is] now to be added—Woodstock." In line with fancying themselves quite the Barbizon on the Hudson, Woodstockers were tightly knit and self-congratulatory. They mentally appropriated any prize or honor an individual artist received for the group as a whole; one person's success accrued to the greater glory of Woodstock. Gossip, transmitted in the form of drop-in visits and letters to neighbors who were out of town at the moment, was a thriving leisure pursuit, and dispatches relaying accounts of the latest public acclaim usually closed with the smug exclamation, "Pretty good for Woodstock!" This musketeering attitude fostered a team spirit necessary for mutual survival in pursuing an uncertain livelihood, but it also sanctioned a kind of slickness. Artists grew canny in the marketing of their pictures, and one of the main objects of their self-advertising was Juliana.

Juliana first started going for weekends at Woodstock in the early 1920s. She had been close to Speicher for some years and had gotten friendly with another Woodstock painter named Charles Rosen. Alexander Brook spent several summers in Woodstock, so naturally he was very partial to it. After he started working at the Club in December of 1923, he must have introduced many of his cronies to Juliana. By then, more than 100 artists lived in the Woodstock area at least part of the year, and Juliana knew and showed most of them at the Club. Many of the artists in the colony had merit or promise, and it would have been obtuse and mistaken to ignore them all. However, a Woodstock address did seem to ensure special treatment.

Woodstock was bliss for Juliana. Since she was one of the rare breed who did buy pictures, her visits there resembled an imperial processional. She would stay with the Speichers or Dorothy Varian, and as the powerful Woodstock grapevine passed along the news of her coming, the invitations would pour in. "In those days," recalled the sculptor Hannah Small,

> we had a wonderful telegraph operator and postmistress who took a personal interest in all the artists. As soon as she knew Mrs. Force was coming, she'd get into her Model T and drive madly through town, waving the telegram and blowing her horn. As we ran outside, she would yell, "Mrs. Force is IMMINENT!" That would be the signal to bring out our work. We were all very poor, and the ones who grabbed her first often got the best of it.

It was inevitable that the hustlers would play up to her. Arnold Blanch often chauffeured Juliana from studio to studio when she came to town, and he saw her in action. "She bought spontaneously," he reminisced. "She would see a painting and she'd say, 'I'll buy it.' Quick. She never said, 'I'll think it over.' She never haggled with the price. You told her the price and she paid for it." Juliana's appearance on the horizon was like the second coming to most of the artists, but with so much hope riding on that visit, it is easy to see why she was also regarded with apprehension. It was in Woodstock that "Mrs. Force" was secretly permuted to "Mrs. Fierce."

Arnold Blanch and his wife, Lucile, did very well by their association. Lucile Blanch admitted that in their youth she and her husband were extremely ambitious and that they courted Juliana, who responded by giving Lucile her own show and sending both of them to Paris. "She took to us right away. We were in all the early exhibitions, and those breaks began to add up," Lucile Blanch said. "We went to the parties, too. We were poor, and it was always nice to go to places where there were drinks. Juliana would come to Woodstock because there was a large artist population that she liked. She was interested in our opinions and differences of opinion, and you could never get away with hedging with her. She would say, 'Come on, tell me what *you* think,' and she would quicken bodily when the discussion heated up. She allied herself with our generation, and we bloomed because of her and her connection with Mrs. Whitney. Otherwise who knows what our destinies may have been."

The Blanches and their peers emerged as the Club's new stars. Speaking about Woodstock in the middle and late twenties, the sculptor Eugenie Gershoy said, "Mrs. Force *made* that whole generation of artists. We couldn't have been what we were without her or Mrs. Whitney." In an essay tracing the colony's history, Karal Ann Marling confirmed Gershoy's assertion. "While Woodstock was not the creation of the Whitney organization," she wrote, "the national prestige of Woodstock modernism in the decade just prior to the Depression rested heavily on Mrs. Force's enthusiastic support." The top-heaviness of Woodstock on the Whitney exhibition roster and in the permanent collection was so pronounced that in a 1953 speech Ad Reinhardt could run them together as one: "Very familiar to everyone over forty, is the image inherited from the twenties, the original Whitney artist and old-time Woodstock post-impressionist, the Ash Can Armory Regionalist who finally got the *Ladies' Home Journal* cover job, the crackerbarrel sophisticate who also designs silk handkerchiefs, the real 'professional.' " Despite the cumulative twists and catch-all categorizations of Reinhardt's gibe, his audience would have understood every word of it. He was ridiculing what Juliana should have reckoned with: Her attachment to Woodstock, although not very well-considered, was her prerogative when she directed the Club. But when she was at the helm of a museum, it would not do.

CHAPTER SEVEN

THE TOP
OF THE
VOLCANO

❧ (1926–1929) ❧

D ESPITE the creeping domination of Woodstock over the Club's exhibition program, independent artists and progressive art ventures were supported by the Whitney largesse. With a membership surging beyond 300, the Club could not help but be as open-ended as it was sheltering, and its director's knowledge and sense of exploration helped offset the Woodstock circle's prominence. Emerson's adage that an institution is but a lengthened shadow of a man still applied to the Club. Juliana continued to transmute whatever she touched into something peculiarly her own: Eighth Street remained lighthearted, loose-jointed, unwearied, and unsystematic, a stimulating place where persiflage and sympathy were served up in charmingly upholstered interiors, and obstacles could be removed by a well-placed telephone call or letter of introduction.

The late-1920s were also a time of peak closeness between Gertrude and Juliana. Commissions for monumental public sculpture were heaped on Gertrude, and she relied on Juliana to manage them. The two women's already strong working relationship was tested repeatedly and found invulnerable to artistic, political, and social maelstroms. Their teamwork was the foundation of a new level of endeavor, one sturdy enough to support a permanent home for American art.

The year 1926 started bleakly for Juliana, who was in bed with bronchial pneumonia for six weeks. The Whitney Studio was largely dormant, and most of the exhibitions took place at the Club. However, Jan Matulka, Harry Hering, Dorothy Varian, Glenn O. Coleman, Henri Burkhard, Mabel Dwight, and

Isabel Bishop did get their own shows, and the spring annual, with Juliana well again, exuded its usual carefree air. Bryson Burroughs dropped by the opening of the members' annual and wrote to his son-in-law, Reginald Marsh, that the display was "vigorous, fresh, and mighty little flub dub. Everything is—most everything is, I shd. say—straightforward and keen and good-humored. . . . The place was crowded—everybody talking and laughing as they should at such an exhibition, not like the funeral solemnity—The viewing-of-the-corpse-expression of the Academy visitors."

As Burroughs implied, artists packed these openings and hoped to be spirited away to Juliana's apartment afterward for further entertainment. Louis Bouché remembered the openings as great events.

> These parties . . . became more and more festive, and eventually all the intelligentsia flocked to them. You could hardly move. At some time during the evening, Mrs. Force having done her duty nobly would disappear from the scene and certain artists would be quietly informed that they were invited to her apartment. [The custom became known as "tapping" among the initiated.] They were taken up there by a secretary. This of course was a signal honor. . . .
>
> Almost invariably Alex Brook and his wife Peggy Bacon and Marian [Mrs. Bouché] and I were invited. Once, we four were overlooked, so we sneaked up and stuck a note under the door which read, "What's the matter with us, Have we got leprosy?" Whereat, the door was opened with laughter and greetings.

One of Juliana's favorite anecdotes about these big, noisy artists' parties she gave, however, hinged on a different reaction. At one such gathering, she came in a little late, just in time to find Edward Hopper going out the door. "Leaving so soon, Mr. Hopper?" Juliana inquired. "Yes," rumbled the deep, solemn voice. "No life there."

Juliana's summer revolved around the dedication of Gertrude's memorial to the American Expeditionary Forces, rising out of the harbor of Saint-Nazaire, France. The ceremonies were set for June 26, 1926, nine years to the day after American soldiers first landed there under the command of Gen. John J. Pershing. Juliana renewed her passport, adding some inches to her height (a fictitious 5 feet 6 inches) and subtracting both four and six years off her age. With her usual disdain for details, she stated under oath that she was forty-three years old, while in the same application giving her year of birth as 1881, which would have made her forty-five. In truth she was forty-nine.

As would happen each time she saw one of Gertrude's public sculptures through from germination to completion, hard and frustrating work was in store for Juliana, who had to convince, placate, or circumvent committees and officials as conditions required. For the Saint-Nazaire statue to proceed, authorizations for the site and design had to be obtained from the American Battle Monuments Commission and the French government. President Coolidge and General Pershing, the head of the Battle Monuments Commission as well as the leader of the American Expeditionary Forces, had to give their personal approval to enable the Saint-Nazaire Association, the veterans' body responsible for sponsoring the memorial, to raise enough money. This web of agencies and permissions meant endless letter writing and cabling and cross-cabling for all parties

concerned, with Juliana coordinating communications and movements between New York, Washington, and Paris.

Unfortunately for Gertrude, the Saint-Nazaire Association was ignorant of the need for approval from the National Commission of Fine Arts, a bureau within the U.S. Department of Interior. Once the Battle Monuments Commission learned that the fine arts commission had not been consulted, it withdrew authorization because it could not act without the prior vote of the federal body. In August of 1925, all proceedings came to a dead halt, from the telephones and typewriters in Washington to the construction of the pedestal at Saint-Nazaire, as each agency canceled its approval. By then Gertrude had already been working on the memorial an entire year. The setback put Juliana and Gertrude on tenterhooks, because each day's delay from the authorities meant postponing the completion of the memorial: No one seemed to understand that work in the harbor was perilously dependent on weather conditions.

Even more ominously, the delay gave fine arts commission officials in Washington, who were already testy about being overlooked, the chance to discover that they did not *like* the statue. Washington started asking Gertrude for significant changes in the design; since she declined to make them, some members assumed that her refusal would cause the project to wither quietly away.

The dissatisfied pooh-bahs had a point. Aesthetically the Saint-Nazaire memorial was atrocious. The underlying concept and appearance were feeble, especially when compared to the bluff vigor of *Buffalo Bill*, its immediate predecessor. From the plain and the actual, Gertrude reverted to idealizing symbolism. She based the new work on the same tired cruciform design she had adopted in 1914 for the *Titanic* memorial. As the subscription brochures distributed to lure contributions put it, the statue depicted an American doughboy, in war kit, "with a crusader's sword in his hand, borne on the back of a great eagle." The doughboy and eagle were to stand on a forty-foot shaft of natural rock about 100 yards from the shore. It would be visible from all ships entering or leaving the harbor and tower above the town.

By November of 1925, the voting had gone in Gertrude's favor. Too much publicity about the monument had accrued for anyone to want to take responsibility for canceling it. General Hersey pulled every string he could in the military for the sculpture, and Juliana and Gertrude pressed their advantage with a letter to General Pershing, informing him of their refusal to make changes or otherwise yield. On December 11, 1925, the contingent approvals came through, and from then on the haggling was confined to the wording of the inscription on the tablet. However, in spite of the four-month hiatus, no extension of the deadline was given. Juliana's liaison in Paris was the dependable and well-connected Andrew O'Connor. In charge of supervising the physical synthesis, enlargement, and casting of the sculpture and the readying of the site, he dealt smoothly with French engineers and expended considerable effort and guile in speeding papers through the right offices.

In counterpoint to the quality of the monument were the impressive rites celebrating it. On June 5, Gertrude, Alice Vanderbilt, Flora Whitney, and Juliana sailed for France. Aboard ship their fellow passengers included the play-

wright Charles MacArthur and *New Yorker* wit Alexander Woollcott. To be her guests on land, Gertrude invited a band of loyal artist-friends to the ceremonies. On June 25, Gertrude, Juliana, Forbes, O'Connor, du Bois, Davidson, the American ambassador to France, General Pershing in full regalia, and about thirty other dignitaries rode a special train from Paris to Saint-Nazaire, but Harry Whitney stayed home and skipped it all. Two of his horses were racing on June 26, and he didn't want to miss a double chance at the winner's circle.

At Saint-Nazaire, over 30,000 people took part in the ceremonies. All the houses and public buildings were festooned with entwined French and American flags, and the spectators alighted to a parade of American and French militiamen, followed by a twenty-one-gun salute as ships from the two nations entered the harbor and ran up their colors. The crowd sang "The Marseillaise," and as Gertrude's monument was unveiled, 100 carrier pigeons bearing small French and American flags were released from their cages and soared out to sea. Aerial bombs bursting into red, white, and blue paper streamers spun through the air. Gertrude was made a Chevalier of the Legion of Honor by the Minister of the Marine, and du Bois recorded her decoration in some droll sketches. Concerts filled the afternoon, and fireworks lighted up the night. (The townspeople were content with the monument, and its symbolic value was considered potent enough for the Nazis to dynamite it in 1941.)

In late September Juliana was arranging the fall season. She offered Reuben Nakian and Bob Chanler solo shows, and in early November eight pieces of Nakian's sculpture were surrounded by Chanler's satiric portraits of Richard Le Gallienne, Jane Heap, Iris Tree, Raoul Hague, Louise Hellstrom, and Joseph Stella. While the exhibition was on, Juliana and Nakian discovered that they had a great passion for Fragonard in common. As a joking homage to Fragonard and the Rococo, Nakian modeled Juliana a terra-cotta sculpture of a child playing with a spaniel that he copied from a Fragonard drawing, the entire sculpture just 10 ½ inches long. When the museum collection was established, Juliana put the piece, entitled *The Lap Dog*, into it, along with the drawings Nakian had given her earlier and a carving of a seal she bought in 1930. Nakian completed the circle in 1963 when he donated *Pastorale*, a terra-cotta of 1950, to the Whitney in Juliana's memory.

In November of 1926, as a further incentive to support artists seen at the Club, a shop opened on the premises for the sale of graphic works. The procedure, as would be expected, was casual, and no commissions were taken. Artists left their portfolios of watercolors, drawings, and prints on wide shelves ringing the room. Visitors browsed through the selections themselves and paid Brook. One of the early customers was Joseph Cornell, who bought a work by Peggy Bacon and later said that the shop and the Club were part of his itinerary during his "golden age of gallery trotting." The prices were low—between $5 and $25 was the norm—and most of the artists, who were not exactly brisk sellers in the first place, had no qualms about consigning their art on a long-term basis. Some saw the shop as a spot for free storage as well as potential sales. It is safe to say that quite a few unretrieved works were swept into the Whitney-Force collections and tumbled into the museum in that way.

The inauguration of a shop for prints and drawings may have spurred Juliana to help artists create more of them. In 1927 she hired the master printer George Miller to demonstrate lithography at the Club. Miller installed his press and handed out zinc plates. Louis Bouché, Edmund Duffy, Niles Spencer, and Yasuo Kuniyoshi drew on theirs, and Miller pulled proofs of the images on the spot. A party followed, of course, and afterward they all exchanged prints. To draw customers into the shop, Juliana planted more advertisements in *The Arts*. One, headlined "THE BARREN PERIOD," explained, in essence, the Club's reason for being and its distrust of art bought or exhibited for prestige.

> Did you ever notice how much more often the names of artists come up in conversation than the character of a given picture or given piece of sculpture? . . .
>
> The greatest artist that ever lived has had his failures. The artist of whom you have never heard has made his masterpieces. It is not the name, it is the work itself that counts. . . .
>
> There is a barren period in every artist's career. It is the period when the dealers, the directors and the exhibition managers know his name well enough to invite his paintings and sculptures everywhere while the public does not know his name well enough to buy his work.
>
> The artists need more people brave enough to purchase what they like for themselves and careless enough of whether their neighbors will praise them for the purchase. They need to be spared the barren period.
>
> Buy the works of young artists, of well known artists, of famous artists. Do not buy the name.

That fall, while out driving with Juliana, Gertrude got so sick she had to be rushed to a hospital. After many tests and treatments the doctors learned she had phlebitis in both legs. Throughout November Juliana was worried about Gertrude and hurt by the Whitney family's solicitous determination to prevent Juliana from visiting her. Jo Davidson wrote to his wife, "I saw Mrs. Force yesterday. Mrs. Whitney is not well at all & has not been back to the Studio since I saw her there—and she did not look very well then—if she has not I wouldn't be surprised—and Mrs. Force says that she is quite ill—and under doctor's care. I don't know what's wrong with her. Mrs. Force doesn't say . . . and Mrs. Force is worried, because the family Mr. Whitney wouldn't let her come near her. So she hasn't seen her for a while—Nobody knows this. So say nothing about it." Davidson was as loyal as Juliana to Gertrude, and after he left New York, they exchanged anxious telegrams about Gertrude's health; with palpable relief she wired him on November 18: SAW GERTRUDE FOR FIRST TIME AND DELIGHTED TO REPORT REAL PROGRESS. Two weeks later, Juliana was allowed to visit her in the country.

The Club's most important exhibition of 1926 took place in December: a retrospective of paintings and watercolors by Stuart Davis, consisting of at least thirty works. Davis guessed that his friend Joseph Pollet, a Woodstock painter Juliana liked, suggested it, as she had given Pollet a top-floor studio at 14 West Eighth Street, and Davis was storing many of his canvases there. Juliana helped Davis out "handsomely," for the show, he said, "came at a lucky time for me.

I was dead broke and had no place to work. I lived in 8 × 11 foot room on 7th Avenue near 14th Street."

The show began with works from 1911 (street scenes done under the influence of Henri) and went to 1926. Once again the incisive cigarette pictures were shown—*Lucky Strike, Bull Durham, Sweet Caporal,** and *Cigarette Papers.*† Several paintings registering an overtly Picassoid influence (possibly *ITLKSEZ*‡ and some abstractions and still lifes from 1922) as well as canvases from the artist's 1923 trip to New Mexico, and a small group of more recent works from 1924 to 1926 rounded out the exhibition. Except for Henry McBride, who applauded the boldness, humor, and "genuine talent for painting" displayed, the critics disliked the diversity of Davis's output and pounced on it as a sign of instability. Even Forbes simplistically termed the pictures "laboratory work." Juliana, however, was not disappointed with what she saw. The retrospective convinced her that Davis deserved extended help. "Right after my exhibition she gave me an allowance of $125 a month and that was what I lived on for a year," Davis recalled. During that time, he "nailed an electric fan, a rubber glove and an eggbeater to a table and used it as my exclusive subject matter." This was the artist's terse description of the genesis of his Eggbeater series, the epochal canvases that helped spur American abstract painting. Davis believed that the Eggbeaters, in which he leapt clearly and irrevocably into geometry, were his most pivotal works. "What led to it," he said, "was probably my working on a single still life for a year, not wandering about the streets. Gradually through this concentration I focused on the logical elements. They became the foremost interest and the immediate and accidental aspects of the still life took second place. . . . So you may say that everything I have done since has been based on that egg beater idea." A year's financial independence had given Davis the liberty—in the form of an almost hermetic period of confinement—he needed to distill his thoughts, lose track of the objects as subject matter, and investigate and reinvent them as purely plastic elements.

In late 1926 Juliana's appraisal of Stuart Davis was not a discovery, but a culmination of nearly ten years of observation and camaraderie. About the same time as Davis began getting his stipend, Alexander Brook spotted and launched a likely unknown. He found him not on his gumshoe rounds but a few yards from his office during the winter of 1926–1927, on a rainy afternoon in which friends, spectators, customers, and other signs of human company were scarce. He was dead bored, and the gallery seemed like a prison cell. When the buzzer sounded downstairs, he jumped to answer it.

At the head of the stairway Brook could see a slight, gray-clad figure.

He wore an overcoat that reached to his shoes, or so it seemed from where I was, those shoes' tips merely showing, the ends of his fingers scarcely protruding from his sleeves weighted down by heavy cuffs. When I descended to where he waited, he

---

* Now in the collection of the Baron Thyssen-Bornemisza.
† Now in the DeMenil Collection.
‡ Now in the Lane Foundation.

was five or six inches shorter than I, and I am only 5′ 9″. His answer to my greeting was almost inaudible, and the expression on the face he presented, with eyes that looked straight at me from under George Washington lids, was appealingly woebegone.

His name, I soon found out, was Raphael Soyer.

Soyer extracted sketches of his Lower East Side neighborhood from a portfolio, and Brook was overjoyed.

The gloomy little artist with his gloomy pictures suddenly turned the gloomy day into a sunny and hopeful one for me, because I knew that here I had found, or had been found by, a talent real and big enough to gain recognition as a potential force. I was in the honest and happy position of having a new friend whose work I would be able to ballyhoo wholeheartedly. At the very least, I thought, what little I could do might make him smile once or maybe even twice more.

When Brook showed Juliana Soyer's drawings, she bought one and asked to see the paintings. A week later Soyer brought them by, and Juliana made another purchase. Then Brook independently wrote to an Iowa collector he knew and recommended that she buy a Soyer painting. Her check arrived in the next mail.

Soyer himself realized the significance of being noticed by the Whitney staff. "Thereafter," he wrote in his *Diary of an Artist*, "whenever I finished a painting in my spare time (I still had to do other work for a living), I would take it to the Club. Mrs. Force . . . would emerge from her office . . . and ask, 'How much do you want for this, Mr. Soyer?' I would mumble, 'One hundred dollars,' and she would pay it. One day, for a very detailed painting upon which I had worked many weekends, I asked for $200 and she gave it to me without hesitation. I went home and told my mother that now I feel like a real artist, people were paying good money for my pictures."

Starting in 1927, Soyer was regularly included in the Club's exhibitions. McBride saw him for the first time in Portraits of Women by Men, a show organized by Brook in January of 1927 that featured established artists: Ault, Demuth, du Bois, Wood Gaylor, Kuhn, Kuniyoshi, Maurer, Pascin, Man Ray, and Sloan. In "an exhibition not to be missed," the critic's gaze fell upon "a newcomer, Raphael Soyer, [who] distinguishes himself with some excellent drawings." Soyer also attended the sketch classes and later remembered feeling very young alongside Hopper, Kuniyoshi, and Marsh, the other painters clustered around the model. By 1931 Juliana had purchased five paintings and a drawing from him.

The next exhibitions of 1927 shepherded by Brook were noteworthy. Leon Hartl had his second one-man show and sold fifteen pictures, netting him $638.90. The Club also presented another show of folk arts and crafts, displaying naive paintings, prints, pottery, rugs, and textiles from the collection of an early dealer in folk art, Isabel Carleton Wilde. Brook was an asset to the Whitney, and he would have been happy to remain there. He later said that he had the

best time of his life while working at the Club. The job had given his career a prodigious boost because he met most of the reigning critics and dealers, and his power to determine the content of exhibitions had made him one of the elite in that tight little world. Juliana enjoyed his company, was satisfied with his performance, and gave no indication of dispensing with him. But in the spring of 1927, Brook committed an irrevocable blunder. That May, when he resigned from the Club, Juliana did not dissuade him.

The trouble started at, of all places, the National Academy of Design. Within those sleepy precincts the members had awakened to the discovery of their fading influence. Watching the artists they once rejected emerge as painters of stature, it dawned on the less groggy academicians that there existed a large body of able younger artists who preferred to stay away from their group rather than join it. Juliana and Gertrude had played no small part in this change. McBride wrote of the Academy's self-acknowledged loss of prestige:

> It is impossible at this point to disentangle the success of the Whitney Studio Club from the situation. This club used to be composed of negligible fledglings, but fledglings have a way of growing up, and those of the Whitney Studio Club have at last become adult, and not only adult, but full of cleverness, independent ideas of gayety. It seems to be fun to belong to the Whitney Studio Club. So much so that now there is as much of a crush to belong to it as there used to be years ago at the academy. And the journalistic critics all agree that the exhibitions that occur in the rooms on West Eighth street are the most exhilarating and pleasing in town.

After the Academy digested this turn of events, some of the members wanted to try a compromise. As a "concession to modernism," the organization would ask some of the younger and more progressive artists to their spring annual without subjecting them to a jury. Schnakenberg, whose sedate style and trusted position in the Studio Club made him acceptable to both camps, was deputized as curator. His first invitations went to Allen Tucker and Sloan, the old fighters in the frontline for artistic independence. They refused to budge an inch toward accommodation with the Academy, as did Davis, who said he had nothing suitable to submit. But a host of others known to be affiliated with Whitney activities, including Brook, agreed to exhibit. Schnakenberg also wanted Gertrude in the show, but several artists loudly opposed it on the grounds that her work was too academic. One of those speaking against her was Brook, a Whitney employee on the Whitney payroll. Juliana wouldn't stand for insubordination toward herself, let alone ingratitude or disloyalty toward Gertrude. When she heard about what Brook had done, she became noticeably frosty toward him. The Academy's exhibition opened on March 21, 1927, and Brook, feeling Juliana's displeasure, told her that he wanted to spend all of his time painting once the Club's season was over and then resigned.

Brook went on to fame in the late 1920s and early 1930s, but after a few years in the limelight, he was spurned by critics and museums, and turned against the art world. But even at his most embittered, Brook did not speak ill of Juliana. In 1977, after admitting in an interview the cause of his departure from the Club, he used the words "delightful" and "marvelous" to describe his old boss. Juliana stood high in his estimation because

[s]he was interested in only one thing, and that was in the artist. She always impressed me by saying, "The artist is always right," or words to that effect. In other words, if there was any discussion or any controversy in anything, she always took the part of the artist. And of course I felt the same way. . . . I would never say anything but words of admiration for her.

The best part of his job, Brook emphasized, even surpassing the hilarity, the parties, and the intrigues, "despite hazards encountered and hurdles stumbled over, hurt feelings and misunderstandings, surfacing envy and uncontrolled tempers—was working with Juliana Force."

Brook's adoration of his old Whitney job was not unique. Secretaries, curators, and other museum employees hired by Juliana remember the dazzling color of their working lives. Whether they were logging grueling hours or joining in a celebration, they were not bored. This sense of excitement comes across so convincingly and in such sharply etched detail that the feeling rings with a truth beyond nostalgia.

Like Brook, William Robb, who was the business manager of *The Arts* in the 1920s and thus worked both for Forbes and for Juliana, said these were the most enjoyable years of his life. Since it rankled Forbes to have to report to Juliana on the financial status of *The Arts*, he began sending Robb to meet with her once a month to inspect the previous month's operating statement. *The Arts* always lost money, and because of all that red ink, Robb had expected these meetings to be solemn, cringing occasions. But Juliana's door was open to him, and she was ever the amiable hostess. At the beginning of one glorious month, Juliana inquired, "Mr. Robb, how much do you pay Mr. Watson and how much do you draw yourself?" When he told her that he got $40 a week and Forbes made $75, Juliana replied, "I am shocked. How can you possibly get along on that? Double both of your salaries immediately!"*

Ethel Renthal, a secretary who started with *The Arts* and then transferred to the Club, savored her years with Juliana. "No two days were alike, because Mrs. Force was always on the go. She wore hats indoors, as if she were about to dash away, and she never stayed in for the full day. When she was in, she would pace back and forth, or she would sit on her desk, which was a long table covered with books, papers, and folders, and dictate letters to me. She swung her legs, gesticulated with her hands, and smoked cigarettes from a long holder." Edith Goodrich cited Juliana's kindness to her children and her acts of thoughtfulness, saying, "The winter of the Public Works of Art Project [1933–1934], Lloyd worked night and day, and he was never home. He missed our tenth wedding anniversary, and I was sitting around by myself when an enormous bunch of flowers arrived. Mrs. Force had sent them for Lloyd."

But Juliana was at her best creating jobs for artists who needed an extra hand

---

*This incident most likely took place in 1927. In that year, according to Forbes Watson's records, subsidies to *The Arts* from Gertrude and Juliana jumped from the $4,000 contributed in 1926 to $12,600. In 1928 they gave a total of $9,100, but during that year several employees resigned or were fired. In 1929 the donation was back to $12,600.

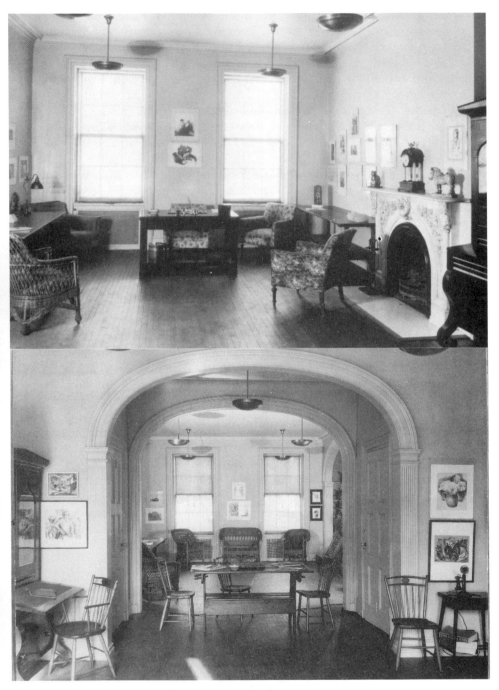

An office and sitting room in the Whitney Studio Club photographed by Charles Sheeler, ca. 1925–1926. Behind the desk, top: a work by du Bois; right: a ceramic horse by Carl Walters on the mantel and an alabaster cat by Duncan Ferguson on the long table.

to keep going. She offered subsistence in such a quick and happy tone that its recipients suffered no loss of dignity. Dorothy Varian had just quit a job that kept her too tired to paint. She progressed to another one requiring her only to supply bouquets to a local church every Sunday. "I realized that if I could get one more account like this, I would have enough to get along on. I would only have to devote two days a week to it, and the rest of the time I could just paint," Varian said. "I went to Juliana and said that I'd been getting paid for providing bouquets to a church. 'I wonder,' I said to her, 'if Mrs. Whitney might like a bouquet of flowers left once a week, every week. I would arrange them and bring them in a vase.' 'Oh,' Juliana said, 'it's a marvelous idea, and I want two for myself! I don't have time to go to a florist and neither does Mrs. Whitney.' So then I was set. With the church and those three orders, I didn't need to hold a job. Juliana just saw it immediately. I did that for a couple of years, and I had the time to paint."

It was Brook's bad luck to test Juliana's tolerance at a time when she was unusually sensitive to artists' being excluded and mistreated. For Juliana, 1927 would be the year of the embattled sculptor, one in which many hours would be logged defending two of them against assault. The artists, an implausible pair under ordinary circumstances, were Constantin Brancusi and Gertrude Whitney.

Brancusi's troubles began with some comments he made to the *New York Times* on October 2, 1926. Preparing for an exhibition, he was in the city on an extended visit, living gregariously and socializing in the Brevoort. In the interview, he ventured the opinion that many of the big civic monuments (those plum commissions that usually went to members of the Academy and its ideological twin, the National Sculpture Society) were "ridiculous." The true sculptural works of New York, he maintained, were its tall buildings, which communicated "the sensation of a great new poetic art." He also added, "I have found the Grand Central Terminal one of the most beautiful specimens of modern architecture. The varying decorations give me as much pleasure as if I had done them myself, although some of them remind me of a peasant woman who puts a basket of vegetables upon her head in order to be beautiful."

These observations did not overjoy the sculpture establishment, bloated with reputations based on the statuary Brancusi dismissed as inconsequential. Their anger was further inflamed by the standard Coolidge-era prejudices against foreigners. Throughout the 1920s, certain conservative artists who felt threatened financially by the ascendancy of the School of Paris tried to restrict the quantity of foreign art coming into this country, but they had been thwarted repeatedly by petitions signed by less selfish artists and the legal briefs of John Quinn, who often put his law practice at the service of artists and their rights. But Quinn died in 1924, and his enemies were persistent. In the spring of 1926, the antimodernists came up with a wily new tactic that was simultaneously an aesthetic insult and an economic harassment. Authoritative sculptors with official laurels would persuade New York customs agents that avant-garde sculpture should not

be classified as duty-free art at all, but as a species of utilitarian object subject to the same taxes as commercial manufactured goods. Although the scheme originated among academic sculptors, any action would *appear* to have been brought by the federal government.

In the autumn of 1926 three events set into motion what the sculptor himself nicknamed the Brancusi brouhaha. First, his remarks were published in the *Times*. Second, the photographer Edward Steichen returned to New York after several years' residence in France. With his belongings was *Bird in Space*, a polished bronze sculpture he had bought from Brancusi for a few hundred dollars. Steichen declared it as a work of art priced at $600, but Customs entered it under "kitchen utensils and hospital supplies." And under kitchen utensils and hospital supplies, Steichen was subject to a $240 duty. He paid the money under protest, and *Bird in Space* was liberated from the Customs House.

From there it went to the Joseph Brummer Gallery, as part of the big Brancusi exhibition opening on November 17, 1926. The art earned rave reviews, and Brummer sold $10,000 worth of work. The show became the third incident in the brouhaha in February of 1927, when a customs appraiser named F. J. H. Kracke slapped a $4,000 tariff on the pieces sold, on the grounds that they were not art. He based his decision on a definition of art as representing "objects in their true proportions of length, breadth and thickness, or of length and breadth only." Appraiser Kracke thought that his ruling would apply only to modern painting and sculpture. He did not know enough to realize that by basing a ruling on a supposed inartistic distortion, he would be disqualifying not only a Modigliani, but also a Parmigianino or an El Greco from duty-free admission.

In the early stages of this mess, Steichen complained at a party about the customs agents declaring *Bird in Space* "a manufacture of metal." Gertrude was one of those present, and she listened intently to what he had to say. Later she sent for him and wanted to know what he was going to do about the ruling. Steichen said, "Well, I'm going to try and get my money back." Gertrude answered, "Let me take over that case. This is an important precedent to be established, and I would like to have my lawyers handle it." Steichen gratefully acceded, with Gertrude also stipulating that she would agree to finance all costs of the case if Brancusi could be listed as the plaintiff. He consented, and C. Brancusi v. The United States was filed by Charles J. Lane, a Whitney lawyer who had already proved himself adept in deflecting shakedowns for money by the Buffalo Bill promoters in Cody.

Stepping into a breach that once would have been filled by Quinn, Gertrude made a complete and honorable about-face from her post–Armory Show statement that Brancusi's sculptures were no more than "chunks of marble." Unlike her more conservative colleagues, she now could accept radical abstraction, even if she did not wish to pursue it herself. Furthermore, she despised ostracizing another artist because his work seemed incomprehensible and his success seemed unfair. Knowing of Gertrude's broad-mindedness and her volunteering to help one of the great modernist innovators, it is no wonder that a month or so later Juliana was irritated by Alexander Brook's wanting to keep Gertrude out of the

group show at an unregenerate and increasingly irrelevant institution like the Academy.

Gertrude sailed for Europe on January 6, 1927, and stayed abroad for three months, but Forbes and Juliana looked after Brancusi's interests for her. Forbes, as usual, was raring to deliver a neat uppercut to the collective academic jaw. He reported in *The Arts* how he, Marcel Duchamp (who had arranged the exhibition at the Brummer Gallery), and McBride went to the Customs House to protest against charging Brancusi duty. The protest having been made—and ignored by the government—Forbes spent the rest of the time talking with the officials. He was thus able to ferret out that the position taken by Krackc and company was "based upon the advice of the 'highest authorities' in art," although they refused to say who those authorities were. He also confirmed the rumors that malicious artists were working behind the scenes and using the customs inspectors as puppets. None of the so-called authorities would speak openly, and Forbes was determined to find out who was responsible. In the meantime, he and the other members of the art press savaged the customs officials and awaited *Brancusi* v. *The United States*, set for trial in October of 1927. The case was also publicized in the popular press, and Brancusi reaped a spurious notoriety from it.

With the Brancusi case in limbo until the fall, Juliana returned to negotiating for Gertrude and improving the Club. While Gertrude was pondering an offer from the Daughters of the American Revolution for a monument to their founding mothers for the national headquarters in Washington, D.C., Juliana whetted the society's appetite for her. She wrote to Aline Solomons, the chairwoman of the committee on memorials, in April of 1927, "I . . . [know] she [Mrs. Whitney] could do your monument better than anyone else; because she does get fired with an idea of which she feels herself to be a part." This was as much a description of herself as of Gertrude, as demonstrated by the very next things Juliana did. Suddenly wanting to give her artist friends an escape from the coming hot months in New York, Juliana introduced her version of a fresh-air fund. In June of 1927 she rented Maxstoke, a large, tree-shaded house in Charleston, New Hampshire, as a summer residence for the Whitney Studio Club. Two of the drawing rooms were turned into exhibition galleries, and the shows were changed every three weeks. Marie Appleton, the sales clerk at the Club, minded the galleries, and Schnakenberg, Sheeler, Blendon Campbell, Ernest Fiene, Edward and Jo Hopper, and Mungo were some of the artists who vacationed there. The experiment was so successful that Juliana wanted to buy the house as a permanent summer extension for the Club. But the plan fell through, and Maxstoke was available only for one summer.

That May Juliana also spearheaded a drive to rescue Sloan from a financial crisis. Dolly Sloan and Dr. Mary Halton, the couple's family physician and friend, came to Juliana with bad news. Sloan suffered from recurrent stomach trouble, and in 1925 he had undergone surgery for a hernia. The operation and his intermittent colic rendered him temporarily but gravely disabled, and while

he was recuperating, he had to give up his teaching job at the Art Students League. He hadn't sold a painting in months, and he was facing a pile of medical bills. Could Juliana do something? In reply, she proposed buying *The Lafayette*, Sloan's painting of the atmospheric Village hotel beloved by artists, and offering it to the Metropolitan. The picture was quickly dispatched from Kraushaar's to Bryson Burroughs, who delightedly told her that it "would be accepted if offered." Juliana then enlisted Duncan Phillips as chairman of a committee to raise the $5,000 purchase price from friends, admirers, and former students. This was the first time the two worked together, and the collaboration led to a warm collegial and personal friendship.

Not only Phillips but the DAR commission, which Gertrude had accepted, was taking Juliana to Washington on various persuading missions during the fall of 1927. After one visit, Aline Solomons wrote, "As usual, you came, saw and conquered." The officers were so impressed by Juliana that Gertrude suggested she should join the DAR herself. Somehow Juliana wriggled out of applying for admission. Her invented antecedents almost got her into trouble, but she had the satisfaction of knowing that even Gertrude had forgotten the real ones.

Presenting *The Lafayette* to the Metropolitan would take seven months and nearly founder on the shoals of trustee resistance. But that buffeting was mild in comparison to the obstacles that would develop in piloting one of Gertrude's monuments into the harbor of Huelva, Spain. The commission was carried out simultaneously with the DAR's amid the most taxing circumstances of her career. Almost a year before, in August of 1926, a Wall Street lawyer named William H. Page wrote to Gertrude about the absence of a monument to Christopher Columbus in Palos, the Spanish port from which he embarked for the New World. Page envisioned a dramatic statue dominating the shoreline. As he admired the Saint-Nazaire memorial and wanted something along the same lines in Spain, Gertrude was his ideal sculptor. Page asked for her permission to secure sponsorship and contributions from the Knights of Columbus and form a Columbus Memorial Fund. Gertrude said yes, and the preliminary work began. The basic components of the design were a standing figure of Columbus with his arms resting on one of Gertrude's all-purpose transverse crosses, seated figures of Ferdinand and Isabella, and reliefs of the hemispheres.

The procedures were all fine and regular, but no one knew what Page and the other key personality promoting the monument—Alexander P. Moore, the former ambassador to Spain and the newly elected president of the Columbus Memorial Fund—were like. Page devoted himself to scrutinizing every detail of the project. Throughout 1927 and 1928, he called or wrote Juliana daily or close to it, and then called or wrote again to find out why he had received no answers to his previous messages. Because Page was new to public sculpture, he seemed to think everyone else connected with the project was, too. He felt it necessary to inform Juliana that photographs of Gertrude's maquettes would be required and, in another letter, he told her to put sealing wax on the envelopes of her correspondence and then instructed her how to do it. However officious, Page was a harmless spout overflowing with ink, but Moore, a political hack who had been married to Lillian Russell, commuted between the United States

and Spain, and was an uncontrollable self-promoter. From the moment he could call his first press conference, he caused trouble, and Juliana and Gertrude privately code-named him Mud. Moore fomented a nasty rivalry where one had not existed by pitting the towns of Palos and Huelva against each other for the site of the monument. He also managed to insult several influential Spanish aristocrats, and his unabashed egotism nearly entangled both governments in a minor international incident. After a clash between Moore and the Spanish monarch about the statue's proposed site, Gertrude warned Juliana, "If questioned by the newspapers, you know nothing." To smooth relations, Gertrude had to meet many times with the Duke of Alba and have him arrange an audience with King Alfonso himself. By the summer of 1927 Gertrude and Juliana were worn out by Page's mania for trivia and Moore's selfish bungling. They trusted only each other for counsel and support, and their letters and wires about the tribulations of the Columbus monument demonstrate their closeness and their dependence on each other's strengths more vividly than any other time in their partnership.

Believing that Gertrude should be in Spain to guard against Moore's trying to get the site changed from Huelva (her first choice and that approved by the king) to Palos, which Page once wanted but was now wavering about, Juliana advised her to station herself there for the summer. On July 15, 1927, Gertrude wrote to her:

> Thank goodness you saw the dangers of my not being on the spot, for aside from his [Moore's] underhand methods I had to push matters all along the line. . . . I presume Hammond* and Alba will help with the permission as it will be merely completing the work which they so far have done for me.
>
> I would like to see the man's face when he hears the actual work has been begun! . . . But I see no reason why he should know anything about what I am doing until after the first week in August. . . .
>
> Then it's such fun feeling the whole thing is progressing and though my evidence against M. is circumstantial it would be pretty convincing to anyone under the circumstances which amuse me. . . .
>
> Good bye & thank God you saw the importance of my being on this side of the ocean.

Four days later, after receiving a batch of cables from Page, Gertrude again wrote to Juliana about the continuing seesaw between Palos and Huelva and Hammond's mediating among the Minister of Public Works, King Alfonso, and the Duke of Alba. As gratuitous hurdles were erected on both sides of the ocean, Juliana crafted a plan for deposing Moore and electing as chairman Anne Morgan, the Paris-based daughter of J. Pierpont Morgan and a philanthropist of commanding executive ability, as the best means of stopping the nonsense. Gertrude remained in Europe and Juliana in New York, the latter never far from Page's tireless dictation of telegrams and letters. Juliana was so bogged down in the Columbus monument that for the first time in years she didn't make the ritual trip to Europe. On September 1, 1927, she wrote wearily to Gertrude:

*Ogden Hammond, the American ambassador to Spain.

You told me years ago that we were living on the top of a volcano & so I've grown used to the quick step which avoided the scorching & to the smell of sulphur generally. But none of these eruptions was any kind of preparation for the particular hell of these last few months. You were so far away & I had to be wise all alone & quite useless—while you were in the midst of it all & ill too! The weather has been weird & the riveting on the skyscraper & on our own studio is the only sure thing I know. Mr. Page has worn out his secretary, likewise Spring 5432.* And when Mr. Draper† called me & said he was sailing today & seeing you soon I shed a very bitter tear. However, it was in the telephone booth & the tear soon dried, especially as I had to come out & face Mr. Page. . . .

It is quite impossible to tell you this way any of the things you would be interested in knowing. It can all wait, since you have accomplished a great thing & have still to accomplish more. Only you must know that the Committee here has been entirely with you all the time and believe that your work there has avoided a catastrophe for them. They are though a Body & move slowly & cautiously. Besides which it is summer & almost impossible to locate members enough for action. They await now the actual "document" of the official acceptance of the site.

I am so glad about all you have so splendidly done & that you are still improving. It sounds sensible & of course is the thing to do—to stay so long. I miss you desperately & think of you always with such real affection that sometimes it must reach you far away as you are.

Yrs

J.

A few days later Moore was neutralized by Anne Morgan, and Juliana cabled Gertrude: CONGRATULATIONS. NO MORE MUD. BLESS BIRCH PRAISE PAGE AND ABOVE ALL MOVE MORGAN SPAIN WITH YOU. The troubles in connection with the Columbus monument were not yet over, but its placement at Huelva was now beyond argument. Much of the maneuvering for the erection of the monument and its attendant proceedings was now in the domain of the Machiavellian Andrew O'Connor, who laughingly told Guy Pène du Bois "of having discovered and taken the marble from an old Roman quarry and of having stolen a shipload of something or other because the failure of his own to arrive was causing a delay in the completion of the monument." Du Bois observed, "Andrew had been in his element playing uncanny politics, injecting the virus of speed into languid Spaniards, accomplishing the impossible."

As if on cue, the Columbus contretemps resolved itself in time for the fall season, but its headaches would only be replaced by others. Gertrude and Juliana had decided to move the Club back to 10 West Eighth Street, which shortened the season and required more renovations. Juliana had neuritis in her arm and was tied up trying an assortment of cures. With no replacement for the energetic Alexander Brook, the Club did not open until December. Other exhibitions and causes needed her attention.

*Juliana's telephone number.
†Charles Draper, an old friend of Gertrude's and a brother of the actress Ruth Draper.

While Juliana was nursing her arm, the gleaming *Bird in Space* was hauled into court to be declared either a work of art or a manufacture of metal. Two meetings at Gertrude's studio were quickly organized. That a ruling against Brancusi would constitute a dangerous threat to artistic expression was recognized by the spectrum of people who attended the first session, including figures as diverse in outlook as Leopold Stokowski, Charles Sheeler, Frank Crowninshield, Frederick MacMonnies, Duncan Phillips, George Grey Barnard, Gaston Lachaise, Elie Nadelman, and Paul Manship—their concern cut across the standard boundaries. In preparation for the trial, which took place on October 21, 1927, Charles J. Lane consulted Forbes, who advised him on cross-examination and helped him line up expert witnesses to testify. Steichen, of course, would testify, as would Forbes himself. He had visited Brancusi's studio in Paris, published sympathetic articles about him, and provided useful letters of introduction when the sculptor was in the United States. The other witnesses were McBride, Jacob Epstein, Crowninshield, and William Henry Fox (director of the Brooklyn Museum).

Against this arsenal of culture, the government could only drum up two limp and easily discredited witnesses willing to swear that Brancusi wasn't a serious professional artist and that his productions were not art. One of them, Robert Aitken, was a reactionary academic sculptor who hated modern art. He testified that he hadn't "read of" or "heard" of Brancusi "for a number of years." He did not "consider it [*Bird in Space*] a work of art or a sculpture." Forbes later discovered that Aitken was one of the covert agitators at the Customs House. If Brancusi could be robbed of his standing as an artist and if his work were reclassified as utensils, Aitken believed he would succeed in diminishing the public taste for modern art. (Did he suppose that buyers, prevented from acquiring Brancusis or Gaudier-Brzeskas, would turn instead to Aitkens?) The other government witness, an art instructor at Columbia University who stated that *Bird in Space* "wasn't the professional production of a sculptor," made equally unimpressive statements. Lane was confident he had won the appeal, but the case was left under advisement for thirteen months. On November 26, 1928, more than two years after Steichen first confronted American customs inspectors, the court concluded that *Bird in Space* could indeed be called sculpture.*

In November of 1927, just a few weeks after the Club returned to 10 West Eighth, the International Composers' Guild left it for good. Varèse wanted to live in Europe, and he felt that much of his job had been done. Experiment, he said, had been established "as a valid and indispensable artistic principle" and in the words of the critic Paul Rosenfeld, the Guild "was cardinal in producing here in New York an audience capable of receiving new impressions." It had exposed audiences to Bartók, Berg, Hindemith, Milhaud, Poulenc, Prokofiev, Respighi, Satie, Schoenberg, Stravinsky, Webern, and more. The con-

---

*Yet it remained difficult to bring modernist art into the country. In 1936, when the Museum of Modern Art borrowed nineteen sculptures from foreign collections for its exhibition Cubism and Abstract Art, the pieces were held up for a week by customs examiners.

certs had been conducted by Varèse, Otto Klemperer, Fritz Reiner, Artur Rodzinski, Vladimir Shavitch, and Stokowski. Thus the disbanding of the Guild was termed a "happy euthanasia," and Varèse and Juliana parted on the best of terms.

Brancusi and Varèse had been vindicated, but Gertrude was still perched on top of an active volcano and in danger of being scorched. Strangely, the next eruption came not from Moore and the Columbus monument, but the DAR. Until now its representatives had been acquiescent and handled easily by Juliana. In late November, however, it was time for the memorial committee to pay a visit to the studio to inspect the model, a thinly draped female figure with outstretched arms (Gertrude's formulaic crucifixion figure again). Mary Schuyler, one of the officers, was shocked by what she saw. The diaphanously gowned figure appeared to be more nude than clothed—accepting it as a symbol of the DAR would sully its pristine heritage. No sooner did Schuyler march out of the studio than she called the papers and convened a press conference to denounce the indecency she had just viewed. A catastrophe seemed imminent, and Juliana was required to restore sanity. Staying on the phone until 1:00 A.M., she reached every reporter who was present during the diatribe and persuaded him to kill the story. She wrote to Aline Solomons:

> I think I succeeded—as a great many of the reporters were men with whom I have had other dealings and I have always found them ready to help me out. I sifted the whole story thoroughly, and it amounts to this, that Mrs. Schuyler wanted some publicity for herself and also a certain prudish delight in crediting herself in standing out for "morality in art.". . . I consider it treacherous to your Committee and disloyal to the D.A.R. organization, for I know positively that had it not been for your help and my own efforts and influence with the press, also Mrs. Brosseau's* wise statement, the whole organization would have been the laughing stock of the country.
>
> This, of course, is my personal expression to you. My surprise and contempt must be swallowed with the matter; we were lucky to come off so lightly. Mrs. Brosseau, you and I, all three of us, adopted the same attitude with the reporters; first, that the meeting was entirely an amicable one, second, that the model was accepted with slight recommendations to the sculptor, third, that the question of drapery was trivial. †

Also preoccupying Juliana that winter was an important traveling exhibition of forty-two new works by Club artists that she was sending around the country for a six-month tour. Beginning in December, the exhibition circulated to the Minneapolis Institute of Arts, the California Palace of the Legion of Honor in San Francisco, the Denver Art Museum, the New Orleans Arts and Crafts Club, and Harvard's Fogg Art Museum in Cambridge, Massachusetts, before terminating at the Art Students League in May of 1928. Juliana strove to line up museum galleries because she wanted to confer prestige on contemporary American art and, by implication, the Whitney Studio Club. As it would be the first time that many in the West and South had seen these painters, she believed they needed public institutions backing them. Sales were always crucial to Juliana, and as she was determined that at least one painting be sold at each

---

*Grace Brosseau, president general of the DAR.
†Nevertheless, in the finished version, the figure was heavily draped.

location, a museum's imprimatur would reassure local buyers. Juliana offered to be at the December 3, 1927, opening in Minneapolis to inaugurate the tour, and proposed that Forbes be invited at the same time to deliver a lecture.

Because many of the records were saved, the exhibition documented Juliana's solicitude toward artists and the touch that endeared her to her peers. Not only did she write letters congratulating each painter who made a sale, but she went over all the press clippings received from each city, copied out any favorable criticisms, and sent them on to the artist. Juliana also wrote warm messages to anyone who bought something. Delighted by the news of a sale, she asked the director of the New Orleans Arts and Crafts Club to "tell me something about this lady's collection, because it interests me tremendously that a purchaser could be intelligent enough to buy a picture instead of a name." To a buyer of a still life by Nan Watson in San Francisco, she wrote, "I believe you have the best that this artist has ever painted, and hope that it will stimulate you to see some of her things when you come here to New York. I shall be very glad, indeed, to show you the five or six which I own, if you . . . can spare the time to come down to the Studio."

These actions were all part of Juliana's fundamental drive to protect and fight for artists and win them a public. If she did her job well enough, the artist might stay out of the fray. As she wrote to the painter Beulah Stevenson:

> I think it is a good thing you are too busy to go hunting and persuading dealers and buyers. I believe that is one of the artist's greatest limitations. I know usually it is a fierce necessity which prompts them to do it, but nevertheless, if he can resist and do as you say, his work is bound to be of value; but it takes a life time to make it so. I believe that you are going ahead and I think a gradual growth is much more healthy, especially at this time.

Juliana was constantly inventing, sponsoring, and nurturing projects, but she preferred buying art over every other method of reward. Around Christmas of 1927 she emphasized that preference by aiding José Clemente Orozco. The Mexican artist had recently moved to the city and was living obscurely and drearily in a basement room on Riverside Drive. Orozco had arrived with enough money to last him three months, but no sales or exhibitions were in sight, and no one seemed to know he was in New York. Eventually the painter Maurice Becker, an old friend of Stuart Davis and a member of the Club, stumbled across him and told Juliana. She immediately bought ten drawings for $350 and thus became the only person who supported him during those miserable months. Orozco's biographer wrote of the sale, "As though miraculously sent, this sum reached Orozco at the very moment his funds were completely exhausted. . . . The sale to Mrs. Force, the only one he had made in New York before our meeting [in the summer of 1928], served to defray the artist's living expenses during the three-month period just ending."

Juliana's own Christmas was brightened by a two-week sea voyage to Panama with Gertrude. Their main reason for going was to inspect a site in Panama City for a prospective Theodore Roosevelt memorial, but Gertrude also wanted Juliana to get a good rest. Juliana had developed a spastic colon that acted up

in times of stress, and there had been no shortage of that over the last few months. On December 29, 1927, the two women boarded a ship bound for Havana. In Cuba they went to the races and the casinos and dined New Year's Day on the roof of the Sevilla Biltmore Hotel. Four days later they docked in Colón, passing through the locks of the great canal en route to Balboa. They made the rounds of sights and receptions, but the real excitement of the trip came when Charles Lindbergh, flying in from Costa Rica, touched down in Panama. As soon as they could, Gertrude and Juliana hurried away from their hosts to meet the newest American idol.

The leisurely return cruise having rested her, Juliana dived into the problems awaiting her at home. *The Lafayette* was not yet lodged safely within the Metropolitan, and Sloan was still in a financial bind. By January 31, 1928, she had gotten the painting's acceptance confirmed by the museum, raised the $5,000 required, and sent the money to Duncan Phillips. She asked him to send the check and his congratulations to Sloan because she felt the appreciation would mean more if it came from him. Phillips, equally gallant, wrote to Sloan, "The credit [for the gift] should go to the active workers on the Committee and especially to Mrs. Force."

The Club could always do with some tinkering, and Juliana could not bear stasis in anything under her control. She and Gertrude had come to the conclusion that sculpture had been done an injustice at the Club: Its representation had been inadequate in the galleries and circulating exhibitions. Their remedy was to split the spring annual of 1928 into two sections, the first entirely given over to sculpture. Opening on March 6, 1928, the show had eighty-seven works by fifty-three contributors. A blistering review was filed by Marya Mannes.

> Judging from this first Annual Sculpture Exhibition, American sculpture in general is pretty inept and embryonic. Only a few things are the result of talent and real care; only a dozen have the breath of beauty in them [e.g., works by Paul Fiene, Duncan Ferguson, Carl Walters, John Flannagan, Reuben Nakian, and Dorothea Greenbaum]. . . . The rest of the sculpture falls into three classes: Imagination without Technique; Technique without Imagination; neither Technique nor Imagination. The first causes granite blocks to be hacked incompetently into the semblance of strange faces; the second results in perfectly smooth and perfectly meaningless torsos, in faithful portraits after the manner of Jo Davidson; the third is embodied in works like the Columbus Memorial model by Gertrude Whitney.

Hand in hand with new ventures at the Club went the perennial concern: artists in need. They needed work, they needed supplies, they needed studios, they needed recommendations, they needed money, they needed rest. And equally crucial to Juliana, they needed joy. Never the cold dispenser of funds, she issued checks for stipends or purchases not just as compliments and actualities but "declarations of love." By now she was so conversant with the artists around her that Forbes was to say, "her lines of communication became so crisscrossed that they formed a net which caught everything." Yet she hated to think she

might be overlooking someone. Writing to Royal Cortissoz about a charitable contribution Gertrude would be making, Juliana appended almost as a matter of reflex, "If there is any moment of your time available, would you help the Club by sending word of any 'new' art you discover? I want to make the place more useful to the artist & more entertaining to the public & I hope I'm not a bore to you in the process."

Just how efficiently this crisscrossed net functioned is traceable in a deed or two. In March of 1928 she briefly employed Harry Gottlieb as a frame maker, advanced money to Myron Lechay, bought a painting by Kenneth Hayes Miller and donated it to the Cleveland Museum of Art, and recommended Jan Matulka for a teaching job at the Art Students League, a post he didn't get until September of 1929. During this same spring, Juliana also wanted to do something else for Stuart Davis. After he turned down a rent-free studio in the Eighth Street buildings, she suggested that he go to Europe, as he was the only major American modernist who had had no direct experience of French art. As part of his arrangements, Davis was to rent Matulka's studio in Paris. As the two men were not friends, the only possibility suggesting itself is that Juliana, knowing of both Matulka's and Davis's plans, arranged the transaction, thus funneling a little money toward Matulka and guaranteeing Davis a place to live upon arrival. Juliana gave Davis $900, and in May of 1928 he was on his way to Paris. "What with a little more money [around $500] she gave me later," he recalled, "I was able to stay in Paris for over a year and I really worked hard. . . . I . . . managed to produce about a dozen paintings which were decent enough to be looked at, as well as some lithographs. It was a very profitable experience and I gave Mrs. Force three of my best pictures when I came back [in August of 1929]." The stipend was one of Juliana's best bargains, for Davis gave her *Eggbeater, Number 2, Place Pasdeloup*, and *Early American Landscape*.* For his part, Davis's artistic vocabulary was broadened by his sojourn abroad, and references to Paris appeared throughout his painting for the rest of his career. During this same period, Juliana sent Lucile and Arnold Blanch, Andrée Ruellan, Joseph Pollet, Emil Ganso, and Clement Wilenchick to Europe, too.

While Davis was preparing to leave New York, Juliana contended with a sudden intrigue enveloping the traveling show, until then plying its uncontroversial and generally applauded way around the country. In April of 1928 the pictures were scheduled to be hung in the Fogg Art Museum, until they came under the jurisdiction of the institution's associate director, the meticulous and imperious Paul J. Sachs. Sachs taught Harvard's distinguished museum course at the Fogg, and he was responsible for educating a generation of influential directors and curators in American art museums. His reputation for connoisseurship was deserved, and his standards were punctilious. A collector himself, he refined and re-refined his holdings until no better examples could be had. Sachs would not countenance the ordinary, and to his finely trained eye, several of Juliana's selections belonged in that category.

After the Whitney pictures were uncrated at the Fogg, Sachs looked them

* All in the collection of the Whitney Museum.

over and was unimpressed. Of the forty-two, he disliked sixteen and eliminated them from the exhibit. Although he had accepted the full exhibition, he would hang only the twenty-six pictures he thought were minimally acceptable. When this news reached Juliana—the Boston art critics were reporting that Sachs "censored" the show—she could hardly contain herself. She flashed an ultimatum to the Fogg: Either exhibit all forty-two paintings as agreed or send them back to New York. Sachs's reply was unsatisfactory, and Juliana was soon on a train to Boston to survey the eviscerated show with her own eyes. If the full complement of paintings wasn't on the walls by the time she reached the Fogg, she informed him, she was ready to remove every picture from the building with her own hands. Astonished by her challenge to the exercise of his famous taste, Sachs doubted Juliana would go this far, but on the day she roared into the museum he had taken care to be out. After Juliana left with a promise that the show would be dismantled, Sachs wrote to say that the paintings would be shipped immediately. He professed to be surprised by her actions.

Juliana and Gertrude might have derived some cheer from having outlasted or outwitted their various opponents, but the strain also took its toll. On September 7, 1928, it was announced that the Whitney Studio Club was closing. Gertrude was said to be withdrawing her financial support, and even Juliana's fighting spirit seemed subdued. There was talk of her retiring to Bucks County to write, although she had just bought herself a house in South Salem, New York, a rural village near the Connecticut line and just a few miles from where the Sheelers and the Brooks now lived. She named it Shaker Hollow, and installed her sizable and still-growing collection of Shaker furniture there.

The primary reason for closing the Club was that it had outgrown itself. Over 400 men and women had joined, and there was a long waiting list. To enlarge it further was impossible, but to refuse worthwhile new artists would be contrary to its principles. The Club had also fulfilled its purposes as a gateway. Younger independents had gained a foothold in the profession, the Academy had lost ground, and dealers were not so slow to recognize emerging talent. The established Rehn, Kraushaar, Dudensing, Daniel, and Weyhe galleries now represented Club artists, and new galleries for independent Americans had opened. The most important of these was the Downtown Gallery, founded in 1926 and located on West 13th Street. Its director, Edith Gregor Halpert, was married to Samuel Halpert, a charter member and frequent exhibitor at the Club, and Edith, a former art student, had shown her own work at the Whitney once or twice. Thus she knew the Whitney group, and when she launched her gallery, the artists she asked to join her—Davis, Nakian, Brook, Bacon, Kuniyoshi, Varian, Sheeler, William Zorach, and Spencer—came out of the Club. Juliana released a statement explaining:

> In the belief that a useful purpose could be served by opening a gallery devoted to the free expression of non-partisan American artists, the Whitney Studio Club was organized. Many of the artists who showed their pictures and sculpture publicly for

the first time at the galleries of the Club have since found the doors of other galleries hospitably open to them.

During the period in which the Whitney Studio Club has aimed to promote liberal American art, the attitude of the public has changed. Art dealers and Directors of great official exhibitions have also changed their point of view. Opportunities for showing work by young American artists have increased tremendously, and academic restraint has become almost insignificant.

The Club, which now consists of four hundred members, is proud to have played its part in bringing about this invigorating change. But this very change makes the Club no longer a pioneer organization. Artists for whom twelve [sic] years ago it was necessary to fight are now in high favor. More than this, a general liberal movement in art is in high favor.

The pioneering work for which the Club was organized has been done; its aim has been successfully attained. The liberal artists have won the battle which they fought so valiantly, and will celebrate the victory as other regiments fighting for liberty have done—by disbanding.

The Club would be renamed the Whitney Studio Galleries and become a slightly more commercial operation (in that a 25 percent commission would be taken on sales) devoted to individual and small group shows. Juliana was quoted as saying, "I will show the work of artists whom Mrs. Whitney and I believe in. We are interested from a personal point of view in certain artists, just as we believe other galleries are interested personally in the men whom they represent. The gallery will revert to and carry on the idea which was originally behind the Whitney Studio Club. That was the idea of an exhibiting gallery for contemporary art, rather than an organization of artists, philanthropically inspired." The huge, heterogeneous annuals and the membership apparatus were eliminated as unwieldy, but otherwise the enterprise hardly changed at all. Replacing the Club with a gallery was supposed to curb some of the bountiful aspects that had gotten out of hand, but Juliana continued to go where her generosity led her. "Mrs. Force had complete financial authority," said Ethel Renthal, her secretary between 1927 and 1929, "and the first of every month a pack of checks went out to artists and other people." But with fewer artists to look after, Juliana could be more creative in organizing exhibitions.

Two weeks after the Club was dissolved, a demise of a very different sort took place. On September 21, 1928, Willard Force died in his sleep of a cerebral hemorrhage. Doctor's death, which occured while he and Juliana were at the farm with the family, was quick, quiet, and unexpected. Juliana was stunned and took the death hard. The Forces' lives and interests had diverged, but they anchored each other, and there was a sense of devotion between them. Doctor had behaved well toward Juliana, letting her do as she wished, and he was happy to embrace her family as his own. He had been blessedly free of spite or unkindness. Juliana felt his loss keenly, and her nephews remembered her distraught tears lasting for days.

Doctor's death altered Juliana's feelings toward Barley Sheaf Farm. He had loved the farm better than any other place, and it was inextricably bound up with his image and presence. Now that he was gone, Holicong and its memories

made her feel morose, and she began spending less time there. She contemplated selling the farm if the right buyer could be found, but did nothing. Shaker Hollow, unshadowed by her past and requiring the extensive renovation she relished, was more congenial.

Juliana was, for the first time in many years, financially pinched. The Forces' habit was to spend, and they used their two incomes willingly for the upkeep of the farm, for Doctor's Packards and her clothes, for art and artists, for trips and presents and antiques and hospitality. Doctor had prudently put the farm in Juliana's name some years before, thus avoiding estate taxes. When he died, his estate consisted of his personal effects and a cash bequest of $3,000 to Juliana. Living on one salary, when she had grown used to the extravagances afforded by two, was too difficult for her, because she was unwilling or unable to economize. She received a salary of at least $1,000 a month from Gertude, but because she controlled the financial aid to artists, Juliana also had access to a drawing account to pay her expenses and the Club's bills. According to Ethel Renthal, after Doctor's death Juliana wrote checks on this account to renovate her house in South Salem because her salary did not cover all her bills.

The Whitney Studio Galleries opened in November of 1928 with Glenn O. Coleman's lithographs (which Juliana sold to the Brooklyn Museum and the Art Institute of Chicago for $15 apiece) and gouaches by Ernest Fiene. Julius Bloch, a Philadelphia painter who came up for the opening, met Juliana for the first time. He later wrote about the encounter, "I am so happy in knowing this very vivid and powerful personality. . . . I recall after Fiene introduced me, how she engaged me in conversation at once with a view to determining what sort of mind and temperament I might possess. How much her friendship has done for me. . . . [It has] shaped my life to a great extent."

Harry Gottlieb and John Flannagan were the next artists to benefit from Juliana's shaping hand. In October of 1928 she and Forbes paid a visit to Woodstock. Flannagan, working there at the time, commented, "Everyone is excited just now over an impending visit of the Dowager Queen and the Crown Prince otherwise Mrs. Force and Forbes Watson." Making the rounds, the royal pair stopped in Gottlieb's studio. Juliana bought two paintings and offered him his first one-man show in January of the new year; Forbes would follow with an article in *The Arts*. Learning in December that Gottlieb's wife was making a slow recovery from a miscarriage, she sent him $250 and wrote:

> I am distressed to hear that your wife is not doing as well as you had hoped, and I want you to understand my attitude toward you in sending the enclosed check. It is only that I feel you might use it better at this time than later on. I am sure that during your exhibition we will sell some of the pictures, and I am sending you this on account of that.
> Hoping that you and your wife will understand that this is only an expression of my sincere sympathy at this juncture and my great belief in the fact that things are going to be very much better. . . .

Artists exhibiting concurrently with Gottlieb were Blendon Campbell plus fellow Woodstockers Emil Ganso, Paul Rohland (who was lent $200 by Juliana

and had asked if the debt could be taken out in pictures or sales), and Flannagan, who was added at the last moment. (The Whitney Galleries contained four rooms, one for each artist; to accommodate a fifth exhibitor, Flannagan's pieces would have to be distributed throughout the rooms.)

In late 1928 Flannagan and his stones were evicted from his rooms. The sculptor happened to run into Alexander Brook, who said he could stay in his studio in the Village until he found a place to live. Brook gave him ten dollars, but Flannagan, a woeful alcoholic, spent the money on gin. When Brook checked on his guest some days later, he was dead drunk and in no condition to go anywhere. But at Brook's next visit, Flannagan promised to finish the carvings in progress if he were assured of having a show.

Brook went to Juliana and told his story. Touched by his kindness to Flannagan, she forgave him, and the two were friends again. She said that the extra studio Gertrude leased on MacDougal Alley (the one formerly shared by du Bois and Davidson) was vacant, so Flannagan could have it. In January he would have a one-man show. Brook was so elated that he went out at once and sold two of the sculptures to a wealthy friend. During the exhibition, Juliana purchased three: *Elephant*, *Colt*, and *Chimpanzee*.* (She must have been partial to Flannagan's monkeys because she also bought one the year before.) The exhibit was a financial success for at least half the artists. Rohland paid off part of his debt; of the fifteen carvings Flannagan had ready for the show, nine were sold, as were six oils by Gottlieb. Afterward Juliana chose another six of Gottlieb's paintings for traveling exhibitions she was circulating to midwestern museums.

The Galleries' critical and social smash of the spring season was The Circus in Paint, a festive group show on the theme of the big top. Opening on April 1, 1929, the exhibition, with an atmosphere devised to match the art, was deliriously received and made the papers from coast to coast. Juliana was tickled to be planning this kind of event, and the results testified that the exhilaration and cleverness synonymous with the defunct Club had not been extinguished.

To make the show more diverting, she asked Louis Bouché to create special decorations. Bouché, who'd cultivated a bit of a reputation as a homegrown Dadaist in the early 1920s, was at his most *sportif*. He painted wild-animal wagons on the walls of the entrance hall and installed gaudily striped stands. Banners trumpeting, "W.S.G. World Famous Circus" directed visitors into the galleries, which were set up to look like circus tents. The ceilings were draped in white muslin scalloped with bright red trim, and clusters of balloons floated in the corners. Sawdust was strewn over the floors, colorfully saddled wooden ponies were planted in the center of the rooms, and chairs were replaced by elephant tubs. Big barrels were filled with popcorn and roasted peanuts. The enchanted McBride said the show "should promptly be seen by all," but not before noticing:

> It is, among other things, a tour de force in picture presentation; and although I detest the shadow of a suspicion of a pun I must let the phrase pass in spite of the

---

* *Elephant* and *Chimpanzee* are now in the collection of the Whitney Museum.

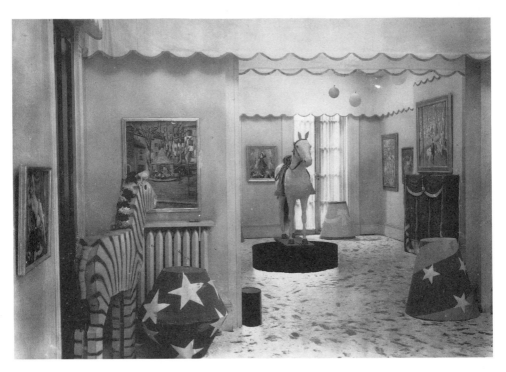

The entrance to The Circus in Paint.

fact that it is Mrs. Willard B. Force, of the Whitney Studio Club forces, who is the genius back of the presentation. . . .

Mrs. Force has a talent, long since recognized but never widely enough heralded, of placing pictures and art objects in such a way that all their virtues shine forth glamorously. Consequently all the pictures in this exhibition look attractive and any one of them seems to insinuate that that spectator is an idiot who does not start in immediately to collecting circus pictures.

The *Times*'s art critic, Edward Alden Jewell, also addressed his congratulations directly to the source. "Yes, Mrs. Force," he wrote, "they don't do things any more expertly at Madison Square Garden, and thousands are going to remember your show with heartfelt gratitude."

The exhibition's catalog was written by Lloyd Goodrich, then a critic for *The Arts*. In a brief but thoughtful essay touching on the visual and psychological appeal of the circus for contemporary artists and citing precedents from Watteau and Hogarth to Daumier, Degas, and Picasso, he introduced a note of scholarship and historical perspective previously absent from Whitney productions. Goodrich had known Juliana for several years, but this was the first time he had done anything directly for her. Through Brook's recommendation, he had begun writing for the magazine in 1924, and became an associate editor a year later. For the 1927–1928 season, Goodrich was made European editor and lived

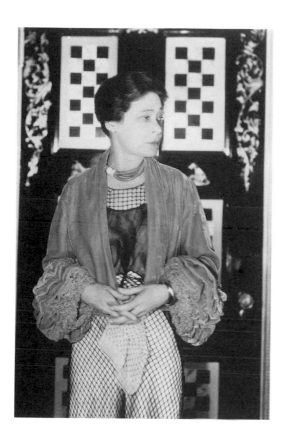

Juliana, very much in command as master of the Whitney revels.

abroad. Back in New York, he was now a contributing editor to *The Arts* and thoroughly a part of the art world.

The Circus in Paint was a triumphal sendoff for Juliana. Shortly after the opening, she sailed for the dedication ceremonies of Gertrude's Columbus memorial sculpture, which was completed without further help from Moore or Page. The celebrations were destined to be just as lavish as those for Saint-Nazaire, and they began well before April 21, the official date of the unveiling. The celebrants began assembling in Madrid, in Gertrude's private train, and O'Connor, Davidson, du Bois, Schnakenberg, Watson, the Cecil Howards, Charles Draper, and Flora Whitney and her new husband, G. Macculloch Miller, made up some of the party. They rested a day or two at the Ritz before proceeding to Seville. There Guy Pène du Bois, Forbes, and Juliana went to a bullfight, and Juliana nearly fainted from the gore. Du Bois remembered her "running away . . . so quickly and quietly that we didn't miss her for some time."

In Seville Gertrude's guests were quartered on a chartered cruise ship, which then ferried them down the Guadalquivir River and along the Spanish coast to Huelva. They were joined at some point by the Duke of Alba, Primo de Rivera, and Ogden Hammond and his family (including his daughter, the future Con-

gresswoman Millicent Fenwick). En route Cecil Howard played the guitar and improvised songs about his fellow passengers and the sights they saw on the banks as they cruised by. At night an unknown miscreant among them raced through the first-class cabins, soaking and tying knots in all of the pairs of men's pajamas the valets had so carefully laid out for a late retiring.

Sodden clothing turned out to be a portent of what was to come in Huelva. The dedication of the monument took place on a wet morning under hundreds of unfurled umbrellas. The dripping spectators repaired to spreading tents where a tremendous lunch was served and shook themselves off as best they could. Amid the damp crowd of dignitaries, Gertrude maintained, said du Bois, a "constantly calm demeanor, the ease with which she stood being the center of the whole proceeding."

Juliana spent the latter part of the summer of 1929 in England. She passed much of the time in the Cotswolds and in Buckinghamshire indulging her ardent Anglophilia. In August she bought a two-story thatched cottage with an adjoining garden in Haddenham, a small village not far from Oxford. In its previous lives, the upper part of the house had been a pub and the ground floor was a cart shed and bakery. The legacy of the bakery was its five tall chimneys shooting up from inglenooks and walk-in fireplaces. Juliana named the house Cobweb, because it lay tucked away inside a maze of footpaths and high-walled lanes. Cobweb stood in the romantically named Rosemary Lane and was itself the quintessence of quaintness. The thatched roof swept down to the ground-floor windows, which were paned in leaded glass, and the walls were not stucco, but wychert, a local variant of limestone that went back to medieval times. Jasmine vines had been trained to grow up the cottage walls, and yew hedges edged the yard. The garden led into an apple orchard.

By American standards, however, the cottage was primitive; it may not have had electricity, and it certainly lacked modern plumbing. So in most un-English fashion, Juliana ordered elaborate fixtures from Germany and installed two full bathrooms. She also built a wall around the front of the house and in the process razed some tenements on the property. Three or four elderly villagers had been living in these rough outbuildings; Juliana helped find them habitations elsewhere and paid their moving expenses.

She upholstered the cottage with thick fur rugs and throws and mixed Bauhaus, Queen Anne, and Georgian furniture. But her outstanding decorating coup was the chimneys. Cobweb's chimneys needed fixing, and having the right kind was a matter of no small importance because with a thatched house, the taller the chimney the less the likelihood of sparks igniting the roof. At a builder's works in a nearby village, Juliana saw exactly what she wanted: handcrafted spiral smokestacks meticulously copied from originals in Tudor monasteries. They had been ordered by the Spencer-Barnards, the ruling gentry in the area, for their manor house. Juliana offered on sight to double the builder's fee if he would deliver the chimneys to her instead of the original customers. He consented, and suddenly Cobweb had five tall twisted chimneys in working order while the Spencer-Barnards were fuming sulfurously, independent of fireplaces or flues. (This story, "of the American woman who purloined our chimneys," was told

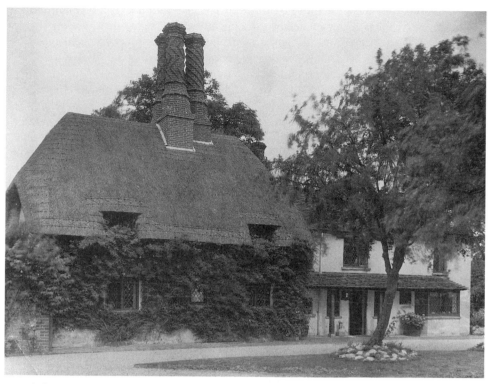

A front view of the English cottage Juliana bought in 1929. She named it Cobweb because it seemed caught in a network of lanes.

to Cobweb's present owners by Robert Spencer-Barnard, who lives in the manor now. Nearly six decades after the incident, the Spencer-Barnards have not forgiven the builder his treachery. On account of it, they refuse to trade with his descendants, who run the business today.)

As would be expected, in September 1929 Juliana was pushing ahead with the Whitney Studio Galleries. She had gotten as far as persuading the Art Institute of Chicago to take a show of Cecil Howard's sculpture when Gertrude made an extraordinary suggestion.

The Galleries, although functioning effectively as a setting for artists to be noticed, were a stopgap measure. They were more an escape from the cumbersome size of the Club than a fresh new venture in themselves. Neither Gertrude nor Juliana would have suffered their pet project to become a backwater; they preferred creating something new and dynamic to functioning smoothly and perpetually in an established system. Moreover, the expansion of commercial galleries was lessening the Whitney impact. Du Bois, who lived in France from 1924 to 1930, commented about the change: "I was particularly astonished upon

my return to New York by the number of its art galleries, the tremendous spread of its art market. . . . In 1924 when I left for France the increase in the number of galleries scarcely kept pace with the increase in the city's population. In 1930 two critics must have had some difficulty in covering the galleries in three or four days."

Then there was the question of the collection—that heterogeneous, uncataloged entity whose objects would be labeled "Collection of Mrs. Harry Payne Whitney" or "Collection of Mrs. W. B. Force" when they were reproduced for publication. These holdings had grown to about 500 paintings, sculptures, drawings, and prints, and almost every piece was in dead storage. With their art stuck in closets, the point of the women's efforts was getting lost. The collection having overwhelmed the exhibition space, they had two choices: to give the collection to an institution with room to show it or to build a museum of their own.

Gertrude's proposition, then, was to offer her entire collection of American art to the Metropolitan Museum, where she had reason to suppose it would be accepted. Her parents, like so many of New York's wealthy, had been prominent donors to the museum, and she in turn had been cultivated by its curators and other officials. They had been aware of the advantages of being on her good side as early as 1916, when Daniel Chester French bought her *Head of a Spanish Peasant* for the sculpture collection. He wrote to several trustees, "I feel that for artistic reasons we should have an example of her [Mrs. Whitney's] work in our collection of American bronzes, and I think, aside from this, that it would be valuable to enlist her interest in the Museum by the purchase of something of hers for the collection." At the curatorial level, Bryson Burroughs and Juliana were in sympathy with each other and together had maneuvered American pictures into the Met. There was a precedent of cooperation between Greenwich Village and uptown, and Gertrude was enough encouraged by it to ask Juliana to represent her at a meeting with Dr. Edward Robinson, the Metropolitan's director. Juliana was empowered to offer the entire collection to him, as well as $5 million for a wing to house it.

Juliana was, according to her secretary, less than enthusiastic about this errand. Ethel Renthal said that Forbes and Juliana had been dreaming about the idea of a museum for years. A folder marked "Museum" held a thick sheaf of papers; she remembered it on Juliana's desk well before the fall of 1929. In a letter to Glenn O. Coleman, dated December 5, 1929, Juliana said she had been making plans along the lines of a museum "for six years." A date of 1923 for germination seems premature—1926 or 1927 seems more probable—and must be attributed to Juliana's utter inaptitude for dates, although Hermon More, Juliana's successor as director of the museum, vouched for a date close to hers.

By 1929, starting a museum of one's own was no longer a novel act. The dizzying prosperity of the last few years led to a conviction that the economy was going nowhere but up, that the boom would last forever. More Americans than ever had extra money to spend, and the established millionaires had unalloyed confidence in the security of their revenues. It had become almost a fad among the great New York collectors of twentieth-century art to make their acquisitions available to the public on a permanent basis. To show his superb

Picassos, Légers, Braques, Arps, Mirós, and Mondrians, Albert E. Gallatin opened the Gallery of Living Art on the premises of New York University in 1927,* and the place promptly became an invaluable resource to artists. During the summer of 1929, Solomon R. Guggenheim began to collect art for the specific purpose of presenting it to a public institution. Most pertinent—and provocative—to Gertrude and Juliana, however, was a decision by three other New Yorkers. Throughout the winter and spring of 1929, Abby Aldrich Rockefeller, Lillie P. Bliss, and Mary Sullivan had conferred many times about the city's lack of a public gallery for viewing the latest developments on the international art scene. By May, they were in the museum business, complete with board members; in June, they had their director, the brilliant young scholar, Alfred H. Barr, Jr. The Museum of Modern Art, as the three women's inspiration came to be called, would open on November 8, 1929, with the backing of the Rockefellers. These three great undertakings had in common an international scope and an emphasis on Europe. There was still no institution devoted *exclusively* and authoritatively to twentieth-century American art. This was the "amazing gap," as Juliana later put it, that she and Forbes wanted to be the first to mend.

Gertrude's approaching the Metropolitan testified not only to her staunch belief in the native product but to the strength of her own position as an art patron. She possessed the largest private collection of American art then in existence. That she believed she could prevail, her good relations with the Metropolitan notwithstanding, was astonishing, for the museum's unfriendliness to recent nonacademic art, both American and foreign, was long a matter of public record. Sculpture was under the control of Daniel Chester French, who favored salon work. Painting, despite occasional victories by Burroughs, fared little better; the trustees' horror of modern art and their general hesitancy about buying anything not officially certified as important had been pilloried in the press for years by Watson and McBride. And in 1927 and 1928 in particular, there erupted a ground swell of dissent against the disposition of the Hearn funds, a large sum of money meant to be spent on contemporary American painting.

The first of what were to be two combined funds was established in 1906 by George A. Hearn, a department store magnate and a collector of Blakelock, Inness, and Theodore Robinson. Besides giving over 100 pictures to the Met, he donated $250,000. The income from this sum was earmarked for paintings by living American artists. As the Met had not established a department of American painting—nor would it, until 1949—the Hearn funds represented the museum's primary statement about the country's cultural coming of age and were perceived as such by local artists. Yet to the conservative trustees, this progressive gift proved embarrassing. Hearn died in 1913, and once he was no longer there to argue, they reinterpreted the terms of the bequest to mean that it could be used to buy works of artists *living in 1906*—the year he made his first contribution. (This convenient rephrasing of Hearn's wishes was in effect

---

*Gallatin later credited the inspiration for his gallery to a 1926 editorial by Watson in *The Arts*.

as late as 1958, when the income was used to buy a painting by Henri, who died in 1929. One feels that Henri, the firebrand and friend of young art, would have objected.)

American artists immediately protested the implications of this policy, and the trustees unbent slightly in 1921 in buying canvases by Glackens, Luks, and Sloan.* But modernism remained indigestible. Although the Metropolitan approved memorial exhibitions for George Bellows and for John Singer Sargent (who both died in 1925), they would not sponsor one for Maurice Prendergast, who died in 1924.

As a result of trustee stubbornness, the unspent Hearn funds piled up, at the rate of approximately $10,000 a year. In February of 1927 a letter in the *Herald Tribune* flayed the Met for ignoring younger artists. Its author, the architect Charles Downing Lay, wrote, "So far as one can judge from the Hearn collection, American art might have ceased in 1913." The museum's president, Robert de Forest, admitted to a surplus and agreed to disperse it. A month later, the entire sum of $90,000 was spent on one picture—the *Portrait of the Wyndham Sisters*, painted in 1900 by the late John S. Sargent.

The widespread institutional antipathy and apathy toward the new was enforced by director Robinson. A by-the-rules Bostonian and a classical archaeologist educated in the German university system, Robinson was tall, thin, precise, and dry. He was a professional museum man and a disciplined scholar in his field, but he had no sympathy for art not based on the classical canon as he saw it. Accordingly, he could discover nothing of value in American art. Forbes said that Robinson was a complete authoritarian, writing that he "was old school in his own day. He was not a modern director but a guardian of sacred premises. . . . In the Robinson reign to criticize anything done or acquired by the Museum was looked upon him as *lèse majesty*. He indicated clearly what he thought of such treasonable behavior." This was the man who would be offered Gertrude's unorthodox, uneven, upstart collection.

On that October morning of Juliana's appointment with Dr. Robinson, Forbes, who knew about the meeting, joined Gertrude at her studio to await the outcome. They were alone for an unexpectedly short time. Juliana returned to MacDougal Alley in a sputtering fury, and the whole story tumbled out. After some polite conversation, Juliana disclosed Gertrude's wish to join her collection to the Metropolitan's. Before she could say a word about Gertrude's willingness to build a wing to house her gift, Robinson stopped her from going on. Mrs. Whitney, of course, was a charming woman and a great philanthropist, but her request was impossible. There were practicalities to be considered. Dismissing the thought once and for all, Robinson sniffed, "What will we do with them, my dear lady? We have a cellar full of those things already."

Juliana heard no more. She stalked angrily out of the office, barely containing her rage. She had been flatly and mockingly refused and Gertrude had been treated with stunning condescension. She had failed in this, the great mission.

*See Chapter 5, p. 173.

Or had she? Was her failure a defeat or a canny victory? After all, Juliana's dream was to start an independent institution, not become a component of another. It is very possible that Juliana broached the subject with Robinson in such a way that she could hold off mentioning the proposed endowment until the last moment, gambling that the collection would be turned down, and she could exit before bringing up the big prize. Juliana was guileful enough for that, and it is extremely tempting to believe that her presentation, by artful arrangement and omission, sabotaged its chances of acceptance. But both Forbes Watson and Lloyd Goodrich stated that Robinson's dislike of American art was so pronounced that nothing would have induced him to take the Whitney collection. Citing the "pontifical manner" and "schoolmaster methods" of Robinson when he met the press, Forbes wrote, "During many years of covering Dr. Robinson's press conferences at the Metropolitan I did not once hear him mention a living American artist. . . . He would have had to look up the artists whose work was included in the [Whitney] gift." Goodrich, who also attended those conferences, said that they were terribly stuffy. He would go in hopes of expecting to hear some real "news," but Robinson would read a report on the latest addition to the Assyrian holdings. "Why don't you ever say anything about modern art?" Goodrich would wonder.

Forbes, however, did confirm that Juliana was not above using sharp rhetorical strategy when she needed it. After Juliana recounted the details of the Metropolitan's rejection, she, Forbes, and Gertrude adjourned to a nearby restaurant for a lunch that would stretch on into the afternoon. Watson wrote about that day:

> Dr. Robinson treated the offer with the surprised disdain which Mrs. Force described, on her return to the studio, with such sharp wit that we were hilarious throughout lunch.
>
> The wit was neither kindly nor innocent. It had a purpose—to keep the collection going in spite of the lack of space in which to show it.

Forbes said that neither he nor Juliana brought up the idea of a museum at first. Perhaps they felt that Gertrude, once she had adjusted to Robinson's refusal, needed time to regroup and think positively again. "Then," Watson wrote, "it [establishing a museum] was tossed back and forth between us three like a bean bag and each time that one of us caught it we put another bean into it. Before we parted in the late afternoon the idea had jelled and become serious. We were all excited, for this seemed to be a historic event in American art."

The accent on American was put there by all three at that long lunch, but it was Forbes who came up with the title. Maria Ealand, one of Watson's secretaries, said, "I'll never forget the time when Nan Watson fixed me with her long, stern stare and said, 'Don't you ever forget that it was Forbes's idea that it should be called the Whitney Museum of *American* Art.'"

The succession of emotional states—devastation, resentment, determination, resolution, jubilation—that Juliana and Gertrude experienced over those few hours seemed to rekindle their passion for experiment and their obligation to their own accomplishment. They recognized the need to regain the initiative

that had somehow been lost in the Whitney Studio Galleries, an initiative rapidly being seized by the new Museum of Modern Art. In Forbes's words:

> The great adventure of a museum would raise the collection out of storage darkness into gallery light for the world to see. Also, and I think the thought excited them with a sense of daring, it would jump the place out of the amateur class into the professional. This would really be doing something for the artists. And for the ladies what fun! Not how noble! No saving the republic! No righteous godliness! Only the daring and excitement that makes life living. For the first time they could see as a whole their achievement which now they saw piecemeal. Mrs. Whitney made up her mind swiftly and gaily.
>
> Before lunch was over Mrs. Force was made director. She was delighted and a little stunned. When she protested Mrs. Whitney said to her: "Either you'll be director or we won't do it." That was perhaps the happiest second in Mrs. Force's life. Half a dozen artists were suggested as preliminary informal advisers. It is noteworthy that neither Mrs. Force nor Mrs. Whitney thought of getting advice from the officers of established museums. Later they may have. At the moment they only thought of help from the artists.

Forbes, in this tribute to Juliana written in 1949, avoided mentioning his own expectations of a formal role to play in the future Whitney Museum. Just as Juliana was proclaimed its director, he believed that he would emerge as more than an unofficial adviser. At the end of that heady day, climaxing in the birth of a new institution, he went back to his editorial offices at *The Arts*. Lloyd Goodrich, who was there working when he arrived, remembered, "Forbes walked in that afternoon and the first thing he said to me was, 'There's going to be a new museum of American art, and we're going to be right in the middle of it.' " The prophesy was only half-right. Forbes assumed that he, Goodrich, and *The Arts* would be crucial to Juliana's plans. What he could not know was that the nation was scarcely two weeks away from economic disaster.

CHAPTER EIGHT

DISTILLING THE AMERICAN FLAVOR

❦ *(1929–1932)* ❦

URING THE AUTUMN OF 1929, Juliana and Gertrude kept their momentous decision largely to themselves. It was business as usual at the Whitney Studio Galleries, while the particulars of the museum were worked out in secret. Gertrude needed to confer quietly with Harry and the Whitney business managers about bankrolling the institution, and there was little publicity value to be gained by an immediate disclosure: The critics were preparing for the premier art event of the season—the opening of the Museum of Modern Art. Moreover, the repercussions of the stock market crash on October 29, 1929, which plunged New York into panic and confusion, had to be gauged and adjusted for.

Traumatic though the Crash was, the *direct* involvement of most Americans with the stock market was less drastic than might be supposed. Out of a population of 75 million adults, 1.5 million were in the market; of these, about 600,000 traded on margin. The majority of artists affiliated with the Whitney, for example, were not personally touched by the initial debacle. But once the Crash deepened into the long economic slide of the Depression, their existence was threatened. By the end of 1930, more than 6 million people were out of work, art galleries were failing, and commissions and sales had dried up.

For Gertrude, Harry, and their wealthy peers, the situation was the opposite: The Crash struck them with the suddenness of the iceberg splitting the *Titanic*. The Whitneys took a beating in the market; B. H. Friedman estimated that Harry's stock portfolio was reduced from $200 million to $100 million and Gertrude's from $20 million to $10 million. But these sums did not reflect the

couple's other holdings in mines, industrial plants, residential and business real estate, antiques, art, and jewelry, which enabled them to ride out the disaster. And because of the demand for hard currency and precious metals, Harry's extensive mining interests, especially in gold, rose in value. In 1930 he was reported to have told his family, "One day you can tell your children that I'm one of the few who made money during the Crash and the Depression." No one, however, would have faulted Gertrude for giving up her art activities in reaction to the Crash; the museum was going to cost $100,000 to $125,000 a year to run. But she was determined to forge ahead, and Harry seconded her without objections. By 1929 his domination of their marriage had been over for some years. Now Gertrude was much the stronger, more vital, more outgoing figure, and Harry the dependent one. His health was chronically poor, and many of his physical complaints, such as liver disease, were alcohol-related. He was said to drink alone, behind locked doors.

To the best of her nephews' knowledge, Juliana did not play the stock market or make investments in bonds or securities. Doctor had been the wild speculator who fantasized about overnight wealth, but investing money was as unnatural to her as saving it. Whatever passed through her hands, she spent or gave to others. If emergencies came along, she sold what she had put her money into —art, antiques, and houses. (Because prudence was the last thing on Juliana's mind, her possessions were bought without thought for their future economic performance, but because of the acuity of her taste, they turned out to be far better buys than shares in such popular investments as the artificially booming industries and pyramid-based holding companies that evaporated early in the Depression.) During the 1930s, whenever the need arose, Juliana was able to sell, in small or large lots, her furniture, glassware, china, paintings, and properties. She did not always make a profit in her transactions, but at least she could retrieve her money from them.

Throughout November of 1929, Juliana proceeded as if she were trying not to notice that anything extraordinary had happened. She may have been registering the sense of unreality about the sudden financial collapse: Could a decade of prosperity and the greatest bull market in history be obliterated within the course of a week? More knowledgeable persons than she refused to believe that a catastrophe had occurred. Newspapers were running optimistic editorials, President Hoover and Secretary of the Treasury Andrew Mellon were giving assurances that the nation's economy was sound, and the governor of New York, Franklin D. Roosevelt, referred to the crisis on Wall Street as "the little flurry downtown." The distress, the authorities said, was only temporary.

Thus Juliana went on with what was expected of her: doing her unstinting best to aid and comfort independent artists and promote their work. As long as an artist could be at least *suspected* of merit, the principal criterion was financial hardship rather than aesthetic preference, but she remained open to the new and the individual, wherever it surfaced. About this time she befriended R. Buckminster Fuller, the inventor and self-appointed explainer of the universe, whom she met at Romany Marie's café, a Village restaurant much favored by artists. Then thirty-four, Fuller was recovering from a depression that had brought

him to the brink of suicide two years before. By 1929 he had evolved his Dymaxion house and had done some lecturing and writing, but he tended to be dismissed as an incompetent, a failure, and a crackpot. Short, sturdy, with owlish eyes blinking rapidly behind thick glasses and talking nonstop—Fuller liked to say that he averaged 7,000 words per hour—about his plans for improving the earth, Juliana's new acquaintance did have an element of the crank to him. But he was just as certainly an original of a classic American type that Juliana at once recognized and relished. She didn't subsidize him, but she warmed to him as someone who needed kindness and emotional support.

Fuller was then living on the top floor of an industrial building that spread over a city block. The space was huge—reminiscing in 1978, he likened it to a football field—and it rented for $30 a month. The catch was that the elevator was turned off after the office workers left, and Fuller had to walk up twenty stories every night. He would take whole parties of unsuspecting regulars from Romany Marie's there and remembered Juliana as being good sport enough to make the trip. Juliana, accustomed to hiking up many flights of stairs to top-floor studios and cold-water walk-ups, had experience in such matters. Attaining the summit, she would comment, "Artists live nearer heaven than anyone else."

Juliana's invitations to tea in her more accessible quarters and her general effervescence kept up Fuller's spirits when he was still unsure of himself and doubtful about reaching the public with his message. He said of Juliana, "I was one of the rather lucky people that she liked. She never picked on me, that's for certain. She defended me. She was interested in my ideas [the Dymaxion designs] and tried to draw me out. She didn't lecture. She put you on your mettle and she brought out the best in you. If she liked you, she was friendly and enthusiastic and let you show your best."

Like Fuller, Joseph Pollet, who had one-man shows on West Eighth Street in 1924 and 1929, was thankful that Juliana was not one to deliver sermons. Writing to her in 1930 about his past conduct, he said, "You've been patient with me a long time. I remember telling you . . . that if the country wouldn't support a genius like me, I would leave it flat. You must have grinned somewhere inside of yourself at so much presumption. You didn't bat an eye as I remember—I hope because you felt the sincerity of my belief. . . . Nevertheless, perhaps you won't mind that I'm through with that phase. I shall become very silent now and let canvases make my arguments."

Emlen Etting, a tall, elegant Philadelphian who later became one of Juliana's most trusted friends, made those same arguments to her in November of 1929. He left a portfolio of wash drawings at her door and came back a few mornings later, whereupon he was taken upstairs to her bedroom. Juliana, Etting was to write,

> had looked over my drawings, found them interesting and asked to keep them to show to a publisher. Then she told me to return, bringing a few canvases for her inspection. This was the first sign of significant interest anyone has shown in New York, so I left exhilarated, running up Fifth Avenue through an early snow flurry.

When he saw Juliana again, he asked her what had happened. She didn't say anything, but showed him a book of Japanese calligraphy. "It was," Etting explained, "her way of telling me that I needed more depth, and she was right. She had a way of twisting things around that was like lightning, as well as encouraging." Reflecting on this period of his life, he observed, "It was great people like Maxwell Perkins [from whom Etting also received advice] and Juliana Force, who through the mere fact of their attention did not squelch me, but made me realize the most important thing was to go out and achieve a body of work of some significance before expecting anyone to take notice."

Juliana expended a good amount of money and faith on Oscar Bluemner, one of the original American modernists. He had been associated with several galleries, was an intimate of the Stieglitz circle, and lived in Massachusetts. He had shown with Stieglitz in March of 1928, but later that year he turned to Juliana, who stored his unsold works and included him in the Whitney Studio Galleries' first Christmas sale. (Whether coincidental or not, after being assisted by Juliana, Bluemner never again showed with Stieglitz. In a letter dated February, 14, 1930, Bluemner reported to one of Juliana's secretaries, "Even my old friend Stieglitz has served notice on me to get out," but he didn't explain why he was expelled.)

Bluemner was a difficult man, but he and Juliana maintained an epistolary friendship. She respected Bluemner's powerful work and was extremely sympathetic to his long struggle. She approached his spiky, Teutonic personality and rambling manifestoes with delicacy, evidently sensing the mental turmoil beneath. (In 1938 Bluemner, depressed by ill health and poverty, cut his throat.) But Juliana brought out the artist's sense of humor: He once drew a miniature silhouette of her, in which she is seen at one of his exhibitions. Hat pitched forward at a 45-degree angle, she puffs smoke from a cigarette in a long holder and says, "I told him."

Bluemner, in short, thought Juliana was a "grand lady"—she won him over by providing help that did not bruise the ultrasensitive artist's dignity. From November 4 to 29, 1929, the Galleries presented twenty-five of his paintings, twenty of which were new abstractions remarkable for their emotive symbolism. She then purchased the 1929 *Last Evening of the Year* for $500 and *Old Canal Port* of 1914 for $1,000, marked down from $1,500 especially for her.* Both were superb bargains, especially the latter painting, an emphatic composition in the artist's characteristic reds and yellows. Bluemner was an important artist not yet represented in the Whitney collection, and these acquisitions are evidence

---

*The records kept for the Bluemner sales—which were better than the norm because they *exist*—illuminate the difficulties in ascertaining how or why works of art were assigned to the Whitney-Force collections. *Last Evening of the Year* was recorded as being sold to "Mrs. W. B. Force," whereas *Old Canal Port* was recorded as sold to "Mrs. H. P. Whitney." Yet it was Juliana who bought both paintings, and they, in turn, immediately entered the collection of the new museum. Bluemner, who as a rule kept obsessively careful records, is equally unhelpful in this instance. He wrote in his catalog next to the listing for *Last Evening of the Year*, "Mrs. Force bought and gave it to the Museum."

that although not yet publicly advertised, the museum and the need to buy for it were foremost in Juliana's mind. The future institution took precedence over the tempestuous economic climate.

Juliana went even further for John Steuart Curry, whose name would soon be linked with those of Thomas Hart Benton and Grant Wood as the leading exponents of Regionalist painting. Born on a Kansas farm, Curry was a professional illustrator who decided in 1925 to become a painter. He was one of the last to join the Whitney Studio Club, becoming a member in 1928. Curry had difficulty with draftsmanship: He drew slowly and worked laboriously over his studies of the nude. He attracted notice at the Club's sketch classes because of his arguments with Reginald Marsh, whose pencil skimmed over sheets of paper as fleetly as the wind, about the length of time the model should hold a pose. Juliana saw something in Curry's awkward sketches that showed promise. * She offered him an allowance of $200 a month so that he could not only work unhindered, but spend more time in the Midwest. Curry thought that if he returned to his parents' farm in Kansas, he might find inspiration in his rural roots. His stipend commenced in 1928 and lasted for two years; it was subject to renewal every six months.

As Curry realized, studio nudes were not his métier. His true subject was the plain folks at home. Especially drawn to religious rituals and social customs of farming families, he painted *Baptism in Kansas*, which portrays a young woman being baptized in an open horse trough, surrounded by a crowd of hymn-singing neighbors. Dramatic and homespun, the picture excited critics when it was exhibited at the Corcoran Gallery of Art in the summer of 1928. Curry suddenly acquired a name and a reputation, and *Baptism in Kansas* became the first well-known emblem of the burgeoning movement known as American Scene painting. Curry's painting and its reception earned the American Scene a wider public, but the movement's true icon would not appear until 1930—that would be Grant Wood's *American Gothic*, owned by the Art Institute of Chicago.

Baptism in Kansas touched off a wave of positive response, one that been gaining in momentum since the middle 1920s. In parallel to the country's political isolation, native artists were exhorted to "Paint America," especially the regions other than the Northeast. The American Scene, particularly when it encompassed the Midwest and was labeled Regionalism, radiated not only an aura of self-conscious virtue attached to ruralism, but an intolerance of internationalism. Its partisans spelled out their opposition to other cultures in an excess of rules and rhetoric: Painters were to cleanse their brushes of big-city ways and foreign influences, especially the poisonous taint of Cubism. Chauvinist critics accused the School of Paris of being a corrupt old libertine sapping the vigor and personality of healthy, red-blooded Americans trapped in its pes-

---

* In an interview, Mrs. John Steuart Curry said that her husband told her that it was Gertrude who admired him and initiated the stipend, not Juliana. Curry felt that Juliana was not very interested in his work. However, all the surviving correspondence, which commences in 1929, is between Juliana and Curry and relates to judgments made by Juliana.

tilent foreign grip. Modernist art and American art were redefined as mutually exclusive: To make a truly national art, painters should depict the hinterlands in realistic, easily readable styles. These demands, which reduced art to a social message and implied that abstraction was unpatriotic, began to make inroads because they came from influential voices. Peyton Boswell, Sr., the editor of the *Art Digest*, and Thomas Craven, a xenophobic critic who took pride in becoming the chief ideologue of the period, were the busiest and shrillest supporters of the movement, but other critics indulged in some eagle-screaming, too. Even Forbes, normally so liberal and fair-minded, began to take a disappointingly more conservative and dogmatic position toward the French. Disgusted by the numerous Americans he saw turning themselves into secondhand Parisians and the French dealers who were dumping inferior wares on the New York art market, he ascribed such opportunism and cynicism to the art itself. Being less subservient to Europe and avant-garde experiments, he believed, would do most American artists some good.

Forbes's embrace of nativism signaled that he had evolved from a formalist critic who learned from Roger Fry to one who judged art primarily on the basis of how it fit in with his activist positions, but his judgment was not completely obscured. For an antidote to French painting, he recommended not the folksy narratives of Curry, Wood, and Benton, but the outdoor scenes and architectural portraits of Hopper and Burchfield, who were the real pioneers in the rediscovery of small-town America.* Forbes knew too much about art to be seduced by strident jingoism and painters whose pictorial processes were subsumed to nostalgic local anecdotes. Burchfield and Hopper, with their subtle formal qualities and more complex attitudes toward their motifs, seemed to him the immutable and authentic figures.

Juliana avoided formulating any narrow definition of American art in her public statements. Her concern was for artists as individuals, but because of the power she held in the art world, her early assistance to painters who would *later* become two of the movement's leading lights was interpreted as a vote of confidence in the broader Regionalist movement. Juliana's patronage enhanced the prestige of American Scene painting as a whole and gave it extra visibility. She was not only a benefactress of Curry, but of Thomas Hart Benton, who had exhibited his first American historical murals† at the Whitney Studio Club in 1925. Beginning in 1930 and culminating in 1932, Juliana's furtherance of Benton's reputation would surpass in importance anything she had done for Curry. However, the art of Grant Wood, the third prominent Regionalist painter, did not appeal to her. Wood was also at a disadvantage with Juliana because, unlike Benton and Curry, he had never lived in New York or joined the Club, which meant that Juliana did not get to know him. She first declined to buy one of Wood's pictures in January of 1931, several months after he had

---

*Both Hopper and Burchfield vehemently disliked being linked with Regionalism in any guise. For that matter, Curry did not enjoy being typecast as a Regionalist either. He would frequently (and correctly) point out that his ideas had crystallized well before the movement had coalesced.

†The *American Historical Epic*, now in the collection of the Nelson-Atkins Museum of Art.

achieved instant fame with *American Gothic*. Wood was included in the museum's first invitational show in 1932, but when he offered her two paintings, she refused point-blank to buy either of them.* Juliana was unswayed by the phenomenal success of *American Gothic*, but in 1933 she bought two of Wood's drawings. †

Now, in the fall of 1929, Curry was hoping to have his allowance renewed. He sent *Baptism in Kansas* to Eighth Street for Juliana to inspect and possibly buy. (In return for financial support, she probably had the right of first refusal.) Juliana's response was positive: Curry's allowance would go on, and he would be given his first one-man show, to open in late January of 1930. From the Whitney show, Juliana bought *Baptism in Kansas* for $300, as well as *The Stockman* (a portrait of the artist's father) for $500, *The Ne'er-Do-Well* (migrants crossing the plains in a covered wagon), and a watercolor of horses running in a storm. The critics fell over themselves in applauding Curry's stories of the farm belt, and several other paintings first seen in the Whitney show would enter public collections. Later that year, the *Times* went so far as to announce that "Kansas has found her Homer." As Curry's biographer observed, the purchases and rave notices were "not a recognition of the artist alone, but a reflection of the rising tide of social conflict and consciousness that characterized the period." To these reasons might be added that of a hunger for reassurance in an increasingly alarming world.

Rabid flag-waving for art became so pervasive that even Henry McBride, a stout internationalist, could be seized by it. This was demonstrated in the course of another exhibition Juliana arranged. On November 25, 1929, she opened an exhibition of watercolors by Stuart Davis, Mark Baum, Richard Lahey, and Paul Rohland—a typically Whitney mixture that hung the accomplished with the promising and the experimental with the conventional. McBride, in reviewing the show, devoted most of his space to Davis, saying that he was "the best delver into the abstract that we have." But he scolded Davis for being too Parisian. "[I]f Picasso and Braque had never lived this artist of ours would have had to think out a method for himself," he wrote. "It sticks in my gorge a trifle to see a swell American painter painting French."

These words elicited a reprimand. That a confirmed and sophisticated member of the avant-garde like McBride was susceptible to such chauvinist nonsense was too much for Davis to accept in silence. In an open letter to *Creative Art*, a magazine McBride edited, he wrote:

> In speaking of French art as opposed to American the assumption is made that there is an American art. Where is it and how does one recognize it? Has any American

---

*Juliana was offered the lackluster *Arnold Comes of Age* (now in the collection of the Sheldon Memorial Art Gallery, University of Nebraska–Lincoln) and the better yet nonetheless overdetermined *Stone City* (now in the collection of the Joslyn Art Museum).

† Studies for *Dinner for Threshers*, or at least labeled as such. Wood drew them so he could have something to submit to the Whitney.

artist created a style which was unique in painting, completely divorced from European models? To soften this flock of hard questions I will answer the last,—no, J. S. Copley was working in the style of the English portrait painters and to my taste doing better work than they did. Whistler's best work was directly inspired by the Japanese while he was housed and fed in England. . . . I have never heard the names of the European masters that Eakins particularly admired but from his work I should say they included Rembrandt and Velasquez. These painters are now regarded as the best that America has produced. Suppose a selected show of the painting of Europe and America for the last four hundred years were held, would the American contribution stand isolated as a distinct point of view, unrelated to the European? Again the answer is, no. . . .

[Picasso] has been the dominant painter of the world for the last twenty years and there are very few of the young painters of any country who have not been influenced by him. The ones who were not, simply chose some other artist to be influenced by.

I did not spring into the world fully equipped to paint the kind of pictures I want to paint. It was therefore necessary to ask people for advice [and seek other sources of information]. . . . This process of learning is from my observation identical with that followed by all artists. The only variation lies in the choice of work to be studied. . . . But why one should be penalized for a Picasso influence and not for a Rembrandt or a Renoir influence I can't understand.

Davis's rebuttal is worth quoting because it seizes on the basic inconsistency of American Scene painting. Benton, who spent many years in Paris, dabbled in Synchromism and other variants of color abstraction in his youth; in his mature "American" phase, the knobby, elongated figures that writhed across his canvases were a cracker-barrel translation of Tintoretto. Wood first painted in an uninspired Barbizon style. He did not take on his tight, neat "Regionalist" look until after a trip to Europe, where he studied the Flemish and German masters. Curry owed a debt to Courbet, Rubens, and Baroque painting. In all three instances, the Americans were responding to the Old Masters' formal qualities, not their subject matter, thus undercutting the American Scene's central premise that local or national content had priority over aesthetic factors. Why then were these painters who borrowed from the past certified as "free of foreign influences" and 100 percent American, while those who looked to Picasso, Léger, and other modern masters were labeled as epigones and slaves? Davis's question, "Why should one be penalized for a Picasso influence and not for a Rembrandt or a Renoir influence?" was an astute one, but it was ignored for the rest of the decade.

By December of 1929, the long-term economic decline provoked by the Crash began to sink in, and Juliana was curtailing the Galleries' exhibition schedule. The show she had arranged for Cecil Howard was canceled because of the expense of transporting his work from Paris, as were two group exhibitions. In canceling another one-man show, Juliana wrote to the painter who was dropped that she had to renege "on account of the financial state of affairs which seems to be growing worse instead of better. . . . It costs so much to put a show

over, and so little can be expected as returns, because of the existing financial conditions." But Juliana being Juliana, her human impulses once again overcame practical exigencies. She could not bring herself to give up a show of Gerard Cochet's paintings, an exhibition for which there would be very little public. Cochet was a French painter who had been gravely wounded during the war. He had lost one eye in combat and the vision in the other one was severely impaired, but he was still attempting to work. Juliana met him in Paris during the summer of 1929 through Cecil Howard and had a group of canvases sent to West Eighth Street. Not one was sold. Juliana, who had all the works framed at the Galleries' expense, then bought two works and got some friends of hers to do the same.

During the last two months of 1929, Juliana walked a secret and delicate line. The belt-tightening necessitated by an unstable economy alternated with the excitement, enlargement, and newness a museum promised. Her own natural expansiveness and enjoyment of disbursing funds had to be restrained while money went to the expenditures demanded by a museum. In the midst of denying artists their shows, she hired a staff of four, three of whom would be practicing artists.

The man Juliana chose as head curator was Hermon More, a painter of romantic landscapes who joined the Whitney Studio Club in 1924 and had some practical experience in running an art gallery. From 1928 to 1929, he was director of the Davenport (Iowa) Municipal Gallery, where he had also taught for some years. He lived in Woodstock during the summers and was identified as a Woodstock artist. Tall, heavyset, and extremely shy, More was esteemed by his fellow artists for his sensitivity and judgment. He was remarkable for a self-effacement unusual to someone in his profession—he was glad to spend most of his life advancing the careers of other artists. More's modesty was matched by his physical stoicism. He had contracted encephalitis after World War I, which left him severely lame and partially paralyzed, but he put in long hours at the Whitney caring for the collection, arranging loans, and planning exhibitions. He also made the rounds of galleries and studios, no matter how many flights of stairs lay ahead of him. More's forte was the hanging of shows, and he was responsible for the layout, disposition, and general appearance of the galleries after 1930. He shared Juliana and Gertrude's conviction that exhibition spaces should not be halls but intimate rooms. During its years on Eighth Street, the museum was lauded for the expressiveness of its installations, and the credit for it should go to More.

Juliana became very fond of Hermon and his wife, Edna, and when she visited Woodstock, she often stayed with them. In the city, Juliana would have dinner with the Mores about once a week, according to Donn Mosenfelder, the Mores' nephew. He remembered the three of them—"all compulsive smokers"—sitting around and talking as the cigarette butts overflowed their ashtrays. Put more accurately, Juliana and Edna would chatter away, waving their cigarettes like batons as they conducted their conversation. Hermon occasionally inserted a word but was content to blow smoke and listen. His affability and equilibrium ensured his suitability as Juliana's second. Much as she liked

to have dashing people around her after hours, Juliana could not have worked with her flamboyant friends for very long. She herself had more than enough vividness to go around. Her autocratic ways sometimes grated on the Mores, but they knew how to avoid antagonizing her. Thus Juliana and Hermon remained a productive team, and the three of them enjoyed a personal and professional friendship that grew richer and closer with the years.

In addition to Hermon More, Juliana hired two other painters—Edmund Archer and Karl Free. They were made assistant curators, in charge, respectively, of drawings and watercolors. Both men had exhibited in various Whitney shows. Eleanor Lambert, who had worked as a free-lance publicist for the Club and the Galleries, continued as a part-time publicity manager. Mungo, who'd been getting $100 a month plus a 5 percent commission on any sales she made at the Galleries but was no one's idea of museum material, would be transferred to Juliana's personal retinue.

Everyone's responsibilities were discussed and apportioned, but Juliana took care to keep most of the power concentrated in her own hands. The curators were to be on the lookout for art, and they might make suggestions, but they could not buy anything independently. A letter written to Edith Halpert from Juliana's head secretary makes this plain. "Since Mrs. Force has the entire responsibility of purchasing pictures for the Museum," the dealer was told, "she would like you to please address all correspondence pertaining to purchases to her. She has instructed all the members of the museum Staff to refer to her any pictures of interest that they discover during their Gallery rounds, but she wants them to be relieved of the burden of the financial phase of these matters."

Beyond collecting and showing, the museum would embark on the previously ignored areas of research and publication. One such program, presumably suggested by Forbes but dear to Juliana's heart, was the commissioning of illustrated books on living American artists, which was then an innovative proposal. Juliana would ultimately recruit sixteen different authors to write the essays for the twenty-one books making up the series, but at first she hoped to find a staff writer responsible for them all. The ideal candidate seemed to be Lloyd Goodrich, the editor at *The Arts* who had written the graceful catalog for The Circus in Paint. Goodrich remembered:

> Mrs. Force asked me to come see her and invited me to join the staff of the museum to write monographs on living American artists. Reg Marsh had just lent me $500 to write my book on Thomas Eakins. I told her I had started my book and I had an obligation to finish that, and I wasn't so sure I wanted to write on some of those artists anyway. I declined the position and thought that was the end of that. Then about a week later, Mrs. Force asked me to come over and see her again and said, "Would you accept a salary of $5,000 a year to write your book on Eakins?" This was really a godsend—$5,000 a year, in those days was a fortune. At *The Arts* I'd been getting about $75 a week. So for about three years, I was in the fortunate position of just writing and being paid a salary for it.

Juliana was rampantly unscholarly herself, and the resulting "monographs" were not full treatments of the artists under discussion but impressionistic reviews

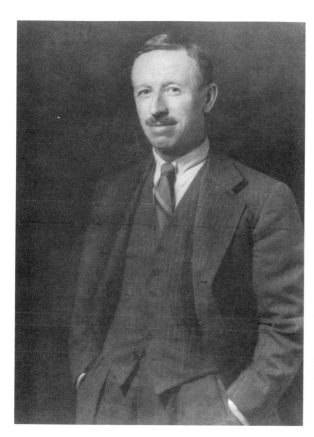

Hired to do some writing at the Whitney by Juliana, Lloyd Goodrich worked at the museum until 1968, when he retired as director. As director emeritus, he was an active presence at the Whitney until his death in 1987.

accompanied by reproductions. Yet in hiring Goodrich and letting him pursue his research in nineteenth-century painting, she did much to stimulate scholarship in American art. After accepting the job, Goodrich suggested the title of "research curator" for himself. One cannot curate research, but the ungainly title stood until 1947.

Word was evidently leaking out about the museum, for on December 2, 1929, Glenn O. Coleman wrote to Juliana about some stories by McBride on the Museum of Modern Art in which he invoked the Whitney Studio Club. McBride praised the Modern's inaugural exhibition of Seurat, Van Gogh, Gauguin, and Cézanne and the high standards of the entire enterprise, but he wished that an institution would stand up for American painting as impressively as the Modern had for the pillars of European modernism. "Except for its lack of a permanent collection of works of art," he remarked, "the Whitney Studio Club has been doing Luxembourg work for quite some time, and doing it well. Also, it seldom forgets to be American." Asking Juliana if she'd read the review, Coleman wondered if Gertrude might consider starting such a museum as she had done so much in that direction already. The purpose of the letter seemed

to be to get confirmation that the rumor of a nascent museum of contemporary American art was true. In reply, Juliana permitted herself a discreet but promising hint. "If you will have just a little more patience," she wrote, "I think you will see something that will please you. This is all that I can say at present."

But to museum men, Juliana was more forthcoming. George William Eggers, the director of the Worcester Art Museum, was organizing an exhibition of American paintings traveling to the Swedish Royal Academy of Art. He wished to borrow eight pictures from the Whitney collection, and in early December he came down to New York to speak with Juliana about the loans. She obviously told him about the museum, for in writing to her on December 17 to seal the loan agreement, he added, "You have quite opened my eyes to some new values in American art. The new scheme for 'distilling the American flavor' in a specialized museum is an inspired idea and I know it will meet with the success it deserves."

An exchange of confidences was not known to have occurred between Juliana and Dr. Albert Barnes, who showed up unannounced one stormy afternoon shortly after Goodrich had signed on as research curator. On presenting himself at West Eighth Street, he was escorted upstairs to Juliana's apartment. Astonishingly, the pugnacious Philadelphian was trying to be sociable. Juliana had still never visited the Barnes Foundation, but she knew what it contained. Aware of Barnes's interests, she pointed to her two paintings by Henri Rousseau and said, "If ever you want Rousseau, well, there you have him!" The parlor congenialities were suddenly terminated. Barnes picked up his coat and umbrella and lumbered grumpily downstairs. The large, bearlike form stopped at Goodrich's office to roar, "I came to pay a call, and she tried to sell me a Rousseau!"

Another indicator that something was afoot was an increase in Juliana's buying during November and December of 1929. From the Bluemner show, the four-man watercolor show, and a Christmas sale of small works by 150 different artists, she bought thirty-four works from eighteen artists for a total of $2,490. The most important of these purchases were the two paintings by Bluemner, a gouache and four lithographs of Paris city scenes (at $15 each) by Davis, and a gouache by Coleman. Augmenting what she selected from her own galleries, Juliana bought graphic works by fourteen artists from the Downtown Gallery for just over $400.

Juliana's acquisition of a significant group of prints and drawings that were not on view at her own galleries was too suspicious for the art world to ignore, and the long silence was over. On January 3, 1930, she held a press conference. Juliana announced that Gertrude had decided to endow the first museum dedicated exclusively to native—and predominantly twentieth-century—art. Her collection, numbering close to 500 objects,* would form the nucleus of the museum's permanent holdings. Gertrude was not there at this historic

---

*On account of the scanty records and the pooling of Juliana's and Gertrude's personal collections, an exact figure for the Whitney holdings before 1930 cannot be determined. However, the number of works was probably close to 500. By the time the museum opened, another 200 works had been added to the permanent collection.

moment—she had just sailed for France to do research for a memorial to Marshal Foch. Juliana read a statement in Gertrude's name and credited her with the prospectus and impetus for the new enterprise, to be called the Whitney Museum of American Art. First making it clear that the Whitney would attempt to survey and examine three centuries of the fine arts in America, she then went on to explain a crucial difference between the new museum and other institutions. The Whitney would not fall victim to the cold, unfeeling relationship that so often existed between artists and museums:

> Ever since museums were invented, contemporary liberal artists have had difficulties in "crashing the gate." Museums have had the habit of waiting until a painter or sculptor had acquired a certain official recognition before they would accept his work within their sacred portals. Exactly the contrary practice will be carried on in the Whitney Museum of American Art.
>
> A vigorous campaign of acquisitions in the effort to discover fresh talents and to stimulate the creative spirit of the artist before it has deadened by old age is perhaps the chief object of Mrs. Whitney in founding the new museum.

Reactions to the announcement ranged from satisfaction to euphoria. Approval was unanimous because it was the logical conclusion of what had gone before; furthermore, the art world had grown used to Gertrude as a patroness of the arts. And overall, with the country turning inward, Gertrude and Juliana's pioneering belief that the art of a nation was of great importance to the life of its people had attained respectability.

In Greenwich Village, the artists were going about in a blissful daze, their feet barely scraping the ground. Their reason for being would be validated by the dignity and prestige of a museum. As Juliana would write in 1931:

> The word "museum" has an awesome sound. It frightens and intimidates on the outside and it paralyzes thought on the inside. Horace Walpole defined a museum as "a hospital for everything that is singular." Yet the general impression which the word museum leaves is one of dignity and authority. To the onlooker there is a vast difference between a picture in a museum (if it is not in the cellar) and a picture in a studio or in a gallery. The public is impressed, and rightly so. For, ordinarily, a work of art is acquired by a museum with deliberate intent to add to the importance and usefulness of that museum, and the public is duly impressed with the weight of the authority which sees when a painting is good and by the act of acquiring it pronounces it so.

American artists, even as they flocked to the Museum of Modern Art's compelling exhibitions, recognized that its international aims and sharply argued definition of modernity would by nature preclude extensive concentration on the home talent. In the Whitney lay their hopes for a place in the pantheon. And if the Modern was too advanced, the Metropolitan, a bastion of the official art world, was still unready for even the liberal. Director Robinson, whose rejection of Gertrude's collection goaded her museum into being, pronounced the new venture "a very interesting scheme."

With the secret out and congratulations warmer than Dr. Robinson's pouring in, Juliana turned once more to striving artists and the final season at the Whitney

Studio Galleries. Two shows seem to be vigorously hers, as if she wanted to stamp her own signature on the Galleries one last time before the advent of the museum, when her efforts would be commingled with her staff's and the achievements no longer hers alone.

The first exhibition, which ran from February 26 to March 8, 1930, was called Four Sunday Painters and reflected Juliana's interest in naive and self-taught artists. Of the group, the notable discovery was Beauford Delaney, a young black artist who would later become known for his portraits and lyrical abstractions. Delaney had come to New York in 1929, and Juliana was one of the first to buy his pastels. He was not a naive or Sunday painter in the conventional sense of the phrase, but a trained artist who, because of his race, could get only low-paying jobs. He had to work more hours to support himself, and he had correspondingly less time to paint. But at the Whitney Galleries he had three oils and nine pastels to show. Juliana purchased two pastels and offered him a longer-lasting source of income. The museum would need a guard, and Juliana asked him to take the job. Besides his salary, he would receive free studio and living space in the basement. Delaney worked at the Whitney for about three years. Depending on what was required, his duties were those of a guard, gallery attendant, telephone operator, and caretaker.

The second exhibition, the last the Whitney Galleries would ever hold, was a group show of flower paintings by forty-nine artists long associated with West Eighth Street. Romantic, decorative, and felicitously presented, the show was pure Juliana. Before its opening on March 17, 1930, Juliana worked hard to make Flowers in Art a success equal to The Circus in Paint, its model in gaiety and tone. She turned four galleries into a garden party—a bower garnished with rustic lattices, green hedgerows, and Victorian cast-iron benches. The ceilings were hidden by tented hangings, the floors were laid with a grass-green covering, and the walls were painted pink. After the flower show closed on March 29, 1930, there were no more exhibitions for another twenty months. When the building reopened, it was as a museum with selections from the permanent collection on the walls.

The shift from the autonomy of private patronage to the accountability of a stringently scrutinized public institution was to be a wrenching one. Juliana "had no fears in her amateur days," said Forbes, "but a great fear attacked her when she was called upon to act like a professional." She and Gertrude were moving into untraversed and unique terrain. The Addison Gallery of American Art, which collected and exhibited contemporary and historical work, was still in the process of being formed. The places closest in spirit to the Whitney but by no means identical to it were the Newark Museum, long active in native art and design, and the Phillips Collection, which showed nineteenth- and twentieth-century works in a gracious, homey setting. There were bound to be about-faces and contradictions, as the women's next foray into policymaking would demonstrate. Two months after her initial announcement, Juliana had to issue her first retraction.

In March of 1930, Juliana held another press conference. She announced the curatorial appointments and confirmed that the museum would remain in

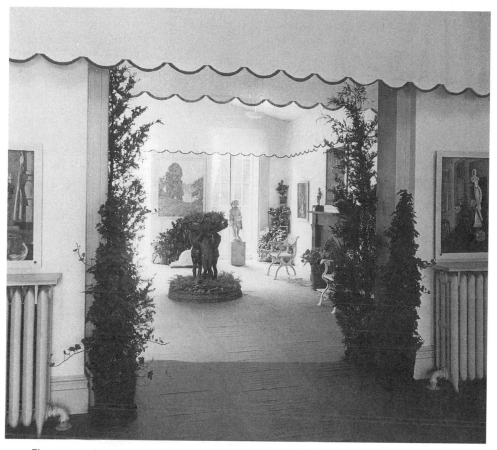

Flowers in Art, Juliana's farewell bouquet to the Whitney's informal past. Right of door: *Soap and Wax* by Glenn O. Coleman; left of door: *Arrangement* by Louis Bouché; center: Arlington Fountain by Gertrude Whitney.

remodeled quarters at Nos. 8 and 10 West Eighth Street. The primary purpose of the gathering was to correct an earlier impression that the museum would continue to be a threshold for young artists. Juliana now stated, "While this museum will emphatically not be a repository for relics, no museum can be a place for experiment. It is no longer necessary for this organization to help young artists to gain a hearing. What is now needed is a depot where the public may see fine examples of America's artistic production, and it is this need which we hope to fill. The purchasing fund is to be a large part of our endowment and acquisition one of our most important functions, but our objective will be the formation of a collection of pictures and other works of art whose merit alone make them worthy of being preserved in a public collection."

Juliana and Gertrude amended their original statement in order to make it understood that the museum could not merely reprise the Studio Club. Their modification tacitly acknowledged that the Club had more often been interesting

than good. They now had to effect a transition from their former agenda of art collecting, which had been ruled by emotion and personal impulse (Juliana, without regard to order or system, buying objects because she liked them or because the artist was in distress), to a more cerebral enterprise (Juliana, with an eye toward posterity, buying objects for their historical and aesthetic significance because the museum should have them). Encouragement, the women now proposed, was not the duty of a public institution.

Even as Juliana announced this, the spadework she and Gertrude had done over the last decade was being vindicated by the Museum of Modern Art, which mounted two group shows of American art in quick succession. Of the nineteen painters in the first exhibition, twelve were Whitney regulars. In the second show, which was devoted to painters and sculptors under the age of thirty-five and mounted "to prove the artistic vitality of the younger generation," one third of the participants had received earlier exposure at the Whitney. Thus Juliana and Gertrude, who had been known to buy and show for all kinds of extra-artistic reasons and whose record of generosity was unequaled, could assert that it was time to put a premium on quality while reveling in the fact that their "amateur" instincts were now crowned by approval from the Museum of Modern Art.

No one would quarrel with the idea of making fewer but better purchases, but the degree of experiment and alignment with the new to which the museum could lend itself was an issue that was never satisfactorily resolved. Juliana changed her second, sterner statement in 1931. Allowing that topicality could be ignored only at the expense of vitality, that the Whitney could not be divorced from the art life bubbling around it, she would write, "Art, like history, is made in the present, and the historian adds to his true value if he has lived and felt in the epoch which he records." Paradoxically, in trying to be more discriminating and authoritative, the museum sometimes regressed. It became less innovative and more prescriptive in the handling of contemporary art. The original organizing principle—to create an exclusively and unabashedly American museum—and then persevere with it during the depths of the Depression was the great and valorous goal, and the one that endured. Most of the verve, vision, and daring of that idea was spent on the overall conception of founding a museum of national art where none had existed and making that museum stand for something. Less reflection was given to the fine points within the larger framework. This way of thinking—scanting the melancholy but crucial details—had serious limitations. The implications of adopting certain policies were not foreseen, which boxed the museum into unnecessary traps of its own devising.

One assumption that was not sufficiently reevaluated was the setting of the museum's boundaries. The Club and Galleries had followed the traditional rankings of the fine arts: Painting and sculpture were treated as the major art forms, and prints, drawings, and watercolors were adjuncts to be pursued more modestly. Neither Juliana nor her curators saw fit to expand their concerns into a richer and more informative presentation of the visual arts. They neglected American architecture, design, and photography, so their perspective on American culture was not as lively, exploratory, or wide-ranging as it should have

been. And as a consequence of these blind spots, the museum also missed some spectacular buys offered by artists in bad straits during the Depression. In 1936, for example, Edward Weston volunteered to print 250 of his best photographs for the Whitney at the bargain-basement price of $1,000. Hermon More, in rejecting the offer, wrote to Weston that "we have not attempted to inaugurate a collection of photographs and have not given the matter of forming such a collection sufficient thought to enable us to give a definite opinion as to the advisability of such a course."

The museum backed itself into another unfortunate corner in trying to avoid pressure from dealers, donors, artists, and others eager to push their own interests. Shielding the museum from improper influence was not an insignificant problem because the Whitney was wrapped up with living artists, many of whom resided within blocks of its doors. Furthermore, the museum lacked the protection of trustees. The latter arrangement, from Juliana's point of view, was a glorious blessing and was perceived as such by other museum directors and curators, who practically swooned with envy when they learned of it. Several of them, in sending messages of goodwill to Juliana on the founding of the museum, told her not to let any trustees ruin it. While Juliana and the Whitney enjoyed a freedom that only a trusteeless institution could enjoy, Juliana had no recourse to the shelter that trustees afforded. If she chose wisely, the credit accrued, but every mistake was all hers. Gertrude was an exemplary founder in that she stepped aside and left the administration of the museum to her staff. In 1930 her main interests were sculpting, writing, travel, and family, and they, rather than the directing of the museum, were what engaged her. She watched over the museum, of course, and very occasionally she selected a work of sculpture for purchase, but the Whitney's institutionalization and public nature allowed her to detach herself from it in all ways but the financial.

Juliana had the courage to be seen as a principal author of the museum's policies, well- and ill-considered. She reported to Gertrude and Gertrude alone, and Gertrude's money was to cover all expenditures. The Whitney refused to accept gifts, which kept the museum from having to sell itself to collectors and patrons by organizing or receiving opportunistic shows. Yet to be enjoined from accepting bequests and donations, especially works of art, was falsely prudent. This decision was probably made by Juliana, Gertrude, and possibly Forbes, who was vehemently against external bodies, especially the rich, having any influence on museums.

The prohibition on gifts (other than those from Juliana, Gertrude, or the Whitney family) was not reversed until 1949. The embargo very likely caused some important losses to the collection, but another policy put into effect to counteract pressure was a worse hindrance. The exhibitions mounted of individual artists' work had in the past provided the two women with some of their finest moments: In giving artists one-man shows, for many of them their first ever, Juliana and Gertrude demonstrated prescience, discernment, and belief in Hopper, Sloan, Joseph Stella, Flannagan, Nakian, Dasburg, du Bois, Sheeler, Marsh, Glackens, Davis, and Coleman. Once the Whitney became a museum, one-artist shows were eliminated. This was a ghastly error, for it cut off the

museum from a vital means of documenting and paying tribute to creative achievement. Retrospectives now went only to the dead—Colonial, nineteenth-century, and recently deceased painters—so they took on a marmoreal quality. Because of the Whitney's inflexibility, it was the Museum of Modern Art in the 1930s and 1940s that mounted the major retrospectives of living American artists. The Modern showed several painters (e.g., Hopper, Sheeler, and Davis) whom the Whitney had backed when they were young and unknown. Meanwhile, the Whitney, prevented from honoring its own discoveries, was deprived of deserved credit. This crippling policy, probably the brainchild of Juliana and Hermon More, was not rescinded until 1948, when retrospectives were scheduled for Kuniyoshi, Weber, and Sloan. These painters were estimable candidates for one-man shows, but they should have had them in the museum's formative years. In 1948 the curators should have been free to organize retrospectives of younger artists still in the process of redirecting the course of American art, but they felt obligated to begin by paying homage to Whitney stalwarts now at the close of their careers.

If the Whitney removed itself too much from artists by its ban on solo shows, it was sometimes done in by the very lavishness of warmth and egalitarianism that made the Whitney-Force activities of the preceding two decades so memorable. The Whitney Studio Club and Galleries were run by artists for artists to stiffen their resolve, nurture their creativity, and aid their reputations, and neither Juliana nor Gertrude could bear to make the museum tremendously different. With the exception of Juliana herself, everyone involved with the museum, from the founder to the watchman, was or had been an artist.

Intent on keeping the museum a place for artists, Juliana would not countenance an intimidating gallery atmosphere or the enthroning of art on a pedestal of grandiloquent gloom. Through the intimate environments she always chose for the showing of art, she tried to replace sacrosanct attitudes with real human interest. She once wrote, "Is it too much to suppose that some of the mystery of the museum will vanish into thin air and we will come to look a picture in the face?" The early Whitney was sometimes the most un-museumlike of museums in its practices. Lloyd Goodrich, who started advising Juliana in early 1930, explained that at that time "I used to take her out to lunch and she was wonderful company. We'd talk about the coming museum, and we talked about lots of things. I gave her a list of artists that I thought were important to be collected, and she practically paid no attention to them at all, may I say. It wasn't that she didn't care about this kind of thing, it was just that she'd rather talk and get a person's ideas through talk than get something in writing or anything formal at all."

The museum was what it was because of its past, which was grounded in philanthropy, and because of Juliana, who chose to be artist-oriented rather than art history–minded. She often judged people, not pictures, valuing the artists as much as the objects they created. She could not, in her fifty-fourth year, stifle her emotional impulses for the sake of the permanent collection or pared-down exhibitions. Her cardinal priority was the support of the artist's creativity, and she was prepared to sacrifice a lofty institutional image for it.

Juliana was knowledgeable, and she tried her best to be objective, but it wasn't in her nature to act with cool neutrality or be impersonal in her professional demeanor because she cared so much about artists as people. In Forbes's words, "They [Gertrude and Juliana] had many years of working with artists personally. Hence, as long as they lived personal relations counted in all their art activities. Especially was this true of Mrs. Force. . . . In her museum direction Mrs. Force tried to be impersonal and rather believed she had become so. The cocktail hour always brought forth the evidence that she could not be neutral or impersonal." Juliana's rush of feeling for an artist for whom she felt sorry was heartwarming, but as a consequence of so much heart, many negligible works of art were added to the museum. This was indulgence in her own power, and it went hand in hand with her habit of making snap judgments when more measured appraisals would have served the collection better. Juliana's Lady Bountiful leniency came out in full strength when she dealt with Woodstock, her pet art colony. Its residents were rewarded by too many purchases and too many invitations to exhibit. Although such advanced and idiosyncratic artists as John Storrs, Arthur B. Carles, John Graham, Ivan Albright, Peter Blume, Arnold Friedman, Arthur Dove, Florine Stettheimer, and Arshile Gorky were sought out by the museum in its first few years, they are not the names commonly associated with the Whitney nor is there a sense that any of them were among its durable enthusiasms. In 1932 Henry McBride accurately commented that most of the Whitney's younger artists "seem to have studied with Kenneth Hayes Miller, [and] certainly spend the summers at Ogunquit or Woodstock."

A perennial dilemma for the museum lay in arriving at the composition of its mammoth biennial exhibitions of painting, sculpture, and graphic works, which would be inaugurated in 1932.* These shows were the descendants of the large, mixed members' shows the Club put on for ten years. Like the Club, but counter to the practices of other museums, the Whitney annuals and biennials had no juries and no prizes. Juliana and her curators endorsed the diversity of American art by inviting works by individuals representing all notable tendencies and schools. The Whitney wanted to recognize new talent, retain its commitment to older painters in "the Whitney family" as well as those not affiliated with the museum's history, and find contemporary and historical masterworks. For in the biennials, the main questions were, Should the museum report on or confront the present? Should it editorialize or present an inventory? The museum chose to recapitulate what had been going on around the country. The biennials and annuals could at best purvey a useful catholicity of taste and at worst produce a view that was middle-of-the-road. A little of everything was shown, and therefore everything was accorded the same weight. During his tenure as curator of twentieth-century art at the Metropolitan Museum of Art, Henry Geldzahler recalled his impressions of past Whitney annuals. He tactfully

---

*Biennial exhibitions of contemporary American art, one of paintings and one of sculpture, watercolors, and prints, were held from 1932 through 1936. In 1936, the latter exhibition was divided into two parts—sculpture, drawings, and prints, and watercolors and pastels. From 1937 to 1948, the biennials became annuals.

suggested that the museum's universal coverage was an abdication of its responsibilities because it did not provide enough guidance to viewers.

> From its founding, the Whitney has had a sense of responsibility and fairness to all the styles that at any moment make up the totality of contemporary art. This sense of fairness has always made the annual exhibitions of painting and sculpture at the Whitney anthologies rather than attempts to define styles and emphasize quality. . . . The Whitney Annual was always a much-anticipated event, for it allowed us to see in one large exhibition much of the best that was being produced along with the most stagnant, least provocative art imaginable. Thus the viewer was thrown into the healthful turmoil of doing what some consider the museum's job—of deciding, comparing, rejecting, and accepting until he felt, often after several visits to the same Annual, that he was able to find his own way to what constituted quality in contemporary American art.

A rule that severely handicapped the biennials and annuals was in effect until 1940. Invited artists were allowed to select which works would represent them in these exhibitions. Lloyd Goodrich said this sounded like an artist's idea, and he guessed that the policy, which was a sweet gesture of faith in the artists, originated with the other curators. Artists usually think that their best work is their latest one; the most recent painting was often the one sent to the Whitney. Some artists baldly submitted work they wanted to sell. Juliana and her staff trusted to the artists' honor, and sometimes their trust was abused. As she told the *New York Times*, "We send out our invitations and each artist wears what he pleases to our party."

In December of 1932, after seeing the first biennial, Oscar Bluemner was sure that some of the artists had exploited the Whitney's idealism. Bothered by the affront to the museum's "broadminded, impartial and generous call" made "with such splendid hospitality, unstinted money sacrifice, in these cataclysmic days," Bluemner protested in a broadside he sent to fifty people, "many of us forerunners could and should have sent much better work. . . . The Whitney Museum . . . was sincere. Are the painters, in reply, sincere? Said a highly gifted painter friend of mine: 'I sent a pot-boiler, hoping for a sale.' That I believe to be the attitude of many. . . . I say we painters have not deserved the free lunch at Mrs. Force's reception." Bluemner also worried over the Whitney's pledge to acquire chiefly from the biennial exhibitions instead of the best and widest selection possible. His observations were seconded by the art press. In their reviews, Henry McBride, Forbes Watson, and several other critics were outspoken in their disapproval of artists being allowed to choose what they would send to the biennial.

The Whitney was established primarily as a shrine to the progress of contemporary art, but it was to perform impeccably in fostering an appreciation of the American past. One of its stated purposes was to shed light on the preceding two centuries, from the Colonial period through the Gilded Age, and Juliana's letting Goodrich follow his interests in historical art involved the museum in a steady exhumation, rediscovery, and reevaluation of earlier artists, many of whom were then little known or underappreciated. At that time, such institutional acknowledgments of the validity of research about American artists were

rare. John I. H. Baur, who was the director of the Whitney Museum from 1968 through 1974, said that when he began his career as an art historian during the early 1930s "it was one of those anomalies where really much more was known about fourteenth-century Italian painting than was known about nineteenth-century American painting or [the art] of our own century."

Just as it is always easier to work with the certainties of the past than the conflicts and flux of the present, it is always easier to criticize when one is aided by hindsight. Juliana unquestionably made some key blunders in setting up the museum, but she was the right person for the job, and there was no one who could have done it better. Under the circumstances, working without benefit of established traditions or precedents, what she accomplished was remarkable. She was not meeting previous standards, but setting new ones. Her budget was limited, her staff, although dedicated, was tiny, and she was operating in a climate of economic desperation. As the first of its kind, the Whitney became a prominent cultural institution from the moment it opened, and it is a tribute to the reputation Juliana had made that nothing but the largest responsibilities and obligations were stipulated for her. Her critics expected her to make up for the neglect of three centuries of the country's artistic patrimony and to sort out the welter of the contemporary in a few short seasons and within the physical space of a few small rooms.

Flecked with faults though it was, the Whitney was more lively and progressive than most other art institutions around the country. From the day she announced that the Whitney Museum of American Art had come into being, Juliana was accepted as a leader in the museum world. In those days, the museum profession as we know it was in its infancy, and the disciplined study of art history lay in the future. The instinct for art—a combination of experience, memory, taste, and insight—was then qualification enough for heading a museum, and instinct Juliana had in abundance. Before 1930 she was already working on a close and equal footing with the directors of the Phillips Collection, the Cleveland Museum of Art, the Denver Art Museum, the California Palace of the Legion of Honor, the Newark Museum, the Art Institute of Chicago, the Carnegie Museum of Art, the Museum of the City of New York, and the Philadelphia Museum of Art. Once the museum was under way, she became friends with the brightest and most adventurous of the younger generation of directors: Alfred Barr of the Modern, Charles Sawyer of the Addison Gallery of American Art, A. Everett (Chick) Austin of the Wadsworth Atheneum, Gordon Washburn of the Albright Gallery, Daniel Catton Rich of the Art Institute of Chicago, and David Finley of the National Gallery of Art.

As their correspondence with Juliana shows, these men believed she was doing an excellent job. Charles Sawyer said, "In 1931, at age twenty-four, I was appointed director of the Addison Gallery of American Art in Andover, Massachusetts. The opening of the new Whitney on Eighth Street pretty much coincided with ours, and while the Addison Gallery was smaller and off the beaten path, its collections, especially in the art of the nineteenth century, were excellent, and received considerable publicity at the time. Mrs. Force could have regarded us as a competitor, but quite the contrary, welcomed me as an

ally in the cause of American art and was very generous and hospitable to a very young and ignorant colleague. I usually stopped to see her on my trips to New York, and we exchanged impressions of colleagues, artists, pictures." Barr, who was always modest and deferential toward Juliana, once wrote charmingly to her, "I look forward with keenest anticipation to the opening of the Whitney Museum. Everywhere I go among dealers I pick out what seems to me the best things only to discover that you have already bought them. This is very annoying. I congratulate you."

But in arriving at any fair reckoning of the Whitney's stature in its early years, it must be measured against the one institution that consistently surpassed it—the Museum of Modern Art. Indeed, because they were inaugurated at about the same time, the Whitney from its advent was doomed to debilitating comparisons with the Museum of Modern Art and Barr's unmatchable legacy of connoisseurship and erudition. Besides overpowering the Whitney in depth, breadth, and scholarly ambition, the Modern had the advantage of being able to overlook the indigenous product if it chose. (And it chose to do so often. In a letter of 1934, Barr stated that he wanted to concentrate on European art for the permanent collection and confine American art to loan shows. He was also apprehensive about the social and financial pressures of the American art world, "with its problems of personal jealousy and prejudice on the part of artists and their supporters.") Juliana of course would never have viewed the Whitney's mandate to give opportunities exclusively to American artists as a liability—the staunch endorsement of a national art was the whole point of the Whitney enterprise—but there was no avoiding the reality that Picasso, Léger, Matisse, Miró, Kandinsky, and Brancusi were producing stronger art than any American. Relations between the Whitney and the Modern were always cordial, and Juliana admired Alfred Barr immensely, but after years of working just to make art visible to the public, she was suspicious of intellectual concepts and categories that might detract from the direct experience of looking "a picture in the face." This was an attitude she had absorbed directly from artists: Viewers should get their pictures—straight. She would not run after the Modern like a sheep, bleating "me too" as she went. As C. (Cooke) Adolph Glassgold, a curator at the Whitney Museum during the early 1930s, said, "Juliana Force recognized the fact that the Modern was going to exploit what the Whitney was not prepared to exploit."

Forbes later wrote that Juliana wanted the Whitney to retain its identity even if that identity appeared to be provincial. In building truly representative holdings of what serious American artists were investigating, she believed that the museum would have to include conservative and traditional as well as modern artists. Furthermore, she did not want to lose touch with American Realism—the governing taste on which the Whitney collection had been founded. But Juliana could have learned from the Modern's elasticity in regarding all the visual arts as subjects of investigation, its retreating from positions and procedures that hobbled it, and its awarding of one-artist shows. When Katherine Schmidt, a Whitney loyalist and a regular exhibitor there for decades, was asked which museum exerted more influence on American painting, she said that although the Modern was relatively uninvolved with American art, "I think the Whitney

was more important in the beginning in maintaining, buying, supporting people. But the Modern is *far* the greater influence and is more meaningful as an expression of the time." Even a Whitney admirer could see why the Whitney Museum, constituted as it was, could be good and even powerful—and at its best, it was often very good—but it could never be great.

Juliana continued to make additions to the Whitney collection of artists whose work was not yet sufficiently represented in it. In May 1930, she paid $400 for Thomas Hart Benton's *The Lord Is My Shepherd*, an uningratiating double portrait of a husband and wife that the artist considered his first realized painting in a Regionalist style. With its dour subject matter and somber colors, the painting dares viewers to like it. (*The Lord Is My Shepherd* was the second picture by Benton that entered the Whitney collection; in 1927 she had bought a small landscape of Martha's Vineyard.) Then, on a visit to the Rehn Gallery, she purchased the painting Edward Hopper had brought in to his dealer just two months before. The work was *Early Sunday Morning*, for which she paid $2,000—then the most expensive contemporary painting ever purchased for the Whitney collection. The painting was and is one of the museum's masterworks, and Forbes proudly reproduced it in *The Arts* as an example of the star-spangled standard to which the new museum should aspire. Before this, Juliana had bought several of Hopper's prints but no oil paintings.

Following her usual pattern, Juliana sailed later in the month for France, where she went over business with Gertrude before going to England. Cobweb was in for the full decorating treatment. The kitchen and drawing room were done in yellows and pinks. A gardener-handyman was hired to lay out fruit, vegetable, and flower gardens and watch over the place during the winter months. The gardener, who drew a salary all year round, was very happy with this arrangement, although supplying produce to Juliana's tastes was, he said, "a full-time job." He remembered her throwing "some fabulous parties, which very often included actors and actresses. . . . In every room there were very large fireplaces, and it didn't matter how hot the weather was, when Mrs. Force was at home there had to be large log fires." Every year Juliana closed Cobweb with a farewell party before she sailed, and at the final minute, the glass in which she had her last drink was always thrown into the fire and smashed. This permissiveness scandalized her charwoman. Fifty years later, she described Juliana as "a fast woman" because she preferred cocktails to temperance beverages at teatime and had her bed made up with satin sheets.

Juliana left England early because she had to be within call during the final negotiations over the purchase of more space for the museum. Gertrude had control over Nos. 8, 10, and 14 West Eighth Street, but No. 12 and its studio on MacDougal Alley were still owned by Daniel Chester French. French was now eighty years old and spending most of his time at Chesterwood, his property in the Berkshires. As he was not using No. 12, it was the perfect and logical addition for the museum. Gertrude offered to buy it, but wanted her identity concealed. French, after learning who the buyer was, felt that Gertrude, a

colleague and a neighbor, had behaved shoddily in posing as an anonymous purchaser. On July 15, 1930, he wrote to a friend:

> It looks as if I should have a lot of money to stow away in a few days, as the balance for my studio building will become due. What can we do about that? It transpires that Mrs. Whitney is the purchaser, but I suppose her money is as good as anybody's. Her secretary [presumably Juliana] declared positively to Robert Bush [French's real estate manager] that Mrs. Whitney had nothing to do with the purchase, but women were deceivers ever!

The four town houses would be renovated and joined together by the architectural firm of Noel & Miller, which meant that even the design and construction of the museum would be a family affair, as G. Macculloch Miller, Flora Whitney's husband, was the second partner in the firm. The contract for the interior, which consisted of galleries and offices on the first three floors, living quarters for the curators on the fourth floor, and Juliana's expanded apartment on the fourth floor and part of the third, went to Bruce Buttfield, a decorator who collaborated with Juliana on the design and found some of the antiques. The remodeling required to join four old residential buildings into one unit and subdivide it into twelve exhibition galleries that retained the houses' original character was so extensive that the museum could no longer open in November of 1930 as planned. A new date was set—April of 1931—but that also would prove optimistic, and the opening later was pushed forward to November of 1931.

The results of the renovation were a handsome adaptation of modern and historical elements. The old brick facades were united, and the walls were covered with a salmon-pink stucco that was set off by lintels, band courses and moldings of white stone. Reeded motifs were added to balance the fenestration. Artists liked the museum's out-of-the-ordinary color—as Charles Demuth wrote to Juliana, "It's [sic] pink face is grand!"

The main entrance to the museum was classical. The entablature and pilasters were Greek Revival, and made of white marble. A large bas-relief of a white metal eagle, a guardian figure designed by Karl Free, crouched protectively above the door. (A slightly different version of Free's eagle would also be adopted as the insignia for the museum's stationery.) The aluminum outer doors were set into red Numidian marble. The two inner doors, designed by Carl Walters, were made of molded glass and divided into sixty sections containing reliefs of figures and animals. Juliana asked Walters to make the doors, not knowing what lay in store for the sculptor—it took him thirteen months of experimenting to perfect them.

The interior of the museum was designed to look like a private home— Juliana's home, to be exact—with most of the furniture removed. The entrance court, which held a free-standing fountain by Gertrude and nude nymphs in niches by John Gregory, looked like the foyer that it had been. A double staircase of marble led to eleven galleries for paintings. At least two were painted white and accessorized with blue rugs and curtains, two more were yellow, two were painted and furnished in a dusty-rose pink, two were lined with cork, and one

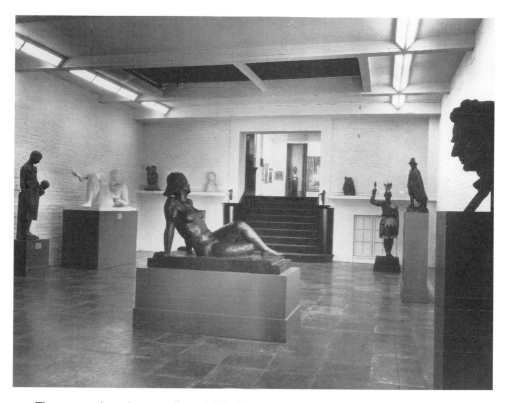

The museum's sculpture gallery, 1932. Foreground: *The Awakening* by Robert Laurent; right: cigar-store Indian; *The Pilgrim* by Augustus Saint-Gaudens; *Head of Lincoln* by Andrew O'Connor.

was gray. The galleries were connected by passages and stairways whose walls were stenciled with eagles, stars, and stripes. As further assurance that the environment would not be bleak, thick carpets covered the floors. In some rooms, Juliana installed tubular steel sofas and chairs; in others, she preferred the curvaceous Rococo Revival settees similar to the ones in her own drawing room. The second floor had a room for prints; the ground floor contained a sculpture gallery. The latter had been French's studio, and it was repainted in a blue-gray.

The plan also called for a library, a director's office, various small offices for the rest of the staff, and a shipping room. Because of the structural dissimilarities of the four town houses from which the museum was being carved—the floor levels were uneven and the ceiling heights varied—the interior layout was discontinuous. Only on the first floor were doorways cut into walls; the upstairs galleries were kept as small rooms whose size and shape conformed to the walls of the old houses and which were reachable by narrow stairways. This was an ingenious solution to a difficult conversion, but the setup worked inefficiently for the third floor, where the offices were located. For a curator working in the

offices in No. 14 to see Juliana, whose office was on the opposite end of the floor once belonging to No. 8, he had to walk down to the first floor, cross it, and climb the stairs leading to her room. This arrangement was inconvenient, but it did give more privacy to all concerned.

On October 15, 1930, the staff of the Whitney Museum held its first meeting. Juliana, Hermon More, Edmund Archer, Karl Free, and Eleanor Lambert were present. The main business at hand was the setting of the public hours. The museum would be open from 10:00 A.M. to 6:00 P.M. daily and 2:00 P.M. to 6:00 P.M. every Sunday, admission free. The staff thereupon adjourned for lunch, which was served in Juliana's apartment. This pleasantry became a custom. Throughout the 1930s, the staff met once a week around noontime and finished up with a meal at her table.

Gertrude did not attend this first staff meeting. At the time, private matters were more pressing. For the last three months Harry Whitney's liver disease had worsened. Gertrude was by his bedside as his condition deteriorated. He developed a bad fever and heavy cold that was eventually diagnosed as pneumonia. On October 27, 1930, Harry lost consciousness and died. He was fifty-eight.

Gertrude was reported to be in a state of shock and was sedated by her doctors, but she asserted herself enough to order a death mask of her husband. After the funeral, Gertrude moved into Harry's bedroom at Old Westbury, and secluded herself there for six weeks. She dealt with her grief, facing her ambivalent emotions about her husband while mourning the loss of a person who had been part of her life for thirty-five years. Schooled to her duty, Gertrude answered the hundreds of condolence letters she received and took over Harry's estate, initially valued at $72 million in cash, real estate, stocks, and other assets. She also took solace in reflecting on the museum. When Royal Cortissoz referred to it in his letter of sympathy, Gertrude replied:

> It means a great deal to me personally as to the success of the undertaking to know that you are in back of us and approve the venture. For it is a venture in a way although to me it is the logical continuation of what I have had in my mind for years. It seems a perfectly natural evolution. Not that I minimize the pitfalls and easy dangers ahead. It is not enough only to have something very much at heart but if besides that one has the intelligence of a Mrs. Force, with the sincere approval and aid of people who really care about what goes on in the art world, I am sure that with time the Museum will become what I dream of. It took a long time and a great deal of thought to build the Gallery from what was considered the whim of a woman who could spend money, or a charity organization, into a serious undertaking. It will take a long time to build the Museum into the important place I want it to occupy, but it is fascinating work and never ending in its multiple sides.

In mid-December she was ready to appear in public, although not in New York. Gertrude sequestered herself in a villa in Havana for the winter.

If Forbes seems strangely absent from all this, it is because he was. After the showdown at the Metropolitan, he, Juliana, and Gertrude seemed to be an indissoluble triumvirate, marching three abreast into an exciting new frontier.

As he had hinted to Goodrich, Forbes expected to be involved not only behind the scenes, but in an official capacity. Of course, the position of director, for which Forbes was qualified, was taken, and since Juliana would not have shared the throne, even with her prince consort, nothing else suitable for him was left. Ethel Renthal was sure that her ex-boss was in line for the job Hermon More eventually got, but both Forbes and Juliana were realistic enough to know that he could not have settled for being second to her.

By the end of 1930 Forbes had disappeared from his place at Juliana's side, but not for professional reasons. Their personal relationship, under heavy strain, was to buckle in a public and private quarrel that would destroy it. Forbes and Juliana's involvement was not the amorous engagement it had been. They had been intimate for twelve years, and the connection was chafing Forbes. Although he still enjoyed Juliana as good company, he had tired of her, grown careless, and crossed her in several dangerous ways—a risky move as their relationship had always had its competitive edge. However, since they seemed to look on their affair as something of a game of skill, the aggressive component within that competition had normally been defused, either by passion or by equalizing circumstances. When the two met, Forbes was not only an important critic, but the first knowledgeable and cosmopolitan art professional who cared enough to challenge what Juliana was doing. In advising her to revamp the Whitney Studio and through his later guidance, he became her preceptor and mentor in European and American art. For her part, she was not only intelligent, amusing, and eager to listen, but a fresh conquest—all of which flattered Forbes immensely. Juliana wanted to be tutored, escorted, and bedded, and Forbes was willing to oblige. As Juliana's authority as Gertrude's representative increased, she could make life easier for him. By showering him with irresistible opportunities, she redressed the balance of power by repaying his knowledge with financial rewards. With the Whitney checkbook at her disposal, Juliana could buy Forbes *The Arts* and underwrite lectures and trips abroad for him. She was also a steady customer for Nan's paintings. This was done benignly, but it was patronage nonetheless, and although he would have denied it hotly, Forbes was tethered on Juliana's leash. During the mid- and late 1920s, no battles for control were necessary. Forbes and Juliana were emotionally and intellectually united—they were frequently together, he would boom the Club and American art, and she would support Forbes and create opportunities for him whenever she could. Having a main source of his income derive from Juliana sometimes told on Forbes, but he liked the good life and accepted the situation.

But now that he was not so enamored of Juliana, this check on Forbes's independence was less easy to tolerate. And he no longer had any counterbalances against conditions he found grating. In the position of a museum director, Juliana had attained a summit of power Forbes could not match, and she was acting like it. Since both of them were advocates of the slash-and-burn style of argument, one incident, which putatively concerned an editorial disagreement at *The Arts*, was really a telltale crack that was soon to widen into a chasm. In 1930 Thomas Hart Benton received his first major mural commission—*America Today*, a

series of panels for the boardroom of the New School for Social Research's new premises at 55 West 12th Street. * Lloyd Goodrich visited the site, was impressed by Benton's unconventional mural style, and thought the work deserved coverage in *The Arts*. He wrote an essay and submitted it to Forbes. To Goodrich's surprise, Forbes told him that he had praised Benton too much, that the murals were overpublicized and overrated, and that he would not print the article. None of Goodrich's arguments could budge him. Not long after this, the two men and some other guests were up at Juliana's having drinks, and Goodrich reported their disagreement to her. Juliana then walked over to Forbes and asked what he meant by not using Goodrich's piece. She then drew Forbes aside and said she wanted to speak to him privately in another room. Some minutes passed, and after the two emerged, Goodrich was informed by Juliana that his article would indeed be published. (It was, in the March 1931 issue.) Forbes said nothing, but his thunderous expression spoke volumes.

Juliana's insistence might have been less adamant had it not been rooted in another discord. Forbes was seeing another woman and took no pains to hide it. He had womanized before during his long intimacy with Juliana, but he had been discreet and in attendance when she needed him. This new affair was an engulfing one, and Forbes had become flagrant about it. He was neglecting his work, and he was neglecting Juliana, who was driven into a frenzy by the defection.

The other woman was an artist who had been a member of the Whitney Studio Club and had even exhibited in the Armory Show. Most mortifying to Juliana was that her rival lived on East Eighth Street, a few hundred yards across Fifth Avenue from the Whitney and in full view of Juliana's apartment. The woman ran an antiques store on the ground floor of her building and lived upstairs. Therefore Juliana stood the constant risk of running into her, and the shop and apartment were constantly before Juliana's eyes. Choked with jealousy, Juliana could not tear herself away from the window after Forbes exited from the building. She would position herself there after he left her drawing room and watch him walk down the street to visit his new paramour.

In the course of her involvement with Forbes, Juliana had not been saintly herself. There were occasional rumors of her making up to artists—"she got teary, she said she was lonesome, and she wanted someone to comfort her," remembered one painter whom she approached—but in none of these tales did anything ever happen beyond talk. Buckminster Fuller said that Juliana had quite a flirtation going with his great friend Christopher Morley, the author and bon vivant, whom she knew by 1931, but their relationship probably stopped short of sexual activity. And since both Juliana and Forbes were unfaithful to their spouses, neither one was in a position to insist on monogamy or fidelity. Yet Forbes was the central man in Juliana's life. She would have been unhappy to lose her hold on him at any time, but at this moment she was singularly bereft. Forbes and Gertrude were the two most important emotional attachments

---

* Now in the collection of the Equitable Life Assurance Society of the United States.

in Juliana's life; she had temporarily lost Gertrude, who was locked away in mourning for Harry and then off to Havana, and now her lover was slipping away from her.

With Forbes bridling at Juliana's high-handedness and Juliana's own resentments stoked by jealousy, a confrontation was inevitable. It took place in the winter of 1930, in full public view, at a dinner party given by the dealer Frank Rehn. The Goodriches, the Watsons, Juliana, and several other guests were there. At the table, the crowd apparently was complimenting Juliana on the astuteness of some decisions she had made. Forbes by then was a little the worse for drink, and it seemed to him Juliana was taking too much credit for her wisdom. He leaned over to her and remarked loudly enough for everyone to hear, "Everything you know, I taught you." This was not the thing to say to Juliana in front of a group of people, and she exploded. In Lloyd Goodrich's words, "Mrs. Force started saying things to him that men and women do not say to each other in public. Then Nan stood up and said, 'Forbes, we're leaving.' That was the end of that dinner party."

The next day, Forbes told Goodrich, "That does it! I'm never taking money from that woman again!" His statement came true, but not because Forbes initiated it. Money, as Juliana knew, was a means of holding Forbes, who lived by his wits but needed her to live well, and it was a means of revenge. Juliana, wounded and blinded with pain, would not forgive him; more than that, she was determined to humble him. She would hurt him professionally by making it come to pass that Gertrude withdrew her support from *The Arts*. Perhaps Juliana also hoped that if Forbes lost such an influential pulpit, he would become less attractive to his woman friend.

From 1923 through the first half of 1930, Gertrude and Juliana had been the principal benefactors of the magazine: The two women had contributed a total of $65,490. Setting up the museum necessitated some cost cutting, and Lloyd Goodrich believed that Gertrude stopped funding *The Arts* because all her money had to go toward the museum. This is a logical assumption, and his view is backed up by a letter Forbes wrote to Gertrude on September 30, 1931, to thank her for keeping *The Arts* afloat for so many years. In it, Forbes notes that Juliana had *recently* told him that all of Gertrude's money now had to go into the museum. However, the last time Gertrude had donated money ($12,600) was for the 1929–1930 season. According to Forbes's records, *The Arts* had received nothing from Gertrude or Juliana after 1930; he also mentions in the letter that he had been trying throughout 1931 to raise money from other sources, which makes sense only if support had been withdrawn during that year. The letter seems too late in relation to other events. It might best be interpreted as a gentlemanly if belated expression of gratitude, and it was possibly a ploy to get Gertrude to reconsider her decision now that the museum was almost ready to open. Just as Forbes would not have begged Juliana for absolution, he would never have spoken of his quarrel to Gertrude, and soon after their fight, Juliana could have raised the question of stopping the subsidy as a cost-cutting measure. She may not have informed Gertrude of her rupture with Watson at first, in

order that Gertrude herself would have entertained the proposal as a disinterested, necessary economy and continue to see it as such.

If *The Arts* was simply a casualty of the mounting expenses of the Whitney Museum, Forbes would have been informed of the loss of support in a manner different from what actually occurred. In a parallel situation, Gertrude had been forced to stop contributing to the Society of Independent Artists. In April of 1931, when John Sloan, the organization's president, wrote to Juliana and asked to be bailed out once more, he was candidly and courteously told why it was impossible. Juliana wrote to him:

> Before Mrs. Whitney went away she and I discussed every possible phase of the work here together with the expenses of the same, and as it appeared the amount found necessary was almost double the cost she had intended allowing for this tremendous project. Since then, in actually organizing the work, I find that I have exceeded even that amount. It is a big job, and Mrs. Whitney said that for the first two years every other expenditure that she had been accustomed to making in the interest of Art would have to be eliminated, and that we would have to concentrate everything on this very important work. This was Mrs. Whitney's request at the end of our interview and I must carry it out. . . .
>
> It is simply a question of doing this big job well, and concentrating every effort towards it, because in the end we believe this Museum is going to help everybody.

No such softly cushioned explanation was readied for Forbes and *The Arts*. William Robb, who was with Forbes when the end came and witnessed it, said, "Mrs. Force called me and Watson down to her office. There was no mistaking her mood or what she meant. She started on a tirade, she knew where she was going and wouldn't be interrupted. She read the riot act to us, but she mostly ignored me. She said something, and then I disputed it. She told me to stop talking and not to interrupt her. She was angry and determined, and I realized that jealousy was involved. I don't remember what she said to us on that awful occasion, but she was hell-bent and we had to sit there and take it. Nothing was ever mentioned about the museum as the reason *The Arts* was folding." In his correspondence with Abby Aldrich Rockefeller, Lincoln Kirstein, and other prospective donors he solicited after the Whitney money stopped, for purposes of discretion and out of gratitude to Gertrude, Forbes's public position was that the museum had to take precedence over *The Arts*. The embarrassing reality was not admitted.

A final piece of testimony that a personal motive rather than economic exigency determined the ouster of Watson from *The Arts* was supplied by Goodrich. In 1932, when the same budgetary restrictions would have existed at the Whitney, Juliana asked him to revive the magazine with himself as editor. She told him that Gertrude was prepared to continue the magazine, but not with Forbes in charge. Goodrich, however, refused to take the editorship. "I couldn't cut Forbes's throat, I couldn't do it to my former colleague, although I gave as the reason the books I was writing," he recalled. But Juliana knew the truth. Goodrich continued, "She said to me, 'I don't question your ability, I question your courage.' But personally it was not acceptable to me."

Forbes's troubles multiplied after Juliana turned away from him. In March of 1931, the *World* merged with the *Telegram* and he lost his job on the paper. Before that took place, he thought he might be able to keep *The Arts* going by not taking a salary and staying one step ahead of the bills with contributions from other patrons. With their help, Forbes put out *The Arts* until November of 1931. In 1932 he briefly rejuvenated the publication as a newsweekly, but this venture, underwritten in part by Lincoln Kirstein and his friend Edward Warburg, was undercapitalized and failed quickly. Forbes, now one of the unemployed millions, was scrambling for assignments like any junior reporter. By the time the museum opened in November of 1931, he and Juliana had mended their differences to some extent, and in April of 1932, she gave him $600 toward the magazine despite her conversation with Goodrich. Forbes was consulted in his professional capacity and invited to the soirees, but the two were never close again.

In 1933 Watson moved to Washington, D.C., to take a job with the federal government. He resented leaving New York, but he needed financial security. Juliana missed Forbes, and it took her many years to get over him. Ethel Renthal, who was Juliana's secretary until 1930 and then returned to work at the museum from 1933 to 1936, remembered that shortly after she was rehired, Juliana called her and Dorothy Freeman, another Whitney secretary who had once worked at *The Arts*, into her office. "She was subdued and sad. She needed to confide in someone. She wanted to talk about Forbes Watson, and we were the only ones who knew him well enough to talk about him. She was suddenly like a girl letting her hair down. She blurted out her love for Forbes. She said, 'I was in love with him. I was mad about him,' and she began to cry."

From the time her affair with Forbes was terminated, Juliana had favorite escorts and friendships with men, but she never again had a serious love interest or, in Allan Rieser's view, "much use for them. She frequently referred to them [men] as vain, absurd, dull or—her favorite term for them—'spoiled.' When she thought they were particularly foolish, she became coy in a manner which I knew was quite false." She liked homosexuals as escorts because they were always safe and usually sophisticated, clever, and charming. In the public eye, they were a claque of loyal, available bachelors who hung on her every word and never betrayed her with another woman; with them, Allan Rieser said, she was at her ease and "took on a tone of intimate banter." There was also a defensiveness behind the preference. Juliana once told Ira Glackens that she went around with homosexuals to keep artists favored at the museum from being accused of getting into the collection because they were sleeping with her.

No one knows if Forbes repented his break with Juliana. Although he applauded her in print and would come to her rescue if the museum needed a defender, he was often condescending in his private asides to friends. In correspondence, he mocked her frivolities and derided her professionalism, but his behavior must be seen in relation to his own disappointments. The painter George Biddle, who worked with Watson in the 1930s, characterized him as a "bitter" and "frustrated" man, and attributed those feelings to the loss of *The Arts*. Watson felt that a government job in Washington was a comedown after

a trailblazing editorship and vivacious life in New York. He and Juliana were reconciled a few years before her death, and in a 1950 photograph of Forbes in his study, hung behind his chair and taking up the most conspicuous spot on the wall, is an enlarged portrait photograph of Juliana.

The facets of Juliana's character that predominated during her conflict with Forbes—those of the vulnerable woman whose insecurities and hypersensitivity to criticism could not always be contained below her burnished surface and the fearsome autocrat who sometimes got her way through sheer terrorism—are seen in three representative portraits of her, all done around January of 1931. Two were photographs taken by Cecil Beaton, and one was a caricature in pastel by Peggy Bacon.* Whereas Beaton's glamorous images alternately portrayed Juliana as sleek and subdued or as tense and romantically vulnerable, Bacon's brutal representation showed a hardened old battle-axe who hatcheted a path through life with deadly bluntness. In a caption accompanying the picture when it was published, Bacon wrote that Juliana was a woman who spared "no feelings, letting people know exactly where they stand."

In Bacon's portrayal, Juliana is sitting straight up in an overstuffed chair, not relaxing into its heavily cushioned arms or base. She seems to be evaluating something she hears, and her expression—gimlet-eyed, skeptical, and devouring—is as explosive as the overall likeness is merciless. Juliana is drawn in profile, so that her nose, which appears to have been molded from blobs of putty, is seen in the fullest oddity of its size and shape, and her chin juts forward at a bellicose angle. Both of Juliana's hands are in her lap, and the smoke from a lighted cigarette in her right hand is wafting upward in a hazy trail. The position of the fingers holding the cigarette suggests that she is waiting for something—for an answer, perhaps, or the effect of a devastating remark. Here indeed was the art-world empress who would have chopped Forbes down to size without explanation or apology, the Mrs. Fierce that artists dared not offend.

Bacon considered the portrait, which she subtitled *The Ugly Duchess*, to be one of the best she ever did. She had succeeded in her objective—to catch Juliana as "a chic [as seen by her perfect carriage and sleekly coiffed, coppery-red hair], sharp-tongued and highly critical woman. But she was very astute, very quick-witted and quick-tempered." In its aggressiveness, the caricature conveyed the subject's strength and directness—nothing that Juliana watched over, the portrait implied, would go unprotected or fail to be provocatively alive.

Juliana, however, didn't appreciate any interpretation of the picture. Florence Cramer saw Bacon's show of art-world caricatures at the Downtown Gallery and afterward went to dine with her and Brook. "Peggy had a biting caricature of Mrs. Force over the mantel," Cramer wrote in her diary, "which she said she was advised not to send to the show." Whenever Juliana visited Bacon and Brook at their house in Westchester, they took *The Ugly Duchess* off the wall and hid it from sight.

Juliana Force, now in the collection of Texas A&M University.

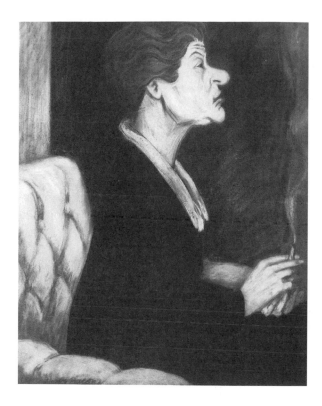

Juliana posed for Peggy
Bacon for this devastating
caricature, but she was
nonetheless shocked by the
results.

The likely reason that Juliana sat for Cecil Beaton was the then-imminent opening of the museum in April of 1931. Official publicity portraits of both Gertrude and Juliana were needed. Gertrude's portrait was eventually taken by Edward Steichen; Beaton, in New York in January of 1931, was the ideal photographer to capture Juliana in situ, in her most grand apartment to date. Construction on the upper floors was completed and her suite of rooms now stretched across the entire breadth of 8, 10, and 12 West Eighth Street. Beaton spent a day setting up many shots of Juliana, but only two have survived.

The more arresting image of the two presents Juliana as a soulful being— someone who is very emotional and easily hurt in the exercise of those emotions. In the photograph Juliana is standing to one side of a decorated door in her apartment. The assymetrical composition contributes to the mood of introversion and hypersensitivity, as does Juliana's downcast gaze.* Displaying an egotism at odds with the shrinking violet presented in the photograph, Juliana used to hand out prints of it to artists as Christmas gifts.

The second surviving image has a more formal and impersonal look to it, and it is the one the Whitney Museum still uses as the standard portrait of Juliana. Wearing satin lounging pajamas and her hair glowing with light, she is poise and fashion incarnate. This impression is further reinforced by her

*See Chapter 9, page 331.

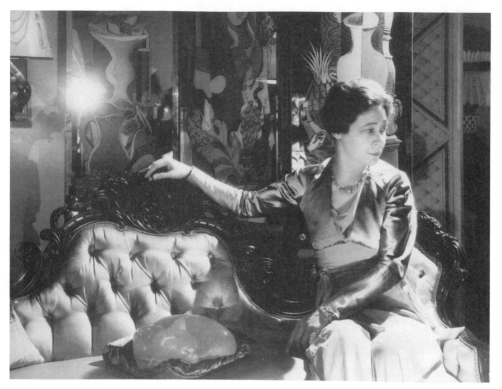

Of the same vintage as the Bacon portrait, this photograph of Juliana by Cecil Beaton highlights her poise and chic.

sidelong glance and air of nonchalant hauteur. Beaton took the utmost advantage of Juliana's decor by draping her arm over a Belter sofa, deep-buttoned in satin. Arranged behind her is a painted glass screen by Louis Bouché that adds to the gleaming quality of the setting. On a pillow next to her sleeps an alabaster cat carved by Duncan Ferguson. The whole composition, stylish but not mannered, is a tribute to Beaton's mastery of lighting, scene arranging, and fey artifice. Beaton must have applied some subtle retouching to the portrait, too, because Juliana never looked handsomer than when she sat for his camera. Beaton later wrote of his session with Juliana, "I cannot remember anything of her except her striking appearance. Her clothes were very remarkable & she wore many of them! . . . She was very hard to take as she had such a preposterous nose, but the effect, with red-dyed hair,* was very gratifying."

The real twist of the pose is not Juliana's nose, but her docile positioning next to the carving of a cat. A sculpted stand-in was as close as she would ever get to a feline, either in or out of photographs, for she had a horrific phobia of the species. Even the sight of a cat aroused Juliana, and she would become

*Beaton's reminiscence shows the keenness of his visual memory, for the photographs were in black and white. Furthermore, he had no prints or negatives of Juliana in his archives.

deathly afraid. Sometimes she flew into a state of nervous panic and tried to escape; at other times, immobilized where she sat or stood, she was trembling and white-faced.

All of the cat owners in Juliana's immediate circle knew to shut their pets away if she was coming to call. (The phobia was so well-known that it was even cited in Juliana's entry in *Current Biography*, published in 1941.) Edith Goodrich remembered that Edna and Hermon More kept a cat in their apartment, which they were careful to lock up when Juliana was about. One evening the Goodriches, the Mores, and Juliana were happily socializing, when suddenly there was a shriek. The cat had escaped and was making straight for the guests. Within seconds of the animal's appearance, Juliana climbed onto the sofa and from there to the top of an adjacent bookcase. The onlookers were amazed to see that she had squeezed herself into the narrow space between the cabinet and the ceiling and lay there, quivering. At another time, Juliana and Lloyd Goodrich were eating in a restaurant together when a cat chanced to enter the dining room. Juliana became distraught and was on the verge of hysterics; she could not be calmed until the cat was removed.

Juliana exhibited the classic phobic reaction—an excessive, involuntary response out of proportion to the reality of the situation. Her phobia was simple and monosymptomatic in that it was precisely identifiable and extended only to cats: She was a great dog lover, and Barley Sheaf Farm was home to all kinds of domestic animals. One-object phobias are usually related to a specific, frightening incident in early life, and Juliana's experience was no exception. According to *Current Biography*, her fear dated "from a childhood episode when her brother asked her to touch one, and she did so without looking. Much to her horror it was a furry animal, and alive." Juliana evidently transferred the unpleasant shock of the experience to the animal associated with it. From then on, cats themselves could elicit anxiety on their own.

The fact that Juliana never overcame her fear could be linked to the theory that children who are intensely emotional, whose feelings are easily aroused, or who are subjected to severe or prolonged stress at home are less likely to conquer extreme fears. These generalizations do fit Juliana. Another reason that Juliana's phobia never evaporated is that she was able to tolerate it. In Juliana's case, being a cat phobic was not disabling and didn't interfere with her normal activities. Indeed, she was so successful at protecting herself from encounters with cats—no one knowingly exposed her to one—that there was no pressure on her to overcome her fear.

When Juliana made up her mind, things happened, and in late 1930 she was assiduously broadening the Whitney collection with shopping trips to galleries and studios. In the sculptor Dorothea Greenbaum's words, "Juliana was dead set on buying," and in December of 1930 her buying could not be faulted. She had just bought Eakins's *Portrait of Riter Fitzgerald** from Fitzgerald's niece

---

*Now in the collection of the Art Institute of Chicago.

in Philadelphia. Juliana had undoubtedly been alerted to the picture's availability by Goodrich, and when she went to see Reginald Marsh, she took along Goodrich, who had grown up with Marsh and was his best friend. Goodrich later recalled:

> Marsh had a picture on his easel that he had just finished, titled *Why Not Use the "L"?*, one of his best pictures. Mrs. Force looked at it and didn't ask him the price or anything else. She just said, "I'll take it. Send it around to the museum." After we left, Reg called me up and said, "What am I supposed to ask in the way of a price?" "Listen, you can't ask me that. I'm with Mrs. Force." "Do you suppose $1,500 would be too much?" "Send the bill in and see what happens." It was paid without question. She was like that—she would skip the details and she didn't worry. She trusted the person.

Within two weeks of seeing *Why Not Use the "L"?* Juliana acquired paintings by Samuel Halpert, Bernard Karfiol, Max Kuehne, and most important, Max Weber's kaleidoscopic *Chinese Restaurant*, the finest canvas of his Cubist phase. Juliana was so pleased with the Weber that she hung it in her drawing room, where it stayed until the museum opened. She then bought four of Weber's gouaches (for $450, a 25 percent discount) that were immediately lent to the Art Institute of Chicago for a show being organized there.

The next recorded discussions of acquisitions took place at the staff meeting on January 14, 1931, a day on which Juliana happened to buy *The Trapper* by Rockwell Kent. The minutes read:

> Mrs. Force asked that each member of the Staff make a list of artists not represented in the Museum collection whose works they consider to make the collection thoroughly representative. The acquisition of works by the following artists was considered advisable: Glackens, Marin, Kroll, Hartley, Demuth, Lachaise, Boardman Robinson (painting), Walt Kuhn. The names of Gus Mager, Saul Schary and Noguchi were considered worthy of investigation for possible inclusion in the list. Peter Blume's name was considered, but no decision to include his work [was] made.

On January 28, a group of works was inspected. Kraushaar Galleries sent seven works by Charles Demuth, out of which Juliana bought the painting *My Egypt*, a monumental view of grain elevators in Lancaster, Pennsylvania, and an irreplaceable masterwork in the permanent collection, for $1,500. She and Hermon More also decided to buy a lithograph and thirteen drawings by Benton for his New School murals.

Juliana's next offer was $3,500 ($1,000 below the asking price) for *Yellowstone in Winter** by John Twachtman, and the bid was accepted. The buying ceased only because Gertrude asked Juliana to join her in Havana in mid-February for a brief visit. As soon as she returned, she bought, among other works, *Coryell's Ferry, 1776* by Joseph Pickett, Luks's *Mrs. Gamley* for a steep $8,000, plus paintings by Ryder, Alexander Wyant, Glackens, Hartley, and Prendergast, a watercolor by Demuth, two paintings and eight drawings by Guy Pène du Bois, sculptures by Robert Laurent, Reuben Nakian, and William Zorach, and more

---

*Now in the collection of the Buffalo Bill Historical Center.

than 100 of Sloan's etchings. From her own collection, Juliana gave the museum a landscape by Eugene Speicher and six ceramic plates by Henry Varnum Poor.

It is telling that the Whitney's Demuths came from Kraushaar's rather than Stieglitz's gallery. Otherwise they might not have arrived at West Eighth Street so quickly, so painlessly, and in such plenitude. Demuth, Marin, Hartley, and Lachaise—the men the staff deemed as not sufficiently represented in the collection—were all associated with Stieglitz, as were Arthur Dove and Georgia O'Keeffe, two names not on the list. No longer did the breezy days of the Club prevail, when Juliana could ignore Stieglitz without forfeit. She now had to ask Stieglitz to sell to her, yet she had never publicly paid tribute to him as a prophet or sage—a failure which, one can assume with confidence, Stieglitz held against her.

The upgrading of the Club and Galleries into an entirely American museum did not make Stieglitz any fonder of the Whitney. It probably influenced things for the worse, because he had a horror of institutions, especially if they were run by women. Sue Davidson Lowe, in her memoir of Stieglitz, who was her great-uncle, spoke of his annoyance with the " 'control' over American art exercised by wealthy woman, particularly Mrs. Whitney and Mrs. Rockefeller [a reference to the Museum of Modern Art]." Any endeavor in which he was not an initiator or prime mover could strike Stieglitz as crass commercialism or an irritating exercise in intellectual exhibitionism. The Whitney Museum, as a promoter of American art, was doubtless looked on as a usurper by Stieglitz, who was now only showing Americans himself, but there was plenty of venom left over for other institutions. The Museum of Modern Art solicited his advice and blessing, but he declined to give either. "[T]he politics and the social set-up come before all else," he wrote. "It may have to be that way to run an institution. But I refuse to believe it. In short, the Museum has really no standard whatever. No integrity of any kind." Stieglitz also tried to persuade O'Keeffe not to lend her paintings to the Modern's second exhibition, but she wanted to be in the show and made the loans.

Nevertheless, Stieglitz handled important artists whose work was indispensable to the development of American art, and their absence from the Whitney would have been inexcusable. The wily old man had Juliana where he wanted her—in the role of suppliant. This was not a role Juliana played with grace, and she was determined to avoid it until all other strategies had been attempted. Her plan was simple and obvious: She would make an end run around Stieglitz by acquiring works of his artists that were in the hands of other dealers.

For the most part, Juliana was successful. The two Demuths came through Kraushaar's, and the Hartley was acquired from the Downtown Gallery for $600. Lachaise was already in Gertrude's collection with several pieces of sculpture, and they went to the museum; in late 1931 Juliana supplemented them with some drawings bought directly from the artist. In an egregious omission, she did not acquire anything by Arthur Dove, who would exhibit at the museum but whose work did not enter the collection until 1951. Juliana's efforts were

thus trained on John Marin and Georgia O'Keeffe, whom she wanted respectably represented in the permanent collection before the museum opened. With Marin, Juliana was in luck. In 1930 she had been able to pick up an important etching (*The Woolworth Building*, for $36) from the Weyhe Gallery, which was run by her friend Carl Zigrosser, but it was essential to obtain some of the artist's watercolors. She and the curators looked over a selection sent from the Weyhe, Downtown, and Reinhardt galleries. Juliana made a point of requesting that the following be read into the record: "Mr. Stieglitz of 'An American Place' was invited to submit examples of Marin's work. He however made the stipulation that the museum should accept all responsibility in regard to the works submitted and that he should be the sole arbiter of whether or not they had suffered injury and if so what indemnity should be necessary. Mrs. Force stated that the museum would be unable to receive work under these conditions." Of the watercolors seen, *Sunset*, for $450, was chosen from the Weyhe Gallery, and *Deer Island, Maine*, for $900, from the Downtown Gallery. The Marins were bought in December of 1931, a banner month at the Whitney for watercolors, for Juliana also bought three Prendergast watercolors of Central Park for $2,500.

Juliana first mentioned that she wanted to buy an O'Keeffe in February of 1931, and in April she was able to get one. *Skunk Cabbage,** an early painting, was available from the Reinhardt Galleries for $450. But Juliana knew that the one example wasn't sufficient or recent enough for the museum. An impasse had been reached, and she had to concede the inevitability of Stieglitz. Normally every knee was bent to Juliana as she made her rounds: There were so few customers for pictures, not to mention American ones, during the hard-pressed 1930s that dealers received her with hosannahs and bowed to her terms. Not so Stieglitz, who was at least as imperious as she was, and often excruciatingly indirect in regard to a painting's availability. Juliana acquiesced to him for the good of the collection, as can be seen by what she went through to get O'Keeffe's *The White Flower* and *The Mountain, New Mexico*.

Juliana first approached Stieglitz in late 1931, and the surviving correspondence dates from 1932. For all his professed indifference to exchanges of money, he was the sharpest and most intransigent opponent she had faced. Most dealers automatically gave Juliana a discount that ranged from 10 percent to 25 percent, and permitted the bill to be paid within one to six months after the purchase was approved. Stieglitz, however, would only allow the discount if she paid up—and on the schedule he ordained. His letters discuss money, prompt payment, and nothing else. In reply to Juliana's expression of interest, he wrote:

> My dear Mrs. Force: I am not going to go into a long harangue of pretty phrases but come right to the point. I have spoken with O'Keeffe in regard to herself & the Whitney Museum.—
> I have the following proposition to make to you.
> The White Flower valued at $3500.00 when you asked its "price" your Museum can have for $2500.00—the Museum to pay O'Keeffe $1000 on or before July 1st

---

* Now in the collection of the Williams College Museum of Art.

[1932], a second $1000 on or before Jan. 1/1933 & the remaining $500 on or before July 1/33. 6% for cash on the $3500 [sic].

Secondly. The Orange Mountain quoted at $4800.00—O'Keeffe will let you have it for $3500 payable $1000.00 on or before July 1/32—second thousand on or before Jan 1/33—the third payment $1500—on or before July 1/33. 6% for cash on the $3500.

Thirdly. Should you want the two pictures you can have them payable as follows. . . . [Schedule of installments given.] If cash be paid by or before July 1st/32 a discount of 6% will be allowed on the lump sum.

I feel this is a more than liberal suggestion. The offer remains open for three days, as there are constant inquiries for both pictures. No one has been offered either picture under the prices quoted to you.

Juliana bowed to Stieglitz's terms for both paintings. To qualify for the discount, she would pay the entire amount before July 1, 1932. In acknowledgment, he unbent enough to write, "Naturally I am glad that O'Keeffe is so well represented in your Museum. My congratulations to every one." The next gracious note Juliana received from Stieglitz consisted of the instruction, "Please don't overlook *registering* the letter containing check due me on or before July 1/32."

The Whitney bought another O'Keeffe from Stieglitz in 1933, but putting up with him was not any easier on the museum staff. For the curators dropping by his gallery, the logorrhea that Forbes found so unbearable had not ceased. Goodrich and More purposely would go there together and pay at least two visits per show. On their first visit, one would get to look at the pictures in peace and the other would have to talk to Stieglitz, who would lecture for the duration of their encounter; at the second visit, the assignments would be reversed. Goodrich later said that the two of them would keep careful track of whose turn it was to keep Stieglitz company.

Goodrich also made a passing attempt to buy O'Keeffe's *Pelvis with the Moon, New Mexico.** In 1943 O'Keeffe began to use the pelvic bones of cattle as a central image in her canvases, and this particular example was shown in the Whitney's 1944 annual. Goodrich, who had long admired O'Keeffe's work and was probably the one to select the painting for inclusion in the show, was struck by the formal power of the skeletal configuration and wanted the museum to acquire the picture. He went up to O'Keeffe at the opening and asked her the price. In answer, she said, "How much was the most expensive painting this museum ever bought?" To which Goodrich discreetly lost his memory, and that was as far as the two got. Talking of O'Keeffe many years later, Goodrich said she was "as cold as stone" and that she had learned well from Stieglitz. Of this incident, he commented, "She was a great artist—and also a great businesswoman."

While Juliana was in Cuba, the fashionable public got its first glimpse of how she lived. On February 15, 1931, her enlarged and refurbished duplex

---

*Now in the collection of the Norton Gallery and School of Art.

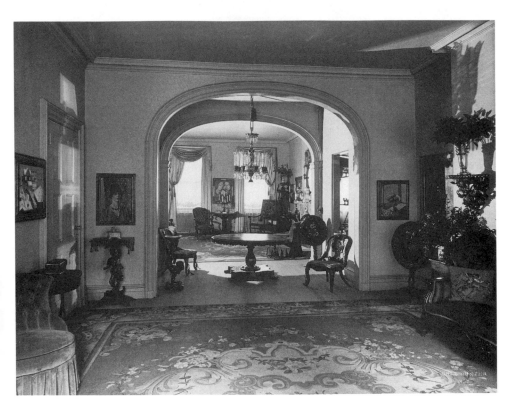

Alcoves and double drawing room of Juliana's apartment spanning the top of the museum. Paintings in the front room, from left: *Winter* by Abraham Walkowitz; *Girl with Black Hat* by Ernest Fiene; *Still Life* by Henry Schnakenberg; and *The Mirror* by Glenn O. Coleman. Back room, far wall: *Peonies* by Paul Rohland.

apartment was featured in *Town & Country*. The article was envisioned as another note of the preliminary fanfare for the opening of the museum that spring. (On March 1, however, it was announced that the buildings would not be ready until November. The staff had just learned that the galleries were never fireproofed.) The story conveyed to society Juliana's standing in the art world: Readers were encouraged to view the decor as an expression of her originality. Once viewed in this astonishing setting, Juliana was never forgotten. As the critic Mary Fanton Roberts would write in 1934. "Even if you have never seen Mrs. Force, these rooms give you an impression of her varied interests, her dramatic temperament, her artistic integrity, and the force of character which has made her one of the foremost women of her generation."

Visitors now reached the third floor in a tiny wrought-iron elevator that was painted in shiny Chinese red. Lloyd Goodrich said that it was the smallest elevator he had ever seen, and that the painter Charles Locke, after emerging from it, exclaimed, "What a place for a bull with claustrophobia!" Guests approached a black door, rapped on it with a brass-mermaid knocker, and stepped into a long hallway. Its floor seemingly was strewn with primroses and meadow grasses,

and when Juliana met her guests there, she would say, "Won't you stroll down my primrose path?" The creation of Bruce Buttfield, the floor covering was lacquered chintz. The primrose path led into successive public rooms: a row of spacious parlors and recessed alcoves, cut from the original buildings and rejoined with wide, flat archways. This panorama of rooms, playfully arranged and exuberantly decorated, was described by Ira Glackens as "one of the sights of New York, elegant, handsome and amusing."

The centerpiece of this floor was the double drawing room, painted in vivid colors, garnished with rococo drippings, and bordered in a floral frieze. The place of honor on the marble mantelpiece over the fireplace belonged to an alabaster bust of Queen Victoria. To its right and left were alabaster candlesticks and compotes; another mantelpiece held an alabaster clock tiered and filigreed like a wedding cake. Flanking these ensembles were carved Venetian blackamoors. One pair balanced urns filled with bunches of drooping tulips on their heads and the other held lamps with parchment shades in their outstretched arms. Aubusson rugs with swirling floral designs were joined and extended by turquoise ingrain carpets. Upholstered shell chairs of the Regency, gilded Victorian papier-mâché chairs, tufted velvet *fauteuils*, petticoated hassocks, and loveseats covered in pink or red satin convened in friendly groupings. They were complemented by lacquered papier-mâché side tables inlaid with mother-of-pearl and gilt tracery down to their little splayed feet. Separated by a long gilt-framed mirror, the windows were framed by sky-blue satin draperies that puddled to the floor and were trimmed and looped with ropes of pearls. Against this arch backdrop, Juliana's art collection—Ingres, Sheeler, Audubon, Henri Rousseau, Picasso, Brancusi, Rufino Tamayo, Abraham Walkowitz, Preston Dickinson, Glenn O. Coleman, and many anonymous eighteenth- and nineteenth-century provincials—was shown in an unembarrassed and harmonious manner. Juliana's affection for the starchy absurdities of period and place unified everything, and the extravagant parlor was conducive to advocacy as well as hospitality. As Lloyd Goodrich put it, "Those parties were more than just sociability. Many of the people invited to them had importance in the art world. They helped to establish the fact that the first museum of American art was not a down-at-the-heels, bedraggled operation, but an upper-level one. More than one project for the good of American art was settled over the coffee and scotch in her Victorian drawingroom."

The study, library, and bedroom were on the fourth floor, and in them Juliana took just as many liberties in using styles and colors, blending whatever suited her purposes. The library had pale pink walls and a dark-brown carpet and curtains. She mixed modern and Biedermeier furniture and topped it with a dollop of Americana in the lighting fixtures suspended from the ceiling: Gilded wooden eagles caught with white-and-gold silk cords clutched milk-glass globes in their claws. The cords were operated by pulleys, and they could be raised and lowered at will. The study was filled with American Empire furniture and had a florid Victorian carpet of red roses splashed on a white ground. Louis Bouché had painted the doors in fine trompe l'oeil, and he rendered them to look as if they had been fitted with quilted padding pounced with minuscule

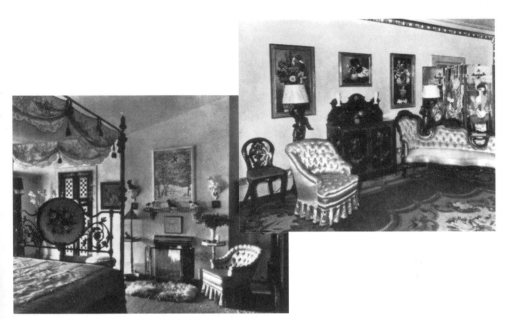

Left: a section of Juliana's bedroom showing the tester bed and the marquetry and gilt doors; right: another corner of the drawing room. The black lacquer cabinet is English, ca. 1850; displayed on it, *Prometheus* by Brancusi.

navels. Indeed, all the rooms on the upper floor had doors that were fantastical decorations in themselves. The ones not executed by Bouché were designed by Buttfield. He took black lacquer and white mother-of-pearl and applied them in a checkerboard intarsia pattern. Along the border enclosing the squares, the gilt and nacre inlays were incised in a scroll motif.

Juliana's bedroom, which was entered through one of those checkerboard doors, was as colorful and elaborate as the rest of the apartment. She slept in a curlicued brass-and-iron tester bed, varnished in black and canopied with pale pink embroidered mull hangings, and a bedspread of quilted pink taffeta covered the blankets and pillows. The curtains, designed by Robert Locher, were purposely made of quotidian black oilcloth, but the fabric was sprinkled with bouquets of opalescent beads picked out with gold thread. An adjoining dressing room was painted and lacquered in six different shades of chartreuse.

It is essential to understand how outrageous and peculiar Juliana's revival of furniture and objects straight from the Grant and Garfield eras must have looked to her contemporaries. Unlike the present, when a liking for the cozy profusions of late-nineteenth-century domesticity might be fashionable or nostalgic, endorsing such démodé styles then was a clarion challenge to prevailing tastes. At the time, the word "Victorian," applied to anything, was a term of withering reproach.

While reveling unabashedly in the foibles of old-fashioned interiors and enjoying the tease her preferences caused, Juliana also significantly updated

Victorian decor by leaving large open spaces where there had been clutter and employing bright, clear, and brilliant color in place of dark, somber shades. Yet even her edited version of the period would have struck the average person as grotesque. The sophisticated journalists assigned to write on the apartment at 10 West Eighth Street were aware that their audiences were not ready for it, and they shaded their essays accordingly. In the feature in *Town & Country*, an inordinate amount of space was spent on reassuring readers that these admittedly bizarre tastes really did possess a certain offbeat charm. The reporter allowed, "It is interesting to see how boldly a virtue has been made of ugliness in the case of the more ornate pieces." *House & Garden*, which ran a spread on the apartment in 1932, cautiously headlined the story, "An Experiment in the Rococo." The author was the art critic Helen Appleton Read, who wrote that the bedroom created "an opportunity for proving that objects and accessories, unlovely in themselves, can, by selective arrangement, form an attractive ensemble." Magazine editors recognized Juliana's exceptional instincts for color, materials, and design, but they were more attracted to her rooms for their sensational oddness.

In 1935 the apartment was still considered strange enough for the newspaperman Stanley Walker to cite it in *Mrs. Astor's Horse*, his consciously "man in the street" report on the screwball antics of the Prohibition years. To illustrate his theme of foolishness in high places, Walker devoted a chapter to the resurgent cult of the Victorian among the arty set. Walker fingered Juliana as belonging to this benighted group, which was eagerly resurrecting the worst atrocities of the previous age. They were all, in his opinion, the victims of slick decorators who had fobbed off irredeemable junk on gullible and trend-mongering aesthetes. The results, Walker snickered, had "produced some rather startling and daffy effects." To Walker, Juliana had made a ridiculous mistake.

No arrangement or layout stayed the same for long. Juliana was a constant redecorator and a restless mover of furniture. It was part of the same churning impulse that operated when she bought, renovated, and maintained several houses at once; it was connected to the hatred of dullness that compelled her to improve on anything she touched or any scene she entered. It was also a matter of energy. Lloyd Goodrich explained, "My wife and I would go off on a trip with her and stay in the same hotel. But in about ten minutes her room would look entirely different because she would have already moved the furniture around. Even when driving in a car, she would make it seem more decorative or more liveable." Edith Goodrich remembered a visit to Martha's Vineyard. "We stayed at a local boardinghouse, simple and stark. Each room had an iron bedstead, a pitcher and washstand, and not much more. We checked in and Mrs. Force said, 'I'll be ready in twenty minutes.' We joined her then, and in that time, she had unpacked her bag, moved the bed, gotten flowers from the garden, laid her dressing gown over the bed, draped a shawl over a chair in the corner, and put some books and magazines on the night table. She had transformed a dull room into something completely hers."

Juliana did prefer the relics of the brownstone-front era, but just as choosing them did not make her conventional, living with them did not make her illiberal

or rule out modernist architecture or design. She was interested in any development or movement that reflected the progress of an individual sensibility. In early 1931, she was working closely with the great architectural renderer Hugh Ferriss on a possible collaboration between him and Gertrude, and she had also asked Herbert Morgan, a painter friend who had become an architect, to design her a modern house for a plot of land she had bought in Woodstock. Morgan, who had lived in France in the 1920s, was strongly influenced by Le Corbusier, and his design reflected this. He drew plans for a plain white Cubist villa in which rooms and balconies flowed into each other. Its construction was based on cantilevers and pilotis. Juliana approved of the smoothly functional interior and stark outer skin, and Morgan built two scale models. But when she and Morgan began discussing the budget—the house was to have a dining balcony, a large art gallery, a spiral staircase, and an indoor swimming pool—she saw that the costs would be prohibitive. The project was abandoned, and Juliana later deeded the property as a gift to Hermon and Edna More. Had this modernist house become a reality, it would have been one of the first buildings in the United States not only to be designed in the International Style, but constructed in it.

The money required to execute Morgan's design must have been an impressive sum, because otherwise there were few signs of Juliana's personal spending being deterred by the Depression. She continued to live lavishly, using up her salary and supplementing it with her expense accounts, although in April of 1931 she conducted a public sale at the farm of some of her Pennsylvania-German and Shaker antiques. The sale, which netted a few thousand dollars, may have been held to weed out duplicates and lesser examples as much as to make money, because records from the Downtown Gallery list fifteen quilts and twenty hooked rugs as among the things offered. Thirty items were bought by Edith Halpert, who promptly resold them to Abby Aldrich Rockefeller for Bassett Hall, her house in Williamsburg, Virginia.

If relatively unscathed herself by the Depression in 1931, Juliana was actively concerned about the problems artists were having. Most of the painters and sculptors she knew had become acutely impoverished because their services were the first to be dispensed with in a moribund economy. As Moses Soyer put it, "Depression—who can describe the hopelessness that its victims knew? Perhaps no one better than the artist taking his work to the galleries. They were at a standstill. The misery of the artist was acute. There was nothing he could turn to." To make matters worse, the general public looked on artists with suspicion—they appeared to be deadbeats who scorned to hold real jobs. For some time Juliana had been trying to help needy artists, and throughout 1931 the responsibility would preoccupy her almost as much as the opening of the museum.

By the summer of 1930, most of the artists who lived in Woodstock were out of cash. No credit was extended to them because the banks were closed or had failed. The artists couldn't even get groceries. Sidney Geist, in an article

about the plight of American artists during the Depression, reported that during the summer of 1930, "In what remains a memorable gesture in that time of crisis, Mrs. Juliana Force . . . rushed to the scene, and bought paintings to a sum rumored to be twenty thousand dollars. It saved the day." Juliana did rush to the scene, but it is improbable that she disbursed this much money to Woodstock. The amount is too great to be convincing. Asked to confirm this figure many years later, Geist said that the source of the story was the painter Ben Benn, whose memory he had found from experience to be absolutely reliable. However, $20,000 was exactly the amount of money established by Gertrude as a purchase fund for the early biennials. Benn could have conflated or latched onto this figure because $20,000 was a well-known and set sum associated with the Whitney during the 1930s. Juliana could easily have arrived in Woodstock with two or three thousand dollars and done quite a lot of good. (She also did it in her own distinctive way. Eugene Ludins, who benefited from the visit Geist described, said, "I had a shack on the Maverick, and Hermon More and Mrs. Force came by while I was out. They climbed in the window and bought a picture.* They left a note.")

Juliana met with Abby Rockefeller on April 15, 1931, and asked her to join a pool she was organizing to set up a fund of $50,000 for needy artists. Mrs. Rockefeller agreed and immediately pledged $5,000 (which turned out to be $4,500 spread over four years). Heartened by Juliana's activism, she wrote to her, "I cannot tell you what a pleasure and comfort it was to me to have you here yesterday. My talk with you has cheered me greatly and has given me confidence to go ahead." Juliana received the first installment of $2,500 in December of 1931; with it, she was to purchase prints, drawings, and similarly inexpensive works for the Rockefeller collection, spreading the largesse among as many artists as she could. In addition to spending the Rockefeller checks, Juliana would also buy works of art out of her own money and later, as the budget allowed, "sneak" them into the Whitney collection; if the budget did not allow it, she would often donate them. Besides buying works of art, Juliana also used the Rockefeller donations to make sure artists kept working and kept eating. She reported to Abby Rockefeller that she had underwritten an artists' cooperative:

> With the help of your money these four hundred men are assured, until the first of April, of a building, heated, lighted and equipped for selling of their work at low prices. I am also taking care of a number whom I know to be without homes and without food or clothes. Just now I am planning a Christmas Dinner for those who have no other place to go on that day.
>
> I am sure that no money you have ever spent would gladden your heart more, if you could know of the many people who, by this money, have been raised from the paralysis of despair to at least make an effort to help themselves and thus keep their self-respect.

But no matter how much they did, nothing was enough to counter the universal deprivation, and Juliana received dozens of pathetic letters from artists known

---

*Landscape, in the Whitney collection, for $300.

and unknown to her, all begging for relief. For every artist she aided, there were too many more that she was powerless to help.

Concurrent with these charitable efforts, as well as the ongoing stream of acquisitions, Juliana was readying the museum for its public opening, which would take place on November 18, 1931. Four days before the Whitney opened its doors, she concluded negotiations for one more painting that she felt she had to have on the walls in time for the great event. The museum did not have a significant figurative painting by George Bellows, and Juliana wanted *Dempsey and Firpo* of 1924, his brash and energetic rendering of one of the most famous prizefights of the day, and a canvas that epitomizes the strenuous masculine exertions that Bellows and his master, Henri, favored as subject matter for American art. Bellows had died in 1925 with a big reputation, and his widow, Emma, was well aware of his standing in managing the estate. She put a budget-wrecking price on the picture—the final cost for the Whitney was $18,750, which had to represent a 25 percent reduction from $25,000. Even with the discount, *Dempsey and Firpo* brought the highest price ever paid by the museum for a work of art, a sum that was not exceeded until 1960. Not only did Emma Bellows name an astronomical price, but she insisted on being paid at once. It seems all too likely that the conditions she imposed led Juliana to make what became an oft-quoted remark: "Artists' widows should commit suttee."

Dempsey and Firpo was hung on the main staircase, where it could not be missed. The new museum now possessed nearly 700 works of art of the present and recent past; it was painted, scrubbed, and upholstered; its sales desk was filled with catalogs and reproductions, and its curators were ready to guide and explain. Beginning on November 16, 1931, it was the scene of several days of luncheons, cocktail parties, receptions, speeches, and coast-to-coast radio hook-ups. Only one hoped-for publicity coup eluded the Whitney—Juliana tried to get Herbert Hoover to attend the opening, but she had to settle for a telegram from the White House.

November 16 was given over to the press, and the high point was a luncheon in the sculpture gallery for thirty art critics from different parts of the country. Forbes, Royal Cortissoz, Hugh Ferriss, and Christopher Morley were called upon to make speeches. Morley, bowled over by *Dempsey and Firpo*, said the picture was a reminder that "[h]ere in this brilliantly controversial place the art which is merely correct, genteel, and sterile gets a tough one in the midsection. This is not just a museum; it is a ring; not a ring-around-the-rosy but the squared circle of combative and contemporary talents." Then it was Juliana's turn. "[I]n a frank little speech," McBride said, "she spoke of the enterprise as a 'gesture,' and added that the true test of the gesture could be made about twenty-five years hence." Bargaining with posterity, Juliana reserved for the museum the right not to be wholly right. On this subject she would also write, "The Whitney Museum of American Art enters the field with a little bow of apology for its inadequacies, but no hesitancy." The statement was characteristically Juliana —she may have occasionally had qualms about certain policies (for which she

herself was responsible), but she entertained no doubts whatsoever about the advocacy of a permanent institution that would give American art a new stature.

On the following afternoon of November 17, the ceremonies culminating in a private reception for the friends of Gertrude, Juliana, and the museum began. Starting at 4:00 P.M., CBS broadcast the inaugural speeches from Juliana's office. The presidential message was read, and then Gertrude welcomed the general public to the museum. After she spoke, former Gov. Al Smith and Otto Kahn offered up some bromides instructing the public to give thanks for what it was about to receive. Meanwhile, between 3,000 and 5,000 invited guests were converging on Eighth Street, undeterred by a day that was wet, foggy, and dismal. The road was jammed with cars, and the detail of police officers assigned to keep traffic moving couldn't keep up with their duty. The area was impassable for hours, and local storekeepers gave up on doing any business. The line of people waiting to get into the building stretched several blocks up Fifth Avenue.

After the speeches were read, Gertrude, in black velvet and chiffon, and Juliana, contrastingly attired in a vermilion dress and hat, went to greet the waves of happy guests—artists, museum directors, dealers, publishers, collectors, writers, actors, musicians, friends, family—who had been listening to the broadcast downstairs. Gertrude and Juliana, founder and director, partners and friends, promenaded in gala formation as they had for twenty-five years, receiving homage from uptown and downtown. Julius Bloch, who watched the two as they walked around, wrote in his diary the next day, "Mrs. Whitney, somehow veiled in a half light, no definitions, but yet the bounteous, generous source of this beautiful home for works of art. Mrs. Force, . . . strong in spirit, ever buoyant, doer of wonders."

On November 18, the public got its first chance to visit the museum. An estimated 4,000 persons attempted to enter, not all of them artists and art lovers. As the head of a secretarial agency wrote to Gertrude, she immediately began sending despairing job seekers to the museum. The agency had no work for anyone, and the Whitney, with its deep carpets, plush sofas, and free admission, was an oasis of comfort for these unemployed men and women. "[I]t has helped so much," she wrote. "If I may send these poor souls to your building [I] hope you will not mind." Gertrude, of course, could not have minded. She would have been gratified that her museum might offset such bleakness. As Juliana wrote in her Christmas card for that year:

> Dear Gertrude,
> A crown you've won
> For all you've done
> A dove for peace &
> joy and love.
> From Juliana

"My fears that the Whitney Museum of American Art would not be sufficiently criticized proved groundless," wrote Henry McBride, and he was right. The museum was now the preeminent symbol of the claims made for an Amer-

ican renaissance in the arts, and commentators could not resist turning their appraisals of the collection into a referendum on the prestige of native painting, especially with respect to the challenge it issued to the French. With the advent of the Whitney, declared Edward Alden Jewell, "the vogue of the so thoroughly press-agented Ecole de Paris is on the wane." Negative criticism addressed the collection's inadequacies as well as the degree to which it did or did not embrace modernism and tradition. Speaking for the conservatives, Cortissoz felt that the pictures had a sameness about them, and that they lacked a poetic touch. "[T]he bulk of the painters have a kindred aim," he noted. "It is that of a literal transcription of fact. . . . The typical painter will have nothing to do with drama or symbolism. The late Arthur B. Davies seems very lonely on his eminence of imaginative contemplation. . . . The majority are content to fasten upon some ponderable object and then keep their eyes glued to it." Speaking for the progressives, Samuel Kootz, after several days of "trudging" through the museum, "was unable to find any final evidence of the arrival of native art at any maturity. . . . For though most of our important men were represented, a herculean effort must have been expended in rounding up such uniformly inferior examples of their work." The only recorded reaction from Juliana to all of this was a remark for the *Times*: "There may be pictures here that you do not like, but they are here to stay, so you may as well get used to them."

The longest and most scabrous verdict was rendered by an important critic— Paul Rosenfeld, writing in *The Nation*. Rosenfeld made several salient points, but he was also one of Stieglitz's inner circle, and that affiliation colored his view of the Whitney. Rosenfeld astutely stated that the museum's collection, formed to support the young and striving, was "bought with an eye bent more to the struggles and promise of the artists than to the completeness of their expressions. Later, when the idea of a museum began to obtain, the collection appears to have rather hastily been augmented to fit the new purpose." Calling what he saw "secondary and provincial," Rosenberg accused the collection of being "sadly unfaithful to the work it pretends to represent." He felt that Stieglitz's artists weren't represented well enough and pounced on the work of the Henri school, for which there was a thorough selection: "Of all ambitious American painting, it seems least deserving of a place in a museum of art." He concluded sourly, "One could almost wish that the Whitney Museum had never opened its pompous doors."

A review that meant more to Juliana—the museum "was much pleased to receive it," as it "came at a time when we have been busy dodging brick-bats" —was filed by a young Harvard man. He was A. Hyatt Mayor, a future curator of prints at the Metropolitan Museum of Art, but then a student writing for *Hound & Horn*, the lively little magazine founded by Lincoln Kirstein. Mayor, who thought the opening of the museum a "miracle" and its inauguration "the most important thing that has happened to American art since the foundation of our now useless academies," dismissed the Franco-American controversy that obsessed all the other critics with, "The question is not: 'How must I, as an American, paint this?' but: 'How *must this be painted?*'" He went on to say, "If any institution can help American artists, the Whitney Museum is that

institution. It can help because it is not yet an institution, but two women of remarkable flair and energy. When they choose artists to exhibit, they will not consider what will sell, as dealers must; and the best things are often slow to sell. . . . Since it is only a growing 'nucleus' of what will be, it will help certain artists by buying their works (the only real help there is). . . . It may also help artists by showing them each other's work and so making them aware of some common movement."

Along with acting as a lightning rod for informed critical opinion, the Whitney was bringing American art before a largely uninitiated public. Sometimes the effort was not repaid until many years later and in ways not easily predicted. The museum could be a revelation to someone unfamiliar with American art, as the following account, published in 1977, suggests. In the early 1930s, James Michener, who would not only become a best-selling author but a collector of American art, was working in a publishing firm four blocks away from the museum. Each day he would walk down to Eighth Street to eat lunch at one of the restaurants there. After a while he noticed "the severely handsome facade of the Whitney Museum." One day he decided to go in. Michener saw "a selection of paintings by Marin, Weber, Kuniyoshi, Hopper, and Burchfield. They quite staggered me with their beauty. . . . I formed then my basic taste for American art and have merely modified it as the years passed. . . . The great virtue of the Whitney Collection was that it specialized in American artists and showed a wide cross section of the work then being done. . . . If I were to specify the one influence which had the most profound effect upon my attitude as an amateur in the field of American painting, it would have to be the Whitney."

Being the center of debate didn't affect the museum's course one whit, and 1932 opened with more of the permanent collection on display, as well as work by members of the American Society of Painters, Sculptors, and 'Gravers, an artists' "organization which, at the time, was the nearest thing to a labor union in the art world." As the society existed to fight for artists' rights, its membership entertained a broad spectrum of political views and aesthetic stances: Stuart Davis, Florine Stettheimer, Edward Hopper, Peggy Bacon, Charles Sheeler, Yasuo Kuniyoshi, and Charles Demuth, to name a few, were all in it. Another member was George Luks, who had lost none of his blowsy charm over the years. At the party given for the show, Luks trailed after Gertrude wherever she went. Finally she asked him, "Mr. Luks, why are you following me around?" "Because," he sighed ecstatically, "you're so goddamn rich!"

Shortly after this encounter, Gertrude invited Juliana, Charles Draper, and Robert Locher on a two-week cruise to Cuba. They sailed on March 19, 1932. While they were gone, the museum opened a show of nineteenth-century provincial paintings that received rave reviews. The pictures were hung in tandem with cartoons by Thomas Nast and prints by Audubon and Currier & Ives. Almost all of the folk art came from Juliana's huge personal collection, and after the show (which went on to two other museums) was dismantled, she donated about sixty oils, pastels, and watercolors to the Whitney.

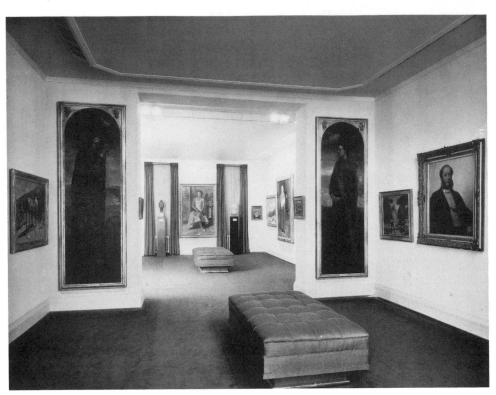

An installation of the museum's permanent collection, summer 1932. Front panels: *The Virgin Mary* and *St. John* by John La Farge; back wall, center: *Portrait of a Girl* by Eugene Speicher; back right wall: *Mrs. Gamley* by George Luks.

To give New Yorkers a free place to visit, the Whitney stayed open during June and July of 1932. Juliana, however, after a midnight sailing and a send-off attended by "endless guests," left on May 5 for Europe. There, she told Abby Rockefeller, she "hoped to find peace and rest and regain . . . [her] strength." England was still the same place she knew, but the Continent had changed. In Venice for the 1932 Biennale, she was "horrified," as she told Allan Rieser, by Mussolini and the hold fascism had on Italy. She was also distressed about the conditions in Germany, and she spoke of them to several artists in Woodstock in 1933. One of them recorded Juliana's report in her diary. "Such changes she told of—one can hardly believe—German women not smoking—no make up —no nightclubs—no liberty of any kind, it seems to us." The Nazi threat continued to disturb her. A year or two later, Lloyd Goodrich remembered being at the farm one weekend, and Juliana insisting that she read aloud to her guests a short story about the effects of the Third Reich on relations between friends.

The universal shortage of money was still Juliana's reigning reality that autumn. How to do enough? On September 4, 1932, she was in Manchester,

Vermont, at the opening of the Southern Vermont Artists Association. Also present was Laura Bragg, the director of the Berkshire Museum in Pittsfield, Massachusetts, which led to Juliana being invited to a new show at the Berkshire Museum.

The museum was exhibiting several rooms of Shaker furniture and artifacts—objects familiar to Juliana, who had been collecting such pieces for years. The show was organized and curated by Faith and Edward Deming Andrews, a husband-and-wife team who visited a Shaker community in 1923, were overwhelmed by what they saw, and had become students and devotees of the sect and its culture ever since. The Andrewses bought and sold Shaker furniture and objects; they were considered "junk dealers" by the less imaginative antiques sellers in the Pittsfield area. "Most people thought we were out of our minds, bothering with such poor people," Faith Andrews said many years later. "Very few people understood the value of what we were doing."

At the Berkshire Museum, Juliana demonstrated that she was someone who did understand. "She saw rooms all together," Faith Andrews recalled. "She was swept off her feet. She was the first person to use the word 'elegant' in reference to the furniture. You can imagine what a boost that was to us." Besides sharing a belief in the formal sophistication of Shaker craft, Juliana and the Andrewses were already unwittingly connected by business transactions. As Edward Andrews wrote, "Mrs. Force had a collection of Shaker furniture which she had obtained from a dealer in Ridgefield, Connecticut, who had bought certain pieces from us at a time when we were under obligation to sell. The dealer, naturally, had not revealed the source of his purchases, so it was with great surprise . . . that Mrs. Force learned that we were the original owners. Deeply interested as she was in promoting American art and craftsmanship, she was avid to know all about the Shakers and their work."

After this, said Faith Andrews, "the Whitney Museum became part of us and our work." Many of the items in the Pittsfield show had come from the Andrewses' house, and Juliana visited them as soon as the exhibit was broken up and everything back in place. She took the 5:00 A.M. milk train to Pittsfield from New York. The Andrewses then drove her to the small but surviving Shaker communities in Hancock, Massachusetts, and New Lebanon, New York. Faith Andrews remembered, "The first place we took her was out to Hancock because we wanted her to meet [Sister] Alice and the people there and where we had our own start. There were buildings empty, all except the dwelling and we went into every building—the laundry, the dairy, . . . the church, everywhere, and Juliana Force was like Alice in Wonderland. She just could not believe that this was real. . . . She was so shocked that this situation, this separate culture existed. . . . She felt it was a great opportunity we had given her." Juliana "loved meeting Sister Alice and asked questions about everything. She had vision. She saw what this was in a glance and knew it had to be shown as a special contribution to American culture." After that, the three of them talked from early morning until late at night about what they could do to preserve and document the Shakers' secluded life. Juliana wanted the Andrewses to assemble a show for the

Whitney (which would not take place until 1935) and discussed the possibility of a permanent Shaker room and collection for the museum (which never came to pass). For the present, convinced of the value of the couple's work, Juliana offered to sponsor their labors, granting them a subsidy that continued for two years. Said Faith Andrews, "It [her visit] was quite, quite an event. Juliana Force was a force herself. Once was enough—that's all she needed." In November of 1932, the Andrewses began receiving $200 a month, plus the services of a photographer. (No matter how strictly the museum's budget was calculated and allotted, Juliana would override it if she believed the cost—or the cause—was justified.) The research and pictures resulted in *Shaker Furniture, The Craftsmanship of an American Communal Sect*, published by Yale University Press in 1937. In pursuing their studies, the Andrewses established themselves as experts on Shaker culture and became further involved in a long-term campaign to preserve Shaker communities. They also worked as Juliana's agents, locating additional Shaker objects for her house in South Salem.

In late October of 1932, Juliana wanted Charles Sheeler's *River Rouge Plant*, one of his best industrial landscapes, for the museum. Finished earlier that year, the picture was first exhibited at the museum itself, during the run of the Painters, Sculptors, and 'Gravers exhibition. Juliana began negotiations with Edith Halpert, who had originally priced the picture at $1,000 and then raised it to $1,200. As Juliana was one of the Downtown Gallery's best customers and had been responsible for subsidizing quite a few of its artists, Halpert was quick to telephone Sheeler about a price reduction. Juliana got the painting for $900.

Juliana continued to nurture artists vigilantly. With the backing of Abby Rockefeller, she kept an artists' cafeteria going. She also endorsed the Washington Square Outdoor Art Exhibit, a temporary outdoor fair initiated by Vernon Porter, an art administrator. The first exhibit took place in May of 1932, with artists selling their work directly to the public in designated areas along the perimeters of Washington Square. Juliana had written recommendations to the proper municipal departments to enable Porter to get the necessary permits, and she let her name be used for publicity purposes. The exhibit was successful enough to encourage another, which would open on November 12, 1932. This time, 300 artists signed up; among those registered were Burgoyne Diller, Palmer Hayden, Joseph Solman, Francis Criss, John Gregory, and Alice Neel. Unfortunately, winter came early to the city, and passersby were not prone to linger among the shivering men and women huddled against their pictures. Juliana took one look at the freezing artists and arranged to take all of them, in groups of fifty, to a hot lunch at a nearby restaurant for the rest of the week. She then bought fourteen works of art from various exhibitors (for $108.50), and on the evening of November 20, which was the last day of the show, she invited all the exhibitors to a tea at the Jumble Shop for "a round table discussion concerning the problems of the winter." Juliana spoke first at this gathering, and almost before she finished, some of the artists shouted, "Down with private capital!" Nevertheless, she hired Porter, because of his knowledge of the worst cases of privation, as a part-time confidential assistant. He was to make sure that needy

artists received money (private capital from Whitney and Rockefeller fortunes) for food and shelter that winter. He also helped Juliana plan a Christmas dinner for seventy-five artists who had nowhere to go that day.

At the museum itself, the first biennial exhibition of contemporary American painting opened on November 22, with 157 paintings submitted by as many artists. Given the conditions of the art world, Juliana felt that the biennial was an occasion for which every effort should be made to *sell* pictures as well as show them. The entries were frankly publicized as being for sale, and a special salesperson was hired for the purpose. The museum was taking no commission, so Juliana asked the artists to put low prices on their canvases. Seven were sold, four of them to the Metropolitan. In turn, out of the $20,000 purchase fund earmarked for the biennial, Juliana bought twenty-eight paintings. The ones that seem of most interest today are Peter Blume's *The Light of the World*, Bluemner's *Composition*, Ault's *Hudson Street*, and Curry's *The Flying Codonas*.

As already noted, the first biennial was pilloried in the press because each artist was asked to send a work of his or her own selection. However, in terms of the artists who were invited, the Whitney had spread beyond ex-Club members. Stefan Hirsch, Dove, O'Keeffe, Karl Knaths, Ivan Albright, Hartley, Grant Wood, Ben Shahn, Theodore Roszak, John Kane, and Louis Eilshemius made their Whitney debuts; Mark Tobey and Kenneth Callahan were also invited for the first time, but they did not send work. Other veteran exhibitors previously shown at the Whitney were Joseph Stella, Oscar Bluemner, Konrad Cramer, Arnold Friedman, Bradley Walker Tomlin, Florine Stettheimer, John Graham, Abraham Walkowitz, Max Weber, and Isabel Bishop.

Each artist reacted differently to being chosen for the first biennial. Dove, then living in western New York, stated only that he couldn't afford to come to the city for the show, but made no substantive comment. Stieglitz then told Dove that he sent his painting (*Red Barge, Reflections*) in only because McBride and others said "it ought to be in the Whitney Museum," as he himself scoffed at the possibility of a sale. After Dove was bypassed, Stieglitz wrote to him, "I see the Whitney Museum has remained true to its blindness. And I fear ever will." However, some good did come out of the biennial for them. Duncan Phillips attended the show and liked *Red Barge, Reflections* better than any other picture he saw. Stieglitz sold it to him for $700.

For the younger, lesser-known artists entering the Whitney as first-time exhibitors, to be shown side by side with Hopper, Sloan, Davis, Stella, Dove, or O'Keeffe was thrill enough. In the words of Harry Sternberg:

> I was a relatively young artist when I was included in that first Whitney biennial. It was one of the most exciting moments in my life. For the first time, one of my paintings was hanging in a *museum*. I think I was one of the first to arrive for the opening—and one of the last to leave. I guess I spent most of my time casually lounging near my painting.
>
> Juliana Force presided regally, the building was indeed beautiful, warm and friendly. Our paintings looked magnificent. And there was an unlimited flow of booze! By midnight the artists and the place had become a glorious shambles—sandwiches ground into the carpets, cigarette butts everywhere, even in the outstretched hands

of some sculptures, and happily drunken artists passing out. Mrs. Force had two big strong men in livery standing by—and at a nod from her, these men began carrying drunks out of the 8th Street entrance and stacking them on the sidewalk like cordwood.

But Juliana's most large-hearted extension of support, which climaxed during the winter of 1932, was an ongoing adventure that had swerved in an unfriendly direction. She had embarked on it trustingly enough, in early 1932, with no inkling of how she would be punished for her generosity. Both her beneficiary and her antagonist were Thomas Hart Benton. After the New School commission, which met with critical acclaim, Benton had become the most conspicuous muralist in the country as well as the dominant painter of the American Scene movement. The prices on his paintings went up, and Benton began spending the money that poured in. He and his wife, Rita, moved into a better apartment, hosted big parties, and looked into buying more real estate on Martha's Vineyard, where they had a cottage. But sales declined as the Depression wore on, and by the end of 1931 the couple was in danger of losing their property on the Vineyard. Rita, who was a shrewd business manager when she could intercept their income before her profligate husband squandered it, had a fine grasp of the art market. Indefatigable in advancing Benton's career, she reminded him that Juliana Force had not only commiserated with him about his lack of recompense for the New School murals, but then did her best to make up for the inequity. Benton said that Juliana, upon learning that the artist had not been compensated for painting the New School murals other than reimbursement for his expenses, "was outspoken in her condemnation of people who would let an artist do such a work for nothing. She made up for the matter somewhat by purchasing a lot of my preliminary studies for the Whitney Museum, paying a good price for them." Whitney records show that Benton received $840 for the fourteen works, which was generous.

Rita Benton went to see Juliana in early 1932 and explained that she and Tom were going to lose their Vineyard house unless they could come up with $12,000. Juliana must have been asked to buy some pictures, but the museum had no budget for acquisitions. Yet Rita pleaded so effectively that Juliana, anxious to be of assistance, offered to lend the couple $3,000 of her own money, free of interest.

The Bentons took the money with alacrity, and their real estate was saved. However, they were unwilling or unable to pay back Juliana, and this time it was Benton who asked Juliana to accept either easel paintings or his *American Historical Epic* murals in lieu of repayment. The latter had been intended for the New York Public Library and thus were not the right size for the Whitney's walls, so Benton suggested creating a new set of murals especially designed for West Eighth Street. The museum did not need any murals, nor did it have the money to commission artists to make them, but Benton was so insistent that Juliana consented. The project seemed to be the only way to absolve him of his financial obligation to her. According to the minutes of several museum staff meetings, the commission was approved in January of 1932. In February, Juliana

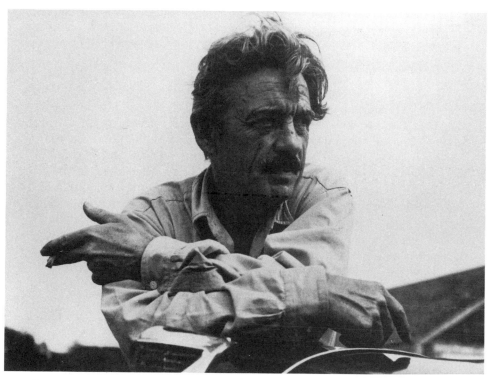

Thomas Hart Benton in a seemingly pensive mood—a side that not many people saw.

consulted with Gertrude on a suitable location. The murals would be hung in Juliana's library, which would become a public reading room after they were finished.

Juliana let Benton know that he could proceed and gave him free rein as to subject matter. He left the city that spring, as he was in the habit of doing, for a sketching trip to Georgia. These journeys into the countryside, Benton felt, kept him in touch with American life. Nothing was heard from him for several months.

Benton's excursion to the rural South was probably Juliana's last moment of peace regarding the mural commission, for the turmoil visible in Benton's paintings was nothing to the turmoil generated by his personality. Benton relished controversy, and he had a talent for provocation exercised without restraint. By 1932, Benton had many enemies, most of them earned. Maynard Walker, one of the artist's dealers during the 1930s, said, "Benton always repaid people who helped him with a kick in the pants." Always contentious, Benton cast himself as the savior of American painting and displayed the stigmata of notoriety to prove it. In this role, he could not fail to draw attacks—or gain fame. His impolitic remarks kept him and his art in the public eye and attracted extensive coverage in both the art and popular press. Even the denunciations were welcomed.

Benton, however, was abnormally combative, even for someone who was a master at profiting from polemics. Some portion of his aggressiveness might be laid to an obsession with his height. At 5 feet 3 inches tall, he was the classic example of the hard-driven runt who tries to compensate for his smallness with outsize energy and pugnacity. Swarthy and square-set, with a lined face and a bristling mustache, Benton had a face like a Gypsy and a body like a gnome. However, in several self-portraits, where he was free to fashion his image as he liked, he represented himself as towering over his companions—all of whom were taller than he in real life. It cannot be accidental that Benton's figures are characterized by their extreme height and elongation.

Benton was expected to become an illustrious lawyer, politician, or businessman. In his parents' eyes, drawing was a waste of time for a healthy, red-blooded man. His father "was profoundly prejudiced against artists, and with some reason," recalled the artist in his memoirs. "The only ones he had ever come across were the mincing, bootlicking portrait painters of Washington who . . . lisped a silly jargon about grace and beauty. . . . He couldn't think of a son of his having anything to do with their profession." The resolution of these conflicts—the pressure to add luster to the Benton name by becoming a public figure headed for a place in American history and the virulent bias against artists as fairies and shirkers—was to plague Benton throughout his career. In pursuit of immortality, he courted controversy and tumult. To advertise that he was not an overwrought aesthete, he paraded his masculinity by fighting, cussing, and drinking. He made slurs about "the pretty boys in museums" on the wispiest pretext.

Benton also augmented his he-man image by a splendid impersonation of a tobacco-spitting, whiskey-guzzling, butt-kicking mule from Missouri. Benton had been groomed to be a sophisticated cosmopolite, but these details of his history he kept to himself. Born in 1889 in Neosho, Missouri, of eminent ancestry, he was the grandnephew and namesake of the state's first senator and the son of a prominent congressman known as the "little giant of the Ozarks." The Bentons were the first family of Neosho, and they entertained the famous in a big mansion where the likes of William Jennings Bryan came to call. Having the name Thomas Hart Benton in Missouri was comparable to having the name Paul Revere or Henry Cabot Lodge in Boston. Even as a child, Benton was scarcely a rube—as the son of a congressman, he spent most of his youth in Washington, D.C., where he studied at the Corcoran Gallery. As a young man, he was happy only in metropolitan environments—whenever he could, Benton fled rural Missouri for Chicago, Paris, or New York. In each city, he was involved in the most advanced art movements. But in tune with his purveying of his old-time, just-folks narratives of America and his debunking of much modernist painting as a passel of fancy foreign tricks, Benton assumed the language and demeanor of a roughneck. In countless interviews, he successfully presented himself as an unlettered populist, a harmonica-playing hillbilly only at home in the bucolic Midwest where the true America lay.

Reporters were always swarming around Benton because of his easily loosened tongue. The painter was an abusive, raucous drunk who seemed proud of it—

in his self-portrait for the New School murals, he showed himself with a brush in one hand and a glass in the other. Benton couldn't handle liquor, and he would insult anyone after imbibing. Later in life, he admitted, "One highball and one newspaperman and I was off." But in 1932, as Juliana soon would learn, Benton was not so rueful.

In May of 1932, he returned from Georgia and was ready to begin the murals. During his absence, he forgot that the $3,000 he received was a loan —Benton had mentally converted the money into a very partial down payment. Then, since he'd made sketches on his travels that he could use for the Whitney, Benton asked the museum to pay his living expenses for both his spring trip and the ensuing summer when he would begin to paint. This had not been brought up in January or February, and Juliana informed him that he'd have to give up the whole project. Typically, Benton had lost sight of just who had instigated the commission. When he had earlier complained to Juliana about the New School's failure to pay him, he neglected to mention that to get an expanse of public wall and the visibility it promised, he had offered to paint those murals for nothing save the cost of materials. He was reported to have said to Alvin Johnson, the director of the New School, "I'll paint you a picture in tempera if you finance the eggs." Johnson took him at his word, and Benton groused about it afterward to anyone who would listen. This time around, Benton did not want to lose the Whitney job, but he did need more money. On May 5 he asked Juliana to guarantee him another $1,000 for the murals upon completion; if he had that guarantee, he could borrow another $1,000 from someone else to secure the property on the Vineyard. He volunteered to curtail his living expenses if she would advance him $600 for materials; he would take care of the models and assistants. Not waiting for a reply, Benton announced he was going ahead with the project. It would consist of four wall murals and four ceiling panels.

The subject of the murals was "The Arts of Life in America,"* which Benton defined as the leisure pastimes common to different regions of the country. These arts were not genteel but popular, he took care to point out, "in contrast to those specialized arts which the museum harbors." Just as sententiously, he said, "The local pursuits here represented the peculiar nature of the American brand of spirituality." In other words, the murals exalt the frontier and agrarian spirit, as well as mass culture, although the glorification is undercut by the artist's exaggerated manner. They are based on Benton's observations, either stereotyped or merely generalized, depending on one's point of view, of rural and urban types. The South is symbolized by Holy Rollers, black singers, crap shooting, and mule driving; the West by bronco busting, poker playing, horseshoe pitching, and square dancing; and American Indians by dancing, weaving, hunting, and chasing the Great Spirit. The arts of the city are cosmetics, comic strips, jazz, war, radio, politics, gin, love, and men needing a handout. The ceiling panels depict radical protest, folk and popular songs, and "political business and intellectual ballyhoo." The paintings are executed in Benton's trademark hyperem-

---

*The murals are now in the collection of the New Britain Museum of American Art.

phasized style: Arbitrarily undulating contours and a crowded, tabloid format convey a sense of raw and explosive energy. The figures gyrate frantically, their heads and torsos seeming to surge out of the framework of the canvas.

Juliana assented to paying Benton another $1,000 upon completion of the job, plus the $600 for materials, for a total of $4,600. But she was aware that trouble was coming, for she felt constrained to remind him on May 25, 1932:

> As I stated when the agreement was made between us for those murals, the museum could not contract for such work for some years to come. But as I had already—and at considerable embarrassment and sacrifice—loaned you $3,000 in order to save the $12,000 interest which you had in your country house; and also, in view of the fact (as we both agreed) that a psychological moment had arrived for the painters of mural decoration; I acceded to your proposition that you proceed with the work. . . .

Maynard Walker said that Benton did not live as frugally as he promised during the summer and fall of 1932. Liquor and girls were in abundance, and his total expenses, which the Whitney paid without demurral, came not to $600, but $1,676.25. (The museum also picked up the tab for the models and assistants, for whom Benton was supposed to be financially responsible.)* In addition, the library had to be refurbished with lamps, tables, and chairs to make it a public room, and an illustrated catalog with an essay by Benton was published.

As the opening approached, the museum promoted Benton's work, and Juliana invited 200 people to the unveiling, which took place on December 5, 1932. Benton arrived drunk and got worse from there. After a few cocktails, he was just coherent enough to accept Juliana's check for the promised $1,000. He recounted the event as follows:

> Parties at the Whitney Museum are thoroughly taken care of. Before this one was half started I was thoroughly taken care of myself. I was as tight as a jay bird in blackberry season. Mrs. Force came over to me. I recognized her even though she had several heads and seemed to be dancing some kind of shimmy. She held out a slip of paper. I knew it was a check and took it. I couldn't make it out for sure but it looked like ten thousand dollars. I nearly fell over. I controlled my impulse to shout and sticking the paper in my pocket proceeded to get as tight as I could.
>
> Somebody was giving a supper party for me that night. I discovered when I started out to it that I couldn't make the grade. I went into a drugstore, got a zinc emetic, and spilt my mural party in the gutter. When I could see clearly I looked at my check again. The check was for one thousand dollars. The sight of it ruined my supper party. The next morning I sent the check back to Mrs. Force with a note to the effect that I would feel better in making my mural an outright present to the Whitney Museum.

Benton had repressed the original circumstances and price for the murals. The story he began giving out was that his year's labor for the Whitney—during which he neglected other propositions—hadn't profited him a cent. Afflicted again with selective memory or perhaps still in an alcoholic haze, Benton was indignant that the Whitney hadn't reimbursed his summer living expenses. He ignored the fact that the museum's absorption of his cost overruns ($1,076.25)

---

*One of the young men who helped Benton install the murals was Jackson Pollock.

meant that the final $1,000 was that much above the $4,600 agreement. Benton claimed that the $1,000 was to cover his summer living expenses, making it appear as if the Whitney had not given him any extra money for the paintings themselves. Juliana's check, accompanied by this explanation of how things stood, was returned on December 8. Flabbergasted by the construction Benton put on the affair, Juliana sent the check back, writing:

> The Museum does not look upon these murals as a gift from you, although I agree with you that the price we have paid is very small.
> May I take this opportunity to remind you that the $3000 which I gave your wife last spring was not given as a payment on the murals. It was given, at great sacrifice to myself, because at that moment you needed the money to save your $12,000 house. It later became a part payment on the murals, at your suggestion, and I, in good faith, feeling that I understood your gesture, allowed it.
> It is extremely embarrassing for me to remind you how deeply grateful you were for my help at the time. I am sure you understand my reference to it is made only in justice to myself and because of your evident misunderstanding.

Benton countered that he did not distort the facts, but construed them as he understood them. He acknowledged the check—and cashed it. This is contrary to what Benton maintained in his autobiography, in which he implied that his renunciation of the money was final, as if he had sacrificed it forever in a gesture of extravagant and noble insouciance.

Benton was not going let the matter drop. He fed his version of events to Anita Brenner, who reported it in *The Nation* on January 18, 1933. "[A]las," she wrote, "the painter was paid just about what the job cost him, and less than the rate per foot paid to commercial decorators for restaurants and hotel jobs."

Brenner had accepted Benton's side of the story without checking it with the Whitney. Juliana protested the misstatement to the editorial board of *The Nation* and asked for a retraction. When Brenner continued to take Benton's part, Juliana met her in person, armed with canceled checks and receipts for bills supposedly unpaid. Juliana received an apology, but never saw a retraction.

Now that Brenner was contrite, Juliana wanted to confront her accuser. She summoned Benton to her office, but he had already left for Indiana on his next mural commission. He was unwilling to return to New York because he still believed he had been cheated. As a compromise, Benton suggested that Rita appear in his stead. He asked Juliana to look on their quarrel as a minor difference, to be viewed with indulgence and humor. "Try to get something out of the murals," he counseled, "and in return I'll forget I ever did them or had any illusions about what they might be worth to me." This breezy advice, coupled with the cowardly proposal that Rita take the tongue-lashing meant for him, infuriated Juliana almost more than Benton's previous transgressions. She wrote him a letter saying as much, but Benton would not come back.

Juliana did not pursue the apology any further, but the denouement of the Benton affair enraged her for some time to come. "After the incident," said Edward Laning, "she treated the murals as if they didn't exist. [A few months after the opening, the reading room was closed to the public.] To soothe her, I

said, 'Oh, Benton's just like the Platte River—a mile wide and an inch deep.' Juliana roared at that, and then she said, 'I wish I'd said that. Never mind, I will.' " Talking to other artists, Juliana wrote the murals off to her own gullibility and Rita Benton's suasion. "She felt she had been conned by Rita Benton," Eugene Ludins remembered. "She said, 'That woman did a job on me.' "

Benton was unable to let the feud fade away. In his memoirs, published in 1937, he spouted the same charges he had made in 1932. Juliana learned of this through Goodrich, who had solicited advance galleys of the book because he expected that Benton would not tell the truth. Goodrich assembled a detailed financial dossier on the murals, and he wanted Juliana to let him block publication of the book until the erroneous portions were amended or omitted.* She declined. "I don't want to do it," she said. "I don't want to quarrel with an artist." But if Juliana thought she could avoid public skirmishes, she was gravely mistaken. The clash with Benton would be nothing to the mudslinging soon to come.

* Benton never recanted. He believed what he wanted to believe, overlooking the bulk of evidence to the contrary. As late as 1973, two years before his death, he stated in an interview that the Whitney Museum commission "was done for nothing, too, in fact."

CHAPTER NINE

A FINE
OLD
WARHORSE

❧ *(1932–1935)* ❧

W ITH THE MUSEUM a full year old and a working concern, Juliana
was ready to look beyond New York and represent the rest of
the country—a geographic entity she and her curators referred
to as "out of town." She wanted to bring artists from around
the country into Whitney exhibitions; she hoped to make the Whitney collection
available to smaller towns and cities that had less access to contemporary American art and were unconvinced of its merit. A public forum for contemporary
work had been established in New York, but not so in many places west of the
Alleghenies. Stuart Davis summed up the problem of the provinces by saying,
"We have the talent right here now but [we] could do with a trifle more support
from the bleachers."

Juliana's desire for the museum to assert itself in this way did not spring
from a pedagogical motive. Unlike the Modern and the Metropolitan Museum—institutions that took great pains to bring young people into their
galleries—the Whitney made scant effort to attract children or provide art interpretation. The museum did not establish an education department or hold
classes. The curators occasionally led adults through the exhibitions, but docents,
sporadically tried as an experiment, were found to be of doubtful value. Juliana,
eyes rolling heavenward, often repeated what she heard imparted by a docent
at the Metropolitan. In the course of conducting her audience through a gallery,
the elucidator stopped in front of one painting and intoned, "This artist certainly
took a whack at his epic."

The Whitney, with little tolerance for epic-whacking in the toils of art
appreciation, concentrated on its duties of collecting, preserving, exhibiting, and
publishing. Juliana felt that the best art education lay in the sustained and direct

contemplation of objects. As far as she was concerned, the Whitney's first constituency was always its artists, and indeed she felt that all museums should take more responsibility for the care and preservation of artists. One of her museum's primary purposes, she said, was "a ceaseless endeavor to meet the need of the artist, i.e.: an audience for his work." That is, the Whitney should be garnering more support from the bleachers.

The Whitney had a long record of sponsoring traveling shows, and Juliana never stinted on lending works, feeling that the circulation of a museum's major works of art was a matter of personal and institutional honor. In 1933, when she sent a group of important paintings to the Dallas Museum of Fine Arts, Juliana would write:

> The aims of the Whitney Museum of American Art in its field work are, in essence, not to be distinguished from the purpose which animated its founding. Any activity of an organization bespeaks the meaning of the whole.
>
> Therefore, to describe the broader aims and purposes of the Whitney museum is to describe as well its more specific intentions, chief among which is the idea of traveling exhibitions. . . .

Thomas Carr Howe, director emeritus of the California Palace of the Legion of Honor, had reason to know that Juliana meant every syllable of those words. He was present at a meeting of the Association of American Art Museum Directors when he saw Juliana leap into action over this issue. He later recounted:

> At one of the afternoon sessions, on a very hot and muggy day late in May, Herbert Winlock [who became director of the Metropolitan Museum of Art after Edward Robinson died in 1931] was drowsily presiding and nearly all in attendance were dozing. He brought up the subject of membership qualifications and also the matter of loans to smaller museums in the U.S., making a pretty clear implication [that] only the major museums warranted consideration as recipients of the loan of major art works. Then lightning struck—Mrs. Force was on her feet and the place came to sudden life. "Mr. Winlock," she began, "I think what you have just said is the most *damnable* thing I ever heard. You know perfectly well that we take into this organization only those whom we like—be the museum large or small—and we blackball the others. And, as to loans—for you to suggest that second-rate works of art will do for the provinces, I consider the suggestion positively *immoral*." Then she sat down, leaving a rather sheepish Winlock to get out of his predicament.

Juliana's field work took a variety of forms. Artists from Philadelphia, Pittsburgh, Cleveland, Chicago, Santa Fe, Seattle, and San Francisco had been invited to show in the first biennial, but of the 157 exhibitors, 133 were from the New York area. At about the same time (in late 1932), it was decided that the Whitney would mount several shows featuring artists working in different parts of the country. The first exhibition would be devoted to paintings and prints from Chicago-area artists, and it was planned for February of 1933. Perhaps the heightened publicity about the Midwest as a center for Regionalist art was having its effect on the East Coast.

The interest in Chicago-area artists was fanned by Juliana's amicable relationship with Robert Harshe, the director of the Art Institute of Chicago, which

went back to the early 1920s. Harshe introduced her to a protégé of his, an art student named Theodore Roszak, then a painter. Juliana looked at his work, liked it, put him in the first biennial, and invited him to show in many exhibitions thereafter. Roszak later said, "[I]t was Juliana Force and the Whitney Museum that were the first source of real encouragement I met in my early years in the city." Her favor "did lead to my showing in New York City officially, and from then on, I was able to see my way clear to jobs that ordinarily would not have been available to me." The biennial itself was "an exciting time" for Roszak, who had not been to such openings and parties before. He remembered Juliana greeting him "with, 'Well, now what will you be drinking, rye or Scotch?' I finally blurted out a hesitant 'Scotch' (my first, by the way), and have been grateful among other reasons to the Whitney Museum ever since."

The focus of Juliana's next forays was Philadelphia. She spent December 16, 1932, flying in and out of galleries and studios and making the local dealers very happy. Julius Bloch wrote in his diary for that day that he met Juliana

> at the opening of George Biddle's show at the Mellon Gallery, which is across the street from my studio. There were perhaps a hundred people present, endless Biddles turned out. Mrs. Force walked around to see the pictures with me, and told me that [my] "Lynching" had been acquired for the Whitney Museum, also "Kingston," a gouache. . . . I am so dazed that a picture dealing with such a grim situation was so readily acquired by a museum.

At the Mellon Galleries, Juliana also bought a watercolor and a drawing by Biddle and two woodcuts by Salvatore Pinto; at the Warwick Galleries, she bought a watercolor by Hobson Pittman. Juliana would later have reason to regret her dealings with the Mellon Galleries for another purchase she made. Unknown to her or others in the New York art world as yet, the director, C. Philip Boyer, was in debt and embezzling from his artists and other dealers. (He slipped in and out of directorships; within a few months he would be gone from the Mellon Galleries and open the Boyer Galleries, which would also go into the red.) The Downtown Gallery had recently consigned several works by Charles Demuth to him. One, an architectural painting of Lancaster, Pennsylvania, called *From the Garden of the Chateau*, was bought by Juliana for $1,000. After receiving the Whitney's check, Boyer never paid Edith Halpert or Demuth their fair shares, stalling them by saying that Juliana was the delinquent party. The fraud was not discovered for another two years, partly because—and Boyer must have counted on this—neither Demuth (who was very sick and desperately short of cash) nor Halpert wished to risk offending Juliana by complaining that she was holding up their money.

In January of 1933, Juliana, Hermon More, and Karl Free boarded a train for Chicago to make selections for the group show of Midwestern painters and printmakers. Their trip was timed so that their first stop, on January 20, would be the Art Institute's annual exhibition of 193 local artists. (This was a juried affair, and the staunchly antijury trio from the Whitney insisted on examining the rejects, from which they plucked four oils and two watercolors.) Later in the day, the visitors went to some of the more progressive commercial galleries.

On January 21, Juliana and Hermon More were brought to several studio buildings that had many artists as tenants. Aaron Bohrod recalled:

> She and Hermon More, shepherded by Robert Harshe and Dan Rich [Daniel Catton Rich, who succeeded Harshe as director in 1938], came to my studio to see my work. They simply knocked on the door and let themselves in. She *was* interested and encouraging to the extent that I exhibited regularly and my work was purchased by the Whitney. . . . I was invited to be in the next annual and the *Art Digest* reprinted a good notice I got. Being singled out in the big town helped me as a local artist in Chicago. New York showing appreciation helped transform an ugly duckling into a respectable swan.

Along with Bohrod, some of the others whose work Juliana selected and perhaps helped elevate to swanhood were Roszak, Ivan Albright, John Storrs, Francis Chapin, Archibald Motley, Boris Anisfeld, Emil Armin, and Paul Kelpe.

In February, Juliana was back in Philadelphia, looking, buying, and appraising. She stopped at one-man shows of Ryder, Pavel Tchelitchew, and Emlen Etting. She bought a sculpture for the museum and a chess set for herself by Wharton Esherick, the modernist woodcarver, as well as ceramics by Carl Walters. Another reason Philadelphia was prominent in her thoughts was that the Whitney was publishing Lloyd Goodrich's pioneering study of Thomas Eakins in February. That month she further celebrated Eakins's achievement by purchasing the painting *The Biglin Brothers Racing* and a preparatory drawing for it* from an exhibition at the Milch Gallery.

In early 1933, the Whitney was making purchases whenever it could be managed, although directives to reduce expenses were constantly being issued. Yet such cutbacks, as Juliana understood them, were not meant to apply to her personally. Gerald Kelly, a friend of hers who had been director of the exhibitions department at Wildenstein's, was in Europe in 1932 and 1933. In his letters to Juliana, he mentions picking up clothes she had ordered from Schiaparelli (including one gown of "poison green" velvet and another of "flaming gold" net) and reminisces about her parties. At one soiree, the two of them sat in the bathtub and drank champagne. In April, Juliana bought a chest of drawers decorated by Max Kuehne, for $400. And in planning the opening of a show for April, she directed that there be two orchestras: a string quintet for chamber music during dinner, followed by a jazz band for dancing that would go on until 4:00 A.M. Marchal Landgren, an art historian who met Juliana about this time, loved her gaiety and "her terrific sense of humor," but he was sometimes put off by them. He said:

> Juliana was in my mother's generation, but she seemed so much younger. At one opening, she was wearing a little pink straw hat with two spines of feathers in the back. I went in, and after she greeted me, I said, "If you turn that hat around, you'll have antennae." Without a word, she took her hatpin out, turned the hat around,

---

* Both are now in the collection of the National Gallery of Art.

and wore it that way for the rest of the party. Another time after an opening, she gave me a photograph of herself by Cecil Beaton.* About a dozen of us were up in her sitting room and when Juliana went downstairs to say goodbye to her other guests, Emlen Etting and I decided that for some outrageous reason or another we would stretch ourselves across her bed and lie there until she returned. I put the photograph on my chest. Juliana came back, saw us there, and, quick as anything, said, "Whoops, my dear!" and threw herself bodily on top of me. She crushed the photograph—she just fell on it.

She was great fun, but I never took her very seriously because she was so exaggerated, because she'd turn her hat around. She wore fantastic clothes, she liked people, she liked crowds around her, she liked the smart world. At her parties, the liquor flowed and Corona-Coronas were always passed around.

But frivolity, fun, and indulgence coexisted with deep concern. Juliana was conscious not only of the museum's role as a repository of contemporary art, but its power to tide an artist over during the continuing harshness of the Depression. Besides visiting studios and galleries, the staff also instituted specified viewing days when artists could submit examples of their work. Juliana and her curators looked at the work and then marked it A, B, C, or D. "A" meant that the artist should be invited to exhibit, "B" meant that the artist should be kept in mind as a possibility, "C" meant that the artist should be asked to submit work in the future, and "D" meant that the voter never wanted to see the work again.

The import of a purchase in the life of an impoverished artist in the early thirties is made concrete in a letter to Juliana from the sculptor Richmond Barthe, dated January 17, 1933. "First," he wrote,

> I want to thank you for the purchase of the figure "The Blackberry Woman," and for the bronze cast of it. I'm so happy to see it in bronze. I was so afraid that it would always have to remain in plaster. And thanks also for allowing me to use your name in applying for a Guggenheim scholarship.
>
> Just at the time that you bought the figure—I was feeling pretty discouraged. I had to give up my studio, and couldn't find work of any kind—so I thought I would have to give it all up and go back home for a while. But when I sold the figure, I felt so encouraged. I rented another studio and decided that I would *not* give up my work. And later I found a porter job and have been able to hold on. Things are beginning to move along much better now.

For the moment, Barthe was one of the fortunate. In another instance, Juliana, in apologizing to a painter she could not assist, told him that seven other despairing letters similar to his own arrived the same day. The museum was also soliciting cash contributions for unemployed artists, but too many people were out of work for an ad hoc fund to go very far. Willing to consider any practical endeavor, Juliana discussed a plan for a sales gallery at Rockefeller Center with Edith Halpert and Nelson Rockefeller, but she pulled out of it when she saw it was to be a commercial venture that would probably end up under Halpert's control. Halpert, thirty-three, had always looked up to and curried

* See Chapter 8, p. 298.

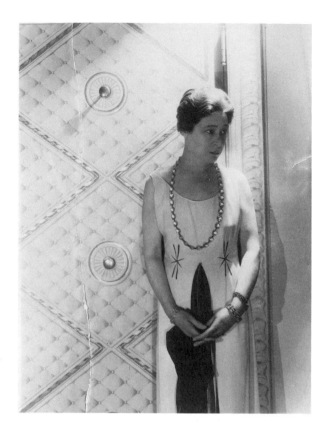

Marchal Landgren playfully stretched himself across Juliana's bed with this print across his chest. Juliana reacted by throwing herself on him, which crushed the photograph and left a permanent crack.

favor with Juliana as a Downtown Gallery customer and as a cynosure of taste. Juliana had gone along with her because she was determined to succeed as a serious dealer who specialized in living Americans. In addition, Halpert, an attractive and quick-witted woman, was a superb saleswoman who did very well for her artists, many of whom were Juliana's friends. But from about this time onward, Juliana was less sanguine about Halpert—she felt that much of the dealer's public-spiritedness masked a shrewd self-interest.

Juliana's experiment with a cooperative gallery for artists, the venture she had discussed with Abby Rockefeller, did come to pass, but it was pitifully short-lived. From December 8, 1932, to January 31, 1933, she personally financed a salesroom for artists to display and sell their works directly to the public. It was run by Vernon Porter. The smallest possible commission (5 percent) was taken to cover the overhead. Any artist was eligible to bring in work, and 480 of them did so. Of these 480, 150 sold 410 pictures, for a total of $4,267.50. The income from commissions amounted to $201.31; for the fifty-five days the gallery was open, expenses came to $1,288.68. Juliana absorbed the deficit of $1,087.37, but she had hoped that the gallery would be closer to self-supporting than it was. She couldn't afford that substantial an obligation every month and closed the gallery.

Except for getting help under Whitney auspices in these ways or through a "private" and "all very secret" relief project underwritten by Gertrude in which "quite a few artists . . . received $50 a month by check," artists could apply to a temporary employment authority that placed nearly 400 artists in New York State in jobs as art teachers, or to the College Art Association, which was sponsoring limited relief programs. But the majority of painters and sculptors had no work, no supplies, no patrons, no clients, and nothing to look forward to. In Delmore Schwartz's phrase, "hopes . . . were worn thin like a cloth." But on March 4, 1933, Franklin D. Roosevelt took office as President of the United States, and during his first 100 days the Congress passed a raft of social and economic legislation designed to bring economic recovery to the Depression-ravaged populace.

Unfortunately, no provision was made for artists in the alphabet soup of jobs, agencies, and other relief measures of the New Deal, and they might have remained the forgotten men and women of the Depression had it not been for the inspiration of George Biddle, the Philadelphia painter. Biddle was not alone in believing that artists should be subsidized by the New Deal, but unlike most of his peers, he was someone whose appeal would be heard. Not only was he one of the eminent Biddle tribe, a family as patrician as Roosevelt's, but his brother Francis was an adviser to the President and would soon be made Solicitor General. Furthermore, George Biddle had been a classmate of Roosevelt's at Groton, a fellow graduate of Harvard, and now lived in the New York suburb of Croton-on-Hudson, not far from Hyde Park. He must have been the only painter in America who could write a letter to the White House and legitimately begin it "Dear Franklin."

In late April of 1933, Biddle started conferring with other painters about how to put artists on the national payroll. He also spoke with Juliana, who gave him advice and was kept informed of developments throughout the summer. On May 9, Biddle wrote to the President suggesting that artists might be hired by the government to paint murals in public buildings at a small, regular wage. This, he assured Roosevelt, would turn mural art into "a vital national expression." On May 19, the letter was answered.

DEAR GEORGE:

It is very delightful to hear from you and I am interested in your suggestion in regard to the expression of modern art through mural paintings. I wish you would have a talk some day with Assistant Secretary of the Treasury Robert, who is in charge of the Public Buildings' work.

"As I read his letter," Biddle would write, "walking down our wood road from the post box to the house through the heavy-laden glory of the dogwood blossoms, my heart beat with excitement." And no wonder—for this was the germ of all the federal art projects, which were broadened beyond mural commissions to encompass easel paintings, sculptures, prints, drawings, photographs, designs, and teaching jobs. These programs, which ran from 1933 through 1943, would sustain thousands of artists and artisans and allow them to survive, experiment, and remain in their chosen profession whether they sold anything or not.

But this valiant accomplishment was years away. In the meantime, Biddle found, his was a "frail purpose" that had to be guided "over many ominous hazards and through hostile forces which stood directly in our path." Opposition, voiced immediately, never let up, and Biddle began devoting all his time to forwarding his proposal. He canvassed artists for their ideas and lined up every influential friend he could. This was a considerable roster—Eleanor Roosevelt, Secretary of Labor Frances Perkins, Secretary of the Interior Harold Ickes, Assistant Secretary of Agriculture Rexford Tugwell, Walter Lippmann, and the editors of *The Nation* and *The New Republic*. Lawrence W. Robert was enthusiastic, and after undergoing some moderation, the project was about to take off.

But in July, activity ceased. The President's private secretary had forwarded the proposal to Washington's Commission of Fine Arts, a notoriously rigid organization with jurisdiction over the placement of art in the capital. The group was headed by the archconservative Charles Moore, who believed that American art and architecture had reached their zenith at the World's Fair of 1893 and found Biddle's idea frought with "controversy," "embarrassment," and menace. As Forbes Watson would later remind Biddle with his customary directness, "on July 28, the Commission, then under the chairmanship of that old fathead Charles Moore, turned down your suggestion." Moore had endorsed a critical report downgrading the idea and implying that most of the artists committed to it were incompetent. The report, which was sent to Roosevelt, concluded, "I think the Government would be glad to avoid such experiences."

The Commission's action succeeded in delaying the project for months, but Biddle and Robert were as stubborn as their enemies. After all, it was the President himself who had used the phrase "modern art" in defining what was suitable for public buildings. Biddle read this as an espousal of individual expression, and not, as he put it, "the mephitic odors of the Fine Arts Commission." As Henry T. Hunt, Harold Ickes's general counsel, would write, "We have broken away from the Republican regime in other particulars. Why not in art?"

In October of 1933, the advocates of the mural movement made progress. They were allowed to quote Ickes as saying that art, architecture, and crafts must be kept alive during the Depression, and at the end of that month they found a means of doing so. Robert asked the advice of a recently hired Treasury official, Edward (Ned) Bruce. Bruce had a background in business, law, and diplomacy, with political and social connections in all three fields, but he had also studied painting seriously and been successful at it. His imagination was fired by the idea of federal sponsorship of the fine arts, and he pledged his enthusiastic support. Bruce also thought big, envisioning the program as more than a plum for a small group of preferred artists painting three or four murals in Washington. He suggested something more politically viable—a national agency that would prove artists were a necessary part of the culture by bringing art to people all over the country. It was his formulation that would prevail. Bruce understood the machinery of Washington well—he was a master of balancing weight with counterweight. He lobbied such influential powers as Supreme Court Justice Harlan Stone to help shield L. W. Robert, who had decided to ignore the Commission of Fine Arts and forge ahead. Just as sagaciously, he suggested that

endorsements of the project be sought from leading art critics and administrators. On November 8, Bruce and Biddle approached Ickes for an appropriation, with Biddle asking why artists shouldn't be treated as well by the government "as the farmer or the bricklayer." Only twenty minutes were needed to convince Ickes. Afterward, Bruce confided to Biddle that he was going to assemble a large committee of highly respected figures in the art world; with their backing, he would press on. It became clear to Biddle that his original modest proposal, suddenly enlarged almost beyond recognition, was out of his hands and under Bruce's thumb. Although his title was secretary, he would be supervising overall policy and hence be directing any program under Treasury Department auspices.

On November 9, 1933, Civil Works Administration (CWA) Relief Administrator Harry L. Hopkins was ordered to transfer $1,039,000* to the Treasury Department for the employment of artists. The project, in which artists would be paid regular wages in exchange for works of art executed for the government, was designated as a short-term experiment, but at least it was a concrete reality. There was still Charles Moore to placate, and Bruce, who was no more in sympathy with him than Biddle or Watson, endeared himself to both men when he said:

> [T]here are a lot of old dodos that have never done a thing for American art or American artists. Now we want to get rid of the sort of academic art that paints a lot of semi-nude ladies, draped in cheesecloth with a ribbon under their nipples, holding scales in one hand and a lamp in the other. But perhaps . . . it's better to have that old dodo Moore on the Committee, as he won't play ball with us. Better to have him peeing from the inside out than peeing from the outside in.

With the pragmatic Bruce in charge, Biddle moved largely out of the picture, although he remained active behind the scenes as an adviser. Bruce named the new agency the Public Works of Art Project (PWAP) and set it up with a view to aid roughly 3,000 artists working in all genres in all sections of the country. He would be heading the central office in Washington, which would require a staff of energetic men and women who wouldn't wilt under the glare of controversy. In particular, Bruce was looking for someone knowledgeable about art and able to defend and explain the government's position through articles, speeches, and press releases. On a trip to New York shortly after his appointment, Bruce bumped into Forbes Watson and realized he had found his man. Although Forbes did not want to leave New York, he knew that he had been offered an important job. For that matter, it *was* a job, which he did not happen to have. Forbes became technical director of the PWAP, at $300 a month, and he and Nan moved to Washington.

Bruce devised an organizational plan designed to deal with the prickly matter of judging an artist's qualifications for being put on the project. He adopted the CWA's division of the country into sixteen geographic sectors, each of which

* Later, $1,312,177 for 3,749 artists and 15,663 works of art, or about $350 per artist. However, most artists would not have made $350, because of the wildly varying lengths of time they were employed.

would have its own PWAP regional branch reporting to the central office. Each branch, which would be responsible for screening applications and hiring and supervising artists in the area, was to be run by a chairman and advisory committee of art experts chosen by Bruce. By mid-November, Bruce, aided by Biddle, had compiled a list of recommended candidates and submitted it to L.W. Robert. Number one on that list was Gertrude Whitney, whom Bruce praised as having "done more for the development of American art than any other influence in America. I believe the invitation should go to Mrs. Whitney to be a member of the committee, but it might be that she would desire to appoint as her substitute Mrs. Juliana R. Force, the director of the museum." Bruce invited Gertrude and other prominent members of the museum world to a meeting in Washington on December 8, 1933, to discuss the aims of the project and his proposed division of the administration into territories. The PWAP's most important region was, of course, the one encompassing metropolitan New York, northern New Jersey, and southern Connecticut. And as Bruce guessed, Gertrude deferred to Juliana in heading it.

Juliana's experience with patronage and art administration, plus her familiarity with hundreds of American artists, made her an obvious candidate for chairing the regional committee. Professionally she was a perfect choice, although privately she was a Republican and opposed to the Roosevelt Administration. Because of her association with Gertrude, Juliana could not help but hold the aristocratic view that philanthropy should come from the moneyed elite, who justify their wealth by quietly helping worthy individuals. This fed into her own dislike of enterprises that smacked of collectivism or, indeed, any theorizing at all. However, she respected the practical wisdom of Bruce and Watson, and many of her close colleagues—Duncan Phillips in Washington, Homer Saint-Gaudens in Pittsburgh, and William Milliken in Cleveland—had agreed to serve. She also recognized that the times demanded something new —the economic dislocations were too violent to be corrected by private citizens, the artists were in need, and if the government was the body to subsidize them, so be it. (One suspects that if the devil himself had shown genuine concern for artists, Juliana would have had a few kind words for hell.)

A rescue operation for the artists was Juliana's top priority, and when Bruce asked her what she thought of his undertaking, she could not help but write of their pervading despair.

> As you might know, this matter has been concerning me for some time. I have been working all year on some scheme to present to the Government with the same project in view as expressed by you. Your whole plan, however, is so much more practical, so much better presented and altogether so constructive a proposition, that I resign my feeble efforts and will throw [in] all my time, energy and if possible money, for furthering this project. Perhaps you do not know as well as I do the utter destitution of the artists, and how their courage is failing at the thought of facing another winter! . . .
>
> I am eating my heart out over this inactivity! The little I can do with our reduced budget is wholly inadequate and makes me feel almost useless in a situation where my experience and knowledge and awareness should be operative.

In telegraphing her acceptance of the chairmanship to Bruce, Juliana added: OVER THREE HUNDRED FIFTY PAINTERS AND SCULPTORS OF FIRST RATE IMPORTANCE DESPERATELY IN NEED OF JOBS. THIS LIST IS PERSONALLY KNOWN TO ME.

Even if Juliana's opinions were not politically correct for the job, her temperament, like her professional knowledge, certainly was. As Watson knew, if not Bruce, the New York chairman was a tenacious fighter. She thrived on the battlements, and with the welfare of American artists at stake, she would stay on the job through the months of vehement and unabated criticism to come. James Thomas Flexner, who met Juliana at about this time, said that she impressed him as "a fine old warhorse of a woman." Given her history and what was about to transpire, the description couldn't have been better.

On December 3, 1933, the museum's first biennial for sculpture, watercolors, and prints opened with a viewing and unlimited cocktails, followed by a midnight supper and dancing. Over 200 artists were represented, with Milton Avery and James Brooks exhibiting for the first time. Forty-seven works of art were bought from the biennial, for just over $17,000. The most important purchases were a terra-cotta sculpture by Jo Davidson, *Interior, Bucks County Barn*, a conté crayon drawing by Charles Sheeler, and Gaston Lachaise's *Man Walking*, a full-length nude bronze of Lincoln Kirstein. Lachaise was also working on a portrait bust of Juliana, which he hoped to complete in the early part of 1934. No correspondence survives as to how or why the agreement came about. Juliana could have commissioned the bust. Or Lachaise may have suggested it—the planes of her face, which made her homely and handsome, could have intrigued him, because he told his friend Ernest Fiene that she would make a "very fine" subject for a portrait. Besides, Juliana had so much presence that Lachaise could see that posing came naturally to her. Another reason for thinking Lachaise initiated the portrait is that, in his biographer's words, he "did not ordinarily agree to do a portrait unless he admired the sitter." There was no question of the sculptor's respect for Juliana. Isabel Lachaise said that "[a]ll through the years both Lachaise and I admired her valiant stand," and Lachaise himself thanked Juliana for "the interest which I feel you have alway[s] given to my work."

Biddle was at the opening of the biennial, and that evening he made arrangements to meet Juliana the next day for dinner at Ticino's, a low and lively Village restaurant popular with artists, to plot strategy for the PWAP and the coming conference. To Biddle's delight, she revealed that she had asked Bruce to let him be present at the meeting. The administrators in Washington had been against inviting any artists to their deliberations, but because of the part Biddle had played, Juliana felt that an exception should be made.

On December 8, 1933, museum directors, the PWAP staff, and several members of the New Deal cabinet and brain trust gathered at Edward Bruce's Washington town house for a luncheon of turkey hash, corn bread, baked beans, and pumpkin pie. Eleanor Roosevelt, there to lend her support, declared to the other guests that she thought it "unbelievable that a great nation could fail to utilize . . . its creative talents to the fullest." (The local gossip columnist reported

that aside from Mrs. Bruce, Mrs. Roosevelt was "the only lady present," even though Juliana was not only there but named in her column!) Over coffee in the drawing room, where the First Lady listened quietly and knitted, Frederic A. Delano, the President's uncle, guided the discussions that followed.

After returning to New York on December 9, Juliana asked Lloyd Goodrich to be on her advisory committee, because Alfred Barr and Edward Warburg,* who were not of her choosing, were assigned to it. "Mrs. Force called me up in a state of great excitement," Goodrich recalled, "and said, 'A wonderful thing has happened. The government is going to do something about the artists, and I'm going to be chairman of the regional committee. I want you to be on the committee—it's not going to involve any work.' Whereupon I never worked harder in my life." She also asked Bryson Burroughs, William Henry Fox, Gordon Washburn, and Beatrice Winser of the Newark Museum, to join her. Goodrich cited an uneasy moment between Juliana and Alfred Barr after the PWAP was under way. "I imagine that to some professionals Mrs. Force was a little high-handed," he said. "I think she had quoted me, saying, 'Lloyd Goodrich and I think that etc., etc.,' and I remember Alfred saying rather sarcastically to her, 'Well, if you and Lloyd have decided . . .'" But I think that was a very exceptional thing because Mrs. Force and Alfred liked each other."†

Juliana's pique about being assigned assistants instead of being allowed to choose them went no further than Biddle and Watson, who had witnessed it in Washington. In public, she was part of a united front, and perhaps the high hopes and idealism of the New Deal did affect her when she commented for the benefit of a press release, "For the first time in America the Government is behind the artist, recognizing him not only as an individual but as an important spiritual force. There can be no future without a present, and now the future looks good to me."

The prediction was perhaps premature. Bruce's meeting was held on Friday, December 8, the announcement of the regional committees and their chairmen was released on Monday, December 11, and Juliana was under fire by Tuesday, December 12. The first salvo came from the more conservative art organizations, angry that they had been ignored by Bruce and their officials left out of the process. Eight spokesmen representing twenty-four different artists' societies pro-tested that she would favor the modernist school and give jobs only to the progressives.

Leading the anti-Juliana charge was Harry Watrous, the president of the National Academy of Design, but Robert Aitken, Forbes's and Juliana's old adversary in the Brancusi brouhaha, was also making a fuss. With Forbes and

---

*Edward M. Warburg, a friend of Lincoln Kirstein, who was about to become one of the founders of the American Ballet, George Balanchine's first American dance company.

†Barr held Goodrich in high esteem, too. In 1932, Barr took a year's leave of absence from the Modern for reasons of health. When the trustees were looking for a temporary substitute, Goodrich was Barr's first choice as his replacement. "You are my candidate," Barr told him. But Goodrich declined because he wanted to finish his book on Eakins and because he wanted to stay with American art, not all of it necessarily modern.

Bruce at the central office, of course, the academicians stood little to no chance of being consulted, but that was because their own record was so poor. When the Academy and other societies friendly with it had been more influential in the art world, they had not exactly been champions of fair play. Now they were afraid of being discriminated against. The point was not so much that Juliana was identified with a certain art movement, but that the movement was not theirs. More bluntly put, the academicians, Biddle guessed, were "boiling mad . . . because allowing needy artists to do mural work on public buildings at thirty-five dollars a week may cut into their swill."

Part of the blast directed toward Juliana was in truth resentment of the Museum of Modern Art and its commitment to Europeans. This can be seen in a letter from Leon Kroll to Bruce. Kroll, an urbane wheeler-dealer in the art world, had been offering advice to Biddle about the federal art program for months, but he thought of the Academy as fair and broad-minded, with a right to be miffed:

> I do not, however, see the necessity of the Modern Museum flattered to the extent of two members on the Committee, when their contribution as far as American art is so slight. As I said when I saw you that a conservative member for New York would have brought you the support of the Art world. As chairman, I think Mrs. Force will function better than anyone I can think of. She should have the support of the Academy which will and with justice claim that their support of American artists [is] of over [a] hundred years duration, that they have bought more pictures than the Museum of Modern Art. . . .

Howls of alarm filled the papers about taxpayers' money being delivered into the hands of a single partisan faction. Juliana denied the allegations of favoritism and retorted that her opponents' apprehension was ill-founded. She observed that the appointments of Burroughs (who happened to be a member of the Academy) and Fox should be sufficient balm for the conservatives. As to her own orientation, Juliana said, "That I am very catholic in my tastes is evidenced by the collection of art in the museum over which I preside. It contains modern art but it also contains the work of many academicians." But for the PWAP, an artist's aesthetic stance was supposed to be irrelevant—only financial need counted. "We are interested in knowing only one thing about any particular artist," Juliana continued, "that is, is he in need of employment?" Getting the artists on the government payroll was the issue, she told the *New York Post*. "You understand," she said, "I'm not buying art. I'm not, as people may fear, going to fill the walls of public buildings with bad art. I'm really employing artists. . . . The most important thing about this is that needy artists will be put to work. Their salaries will begin as soon as they are taken on by our committee, and they will be paid regularly each week whether their art ever gets on any walls or not."

At this point, Juliana was unruffled and in complete control—a commander to the hilt. Reporters covering her during this time were struck by her decisiveness and executive bearing. She would talk to them at great length, but she was always careful to say nothing. All the while, the telephone in her office rang and rang. As the ruckus continued, John Sloan, speaking for himself and for

the Society of Independent Artists, was one of the first to come to Juliana's defense. Sloan assured the reporters that she was an excellent choice, telling them about her thirty years of ministering to artists in distress and finding out where help was needed. Queried as to why there should be so many objections to Juliana, he quipped, "This trouble is the natural result of throwing corn in the chicken coop. There are bound to be feathers flying." Juliana, declining to fan the controversy any further, snapped, "If the people who are complaining can get a person better qualified than I to head the New York committee, I hope they will do it. It is an extremely hard job, which I am undertaking only because I love artists and value them more than any other part of the population. I will work to the limit, but I won't waste time fighting."

The academicians' objections to Juliana vanished after Bruce jawboned Watrous into submission, and the other groups consequently agreed to a truce. Juliana and Goodrich further prevailed by defeating for the New York region an order that other regional chairmen had accepted without argument. Bruce and Watson had proposed to categorize artists according to arbitrary standards of merit and ability. Class A artists would be paid $42.50 a week and Class B artists, $26.50. Juliana and Goodrich refused to serve under this system. Washington yielded, allowing all New York–area artists to have a weekly salary of $34, but with the proviso that a distinction would be made between creative artists and assistants.

Juliana also met with an early success in formulating a distinct category of jobs for the academic sculptors who had specialized in public monuments, as they would be unable to carry out such commissions within the financially limited scope of the project. Conferring with the mayor-elect, Fiorello H. La Guardia, on December 20, Juliana explained that these artists were skilled laborers who could renovate the crumbling City Hall building. She then suggested that they also be assigned to clean and repair the city's outdoor statues, arches, and architectural ornaments.

La Guardia, who would take office on January 1, approved the idea, as long as the *Maine* monument at Columbus Circle—the creation of Attilio Piccirilli, a personal friend of his—would be among the first public sculptures to be restored. The deal was struck, and Juliana proposed to Forbes that similar programs be initiated around the country. "If conditions in other cities are like they are here," she wrote to him, "the work accomplished will be a lasting tribute to your efforts and mine."

Unfortunately, 90 percent of the monuments were under the jurisdiction of the New York City Parks Department, and the brand-new city parks commissioner, Robert Moses, saw any overlap of authority as an unpardonable trespass. Furthermore, Moses's own power by now was unchallengeable. Karl Gruppe, hired by Juliana to survey the monuments, said Moses refused to meet with either Juliana or Gertrude; in particular, "he would have nothing to do with Mrs. Whitney." (Moses may have been repaying an old score dating from 1924, when he first attempted to put the Northern State Parkway through the Long Island estates of New York's wealthiest—including the Whitney compound at Old Westbury—and "teach the Wheatley Hills people a lesson." However, it

was he who received instructions in accommodation. Harry Payne Whitney and the other millionaires who owned property on the North Shore were ready to fight Moses to a standstill. They used their influence to delay construction of the road for years; when the parkway could be deterred no longer, they forced Moses to plan it with a five-mile detour around Wheatley Hills.) Moses, who was directing a massive overhaul of the city's parks, made so many difficulties for the PWAP that the appropriation for the cleaning and repair of public sculpture had to be transferred to him. Any improvement involving the park system had to be *his* improvement. Thus Gruppe, as well as the other artists, had to go to work for the parks department, and Moses got the credit for the restoration.

Juliana jumped into her appointment by phoning or writing all the artists she knew who needed jobs and told them to come register at once. Her first payroll dates from December 12, and Florence Cramer recorded in her diary for December 16 that "[a]lready a dozen of the Woodstock artists have been called to New York—to see Mrs. Force . . . and have received jobs. . . ." Dorothy Varian corroborated this. "I was stuck in Woodstock in my house, which wasn't winterized, and I was staying there," she said. "Juliana put us all on, and I was one of the first ones. I put an easel and a folding bed in my car and came to New York at once."

These stories were much the rule. Another artist to receive an early call was Chaim Gross, who was then supporting himself by tracing embroidery in a sweatshop. He remembered that Juliana told him to report to her office at once, and she gave him a job during the first weeks of December. This was the first time the sculptor had ever been able to work at his art without interruption. Ben Shahn, who had shown regularly at the Whitney in 1932 and 1933, recollected, "Suddenly they set up a project called the Public Works of Art Project. . . . I was on a salary for two weeks before I knew why." Stuart Davis, then living in Gloucester, Massachusetts, tuned in to a radio program explaining the new government initiative in art and was "amazed that such a thing could exist." He wrote to Juliana on December 13 asking for information. Once he knew about the PWAP, he quickly went down to Manhattan and was hired within one day of his arrival. Such scenes were repeated, as Juliana was seeing thirty to sixty artists a day and collecting names of worthy candidates from various sources. Ben Benn, Alexander Stirling Calder, Blendon Campbell, Elsie Driggs, Mabel Dwight, John Flannagan, Harry Gottlieb, Harry Holtzman, Edward Laning, and Joseph Pollet also got jobs soon after the PWAP was launched.

Juliana also listened to her network of artists and colleagues. Lincoln Kirstein recommended hiring Martin Craig, Duncan Phillips recommended John Graham, Sloan recommended Philip Evergood, Cooke Glassgold recommended Louis Lozowick, and Kuniyoshi recommended Paul Burlin. When Raphael Soyer, who felt he should not apply for relief because his wife had a teaching job, wrote to Juliana asking her to put his brother Moses on the project, he added, "I write this unofficial letter to you because you've always been unofficial in your dealings with artists & because of the high esteem in which I hold you." Meanwhile, Goodrich, who was in charge of interviewing, processing applica-

tions, matching artists with assignments, collecting blueprints of public buildings with spaces that could be embellished, deciding what constituted allowable expenses, and signing payrolls, said, "Every day, Saturdays, Sundays, holidays, everything else, from 10:00 A.M. and frequently until midnight, I was there."

Because she was working unofficially, within one week of her taking office, Juliana could announce that she had put eighty artists on the payroll at a uniform wage of $34 a week (later, $38.25); 300 other artists were on the waiting list. Funds would be available to employ a quota of 600 artists until February 15, when the project was slated to end. After reporting these statistics, Juliana said, "I believe that the government will be well repaid for the money it is spending in this undertaking. I can't recall any other time at which artists were willing to work for so little." A reporter then asked her the ratio of "modernists" to "conservative artists." Juliana facetiously exclaimed, "Oh, this so-called modernism! Goodness, you should see some of the wild works of the academicians. There might be seven men on the list you would call modernists, but I'd only classify two in that category. The public's meaning of the term is radical and there are perhaps three in the group. There isn't one surrealist, however." She also stated that she would have the final say on the selection of artists and projects. "You see," she purred, "Mr. Roosevelt says I'm the Czar."

Juliana was operating as she always had: by direct, often autocratic, one-to-one actions based on personal knowledge. Her hasty methods—the opposite of the careful accumulation and stapling together of vouchers, applications, and forms in triplicate—played hell with government procedures, and Washington admonished her for those fast, informal decisions. To process the artists in a more businesslike fashion, Juliana hired—at Gertrude's expense—Vernon Porter, Robert Locher, the architect Paul Chalfin, and Lloyd Rollins, who was an experienced art administrator. Juliana and the other museum personnel were serving as volunteers, their salaries covered by their institutions. Even though the volume of work was greater at the New York office, the government would not put anyone other than clerks, secretaries, and bookkeepers on the federal payroll. Goodrich recollected that during one conflict with Washington, a member of Juliana's PWAP professional staff said, " 'We'll all rebel. We'll quit.' Mrs. Force looked around and replied, 'I don't think I can afford it.' She knew she would have to support all those out of work. She always had a great deal of wit and it always had a little edge to it—quite a lot of edge to it, sometimes."

The central office wasn't making life any easier for Juliana, who was blamed locally for their switches in policy. The PWAP was a program without precedent, and Bruce and his staff were making much of it up as they went along. The regional chairmen could not help but be criticized for what seemed like incoherence. In the first days of the PWAP, it was conceived of as a relief measure. The committees were told to focus on financial need and not worry about the artist's aesthetic stance or merit as long as he or she was a professional working artist. Hence Juliana's public statement that she and the government didn't care who was the best artist, but who was the unemployed artist. Scarcely had that dictum been reported when on December 18 Bruce cabled the regional chairmen new and contradictory orders: They must eliminate the use of the words "relief"

and "needy" in connection with the PWAP, thus invalidating all previous declarations. There was also an order to be more selective. On December 22 Juliana was pushed to recant, having to make a public announcement that on instructions from Washington the project was no longer open to any unemployed artists, but the *best* unemployed artists. She told reporters, "My instructions are that the work is to be done by the best material available, and by available is meant unemployed." After this switch, Juliana invited Sheeler, Jerome Myers, Sloan, and William Zorach to be on the PWAP so as to ensure the enrollment of some well-qualified artists. By now she had some idea of how tempestuous her term of office was to be. When Edith Halpert wrote to congratulate her on this latest honor, Juliana replied, "I appreciate very much what you say about my appointment. It is, so far as I can see, a doubtful compliment on the part of the Government."

Unemployed New York artists were incensed at the flip-flops. They were behind the next cannonade of protest against her, which this time came from the Left. These artists noticed that Juliana's selection processes did not have the appearance of the much-vaunted impartiality promised by all. In Lloyd Goodrich's words:

> Our enemies said it was very personal. That we took on artists who were friends of Mrs. Force and the Whitney Museum. There was a certain element of truth in this, because they were the first people we knew, and we knew they were hard up in many cases, in almost all cases. We never tried to have a means test, to have any artists fill out a financial statement. All we asked was that they sign a simple statement saying that they needed money.

The difficulties in establishing criteria for employment, which led to Juliana's personal invitations to established artists to join the PWAP, led to one grievance; another, an omission on her part, catapulted her straight into another controversy.

As one of her first acts as chairman, Juliana sent a letter soliciting the names of unemployed members from twenty-three local artists' societies, but she neglected to write to a twenty-fourth because, she later said, it had no known address. This was the Unemployed Artists Group, founded in September 1933, and spearheaded by Ibram Lassaw, Max Spivak, Philip Bard, and Bernarda Bryson (later Bernarda Bryson Shahn). As many of its members had been active in the John Reed Club, the organization was seen as a cell of radicalism, and, indeed, it was more militant than any other artists' group opposing Juliana and the PWAP. The leaders knew how to organize, and they were adept at portraying the government program as a capitalist sop. Even though they didn't hear from her, the officers sent Juliana a list of unemployed artists, very few of whom were hired. They were furious, and charged that artists personally acquainted with Juliana had been hired without going through the same channels as everyone else.

Disgruntled with her administration, 150 artists in the group held a meeting on December 28 on the subject. The next day, a delegation of fifty, led by Bernarda Bryson, handed Juliana a series of "open questions" for which immediate answers were demanded. She could do nothing but repeat Bruce's

insistence on proven quality. "I am deeply sympathetic with all unemployed artists," she began, "but I cannot violate the instructions given me by the government, which are that the committee must select artists best fitted to carry out definite art projects." Although Juliana did have to secure the approval of city officials for certain commissions, such as murals, her contention was not entirely true. Many artists were painting easel pictures for an unknown destination. The dissident artists could not accept her reply, they said, because of their great need. "Need," retorted Juliana, "is not in my vocabulary." Regrettably, her distillation of Bruce's revised orders made her sound utterly uncaring and isolated her from young, struggling artists, perhaps for the first time in her life.

In mediating between government red tape and the rare group of artists who were not convinced that she was on their side, Juliana felt threatened. At this point, she was needled more by her own insecurities than nettled by external pressures, although she doubtless was unhappy about being disdained by the young. "You admit," she counterattacked, "that you came with a preconceived idea that I play favorites. . . . I tell you that is an accusation I will not tolerate and I will answer no more questions."

On January 7, 1934, Juliana announced that 356 artists were now employed, reiterating that artists had to be "thoroughly qualified for the particular work to which they are assigned." She also asked Bruce to enlarge her quota so she could hire another 250 artists. That same day the Unemployed Artists Group, now renamed the Unemployed Artists Association, picketed the Whitney. A hundred protesters gathered in Washington Square and marched over to the museum, waving placards reading, "THE WORD 'NEED' IS NOT IN MY VOCABULARY," "ART WORK FOR NEEDY ARTISTS OR IMMEDIATE CASH RELIEF," and "WE PROTEST AGAINST THE 'MERIT' SYSTEM." Juliana called the police to protect the museum, but allowed Philip Bard, Bernarda Bryson, and three others inside. Bard denounced the criminal treatment and the use of police intimidation. Juliana refused to debate Bard unless he retracted the word "intimidation." After doing so, he presented the association's demands—principally, that Juliana hire all hungry artists and put one of its members on the PWAP screening committee. Juliana insisted that the artists stop picketing the Whitney and submit their grievances in writing. When Bard refused to discontinue the demonstrations or accede to her requests, Juliana abruptly terminated the interview and set about preparing a brief against the Unemployed Artists Association for the district attorney's office.

However, writing up a document was as far as she went. She took no legal action, nor did she make reprisals against the picketers. Max Spivak, Ibram Lassaw, and Bernarda Bryson were employed by the PWAP. Another artist on that picket line was Ilya Bolotowsky, who had just gotten on the project, but felt "it was a matter of duty" to join the dissenters. "People told me I was crazy," Bolotowsky said many years later, "because Mrs. Force was looking out the window and she would recognize the mustache. . . . [Bolotowsky cultivated long, drooping mustachios that stood out in any crowd.] Anyhow, I walked to and fro until I finally got tired and then everyone got tired and left. . . . That was the beginning of the PWAP."

Juliana maintained in all public discourse that Washington was responsible for pitting the competing claims of quality and need against each other. But on her own, she had moved toward the position that economic and aesthetic issues should be separated. Artists of dubious ability whose main qualification was poverty, she had concluded, should apply to a relief agency for aid. Barr and Goodrich agreed with her, but the other regional committee members were of the opinion that the program should be chiefly a relief measure. Overriding them and using some recommendations provided by Barr and Goodrich, Juliana advised Bruce that the PWAP hire only the better artists: "The majority of them have not sufficient talent to justify the Government supporting them as artists . . . [they] should not be officially encouraged to pursue art." Although Juliana and Barr were on good terms at this point, she could not rest until she asserted herself on another matter. She was still simmering about having two men from the Museum of Modern Art imposed on her from above. By the end of January, she had nullified Edward Warburg's effectiveness and maneuvered him into resigning from the committee. Warburg wrote Juliana a coldly furious letter calling her on her calculations.

An unfortunate side effect of Juliana's clashes, intrigues, and piles of paperwork was that she became too preoccupied with business to continue her sittings with Lachaise. On January 31, she promised to come see him as soon as she had time, but that time never materialized. The PWAP consumed her until May, she was abroad in the summer of 1934, and when she returned, she let the sittings slide or did not allow enough of them—Lachaise required anywhere from ten to seventy sessions to complete a portrait. When Lachaise died suddenly of leukemia on October 17, 1935, the bust, in the form of a plaster cast, was unfinished and in an unresolved state. The portrait lacks vitality—an anomaly for Lachaise—and neither the bland expression nor the routine articulation of the features conveys any sense of the subject's essence. The nose is unrecognizable as Juliana's—it is flatteringly tip-tilted. Too late Juliana regretted losing the portrait; after Lachaise's death, she had Reuben Nakian supervise the casting and patination of the plaster model as it was. She would write to Lincoln Kirstein after seeing a Lachaise show he organized, "I felt, after looking at his other portraits [the inspired likenesses of John Marin, Carl Van Vechten, e. e. cummings, and Marianne Moore], awfully ashamed that I neglected the sittings with him so that it was never finished. It was a chance to have a portrait done by a great artist."*

Artists who made it onto the PWAP's rolls had their troubles, too, although not from the expected pitfalls. When the project began, Forbes promised that artists could work with complete freedom of expression, but this policy was soon modified by Bruce. He stipulated that artists should be depicting the American scene in all its phases pertaining to the life and setting of the country. As well as being an enthusiast of American Scene painting, Bruce believed that such a

---

*It is now in the collection of the Whitney Museum.

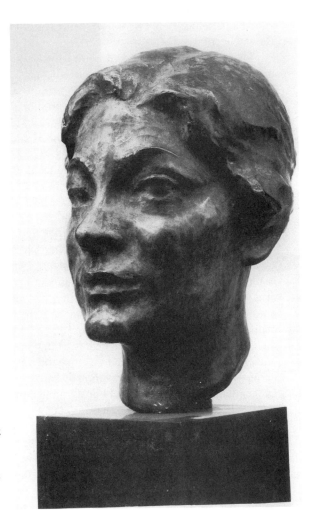

Gaston Lachaise thought that Juliana would make a "very fine" subject for a portrait, but in this unfinished bust his own efforts, as far as they went, were undistinguished.

theme would keep the politicians calm, allow latitude for the contemporary idiom, emphasize observation from life, and keep the nudes swathed in cheesecloth to a minimum.

Prescribed subject matter—that of a national epic showing the aims and aspirations of the people—promised conflict, especially for nonrepresentational artists, but in New York the administrators were able to evade these guidelines and let the artists work as they preferred without rejection or chastisement. Sloan said in 1934 that as far as he knew, none of the artists were given orders, "thanks to the wisdom of the director, Mrs. Force. We were told to do *anything we liked*. The thing this 'did' to our creative spirit was to set it free." And this must have applied to abstract artists, too. Besides Davis, Holtzman, and Graham, such abstract and semiabstract artists as Arshile Gorky, Ralph Rosenborg, José de Rivera, Francis Criss, Werner Drewes, Ibram Lassaw, Jan Matulka, Pietro Laz-

zari, Paul Kelpe, Louis Schanker, Burgoyne Diller, Raoul Hague, and Byron Browne were hired.

These artists may have had complaints about the system—Bolotowsky had to sneak onto the project with a fake appointment card that got him past the guard to a sympathetic application processor, and Browne was summarily on and off the payroll within four weeks—but not about any restrictions on the art they could make. Holtzman, in a letter to Juliana, cleverly finessed the question of the American scene by saying that his work would be called "Impressions and Description of America by a Contemporary Citizen." Lassaw's description, however, was straightforward—his sculpture would be "an abstract composition of two main figures with the feeling of tension between them." It was accepted without comment. Goodrich, who was sensitive to the creative process, wrote to Matulka after the latter had submitted a careful painting, "If you feel like varying the subject, and perhaps painting a freer type of subject, please do so."

Overall, the PWAP's record in hiring advanced artists was uneven, with small victories in tolerance weighed against several disasters of inflexibility. A notorious exception to the sensitive treatment many artists received was the case of Isamu Noguchi, who was penalized for his imaginative reach. Hamstrung by a web of government directives, Juliana and the other PWAP officials felt more comfortable with the competent performance that satisfied government criteria than the work of genius that defied Washington's strictures. As Juliana wrote to one artist, his paintings "should be along the lines which have succeeded before upon which your present reputation is based." Negotiating the maze of rules and regulations had the effect of transforming normally elastic and understanding persons like Juliana and Goodrich into petty enforcers. They had to act against their own better instincts to protect the greater program. Noguchi, although not the internationally renowned sculptor that he is today, was not an obscure artist in 1933. He had been a Guggenheim Fellow, and his work was shown and collected by the Whitney. There was no question of a lack of talent or a lack of need; Zorach had recommended that he be hired in December, but his enrollment was delayed until February of 1934 because he refused to compromise.

Noguchi had no wish to make anything that had "succeeded before"; rather, he thirsted to create something of radical distinction. In his words, he "had a desire to get into another realm, another dimension." Fired by the noble principles of the New Deal and his own social consciousness, Noguchi wanted to design environments that would vitalize open spaces where the public gathered. By government definition, this was not considered "pure sculpture," and Juliana had to deny him a job unless he agreed to conform by carving, modeling, or constructing a discrete and conventional work. Noguchi declined enrollment on those grounds. But after two months passed, he was so desperate for money that he became conciliatory.

Once hired, Noguchi did what he wanted to do—he designed models for large-scale sculptural environments. Incapable of turning out something routine, he responded with plans for *Play Mountain*, *Monument to the Plough*, and *Monument to Ben Franklin*. In short, the artist created three of the finest public

sculptures in his oeuvre and what would have been the most visionary and courageous works of art to have come out of the PWAP—had they been executed. But no one with any power to have the designs realized was ready for them. It is unclear from the correspondence on Noguchi if Juliana, Goodrich, Locher, or Rollins ever understood the designs; they first and foremost saw them as "impractical." However, they did not reject them outright, and Goodrich made a sincere attempt to carry them forward. Because the environments were supposed to be built on thousands of square feet of public land,* Goodrich wrote to Washington for a decision and possible suggestions for placement of the work. The New York office was probably more sanguine about the future of the studies for the *Monument to Ben Franklin* and *Monument to a Plough*. The fate of *Play Mountain*, which Noguchi wanted to put in Central Park, would ultimately be decided by Robert Moses, who would have turned it down flat because, if nothing else, it had emanated from Juliana and the PWAP. But before it came to that, Noguchi saw Moses in hope of winning him over. "Moses," remembered Noguchi, "just laughed his head off and more or less threw [me] out. That was the beginning of my experience with the New York City Parks Department."

Moses needn't have been so cutting, because the designs were aggressively vetoed by Washington. On February 28, Forbes wrote to Goodrich, "Noguchi designs have just arrived, and the Technical Committee in the central office turned their thumbs down on them so hard that they almost broke their thumb nails." The day before, Juliana suspended Noguchi from the payroll because of his willful refusal to do anything "purely sculptural"—as if his efforts had not been honest. She may have reasoned that she had to dismiss Noguchi so as not to endanger the program.

Noguchi gave up and asked to be reinstated. Part of his letter to Juliana read:

> May I ask of you the great kindness to allow me to once more work for the C.W.A. I propose to model weather vanes for public buildings. I have plans for musical and illuminated weather vanes. I will be most pleased to make them according to your specifications. Please give me an opportunity to explain to you that God must come to me thru the C.W.A.

After getting on the PWAP again, Noguchi submitted a bronze head of a woman he had on hand in his studio to satisfy the requirements, but because the piece had not been made for the project, it was rejected. Noguchi then perfunctorily began carving some acrobats in wood, which pleased everyone but him. However, he became embroiled in another spat with the New York office, this time over liability for incurred expenses and the return of the photographs and renderings of the disallowed environmental works. Although the models for the public sculptures had been spurned and the artist had been thrown off the project for them, Juliana wouldn't give them back, saying they were government property. In his final letter to her, Noguchi, although exasperated, gave her the benefit of the doubt in allowing that she had a bureaucratic agency to run:

Play Mountain required a city block, and *Monument to the Plough*, a pyramid designed to be a mile wide at the base, was meant to be placed in Idaho. Neither of these works have ever been executed; the *Monument to Ben Franklin* was not erected until 1984, in Philadelphia.

You then informed me that you were not interested in any new ideas, insisting that I must devote myself 'purely to sculpture.' . . .

I realize that you, personally, are not altogether unsympathetic to the birth and fostering of new ideas.

On the contrary, I am aware that the fault is inherent in a system of a minimum dole and regimentation.

I imagine one might as well abandon the expectation of leadership from those imbued with timid hope.

Noguchi's miserable experiences of having his work constricted and rejected was an anomaly. More often than not, an enrollee's idiosyncratic work habits or unusual hours gave Washington a collective ulcer. Artists who could not produce on schedule were often terminated peremptorily, because the foes of the New Deal were always on the lookout for PWAP shirkers. Even the appearance of malingering or goldbricking was to be avoided, because any hint of "boondoggling" brought on the interference of a congressman or sensational headlines in the Republican papers. One artist who was unable to feign that he put in office hours was John Flannagan—and for that, Juliana dismissed him.

Flannagan had been heavily supported by the Whitney in the past, and he was hired at the inception of the PWAP. Provided with a large piece of sandstone, and later an assistant, he was expected to execute his first monumental sculpture. But Flannagan, who was known for his direct carving of wood and small stones, had never worked on this large a scale before. He slowed down, groping uncertainly toward a solution. He did not make good progress nor meet the completion date of February 15, 1934, and no latitude was allowed for inexperience. In January, administrators from Juliana's office began to drop by to see how he was doing. On one of these inspections, Flannagan was drunk. The artist's alcoholism was always problematic, but the government could not sanction his irregular creative cycle: He alternated marathon work sessions with drinking bouts. Indeed, Flannagan had put in ninety hours one week and then took the next two weeks off, as was his custom. He worked until he was utterly exhausted, and then drank to blot out the fatigue.

The New York office investigated these patterns and ordered Flannagan to work according to the prescribed routine. He promised to do better, but he could not manage it. The PWAP staff stepped up their inspections—one man in Juliana's office went to Flannagan's studio on March 14, March 15, March 16, March 21, and March 26. (Juliana did not upbraid Flannagan herself, but she did give her consent to the harassing visits.) Flannagan, who had a history of mental instability, began to crumble under these encounters. He was separated from the PWAP on March 29, and the strain and tension he had been suffering intensified. Two days later, Flannagan's psychiatrist wrote to Juliana to say that firing the artist had undermined his already fragile mental state. The doctor requested that Flannagan be rehired, but the letter was ignored.

The argument can be made that Juliana carried Flannagan on the payrolls for three months while getting nothing in return, but since the sculptor had a medical excuse it would have been worth covering up for him or fighting to save him from dismissal. However, she couldn't or wouldn't. Evidently the risk

of catering to a "loafer" took precedence. Once more, in the interest of general efficacy, Juliana's natural compassion—had Flannagan been receiving Whitney money, pressuring him or throwing him off the dole would be unthinkable—was subordinated to bureaucratic triage. A few months after the psychiatrist's letter was written, Flannagan had a severe mental breakdown. He was confined to Bloomingdale Hospital, a sanitarium in White Plains, New York, from September of 1934 until March of 1935. There to regain his health, he was forbidden to sculpt because the attending doctors felt that work was too absorbing for him.

Pilot program that it was, the PWAP was supposed to end on February 15, 1934, but funds were found to extend it until April 28. Accordingly, to compare notes and plan the next two months, the sixteen regional committee chairmen met in Washington, from February 19 to 21, with Bruce and the rest of his staff. The main purpose of the conference was to examine what had been done in each region and discuss ways and means of carrying the project forward. As she had worked out with Barr and Goodrich, Juliana presented her conviction that the artistic and purely relief aspects of government support should be separated. Bruce and Watson, assisted by Francis Taylor, the director of the Worcester Art Museum and chairman of the New England Regional Committee, seized on these words as an admission that she had been wrong about the uniform pay scale for all artists. They tried to dissuade her from continuing with one wage, but she wouldn't budge. Instead, Juliana tried to persuade the other museum directors to see the issue as she did. All in all, she confided to Biddle, the conference was "extremely discouraging," with her point of view "for the moment entirely lost."

Even though the PWAP was given an extra ten weeks, the quotas for artists were not increased, and several thousand were still on the waiting list in New York. Juliana, to employ as many people as possible,* began churning their names through the payrolls. Some artists were discharged to make room for others for the duration of the program; some stayed on the PWAP the entire time it lasted; and some were on for as little as two weeks. As before, these cutbacks were based on appraisals of ability and need, a system guaranteed to please nobody. The turnstile approach to employment and unemployment provoked further protests from the Unemployed Artists Association—with dismissal notices mounting, the group stepped up its demonstrations to one a week. Between February 15 and the end of March, eight marches took place. Picketers buzzed the Whitney like dive-bombers, with Juliana as their target. On February 9, Biddle noted in his diary, "Mrs. Force is under heavy criticism, both for poor organization and favoritism. She tells me that she has been sabotaged by both the National Academy of Design and the John Reed Club."

The confrontations escalated in hostility. Lloyd Goodrich recalled:

---

*At one point, she had 719 or 722 artists on the rolls. The total number of artists Juliana was able to employ is estimated to be between 800 and 850.

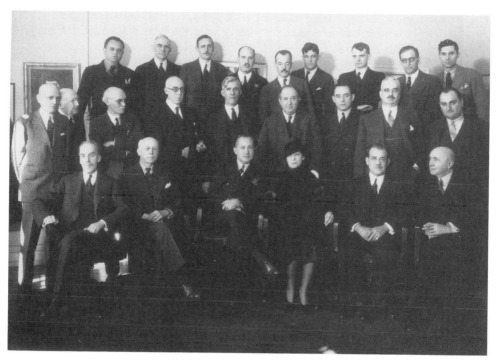

The regional chairmen and Washington staff of the PWAP. Seated: far left, Duncan Phillips; third from right, Juliana. Standing: second row, directly behnd Juliana, Edward Bruce; far right, Francis Henry Taylor; next to him, Fiske Kimball. Top row, directly behind Bruce, Forbes Watson.

We would send word out to pick five people and we'd talk to them. Their whole objective was to employ more artists, but we couldn't do that because we were under the control of the Washington office. . . . On one of these occasions, Mrs. Force started talking to the delegation, saying, "We cannot do anything further. . . . We're powerless, Washington is telling us how many we can employ." But they proved utterly unresponsive to this—they thought it was all a big front. Finally she turned to me and said, "Mr. Goodrich, why don't you take over?" I said more or less the same thing, but nothing would penetrate. . . . Then one of the cops standing around in the background asked, "Should we throw them out?" "No!" we said, and I went to the window to watch the delegation leave. There was a soapbox in the crowd. A guy stood up on the soapbox and said, "Well, we got the same old crap!" And that was all our arguments had done. It was pretty tough.

After another visit from the protesters, Goodrich said, Juliana was so upset that she had hysterics. He had to give her some brandy to quiet her. These encounters were harrowing for Juliana not only on account of the bitterness of the dispute, but because of her remoteness from political issues. Never a political or social thinker, she was moved not by abstractions, but by the direct, human particulars—if one-to-one discussions failed, she took the young artists' discontent personally, as a rebuke to her. Allan Rieser said Juliana told him that while

listening to one of the protesters angrily haranguing her, she noticed that the man had a hole in his shoe. "The thought struck her," he wrote, "that what was making him so unreasonable was that his shoes were worn out and uncomfortable. So she offered him the money to buy a new pair." Similarly, when a newspaper attempted to cause a scandal by disclosing that Juliana had put William Gropper, whose cartoons appeared in the *Daily Worker*, on the PWAP, she declined to be perturbed. She was not offended by the artist's Communist sympathies,* only motivated by her knowledge of the human agonies involved —he and his wife were jobless with two children to support. "His political opinions had nothing to do with us," Juliana informed the editor. "We have even been known to employ Republicans!"

As the weeks wore on, relations between Juliana and the representatives of the Unemployed Artists Association unraveled. She was tired of having to defend herself, and being unable to relate to their politics, she was further estranged from their poverty and tribulations. She reclassified their social grievances as bad manners, and was distraught by them. (At this point in her life, Juliana never would have admitted, even to make peace with the agitators, that she could understand from personal experience their sense of being penniless outsiders. Perhaps she was no longer capable of a such a confession—the humility of poverty was long years behind her, and her grand forgetfulness finally may have served her too well.) Edward Laning, who watched one of the demonstrations, "complete with placards and chants and shouted imprecations," wrote of the incident:

> My friend Karl Free . . . leaned out of an upper window of the beleaguered Museum and called to many of the demonstrators below, "I know *you*, So-and-So, and *you*, So-and-So," implying that he meant to blacklist them forever. Mrs. Force was tough as long as she could play the great lady, but this was no time for ladies. I visited her one day in her fabulous apartment and she told me of the outrages she was experiencing. As I bade goodbye in the entrance room of the apartment . . . she told me of a delegation of destitute artists she had recently received. "They stood on this very spot," she said, "and howled insults at me. And as they turned to go, one of them *spat* here, right at my feet!"

The artists' demonstrations interfered with the running of the museum, which was open for business all this time. (Oscar Bluemner thought it prudent to write a letter about a future exhibition to "Dear Museum," explaining that "I address you thus wholesale having heard or read that your director has been kidnapped by the Federal When Do We Eat association for painters.") For part of February and most of March, the entire building was given over to a comprehensive showing of the work of Maurice Prendergast, who had died in 1924. The Whitney was the first museum in New York City to organize a Prendergast retrospective, † and Juliana was even able to wheedle a painting out of the Barnes Foundation for the tribute. More astoundingly, the dyspeptic Dr. Barnes came up for the

*The Communist party was then a legal political party in the United States.

† Soon after Prendergast's death, Walter Pach urged the Metropolitan to give him a memorial show. He was turned down because the trustees felt that the one Prendergast on the museum's walls, a loan, was enough.

opening. But during the visit, Eugenie Prendergast, the artist's sister-in-law, remembered him marching around and emanating disapproval, his face set in a belligerent expression.

The incessant disruptions the PWAP caused the museum couldn't be ignored forever, and on March 3 the whole PWAP operation was moved downtown from the Whitney to the Civil Works Administration headquarters at the Municipal Building. Although the office gained a measure of freedom and serenity with a change in location, it was now subject to cronyism and political fiat. After the office in the museum closed, someone took the opportunity to replace the chief clerk with a political appointee. The new man couldn't do the job, and he quarreled with the other clerical workers. After three days of chaos, Juliana fired off a telegram to Washington: FIND . . . CHIEF CLERK INCOMPETENT AND IM-POSSIBLE. PREFER GOOD BOOKKEEPER TO GOOD DEMOCRAT.

Tempers were feverishly high in February of 1934, and not just because of PWAP firings and cutbacks. In March of 1933 the Mexican artist Diego Rivera arrived in New York to paint murals in the RCA Building at Rockefeller Center. The commission, instigated by Nelson Rockefeller, was seen as a signal event in the annals of American art—not only was mural making associated with populism, but Rivera was a charismatic figure to many painters. Young artists such as Ben Shahn, Louise Nevelson, Seymour Fogel, and Lucienne Bloch lined up to be his assistants. One panel contained a heroic portrait of Lenin, whom Rivera equated with Lincoln. The Rockefellers asked him to remove the image, and when the artist refused, he was fired. Influential intellectuals and artists flocked to Rivera's cause; nevertheless, the murals were covered up with canvas sheeting and remained so until the night of February 9, 1934, when RCA workmen secretly entered the building with orders to pulverize them to dust.

More was destroyed than Rivera's work. The vandalism sabotaged the reception of the First Municipal Art Exhibition, which opened in the RCA Building on February 28. Featuring the work of 500 New York artists spread out through thirty-three galleries, the event was devised to stimulate picture sales. Although administered by the heads of the New York museums, the show was a gesture of goodwill by the La Guardia Administration, and the committee inviting the artists—Juliana, Barr, Winlock, Fox, Watrous, Holger Cahill, and Kroll—encompassed most of the art establishment. The mayor, however, reaped neither prestige nor rosy notices. On February 27, noisy demonstrations broke out against the Rockefellers and the exhibition itself. Artists indignant about the fate of the Rivera murals withdrew their paintings—among them, Sloan, Shahn, Lozowick, Laning, Gropper, and Biddle. Others formed picket lines. Harry Watrous tried to have Stuart Davis, who was leading a demonstration, arrested.

There was, it would seem, enough vilification of Juliana in the air to satiate even the most voracious adversary, but more strife was purposely fomented by an envious peer. Over the past two or three years, a rivalry had grown up between Juliana and Audrey McMahon, the executive secretary of the College Art Association and the able administrator of its circulating exhibitions and relief programs. She would later become supervisor of the Works Progress Adminis-

tration's Federal Art Project (WPA/FAP) in the New York area and thus emerge as a figure to reckon with in the city's art and politics.

Before McMahon's ascent to power, she attempted to be accommodating, whereas Juliana was often high-handed, dictating terms and doing the minimum that she could without being accused of rudeness or unprofessionalism. McMahon was less casual and quixotic in her procedures than Juliana, but she was just as tough. Edward Laning said that McMahon could inspire an artist to fear and obey; the artists' nickname for McMahon, he wrote, was Arsenic and Old Face. Juliana probably disliked her in the way she reflexively disliked other formidable women (such as Rebecca West) whom she perceived as threatening her unique standing. McMahon, speaking many years later of the "great rivalry" between her and Juliana, said of her old antagonist, "She was one of the most extraordinary women I've ever met. Her will was law. She was . . . brilliant, but . . . she brooked no interference." Another source of the conflict may have been rooted not so much in their competitiveness as in their alikeness—a subconscious recognition by Juliana of traits shared but so very differently channeled, of problems shared but so very differently handled.

McMahon justifiably believed that she was qualified for and entitled to be chairman of the PWAP's regional committee, and she lobbied for the post. She resented it when Juliana was tapped. One reason Juliana got the job was that the Whitney was the institution in closest touch with American artists. Bruce awarded her the position because he thought "the Whitney Museum . . . [was] more entitled to representation on the committee than any other institution in America, and far more than any other of the New York museums." But McMahon and others who sided with her chose to believe it was merely for snob value— Juliana had more social cachet. After Juliana was named as chairman, relations were tense between the PWAP and the College Art Association. "We had an armed truce," McMahon was to say. "We agreed to co-exist. And that is about what we did. She had the upper hand, usually; we had the upper hand, occasionally—as when we would have something very distinguished happen by pure chance and get some public acclaim. But it was co-existence, not coordination."

The truce, to whatever extent it was observed, did not last for long. McMahon made her displeasure known, talking against Juliana and trying to incite artists to do injury to the museum. Ben Shahn, who had no trouble getting on the PWAP and was liked by Juliana, said that McMahon hinted to him, "I wouldn't blame you if you threw a brick through the Whitney Museum." Bernarda Bryson Shahn, notwithstanding her conflicts with the Whitney, preferred Juliana to McMahon. In appraising them both, she said:

> Mrs. Force wasn't the worst of art administrators, believe me. Audrey was a demon and jealous of Juliana Force, and she supported our demonstrations. But Audrey was easier to work with because she was less autocratic in confrontations. Juliana Force practiced a snobbery in art that was rather hard to take. At the end of openings, she selected people and whisked them off to her private parties. In the PWAP, the division occurred between those who had arrived and those who had not. Audrey was a fierce woman, but she was also more capable of grasping the political implications of what

was going on. Juliana had good taste, she reacted well to all kinds of art, and we respected the Whitney, but we were angry at her.

Juliana retaliated against McMahon in kind, although some time elapsed before she could be appropriately avenged. But when she struck, she did so with a dart of poison that demonstrated the absoluteness of her influence. After the PWAP was terminated, there was a few months' hiatus in government support for the arts before appropriations for two other projects were made—a denouement directly traceable to the effectiveness of the PWAP experiment. In 1935, McMahon became the WPA's supervisor of the art division in New York. In essence, she was given Juliana's former job in the new agency, although her authority was greater and her tenure longer than Juliana's, and the scale of her program larger than the PWAP. In 1937 McMahon hired Eugene Ludins to be her deputy in Woodstock. Artists who felt that Ludins was too radical demonstrated against his investiture, and McMahon and her assistants went up to Woodstock to quell the revolt. By coincidence, Juliana happened to be in town at the same time and staying with Ludins. After McMahon and her contingent arrived, they "had the unprecedented experience of not being served any dinner in a public restaurant in which Mrs. Force was entertaining friends. We decided we were doing Ludins no favor by staying any longer and left for the city." Besides sanctioning this power play in Woodstock, Juliana, then no longer connected with government patronage, went on the record with a comment that the WPA was fostering too much mediocre art. She was scornful of the FAP's standards, whereas she approved of the aristocracy of the Treasury Department's art competitions—in that program, she believed, the artists were more carefully selected. Holger Cahill, who became the FAP's national director, did not react kindly to these remarks. He took to calling Juliana "Mrs. Whitney's almoner."

But the unemployed artists didn't need McMahon to inflame them. Bad luck assailed Juliana—little went well on the PWAP, no matter what she did or didn't do. On March 3, the same day the PWAP office was transferred to the Municipal Building, she met with a dozen or so artists on the project, artists she knew and believed would listen to reason. Juliana explained that thousands of artists were still on the waiting list, unenrolled. Would those in attendance and other employed artists agree to accept a lower weekly salary en masse so she could take the new "surplus" and use it to put others on the payroll? Dorothy Varian, who was at the meeting, said that all the artists consented at once. The idea was Juliana's, not Washington's, which meant much maneuvering. But she was still feeling scrappy enough to undertake it.

Before she could suggest this reform, Juliana was derailed by enemies of the New Deal. On March 18, 1934, the *Herald Tribune*, a Republican paper that wanted to smear the Roosevelt Administration, ran a front-page exposé of PWAP malfeasance in New York by reporting that such eminent artists as Sloan, Zorach, and Alexander Stirling Calder, who were not considered to be in need of assistance, were receiving $38.25 a week from the government till. The list of PWAP artists had been a secret, so this was big news. The other papers picked up the story and accused Juliana of impropriety. As usual, she recapitulated that the

PWAP was not entirely a relief measure and that eligibility requirements allowed an artist to have another income, as long as it didn't exceed $60 a month. In addition, the artists' avowals of need were accepted without question. "We are not a detective agency," Juliana said. Sloan, thought to be well-to-do, had a total income of $50 a month from teaching. He was therefore within the regulations, and Juliana felt within her rights to hire him.

Juliana asked all the artists named in the story to turn in descriptions of their financial status. She promised to keep them confidential unless there was an emergency. Their replies, which she did not use even though their publication would have dissipated the abuse directed against her, are poignantly revealing documents of the Depression's impact on artists and their unswerving determination to remain in their profession. Calder wrote:

> During the past two years I have earned only $2000—and spent $5300 of our savings which are now exhausted—Our only income amounts to $518 yearly—and our needs however stringently reduced are ten times that. I am not yet prepared to throw everything overboard and take to the woods, because I have confidence that our President will find a way. . . .

Calder was then sixty-four years old, and in 1934 Social Security had not been inaugurated. Hayley Lever, who was fifty-eight, stated that since October of 1933 his income had amounted to $120. "If I have any reputation as an artist," he mused, "I often wonder how we can exist on it." A. S. Baylinson said that he had been out of a job since June 1, 1933, when he lost his instructorship at the Art Students League. Since then he had made $600, but he owed $150 in back rent and was responsible for a wife and two children. Without the PWAP, Baylinson wrote, "I certainly would be up against it."

Zorach's case was different. He had a teaching job in Greenwich, Connecticut, so he didn't apply for relief. Juliana had come to him, an artist of some stature, and asked him to produce something worthwhile to counteract the great quantity of poor work she was seeing. Zorach agreed to help out, but he didn't want to be compensated—he would work for nothing. But to enroll in the PWAP, he and Sloan, like everyone else, had to sign a declaration certifying their financial need. Juliana, with her cavalier attitude toward detail, brushed off the rule as insignificant. It meant nothing, she assured them—it was just another bothersome government form. Yet it was their signatures on that honor statement that caused much of the ensuing uproar. As the reporters who dropped by Zorach's studio informed him before the story broke, "Boy, are you really in trouble."

Though Juliana might have sat out the latest scandal in silence, Sloan did not. Fearless about speaking out, he also wanted to correct the impression that he had gotten rich by his art. His being perceived as financially comfortable had been fueled by widespread publicity about a supposed transaction between himself and Carl Hamilton, a collector and shady investor with a history of stock and art swindles, made in 1928. Hamilton contracted to buy thirty-two of Sloan's paintings for $41,200. The pictures were put in storage, under bond, until the bill was paid. But when the stock market crashed, Hamilton went bust, the sale

fell through, and Sloan never received a cent. Meanwhile, on the strength of his expectations, Sloan borrowed money from his bank to lend $7,500 to a friend who was broke. The friend only paid back $2,700, and Sloan was having such a rough time that in November of 1933 he wrote to sixty museums around the country offering his paintings at half price. He made one sale through this letter, but not until 1935.*

None of these vicissitudes were known to the *Tribune* when the paper sent a reporter to call. Sloan assured his interlocutor that despite his reputation, he had not been able to dispose of a painting in years. As he was thrifty, he admitted, he could "get along" without the $38.25 a week and exist on $50 a month, but he had entertained the patriotic hope that canvases executed for the PWAP would be considered as his contribution to the nation. "The consumption of my art," Sloan offered, "is as important to the country, I think, as the consumption of the work of the less skillful." And the government was receiving a bargain, to boot. For his few weeks' salary, Sloan had handed over two paintings with a market value estimated at $3,000 each.†

Sensing that these arguments weren't winning any converts, Sloan revealed that he had never made a living from his painting—he had to rely on teaching and illustrating to pay the bills. He then took the man into his studio and said, "I have here nearly ninety per cent of all the work I have done in the last twenty years. . . . Nevertheless, I would be willing to give up all my works here and my complete output during the rest of my life for a steady income of $100 a week." Sloan's words were printed, and the smear backfired. His offer to trade his life's work for a guaranteed wage killed the story, as did Zorach's testimony that he wasn't taking any money for his work, but getting a retraction from the paper took several weeks. But before public reaction quieted down, Zorach said, "We got write-ups and crank letters and telephone calls over our scandalous behavior, saying what an awful, unscrupulous thing it was for us to do—to horn in on government money meant for desperate and needy artists."

When the ranks of the Unemployed Artists Association, which had lately merged into the Artists Union, heard that several of the best-known artists in America were working for the government, they exploded. To this group, Sloan's and Zorach's presence on the PWAP did not seem well-intentioned, and the union was not in the mood to be civil. Over 100 demonstrators quickly assembled in front of the museum and started agitating for jobs. They attracted bystanders, and neighbors were so frightened by the ominous-looking crowd that they called the police. When the squad cars arrived, the protesters pushed their way into the museum. There was no rioting, but one artist was hit with a billy club. The demonstrators who had penetrated inside were escorted out by the police, but four designated leaders—Joseph Vogel, Simon Kennedy, Byron Browne, and Bernarda Bryson—were permitted to return for an audience with Juliana. They

---

Pigeons, bought by the Museum of Fine Arts, Boston.

†*Fourteenth Street, Snow* (whereabouts unknown) and *The Wigwam, Old Tammany Hall*, on permanent loan to the Metropolitan Museum of Art. If either of these paintings were to come on the market today, the assessed value would be in the hundreds of thousands of dollars.

sparred for ninety minutes, after which the artists exited, returned to headquarters, and drafted a list of eleven demands. The union wanted immediate employment for all artists who registered for unemployment, retroactive pay for their periods out of work, elimination of the "merit" clause, continuation of all CWA art projects, and permanent free exhibition space for all artists. In addition, Juliana received a telegram accusing her "of callous disregard for hundreds of destitute artists."

The more extreme forms of harassment were stretching her beyond tolerance and endurance. Juliana told George Biddle that for several nights running, angry artists had been marching back and forth under her bedroom window and shouting, "We want jobs!" and preventing her from sleeping. Biddle knew that unlike Holger Cahill or Audrey McMahon, Juliana couldn't realize "that these boys marching up and down . . . could be politically useful" to her cause if she portrayed them as victims of the Depression. She saw them as Communists, to be despised and ignored.

Although the PWAP office was no longer within the Whitney, the museum remained a target of the Left and the Right. Juliana's beloved institution was disrupted and inconvenienced beyond measure, and she who had given so freely of her time heard herself being maligned as recklessly indifferent to the fates of the artists. These were too many injustices, and Juliana had had enough. Citing the possibility of harm to the building or its objects, she abruptly shut down the entire museum as of March 27, six weeks before the season normally ended. On March 30, Juliana would make a speech marked by jests that were more revealing than she might have thought. "When I started as chairman of the New York Regional Committee of the Public Works of Art Project, three months and three weeks ago," she told her audience, "I was full of patriotism and enthusiasm. After this time I don't feel full of enthusiasm or patriotism—I just feel full of facts and figures. And figures do not lie, except the human figures, sometimes!"

The PWAP was to be disbanded by April 28, and artists were dismissed from the payroll each week until none were left. The liquidation of the project meant that many artists, briefly solvent, were without subsistence wages again. Another item of business for Juliana that month was to sort through the 1,977 works executed in the New York area and send the best ones to Washington. With the PWAP about to run its course, Bruce and Watson knew that they had to create enthusiasm for the art made under its aegis to get another appropriation. They gambled that a nicely culled cross section of PWAP art, tastefully mounted in an established museum, would do much to convince Congress that the taxpayers' money had been wisely spent. The show, which opened at the Corcoran Gallery of Art on April 24, boasted a predominance of accessible, easily recognizable scenes, often of a productive America exuberantly at work. Abstract artists, it turned out, need not apply. Bruce and Watson frowned on the work Juliana sent them by Gorky, Davis, and Burgoyne Diller; out of prudence, they also passed by Ben Shahn's spicy sketches for a projected history of Prohibition.

Bruce seriously underestimated the thinness of Washington skins. An entry he accepted from the New York office nearly did him in. Juliana and Goodrich were proud of a discovery they had made on the project, that of a twenty-seven-

year-old artist named Paul Cadmus. When his finished painting was brought in, Goodrich remembered "our surprise and delight" about it. Juliana sent the canvas to Washington, and it went into the Corcoran show.

Cadmus's painting, called *The Fleet's In!*, is a raucous portrayal of sailors on shore leave. Young men, drunk and rowdy, carouse with willing women; Bruce and Watson must have recognized it immediately as being in the racy and ebullient vein of Hogarth, Rowlandson, the early Sloan, and lately practiced by Reginald Marsh. However, Hugh L. Rodman, a retired navy admiral, was oblivious to the painting's art-historical pedigree. Before the exhibition opened, Rodman saw the painting and immediately pronounced it an insult to the navy. He indignantly called the wire services, and Bruce and his exhibition were the focus of a national outcry. The Secretary of the Navy requested Bruce to pull *The Fleet's In!* from the Corcoran, and he complied. The painting was then confiscated and suppressed, and it vanished for some years.*

The sanitized Corcoran exhibition, attended by President and Mrs. Roosevelt, was a victory for Bruce and Watson. The Roosevelts stayed for an hour and a half, praised the pictures, picked some to hang in the White House, and assured Bruce that he had their backing. The New Deal would renew its commitment to art patronage, paving the way for the establishment of the WPA and Treasury Department projects. Juliana, also at the Washington festivities, was glad for Bruce and relieved at the good reviews the exhibition earned, but her own views no longer coincided with his. Never again would she or the Whitney administer a government art program, and when Lewis Mumford panned the Corcoran show in *The New Yorker*—the art, he said, was "a minor matter . . . amiable but undistinguished, gentlemanly but lacking in guts"—Juliana could not keep her thoughts about the PWAP to herself. Rather than bridle at Mumford's words, she embraced him as a kindred spirit. She drafted the following letter to him:

> The New Yorker has just come and away from the scene of battle, as it were, I read with the greatest interest your review of the P.W.A.P. Exhibition in Washington and agree with the indictment based on the show as hung there.
>
> As ex-chairman of the New York Regional Committee, however, may I tell you what is to my belief the real criticism of the result of this "Public Sanction of Art." Not the artist nor the hopefully banal production, but that old old business of making it safe for Democracy!
>
> The New York Committee was asked and did send about 600 works of Art, as Exhibit A. When I visited Washington at the opening of the Exhibition there were but 150 of these hung. The wall space of course was limited and when I saw the selection I realised that the feast had been spread for Official Washington's stomach.
>
> The men responsible for the safety-first motive are too intelligent and too devoted to have wantonly "canned" some of the really fine stuff. I believe it was fact and not a theory which confronted them. They were under the fierce necessity of justifying this Public money's expenditure, not to the Artist, not to the Critic, not to the world we live in, but to that Official world through whose efforts the whole gesture was

---

* Now in the collection of the Naval Historical Center.

made possible—that world which is not accustomed to look upon any evidence of an inner life.

The Artist did not fail, the work produced was better than you saw in Washington. And I am sure that if Officials anywhere were half as courageous as the men at Dartmouth were we would have other murals besides Orozco's* to talk about.

While Cadmus's lampoon of horny sailors kept the PWAP controversial in April, a more reverent portrayal of the military was in the making. For his PWAP endeavor, the artist Thomas Loftin Johnson conceived of a gargantuan mural —35 feet high and 70 feet long—celebrating the history and profession of arms. The images chosen were based on the English historian Sir Edward Creasy's *The Fifteen Decisive Battles Of The World*. Destined for Washington Hall, the cadets' mess at West Point Military Academy, the design, an echt-kitsch, pseudo-medieval rendering of heroic figures, was in tune with the building—a gray stone fortress in military Gothic style. After the preliminary sketches were approved, Johnson worked on the 10-foot-long oil enlargements in the Whitney's sculpture gallery during the summer of 1934. When she was in New York, Juliana would stop by to see how he was getting along. In this school-of-Rivera pageant of personages and campaigns—Alexander the Great, William the Conqueror at Hastings, Peter the Great, Marlborough at Blenheim, Wellington at Waterloo, and Joffre at the Marne—the one woman included was Joan of Arc. Johnson felt indebted to Juliana for the interest she took in his work, and when he discovered that no actual likeness of Joan of Arc existed, he modeled the head after Juliana. His Maid of Orleans was given red hair, thin lips, and hooded eyes. As Joan, Juliana offers her sword to God, while a company of soldiers kneels in prayer at her feet. Johnson felt that the comparison was apt—for him and multitudes of other grateful artists, she was the Joan of Arc of American art. To Juliana, the analogy must have stung with the kind of irony that would amuse her in less stressful times. Although she might not claim that she had heard voices, she had more than an inkling of what it was like to be burned at the ideological stake.

But Johnson's mural would not be completed under PWAP auspices. The program ended before Johnson finished his oil sketches. Now out of a job, the artist used his remaining savings for a lobbying trip to Washington. Juliana gave him a letter of introduction to the Secretary of War, who was friendly but unwilling to allocate money. Johnson then called on an influential congressman, who told him that if a log cabin was good enough for Abe Lincoln, then West Point without wall decorations was good enough for any cadet.

Johnson was thinking about returning to New York, but on the spur of the moment he decided to visit the Army Chief of Staff. The officer, a graduate and former superintendent of West Point, was Douglas MacArthur. MacArthur read the letter from Juliana and looked at some small sketches and photographs Johnson had brought along. Striding dramatically to and fro, MacArthur turned

---

*In his review, Mumford contrasted the mediocrity of the government-sponsored art with the "passion and drive" of Orozco's murals in the Baker Library at Dartmouth College. On March 12, 1934, Mumford had lectured on "Orozco in New England" at the Whitney.

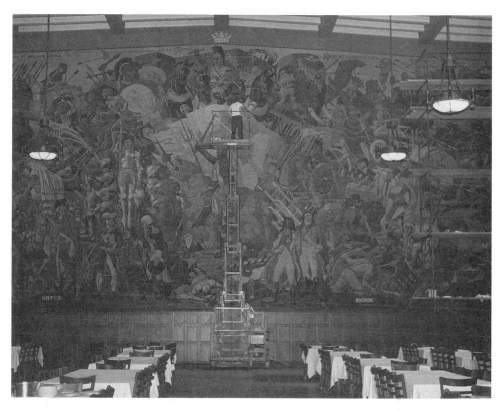

Thomas Loftin Johnson at work on his gargantuan mural in the West Point mess hall; Juliana as the armor-encased Joan of Arc to his lower left.

swiftly on his heel and declared, "West Point must have that mural." After a talk with Ned Bruce, MacArthur set in motion a complex sequence of negotiations that resulted in the transfer of authority for the mural to the WPA in 1935. He also saw to it that $1,750 was donated from military sources. The mural, completed in 1936, and cleaned a few years ago, can still be seen on the vast unbroken wall in Washington Hall. Juliana's armor-clad figure, once murky, is sharp and visible again. She stands eternally vigilant, triumphing over the past food fights of generations of cadets, who found the mural an irresistible target for rolls, preserves, and globs of mashed potatoes.

Juliana was ready for a vacation from the politics and pettifogging of the PWAP. The other members of the New York Regional Committee threw a congratulatory party in her honor on May 15, eleven days before she sailed for Europe on the *Bremen*, but she did not feel very congratulatory herself. Just before her departure, she confided to Leon Kroll, "I could only say, now that the works [sic] is finished, I wish I might have made a better job of it." As usual, Juliana traveled elaborately, with mountains of luggage, hatboxes stacked high,

stores of books, and champagne and flowers for the send-off. With all that she had to do, one task was never neglected—fiddling with her passport. On the back of a photograph she was going to submit to the State Department, she had done some subtraction: 1886 from 1934. She was figuring out what age she should enter on her application if she gave, as she did, her birth date as 1886. This flare of vigor and vanity to the contrary, Juliana was drained. Her habit, intensified during the run of the PWAP, was to go at top speed until she collapsed in exhaustion. Her recuperative powers were excellent, and normally she would be ready to go again after a brief rest. But the rigors of the PWAP had sapped her strength to the extreme, and Juliana was in a despondent mood when she sailed. Six months of controversy and strife and the ceaseless publicity engendered had ruffled Gertrude, to Juliana's great anxiety. Juliana's reactions to the tumult of the last few months, her mental and physical fatigue, and her concern for not dismaying Gertrude are seen in a letter she wrote from her suite on the *Bremen* on May 31, 1934. Writing in bed, relaxed but still tired, Juliana's guard was down.

> Dear Gertrude. Here in this twilight world I call you by your name.
> "On the dim marge of grey
> Twixt the Soul's night & day
> Washing 'awake' away
> Into 'asleep.' " I've just read it in a new book of verse & it sounds to me like an entirely accurate report of my activities on board S.S. Bremen! What a heavenly world it has been. Made in 5 days this one, made of light & air & the sound of swishing waters. Filled to overflowing with flowers & books & "leisure to invite one's soul." I have never been happier nor so at peace. What happened? I really do not know. But when the door of my cabin closed it shut out much which I wanted to forget. And then I opened your letter to me. It was a loving & a tender letter, but it was also a wise one. The great love for you came back again & flooded my heart & the hardness was no more. Life was not something to be afraid of & somehow it seemed to me important how I lived it. . . .
>
> You said you would try to forget the winter* & that made me glad. It has hurt so to stand aside & know that you were suffering. I could not share nor lighten any grief. My part was to see that your work was carried on & that the dignity & the importance of it should not be diminished. I have not failed you in that sense at least. It is my pride & my comfort that only the years will tell that truth to others. You & I know now.

Juliana, rereading the above, may have worried that her words had been too intimate, too plaintive, or needy. She did not like appearing pathetic, especially to Gertrude, and the letter does an about-face. It reverts to Juliana's tried-and-true mode of bucking up Gertrude with an allusive miscellany, cleverly laced with puns, of the latest books she has brought aboard ship to read. It is the same

---

*Gertrude was disheartened by the artists who seemed to turn against the Whitney by their demonstrations. She was also saddened by two personal losses that occurred during the closing days of the PWAP. On April 22, 1934, Alice Vanderbilt died. Less than two weeks later, Jo Davidson's wife, Yvonne, died in New York, and Gertrude had to help with those arrangements, too.

kind of letter as she wrote to Gertrude in 1911, when she was earning her wings as a literary agent.

> This is letter Number I, written in bed where I've stayed the entire trip, not because I'm ill but because I *could*. I have not seen nor talked with anyone—not because there isn't Pierre Matisse on board nor yet an Eyre de Lanux*—but because I like better to hear Miss Nat-O-Dag.† Isn't she delicious! It has given me great entertainment, Seven Gothic Tales. So curiously reminiscent & yet so certainly of our day. What do you think of the style? Firbank, Boccaccio, Joyce & even a dash of Thomas Mann. They each sneak into my mind as I read. Sometimes after an excursion into Greek Peoples I'm sure I smell Russian-sort of half-calf. It's been fun & I'm not yet through. I feel like a child in a sweet shop when I look at all my new books. I do not know which to choose but long to finger them all. I'm that scatterbrained that I nibble first at the Odyssey then peck at Simple Folk. I Breakfast in Bed while Rome Burns[.] The Postman Rings Twice (& doesn't waken me)[.] I'm Here Today & Gone Tomorrow on Modern Art. I lie down with The Lamb in His Bosom & sit up In This Bewildered World!‡ now that tells you the State I'm in—and I like it.
>
> Please give my love to Flora. I hope Pam's§ measles are better & that the innoculations [sic] were effective. It would be nice to hear too how you are.
>
> Lovingly
>
> J.

The first stop on Juliana's itinerary was England, where she wanted to lose herself in her garden and her flowers, but she would not be at Cobweb for long. She had two business matters waiting for her in Italy. First, she hoped to conclude a purchase with Florence Powers, a descendant of the nineteenth-century American sculptor Hiram Powers. Miss Powers resided in Florence, and Juliana planned to visit her there and buy a marble version of *The Greek Slave* that was still in the family.

The central reason for the sojourn in Italy was more in Juliana's usual line of calling attention to contemporary art. In 1930 Edward Alden Jewell, who was in touch with the Italian cultural authorities, had approached Juliana about taking over the American pavilion for the 1932 Venice Biennale and filling it as she chose. The Biennale, an international exhibition of new art that was held every other summer, had become a lively tourist attraction and a place for artists

---

*Pierre Matisse, the son of the painter, had opened an art gallery in New York in 1932. Eyre de Lanux, an American-born artist, writer, and furniture designer, was based in Paris for many years.

†Malin Nat-og-Dag, one of the main characters in "The Deluge of Norderney," the first story in Isak Dinesen's *Seven Gothic Tales* (1934). Miss Nat-og-Dag, although a sixty-year-old maiden lady "of the strictest virtue, believed herself to be one of the great female sinners of her time."

‡Juliana ran together *Breakfast in Bed* by Sylvia Thompson, *While Rome Burns* by Alexander Woollcott, *The Postman Always Rings Twice* by James M. Cain, *Here Today and Gone Tomorrow* by Louis Bromfield, *Modern Art* by Thomas Craven, *Lamb in His Bosom* by Caroline Miller, and *This Bewildered World* by Frazier Hunt. She was also reading the diaries of Alice James and *Three Essays on America* by Van Wyck Brooks.

§Pamela Tower, the eldest child of Flora Whitney Tower Miller, born in 1921.

to gain European exposure. Juliana declined to participate then, feeling that greater réclame would accrue to the Whitney if she waited until after the museum was open and officially established, so the Whitney undertook the running of the American pavilion two years later. In January of 1934, sixty-three oils, thirty watercolors, and a group of etchings were selected from the Whitney's permanent collection. Juliana's intent was to pick works that either displayed the representative character of the collection or that had been done by an American who had not exhibited abroad. Once again, she did not cavil about lending the best. Some of the paintings earmarked for Venice were *Place Pasdeloup, Why Not Use the "L"?, Baptism in Kansas, Light of the World, My Egypt, River Rouge Plant, Early Sunday Morning, The Green Table* (by Niles Spencer), *Winter on the River, Chinese Restaurant, The Blue Clown* (by Walt Kuhn), and *The Mountain, New Mexico.* The accompanying watercolors were by Joseph Stella, Davis, Hopper, Demuth, Marin, and Sheeler, and the etchings by Bacon, Marsh, Sloan, and others. The pavilion was to open on May 12, 1934, but because of her PWAP obligations, Juliana could not leave New York in time to supervise the uncrating or hanging. She asked Gerald Kelly to be her deputy in Italy, and sometime in May, Eleanor Lambert went over to assist him. These two duties —the visit with Miss Powers and the ceremonial viewing of the American pavilion resplendent with the Whitney collection—promised to be the peaceful highlights of an otherwise uneventful summer.

The hoped-for tranquillity would not only elude Juliana, but Italy would become the scene of her latest warfare. Peculiar reports were filtering out of Venice of an unwanted and unauthorized insertion into the Whitney's exhibition. Eleanor Lambert, joining Juliana in Buckinghamshire, verified the strange news. A three-quarter-length portrait of the actress Marion Davies—not owned or sought by the museum—had been clandestinely added to the exhibition, and works from the Whitney collection were moved to make way for the intruder. The painting, by a Polish artist named Tade Styka, hung in the most prominent spot in the pavilion—the vestibule, considered the place of honor. But why Marion Davies? The answer, as both Juliana and Lambert knew, could be traced directly to William Randolph Hearst, Davies's lover, protector, and tireless promoter. When the Whitney collection was being packed for Venice, Hearst offered to pay the shipping costs if Juliana would see her way to including the picture of Davies in her exhibition. Juliana would not, and thought no more of it.

The decision of one lone museum director meant little to a William Randolph Hearst. His ego and influence were not to be denied. Hearst must have been particularly eager to have the portrait ensconced in the center of a large and prestigious show because this summer he, Davies, and a party of their friends would be on the scene in Europe themselves. What could be more joyous for Hearst than to suggest dropping by the Venice Biennale and being greeted by the sight of his own Marion ennobled by dashing brushstrokes and a heavy gold frame? After Juliana brushed him off, Hearst privately sent the picture to Italy. Seymour Berkson, one of his correspondents in Italy, called on the Count Volpi di Misurata, an official in Mussolini's government and the president of the

Biennale. Recognizing what an invaluable ally Hearst could be, Count Volpi arranged with Berkson to smuggle the picture into the pavilion after the show opened.

After being apprised of all that had gone on, Juliana instructed Eleanor Lambert to return to Venice with an ultimatum for the Italian authorities: Either remove the offending portrait at once or Juliana would withdraw the rest of the art and take it back to New York. Lambert was also to say that if this condition wasn't met, she would break the story to the Associated Press, to the embarrassment of the Italian government and William Randolph Hearst. Juliana gambled that Hearst wouldn't want the story to come out, for in public he was a stickler for the proprieties. He maintained to the world that he was happily married to his wife, Millicent, and that he and Davies were just friends. Juliana courteously observed these proprieties during her row with Biennale authorities. Although she knew very well who owned the portrait and where it came from, she never linked Marion Davies's name with Hearst's. Despite Hearst's appalling stunt, she treated him with the same circumspectness she would have accorded the Whitneys—not that it got her anywhere.

Juliana's instincts about Hearst's desire for discretion were confirmed by the policy of his newspapers. After the story broke and unfolded day by day, his chain gave Juliana and the Biennale the silent treatment. Unlike the rest of the American papers, the Hearst press never said a word about the dispute or reproduced the painting. (If Juliana had welcomed Davies's portrait into the Biennale, it is certain that Hearst editors would have responded with glowing stories and deluxe photo spreads.)

However, the sinister realities of the international situation were against Juliana as much as Hearst's own clout. When Hearst used his influence with Count Volpi, this was not some abstract quid pro quo. Hearst had met and admired Mussolini and wrote that "he is a marvelous man. It is astonishing how he takes care of every detail of his job." Two weeks after the Biennale opened, Hearst was quoted as saying that he would be delighted to see Mussolini again, and he wouldn't mind meeting Hitler either. Hearst landed in Spain and went on to Bad Nauheim to take the cure. Before long, a plane and an escort of four storm troopers arrived at Bad Nauheim to take Hearst to Berlin and Hitler. Reaching Rome in early June, Hearst visited Mussolini. Hitler and Mussolini were staging their own historic first meeting on June 14, 1934—in Venice. Juliana could not expect to obtain justice in such a climate—she and the Whitney could only be victims of political snares. Whereas Juliana would risk tangling with Hearst and his empire, Mussolini would not. A world-famous American press lord granting legitimacy to the Fascists by hobnobbing with their leaders was going to prevail.

Juliana was, of course, not privy to the entwined movements of Hearst, Mussolini, and Hitler. She was merely trying to deal with Count Volpi. But the Italians weren't as closemouthed as Juliana or Lambert, and word of Marion Davies's image as the presiding goddess of the Biennale hit the papers on June 22. Someone in the count's office had leaked the story. But Hearst, instead of

being angry, wrote an exultant note to Berkson. Because the Italians were prepared to fight to keep the portrait in the pavilion, it was excellent publicity for Miss Davies. He couldn't be happier.

On June 23, Juliana, as well as Hearst and his guests, were in London, a boon for the reporters shuttling between the contending parties. The press, in covering Marion Davies, bowed to standard practice and did not reveal that she was traveling with Hearst. He was never drawn into the case by name, nor was he interviewed. At first the actress professed ignorance of the affair, but she later had the crust to venture, "So far as I know, the people running the show asked that my portrait be sent." Juliana simply reiterated that the painting had been inserted without her authorization, and as such, was a wrong against all the other artists whose work she had not taken. She kept to the letter of the law, reminding her listeners that the author of the painting was not an American, but a Pole. "In justice and fairness to all concerned," Juliana evenly told the press, "I had to remonstrate when a picture not belonging there was placed on exhibition." While she was firing off telegrams from London, Count Volpi had taken himself to Brussels, conveniently out of reach for a few days. The Italians stalled until the count returned, saying they could do nothing without his permission. On June 23, as a concession to Juliana, Venetian officials helpfully added a sign beneath the portrait. This painting, the card read, was not to be considered a part of the American exhibition. When Count Volpi surfaced on June 27, he ruled that picture would stay where it was. There was a clause in all exhibition contracts stating that the contents of a pavilion could not be removed until the termination of the Biennale; he invoked this to back him up.

Juliana maintained that since the Italians had violated their part of the agreement, her contract was null and void. She cabled a New York broker and asked him to repossess the Whitney collection for her. Italian authorities then barred the packers from the premises. Juliana lodged several protests with Count Volpi, but they were fruitless: He had, in essence, imprisoned the Whitney collection, and he would continue to do so until the Biennale ran its scheduled course. Juliana was refusing to set foot in Italy or do anything that might hint that she had given her blessing to the tainted exhibition, but all that was left to her was a personal appeal. She arrived in Venice on July 15, was stymied, and left two days later for Paris. There she retained a French law firm to sue for the return of the art. A legal action was instituted in Milan, although it was a foregone conclusion that any court proceedings under Italian jurisdiction were not going to be decided with speed. Juliana was beaten before she began, but she could not stand still when her artists were being mocked. Her recent comrade-in-arms, Ned Bruce, wrote empathetically on July 21, "You certainly had the rights in the situation, but I suppose there is no use trying to buck the Hearst organization as far as Italy is concerned. It must have been a damned aggravating thing to have happen."

After the suit was filed, Juliana cruised on the Aegean—close to Italy if necessary, but not in it. On July 28, she wrote another shipboard letter to Gertrude:

Dear Gertrude—

Graduate of the School of Eightwesteight I address you as Founder of the Live
Dangerously Institute, sending you gratitude for the extra course in Gunpowder Plots
which you, the Clear-Eyed, allowed me to share with you in days of old when Nights
were bold & mornings without shyness. For to that knowledge, never learned in
schools, I attribute my survival in the late unpleasantness. . . .

I think of you so often & wish you here in the heat & the glare, but the rapture,
I know, wd be yours too as it is mine & shall be. If life allows the time I shall live
in the hope that your confidence & understanding may come back to you a hundred
fold. If this ever reaches you, because I do not know your whereabouts, my love, if
not there will be enough left over when we meet.

Yrs,

J.

The suit was filed on August 2, but the Italians tied it up in postponements and
other delays, playing for time until the exhibition was over. Juliana was stung
by her failure, her inability to rescue her pictures. She was not living up to the
standards she had set for herself, and the mistakes made on the PWAP may have
been haunting her, too. Gertrude was incommunicado, and Juliana was upset
by that, which led to more uncharacteristic displays of helplessness. When she
was in good fettle, she was not given to exploiting her fears.

By September 1, Juliana was more dispassionate about her defeat. She wrote
tersely to Gertrude and addressed her as "Mrs. Whitney," for the benefit of the
secretary who opened the letter.

Dear Mrs. Whitney.

After everything we had to give up the suit for our property, & I have come back
here [Haddenham] to rest a bit before sailing. Before any statement can be made I
must consult you & get some advice. You are the only one to whom I may tell the
whole disgraceful story. On the other hand, we owe it to ourselves to let the public
know some of the story. Where will you be?

Yrs

JRF

Gertrude, who loathed any kind of personal publicity but was especially shy
of it at the moment, had no wish to have the story told, and it wasn't. The
museum's suit was withdrawn in November of 1934, because it was now
moot—the American pavilion closed in October. Owing to the mess the Biennale
had become and the consequent decision to avoid visiting Italy, Juliana did not
pursue *The Greek Slave*. The only positive outcome of the whole affair is that
Eleanor Lambert ended up marrying Seymour Berkson.

The battle to reclaim the museum's own art collection from the compromised
exhibition in Venice was not the only legal action Gertrude was contemplating.
Juliana had been frustrated and depressed by Gertrude's lack of consideration
for her over the summer. Just when Juliana found herself floundering, Gertrude
slithered behind the portcullis of privilege she had always used to shield herself

when people demanded too much of her. Isolated in England and feeling miserable about her inability to budge the Italian government, Juliana blamed herself excessively for Gertrude's glacial remoteness. She thought Gertrude's silence was a reproof for her failure, but it was more a matter of having only so much feeling to spare. Gertrude had, said her sister-in-law, in a cool but fair assessment, "that same impersonal sympathy of a doctor giving advice to a patient, but I was never to see her compassionate and emotionally tender." Dealing with another, truly uglier affair had to come first. Juliana, who could take care of herself, was left to do so. But after her return to New York on September 27, 1934, she would have learned the worst about Gertrude's dilemma.

Since June of 1932, Gertrude's ten-year-old niece, Gloria Laura Vanderbilt, had been living at the Whitney compound in Old Westbury. Gloria was the daughter of Gloria Morgan and Reginald Vanderbilt, Gertrude's youngest brother. Reggie was forty-two when he married the seventeen-year-old Gloria Morgan, the daughter of a minor career diplomat, on March 6, 1923. On February 20, 1924, "little Gloria," as she was called, was born. Reggie died in 1925 of cirrhosis of the liver, having drunk himself to death and gambled away most of his inheritance. By the time he married Gloria, who was his second wife, Reggie had spent or lost $25 million. All he had left was the income ($217,000 a year, which was not enough to keep him) he received from a $5 million trust that he could not invade. Upon Reggie's death, the income from that trust would go immediately to his children: Cathleen, the offspring of his first marriage, and little Gloria. At age twenty-one, each child would receive her half of the principal.

Producing a Vanderbilt heir should have meant financial security for Gloria Morgan Vanderbilt, because her daughter's portion of the trust yielded an income of $112,448 a year. But Gloria was twenty* when Reggie died, so she was too young to be the sole legal guardian of little Gloria's person and property. She asked George Wickersham and Thomas Gilchrist, lawyers in the firm used by the Morgan family, to be the coguardians of her child. They, together with Justice James Foley of the New York Surrogate's Court, would administer little Gloria's trust. Gloria had to sell Reggie's properties and possessions to pay his debts, and she was left with $130,000. To someone with her history, who was raised to snare a rich man, had never been taught how to handle money, but had grown accustomed to spending it like a Vanderbilt, this was not a great sum. Furthermore, other members of the Morgan family—an unsavory brother, an opportunistic father, and a grasping mother—had all been living off Reggie, and Gloria felt obligated to continue supporting them. Before long, Gloria had gone through what remained of Reggie's estate and was dependent on the court allowance made for little Gloria's upbringing. Gloria came to regard little Gloria's money—$48,000 a year—as her own, to do with as she wished. The monthly $4,000 awarded for the child's upkeep was the only way the mother could receive

---

*Actually, Gloria was twenty-one. She was born on August 23, 1904, but her mother told her she was born in 1905. If Gloria had known the truth, she would have automatically qualified to be little Gloria's sole guardian, and the whole custody trial would never have taken place.

money because the conditions of the trust were so demeaning. Gloria was not granted a separate allowance for herself, creating a tense relationship between a penniless mother and a very rich baby.

Gloria's spending of her daughter's maintenance allowance might not have attracted the attention of her guardians had she not been leading a highly publicized life in the company of flighty and dissolute friends. Weeks and months went by without mother seeing daughter, for Gloria led a nomadic social life. She would migrate from London to Paris, Paris to Biarritz, Biarritz to Cannes, Cannes to New York, New York to Hollywood, and Hollywood to London again. Little Gloria was brought up by her nurse, Emma Sullivan Keislich, and her maternal grandmother, Laura Kirkpatrick Morgan. These two women were the only adults who were consistently with little Gloria, and little Gloria, the center of their lives, adored them unreservedly. Grandmother Morgan was undoubtedly mentally ill, and she became obsessed with her one Vanderbilt grandchild. As an adult, little Gloria would write of her grandmother, "She was capable of blowing up subways if things did not go according to her plan. That she had a plan, and that I not only was included in the plan but, in fact was the heart of the plan, never occurred to me until much, much later."

Laura Morgan persuaded herself and Nurse Keislich that Gloria would murder her own baby to get her hands on that half-share of the Vanderbilt millions. Grandmother Morgan's plan eventually took the form of wresting little Gloria away from her mother. Gloria's extended absences and general inattentiveness fit in with standard child-rearing practices of men and women in society—Gertrude's own children had been raised by upper servants and went months without seeing their parents. (Barbara, the youngest, had been rejected by Gertrude from the time she was born, and a *New Yorker* profile of Sonny Whitney published in 1941 delicately reported that the "elder Whitneys travelled a great deal, and sometimes, when Sonny was at Groton or Yale, he learned of their whereabouts only through the social columns of the newspapers.") But Gloria, besides being self-absorbed, was also resentful of her child because the court guardians made sure that the little girl's desires always took precedence over the mother's. In the summer of 1932, little Gloria, sickly and nervous, arrived at Wheatley Hills to spend a few weeks in the country. She quickly showed a marked improvement, and Gertrude asked Gloria if the child could stay on at Old Westbury. Gloria said yes, and prolonged her travels abroad. She permitted little Gloria to live at Gertrude's estate for the next two years; during that time, she saw the child approximately ten times. However, when Gloria asked for her daughter back, Gertrude and her doctors kept advising her to leave little Gloria in the country. Laura Morgan, who had made a place for herself among Reggie's relatives because she was grandmother to a Vanderbilt, told Gertrude tale after tale of Gloria's glittering life abroad, a life of wild extravagance and dissipation while the child "did without."

By 1933, Gertrude had become convinced of Gloria's unfitness as a parent by Gloria's own mother. Not comprehending the pathological element of Laura Morgan's makeup, she ascribed no motive other than grandmotherly concern to the woman for her to turn against her own daughter. Hence she did not doubt

the veracity of such monstrous charges. Gertrude genuinely believed that little Gloria was being mistreated and had lived in an unhealthy atmosphere until 1932. She wanted little Gloria to stay at Wheatley Hills and continue to attend the Green Vale School, an exclusive private school nearby.

On June 18, 1934, Gloria applied to be sole guardian of her daughter's person and coguardian of the estate. (Wickersham and Gilchrist had neglected to inform her that on attaining her majority it was her legal right to obtain guardianship papers.) Upon hearing this, Gertrude moved to contest the application, but on her own terms. As with the Brancusi trial of 1927, she would not enter into litigation unless she could avoid appearing to be the plaintiff. In this case, Grandmother Morgan agreed to bring the complaint against Gloria if Gertrude engaged legal counsel and paid for it. Gertrude consulted her lawyers and hired detectives to shadow Gloria and collect damaging information. The Whitney operatives had plenty of help. From the first, Thomas Gilchrist, who was supposed to be impartial, was on Gertrude's side. He even got lucrative legal assignments from her. With Laura Morgan as his informant, Gilchrist kept Gloria under constant surveillance without her knowledge. Over the last two years, he had been working with Frank L. Crocker, a lawyer who had served the Whitneys for years, to reduce the maintenance allowance from $4,000 to $750 a month.

Like Gilchrist, Crocker viewed the situation in black and white. He pegged Gloria as an adventuress, one of the countless leeches and gold diggers he had been defending the family coffers against for years. As Crocker saw it, his iron duty was to preserve Whitney capital at all costs, mainly by preventing it from being used by someone outside the family. Anyone not born to money was a dangerous pretender who had no right to a penny of the Whitney or Vanderbilt fortunes. (Reggie Vanderbilt might never work a day in his life and drop $70,000 during one night at his favorite casino, but if his destitute widow attempted to collect what she felt was due to her, this was insupportable.) This was the code of suspicion Crocker enforced for interlopers—and it did not vary, as Juliana was later to find out.

Gloria made her petition for guardianship in Surrogate's Court on July 3, 1934. She then learned that her mother had sworn out a complaint against her. Immediately guessing who was behind it, Gloria sped over to 871 Fifth Avenue to confront her adversary. Gertrude falsely denied her involvement—at this point, she confidently assumed that she could keep her hands clean and remain aloof. Throughout July and August of 1934, while Juliana was filling in Gertrude about the delaying tactics and treacheries of the Italian government, Gloria and Gertrude bargained with each other—Gloria demanded that her child be with her all the time, whereas Gertrude, on the move with little Gloria as they perambulated between Manhattan, Long Island, and the Whitney camp in the Adirondacks, wanted Gloria to adhere to the present arrangement of visiting and vacation rights. While this scuffling was going on, teams of lawyers on both sides prepared for a bitter battle in open court.

To this day, it is amazing that Gertrude consented to the horror of a public trial in which she and her family's intimate secrets would become the common property of the scandal sheets that devoured the misdeeds of millionaires. As

Barbara Goldsmith wrote in her account of the case, "The *Matter of Vanderbilt* was the most sensational custody trial in the history of the United States. It exploded into the headlines on the first day of October 1934, and didn't leave the front pages of the newspapers across the country until the year was out." Initially Gertrude did not think that Gloria would persevere with her petition in light of her own indiscretions. Nor did Gertrude realize how ruinous the widely published revelations of Vanderbilt sex and folly were to be. But given even those miscalculations, only her absolute conviction that little Gloria was terrified of and disliked her mother brought Gertrude to this pass.

Gertrude had good cause to be worried about her niece's welfare. She saw with her own eyes that little Gloria went into hysterical fits if she had to visit her mother; whenever her mother came into the room, little Gloria would shrink with dread at the sight of her. (Not until 1985 did Gloria Vanderbilt disclose that Grandmother Morgan taught her to feign sickness and hysteria. Laura Morgan also dictated the letters ostensibly written by little Gloria that helped destroy her mother's reputation; the child was also instructed to greet Gertrude, whom she hardly knew, with great outbursts of affection. Little Gloria went through with these frenzied performances and wrote the mendacious letters because her grandmother told her that if she did not fool Gertrude and the other adults, her beloved Nurse Keislich would be "ripped away" from her forever. It was Emma Keislich the little girl wanted to live with, not Gertrude.) One of the few remarks Juliana ever made about Gertrude to others, and made repeatedly, related to the messy saga of the custody trial. "Aunt J.'s comment," Allan Rieser said, "was, 'The one *completely unselfish* thing that Mrs. Whitney ever did was the most thankless one.' I remember the wording of this very vividly, because it struck me at the time that it revealed Aunt J.'s final feelings about her relationship to Gertrude, and her assessment of Gertrude's character."

On September 21 and September 22, 1934, a few days before Juliana was due back in New York, Gloria attempted to retrieve her daughter from Gertrude's care at 871 Fifth Avenue, but little Gloria screamed uncontrollably at her approach. Gertrude believed the performance she saw, masterminded once more by Grandmother Morgan. While Gloria was waiting for the child to calm down, Gertrude had little Gloria clandestinely driven away to Old Westbury. "Thereupon," reported *Time*, "with a disregard of privacy which shocked her in-laws, Mrs. Reginald Vanderbilt practically charged her sister-in-law with kidnapping and instituted habeas corpus proceedings to obtain possession of her daughter" on September 22, 1934. Gertrude's official identification with the scandal began. She could no longer gaze "straight ahead as if none of this were happening" to her.

Beginning on October 1, Gertrude was in court for six weeks. To her astonishment, she was not only headlined as a principal in this dirty business, but cast as a villain by the tabloids—in particular, by the Hearst empire. Although the charge was denied by several higher-ups in the Hearst organization, a journalist friendly to Gertrude discovered that Hearst was paying her back for the controversy over the Davies portrait. Juliana's niceties about not naming William Randolph Hearst as a party to the Biennale squabble counted for naught. Ger-

trude could not avoid being muddied by the tar baby that this trial would become, even if she kept to a straightforward complaint of child neglect. She did not realize that Crocker and his associates could win custody of little Gloria only by demonstrating her mother's gross immorality and shattering her reputation. They called ex-servants who testified as to Gloria's partying, drinking, and sexual relationships. The court was in an uproar on the day that Gloria's maid in Paris alleged that she had seen her former mistress kissing the Marchioness of Milford Haven, a member of the British royal family. But Gloria, in her role as the downtrodden widow, remained the sympathetic figure to the crowds outside the courthouse. Gertrude, the impeccable public benefactor and pillar of society so used to being treated deferentially by everyone, felt the sting of censure. She was bombarded with hostile letters and heard mobs of people shouting at her, "Down with Gertrude! Down with her millions! Down with the aunt, up with the mom! Down down down Gertrude!"

On October 22, Gertrude took the stand at the Vanderbilt trial and testified for three days. Crocker's team produced witnesses who stated that Gloria read pornography; Nathan Burkan, Gloria's lawyer, introduced reproductions of nudes in the museum's collection, attempting to establish that the works of art Gertrude bought and displayed were obscene and liable to corrupt little Gloria's morals. Among the works he likened to dirty pictures were sculptures by Lachaise ("a man's torso showing the penis and testicles"), Robert Laurent ("the breasts highly developed, the legs slightly raised but apart, and heavy indentations to show the hair at the very extreme bottom of the abdomen"), a painting by Arthur B. Davies ("seven nude women in various poses"), and an etching by Sloan ("the impression of a married woman cheating in front of her child"). Burkan apparently made an impression with these ludicrous charges, for when Gertrude told the presiding judge, John Francis Carew, that her museum was not only open to the public but visited by women's clubs and school groups, he was startled.

Ever since the details of Gloria's friendship with Lady Milford Haven were elicited, the court proceedings had been closed. In compensation, Judge Carew would feed bowdlerized summaries to the frustrated feature writers hovering beyond the courtroom doors. After Burkan had entered the reproductions as exhibits, Judge Carew told the fourth estate that the photographs showed "a mural of gay life in Greenwich Village in which nudes wearing opera hats play leapfrog"—an explanation even the *Times* swallowed. After hearing that description, the reporters on the case, most of whom had apparently never been in an art museum in their lives, rushed over to the Whitney and begged Juliana to show them this unique art treasure. She broke the sad truth to them. "The judge must have made that one up," she snorted.

The legal battle was over on November 15, 1934. Little Gloria was declared a ward of the court until she was twenty-one. Save for her not being allowed to leave New York State without permission—a real hindrance to Gertrude as well as Gloria—the child's living arrangements were the same as before the trial. In Gloria Morgan Vanderbilt's words, "I was to be given the custody of Gloria every weekend, and for the entire month of July; the remaining days and months of the year, Gloria was to be with Mrs. Whitney. The opinion of the court, in

short, was that I was an unfit mother most weeks between Monday and Friday; but every weekend my shortcomings vanished—and in July I was practically perfect."

What did change was the position of Frank Crocker in Gertrude's life. For his services, he had ascended to the inner circle of her entourage. He was rewarded with increased power over Gertrude's affairs and with her friendship. Crocker's growing influence would have consequences for Juliana. In ways she could not foresee, her future would be gravely affected by the aftermath of the *Matter of Vanderbilt*.

With the trial about to subside, Juliana's immediate task was to put the museum's schedule right and step up her activities. Since government art patronage was temporarily in limbo, she revived her informal philanthropy with Abby Rockefeller and bought small works from needy artists for her. The first exhibition on the Whitney docket was another regional show, this time focusing on the Philadelphia area.

In conjunction with the Whitney show, Juliana made a great effort to stimulate the apathetic Philadelphia art scene. She made more trips to the city's museums, galleries, and studios, but her main activity was the promotion of a new gallery of contemporary art that was about to open in the Philadelphia branch of Gimbels department store. The angel behind the gallery was Fridolyn Gimbel, who was married to the painter Franklin Watkins. But the couple, because they were so enmeshed in the city's art circles, could not figure out a diplomatic way to pick and choose among local artists.

"Fridolyn wanted to open the gallery with a show of Philadelphia artists, but she was afraid of making enemies with the selection," said Marchal Landgren, who came up with the solution. "I said, 'Why don't you repeat the Whitney show and then you can blame it on the Whitney?' She was delighted with the suggestion," and Juliana agreed to send the show to Gimbels after it closed in New York on November 26. But the artists, instead of being elated, were up in arms about this, and not because of the selection process. Philip Boyer, the dealer who was defrauding buyers and sellers in his own gallery, had been hired as the Gimbels Galleries' director. The artists were well aware of his dishonesty, but Fridolyn Gimbel and Juliana brushed off their complaints. Fifteen artists formed a secessionist group and withdrew consent for their work to be shown at Gimbels. Julius Bloch, who was against Boyer, summarized what had transpired in his diary entry for November 26, 1934.

> When I was informed about two weeks ago that the Philadelphia Regional Exhibition of paintings would be brought from the Whitney Museum to the Gimbels' Galleries here, I immediately wrote to Mrs. Force that my pictures were to be returned to me after the New York show, as I had no intention of allowing any works of mine to fall into the hands of Boyer, Gimbels' newly appointed Art Director. . . . This unscrupulous individual has fleeced numerous artists of their work, has pocketed the money received from the sale of the artists' pictures and sculptures. His reputation

for dishonesty is well established here and in New York and yet such a firm as Gimbel Brothers is willing to employ him. . . .

Juliana Force wired me to meet her here last week, with Mary Curran* to discuss what she termed the secessionists' Revolt. But her impassioned defense of what she believed to be a constructive idea—that is, bringing the show intact to Gimbels, and thus letting Philadelphia see its own artists work grouped together by the . . . choice of a museum staff, did not move us. We insisted that it meant our sponsoring Boyer, against whom we had stood our ground for years, and we did not yield.

For Bloch, who hero-worshipped Juliana, to dare oppose her in a face-to-face discussion demonstrated the intensity of his objections as no argument could.

Bloch and Curran to the contrary, Juliana went down to Philadelphia for the opening festivities on November 28, 1934—a sit-down luncheon at which she was to be the main speaker and the guest of honor. Juliana dressed with great fastidiousness, in the latest fashion for the new season. (Her practice was to give away most of her clothes of the previous year to her brothers' wives.) For this occasion, she chose a deep-brown velvet suit with a matching velvet tricorne. In the hat was a brown feather with a tinge of green at its tip, highlighting the orange of her hair. Juliana went to Pennsylvania Station, boarded a car, settled into her seat, and began her journey. At some point, she discovered that her train was on its way to Pittsburgh—whereupon she pulled the emergency cord. The conductors would not stop the train between stations, but they would slow it down. At the agreed-upon point, two conductors each took an arm and dropped her from the moving train. Juliana jumped to the ground and made for the nearest highway, where she put out her thumb and started hitchhiking. A man in a dairy truck pulled up and offered her a ride. Juliana bounced into Philadelphia next to her benefactor, seated on the rim of a large milk can. In all the excitement, it didn't occur to her that velvet absorbed moisture. She swept into Gimbels, a vision in brown—except for a big, white, perfectly formed circle of milk imprinted on her derriere.

Lloyd Goodrich, when he heard this anecdote, was amused but not surprised by the story, for this was not the only time Juliana had misplaced the City of Brotherly Love. "Her sense of detail was very strange, sometimes," he said laughingly. "Jack Baur, Mrs. Force and I were once on a committee, a jury to pick out works of art by men in the Armed Forces. It was sponsored by *Life* magazine, and Mrs. Force and Jack and I flew down to Washington from New York. After about a half an hour from taking off, we passed over a large city and Mrs. Force pointed down and said, 'Providence.' It was Philadelphia, of course. Jack just looked at me."

Milk stains and all, Juliana brought off her Philadelphia visit with élan. Landgren said of it:

There must have been 200 people there. Juliana was the guest of honor and she didn't show and she didn't show and she didn't show. We kept having our before-

* Director of the Little Gallery of Contemporary Art, in Philadelphia.

lunch drinks, and we finally decided to go ahead with the luncheon. While we were eating, she came in, dressed to the teeth, and made the most outrageous apology I've ever heard in my life—about how she got on the train to Pittsburgh and so on —and carried it off beautifully. She was a figure, a very definite figure.

After her apology, Juliana launched into her speech. She delivered her standard message—one encourages art best by buying it—but she aptly couched it in the language of merchandising. "The production of art depends on con-sumption of art," Juliana told them, and went on to plead her case.

We need greater consumption of art. People need works of art just as they need chairs, tables and clothes. What has made Paris the centre of art for the whole world is that people there have the habit of placing in their homes pictures by men alive when those pictures are bought.

How do we know what paintings really matter? We know only that some of them will matter enormously; that some artists are coming along today who will be important centuries hence—provided we do something about it today to enable them to keep on painting.

The artists' welfare was never far from Juliana's thoughts, and after the Philadelphia triumph, the artist in distress was Charles Demuth. Two years after she bought *From the Garden of the Chateau* from Boyer, she learned that Demuth and the Downtown Gallery had not received any money for the painting. Julius Bloch had been right, and she was wrong. Juliana agreed to testify against Boyer in court if necessary, but she didn't give up on him. On the contrary, in late January of 1935, she borrowed works of art from the Boyer Galleries for a Whitney exhibition—even though he was still stalling Demuth and Halpert! Juliana probably would have argued that she was giving the artists some exposure, and any sales of their work would have been overseen by her. Emlen Etting, in talking about Juliana's intransigence even when she was in error, said, "She believed so much in what she was doing, and she was usually so right about people and art that it was better for her to stick to her guns than capitulate. She practically never did."

In 1935, the Whitney curatorial staff was done with the political and other extra-artistic considerations of overseas pavilions, regional shows, and govern-ment service. They were at last free to present a more rounded picture of art in America. As if in joyous relief, the exhibitions mounted that year were some of the most exploratory and imaginative the Whitney had organized to date. The museum made exemplary rediscoveries of neglected artists and presented con-temporary and historical art in enlightened juxtapositions.

January began with exhibitions of two little-known bodies of work: textiles and sculpture by Arthur B. Davies and paintings by Robert Loftin Newman, a then-forgotten nineteenth-century Romantic artist. The Newman show was or-ganized by Marchal Landgren, who had been collecting material on the painter for years. Not surprisingly, the assignment happened by chance. Karl Free dropped by Landgren's apartment one Friday night, saw five paintings by New-

man on the wall, examined his card file, and told Hermon More. By now aware of the dearth of information about this reclusive artist, More asked Landgren if he would do the show. He was given the whole second floor for it; he selected it, he hung it, and he wrote the catalog. The fee was $100.

These two exhibitions were followed by a very important survey that did not garner an admiring public. In recognition of new and diverse developments in the art world, the Whitney became the first museum to mount a show of American abstract painting. This was an act of vision on the part of More and Free, who did most of the work, because they, along with Juliana, Goodrich, and Archer, were much more at home with representational art. Abstract Painting in America, which was on view from February 12 to March 22, 1935, examined two generations of artists. The first encompassed the painters who had shown in or had been directly influenced by the Armory Show; the second consisted of their heirs—younger, emerging painters who were addressing not only Cubism, but Surrealism, Constructivism, and Neo-Plasticism. Thus the Whitney, although devoting most of its space to avant-garde artists who had come of age during the teens—such as Konrad Cramer, Bluemner, Dasburg, Davies, Davis, Demuth, Dove, Hartley, Kuhn, Stanton Macdonald-Wright, Marin, Alfred Maurer, O'Keeffe, Morton Schamberg, Stella, Walkowitz, and Weber—still had room for Browne, Drewes, Gorky, Graham, Balcomb Greene, Stefan Hirsch, Earl Horter, Morris Kantor, Earl Kerkam, Karl Knaths, Matulka, I. Rice Pereira, Roszak, Louis Schanker, and Storrs. Hermon More would have added Carl Holty if he could, but he didn't learn of his work until his deadline had passed.

As can be deduced from the list of the younger artists they invited to show, the curators preferred Cubist works and biomorphic abstractions derived from Expressionism and Surrealism to rigorously nonobjective painting. (However, Greene, a follower of Mondrian, did get in.) As a rule, the Whitney was happier with artists who abstracted from nature than those who invented forms. Even though viewers were more likely to see examples of traditional realism, social protest, and American Scene painting at the Whitney in the 1930s, artists pursuing Magic Realism and varieties of abstraction rooted in Surrealism, Expressionism, and Precisionism made some inroads. But Americans who were investigating geometric abstraction were slighted.

The Whitney's taste had matured greatly since 1933, when a first stab was made at responding to the renewal of interest in abstract art. The outcome of this undertaking, despite the good intentions, was decidedly mixed. Cooke Glassgold was in charge of a symposium on the subject that was held at the museum during the evening of April 10, 1933. Four critics—Goodrich, Pach, Leo Katz, and Morris Davidson—led a discussion called "The Problem of Subject Matter and Abstract Esthetics in Painting." The title itself disclosed that the museum was hedging about art that did not portray recognizable objects or events. This uncertainty was spelled out in Glassgold's injunction to the speakers that they take up "the need or uselessness of contemporary subject matter."

Goodrich, the one representative of the museum on the platform, was then not quite ready to accept that relationships between color, form, light, volume, and mass were in themselves an alternative to identifiable subject matter. At the

symposium, he said that for him, representations of the human figure, as depicted through solid forms in deep space, yielded the greatest formal significance. Many artists were in the audience that night, and one of them, Arshile Gorky, stood up and challenged the critics. "You must analyze abstract art the way you analyze a fugue by Bach," he said, and expounded at length on what he meant. "I didn't understand what he was talking about then," Goodrich said, "so I thought he was being facetious, but of course he was serious. I didn't get what he was saying, and I told him to sit down. He was right, and I was wrong. I never should have talked like that to an artist—I've always felt badly about it." But after this unpromising start, Goodrich became an ardent admirer of Gorky. Through the PWAP, he got to know the artist better, and in early 1937, the Whitney purchased *Painting*, an abstract still life by Gorky. This was his first sale to a public collection.

Goodrich's preferences for humanism and direct observation of nature were shared by the rest of the staff, which probably inclined them toward the more painterly, more sensuous, more allusive, more organic examples of abstract art. By now, the curators would all have come to terms with the modernism of Picasso, Miró, and Léger—minutes of staff meetings record that the curators regularly visited J. B. Neumann's gallery, which showed the great European innovators—but they might have been resisting Mondrian. Neo-Plasticism, judging by how rarely its American practitioners got into the Whitney, evidently struck Juliana and her curators as impersonal, impoverished in content, and too much like industrial design.

It is probably not coincidental that most of the younger painters in Abstract Painting in America had been on the PWAP. Whitney curators easily could have looked at their work in the museum if they had not already seen examples of it during the enrollment process. Artists who were not on the project, artists the curators may not have been used to, broke into the Whitney less easily. Similarly, some artists who lived well outside New York were overlooked completely—Patrick Henry Bruce,* Josef Albers, and Edwin Dickinson, for example, did not exhibit at the Whitney in the 1930s. And so much still depended on Juliana's arbitrariness, on whether or not she liked the artist as a person. The ultimate example of familiarity equaling unconditional acceptance must have been Stuart Davis, who was commissioned to write the introduction to the catalog. It was true, as the foreword said, that Davis was "one of the most brilliant exponents of the movement." Yet there is also a lingering sense that the Whitney was behind him because over the years he had become the house abstractionist, someone that Juliana knew, liked, and trusted. That he was a friend and a former protégé may have counted more than the merits of his work.

It was apparent to the younger vanguard that Abstract Painting in America was not only the first effort of its kind, but a serious and knowledgeable exhibition

---

*In general, expatriates were ignored by the Whitney. Other Americans abroad who did not get their due from the museum were Romaine Brooks, Gerald Murphy, and Mary Callery. Juliana did buy a painting by Man Ray, but as the museum was not collecting photographs, the work for which he is celebrated was passed over.

that would validate them as artists. They strongly wanted to be in it, especially since the Museum of Modern Art wasn't showing their work at all. Commenting on the Modern's remoteness from American painters, David Smith said, "One did not feel disavowed—only ignored and much alone." The painters appreciated the Whitney's more tolerant attitude, yet they also clung to their status as rebels and outcasts as a mark of integrity. One day at Romany Marie's café, a half-dozen artists, including Smith, formed an alliance for the sole purpose of attracting the Whitney's attention. He wrote:

> It was in Marie's where we once formed a group, [John] Graham, Edgar Levy, [Mischa] Resnikoff, De Kooning, Gorky and myself with [Stuart] Davis being asked to join. This was short lived. We never exhibited and we lasted in union about 30 days. Our only action was to notify the Whitney Museum that we were a group and would only exhibit in the 1935 abstract show if all were asked. Some of us were, some exhibited, some didn't and that ended our group.

Other excluded painters found fault with the museum for putting more emphasis on the early American modernists than on the up-and-coming artists. But the painters in the show, both older and younger, also had a right to be disappointed. Even if experimental artists were invited to show their work, that work was unlikely to be acquired. Of the 134 pictures chosen for Abstract Painting in America, more than 100 of them were available for purchase. Not one was bought by the Whitney. Forbes Watson noticed the great number of unsold works, although he did not point a finger at the museum. "Why are so many of these pictures unsold?" he asked in his review. "I can't imagine an American collection thinking it had any historic weight if it did not include many of these paintings, which are evident and, frequently, such handsome reminders of . . . the development of American art."

Forbes also joked that while walking through the galleries he had to remind himself that he was in the Whitney, not the Modern. This was a prophetic jest, for one year later, the Whitney's effort was eclipsed by a landmark exhibition that took place at the Modern. Cubism and Abstract Art, formulated by Alfred Barr, became *the* show on the subject, and justifiably so. Beginning with Post-Impressionism and moving through Cubism, Fauvism, Futurism, Expressionism, Suprematism, and Neo-Plasticism and their offshoots, he traced their genesis and evolution and codified their precepts with such lucidity and authority that his conclusions exerted a lasting influence. Alexander Calder was the only American in the Modern's show, which further sharpened in people's minds the division between American art and modernism, and between isolationism and internationalism.

As for Abstract Painting in America, save for Watson and McBride, who spoke of the art's "persuasive beauty," the reviewers were baffled or derisive. Their allegiance to Regionalism, which was still highly visible and continued to be the standard fare of the government art projects, made them suspicious of abstract art. Thus when the Whitney presented American Genre: The Social Scene in Paintings and Prints (1800–1935) as a bookend to Abstract Painting in America, the reviewers heaved sighs of happiness. The public was comforted,

too—over 10,000 people attended, about twice the number of spectators at most of the other shows. Actually, the genre exhibition was a first-rate historical survey of nineteenth- and twentieth-century scenes of everyday life in America as interpreted by 105 artists. But reviewers saw the nineteenth century mainly as a forerunner of the nationalism of the American Scene and spilled gallons of red, white, and blue ink on the subject.

One of the artists in The Social Scene in Paintings and Prints was Peggy Bacon, who was at work on a witty drypoint that she titled *The Social Graces*. The print shows a scene she had witnessed many times—an evening party in progress at Juliana's apartment. The guests are drinking and gossiping under the light of the eagle-topped globes and the hostess is fox-trotting away, her feet lightly brushing the floor. Although this caricature of Juliana is much gentler than *The Ugly Duchess*, it does convey the impression of a caustic, high-relief personality who liked to amuse and disturb. Of course, Juliana had long been fierce and fearsome, taking over any room she was in and telling the world what she thought whether the world liked it or not. But the conflicts and treacheries of the past few years had roughed her up to a greater extent than perchance she realized. In her various battles, she had used arrogance as a defense, but arrogance is not easily shed, and it had come to fit her.

This was a weakness, but Juliana didn't try to conquer it. Her conversation was unregrettedly more withering, her humor earthier, her retorts more intimidating. Indeed, all of Juliana's remarks gained in aggression by virtue of their being delivered in her clipped, precise, basso profundo voice, ever deepened by cigarettes and Scotch. The soft spot she had for some artists was sometimes contradicted by skepticism or malice toward others. Even her appearance was arranged less subtly. "She looked like a Polish whore, with her elaborate makeup and extreme clothes," said Edward Laning. But to Horace Day, Juliana's taste had "a zest and a wonderful arrogance to it, because she dressed as if she were a great beauty, except that she was ugly." The old warhorse, still combat-weary, was showing, depending on the spectator's point of view, her scars or her medals.

Charles Sawyer, who helped run the New England branch of the PWAP, said that the administering of the New York project and its aftermath "was a distressing period for Juliana. Dealing with a bureaucratic institution on the one hand and artists who were pretty vociferous on the other—she didn't like that at all. The joy of the give-and-take, which was one of her great pleasures with artists, just went out of it for her at that time, and in a sense she never quite recovered from that as far as her own feelings went. She thought that the artists had let her down. I don't think she should have, because there was a new generation of artists, so the whole perspective and rules were changing." Faith Andrews, who also observed Juliana in action during those tumultuous days, felt that her disillusionment sprang not from her previous conditioning as a patron, but her passion for improving and perfecting. "She was always on to new things, well before anyone else," Faith Andrews said. "She didn't wait for something to come along—she found it and then she looked for ways to make

it better. Juliana kept to an ideal of quality about everything she did, and because she had standards, she was bound to be disappointed. She lost faith—you can't go around doing things for people all the time and not get bitten. Any hardness or difficulty she had should be forgiven because she gave of herself completely."

The trouble was, Juliana's victims couldn't always tell when they were about to be tossed and gored. Hannah Small said, "I liked her, but I was scared of her because she was so witty and so sharp. I was afraid that she would come right back at me like a knife." Artists were also the targets of Juliana's comic deflations when she became fed up with what she perceived as empty posturing or ingratitude. Both Stuart Davis and Lloyd Lózes Goff repeated the story she told about one man, although she never betrayed his name. In Goff's words:

> This so-called artist had really taken advantage of Juliana. Over the years he had come to her for hand-outs, she had had to listen to his accounts, in detail, of his sexual conquests, of his sexual prowess. . . . One day he came to her for "a loan," which both knew meant another hand-out. He was engagingly enthusiastic about his fetish: women with long hair, the longer the better as far as his hang-up was concerned.
>
> "Oh, Juliana!" cried the sculptor, "You can't imagine how happy I am! I've just discovered the girl of my wildest dreams! She is THE most exciting of all! She has, she's got hair all the way down to her ANKLES!"
>
> Calmly Juliana asked, "Down from where?"

Juliana's put-downs were famous among her friends and enjoyed and quoted widely. But this was not to say that she had become unapproachable or out of sympathy with artists or their causes, as two of her gestures show. In 1934, Juliana's friend and colleague Bryson Burroughs died, and in April of 1935, a memorial exhibition of his art was held at the Metropolitan. Mumford, reviewing the show for *The New Yorker*, was aghast at the work—"a tasteless jug of syrup," he called it. The paintings were so feeble, he said, that Burroughs should have been disqualified from his job at the museum. The Metropolitan would "need all its reserve power to live down the fact that it not merely harbored Burroughs but . . . actually permitted his lifework to go on view." Burroughs, intimated Mumford, should have been gentleman and critic enough to destroy the contents of his studio in deference to his own artistic incompetence.

While granting the reviewer the right to his opinion of an artist's work, Juliana seethed at Mumford's violent denigration of Burroughs's record as a curator, for she knew he had been hemmed in by a deadly combination of trustees and academicians. There was no choice but to protest publicly. "I could not withhold my defence of a man who had performed a great service, in my estimation," she said, "and who is no longer here to speak for himself." Juliana wrote a disciplinary letter to *The New Yorker* refuting Mumford and praising the Metropolitan for its good sense in "harboring" Burroughs. Her name meant enough that, contrary to the magazine's usual policy, the letter was published.

Although she detested the picketing that took place during the run of the PWAP, Juliana was not necessarily against all artists' strikes or unions—especially if she could have a hand in shaping them. Six years after the Crash, most artists were still poverty-stricken and looking for ways to earn money. Because exhibiting

their work produced no income, the Society of Painters, Sculptors and 'Gravers voted in May of 1935 to ask museums for a rental fee for the "use" of their work during shows. The figure arrived at was 1 percent a month of the selling price of a picture, with a ceiling of $10.00. To enforce this measure, the artists in the organization, led by Katherine Schmidt, agreed to boycott any institution that would not pay them. Most museum directors thought the artists had overstepped themselves—they should be grateful to art institutions for the opportunities created. But Juliana, acting against her economic interests as a museum representative, took the artists' part. "Juliana was a minority of one among the art museum directors at the time in favoring rentals for pictures," Charles Sawyer said. "She was very concerned that the artist wasn't getting his fair share—this offended her sense of justice and equity." Schmidt reported to the first American Artists' Congress in 1936, "With few exceptions (the Whitney Museum may be cited as an outstanding example) the choice [of paying a fee] was forced upon directors by the realities of the situation, and was not made voluntarily from solicitous interest in the American artist."

The dispute over the rental issue went on for the next two years before the boycott was suspended. During that time, Juliana was the spokeswoman for the artists within the museum world, debating Robert Harshe and Francis Taylor, the leaders of the opposition. Taking a pro-rental position put Juliana back where she liked to be—squarely and generously with the artists, fighting for their rights against the conservative and self-interested. In this way, she could reconfirm her relationship to the group of people she was devoted to and whose interests she still had at heart.

While Juliana was fighting for justice and equity, she was also being plotted against. Frank Longfellow Crocker, Gertrude's lawyer, was a descendant of Henry Wadsworth Longfellow, but not a drop of the poet's blood seemed to flow through his veins. Inspired by his victory over Gloria Morgan Vanderbilt, he looked appraisingly at another person he thought was preying on Gertrude's money and trust—Juliana. To Crocker, the keeper of Whitney capital, the museum was a mere frill in Gertrude's life, kept alive on her sufferance and Juliana's spending. In his eyes, the extravagant Juliana, who requested tens and tens of thousands of dollars for the museum, was taking advantage of the Whitney fortune. Although smarter, better educated, purposeful, morally unimpeachable, deservedly in a position of trust, and almost impossible to ensnare, Juliana was not altogether different from Gloria in Crocker's books. Both were intruders in the family bank vaults, and both were obstacles to tight financial management. Both had to be controlled—and, if possible, ousted.

Crocker had been pressuring Gertrude to cut expenditures since at least 1932. He was certain that the museum was costing too much—between $110,000 and $125,000 a year—to run, even though in 1932 Gertrude was worth between $64 and $72 million and had a gross income of $1,093,000. After taxes and all expenses (including the museum), she was left with about $633,000. That year, besides keeping up her silken existence, she could manage, for ex-

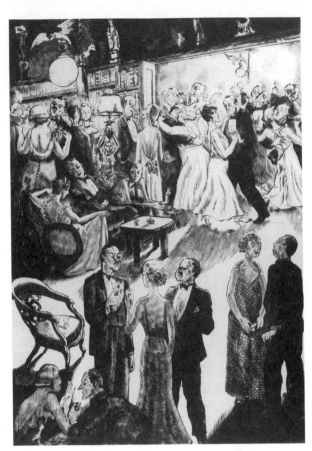

The Social Graces, a 1935 drypoint by Peggy Bacon, shows an evening party on Eighth Street. Juliana is on the upper right, doing a slick fox trot.

ample, an astoundingly generous donation of $250,000 to the American Museum of Natural History. (In 1934, Gertrude was better off, because she inherited $7 million from her mother's estate.) Crocker was closeted many hours with Gertrude during the first six months of 1935, because Gloria Vanderbilt was continuing to file custody appeals for little Gloria. Gertrude was contesting the suit, and she and Crocker were occupied with reviewing testimony from the trial. He was too astute to say that the museum was superfluous, and he knew that Juliana, being indispensable to Gertrude, was impregnable. Crocker could never go so far as to imply that Juliana was a drain on the Whitney purse, nor could he try to get rid of her, but he could argue for sound fiscal management. As had been done with Gloria Morgan Vanderbilt, Crocker could restrain Juliana's power and behavior by limiting her access to money.

Juliana had a salary plus an elastic expense account. The latter she used liberally—sometimes too liberally, because her salary didn't always cover her bills. Gertrude had never minded the overlap, and from 1914 to 1931, the bookkeeping system for Whitney art activities, such as it was, was so spotty and haphazard that mixing personal and professional expenses was standard practice.

By the mid-1930s, the combination of salary and expense account must have given Juliana from $25,000 to $30,000 a year to work with. Crocker evidently persuaded Gertrude—who didn't realize or chose not to realize how much Juliana depended on both sources of money—that cutting off Juliana's access to the expense account would be a painless way to save. He received permission to put Juliana on a straight salary of $15,000 a year. This, Crocker must have argued, was plenty to live on. And in truth, he was hardly advocating a degrading sum. In 1935, $15,000 was a lavish salary for anyone, but a fifty-nine-year-old woman with several houses, multiple dependents, and a habit of going first class was not just anyone.

After Juliana learned that Crocker should be regarded as an enemy, she became so provoked at losing her latitude of freedom—which she read as an egregious personal criticism of herself and her years of service—that she made a few angry remarks about Gertrude, who had once more glided into the steely, silent self-containment that comes from having other people act as executioners. "Mrs. Force was fuming and very upset," recalled Ethel Renthal, her secretary. She said, 'I have devoted myself to Mrs. Whitney, and now they are doing this to me.' " The curtain was also lifted briefly for Carl and Allan Rieser. It may have been at this period, they said, that their aunt seriously considered an offer to head a big New York department store because the salary would be so much higher. They remembered that it was Gertrude who talked Juliana out of quitting by promising to leave her a million dollars in her will.

Economic constriction came as a terrible blow to Juliana, and the diminishment of her own high style of living was the least of her worries. Juliana would not have denied her love of luxuries, but in her hands money was always something to be shared. She had many commitments, and she would not renege on them. For example, in 1935, she was paying Chaim Gross $50 a month over several installments for a sculpture, and she was still sending $200 a month to Edward and Faith Andrews for their research on the Shakers. There were also Juliana's obligations as head of the Rieser family. She was supporting Clara and Mary Rieser in Chatham, and she recently had assumed financial responsibility for her brother Charles and his family, who were also living out there. Charles drank himself out of one job and could not find another one. Irene was working part-time in a linen store, but her salary could not keep four people. They went to Juliana for aid, and she started subsidizing their household expenses.

Of great concern to Juliana was that Charles and Irene could not afford to educate Allan and Carl properly. When the time came, she paid for voice and acting lessons, as well as playwrighting classes at Columbia University for Allan, who wanted to go into the theater. Carl, who was graduated from high school in the spring of 1934, would be ready for college the following fall. The only way he could attend would be through Juliana, who remembered the sacrifice of her early dreams because her family was too poor to send her to Wellesley. She could not bear to see him deprived of such an important advantage and volunteered to put him through Amherst.

Juliana was extraordinarily loyal to take on these burdens, and she did so

with unalloyed pride and pleasure. She wanted to help because she was warm and generous, but being the family's fount of bounty also enhanced her domination of it. She actually got angry at her brother Louis because he sent his son to Cornell without consulting her or asking her for money. She had seen to it that Allan was raised as an artist, whether he wanted it or not. It so happened that he did, but later he had to resist his aunt's complete molding of him to her projections of unfulfilled creative needs. Juliana's actions were perfectly consistent with the larger fiction of her life, the Rieser myth of exiled nobility. At first Carl accepted Juliana's espousal of the family romance of aristocratic entitlement. Of course, he had also seen proof of the myth. During his childhood he had witnessed countless scenes of his aunt operating as a fairy godmother—in moments of crisis, she would sweep in, lumbered with gifts, and rescue the Riesers from distress. Or, they would visit her for weeks at the glorious farm, where life was idyllic.

If Carl thought that money for college belonged to him by birthright, his attitude was not so much callowness as naive belief in his aunt and her ability to provide. Much of this can be gathered from a letter Juliana wrote to Carl from Cobweb that summer after he asked her for $360 for his first tuition payment.

Dear Carl—I am enclosing a cheque for 360.00 the amount you must have by the 12th [of September], & you may go to Bests [Best & Co.] & order your dinner suit & the overcoat. I think the other expenses we will let rest until I get home & we may have an opportunity to talk things over. I think that fifteen a week is much too high for expenses & also that your laundry should be sent home each week. Not only will your clothes last longer but they can be mended & kept in shape better. It isn't that I am stingy with you, but I really cannot afford to give you so much now that I am reduced to almost half my income & also have had very heavy expenses in the way of doctor bills, etc. We must try to cut out everything that isn't absolutely essential, & I am sure you will do it. . . . There are lots of things you simply won't be able to do because you haven't the money to do them. That is awfully hard, especially for you, but the education is the only thing which really counts & that I guarantee, & if the fraternity seems essential, that too must be taken care of. You will find many fellows who will not have an income & who will have a go to make both ends meet, more especially in these days when money is so precarious. I wouldn't bother much taking the advice of anybody else—find out for yourself how little you can get on with; you will need the experience & it will be useful when you leave college & try to earn your own living. It took me a long while to learn that & I wish the ability to "manage" had come sooner. I shall be home the 22nd or 23rd [of September] & we will get in touch immediately. I hate to sound preachy, but you will understand, I know, that I mean this all for your best good & with my own limitations it is all I can do. It's such a pleasure to be able to give you what you want & this shouldn't hurt you a bit.

Love.
Jul

Juliana did not see Carl until he returned home for Thanksgiving. Visits and meetings intervened. John Flannagan, released from Bloomingdale Hospital

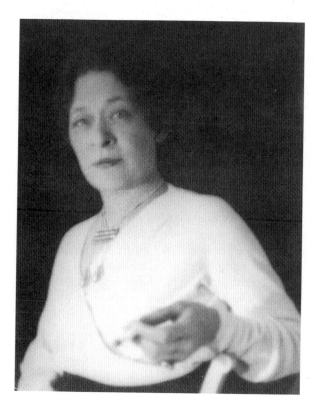

Juliana, elaborately made up and ready for battle.

a few months before and working again on the stone given to him while he was on the PWAP, wrote to Juliana to reestablish their friendly connection. He wanted her to see the progress he had made on the sculpture, hoping that she would be impressed enough to buy a piece of the new work. The artist even managed to make light of his recent ordeals with some gallant black humor. "Bloomingdale," he wrote to Juliana, "figuratively and literally took all the teeth out of me. I am now very well except for the slight discomfort of a very sore mouth which is probably fate's revenge for all the terrible stories I've told."

In November, it was necessary for Juliana to resume her duties as agent and intermediary for Gertrude's sculpture. Gertrude was to be represented in the 1939 World's Fair, which would be held in New York City, with a yet unrealized monumental sculpture. She wanted a dramatic setting, and in preparation, Juliana made arrangements for her to collaborate with four architects on site plans. Gertrude had immediately called in the family architects of Noel & Miller, and Juliana, with her consent, hired the architects Hugh Ferriss and Eric Gugler as well. Gugler and Ferriss were paid $1,000 and $500 a month, respectively, to come up with and render grand designs for pavilions, courtyards, theaters, avenues, and gardens in which her sculptures could be placed.

November also saw the fruition of an idea that Juliana had proposed in the spring. Faith and Edward Andrews had collected enough material on the Shakers

for a show, and Juliana wanted them to put on a comprehensive exhibition of furniture, costumes, drawings, prints, manuscripts, books, and photographs of buildings. The Andrewses were delighted to organize it—"It was a real stamp of approval," said Faith Andrews, "which we never found in our birthplace. We brought in everything we owned—I think all we had at home was our beds— to show the magnitude and richness of the life the Shakers had."

The experience of arranging their exhibition—the most important show of Shaker art and culture New York had seen to date—was "Christmas all the time" to the Andrewses. "It was not just money," Faith Andrews said. "It was Juliana Force's influence and support. Just like that, she would get things, pointing them out with her finger. You could feel her mind going. And she looked for ways to help us. We met Orozco at her apartment, and every now and then she would give me a lovely dress made in France. At the museum, several rooms were emptied for us. We had absolutely free say and no warnings about anything. We were running it all."

The show opened on November 12, and the lively Whitney atmosphere thrilled the Andrewses. "Juliana introduced us to people from the Guggenheim Foundation, and through that, we were able to get a Guggenheim to continue," recalled Faith Andrews. "Our exhibit there was probably the finest that we ever did because we had the audience—a very different audience in New York. I will never forget it. Every day was a new experience, speaking with book dealers, collectors from all over, artists, people who didn't know about the Shakers."

The Andrewses' scholarship was acclaimed, and their efforts stirred up such interest in Shaker handicrafts that Holger Cahill decided that a permanent record of the genius of Shaker craftsmanship should be made through the WPA's Index of American Design. Juliana's confidence in her protégés was justified, and they, in turn, were permanently affected by her insistence on quality. "She had such high standards," Faith Andrews said. "After the Whitney Museum, everything Ted and I did was a comedown. The Whitney experience set certain standards for us. They never left us."

Unfortunately, Juliana's standards and ways of doing things were never understood by Frank Crocker, who was ruled by financial considerations. Crocker had been busy over the summer. While Juliana was abroad, he pragmatically pointed out to Gertrude, who was now sixty years old and pondering the future of the museum, that the Whitney would one day have to be independent of her. She could greatly benefit from the tax laws if the museum were incorporated as a nonprofit, tax-exempt public institution with a constitution, a charter, bylaws, and trustees.

Crocker's proposal, which served Gertrude's interests expertly, is blameless. But he also happened to believe that in conjunction with the new charter, the museum should be made to turn a profit or at least break even, and there he was overzealous. Museums, especially during the Depression, could not be run like a business and expect to be successful in their mission. Crocker, however, was convinced that the Whitney could be self-sufficient.

The plans to incorporate were set in motion while Juliana was in Europe. That the consultations took place during her absence appeared to her as yet

another betrayal, but Juliana was bound to be enraged. No matter what the motivations were, the end result of transforming the Whitney from a private undertaking in which all was between the two women into a legal entity answerable to a board of trustees, was the shrinking of Juliana's autonomy and authority. Characteristically, she viewed the incorporation as a personal rebuke and a professional horror. She had been robbed, and the fortunes of her museum were about to be placed in the grasp of a man she had grown to detest.

Juliana, Crocker, Sonny Whitney, Flora Whitney Miller, and William Adams Delano were named as the Whitney's first trustees. Of these, three would have been objectionable or unhelpful to Juliana. Crocker was hateful, and neither of Gertrude's children then had much interest in art. Flora Miller later said that the only reason she and her brother were brought in as trustees was for tax reasons, and Sonny Whitney, who hardly noticed Juliana's existence, thought of her as a glorified secretary who rendered minor services to his mother. Delano, although genial and knowledgeable, could not be counted on to be a passionate defender of the museum when Crocker wanted to whittle away its operating budget. Since Flora and Sonny traveled extensively and were not often in New York throughout the winter, in day-to-day transactions Juliana would be dealing with Crocker and Crocker alone.

On November 27, 1935, the museum was incorporated during a meeting at 871 Fifth Avenue. Gertrude and all the trustees except Flora, who was at her winter residence in South Carolina, were present. Gertrude donated $100,000 in cash for operating costs for 1936, plus 20,000 shares of R. J. Reynolds Tobacco Co., which had a market value of $1.2 million. The stock would yield an annual income of $60,000. After 1936, the museum would attain financial independence by staying within its yearly budget of $60,000—a 50 percent cut. Deficits were to be made up through sales of catalogs, tickets to lectures, and the like. Admission to the museum would remain free.

The first consequence of the Whitney's changed status and drastic cutbacks was a curtailment of acquisitions and loan and traveling shows. The curators would have to concentrate on displaying works from the permanent collection, but as an economy measure rather than as a felt necessity. The long-term effect was that Juliana was never free from worries—about money and about the museum—again.

THE VALUE OF ALMOST EVERYTHING

❧ (1936–1942) ❧

MONEY—and squabbles about money with Crocker—continued to plague Juliana in 1936. She knew she had to cut back, but economy measures grated on her and represented concessions to Crocker she hated to make. Her expenditures were for principles held and dearly defended, but there was also a determination not to give unnecessary ground. And Crocker, armed with the Whitney's new charter, bylaws, and tax code, was working inexorably to demonstrate just how irresponsible Juliana was.

Crocker could now examine all the museum's books, and he submitted the accounts to an auditing firm. Soon after, he won the first skirmish, which was over insurance. Juliana was the old and dear friend of a couple named Bernice and Harry Farmer. Harry was a partner in Farmer and Ochs, a downtown insurance firm; as a matter of course, Juliana had given the Whitney's fire, accident, fine arts, and liability coverage to his company in 1930. Crocker jumped on her for that—Juliana did not shop around or compare prices, nor would it have occurred to her to do so. Within a month of the museum's incorporation, he had succeeded in showing Gertrude and the other trustees that Juliana was unbusinesslike, if not negligent, and implied that her insurance broker was overcharging Gertrude. Favoritism had cost the museum money, Crocker claimed. He calculated that several thousand dollars a year could have been saved if another firm had written the policies. This assertion was contested by Harry Farmer and seconded by Juliana in some aggrieved letters, but Farmer and Ochs was dropped, and the insurance company preferred by Crocker got the Whitney's business. After this episode, Crocker was also able to impose a stricter system of record keeping. Juliana feared that he would override her on

financial decisions regarding artistic matters—that is, on rental fees and on acquisitions from the 1935–1936 biennial of sculptures and graphic works, which would occasion the next major expenditures. But here she made a stronger, cannier opponent—he could not outduel her, and he was not so incautious as to try.

As a sign of solidarity with the artists who were demanding fees in return for lending their works to museums and as part of her promise, Juliana wanted to pay *all* the exhibitors—not just the ones belonging to the society behind the strike—in the biennial. She had agreed to do this before the Whitney's status changed; in October of 1935, on the eve of that change, she was careful to confer on the rental issue with Gertrude, who gave her approval.

Juliana informed Stuart Davis when inviting him to participate, "We have decided to make an experiment and pay to the artists invited to this coming Biennial Exhibition a rental, for the duration of the exhibition, of ten dollars per month for sculptures, five dollars for watercolors and drawings, and one dollar each for prints." To a magazine editor who asked her about her stand, Juliana was less guarded. "Yes, I am in favor of a rental fee paid to the artists. . . ." she wrote. "I do believe, however, that the matter has not yet been worked out satisfactorily and, if you notice, our only offer is for this coming exhibition. After that—perhaps, the Deluge!"

Juliana got a welcome second when Alfred Barr came out for paying rentals. All other claims, he wrote, were "outweighed . . . by the incontrovertible fact that practically everyone involved in exhibitions is paid except the artist, who is the original and essential producer." Juliana fought to gain more widespread approval for the rental fee, but the idea was defeated overwhelmingly by her colleagues.

The rental payments to biennial exhibitors amounted to $822 and earned the Whitney much goodwill. Ward Lockwood sent Juliana a long letter from New Mexico, part of which read:

> I wish that all of the museum directors of the country could have been placed in my shoes at the time I opened the envelope and found this check. If such could happen, I feel sure that the rental idea would be an accomplished fact in a few weeks throughout the country. . . . It was a sample of your museum's understanding of the artist and his problems. . . . It is this sense of "rapprochement" between the museum and the artist that is so important at the present time. I feel certain that it is this, even more than the actual money involved, that has brought about the present rift in the relations between so many museums and the painters.

Besides paying fees, Juliana of course made purchases from the biennial, although it would have been unwise to spend anywhere near the $20,000 limit, which was discouraged strongly by the trustees. She bought thirty-six items, a quantity attributable to the fact that works on paper were inexpensive. Of these purchases, twenty-three were prints, and they came to $392.

Juliana also made an indisputably great acquisition, spending what was necessary to get it. Gaston Lachaise had been invited to the biennial, and before his death, he had selected a sculpture for inclusion. Juliana wanted to buy a Lachaise, but she also wished the Whitney to have a work commensurate with

the artist's stature and representative of the central source of his art. Accordingly, instead of buying what had been sent to the exhibition, she broke with precedent—of only buying out of the show—and arranged with Isabel Lachaise to substitute a cast of the monumental *Standing Woman*, which Lachaise had worked on and refined for fifteen years. The bronze cost $8,000 and the price, if not the subject matter, probably gave Crocker indigestion, but the curators were solidly behind Juliana.

Two other exhibitions succeeded the biennial that spring, but she was more involved with business pertaining to the promotion of Gertrude's sculpture. Gertrude was having a show at Knoedler's, opening on March 17, and that required some attention. Juliana was also working with Hugh Ferriss and Eric Gugler, who were still on retainers, on the designs for the World's Fair installations. In addition, inquiries had been made as to Gertrude's executing two public works—a memorial to the philanthropist Mary Harriman Rumsey and a statue of Peter Stuyvesant—both destined for New York City parks. Gertrude accepted both of these commissions, which were sponsored by two groups of old-guard New Yorkers, and Robert Moses thought it wise to patch up past quarrels. In turn, Gertrude had come to admire the improvements Moses made in the city's parks, and his friendly overtures reaped the gift of the 16-foot-high wrought-iron gates and fences that had once guarded the Vanderbilt mansion at 1 West 57th Street,* plus Gertrude's promise to pay for their storage and repair. Moses would plant the great grille at the entrance of the Central Park conservatory garden at Fifth Avenue and 105th Street, where it stands to this day.

Meanwhile, the New York art museums—the Metropolitan, the Brooklyn Museum, the Museum of the City of New York, the Museum of Modern Art, and the Whitney—were also going to contribute to the 1939 World's Fair. The Whitney's role would change as time went on, but in early 1936 Juliana was responsible for a loan show of 100 American masterworks dating from colonial times to 1900. It would begin with *Mrs. Elizabeth (Clarke) Freake and Baby Mary*,† one of the most celebrated American paintings of the seventeenth century, proceed through the eighteenth with Smibert, Feke, Copley, Stuart, Trumbull, and West, and cover the nineteenth century with Allston, Morse, Durand, Cole, Mount, Bingham, Kensett, Homer, Eakins, Duveneck, Ryder, Inness, La Farge, Whistler, Twachtman, Cassatt, Sargent, and Prendergast. To have all these names accepted under the "masterpiece" banner without argument was palpable proof of how well the Whitney had done its proselytizing work over the years.

Another edict from the museum's new regime wreaked havoc on Juliana's finances. In 1935, along with her salary, Juliana drew $11,200 for expenditures, some of them museum-related, some of them personal, and some of them entwined. Formerly, Gertrude had paid the income taxes on the drawing account; in future, the trustees declared, any money turned over to Juliana from the account would be reported as compensation. This meant she would be respon-

---

*The house was torn down after the death of Alice Vanderbilt in 1934.
†Collection of the Worcester Art Museum.

sible for the taxes. Crocker unfairly made this ruling retroactive, so Juliana not only had to meet taxes that she had not been expecting to pay for 1935, but a penalty was going to be levied by the government for what looked like unreported income. Crocker did not offer to reimburse her for the penalty, although it was his doing. In addition, since Gertrude paid the insurance on Juliana's apartment because it was within the museum building, Crocker was going to report this benefit as part of her income. Gertrude was aware of these changes—on March 11, 1936, William Delano resigned from the Whitney's board of trustees, and she took his place at all the meetings—but she evidently deferred to Crocker. And as for the cruelty inflicted on Juliana, who was too proud to quarrel over money for herself, Crocker and Gertrude seemed to be unconscious.

Feeling harassed, Juliana took out some of the pent-up fury, which was meant for Crocker and ultimately Gertrude, on Carl Rieser. In her letters, she scolded him for trivial lapses. When he didn't write, she was annoyed. When he did, the letters weren't good enough. After she had trouble reading his handwriting, she complained, "But really, can't you try to write more plainly? It isn't quite fair—unless this is the best you can do."

Juliana came to the sad conclusion that she could resolve her financial crisis only by selling Barley Sheaf Farm. The thought of it devastated her, but it was the one way that she could lay her hands on enough cash to pay her debts and leave her with some extra money. Selling the farm was not a new idea—in 1934 Juliana briefly put the property on the market and then took it off again because the buyer wasn't right or because she just couldn't bear to sell. But in the spring of 1936, a serious and persistent buyer appeared. Beatrice Bakrow Kaufman, an editor at *Harper's Bazaar* and the wife of the playwright George S. Kaufman, spotted the farm on a visit to a friend and liked it. She seems to have looked over the place several times—Allan Rieser remembered her appearing there once with Alexander Woollcott. In any event, nothing happened, most likely because the asking price—between $45,000 and $60,000—was too much for the playwright, who was said to be a skinflint. (Juliana was not out of line asking for $60,000, even during the Depression. She and Doctor had improved the property and refurbished all the buildings extensively—installing the swimming pool cost more than $30,000, and Juliana estimated that they spent about $75,000 overall in renovations.) Kaufman himself did not view the house because he was in Hollywood doctoring movie scripts.

The farm was left unsold and in the local real estate agent's hands when Juliana sailed for England that summer. She left on July 8 on the *Queen Mary*, and took Allan, who had never been abroad, with her. Previously he had gotten only sporadic glimpses into his aunt's world, but throughout the summer of 1936 he had a chance to observe its panache and badinage at length. His introduction really began the morning they boarded the great ship in the usual profusion of champagne, telegrams, flowers, and well-wishers. During the voyage, Allan watched in wonder while his aunt attracted notice without making a visible effort to do so. One evening while they were having dinner, a gentleman at another table sent over an adulatory note addressed to "Madame Nazimova." Juliana waved grandly at her admirer and kept up the masquerade.

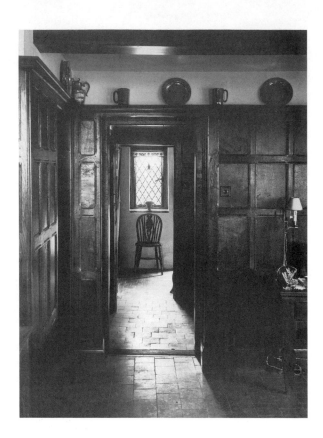

Some of the oak paneling
that Juliana bought from a
ship's cabin and installed at
Cobweb in 1936.

Once they were unpacked at Cobweb, Juliana decided to fix up the dining room. She bought an actual wood-paneled ship's cabin, and then had it removed from the boat, transported, and reassembled into a pocket dining room. This extensive reconstruction was her idea of a little redecorating. After the remodeling was completed, Juliana, learning that none of the workmen had ever seen the sea, hired a bus and arranged to have all the men taken to the nearest beach for a picnic lunch. To her amazement—and later, great amusement—all the men dutifully ate their lunch without ever leaving the bus. But that was fine with Juliana, who loved everything English. One day, Allan wrote:

> There was a fair in Aylesbury, the county seat, and Aunt J. insisted on going there dressed in a very elaborate eighteenth-century costume (she always seized on every opportunity to wear a costume) and for some reason we found ourselves in some local civic chambers where everyone looked very sedate and rather stunned at what must have seemed a sort of apparition. Aunt J., of course, was very happy at the sort of confusion she was creating. She adored being at the center of things and always managed it, in one way or another, although, actually, it was an inborn gift, and she could do it just as well by sitting quite still in a corner. All parties eventually (usually quite quickly) circled around her.

Allan also noticed his aunt's skill at handling men, who flocked to her for her dramatic presence and her deep voice—

a baritone which could always become kittenish if she felt coquetry was in order. If men didn't find her beautiful, they soon forgot it in the charm of her presence. The American ambassador of the time* drove over to pay a visit, which she had been trying to avoid, and stayed for hours, obviously enthralled. She complained to me at odd moments that she was bored to death but didn't know how to get rid of him.

Allan wanted to be alone to work on a play he was writing, so Juliana took a quick trip to Germany and Austria in August, stopping briefly in Berlin for a day at the summer Olympics. While she was there, a Hollywood scandal broke whose ramifications were felt even at Cobweb. The actress Mary Astor was trying to gain full custody of her daughter from her ex-husband, Dr. Franklyn Thorpe. Thorpe sought to paint her as an unfit mother by stealing the star's diary and releasing what he claimed were excerpts from it. The passages splashed across the tabloids divulged lurid tidbits about an affair she had had with George S. Kaufman. Astor purportedly filled two volumes with postcoital moonings about Kaufman's manly prowess. She was quoted as writing of "many exquisite moments" and "thrilling ecstasy." Astor also was supposed to have confessed, on paper, "He fits me like a glove."

On September 2, Juliana received a transatlantic telephone call—an event so unusual that it was the talk of Haddenham—from the Kaufmans. They offered $45,000 for the farm, and she took it. Juliana believed that Kaufman bought the property for Beatrice to make up for the embarrassment he had caused her. But the Kaufmans, like the Forces, had gone their own amorous ways for years. Given the understanding the couple had about pursuing other sexual partners, Malcolm Goldstein, Kaufman's biographer, has suggested that the Mary Astor trial should not be credited too heavily as the reason for Kaufman buying the farm. Yet the purchase of the property, which did not interest him at the time, had something of a peace offering to it, and the transatlantic call hints at a need for urgency. As for Juliana, she gleefully referred to the $45,000 as the price Kaufman had paid for his dalliance. After the house changed hands, she liked to say, "And to think I owe all this to Mary Astor."

Juliana and Allan reached home on September 28, in time for her to be in Bucks County for an October 3 closing. At the farm, Clara, Mary, and the rest of the Riesers started cleaning and packing. Juliana's many antiques were shipped to Shaker Hollow; bedding, linens, and the garden furniture were to go to the Kaufmans. Irene described the removal of Juliana's possessions as "a grand upheaval . . . with trucks lining the highway up to South Salem." The other residents of Holicong resented Juliana for selling her house to a Jew and let the Riesers know it. When Moss Hart, Kaufman's collaborator, bought a house in the area to be near him, Juliana was blamed for this further incursion.

As soon as Juliana arrived, there was another demand. Carl's tuition needed to be paid by September 30, and on September 29 he sent a telegram asking for

---

*Robert Worth Bingham.

it. He had handled this clumsily, but Juliana was so wrapped up in her own emotions that she let him off rather easily.

> Here is the cheque. Please do try & let me know by letter at least two weeks in advance when things are due. I have so much on my mind always & you really should attend to these matters with a bit more graciousness, don't you think?
>
> It sounds a bit as if I were the cashier of the Bank to get a wire like that!
>
> I am off to the "sack of the farm" this morning & it's a melancholy business. It seems quite fantastic that I shall have no real home ever again. You have known it since you were born & I all my best days.

Regrettably for Carl, he misunderstood something about his tuition bill and had to write his aunt telling her that he had bungled things. This time, there was no gentle rebuke. She lashed out:

> Your letter just arrived & I am hastening to send the cheque. If you would make yourself think before you write I might possibly have understood your first letter. Or maybe it was the writing. Anyway it's your own fault & for God's sake learn to spell like a gentleman. "Nite" for night made me violently ill.

Juliana lost her temper again when Carl did not thank her promptly for the check. "Don't you really think," she admonished him,

> that you should acknowledge the cheques as soon as you receive them? Even if as you call it, it *is* your "pay," you must stop to say thank you. It's really not polite & very bad for you to allow yourself to get so sloppy. I realize that you are busy; so is everybody who amounts to anything. I hope that you are not impolite to anyone else. I should be ashamed of you if you were.

Carl, realizing by now that his aunt was not the easiest person to please and that any shortfalls would be greeted with terrifying exasperation, made amends. By the end of the year, Irene was congratulating him for his clear handwriting and the high quality of his latest letters. Aunt Julia, she reported, had forgiven him, and Carl was an angel again—until the next time.

There would always be a next time because Juliana demanded perfection of her nephews. Allan Rieser, who also came in for his share of scalding mockery, said, "No doubt I was one of her disappointments. She had me set down for a poet, and nothing short of becoming Keats would quite have done. I felt the sting myself one day when I said to her, defensively, 'Well, you can only do your best—' 'And it's never quite good enough, is it?' she snapped—almost, it seemed, before I had begun." Carl Rieser, reflecting on his relationship with his aunt, added, "She wanted so much of other people, as you can see from her letters—scolding, always scolding—to me. But it also must be remembered that *she* lived up to what she asked of others. She was punctilious about her obligations and her commitments. She expected others to be."

The 1936–1937 Whitney season began on October 6, and the fare reflected the tension between constriction and largesse that the museum and Juliana were experiencing. The opening show, featuring paintings and sculptures executed for the Treasury Department Art Project, didn't cost much to put on. Forbes

Watson had asked Juliana to hold the show, and perhaps he offered to cover the expenses. Watson wrote the catalog and did some drumbeating in Washington for the show because Eleanor Roosevelt and other New Deal notables came up for the opening. Mrs. Roosevelt plugged the show in "My Day," her famous column, and the President indicated his continued confidence in Ned Bruce and the Treasury Department art programs.

If a display of art made for federal buildings had overtones of favors owed and repaid, the exhibition that followed it was of irreproachable caliber. The Whitney was allowed to step out and mount an expensive loan show—Lloyd Goodrich organized a centenary exhibition honoring Winslow Homer; 170 works were borrowed from sixty-two institutions and individual collectors, and a full catalog was prepared. Goodrich had been doing research for some time, and the show was planned so much in advance that the penny counters could not block it. The Homer centenary broke all previous attendance records.

Crocker, in deciding to push, might have known that Juliana was going to push back. On December 29, 1936, in what can only be construed as an utter defiance of budgetary strictures and an assertion of her former liberty, she walked into Kraushaar's and bought *Backyards, Greenwich Village* and *Sixth Avenue El at Third Street* by John Sloan. Whitney records say that the price paid was a very reasonable $2,040 apiece, but spending that money was a brave step for someone so closely watched and in a position to be harassed. For Crocker, the issue was always how much something cost. Juliana said that he "had no aesthetic understanding," and Lloyd Goodrich was of the same opinion. Among friends, she referred to Crocker, who wore an eye patch, as One-Eyed Dick, but if she had to say his name, Juliana would roll her r's and spit it out—C-r-r-r-ocker—like a dirty word. After the Sloan acquisitions, Juliana announced that beginning in the fall of 1937, the biennial shows would become annuals in order to increase the number of young artists the Whitney could include in those exhibitions. Such a change could not be made without Gertrude's assent, and Crocker, ever looking for opportunities to give grades to Juliana, merely veiled his condescension with two-edged compliments.

The next two Whitney exhibitions—the third biennial of contemporary painting and New York Realists: 1900 to 1914—were more indicative of the state of Juliana's tastes and priorities than budgetary conflicts. From the biennial, eight paintings were purchased, the most notable being *Office Girls* by Raphael Soyer and *The Circle Theatre* by Edward Hopper. The Museum of Modern Art, which rarely went after anything American, bought *The Senate* by William Gropper for its permanent collection. This purchase must have pleased Juliana no end. She would tell Jared French, "I want above all to have work sold from this museum." French also said that when Mrs. Ogden Phipps wanted a picture of his from a Whitney show, but offered considerably less than the price he put on it, Juliana said, "I would like you to sell it to her. I must sell paintings from the museum shows. I shall buy the next painting you do." And, added French, "she did."*

*Summer's Ending, of 1939.

The exhibition of New York Realists traced the early careers of the painters who had taken American art in a forthright new direction at the turn of the century and aroused great storms of protest in doing so. These men were, of course, the artists who had profoundly influenced Gertrude and Juliana: Henri, Sloan, Luks, Glackens, Lawson, Shinn, Bellows, Coleman, and du Bois. The museum was in its element, and the curators were able to borrow such fine examples of the school as *Chez Mouquin,** *The Spielers, Stag at Sharkey's,*† and *Yeats at Petitpas.*‡ The problem, as reflected in several reviews, was that the Whitney regarded the show as somewhat contemporary, whereas the critics looked on it as historical. For Anita Brenner, who was covering the show for the *Brooklyn Eagle,* the art she saw was not so much historical as dead. The paintings were ringed with a "cloud of futility," and they belonged to an era that museums should not be reviving, but doing their best to forget.

Henry McBride, who liked the show, confessed that he still thought of these revolutionaries of thirty years ago as contemporaries, and it would not be wrong to say that Juliana shared that feeling. Her career as a talent spotter and trailblazer began to be overtaken by a gradual but perceptible sense of closure. She kept looking for unknown artists with her old vigor and sympathy, she kept working to make young artists who felt separated from the art world feel included, but the ones she understood and befriended were less likely to be innovators or pioneers. Her humanity, her character, her gusto, and her crusading spirit persisted; her feeling for the sharply new and unfamiliar did not.

Vanguard artists in New York were beginning to comport themselves differently. Their aesthetic assumptions and alliances had shifted, and Juliana was unable to follow where they were leading. Almost everyone who has sustained a public career in the fine arts over many decades has found it impossible to remain consistently in contact with the most vital developments in the field from the start to finish of that career. As a rule, an individual's best and most memorable work is done with the artists of his or her own generation and the one immediately succeeding it, and Juliana was no exception. In these years, her finest moments would involve such artists as Lachaise, Sloan, Stuart Davis, Marsden Hartley, and Louis Eilshemius—artists she had grown up with, battled for, and understood very well.

One reason why Juliana was growing out of touch was her inability to understand how important political activism—the need to take sides and make commitments—was to the artists who came of age during the Depression. Because of her abhorrence of Communist manipulation, she became isolated from some of the younger artists who were vocally on the Left. "Juliana wasn't interested in the merger of politics and art," said Charles Sawyer. "Actually, she had no interest in politics. She couldn't see why artists should be so radical. This was why the PWAP was quite a shock to her. Because everything was very personal to her, what was in her horizon was important and things that were outside her horizon, like the political world, she didn't care very much about."

* Collection of the Art Institute of Chicago.
† Collection of the Cleveland Museum of Art.
‡ Collection of the Corcoran Gallery of Art.

Juliana also lost her edge because she was slow in registering the impact of the various strains of European modernism on vanguard American artists. Regionalism held little interest for these painters. They wanted to be measured against internationally known artists and to keep abreast of the latest advances, whereas the Whitney was catering to Woodstock and other localities and showing nice, inoffensive paintings. It was the Whitney's effort more than the quality of the works of art seen that won renown for many of these artists. (Consequently, after Juliana was no longer there to bolster them, quite a few Whitney regulars disappeared from view.)

Juliana still cared passionately about furthering the interests of American art and artists, and she remained a power in her world. But because the museum did not take enough chances, she would never be a determining factor—as she had been for the previous two generations of artists—for the painters in the process of forming the loose coalition that would be known as the New York School. (When the Whitney began showing Pollock, Rothko, Baziotes, and David Smith in the mid-1940s, they were there through Hermon More. The only member of the New York School she was truly close to was Bradley Walker Tomlin, whom she had known since the 1920s and whose work she saw evolve.) The painter Jacob Kainen, who did not exhibit at the Whitney in the 1930s, but went there regularly to review its shows, was not challenged by the museum's fare. "The Whitney was conservative in retrospect, but not during the period," he said. "It was a middle-of-the-road place that always picked a few that were more advanced, like Stuart Davis. You looked forward to shows, but you didn't expect much. They were not stimulating, but they were something you saw. The further you got into the thirties, the less significant it was." In 1940, Vogue, hardly a mouthpiece for artistic discontent, reported that Juliana's critics charged the museum with being "too pretty, and feminine, and manicured; that it . . . does not have the same old rebellious spirit, the same energy in keeping up with new young work; that what America needs now is the Mrs. Force of thirty-two years ago."

Juliana's nephews thought that her social acquaintances were less vibrant, too. Allan Rieser said that some of the people she surrounded herself with were not on a par with the bright and charming painters who had swirled around her before. Allan was threatened by the general atmosphere because he felt that his aunt was trying to steer him into homosexuality, or at least into the life of an eternal bachelor and permanent escort. "What I would not be," he said, "was one of the effeminate drones I frequently saw around her. Not that there weren't vital people, too—but the drones were very prominent."

Allan was being trained for the post of extra man even though one of those useful creatures had recently come into Juliana's life. Arthur Mayer, a New York osteopath and a closet homosexual, became more or less her regular escort, especially for the operas and symphonies they both appreciated, as he loved music, particularly Wagner and German lieder. Allan Rieser's opinion of his aunt's friend was low. "Mayer and his German-musical circle were a kind of people I'm sure she would have dismissed in earlier years as 'vulgar,' " he wrote, "but in her last rather sad phase when a kind of bitterness set in generally, I

think they answered her need to have activity around her. The more brilliant and interesting art people seemed less and less in the picture. Attrition, I suppose—and also she may have alienated a lot with her increasingly misanthropic tongue, and what amounted to a talent for vituperation."

In March of 1937 the pendulum of Gertrude's judgment swung toward Juliana's point of view and away from Crocker's. In appraising the Whitney's subdued year of 1936, Gertrude could see that the $60,000 annual budget that Crocker tried to enforce had limited the museum too severely, and she increased it to $100,000 a year by donating 10,400 shares of Chemical Bank stock to the museum. Gertrude also raised Juliana's salary to $25,000 a year. Another project she approved was a memorial exhibition for Lachaise. His widow was insolvent, as no one wanted to buy any of the sculptor's work. Lincoln Kirstein asked Juliana if the museum might take over the Lachaise estate. This was an institutional impossibility, but she could arrange for a show of sculptures and drawings that might stimulate sales.

During this period of comparative openhandedness, Juliana aided Marsden Hartley, who was having a wretched time. In April, Hartley had what was to be his last show at An American Place, because Stieglitz was no longer interested in his work. (The art critic Elizabeth McCausland, who was devoted to Hartley and later became an expert on his work, stated that when she came to see the paintings, Stieglitz trailed after her and said, "Oh, Hartley isn't an important artist.") Naturally the show was a financial disaster, with no sales made. Hartley had not sold a painting in over a year, and he was close to suicide. After his show closed in May, Hartley wrote to Goodrich, who had befriended him during the PWAP, pleading with him "to help me out in any way you can to get out of the worst hole in all my life." Goodrich showed this letter to Juliana, and he received permission to buy a painting at once. The Whitney acquired *The Old Bars, Dogtown* for $800, and Hartley, said Goodrich, "wrote to say that it made all the difference in his life. He could go back to Maine and get his teeth fixed." This was the only sale he made during all of 1937.

Juliana's struggles with Crocker were known only to those inside the museum, and her need for money was a Rieser family secret. To the rest of the world, appearances never crumbled, but the signs of difficulty were discernible to anyone who looked for them. Her income taxes were horrendous again, and she was unable to pay Carl's spring tuition bill until May. Now that the farm was a memory, the next group of things to go was her sixty-odd pieces of Shaker furniture. The numerous chairs, tables, counters, chests, desks, stands, sewing tables, cabinets, benches, and oval boxes were all early examples, coming from communal joiners' shops, and they constituted one of the finest collections that had been assembled to date. Juliana first decided to sell in October of 1936, after the contents of the farm were crammed into the already full interior of Shaker Hollow. Edward and Faith Andrews cataloged her collection, and from May 18 to 19, 1937, a private sale was held at South Salem. Not everything was sold, but Juliana did realize enough money to honor an obligation. Years

before, she promised to subsidize the production costs ($1,000) of the Andrewses' book on the Shakers. But in 1936 she had only managed to send $100 to Yale University Press, their publisher. On June 1, 1937, she sent her personal check for the remaining $900, and the book* came out later in the year.

Juliana could not afford to go abroad, but Gertrude, evidently trying to make up to Juliana for the harsh changes of the past season, said that the museum would advance her whatever she needed. Apparently Juliana demurred, too proud to admit that she had mismanaged her money and anticipating Crocker's reaction to yet another drain on the Whitney exchequer, but Gertrude was doing her best to repair the old, easygoing relationship that had been destroyed by Crocker and his strictures. She insisted that she needed Juliana with her in France, and on June 8, she had the trustees vote on a special resolution deputizing Juliana to report on how well the American paintings fared at the Paris Exposition that summer.

Before the trustees acted, Gertrude prepared the way by writing Juliana a warm letter that erased some of the hurt and won her trust again. It began:

> Won't you please go abroad for a short time? After all, you have had a devastating winter and here we are soon to start, so soon, on a very important new season. I am sure that quite aside from me it is considered by the trustees important that the director of a museum keep up with what is happening on the other side besides having a holiday—which you are not having, nor did you propose to. I feel this so strongly that it is hard for me to put it into words, which is all wrong on my part. I can't just be hardboiled as far as we are concerned. If you prefer to be businesslike —I will not mention the matter to Frank—except to state the fact that I think you ought to go abroad (and that the situation is not so tense) to check up on what is happening there.
>
> Don't think I am being nice—I am not—I am only trying to think out something which is so personal that to put it on another basis is almost impossible.
>
> Love,
> G.

The day after the trustees passed their resolution, Juliana wrote to Carl Rieser about her financial woes. Carl, the youngest person in Juliana's family, was developing into her trusted confidante. Juliana's letters do harangue him about money, but they also contain many more revelatory details about her beliefs and preoccupations than would be expected from a sixty-year-old woman writing to a boy forty years her junior. Carl was making an effort at composing serious letters to his aunt, and he offered kind words during some hard moments. Juliana responded to his concern with her own outpouring of feeling, allowing herself to draw sustenance from their exchanges. Her letters to Carl, who was far from the art world, were a safety valve for disgruntlements she could not express to her colleagues or even to her brothers and sisters. In turn, despite the occasional blunder that earned him a show of temper, Carl's improvement as a correspondent and student gave him a new wisdom in Juliana's eyes. This led her to treat him more and more as an equal. Juliana looked on this advance in their rela-

*Shaker Furniture: The Craftsmanship of an American Communal Sect.

tionship as an honor. What she did not sense was how burdensome such confidences and expectations could be to someone who was still so young and inexperienced. She wrote to him on June 9:

> I have suddenly been called abroad & go without seeing you & also with many misgivings. I wanted, after your last letter, very much to talk seriously with you, about money & about yr responsibilities. On paper it sounds quite stupid, but it is very much on my heart & I owe it to you to speak frankly. Besides, you are really a grown man & can face facts as well as any one. One of the facts is that I must change my mode of living because now the Government takes more than one-third of my income each year. To pay the enormous amount this year I was obliged to sell all my investments at a sacrifice & my income now is only what I can earn. For all the money I give to either support or aid in supporting others, I get no exemption. Whether the Government is right or wrong, it is our Government & we must adjust our lives accordingly. In my case it means living without many things I've become used to. More difficult though is the fact that I must reduce my gifts to others in proportion. The aunts are getting older & cannot alter their mode of life. Alan [sic] is not physically or temperamentally fitted. I have great faith in his one day doing something quite great. If at the same time it is not remunerative what difference does it make? I shall always be proud to do what I can for him. His wants are so very few! . . .
>
> There are other obligations which I need not go into but which I cannot shirk. Now we come to you—the point of my long dissertation! I want you to go through College. It w'd be wrong to stop now. But I do think you should work in the summers & save what you can towards yr clothes for the year. It can be done, lots of men have done it & to my mind it is yr obligation & responsibility just now. You know that yr father is trying hard to get on his feet—he has done what few men could have done under the circumstances, & I admire him very much.* It is hellish to work at what you despise doing & especially with nerves that jangle out of time all the time.
>
> You must not accept any help whatsoever from your mother & father until they are in better shape. It's not easy for either of them & they are doing a good job, in my opinion. . . .
>
> It was a bitter disappointment to me, for I had planned to invite you abroad this yr as Alan [sic] had done last yr—but some day it will come.
>
> Do write me & do not ever show this to anyone. It's between you & me & for always.
>
> I leave to the last my congratulations on yr year's progress. It is a fine record & I am more than pleased. My heart is very heavy at leaving, but you must write & keep in touch with me. Goodbye & get some fun out of the summer. Life is quite sweet anyway. Love, J.

Without Juliana's prompting, Carl already had taken a summer job, and he also lined up work during the next school year. Meanwhile, she again shored up Charles financially in hopes that if he felt secure he would be in better shape to keep his job.

On June 11, Juliana and Gertrude sailed for France. In Paris, they visited Jo Davidson's studio, but Gertrude was tired and thin, and Juliana was concerned

---

*Charles was then working in an advertising agency, which he hated.

about her poor health. She was too distraught to leave Gertrude and carried on so that Gertrude wrote to a friend, "I told her before I left that I was going to be quiet here and that unless she would go ahead and do her own things I didn't want her to stay with me. Instead of which she worries all the time (even if she doesn't say anything) and appears with red eyes etc. etc." The women parted company in early July—Gertrude to Pest and Juliana to Venice and then England—but Juliana's fussing was well-founded. When Gertrude left Paris she was down to an emaciated ninety-one pounds (a frightening weight for her height of 5 feet 8 inches), and in Hungary she came down with bronchitis and spent several days in the hospital.

While in England, Juliana came to another sorrowful decision. Her need to economize, plus the instability of the political climate, were imperatives that could not be ignored. Cobweb had to be sold. Juliana, in a letter to her sisters, said she feared that war was imminent. Clara Rieser wrote to Carl about the sale, "I was sorry for that, it was the one Place she could get a rest from every thing."

On August 21, 1937, Juliana sold Cobweb for £ 2,500. Carl wrote his aunt some consoling letters, and Juliana was comforted by them. By the time they reached her, she had vacated the house and was spending two weeks in the Lake District around Buttermere and in Scotland with some unnamed friends. She replied to Carl from Edinburgh:

> We went first to the Lake Country, the home of poets & I can see very well why they were so gentle & so melancholy & so cognizant of all the little things of life which escape most of us. That "inner eye, the bliss of solitude" has always been my goal. I loved it very much, but after a few days we had to move & Scotland's lakes are now my home.
>
> I find that I adopt certain places very easily. Here it is as if I'd always been. And altho' I do not dare to show it, my Wordsworth & my Cowper are my guides. As for conscience, it sleeps. It was the best thing to do to come here & forget what I've lost. Bathe in beauty, is about all I do for exercise. For one thing I'm too tired. This has been a hectic summer, what with exhibitions in Paris, in Venice, etc. & the house business. Life doesn't let me loaf much, but it can't keep me from "inviting my soul."

Juliana sailed in mid-September. She was still apprehensive enough about war to return by way of Canada, where she visited some art museums. In Quebec, she felt "more foreign than in Europe."

At home, the family news was sordid. Charles had gotten into some fights while drinking, and Juliana despised him for the pain he caused Irene. Juliana, not understanding that she had enabled Charles's drinking to go on by coming to his rescue and then continuing to support him in some style, thought that her helping him obligated him to stay righted. Juliana wrote this all to Carl: She was now treating the son as an adult and the father as a child.

> It takes a long time to realize that "only Heaven is *given* away" & that, you see, is after you are dead. . . . [Your] Dad never has [paid] & sometimes it makes me sick! Such a waste! I like him tremendously & admire his brain, but it is almost impossible

to respect him. His attitude toward life is almost childish & certainly entirely selfish. His every thought is of himself. He does nothing to make happiness for others, quite the contrary. . . .

I am no nearer the solution of life than you are. I am only happy at moments & doubt that we are meant to have more—we, I mean, who think. But there is joy in creativity, & giving it to others. There is solace too in achieving a bit of elegance in our own lives. The beauty of graciousness is, more than I can tell you, a great source of happiness to me. I enjoy it in others & try to get some into my own life. It's more important to me than telling others "what I think." I'm quite sick of hearing that. You must not construe this to mean that I do not like to hear what you think. I do & I also enjoy telling you sometimes "what I think!". . .

I do feel sorry for your Dad. I wonder if it's too late.*

The Riesers were not the only family with troubles. Gloria Vanderbilt had been under Gertrude's supervision since the custody dispute over her ended in 1934. Gertrude's idea of child care was to place little Gloria in school and install her at Wheatley Hills with only servants for company. She seemed oblivious to the fact that this child might need extra affection, attention, and reassurance after what she had been through. But Gertrude, who didn't know how to open herself to a young girl, "wasn't," said Gloria, "the kind of woman who could put her arms around a child and kiss it," let alone spend time with one. Now nearly fourteen, Gloria was a lonely adolescent pining for love and companionship. She thought she might feel less alone if she could get to know her mother better and see her whenever it suited them, instead of the strict weekend and holiday schedule mandated by the court. In other words, Gloria wanted a custody amendment. But Gertrude was such an inaccessible and unapproachable guardian that Gloria was not permitted to ask her for such a boon face-to-face. "[I]t was made clear from the beginning," Gloria was to write, "that any questions I had should be relayed to her through her lawyer, Mr. Crocker, or through my legal guardian, Mr. Gilchrist."

That was not at all to Gloria's taste. But then she thought of Juliana. "Like Aunt Gertrude she wore a hat even indoors, and it sat on her tangerine hair as though it were a jaunty crown," Gloria would write. "There were always friends around her and an air of lovely things about to happen. . . . I knew that Auntie Ger listened to what Juliana had to say. Not only that, she could always get to Auntie Ger *immediately*. . . . The fastest way to get a message to Aunt Gertrude was through this most positive of messengers."

Not telling anyone else, Gloria telephoned Juliana, who invited her to tea. The two spent a delightful afternoon together, and Gloria not only never forgot it, but was able to recount it in crystalline detail nearly fifty years after it happened. When Gloria appeared at the door, Juliana greeted her with a big hug and said, "Come down my primrose path."

Juliana's varnished chintz floor was only the first of many wonders. Gloria drank in the alabaster garnitures, the crystal candelabra, the satin sofas, the

---

* It was not, although the recovery was some years in the future. Charles later joined AA, stopped drinking for good, and enjoyed almost thirty years of sobriety.

Bristol-blue glassware, and the lacquered tables. For their tea, they went into a gazebolike room "with trellises and twining Morning Glory vines painted on the walls around us. And on the floor there were cool blue and white tiles, and around, here and there, baskets holding orange trees with plump baby oranges dangling from the branches."

Juliana had planned a Victorian tea party to match the decor and did everything she could to make Gloria feel petted and welcome. The white wicker tea wagon was laden, Gloria said, "with delicacies I had never seen before. There were little soufflés of gruyère with whipped cream on top and a sprinkle of cayenne, round tissue paper–thin sandwiches of cucumber and chopped sweet onion. Centered on another plate were coconut drops surrounded by black walnut lace cookies. But that wasn't all—another dish, heart-shaped, held a coeur à la crème with Bar-le duc jelly close at hand."

Between bites of sandwiches and cakes, the two chattered away, and before long Gloria broached the subject of being allowed to see her mother whenever she wished. Could Juliana get Aunt Gertrude to agree to it? In Gloria's words:

> Mrs. Force nodded, without comment, to everything I said, but I knew she was listening. And later, as we walked along the primrose path back to the front door, she put her arm around me. You'll be hearing something soon, very soon, I'm sure, so try not to worry about it, Gloria, and do come and have tea with me again. I always love to see you. I will, I will, thank you, thank you, I said. For what a lovely time we had had together. And as for tea—why, it had been a banquet!

Juliana lived up to Gloria's estimate of her influence. She discussed the matter with Gertrude, who approved the request and successfully petitioned the court to have the custody agreement amended. In January of 1938, the restrictions were eased on little Gloria's movements, and she could see her mother as she pleased. Gloria, who "felt a great surge of hope," blessed Juliana's responsiveness and powers of persuasion, and Juliana was sanguine about Gloria, too. Impressed by her spunk and determination, Juliana told her friends not to worry about Gloria—despite her traumatic experiences, she was going to be all right when she grew up.

The year 1938 opened with an extensive survey of nineteenth-century landscape painting, a triumphant effort that took up the entire museum, but such expansiveness was illusionary and provisional. Austerity, not lavishness, was once more to be enforced, and Juliana personally started off the new year in a grim manner. First, she heard that Oscar Bluemner had committed suicide on January 12. She telephoned John Davis Hatch, a concerned friend who often looked after Bluemner, and volunteered to pay the funeral expenses. The artist had burial insurance, so Juliana's help was not needed, but, said Hatch, "It was typical of what she did."

Two weeks after Bluemner's death, Juliana took on the officials of the New York World's Fair. She and the other New York museum directors had volunteered to put their services and collections at the disposal of the fair, but the

exhibition proposals they put forth in 1936 were, after much stalling, turned down flat. The fair authorities decreed that there would be no art or fine arts building there—the individual fine arts institutions could hold their own shows on their own premises as adjuncts to the fair. When this decision was made public, it aroused the indignation of Paul Manship, whose protest was printed in the *New York Post* on January 24, 1938. Juliana, equally unwilling to accept the verdict, was the first to join Manship in agitation, and the only museum director who did so. She issued a statement to the *Post* stressing that the fair should sponsor a show of *living* American artists. Otherwise, Juliana declared, the directors of the fair "will indict themselves for lack of vision if they fail to put a democratically selected, representative contemporary American art show in Flushing Meadows in 1939." The pressure Juliana and Manship unleashed on the fair authorities was then increased by dealers and other artists.

While protesting the unfairness of the fair, Juliana quarreled with Faith and Edward Andrews, whom she had been so avid to help. The rupture grew out of the kind of misunderstanding that left her feeling wronged and to which she was excessively prone. In January, Anna Freeman, one of the Whitney secretaries, was making an inventory of Juliana's Shaker holdings. She wrote to the Andrewses asking what had become of some inspirational drawings that were in the Whitney in 1936 and then disappeared from South Salem after the May 1937 sale. Miss Freeman claimed that the drawings belonged to Juliana. The Andrewses countered that they were their property. They had stored the drawings in the museum in 1936 only for safekeeping and retrieved them when Juliana brought them to South Salem in May. Juliana probably forgot how the drawings got into the museum; more important, she evidently assumed that she deserved them after all she had been to the Andrewses. The view she held, which comes across so clearly in her letters to Carl, was that it was shabby not to repay kindnesses, preferably with a flawless act of generosity equal to the original gesture.

Juliana's fix on entitlement was well-entrenched by now, and it encompassed all kinds of situations, both abstract and concrete. If she lectured, she would tell her listeners, "Art is a gift, also a quest, and an achievement that must be earned by the artist." It also became one of her quirks to think that if she conceived a passion for a small object owned by someone, particularly if that someone was in her debt, it was fair to hint at her right of eminent domain. An impulsive and magnanimous gift giver herself, should she not once in a while be the receiver when an especially choice item caught her magpie's eye? Edward Laning once wore an eagle stickpin when he escorted Juliana to a social event. She looked pointedly at his tie and reminded him, "You know I collect eagles." After a soft "Oh," Laning handed it over. Dorothy Varian said that whenever Juliana spent any time at her house in Woodstock, she went on extravagantly about the beauty of a certain Wedgwood platter. After a while, Varian realized that Juliana wanted her to give her the platter. She did.

After an exchange of letters, in which Miss Freeman explained that "Mrs. Force sincerely believes that these drawings are her only tangible result of her large investment" in the Andrewses' work, she, not Juliana, called the couple

and demanded, "We must have the drawings!" The Andrewses tried to talk to Juliana, but she refused to speak to them. The Andrewses were not going to relinquish the drawings in the first place, but they surely would not have done so on the say of a third party. The couple never spoke to Juliana again.

The Shaker inventory was prepared because the private sale at South Salem did not attract too many buyers, and Juliana was letting Edith Halpert handle the collection. Halpert got in touch with Abby Rockefeller, her best client, who thought that Mrs. John D. Rockefeller III (Blanchette Hooker Rockefeller, who later became president of the Museum of Modern Art) might be interested. Halpert wrote to Blanchette Rockefeller:

> I can tell you in confidence that the collection belongs to Mrs. Juliana Force, director of the Whitney Museum. Your rug came from the same collection. Mrs. Force is greatly in need of money at the present time and we convinced her that it would be much more advisable to sell the Shaker collection as a group rather than break it up in single items at higher prices. No similar collection can ever be assembled as this—with few exceptions—represents the cream of the Shaker tradition. . . .

Blanchette Rockefeller bought the Shaker furniture, but afterward Juliana was dismayed by Halpert's conduct, which she saw as slick and unethical. Initially Juliana did not know, of course, the identity of Halpert's client, but her friends said that after she found out her collection was going to a Rockefeller, she felt that she had not received as much money as she should have from the sale. Then Juliana learned from talking to an antiques dealer in the South Salem area that Halpert had prevented him from acting as Juliana's agent by telling him one story and Juliana another. Halpert was caught in a lie that cut out a competitor unfairly, and Juliana never trusted her again. This time Juliana was not mistaken in concluding that advantage had been taken of her. The Andrewses probably didn't wrong her; Halpert probably did.

After these unpleasant transactions came another plea for cutbacks from Crocker. Once more, all purchases and operating expenses had to be entirely dependent on the museum's endowment income. In 1937, the Whitney ran a budgetary deficit of $17,925.02. (Most of the overrun went to security and salaries. Hermon More, as well as Juliana, got a raise, and Alice Sharkey, a capable woman who previously worked for the Treasury Department Art Project, was hired as an executive secretary.) Crocker recommended that salaries and running expenses be reduced and that no more art be bought. He also proposed an alternative demonstrating that he still had no idea of a museum's purpose— for every object bought for the permanent collection, another one should be sold from it. Crocker warned, "I hope that you and I can work this out in some way before Mrs. Whitney returns* because she literally has no more money to give the museum and if she makes up any deficit, it will be out of taxable income and that we cannot permit." Consequently, salaries and the number of exhibitions per season, beginning in the autumn of 1938, would be cut. The museum printed its catalogs on a poorer grade of paper, took fewer books and magazines,

---

* Gertrude was on a forty-day cruise to the West Indies and Latin America.

and scheduled fewer shows that required extensive travel or loans. Juliana estimated that these measures would save nearly $17,000.

However, no expense was considered too great by Crocker or anyone else concerned for Gertrude's contribution to the 1939 New York World's Fair. The amphitheater, courtyards, and gardens she had been planning with Ferriss and Gugler were scrapped, but she was one of several dozen sculptors offered a commission by the fair's authorities for a free-standing work. Gertrude designed a fountain decoration that she titled *To the Morrow*. (The overall theme of the fair was "Building the World of Tomorrow.") Two idealized nudes, male and female, backs arched, toes pointed, and "looking forward and upward, into the future," were poised on the end of a 24-foot-high rainbow-shaped support. Three spreading birds' wings, symbolizing aviation, flapped behind this promontory. (The sculpture was later renamed *The Spirit of Flight*.) The piece, an uncanny throwback to Hendrik Christian Andersen, was the silliest thing Gertrude had done since the Saint-Nazaire memorial. Its pretensions to modernity, technology, and progress were even more outlandish. To provide some perspective, in 1938, David Smith had his first one-man show, in which his epochal welded iron sculpture was exhibited. (Smith also coveted a World's Fair commission, but was not given one.) The fair was paying only a nominal sum to the artists —$2,500, plus some per diem expenses—but for the honor of being in the fair, Gertrude wound up spending about $16,500 to have her model enlarged in reinforced hollow plaster by the sculptor Leo Lentelli and surfaced in platinum leaf by Max Kuehne. The only contemporary element of the sculpture was the base, which was designed by Buckminster Fuller, who also worked at Gertrude's expense.

Although Gertrude's commission was scaled back to one composition, the Whitney's contribution to the fair was revived. Grover Whalen, the city commissioner for the fair and the president of its corporation, opted to avoid more controversy by agreeing to build a fine arts pavilion in Flushing Meadows. The new plans allowed 40,000 square feet for a huge hall of art that would house twenty-three galleries. Whalen then asked A. Conger Goodyear, the president of the Museum of Modern Art, to organize an exhibition of contemporary American painting and sculpture big enough to fill that space. More than 1,200 works would be brought together by artists from all over the country. Goodyear formed a governing committee and invited Juliana as well as Holger Cahill, Laurance Roberts (the director of the Brooklyn Museum), and Herbert Winlock, to serve on it. They then drafted nine artists, including Manship, Eugene Speicher, Stuart Davis, John Gregory, and William Zorach, to help them sort through the thousands of entries they would receive. The governing committee would establish general guidelines, set up regional selection committees, narrow down the final choices, and install their selections. Working on this awesome show —which involved an initial pool of 25,000 objects!—plus seeing *To the Morrow* through its successive stages, would occupy much of Juliana's time in the months to come.

Juliana was also watching over her nephews. She gave a cocktail party for the benefit of an acting company Allan Rieser was in, but she was unhappy

with him. Allan had the temerity to fall in love with Deborah Wood, a young woman he met in 1937, and they became engaged in 1938. Juliana was fuming about this, ostensibly because Deborah didn't understand how frail Allan was. Juliana had gotten it into her head that Allan should be treated as a semi-invalid, and she talked of him visiting a specialist for a revolting-sounding "cure" requiring enemas and a liquid diet. Deborah, who had a mind of her own, looked on Allan as the healthy young man in his twenties that he was. Juliana also worried about Allan and Deborah's ability to support themselves, since they were both in the theater. Allan had a day job, but Juliana didn't think his salary was enough for two. Here she had a justifiable anxiety about taking on another obligation, although any woman attempting to remove Allan from Juliana's control was a natural adversary. There was much head shaking about predatory women and unsuspecting young men being led astray by a pretty face. Allan wrote to Carl, "Aunt Julia writes me that she considers Duty a more dynamic force than Rights." Duty was defined as Juliana's very strong feeling about the way her family should behave.

Allan was given a breather when Juliana went off to Europe in June, on a trip that she said "was about as vagabondish as one could make it." The trustees voted her a $2,500 advance on her salary, and her first stop was Paris to see Three Centuries of American Art, a selection of 380 objects, with sections on painting, sculpture, prints, architecture, photography, folk art, and film, organized by Alfred Barr and shown in the Jeu de Paume. Juliana would have been one of the Modern's few partisans in the galleries because the French treated the show with flagrant condescension. Mrs. Barr described the experience as a "humiliation" for her husband. Did Juliana, observing the frigid reception by the Parisian audiences and art officials, recollect the similar fate of the Whitney's Overseas Exhibition in Venice two decades before?

Juliana then went to England for three weeks, followed by a run through the Third Reich, which had annexed Austria in March and was about to dismember Czechoslovakia. She had no qualms about holidaying there. Appallingly, although she detested the Nazis, Juliana did not put aside her pleasure for moral principle. She found Germany "the most stimulating and comfortable" of the places she had been. She wrote to Carl, "Thinking it might be some time before it could be done again, I made an interesting tour dividing my interests between music & painting. First Munich, Salzburg, then Bayreuth, Dresden, Berlin, Hanover & Bremen & then . . . to NY." Although Juliana chose to take her culture in institutions under Nazi control—and the museums, concert halls, and opera stages were thoroughly nazified by then—she was astute about one thing. The visit was the last she would make to Europe.

When Juliana got back to the United States in August, she was grumbling again about Allan and Deborah's engagement. Allan's fate, she warned Carl, would "be what four out of every ten marriages become—servitude." Relating that Deborah idly floated the idea of the two of them moving to San Francisco, Juliana wrote, "My heart failed me. San Francisco, the home of oranges and banality!" Presumably Juliana was alluding to southern California, but her sense of geography was as scrambled as her remarks were cantankerous.

After venting her complaints, Juliana did an about-face. It helped that she went back to work and the art world. She wrote to Emlen Etting on September 19, 1938:

> Life began again on the 15th & the paintings look good to me, like old friends. And that reminds me of you. So that wonder fills me and next week I plan to come to Philadelphia & hope you are there for me to see. . . . This week I'm off to Andover to see a Prendergast show* & to a dinner with old friends. . . . I love New England, all over, & more now since I can't have Bucks County, P.A. Have you seen the Charles Sheeler opus.† It's not good for a human body to have so much done about him and such a poor much. He pronounces against Ryder, Homer + Eakins, + loves Folk Art!

Juliana then bowed to Deborah and Allan's intention of marrying. Running exactly to form, she decided that if she were going to go along with their wedding, she was going to run it, no matter what the wishes of the bride's family were. Allan and Deborah would be married from Juliana's Victorian drawing room above the museum. Irene wrote to Carl after the the battle over the location subsided, "Score 1 for Aunt J. who didn't want a church wedding."

Juliana was not scoring so well on other fronts. At the museum, she tried to interest the trustees in *The Greek Slave*, which she was still holding with a deposit of $100. Florence Powers remained amenable about selling the sculpture, but Juliana's timing was poor. By the fall, the museum's acquisitions budget was, more often than not, exhausted, and any extra purchases required a special meeting and specific pleading.

Juliana's impatience with artists who took it upon themselves to be her critics rather than her friends manifested itself again in November of 1938. Three years before, a group of rebellious young painters, predominantly expressionist in tendency and without gallery representation, banded together to hold their own shows and perforce get the critics to notice them. The artists called themselves The Ten, but they were more commonly known as The Ten Who Are Nine, because a space was left open for a tenth invitee. The charter members of The Ten were Ben-Zion, Ilya Bolotowsky, Adolph Gottlieb, Louis Harris, Yankel Kufeld, Mark Rothko (then Marcus Rothkowitz), Louis Schanker, Joseph Solman, and Nahum Tschacbasov. In succeeding exhibitions, Edgar Levy, Lee Gatch, John Graham, Karl Knaths, and Earl Kerkam joined the group.

After five exhibitions, The Ten were being taken seriously. Their sixth show, held at the Mercury Galleries (located at 4 East Eighth Street, a quick trot across Fifth Avenue from the Whitney) coincided with the museum's current annual of contemporary painting, and the artists had an idea. In Solman's words, "We were young roustabouts. We wanted to speak our piece . . . and the paintings they [the Whitney] used to exhibit . . . looked as though they were done out of

---

* A retrospective of the work of Maurice and Charles Prendergast, put on by the Addison Gallery of American Art.

† In 1938, *Charles Sheeler: Artist in the American Tradition*, by Constance Rourke, was published. The contribution Juliana, the Whitney Studio Club, and Forbes Watson made to Sheeler's career went unmentioned.

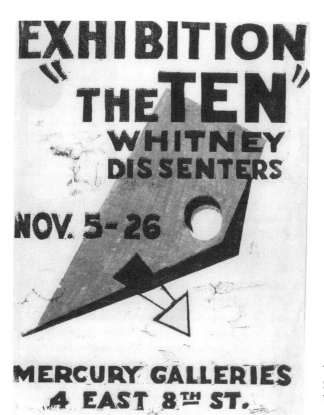

The poster made by Louis Schanker to advertise the Whitney Dissenters show, 1938.

a painful duty." The Ten challenged the museum, defiantly titling their exhibition The Whitney Dissenters and publicizing it as an equivalent of a Salon des Refusés. Schanker, a skilled woodcut artist, made a Whitney Dissenters poster that could be plastered all over the Village. The painters also put out a broadside accusing the Whitney of being overly supportive of the cornstalk and the hayseed. The Ten condemned "the reputed equivalence of American painting and literal painting" and declared that "the symbol of the silo is in the ascendant at our Whitney Museum of modern American art."

The Ten's playing off the Whitney in 1938 was no different from The Eight's playing off the National Academy of Design in 1908, but Juliana could not recognize the parallel or take the more liberal or detached view. Whereas ten or fifteen years before she might have been on the side of the dissidents and gone along with the joke, she wrote them off as malcontents, saw their brashness as an attempt to seize the scepter from her, and defended her institution with a heavy hand. She needed artists to need her, so she was always stung by any form of reproach.

The irony of the "dissent" was that Bolotowsky was in the very annual from which he was supposed to have been so unfairly excluded, and Schanker, Graham, Kerkam, Knaths, Levy, and Tschacbasov had already been in several

Whitney shows between them. Thus the indignant protests of some of the group had a hollow core. Bolotowsky, who agreed to be in The Ten's show before he was asked to the annual, later admitted that he thought the Whitney displayed "extreme tolerance" toward him at that time. Juliana could have charged the artists with the museum's exhibition record if she had only thought carefully about the matter. Instead, she reacted impetuously, and fired off an angry letter to the Mercury Galleries as soon as she read about their impending show. She wrote:

> The New York Art Calendar lists this week at your galleries an exhibition "Whitney Rejects" by The Ten, a title which rests upon the false assumption that the paintings exhibited were rejected for exhibition in our Museum. As we have repeatedly stated, no work is submitted to a jury for inclusion in our exhibitions, which consists only of works by artists whom the Museum invites to participate. We, therefore, must request you to change the misleading title of your exhibition to one more consistent with the facts. "Paintings by Artists Not Invited to the Whitney Museum Exhibitions" would be a truer description of the character of the show, and would meet with our hearty approval.

If part of The Ten's objective was recognition from the Whitney, it was successful, because someone from the museum—probably More or Goodrich—did take note. Gottlieb and Schanker were invited to the 1940 and 1941 annuals. Rothko, however, did not exhibit at the Whitney until 1945, after he had been shown by Peggy Guggenheim, but in fairness to the museum, his work was unimpressive before the mid-1940s.

It was like Juliana to be haughtily quashing opposition at one moment while showing her capacity for tolerance at the next. If she did something that made her look old and tired and outmoded, she habitually seemed to follow it with a word or a deed that illuminated her quickness and curiosity. Juliana alienated certain up-and-coming artists by her abrasive and autocratic behavior, but she genuinely enjoyed cultivating the young, and she could win their gratitude for her embrace of the unconventional. About the time Juliana was earning the enmity of Rothko and Solman and Gottlieb, she was befriending and encouraging Betty Parsons, who in the ensuing decade would become the dealer and champion of many of these artists. Parsons, who looked up to Juliana, said, "I believed in Juliana Force one-hundred percent. She had a great mind in a Victorian age. She was so *positive*, and she had a terrific integrity. I admired her courage, but I was scared of that slashing wit. She wasn't in any way impressed with anything except for great causes and high standards."

The artist Maud Morgan, from whom Juliana bought a painting in 1938, observed:

> She was a very dynamic woman, so I'm sure there were many people who rubbed her the wrong way, but she was extremely open to anyone who interested her. When she cared, she was completely open and she let you be open with her. I had an apartment over a shoe store, and Juliana would come for lunch there. I remember her asking me about what I was doing, and I said I couldn't talk about it or I would lose it. She was very understanding about that.

Isamu Noguchi also benefited from Juliana's openness at this time. In 1938 Noguchi designed the *Radio Nurse*, a short-wave radio transmitter for home or hospital in the shape of a female head, for Zenith Radio Corporation. He believed that the design had aesthetic merit and argued that it deserved evaluation on those grounds, but the only one who would back him was Juliana. She made sure that *Radio Nurse* was seen in the latest annual of sculpture, drawings, and prints, which would open in January of 1939. From then on, Noguchi thought of Juliana as "courageous and outspoken." He later was to say:

> Juliana Force was a formidable lady who seemed to have more imagination and spunk than most people. My regard for her grew as her regard grew for me. She agreed to show my *Radio Nurse*, a commercial product, in a regular art show, which, to my knowledge, was the first time that was done.
>
> The *Radio Nurse* grew out of the Lindbergh kidnapping case. Zenith Radio, then a big, successful company, asked me to design an intercom system so that a parent or nurse could listen to a child's breathing anywhere in the house. They wanted it in the shape of a nurse's hat, but I designed it as I did. I told Mrs. Force about it, and she immediately agreed to show it.

Juliana went out of her way to welcome a young stranger who needed guidance through the mazes of the art world. A Kansas art patron named Louisa Murdock had bequeathed money to the city of Wichita to establish an art collection, with preference given to Americans. The trust went into effect in 1938, and Murdock's friend Elizabeth Navas (then Elizabeth Stubblefield) was given sole authority to form the collection. Miss Stubblefield moved to New York and, although acquainted with no one there, she did know a name— Juliana Force. Juliana was extremely interested in the contents and future of the Murdock collection, as she was in all ventures that strengthened the prestige of American art. Elizabeth Navas remembered:

> I just wrote a note to Mrs. Force and said briefly what I was about to do and, if possible, I would like to see her sometime. I immediately got a note—imagine that!—saying to come and have lunch with her. I went down to the Whitney for lunch and I said I'd been to the Macbeth Gallery. She asked me if I knew any other dealers. I said no. And she answered, "Then I will proceed to tell you about them."
>
> She told me one by one exactly what she thought of every art dealer in New York. I can't remember all these remarks, but I do know that she sat there straight up like a ramrod with her hands folded and simply lectured.* Well, of course, she gave me the most marvelous information, and it turned out to be accurate. I feel I owe her a debt because of that introduction she gave me to the art world.

Navas also said that Juliana steered her toward paintings by Hopper, Burchfield, and some other artists from the Rehn Gallery, but the overriding message was to buy American. The two women maintained a friendly relationship in succeeding years. Juliana may have identified with Navas as a younger version of herself, breaking ground in a section of the country that was still wary of modernism. While Wichita accepted pictures by Eakins, Sloan, Luks, Maurice

---

*This was the pose Peggy Bacon portrayed in *The Ugly Duchess*.

Prendergast, Hopper, and Marsh, Navas's subsequent choices of Hartley, Davis, and Horace Pippin were considered new and daring—and a little bit dicey.

On November 23, 1938, Allan and Deborah were married at 10 West Eighth Street, after several tense scenes between Juliana and the bride's mother, who was said to be Juliana's equal in ferocity of purpose. Irene wrote to Carl after the ceremony was over and he had gone back to school, "Haven't seen Aunt J. since the wedding. Maybe she just doesn't want to see anyone again, as long as she lives, and for that one can hardly blame her." Watching Allan begin his own life away from her, Juliana felt insecure, and two days after the wedding she went out and bought something on impulse to assuage her anxiety. But being Juliana, her idea of an impulse buy was a 1780 house on twelve acres of property in Shelton, Connecticut. Besides representing an extra financial burden, the house was inconvenient, although she could tell herself that she would be near Charles and Eugenie Prendergast, with whom she had become very friendly and who lived in western Connecticut. Juliana, reacting to displacement by replacement, gratified herself with the pleasure of risk. She could still summon up the wherewithal—the house cost about $10,000—and energy to create yet another splendid environment for herself and her friends. Irene wrote to Carl, "It just doesn't seem possible she is buying another house. But then you never can tell."

By the evidence of Gertrude's diaries, the breach between Juliana and Gertrude was completely healed by 1939. Gertrude had worked hard to patch things up, and Juliana had forgiven the indirectness and aloofness, trusting her as wholeheartedly as she had during the old days. Gertrude was especially cognizant of Juliana's value, despite Crocker's campaign to denigrate it. She would write to her sister later in the year, "You say I have accomplished something this winter. . . . The museum I am very proud of, but without Mrs. Force it never could have been accomplished. Other things are largely a question of money." The two women talked almost every day in January about some aspect of the World's Fair, just five months away.

Juliana also had business of a much less agreeable nature. Now that she had another house to pay for, her finances were once more in arrears. She could give Carl only $100 toward his tuition and, as she had done before when about to put up some of her possessions for sale, she spoke wistfully of the need for graciousness in one's life. There was no choice but the auction block, and two sales were conducted at Parke-Bernet Galleries. The first, which was held on February 10 and 11, consisted of European furnishings that had come from the farm and were in storage at South Salem. If this had been the only sale, it would have been seen as a little housecleaning and pruning. However, at the second sale, which took place a week later, many more items—including some of Juliana's dearest American finds—were offered. So much had to go: the Sandwich and Bristol-blue glassware that dazzled Gloria Vanderbilt, the Queen Anne, Windsor, and Hitchcock chairs, the tavern, drop-leaf, and threshing tables, the eighteenth-century pine and maple furniture, the Philadelphia lowboy. Nothing

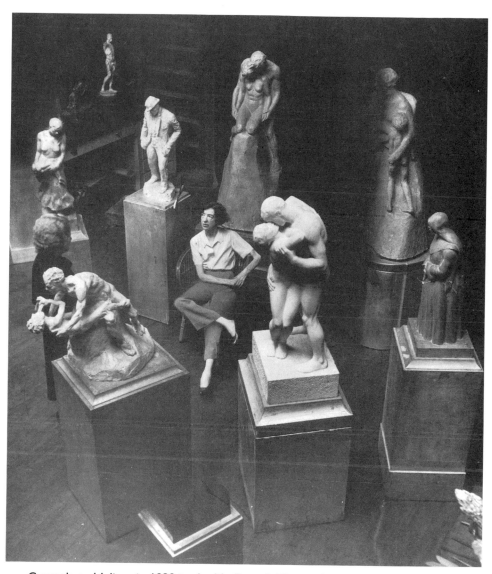

Gertrude and Juliana in 1939 in the MacDougal Alley studio in a telling pose. Juliana saw to it that she and Gertrude were not photographed together unless it was unavoidable. On those rare occasions, Juliana would turn her back to the camera or stay to the side, giving Gertrude the spotlight.

was exempt—twenty-four rare hooked rugs in animal, floral, and geometric patterns, and fifteen quilts were also for sale. The quilts were a hard sacrifice because Juliana recognized them as a brilliant native art form. "I think quilts and bridges are the best things Americans do," she said. Even more disheartening was parting with the majority of her nineteenth-century provincial paintings,

about forty of which were sent to Parke-Bernet. The most prominent buyers were the New-York Historical Society and Abby Rockefeller, who would present her purchases to the folk art museum she was establishing in Williamsburg, Virginia. The sales netted Juliana $20,000, but she was not one to watch the material traces of her life being dispersed with the fall of the hammer. She was out of town during some of the sessions. Afterward, Juliana sent Carl another tuition installment, but not as much as she hoped, because "taxes are due the 15th & I am scraping everything together so that I will not go to jail."

In March, Juliana and Gertrude were acting on plans to alter the Whitney building. The museum had acquired hundreds of objects since 1931 (at a cost of $203,681), over 700,000 visitors had passed through its molded glass doors, and the exhibition areas were cramped. When a temporary show was on, the permanent collection could not be displayed, and in the middle of March the museum closed for renovations. The main construction would be the addition of four galleries, but the front entrance and stairways were broadened, and the lighting system was overhauled.

The New York World's Fair opened on April 30, 1939. In the weeks before, Gertrude and Juliana made many trips to supervise the progress of the site in Flushing where *To the Morrow* was supposed to stand. On April 29, they went to the fairgrounds about noon and did not get home until the late hours of the next morning, but the sculpture was in place. Gertrude skipped the opening, but both she and Juliana were readying themselves for two other ceremonies. On May 25, a fine, sunny day, *To the Morrow* was unveiled. Mayor La Guardia declaimed rousingly about the sculpture, and Gertrude, who ended up having several other works besides this one representing her at the fair, started dropping by there every few weeks for pleasure.

American Art Today, the show Juliana had fought the fair authorities to bring into existence, opened on June 1. As official hostess, she sent out 2,500 invitations. About half of them went to artists, friends, and colleagues in the New York area, and 500 were expected to be at the dedication. Juliana considered her part in the affair important enough to skip a family funeral. Her brother Joseph died at the end of May, and his burial took place on June 1. Juliana went to her sister-in-law's house in New Jersey, but did not go to the family plot in Doylestown for the interment because it conflicted with the reception. Her brief appearance was accepted by the rest of the Riesers without comment or resentment. The fanfare in New York was supposed to begin at 4:00 P.M. sharp, with Grover Whalen introducing La Guardia, who would open the exhibition, followed by short orations from Goodyear and Cahill. La Guardia's speech was very different from his ode to *To the Morrow*. William Zorach recalled his words as a "condemnation of everything modern and calling it distortion. I looked at him, this little man with his big head and his great long torso and his stubby legs—like a piece of African sculpture—up there talking about the distortion of the human figure in modern art. It was fantastic." But almost everyone involved with American Art Today agreed that their efforts were worthwhile, as 1.5 million people reportedly went through its galleries.

Juliana had Gertrude's ear so steadily that it was no wonder one of Gertrude's grandchildren sought help, in much the same way that Gloria Vanderbilt had approached her eighteen months before. Gloria's best friend among her Whitney cousins was Gertrude (Gerta) Henry, the daughter of Barbara Whitney and Barklie Henry. Gerta, like Gloria, was restless and discontented, and, again like Gloria, she realized that Juliana would be her best ally. Gerta was fourteen and wanted to study art. Her parents had already refused her, but Gerta knew that if Gertrude overturned their verdict, they would accept it. Gerta wouldn't risk making a direct proposal to her grandmother, who she surmised would turn her down, so she confided in Juliana. Juliana then spoke with Gertrude, who overruled the Henrys. Characteristically, it was not Gertrude, the artist and the blood relative, but Juliana who volunteered to take the time to look into Gerta's art education. She suggested taking Gerta to Provincetown, Massachusetts, to survey the summer art schools. Juliana, Gerta remembered, was familiar with all the art schools and artists on the Cape. They visited painters from Jerry Farnsworth and Wayman Adams to Hans Hofmann, whom Juliana greeted as an old friend. (Hofmann was a neighbor of hers. In the winter, his classes were held at 52 West Eighth Street.)

Gerta was beguiled by her traveling companion because from the moment they boarded the train, Juliana treated her like another grown-up, and one who interested her greatly. In Provincetown they went to a little café that served artists, summer people, and Portuguese fishermen. "Juliana was outgoing and effervescent and a great drinker," Gerta Henry (now Gerta Henry Conner) said. "She had a few stiff drinks, and in the middle of dinner she noticed one of the sailors. She said to me, 'Are you looking at that man? He looks just like Jean Gabin. Isn't he attractive?' Then she wrote a note to the man asking him to join us for drinks at our table." To a fourteen-year-old in the middle of a fascinating experience, as Gerta was then, Juliana would seem "totally without snobbery—so bohemian and free from convention, so unlike my mother and father." An adult analyzing the episode in retrospect might draw the conclusion that Juliana got drunk and was without judgment.

By the end of her trip, Gerta knew she wanted to study with Hans Hofmann and returned home to get permission. Her parents vetoed the idea, and this time they were the final arbiters, but Gerta remained touched by the interest Juliana took in her. "She went out of her way to be kind to me, and her intervention was a lifesaver," Gerta Conner said. "She was extremely sympathetic to a young girl, and she spurred me on. Later, when I got married and went to Peru, she took the trouble to write to me. She wrote to me until her death."

Gerta adored Juliana after this jaunt together, but the senior Henrys felt otherwise. Juliana was behind Gertrude's intervention in the raising of their child, and her trusted position also aroused feelings of jealousy among the Whitney children—a state that already had been fomented by Crocker. That Gertrude seconded Juliana as frequently as she did fed into his portrait of her as a usurper and a servant who had gotten out of hand. Juliana's intercession for Gerta was yet another proof of her terrible influence. At a family gathering,

when Gerta happened to say that Juliana didn't get enough credit for the museum, the rest of the Whitneys were aghast.

After delivering Gerta to her parents, Juliana rented a cottage in Little Compton, Rhode Island, where Lloyd and Edith Goodrich always summered. She looked at several places with a realtor before taking an old and austerely furnished house. The Goodriches knew that Juliana was not going to like the property, but the prospective tenant pronounced it perfect. Edith Goodrich remembered her exact words as "I'm not going to change a thing." A day or two later, Juliana rolled up in a station wagon packed with leopard throws, fringed lampshades, pillows, stools, chests, and chairs. The stern interior of the house was soon transformed.

Juliana hadn't spent much time at her house in Shelton, and by now she was able to admit how foolhardy she had been in taking it on. She put the house on the market and sold it on August 4, for roughly $3,000. Juliana emerged several thousand dollars poorer from this misadventure, but since she was now free of a mortgage, her extravagant spirit would get the better of her. Nothing gave her more pleasure than making the exquisite gesture, even when she could ill afford it. About this time Juliana became close to Hardinge Scholle, the director of the Museum of the City of New York. Scholle had a penthouse apartment with an empty terrace, of which Juliana made note while visiting. One hot summer's day, a van pulled up to the building. The driver delivered a set of wicker furniture to Scholle's apartment, unloaded it on the terrace, and handed him a card. It was from Juliana, wishing him a Merry Christmas in advance. "Gratitude," she confided to Carl Rieser, "is a terrible word, but . . . graciousness is a beautiful quality."

Juliana had to be in New York for much of August to supervise the final touches on the remodeling of the museum, so she saw a lot of Gertrude, who was in the country at Wheatley Hills and at the World's Fair. The two women may well have been in each other's company on September 1, 1939, when Nazi troops invaded Poland and swept away Neville Chamberlain's assurances of peace in our time. After Britain and France declared that a state of war existed between them and Germany, Gertrude and Juliana discussed whether or not they should reopen the museum and hold their party for it. The answer, they decided, was to go on with their jobs, especially in this case, which was to rejoice that "American art had outgrown housing conditions once deemed quite adequate."

The expanded Whitney Museum, with 288 works from the permanent collection on view, was the setting for two celebratory luncheons. The first, which took place on September 11, was for artists. The second, a day later, was for trustees, museum directors, curators, dealers, and critics. Of the division of the party in two, Forbes Watson wrote, "That the artists took precedence over the trustees in the order of the entertainment was in accordance with the Whitney Museum, where the painters and sculptors have always held first place. As Juliana Force . . . said last spring, in a brilliant speech before The American Federation

of Arts, she owes her most valued knowledge to the artists and the Museum owes them everything."

At both gatherings, Gertrude impressed on her listeners that in a time of world crisis it was more important than ever "to cling to the things of the spirit." Juliana, with her eye on the art she and the curators had chosen to display and the impending reviews of it, was heard to say, "When you judge pictures, remember that the pictures, in turn, are judging you." This was a distillation of a speech Juliana sometimes used with museum visitors, in which she cautioned, "You cannot 'laugh off' a work of art, neither can you destroy it with your scorn. It will live on, enriching life, but it may be that the picture you disregard, your children will rise up and call blessed."

Now that the museum was reopened with the appropriate glory, the two women went looking for a new Manhattan residence for Gertrude, who no longer wished to live by herself at 871 Fifth Avenue. Furthermore, Crocker was making noises about the expense of enlarging West Eighth Street and the carrying costs of the Whitney mansion, which she scarcely inhabited. A smaller place downtown would suit Gertrude better at this stage of her life, and she and Juliana found two connected carriage houses at 58 and 60 Washington Mews, the row of nineteenth-century stables behind the magnificent Greek Revival houses of Washington Square North. The Mews, a small, privately owned and maintained lane paved with cobblestones, equaled MacDougal Alley in quiet, seclusion, and picturesque appearance. Gertrude bought the houses at the end of September, and after the deal was firm, Juliana went to southern Vermont and other artists' haunts in New England for a rest and to fulfill her annual duty as bartender (she shared the job with Charles Sawyer) at the fall show of the Southern Vermont Artists Association.

In October, Gertrude and Juliana began working on the decor for Washington Mews. Juliana gave Gertrude her Victorian tester bed: Its curlicues and lacquered mother-of-pearl insets would be resplendent in her new bedroom. She also introduced Gertrude to John Gerald, an interior designer married to the painter Elizabeth Bart, and he was hired to redo the Washington Mews house. Gerald collaborated with Juliana on the scheme; she was most involved in decorating a room for Gloria Vanderbilt, who would be living with Gertrude during the school holidays. When they started talking about Gloria's room, Juliana pulled out a scrap of silver foil spangled with little blue stars—it had been the wrapping paper around a piece of Perugina chocolate. "What about this for the wallpaper?" Juliana said. "I think it's absolutely perfect, and she'll adore it." Everyone was in agreement and taken with Juliana's ingenuity,* but Gerald thought it couldn't be done. " 'Can't' just fired up Juliana," John Gerald remembered. She said, 'Jack, I want to paper Gloria's room with this,' and I had to track down the makers in Italy to find it." The foil was only 18 inches wide, nicked every time

---

* "Surprise" introductions of silver foil that once graced a bonbon as wallpaper were in truth already in Juliana's repertoire as both a design stunt and a piece of theater. She had covered an upstairs room at Barley Sheaf Farm with a silver and turquoise foil that she first saw wrapped around some Easter candy.

someone's fingernail brushed against it, and, said John Frear, Gerald's assistant, "was hell to put up," but the effect was as magical as everyone had hoped. A gilded handmade bed by Max Kuehne highlighted the delicate palette of silver, blue, and lavender. Juliana was sorry for Gloria, although there was little she could do about it. All Juliana could give to Gloria now was her gift for creating lovely surroundings.

Gloria, who first saw her room at Christmas and didn't know that Juliana had a hand in its confection, later wrote:

> I fell in love with this room and forever after tried to recapture it, but it was hard to define and has always eluded me. . . . It had to do with the two french doors . . . framed by curtains of taffeta of palest lavender spilling from the ceiling onto the floor in pools of silk and rustling across the windows at dusk in a most seductive way. . . . But most of all it had to do with scale, with the use made of space, with the silver tea-papered walls, with the day bed gessoed with water lilies and white butterflies, with the shape of the Venetian bureau between the windows painted with gilded winged creatures, and on it resting a crystal flacon of Chanel No. 5—my first perfume and a present from Aunt Gertrude.

Planning and bringing to completion this shimmering room for young Gloria was great fun for Juliana, as was any act of embellishment or largesse. She had been frustrated in the latter sphere lately, but now that her nephews had reached the stage of being married and through with school, she started doing more for artists again. Juliana couldn't resist lavishing her money on people because living that way was part of her own art, her own creativity. She would have agreed with Robert Frost when he wrote, "In art, politics, school, church, business, love or marriage—in a piece of work or in a career, strongly spent is synonymous with kept." Indeed, Juliana had already made that discovery, and was invariably true to it unless prevented by the most straitened circumstances.

In September of 1939, for example, Stuart Davis wrote to Juliana about his lack of money and asked if the museum would buy a painting. A purchase would make it possible for him to rent a studio, teach an art class, and be independent of government art projects. "You could," Davis said, "get a good picture and return an artist to private industry at the same time." The Whitney's budget was exhausted, as it usually was toward the end of the calendar year, but Juliana asked him to leave a few examples of his latest work with her secretary. "I want to do anything that is possible to help," she wrote, "because I realize the position you are in, and sympathize with your desire to be free and self-supporting." A few months later, Juliana bought a picture—*Radio Tubes**—for herself. Although her friends applauded her spirit, they worried about her inability to rein herself in. After Juliana sent Henry McBride a check for something, he lectured her as follows:

> It's outrageous and I shouldn't allow it—for I know perfectly well you are reimbursing me from your private funds. . . . Why haven't I a strong character? But anyway you haven't either, Juliana, or you wouldn't do these things. Whenever I think of you,

---

* Now in the collection of Arizona State University, Tempe.

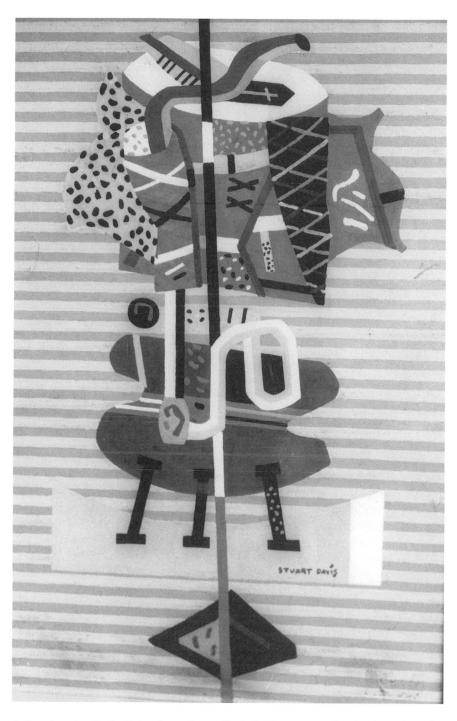

Juliana bought *Radio Tubes* from Stuart Davis for her personal collection when the museum had no money to acquire a work for the institution.

which is often, I feel, as the late Geo. Grey Barnard would say, "two spirits struggling within me."* One is love and admiration for the goodness of your heart and the other is a Scotch horror at your extravagance. I have the secret conviction that you and all the Whitneys will end up in the Poor House, though this doesn't distress me so much as it might for the Poor House† is only three miles away from my Pennsylvania house and then we shall be neighbours. . . .

Just the same it's outrageous!

McBride wrote to Juliana on October 26, 1939, at about the time she was doing what she could for two other suffering artists. Her first effort was simple —an invitation to John Flannagan for the 1940 sculpture annual—but thinking of him had special meaning. In 1939 Flannagan was struck by a car in a hit-and-run accident and had to undergo four operations to relieve the pressure of blood clots on his brain. He left the hospital with a metal plate in his head, and his coordination and speech were heavily impaired. He was not expected to sculpt again, but he was determined. As he was no longer strong enough to carve stone, he learned to work in metal. For Flannagan, drowning in a sea of troubles, any professional encouragement was buoying. He wrote to Juliana from Boston, where he was living temporarily:

> I had hoped to be able to come to the preview of this year's Exhibition of Contemporary American Art—but alas, it seems impossible. One might as well be in South Africa as up here. However, the surgeon who cut my head down to fit me has at last decided to allow me to return to New York and work, so I expect to be there soon and hope to see you.
> I sent in a bronze because it was the one major thing I had. . . . After last summer, I feel like starting all over—as I shall do now in a new medium. . . . Now I still feel unbeaten by circumstances and am going to fulfill another sculptural purpose by working for a complete mastery of metal. The sculpture I sent for your show is the beginning.

Juliana's second activity involved the rescue of Louis Eilshemius. William Schack, Eilshemius's first biographer, discovered that three dealers—most prominently, Valentine Dudensing, but also Henry Kleemann and Philip Boyer, the unscrupulous Philadelphia dealer—had exploited the old painter's physical decrepitude and hunger for recognition. They praised him highly, bought his pictures at a pittance, and emptied his studio. They were selling the canvases at great profit, while Eilshemius was living like a beggar. That October, Schack went to several influential museum people of conscience with his story, including Phillips, Barr, Baur, and Juliana. The New Yorkers immediately united and agreed to exert pressure on the offending dealers. Juliana, who was furious at their shabby behavior at the expense of a pathetic old man, took the lead in pursuing the miscreants. Edward Laning remembered, "She had to have a cause. She had to have battles to fight. One night she didn't want to go to sleep, and she kept me at her apartment all night telling me about poor Eilshemius.

---

* The American sculptor whose *Struggle of the Two Natures in Man* was a fixture at the foot of the grand staircase of the Metropolitan Museum of Art.

† Henry Varnum Poor, a painter and ceramicist.

When she learned what Dudensing had done, she was outraged. She went to Francis Taylor [then the director of the Worcester Art Museum, and an active writer and polemicist] and told him, 'You and I are going to do something about this,' and he listened to her. If Dudensing didn't make an adjustment with Eilshemius, they were going to expose him."

If a threat like that was made, it was in earnest, as anyone who knew Juliana could attest. "Juliana Force didn't want power, but what it conferred," said Allene Talmey. "She could get other people to do what she wanted, but she had aims and principles." Juliana's independent mind, her reputation as a stand-out executive, and her apparent invincibility in the art world led Talmey to select her as the subject of the first of several profiles she was writing for Vogue about New Yorkers in the public eye. Juliana was her first choice for the inaugural article, which would be published on February 1, 1940; she took precedence over the next person the magazine wanted to cover—Wendell Willkie. Juliana seemed like an impregnable little fortress to Talmey, and it was on this occasion she let slip the fibs about her genteel background in Bucks County, her teaching in a private school in New England, and her going to work for Gertrude as a girl barely out of her teens. Talmey didn't realize that Juliana was dependent on a colorfully embroidered family myth for protection and self-esteem. By now, of course, these invented origins were not social pretensions to Juliana, but truths, and therefore she was firm about them.

When Talmey spoke to Juliana, which was at the end of 1939, she noticed that "despite the enormous disparity in size, prestige, and years of operation between the two museums, Mrs. Force had as much influence as the director of the Metropolitan Museum of Art." Early in 1940, Juliana heard from Herbert Winlock, whose health had been fragile for some years. He really had been too ill to go on with his job, but months elapsed before a successor was found. On January 13, Winlock wrote to Juliana that Francis Taylor was about to become the new director of the Metropolitan.

Taylor's arrival in New York meant the enriching of a friendship that had been developing between Juliana and him since the middle 1930s. Their banding together to help Eilshemius was only the latest of many cooperative ventures. Taylor, born in Philadelphia in 1903, was only thirty-six when he was named to the premier job in the American museum world, but his reputation as a prodigy was already secure. Educated at the University of Pennsylvania, Princeton, and the Sorbonne, he had been an excellent curator of medieval art at the Philadelphia Museum of Art and a dynamic director in Worcester. His main goal at Worcester was to make the museum an important factor in the life of the city, and he succeeded brilliantly. Taylor originated exemplary loan exhibitions that were enormously informative but never pedantic, and he did un-heard-of things, like showing foreign films in the museum's auditorium.

Taylor was not only cultivated and erudite, but an enemy of the stodgy and the possessor of a puckish charm. Of medium height, heavyset, with dark eyes deep in their sockets and a great hook of a nose, he could have passed for a Borgia prince. Taylor not only looked as if he had stepped out of a fresco by

Raphael or Mantegna, but he had the expansive appetites of a voluptuary as well. His friend George Biddle, who saw him often in his Philadelphia days, said that Taylor "was such fun over drinks and such fun telling dirty stories. . . . He loved good food, good drink, and was deeply intelligent about everything in the world . . . he was life-enhancing." Biddle summed up Taylor by saying, "He had great charm, he had a touch of genius, and was a naughty boy."

Juliana and Taylor were fun to listen to when they were together. Charles Sawyer said that the two "had a great personal rapport. They were both critical, they both enjoyed raising hackles, and they were both irreverent, with sharp tongues that frequently got the better of their judgment." They also shared the feline pleasure of gossip and amused each other with risqué asides. Although some of his colleagues were offended by Taylor's humor, which featured an endless fund of off-color stories and metaphors, Juliana, who also had a racy side, liked his bawdiness because it was done with remarkable mental agility. Riding in an elevator in the IBM building when a female passenger was pinched and let out a loud yelp, Taylor quipped, "I'm delighted to see that some things around here are still being done by hand."

There was also a comradely exchange after a meeting among museum directors. Juliana, Taylor, and Monroe Wheeler, then the director of publications at the Museum of Modern Art, found themselves on the Boston–New York train together. Taylor steered their conversation in the direction of childhood nicknames. Wheeler related, "Francis said to me, 'I noticed that someone called you Monnie. Is that your childhood nickname?' I said yes, and that everyone who has known me for a long time calls me by it. I asked Juliana what her childhood nickname was. 'They used to call me Ju-lee,' she hissed through clenched teeth."

Now that they had confessed, Wheeler and Juliana turned expectantly toward Taylor.

"Satchel ass," was the instant reply.

For all their camaraderie, Juliana and Francis Taylor had some grave professional differences. They had disagreed at least twice—first on the apportioning of salaries to artists during the PWAP and, second and more seriously, on the issue of rental payments to artists. Juliana didn't think much of Taylor when he opposed rental fees, but she respected his work as a museum reformer. The two stayed friends, even though Taylor remained tough and adamant about drawing the line between art and artists. "There's no special virtue in something because it's been done by someone you've shaken hands with," he stated, and sometimes he went so far as to imply that artists were little more than necessary nuisances. In time, this disparity in philosophy would prove fateful.

Juliana was sixty-three years old to Taylor's thirty-six, but he was the more conservative of the two. Audrey McMahon, whose friendship with Taylor was as enduring as her rivalry was with Juliana, would remark on his lack of confidence in living artists during the 1930s. "With the exception of the Whitney you couldn't get a living artist into a permanent collection [then]," McMahon said. "Even an up-and-coming person like Francis Henry Taylor who was director

of the Worcester Museum never bought for his collection. He wrote about American art. . . but so far as I know, he never bought anything of the contemporary artists. . . . He did understand it, but he didn't risk money on it."

Juliana was limber compared to Taylor. The contrast in attitudes is best seen in their treatment of Stuart Davis, who wrote to Taylor on May 19, 1940. He asked if the Metropolitan would consider buying one of his paintings and enclosed photographs of nine of them. Davis addressed Taylor as the standard-bearer of the new at the museum, but in that assumption he was mistaken. Whereas Juliana, because the Whitney could not assist him, bought a picture for her personal collection as soon as she could, Taylor didn't give Davis a second thought. He dictated an impersonal reply telling the artist he was passing his material on to "the proper committee," which was a euphemism for saying he was going to forget all about it. The reproductions were dumped on Harry Wehle, the museum's curator of painting, along with a one-line note indicating (facetiously, one hopes) that Taylor had not heard of Davis. "Herewith," went the entire letter, "some curious examples of ultra-modern art." Needless to say, with a recommendation like that, nothing by Davis was acquired by the Metropolitan.*

On January, 24, 1940, Juliana and the industrial designer Walter Dorwin Teague, who was one of the guiding spirits of the World's Fair, were the guest speakers at an annual dinner given by the American Institute of Decorators. Because of her passion for decorating and her friendships with decorators, this was a natural thing for Juliana to do, but it exposed her to malicious criticism. Forbes Watson was one of several men who thought she was too much the patroness of decorators, which is to say that he disliked her closeness with effeminate homosexuals. Forbes wrote to Alice Sharkey, whom he looked on as his mole in the museum, about persuading Juliana to put on some historical exhibitions on the evolution of American taste. He wanted to get Juliana "genuinely interested in working on the problem [of organizing the shows] herself. There would always be the danger in the earlier exhibitions of just being *too too* entertaining. That danger must be avoided or the Museum will look as if it had been given over to our sweet boy decorator friends."

Juliana also was blasé about homosexual camp, which, if it simply irritated Forbes, stunned more sheltered types not used to the freer thought and language of the bohemian world. One evening she was caught at a dull dinner given by someone who lived on the Palisades, across the Hudson from New York. From the terrace, a bored Juliana looked at the lights of Manhattan in the distance. They were beautiful, and as she watched, her spirits began to revive. Then a woman rushed to her side, engulfing her in chitchat. Seeing that Juliana was absorbed in the view and inattentive to her, she gushed, "Oh, Mrs. Force, isn't

---

*The Met bought its first Davis—a gouache—in 1948, and that was through Whitney auspices. No painting was acquired until 1953.

New York a veritable fairyland?" "Yes," Juliana replied with mock solemnity, "it is, surely. But I don't see how you can tell from here!" That was a conversation stopper in those days, when no one in polite society alluded to the common slang for gay men.

In February, as he always did, Crocker demanded—and was about to receive—more budget cuts. The museum was deeper in the red because $20,000 had been invested in what turned out to be worthless World's Fair bonds. The fair lost millions of dollars, and its investors were not repaid. The real losers from the investment in the fair were Ned Archer and Karl Free, who were dismissed as of June 1, 1940. Archer, it seems, was fired only because money was scarce. The case of Karl Free was different.

After war broke out in Europe, Juliana, who cared dearly about England, became active in raising money and collecting clothes for British war relief.* She eventually became the chairman of a British war relief fund in New York, and at one point the Whitney was a depot for Bundles for Britain. Free's sympathies, however, were with the Nazis. Edward Laning, who knew Free well, said of him, "He thought that the Germans had received a terrible deal after World War I, and consequently he was pro-Hitler." Free wisely concealed his political views on the job, but he had a self-destructive streak, and he was fed up with Juliana. As he saw it, she was a tyrant and a peacock, and her feminine frivolities were getting on his nerves. When Juliana asked him to design a poster for British war relief, it was an invitation to calamity. In the words of Laning, whose account came straight from Free, "The poster showed the map of England, which he had distorted into a broken-down old horse with its tongue lolling out of the side of its mouth. She was enraged. He couldn't have done anything that would make her angrier." Free's timing was horrible—the poster was made in May of 1940 when the Allies were in disarray. Free later wrote to a friend that his dismissal was his own fault, without going into the details of it. He committed suicide after the war ended. Archer, who remained bitter about his firing, left New York, and thought the worst of Juliana.

The revelation of Free's politics was not the only brush Juliana had with clandestine Nazi involvement. Her servants at Shaker Hollow were a couple (a butler-handyman and a housekeeper-cook) who acted as caretakers in her absence. When Juliana wanted to go to South Salem, either she or her secretary would telephone in advance so the housekeeper could have everything ready by the time she got there. This was the protocol, followed without variation, until one time when Juliana was in Connecticut visiting Charles and Eugenie Prendergast, and the three of them went for a ride near Shaker Hollow. Juliana suggested they stop by the house, but when she rang the bell, the housekeeper opened the door, saw Juliana, slammed the door in her face, and locked it. Juliana was flabbergasted, but ran around to the side of the house and entered through another door. Inside, she couldn't believe her eyes. Her own living

---

* Privately, Juliana sent food parcels to her old friends and neighbors in Haddenham throughout the war.

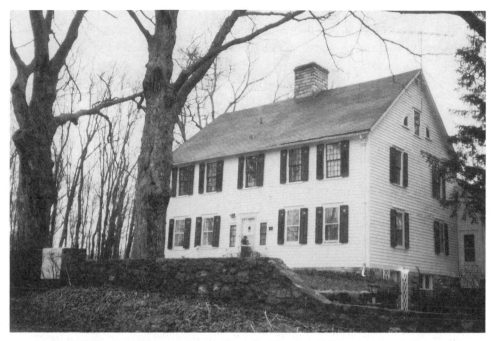

Shaker Hollow, located on a quiet country road in South Salem, New York, was an isolated spot.

room was draped with Nazi flags, and pictures of Adolf Hitler hung on the walls. Juliana ran upstairs, called Rob Rieser, told him what had happened, and asked him to get the police and the FBI. The couple was holding meetings of the German-American Bund in Juliana's house. Shaker Hollow, an isolated house on a quiet country road and in the possession of an absentee owner who obligingly warned the caretakers of her appearances, made an ideal meeting place. The FBI later informed Juliana that the house was also being used as a Bund mail drop. That is, mail from Germany was entering the country addressed to her. The servants' besmirching of her name caused Juliana great worry. She told Eugenie Prendergast that, despite her innocence, she was afraid she would never be able to clear her name if the story came to light. Juliana was primarily concerned about the power of the written word, whether true or false, to tarnish a reputation forever. But she also knew very well that she stood a greater chance of being accused of disloyalty because of her German ancestry. She had done her best to bury that information, but any investigation could exhume it.

Juliana spent most of June raising money for the Red Cross and working with Gertrude on the possibility of making *To the Morrow* into a permanent piece of sculpture that would be installed at La Guardia Airport. She was also looking forward to a two-week swing through the Midwest and Southwest during which she would see shows and meet artists. At the end of July, Juliana was in Chicago, visiting the Art Institute and Daniel Catton Rich. Next she went to New Mexico, beginning with Albuquerque and then moving on to Taos and Santa Fe. She was a guest of the Sloans, who had been summering in Santa

Fe since 1919, and she also stayed with Josef Bakos, an artist who lived there all year. On August 4, Juliana was in New York again and wrote up her impressions for Gertrude:

> I have visited 5 museums & discussed problems . . . with as many directors, but they have all taught me lessons never learned at School. . . . I have paid for it all, as the woman always pays, but would not exchange my experience for 10 times the cost. Thank Heaven, I long ago learned the cost of nothing & the value of almost everything. And all the while the conviction deepens that politics & policies are of supreme importance in a world where there must be so many differences but where, linked together, there must result the closest harmony.

Juliana returned to a cottage with the enchanting name of My Faith Looks Up to Thee. She had rented again in Little Compton, and this time the house she chose, centered on a pretty lawn and looking out on the ocean, suited her perfectly. My Faith Looks Up to Thee was a tranquil spot, but it was close to entertaining company when she was in the mood for it. Besides the Goodriches, the painter Molly Luce and her husband, the art historian Alan Burroughs, had a house there, and Katherine Schmidt, now married to Irvine Shubert, a lawyer for the Hilton hotel chain, was a regular renter. That season Emlen Etting and his wife, Gloria Braggiotti, took a house; they spent the summer making a movie starring Juliana. There were interesting people outside the art world that Juliana liked having over for the evening, too, such as June and Joe Platt. She was a food writer and the author of several cookbooks; he was a scenic designer who had worked on *Gone With The Wind*.

Juliana had a halcyon summer, but even with the Whitney commencing its fall season by marking its tenth anniversary, she was not lighthearted. She clashed once again with Crocker over basic principles. Juliana would say countless times that the Whitney stood for the buying and showing of American art, yet he was doing his best to curtail both. Crocker was strangling the museum's initiative. In her words, "How can we have a future for American art, if we have no present?"

When Juliana remarked to Gertrude in her letter about the woman paying, as she always did, it was her way of saying that she made some purchases during her summer travels. Her acquisitions were inexpensive—watercolors by Carl Ruggles ($100) and Ward Lockwood ($150), a print by Kenneth Adams ($40), and a drawing by Andrew Dasburg ($35). Moreover, the total spent on art for the entire year of 1940 came to a skimpy $2,170—a sum embarrassingly under the $20,000 that the artists had come to expect. This marginal showing, as well as the loss of Archer and Free (who were not replaced), meant that the museum had, in essence, given up on its departments of prints and drawings. In consequence, the Whitney was operating on a scale unworthy of its mission. But those sorts of arguments made no dent on Crocker, and he forbade Juliana to spend any money on art. She did buy, he upbraided her for disobedience, and she had to give an account of her actions. From a letter of October 1, 1940:

> I am sorry you feel I had forgotten your instructions in the matter, but this is what I had intended to tell you.

In the exhibitions which I visited this summer . . . there were opportunities to buy at low price works of art which we needed. The other Museums were on the job and I felt that this Museum had to take some practical cognizance of these occasions. Knowing this beforehand I enlisted the cooperation of my staff, asking them to make definite sacrifices of time and energy toward saving some money which I felt we could use for purchases. Our efforts resulted in the saving of $800.

I am not so sure that it was right for me to expect so much from my staff, but I do know that I cannot do it again, in justice to myself and the Museum. . . .

There is an obligation now on the part of the Museum to enter again the purchasing field, even in a small way, and it has been my chief anxiety these past months. Very soon I should like to take the matter up with you.

Juliana did not meet with Crocker until she had talked to Gertrude about the dispute. When he again attempted to put the brakes on acquisitions, he was jointly told that the Whitney's prestige and influence would suffer. After he saw that Gertrude had taken sides, there was nothing for him to do but come up with a compromise. Gertrude donated more stock to the museum, and the hostilities ceased. But Crocker's setback was not permanent, and he still enjoyed Gertrude's full confidence. Moreover, he was now fanning an ongoing flirtation with her. His letters were addressed to "Dearest Gertrude" and "Darling Di,"* and he flattered her about her writing, which she had begun to pursue again.

The autumn of 1940 brought Francis Taylor's full-scale entry into the New York art world when President Roosevelt asked him to head† a national council to launch Art Week. A booster drive for artists to augment the WPA, Art Week was an extravaganza with the modest goal of placing a work of American art in every American home. This blitz of aesthetic appreciation, which spawned 1,500 art exhibitions around the country, was to be observed from November 25 to December 1, 1940, and Taylor, who was extremely proud of his presidential appointment, threw himself into publicizing the event. He asked Juliana, Barr, Scholle, and Audrey McMahon to work with him on it. As might be expected, Americans did not rush out en masse to buy pictures hot off their local artists' easels, and Art Week, earnestly patriotic, was not exactly a triumph for its organizers. But only the *Daily Worker* advanced the theory that Art Week failed because of the feud between Juliana and Audrey McMahon. Even for that publication, accusing those two of bungling was a wild smear. Regardless of their quarrel, both women wanted American artists to survive, and neither could count incompetence as one of their sins.

After France fell and combat intensified abroad, European artists were in jeopardy. The lucky ones obtained exit visas for America and waited out the war in New York. Their presence would have an unprecedented effect on the local talent, but Juliana's immediate concern was helping more of these men and women to reach the United States safely. Juliana hooked up with the New

---

*An allusion to Diana, the autobiographical heroine of a pseudonymous novel Gertrude wrote in 1932, *Walking the Dusk*.

†George Biddle suspected that Taylor hatched the idea of Art Week and sold it to Roosevelt with himself as chairman.

York–based Emergency Rescue Committee, the valiant group responsible for arranging the escape of more than 1,000 artists, writers, publishers, and political dissidents from Nazi-occupied countries. In November of 1940 she was organizing a meeting on the subject of artists who were trapped in Marseilles and desperate for ships and exit visas, and later she donated and solicited money. Juliana asked emigré artists and Americans who had lived in France for long stretches of time to assist her. On her personal list of contacts and advisers were Salvador Dali, Guy Pène du Bois, Paul Manship, Amédée Ozenfant, Yves Tanguy, Virgil Thomson, Jo Davidson, and Fernand Léger.

That winter, in a patriotic venture loosely classified as war preparedness, Juliana worked with Nelson Rockefeller, who, like Taylor, had received a presidential appointment. Roosevelt desired better relations with Latin America in the event of war, so in August of 1940 he asked Rockefeller to advise the State Department in devising an effective goodwill program. He was appointed Coordinator of Commercial and Cultural Relations among the Americas, which was later shortened to Coordinator of the Office of Inter-American Affairs. Rockefeller proposed shipping art exhibitions around Central and South America. Roosevelt liked the idea, and Rockefeller turned to the New York museum community for expertise. He wanted to send out several exhibitions of contemporary art, with the first one to leave in May of 1941, at the end of the New York season. Nelson Rockefeller, backed by Washington, was not to be refused, and the directors of the Modern, the Metropolitan, the Whitney, the Brooklyn Museum, and the Museum of Natural History all pledged to assist him.

Their work began in December of 1940. The art historian Stanton Catlin, who later became a museum director and an authority on Latin American art, was fresh out of graduate school and had the job of secretary to the committee. He remembered Juliana as the most outspoken person on it. After the first meeting, Juliana realized that she did not like the exhibition plan as it stood, so she telephoned John Abbott, the executive vice-president of the Modern and a man distrusted for his slyness and tale carrying. Abbott would not take the call and made Catlin answer her. "I had a long and very difficult conversation with her," he said. "She was criticizing the plan of the exhibition in a very strong way. She was mad, and she wanted to talk to Abbott—I was just a functionary. She spoke her piece, I listened and answered in an understanding voice. Everyone was hovering outside my door to hear what she had to say. Alfred [Barr] understood her. He listened in his stoical, unemotional way, and when it was finished, he said, 'Good! She's let off steam.' "

The exhibition, Contemporary North American Painting, did become a reality, and seventy-five of the Whitney's best paintings and watercolors—making up one quarter of the exhibition—were lent in the name of inter-American solidarity. The pictures were on tour for a year; they were seen by over 218,000 people in ten cities. Aaron Bohrod, who was in the exhibition, saw Juliana during the run of the show, and recalled that "she wasn't an image of feminine delicacy. She told me, 'Your work [images of rustic, ramshackle buildings] is famous in South America. They call you the Master of the Outhouse.' "

With a new year, money for purchasing was replenished, and Juliana did not hesitate to use it as soon as 1941 dawned. Artists she believed in were in distress, and she could not ignore their misfortunes. Stuart Davis was in the hospital in January, with no money to pay his bills, so Juliana deputized Lloyd Goodrich to pick out a painting for the museum. He selected *House and Street*, a rigorous compression of a corner in lower Manhattan, for $500; she told Davis that she would try to get him a mural commission. Later in the month, David Burliuk wrote to Juliana because his wife had slipped and broken her wrist. He couldn't pay the hospital bill of $54, because, aside from the rare sale of his work, his income was $7 a week. Two days later, he was asked to bring in some paintings and watercolors. The watercolors were priced at $25 each, and Juliana bought two of them for the Whitney.

To benefit the needy of New York, she took complete charge of an endearing exhibition called This Is Our City, a cumulative portrait of artists' observations of the metropolis from 1900 to 1940, which opened on March 11, 1941. The theme was one close to her heart, and was both a crowd pleaser and a subject that challenged most artists to do their best. The exhibition also constituted a farewell to some of the Whitney favorites before they were shipped to Latin America. To make her survey of New York views and impressions complete, Juliana dispensed with her pride and wrote some personal and deferential letters to Alfred Stieglitz, asking him to lend three watercolors by Marin. Stieglitz was cordial in his letters and generous in his loans. He not only gave her the Marins, but paintings by Demuth and O'Keeffe. The show was for a good cause, and Hermon More later guessed that Stieglitz had mellowed a little toward Juliana and the Whitney. The museum had proved itself a staunch if overgenerous champion of American art, his first love, and Juliana's conduct toward Lachaise had been admirable. And although purchases of his artists were not what he would have liked them to be, Marin, O'Keeffe, and Dove were consistently invited to Whitney shows.

Juliana hung over 200 works and surrounded them with the fussy, charming props that she loved. A toy dog was installed near a hydrant, spring flowers bloomed in little carts, and hurdy-gurdies were put in the galleries. Juliana treated the show as an occasion for old-fashioned fun in a tense world, and at the opening reception on March 10, Gertrude and Newbold Morris, the president of the City Council, pulled up to the museum in a hansom cab. The opening also drew Robert Moses, Clare Boothe, James Farley, and Francis Taylor, and 15,000 other people saw the show before it closed.

While This Is Our City was on, John Sloan went into the hospital for major surgery. Juliana heard that the Sloans needed money after that, and she went to Kraushaar's and bought *The Picnic Grounds*, one of Sloan's first fully realized genre scenes, for $2,000. This purchase was followed up by a trip to Philadelphia on April 6, 1941. Juliana went to see Robert Carlen, a young art dealer who represented Horace Pippin, one of the great self-taught American artists of this century. She bought *The Buffalo Hunt* for the museum for $250—a high price for Pippin's work then—as well as a painting by Earl Horter. For herself, she bought a painting by the twenty-nine-year-old Mervin Jules, for $105.

Just before going to Philadelphia, Juliana made headlines for a controversial speech she made. On March 18 and 19, 1941, she was in Washington for a meeting of the American Federation of Arts, which was held in the newly opened National Gallery of Art. She, along with Watson, Daniel Catton Rich, Cahill, and Taylor, were to give speeches on the topic "Can Americans Support an American Art?" The usual bromides were expected and, for the most part, delivered, but Juliana dropped a bomb.

In the eye of the art establishment and with Cahill and Watson, the program's most important spokesmen, in the audience, Juliana, still well-known as a former federal art administrator, blasted the WPA art program with electrifying candor. She charged that it destroyed initiative and produced mediocre art. Her primary target was the WPA, but something else was at work, too. Juliana was fed up with sentimental pity for artists, or persons calling themselves artists, as opposed to the dignified, no-nonsense benevolence she practiced. In line with her view that art was a gift and an achievement that should be earned, Juliana also liked to say, "Don't let anyone pity an artist. Artists are the most fortunate people in the world. They should be proud of themselves." The WPA was not her style of charity, because its coddling subverted pride. Before a group heavily larded with WPA bureaucrats, she declared:

> The Government now gives any man who says he can paint $18 or $21 a week. The basements of our public buildings are littered with the results. Or the administrator finds a blank wall—any blank wall in a public building—and says, "Do you want a mural on that?" The officials say yes—they don't dare say no.
>
> Friends of the Project argue that they have found four or five good artists among the thousands helped, but I believe these would have been discovered anyway. You can't keep a real painter from painting.

Juliana insisted that she was not against the government encouraging artists—she merely disliked the manner in which it was done. After a compliment or two to Ned Bruce and his Treasury Department art competitions, she made it clear that she thought the system should be changed. "I want so much for [American] art to be a part of the important changes that lie before us. Why can't the Government buy the works of contemporary artists, as the French Republic did?" Juliana queried. "Why is American art considered so poverty stricken that it has no museum capable of taking the leadership in a Federal art program?" Juliana was cutting through her audience like a buzz saw with these unpopular ideas, but she persevered with them. "I am glad," she concluded, "that there is no veneration of contemporary American art. What I should like to see is respect—and respect, you know, is founded on knowledge."

In Washington, this address, which criticized Cahill and Watson, won her few friends. After a New York paper asked her to repeat her statements for print, outraged artists picketed the Whitney for two days. Juliana, unfazed, managed a few contemptuous words for them and went on with her work. As one of the Whitney secretaries said of her, "She never gets tired. She has so much ammunition." Malapropism or not, the remark was apt.

Juliana went out of her way to accept speaking engagements, both for the

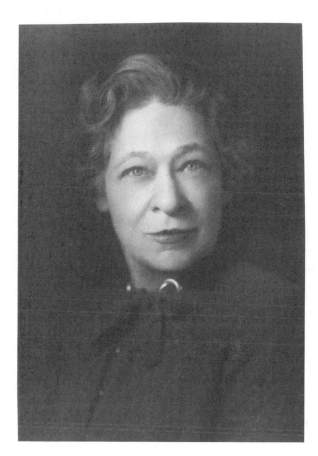

Juliana, ca. 1940–1941, in a
portrait she distributed on
the lecture circuit.

sake of her own reputation and for the further réclame of the Whitney. She was
a popular lecturer, not so much for the content of her remarks, as for the spirit
and energy with which she delivered them. Dr. Kathryn McHale, the general
director of the American Association of University Women and a personal friend
of Juliana's, was entranced by her stage presence and manner of speaking and
described them evocatively.

> Anyone who had ever heard her speak in public had had the certain proof of Juliana
> Force's creative power. When she spoke formally, she had compelling speaking style.
> Her thoughts came into speech in a way which showed perfectly how she was able
> to receive a work of art. The contralto voice, musical, clipped, or conversational at
> will, conveyed thought with the color of the expressionist; wisdom deep in the body
> arranged the thoughts with the precision of the abstraction; the temperament flung
> out overtones of strangeness and mystery; the American vein of bitterness or
> laughter—learned where the rocks are hard—added a line of black, or a surrealist
> image. She was a cryptic speaker because she was almost casually profound. The
> listener had to draw something up in himself to understand her, but even her everyday
> talk twists still in the memory.

Allan Rieser believed that the commanding impression his aunt made was also tied up with "the firm grace and definition with which she performed simple acts—like playing cards or writing a letter, or cutting the pages of a new book. It was always done with the neatness of a rehearsed piece of business on the stage." Juliana, he said, once "cooked a lunch for Deborah and me at South Salem—an extraordinary episode because I think it was the only time I ever saw her in a kitchen. I particularly remember lamb chops, which she explained must always be fried in a little salt—and she did just that, with a wonderful economy of time and motion, as if she'd done nothing else in life. She said to me once, apropos of the Depression and so forth, 'I don't worry, because if there were a revolution, I could always scrub floors. Of course, I would do it very well.' Of that, I was certain!"

In July and August, Juliana was in and out of town. In between trips to Woodstock and Manchester (the latter visited in the company of Royal Cortissoz), she was working on the winter painting annual and worrying about Gertrude, who was not responding to her letters and calls. Instead, Gertrude was engrossed in a futile attempt to collaborate on a Gothic-horror play in Westbury with a resident ghostwriter who, from his sycophantic letters, was doing a lot of sweet-talking and sponging. In addition, Gloria Vanderbilt was disobeying her orders by dating older and unsuitable men—that summer she was going out with Van Heflin. As in the past, Gertrude was unable to communicate with her niece, so she reacted by hiring private detectives to spy on Gloria and Heflin. Gertrude's woes as a guardian, in conjunction with her poor health, led her to reconsider the future, and she conferred at length with Crocker about her estate.

When Juliana saw Gertrude in September, she learned the reason for her silence and doubtless suspected Crocker's connivance in it. Gertrude, in anticipation of the time when death would remove her from overseeing the museum, pondered its fate. She did not think the Whitney could survive on its own unless she bequeathed it more money than she and Crocker thought prudent. However, the museum might live on without her if it were sheltered and absorbed by another institution. She was ready to make overtures to the Metropolitan and the Museum of Modern Art.

Juliana's initial reaction to Gertrude's decision is unknown, but it had to have been one of distress and disbelief. After her head cleared, she told Cortissoz, the critic Gertrude most respected, the story. Not just she, but all the artists needed his help. Could he, a distinguished third party, write something to Gertrude that would keep her from going through with this awful arrangement? Cortissoz saw what had to be done and wrote to Gertrude on October 7, 1941:

> Yesterday when I was calling for Juliana she told me—in a confidence which, knowing me, you will know that I will respect—about the idea that had been broached concerning the Whitney. I mean the idea of it being affiliated with either the Metropolitan or the Modern Museum. Dear Mrs. Whitney I cannot forbear begging you *not* to entertain such fanfaronades. The Whitney has its own roots, its own traditions, and must continue to stand for its own past. Let the beautiful work you and Juliana

have been doing go on under your own banner. The Whitney is not so much a museum as it is a studio, with a character, a personality, which must never be changed. You know how I sympathize with it. I would hate to see its individuality lost. I hope I don't seem intrusive to you. Just think of this letter as simply coming from your friend.

Cortissoz's plea had some effect, because on December 2, 1941, Gertrude declined an invitation to become a trustee of the Metropolitan, a preliminary that would set in motion the transfer of the collection. A stay of execution was granted. It may have been lengthened by the bombing of Pearl Harbor and the uncertainty over what the Japanese attack would mean for the country.

Juliana was under obvious duress at this time, but she went on imperturbably, almost majestically, in matters great and small. Florence Cramer attended a Whitney opening (a memorial exhibition for Emil Ganso), and said that going was "a strain, but I loved it and Mrs. Force was grand and did everything to make it as easy as possible." And when she had so much on her own mind, Juliana changed someone else's life by her capacity for appreciation at, of all places, a fashion house. Juliana was a sporadic client of Mainbocher, the American-born couturier who left Paris during the war and reopened his business in New York. Genevieve Rindner was hired by Mainbocher in 1941 to build the stand-in figures for his customers, and she had reason to remember Juliana. In her words:

> When I was fitting her, all over her small body, she pulled me up (I was kneeling with pins in my mouth) and said, "Child, do you know that you are a sculptor?" Of course, it had never crossed my mind that being able to duplicate the human figure was in any way related to "Art." I was just making a living. Or trying.
>
> Mrs. Force insisted on writing a letter of introduction so I could gain entry to the Clay Club, which was on Eighth Street next door to the Whitney and run by a Miss Dorothea Denslow. . . . However, it took me several months before I could get up enough nerve to join the Clay Club [and take up sculpting]. . . . The fact that I never made the big time in sculpture does in no way ever diminish the satisfaction that I derive from the one or two pieces I do a year, and I'll always be grateful for Juliana's push. Call it guidance if you want. In the interim, I married a fellow sculptor and we had two daughters, so you see how Juliana Force took my dull life and put it in the direction it went.

While devoted to the process of uncovering new artists, Juliana did not forget the older ones. Once more, John Flannagan was asked to exhibit his sculpture at the museum, but his reply was tragically despondent.

> Thanks for your letter. Sorry, but alas, whatever I have is large only in *spirit*. I don't feel the need for mere physical size (mis-called bigness).
>
> Perhaps I'm too sure within myself to feel the need of *shouting* when I could whisper. Jesus and Gautama did with far more to say than I shall ever have.

Flannagan's letter, written in December of 1941, was one of his last. He killed himself on January 6, 1942.

Juliana was cognizant that the Whitney's role as a leader was in danger of being diminished by Crocker's animosity toward her, Gertrude's misgivings about the future, and the certain encroachments the war would bring, but she did what she could to maintain the museum's prestige. A history of American watercolors, covering the years 1800–1941 and the first such survey ever to be presented, opened in early 1942. The show was difficult to mount, because protecting their collections against enemy attacks was of substantial concern to museum directors. Nazi U-boats had been sighted off the Atlantic coast, and the German high command made threats about bombing New York. For instance, in answer to Juliana's request for some loans, Duncan Phillips wrote, "We have been sending some of our most valuable paintings to museums in the middle west for safe keeping during the danger from air raids. And as I consider New York even more dangerous than Washington I really should not be lending you those very distinguished water colors [by Demuth, Luks, Alfred Maurer, and Maurice Prendergast] you asked for. However, I find it difficult ever to say no to the Whitney Museum and to you personally."

To make up for the Whitney's recent neglect of prints, Juliana, after hearing that Carl Zigrosser had received a Guggenheim Fellowship to write a book on American prints, asked him to organize a roundup of twentieth-century American printmaking, which became Between Two Wars: Prints by American Artists, 1914–1941. At the party for him and the artists in the show, Zigrosser said of Juliana, "She has an excellent technique as a director—she picks her persons and lets them go ahead. There is one other thing I should like to reveal about Mrs. Force, something I have found out about her. She likes artists. I found that out 25 years ago. But that is not all: She still likes them, and that is a real miracle."

Juliana also demonstrated her esteem for artists through the furtherance of scholarship. When Lloyd Goodrich informed her that forgeries of American paintings were on the increase and outlined other problems in determining authenticity that he was encountering, she gave him her blessing to form a central information bureau that would become the American Art Research Council. "Although she really had very little sense of art history," Goodrich said, "she took advice about it very well. I had been involved with Ryder, and with all the forgeries—there were about five fake Ryders to every genuine one—I could see how serious this problem was. I talked to Mrs. Force about this once, saying that we should form a body to consider questions of authenticity in American art. I proposed quite an elaborate set-up, and she took it up just like that. It was not at all the kind of thing she was used to, but she saw the necessity and virtue of it and she wanted to be in on it and organize it. I happened to have this idea, and it had expanded to the point of my saying, 'Let's do something about it,' but she activated it. You gave her an issue and she knew immediately what she wanted to do."

In February 1942 the American Art Research Council was established at the Whitney, with Juliana as chairman and Goodrich as director. The council would function as a clearinghouse and registry; its primary objectives would be to locate

and identify American art, separate the genuine from the spurious, and make permanent records of selected American artists of the past *and* present. "We ended up gathering more information from living artists than anyone ever had done before," Goodrich said. "We worked with Hopper, Kuniyoshi, and about fifteen other artists, asking them to give us lists of their work. Our lists for O'Keeffe, Prendergast, and Davis were the biggest records ever made of those artists. In the end, we had about 25 other museums and college art departments participating on the advisory committee for it. Mrs. Force was very proud of it, and it gave her a standing with the other museum directors. The research council became one of her great interests."

The American Art Research Council was predicated on a belief in the Whitney's retaining its independent existence, but Gertrude was again in doubt about that. In late February or early March, she asked Juliana to speak with trustees of the Museum of Modern Art about the possibility of affiliating. From what can be gathered from the few terse notations extant, the representatives from the Modern either did not want the Whitney collection at all or wanted the right to accept only certain works from it. Whatever the conditions set, they did offer a piece of land adjacent to the Modern on West 54th Street if the Whitney wished to relocate. Nothing about the deal appealed to Juliana, who said as much to Zigrosser while his print show was up. "I remember," he wrote, "that on one occasion Mrs. Force had some caustic comments to make about the manoeuvres of museum directors for 'handouts' without equivalent commitments."

Gertrude did not like the sound of the offer, either, and the Whitney's union with the Modern was moot. Juliana went back to mobilizing on the art front with various morale-building schemes. She and Paul Manship planned a future exhibition and auction for the benefit of Russian war relief. She removed a group of watercolors and prints from the museum's collection and presented them as decoration for Army camps and hospitals. When she heard that artists in basic training had no art supplies and couldn't paint during their spare time, she sent them easels, paint, and other studio equipment. At the end of March, Juliana confronted a bleaker reality. The Metropolitan was putting many of its greatest treasures into storage in the event of bombardment, and Francis Taylor offered Juliana space to house 100 Whitney paintings. She would have to respond to his thoughtfulness soon.

Any action would have to wait for a time, because Gertrude was frighteningly gaunt, overtired, and coughing steadily. On April 7, 1942, on the advice of a heart specialist, she checked into New York Hospital for an examination and tests. After a few days, her doctors thought she was making a recovery and were optimistic about her prognosis, so Juliana saw no reason not to hold the first meeting of the American Art Research Council on April 11. Sixteen people convened in her drawing room, including Barr, Goodrich, More, Scholle, Rich, Roberts, Taylor, Edgar Preston Richardson of the Detroit Institute of Art, and Theodore Sizer of Yale. Juliana was all smiles for her guests because the response to her letters was overwhelmingly enthusiastic, and by the end of the discussion, Juliana and Goodrich had the moral support of everyone in the room. Taylor

was the first to say that the identity and sovereignty of the council should be vested in the Whitney, but financial support was not so quickly pledged. If Juliana had been powerful enough to prevail, she would have underwritten the entire project, but her trustees had already informed her that it was impossible. The museums involved would have to subscribe to the council. Working out the responsibilities for funding seemed to be the one real stumbling block for Juliana and Goodrich in an otherwise gratifying day.

But the search for that solution was about to be overshadowed and engulfed. On Wednesday, April 15, Gertrude's condition worsened. She was diagnosed as having bacterial endocarditis, an infection of the heart valves that can cause clotting. On Thursday, an unremovable blood clot went into her upper arm, and on Friday she was so weak that she could hardly speak. At 2:50 A.M. on Saturday, April 18, 1942, Gertrude Whitney breathed her last.

CHAPTER ELEVEN

THE LAST
ADVERSARY

🌼 *(1942–1948)* 🌼

G ERTRUDE'S DEATH, sudden and without warning, was prelude to sweeping and hostile changes for Juliana. Gertrude was not only her employer and friend, but her protector and, even after all these years, the source of much of her power. Gertrude's passing gave Crocker's vindictiveness a license, and the Whitneys themselves closed ranks against the outsider without delay. What was surprising was not that these things happened, but that they happened in such a hurry.

Juliana's changed standing was evident within hours of Gertrude's death. On April 18 and April 19, the body rested in 60 Washington Mews, and the family received relatives and friends. Juliana was grief-stricken by the loss of the person to whom she had devoted herself for thirty-five years. It was noted with disapproval that, unlike Gertrude's relatives, Juliana shed tears. B. H. Friedman, echoing the fatuity of the Whitney point of view, wrote, "Outside of the immediate family, none seem more crushed by her [Gertrude's] death than Juliana Force and Gertrude's personal maid Hortense. They weep freely, expressing their emotion more openly than is permitted by Vanderbilt standards of control." It was not accidental that Juliana was bracketed with a servant, for servitor was the position to which Crocker hoped to relegate her.

Gertrude was buried on April 20, 1942, at Woodlawn Cemetery in the Bronx. The funeral service was held at St. Bartholomew's, at 51st Street and Park Avenue. Floral tributes filled the chancel, and between 700 and 1,400 people were reported to have attended. Lloyd Goodrich said that "everyone in the art world was there," and among the other mourners were family members, leaders of New York society, and a number of doctors and nurses who had staffed her field hospital in France. One of the hymns that was played at the service was "Fight the Good Fight," and none was more apposite for Juliana. Two days after the funeral, Crocker made a formal appointment to confer with her. Her first

436

thought was to organize a memorial show of Gertrude's work as quickly as possible; his was to undermine her authority. Crocker was eager to get rid of Juliana, but for the time being he settled for reminding her of her reduced role. Her office happened to be in the 8 West Eighth Street building, and Crocker questioned whether or not she should continue to use it; because the office was connected to the MacDougal Alley studio, the space was redefined as being part of Gertrude's personal property.

Juliana experienced more shocks when Gertrude's will, which had been drawn up by Crocker, was read. The gross estate was $11,049,838; Gertrude left the museum a legacy of $2.5 million, and forgave any outstanding indebtedness. She left the 8–14 West Eighth Street buildings to her daughter, Flora Miller, who might conceivably sell them. Juliana did not receive the million dollars she might have expected would be hers, but she was bequeathed $50,000, and she gladly adopted Comet, Gertrude's long-haired dachshund. The money Juliana got was still too much as far as the Whitneys were concerned. Although Gertrude's own words in the will were "my friend, Juliana R. Force," B. H. Friedman, once more indicating Juliana's status in his account of the estate, began a new paragraph with, "Smaller gifts include $50,000 to Juliana Force; $15,000 to Marie Pfitzer, Gertrude's personal maid before Hortense; $10,000 to her chauffeur, Fred Stone; and $20,000 to be divided among other servants, including Hortense."

The most revealing aspect of the will for Juliana had to be the clause directing the forgiveness of debts owed. The principal beneficiary was Sonny Whitney, who had borrowed over $2.5 million from his mother, but the second greatest debtor was Crocker, who owed Gertrude $428,518. (The museum, in contrast, had a forgiven debt of $182,895.) If shrewd financial calculations had been at all in her nature and if she had invested in tangible assets rather than people, Juliana would have profited more if she had borrowed extensively from Gertrude instead of selling her houses and possessions. Instead, Crocker taxed Juliana, who had taken advances against her own salary for her personal expenses, with overspending, while he, who was in a position of fiduciary responsibility and trust, had borrowed an enormous sum of money from his client and fixed it so that he did not have to return a cent.

Another provision of Gertrude's will decreed that the remainder of her estate should "be devoted to such charitable and educational purposes including the encouragement of art, as my children shall determine to be most worthy and deserving." Since Sonny Whitney was in the air corps and Barbara Henry declined to be involved in executing the provision, Flora consulted Juliana. She advised that since the Whitney mansion at 871 Fifth Avenue was to be torn down and its contents were shortly to be sold at auction, an excellent first gesture would be to offer certain museums—and here, Juliana was in the luxurious spot of rewarding the generous and teaching the uncooperative a lesson—their first choice of furnishings and fixtures. Fiske Kimball, the director of the Philadelphia Museum of Art, wrote in a journal he kept, "The museums which had cooperated with the Whitney, of which we were fortunately one, were named to the executors [Crocker and Flora] by Mrs. Force—the Metropolitan, Philadelphia, Chicago,

Cleveland, and Worcester—and we were asked first to indicate our preference among major items." Kimball, who was an expert in eighteenth-century decorative arts, picked out and was given a set of four Beauvais tapestries woven in 1761, and he later secured an Italian ceiling. As Francis Taylor had been his protégé in Philadelphia—Kimball once introduced the 200-pound Taylor at an art museum directors' meeting with, "Here he is, my little boy, Francis"— Kimball noted precisely what the Metropolitan took: "a pair of French Renaissance tapestries, a chimney piece of the same period and some intarsia doors and wainscoting."

Juliana was trying to readjust to her sad new state. She could not bear to see Gertrude's name and telephone numbers staring up at her from her address book, so she furiously erased every entry as well as she could. She received letters of condolence from artists and museum directors who knew that she had suffered a devastating loss. A good many sympathizers suggested that Juliana's grief might be tempered if she preserved Gertrude's faith in American art through its embodiment, the Whitney Museum, as if they sensed that there was harm afoot. Royal Cortissoz, who knew intimately of the Whitney's narrow escape from the Metropolitan's clutches less than a year before, exhorted Juliana not to lose heart. He reminded her of Gertrude's

> reliance upon you in the future of the Museum. For it is . . . your guidance of that she count[ed], as upon a strong rock. We all do. And you must know with what warm sympathy I shall continue to back up your doings. It is a great thing to continue her monument. You will do it magnificently, with love and with wisdom. I wish you success with all my heart.

Gertrude had wavered about continuing her monument, as Juliana knew, but she never could bring herself to make a final or irrevocable commitment about placing it in other hands. Juliana took this hesitation as evidence of Gertrude's ultimate attachment to the museum, and she remained vehemently committed to keeping the Whitney a sovereign institution. Juliana's life had been shaped by the prospect of a stronghold for American art and artists, and she was not about to renounce what had become a sacred belief. For the time being, she had extracted a promise from the trustees that they would continue Gertrude's original program.

Nor was Juliana going to rest until Gertrude's account as a sculptor was settled as she would have wished, which now included the attaining of a mark of official recognition denied to her in life. Before Gertrude died, she was taking steps to become a full member of the National Academy of Design. She was elected to membership on April 22, four days after her death, but her elevation was contingent on a portrait of her being created especially for the Academy. (From the institution's inception, associate academicians aspiring to full membership have been required to submit either a self-portrait or a portrait painted by another artist. The practice continues to this day.) Juliana talked it over with Flora Miller, and both women felt that Jo Davidson should be engaged to model the bust.

Yet Academy inflexibility, which had helped forge Gertrude's alliance with

the Henri group back in 1907, prevailed to the end. Hobart Nichols, the Academy's president, said that for Gertrude to qualify as an academician, her likeness had to be *painted*, as opposed to sculpted. He proposed that Charles C. Curran, an Academy member, be hired "at a very reasonable charge" to copy an already existing portrait of Gertrude. Juliana and Flora were insulted by the snub to Davidson and withdrew Gertrude's name from the list of nominees. Davidson nevertheless was commissioned to make the portrait bust for exhibition at Gertrude's memorial retrospective. His fee was $5,000, which was charged to the museum; the cost consumed most of the sculpture budget and only two other pieces were bought that year.

The first official meeting of the Whitney's new trustees was held on June 4, 1942. Flora was made president of the board, taking Gertrude's place. Flora's husband, G. Macculloch Miller, filled her vacancy. Juliana, perhaps in lieu of her diminished expectations from Gertrude's will, was given a $5,000 raise. Her annual salary was now $30,000 a year, paid in monthly installments of $2,500. This money was to come in handy. It would take several months for Gertrude's estate to be settled, and as all museum employees were paid out of one of her accounts, they hadn't received a paycheck since her death. John and Elizabeth Bart Gerald said that during the period between Gertrude's death and the probation of her will, Juliana paid the staff out of her own pocket.

After the Whitney closed for the summer, Juliana went to the tip of Cape Cod, and saw artists in the Provincetown and Truro areas. She visited Hans Hofmann and Fritz Bultman, and Jeanne Bultman, who was a model at the Hofmann school that summer, recollected that both men had great respect for her. Juliana was feted wherever she went, and where she was feted, she bought pictures. As the summer wore on, Crocker had many discussions with the other trustees—that is, the Millers and George Francis, a businessman standing in for Sonny Whitney. He had little trouble convincing them that Juliana was heedless of budgets, that her interests did not serve the family's interests. Furthermore, no matter who the director was, the museum was always going to require many thousands of dollars a year. The endowment would take care of the immediate present, but the Whitney children would eventually have to shoulder a heavier financial burden, which they were unwilling to do. In July, the Metropolitan was paying friendly court to Flora and Crocker, and they were receptive to these advances.

By the end of the summer, Juliana was aware that the Met was flirting with the Whitney again, but the engagement was still only talk. She opposed any union vehemently; to her this was not the ideal romance, but a shotgun marriage made at the trustees' decree. Notwithstanding the terminology of "coalition" and "merger," with their implied promises of an equal partnership, she was certain that the end result would be "amalgamation," in which the smaller entity would be blended and swirled into the larger and lose its individual identity.

Juliana could also advance strong arguments against a merger with the Metropolitan on the basis of historical precedent and her own experience. Although

Francis Taylor was younger and more dynamic than his predecessors, his trustees were as hidebound as ever and he himself made vicious fun of modern art. There was little proof that the Met's attitude toward twentieth-century American art had greatly altered since Juliana made her pilgrimage to Dr. Robinson's office in 1929 and was informed that a gift of the Whitney collection would only clutter up his cellar. In the 1930s, the Hearn funds for buying American art were not fully used. Protesting critics and artists pressured the Met into hiring Lloyd Goodrich as an adviser in 1937, and he got the museum to buy paintings by Hopper, Weber, Gropper, and Eilshemius. But as late as 1940, such modernists as Hartley, Lyonel Feininger, Dove, Sheeler, Joseph Stella, and Davis were not represented.

Charles Sawyer said that Juliana never wanted the Whitney to be a part of the Metropolitan because the Whitney collection was too personal to her, she had no respect for the way the Hearn funds were spent, and the place was not welcoming of artists. The Metropolitan was not welcoming of women either, nor much for elevating them to influential positions, whereas the Whitney was a museum established, managed, and perpetuated by women. The Met's reputation as a stoutly male preserve was not an objection Juliana would have raised, but both she and Flora Miller would have been made to feel out of place. Robert Moses, in an article written in 1949, seven years after the Met's overtures to the Whitney, described the atmosphere and mentality that Juliana and her trustees had to face, which could only have been more rigid in 1942. He characterized the Met as a traditional men's club, sniffy about modern culture.

> This club does not have a single woman trustee, and when I called attention to this gap, I was politely informed that it could obviously not elect one until it could elect two, because one would be lonesome, and it was also hinted that the jolly informal stag atmosphere would never be the same, etc. There is also no active trustee identified with modern art, and the dictum of George Blumenthal, a former distinguished president and generous supporter of this institution, that nothing significant has been painted, molded, or wrought since 1900, is still regarded by some of his associates as a sage observation which grows in authority as we move away from 1900.

Throughout the autumn of 1942, Juliana pressed on as if the Whitney would elude the Metropolitan's grasp. She was determined not to let the American Art Research Council become a casualty of events and took contributions from other museums to keep it going. She was jubilant when Alfred Barr said he would be a special adviser, because work on nineteenth-century Americans was outside his museum's domain and his conviction about many contemporary artists was dwindling. Juliana, who had been working on Barr since the previous May, wrote to him about how glad she was for his cooperation and marveled, "Your list is extremely like mine!"

Juliana was also fighting for any crumbs she could scavenge from Gertrude's executors. At the end of October, she got Crocker and the Millers to release the unspent balance of $20,000 authorized for purchases by Gertrude while she was alive and frozen since her death. After she received word of this, Juliana started looking over work for the approaching annual, which would begin on November

24. Although Hermon More was now doing most of the work on the annuals and was responsible for the inclusion of the majority of newer names, Juliana did make some studio visits on her own, and she greatly enjoyed these direct contacts with artists. Rosella Hartman, a Woodstock painter, said that although she was terrified of offending Juliana when she dropped in, their encounters would always turn out well because Juliana would put her at ease and say the right things. "She knew how to admire something," Hartman recollected. "She looked at one of my drawings a long time and said, 'It's noble.' That's all she said, and I was touched. Another time, I had a gouache and I dared to ask $100 for it, and Mrs. Force answered, 'I would be pleased and delighted to pay $100 for this gouache.' "

In November of 1942, Juliana went to see a young abstract painter named Hananiah Harari. She came to his loft on East 12th Street and left him starry-eyed with faith. Harari said:

> Mrs. Force was very vivacious, full of life. She looked almost clownlike because her face was white from powder, and her reddish hair added to that effect. She came into my loft, and I brought out my latest paintings. She had a warm response, which gratified me very much. She didn't have to give reasons why she liked my work. I knew. She selected my painting* for the permanent collection. It was a highlight of my life. I hadn't sold many things, and it was considered a great honor to be noticed at all.

Harari could not help but observe Juliana's extremely thick makeup, which she had begun affecting lately. It was an attempt to mask the fact that age, plus years of heavy smoking and drinking, had caught up with her. Her face had grown puffy and jowly, and the pouchy area around her eyes was incised with lines. Juliana reacted to her disappointments by drinking more, and in age she could not keep her problems with the bottle under control. For the first time in memory, her acquaintances saw her act visibly drunk.

A few days after Juliana's call on him, Harari received a check for $350 and notification that his work would be in the annual, too. The 1942 annual, although the first really large-scale showing of contemporary American art in New York since the onset of World War II, was not as thoroughgoing as Juliana and More would have liked. The trustees stipulated that for reasons of economy, one show rather than two would have to suffice. Over 200 paintings, sculptures, and graphic works would be exhibited together, about half the number normally given exposure. Clement Greenberg, who wrote for *The Nation* and was in the process of becoming one of the most prophetic and authoritative critics ever to pronounce on American art, wrote that "[f]or the tenth time the Whitney Annual gives us a chance to see how competently and yet how badly most of our accepted artists paint, draw, and carve. But no matter how well these artists paint and model, they do not *affect* us enough." Robert Coates of *The New Yorker* admired

---

* *Diagrams in Landscape.*

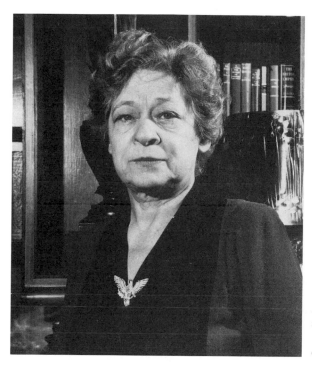

An unretouched close-up of a puffy-cheeked Juliana taken in 1942. Note the American eagle stickpin.

pictures by George L. K. Morris, Walter Quirt, Bradley Walker Tomlin, and George Grosz, but found most of the sculpture section "dull and unimaginative." Pieces by Archipenko, Calder, and David Smith were included in this dismissal. Greenberg liked what he saw by Smith, Theodore Roszak, Harari, Balcomb Greene, Karl Knaths, Feininger, Weber, Marin, and John Heliker, but he presciently went on to say, "The important question is whether contemporary American art is as unenterprising as these two* shows make it out to be. I think not."

The last time Juliana appeared to have been consulted about the question of the Metropolitan acquiring the Whitney was October 20, 1942. She was definitely not invited to attend or even informed of a meeting that took place on November 11. That day Francis Taylor and Frank Crocker met to clinch the agreement whereby the Whitney would be incorporated into the Metropolitan, vacate its Eighth Street premises, and move uptown to the Met into a new wing that would be funded from the money Gertrude left. "Some of the Whitney staff would also be absorbed, one Whitney trustee would go on the Metropolitan board, and the remaining Whitney trustees would serve as an advisory committee on American art," Calvin Tomkins said in his history of the Metropolitan. "Although the wing would be known as the Whitney Museum of American Art, the Whitney collections would be turned over to the Metropolitan."

---

*Greenberg reviewed the annual and a show at the Metropolitan in the same article.

Juliana turned up at the Metropolitan on December 1, innocent that an agreement had been reached. She and several other museum directors were there to select paintings, sculptures, and prints for the Artists for Victory exhibition, an immense show opening at the museum on December 7, a year to the day after Pearl Harbor was bombed. Twenty different artists' organizations with headquarters in New York originated the show and selected 1,418 works from more than 10,000 entries, and the Metropolitan agreed to put up the money to acquire some of them from the meagerly spent Hearn funds. The artists who made up the original jury of admission were, on the whole, extremely conservative, but the jury of award was tilted toward the liberal. Juliana, Barr, Sawyer, Rich, and Henri Marceau, who was the associate director of the Philadelphia Museum of Art, could overrule the Metropolitan's representatives, and this is exactly what happened, Sawyer recalled. "She and I—and Alfred was another—were on the jury for the Artists for Victory show, at which we spent over $50,000 of the Hearn Funds at one whack. To our considerable joy, we were outvoting the staff of the Metropolitan by about five to three on all these choices. It gave us some pleasure, but it wasn't really quite fair to them. But some of the things that were bolder in that collection, we acquired." Sawyer's testimony explains why work by Mark Tobey, Hartley, Feininger, Calder (represented by a mobile that was suspended from the ceiling of the museum), Peter Blume, and Herbert Ferber entered the Met's permanent collection. The judges also voted to buy an Ivan Albright painting—actually, they wanted to award it first prize—but they later learned that it was not for sale.

Throwing her weight around in the Artists for Victory show was probably the last crowing Juliana was able to do at the Metropolitan's expense, and her continuing ignorance of the merger can be seen in a letter or two that she wrote at the time. She used some of the purchase money unfrozen by Crocker to buy a Marin watercolor from Stieglitz. Relations were good between them because he put a below-market price ($1,800) on the work, making it possible for Juliana to get it for the Whitney. He only asked that she keep the price a secret, so as not to sabotage Marin's price levels. When Juliana wrote to Stieglitz on December 9, it was plain that she had no idea that the Whitney was about to go out of existence.

> I want you to know that I appreciate more than I can say, your making it possible for us to acquire the Marin. We are very proud to add it to our collection and I assure you that the transaction will be kept in confidence and known only to the trustees.
> I do hope that you will find some recompense in the thought that you have been most generous.

Stieglitz, replying on December 15, 1942, also thought that the watercolor was destined for the Whitney when he wrote, "I have your very kind letter. I thank you.—I am glad your Museum has acquired one of Marin's finest watercolors." Also in December, Juliana bought an oil by Marsden Hartley for $900, which she believed she was getting for the Whitney.

In the second half of December, Juliana went up to the Metropolitan to

meet with Taylor on some unspecified subject. After some preliminary pleasantries, Taylor started talking animatedly about his plans for "the Whitney wing." Juliana stared at him stunned, and for one of the rare times in her life, she was speechless. It dawned on Taylor that she had no idea what he was talking about. "Good Christ, don't you know?" he said to Juliana. "Haven't they told you?"

"They" most certainly had not, and part of Juliana's anger about the merger, said Charles Sawyer, "was that she felt the trustees, the family were going over her head. This is the way the rich behave. The Whitney staff and Mrs. Force were handed a fait accompli, which they all resented." Sawyer also said that the curators at the Metropolitan "were equally opposed to the merger: Along with the National Academicians, they were concerned that the Hearn Funds would be subject to the whims of the 'Radicals from Downtown.' " Lloyd Goodrich corroborated the fact that the Whitney employees were as cavalierly shut out of the talks as Juliana. He learned about the impending coalition when Howard Devree, an art critic at the *Times*, breezed into his office with the news. "That was the trustees," Goodrich commented.

Juliana had burned with mistrust of Crocker for years, but his meeting with the Met's officials behind her back and her consequent subjection to professional mortification in front of Taylor ignited an inferno of rage. Juliana also blamed Flora Miller for, in her words, "selling the Whitney down the river." What rapport or tolerance Juliana had for Flora vanished, but that would have been inevitable because she was taking a more active, if uninformed, role in directing the museum's affairs.

Francis Taylor was not spared Juliana's vitriol, either—she thought that he too had acted monstrously. Sawyer, who tried to mediate between the two of them, said, "She felt—I think unfairly—that Francis had instigated the merger with the Whitney trustees over her head. But it [the Whitney collection] wouldn't have been a primary interest for him if it hadn't come from the other side. I don't think it was anything he would have ever suggested. This was something Juliana never quite understood." Taylor was genuinely astonished when he learned that Juliana was ignorant of how far the negotiations had gone, but there was something disingenuous in that astonishment, particularly for a man of his subtlety and guile. Juliana's colleague Gordon Washburn, then directing the art museum of the Rhode Island School of Design, reacted indignantly to the prospective coalition and came to the same conclusion as Juliana—that Taylor had been an accomplice by his silence. Washburn wrote to her:

> I am not only saddened but outraged at the thought of it [the merger], and at the thought of the way in which it was done. Even though Francis Taylor had been approached by your Trustees rather than the reverse, he might well have refused to confer with them without your knowledge of the point of the discussion.

Or as Fiske Kimball, who had a touch of the rogue himself, noted in his journal, "It was a great coup for Francis Taylor."

Juliana kept silent and went on, saying nothing that would alarm the artists. Attending an auction for Russian war relief she sponsored, she bought a still life by Milton Avery for herself for $75 and offered to store any unsold works at the

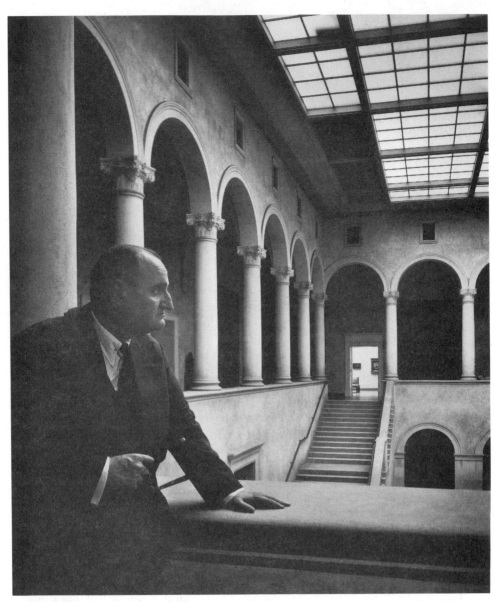

Francis Henry Taylor, fittingly seated amid the classical pillars of the Worcester Art Museum.

Whitney until February. She then retreated to Woodstock to spend a few days between Christmas and New Year's with Dorothy Varian. One evening they had cocktails with Carl and Helen Walters, who lived in a simple, one-story house that the sculptor built himself on a mountain road above the town. After a few drinks, Walters launched into a dirge about how broke he was, and Juliana

offered to buy his house, furniture and all. At first everyone thought she was joking, but she talked and talked about it until she convinced her listeners that she was in earnest.

The alcohol must have spurred Juliana on, but buying the Walterses' house was in character. She felt depleted after Allan's wedding and went on to buy the house in Shelton; she felt desolated and abandoned at the prospect of seeing the Whitney slip away. Juliana's need to be among people who liked her and would reconfirm her place in life was especially great at this moment, and nowhere were there more idolators than in Woodstock. If the Whitney was to be taken from her, she could at least be near artists who were made by the Whitney. On December 30, 1942, Juliana bought the house and two acres of land on Ohayo Mountain Road for about $5,000. Walters kept some of the land from Juliana and promptly built another house next door to hers.

Becoming a resident of Woodstock was a bright spot in 1943, a year that brought sorry awakenings and bad transitions. She couldn't have agreed more when Lee Simonson wrote to her that making the Whitney "an appendage of the Metropolitan is the worst news of the winter." On January 6, Juliana resigned from the Whitney's board of trustees. She wrote to Crocker, "Believing that it will facilitate the meetings of the Trustees in the negotiations for the proposed consolidation of the Whitney Museum with the Metropolitan, I hereby tender my resignation as a trustee of the Whitney Museum."

The news of the merger was leaking out in late December of 1942. Juliana, for one, told several museum directors before they read it in the papers. Someone from the Whitney—presumably Flora Miller or Juliana—spoke to Abby Rock-cfcllcr around Christmas, and she informed the Modern's trustees, who were just about to approach the Whitney again about relocating next to the Modern. By the time Juliana submitted her resignation to Crocker, rumors were flying between offices and galleries, and the art magazines were begging to have them substantiated. The story broke a week later, and on January 18, the trustees of both museums released a joint statement confirming the transaction and ex-plaining that the primary reason for the coalition was to perpetuate the ideals of Gertrude Whitney. A Whitney wing would be erected after the war, and Juliana would be kept on for a while to advise the Metropolitan on contemporary American art and the spending of the Hearn funds. Although the Whitney's collection would not be presented to the Metropolitan until after the new building—which was to be known as the Gertrude Vanderbilt Whitney Collec-tion of American Art—was constructed, the museum would shortly cease to exist. The final art event in the old quarters would be a memorial exhibition of Gertrude's sculpture, from January 26 to February 25, 1943 (later extended to March 14). The press release stated that the Whitney would be shut down to put the collection, now numbering more than 2,000 objects, in order and ship it to the Met for storage.

The announcement was widely condemned, but to no avail. Coates, who was representative of the critics who spoke up, called the merger "the deadliest blow to contemporary art that could be imagined. The Metropolitan, it seems to me, is simply not fitted to take over the functions of the Whitney." The artists

were inconsolable, and they deluged Juliana with letters and telegrams detailing their fear of domination by the uptown colossus. They saw the closing of the Whitney, which they knew was devoted to helping them through their struggles, as the end of a protection and affection unique among museums. They unanimously lamented the passing of the Whitney, both as an art institution and as a Village landmark serving a Village audience with Village zest. The responses ranged from a brief scrawl from Alexander Brook saying simply and accurately, "You did a swell job and it was so right," to anguished commiserations that went on for several pages. However, because Gertrude Whitney's daughter favored the merger, there was nothing much anyone could do. From Philip Evergood:

> I express the feeling of all artists when I say that for years the Whitney has given us the inspiration to go on with our Art in difficult times by showing us that an important institution has confidence in American Art and in us as growing American artists.
>
> It will be very sad never to see exhibitions in the grand and truly American galleries of the Museum again. Also those happy and gay openings and the rare but memorable visits to your own beautiful quarters upstairs which meant so much to us. The only ray of sunshine is the fact that you who have been the guiding light will continue as such when the collection goes to the Metropolitan.

From Yasuo Kuniyoshi:

> The Museum on Eighth Street has been for us, the contemporary American artists who emerged in the past two decades, the institutional cradle that rocked us. Sometimes we disagreed, but never did we doubt either your devotion to art or your courage in fighting for what you believed to be for the best interests of the American artist.

From Herbert Meyer:

> I just want you to know how we [the artists in Vermont] all feel—for I have not spoke to one who does not feel the same. Sorry that the Whitney is to be no more and is to be hitched up to that rather mortuary like place—the Met. Where are those lovely parties to go—where one could so happily greet our fellows in Art—and where the welcome was so warm & genuine—the kind that cheers the heart of all Artists —where are all the Boys & Girls going to get together—surely not at the Metropolitan where I am sure no Artist has been tendered a glass of water—and perhaps a sour look.
>
> No Sir this thing is all wrong—for all will be losers and the future is dark and full of shudders.

From Charles Burchfield:

> Like every-one, who cares anything at all about the future of American Art, I was distressed to hear of the merging of the Whitney museum into the Metropolitan. What every one fears of course is that, the fine Whitney spirit will be swallowed up in the Metropolitan, and not that the Met will be reformed by such a shot in the arm.
>
> I have always regretted that my living so far away [in upstate New York] prevented my visiting the Whitney as frequently as I would have wished. On the basis of cold material facts, the Whitney has been my best patron, for it owns more of my pictures than any other museum, or private collector. Even if that were not so, the very

existence of the Whitney was a rock of strength to us American artists, who have to carry on in the face of mass indifference.

The outlook at the moment for us is very dark, and the disappearance of the Whitney as a separate entity seemed like the last straw.

Juliana could also be proud of the esteem in which she was held by her peers, and there was comfort to be derived from their astute inferences about what had happened to the Whitney. Laurance Roberts was candid in his sentiments and, he assured Juliana, so were Rene d'Harnoncourt, who would presently join the Museum of Modern Art, and John Walker, then the chief curator of the National Gallery. All three were in agreement that her pioneering work should go on under her leadership and said that she *was* the Whitney. She received a handwritten letter from Alfred Barr, which he began by crossing out THE MUSEUM OF MODERN ART NEW YORK on the letterhead and inscribing *Personal* in its place.

Dear Juliana

Of course, before the news came and in the papers I'd heard a lot of rumors—but as you hadn't spoken to me I didn't think I should open the subject—though, believe me, what I heard I didn't like—and some of it I could hardly believe.

What you and the Whitney Museum have done is so admirable and so badly needed—and could I think be done only in a comparatively intimate and friendly atmosphere. Pictures will continue to be bought and shown under the Whitney name I suppose but I'm afraid the spirit will have faded. The Metropolitan is big enough —too big—and its extremities grow cold already.

I do not know how you feel about this event—and perhaps you will think this note irrelevant or that no expression of concern is called for—but I, and many of my friends, feel that we have suffered a personal misfortune.

But there is some comfort in the thought that we shall not lose you.

Sincerely and affectionately,
Alfred

The most fiery letter came from Forbes Watson, who knew the principals and sized up the situation at a glance. He saw that if the Whitney merged with the Met, it would be forgotten. Forbes, with his indomitable sarcasm, was the only one who dared to say that the Whitneys were tired of Juliana, and he was ready to give them—and all the other guilty parties—a good, hard kick.

Dear Juliana,

I can hardly believe it. It's as if a friend had been murdered. And for what? To make an unwieldy octopus more unwieldy? And at this particular time too when the American artists need you more than ever. Good God! What imagination, what love both for living art and for Gertrude, this dreadful illiterate miserliness implies.

We all know what happens when an octopus adds another arm. When the public goes through a so-called collection, the ex-Vanderbilt or the Altman collection, their interest is in the pictures. Not a hundredth part of the public knows that they are looking at a particular collection.

You have given your life to this work. You know the collection, its value and its meaning, what it has meant to the American artist and how it has educated the

American public. So the final tragic decision is made by those who neither know nor care. The strangest barbaric action suggesting weird interweavings of jealousy. Better oblivion than a nickel lost. And as for faith, belief, personality, accomplishment, like procreation they are far too good for the poor, artist or no artist. Better be another arm of an octopus. Better oblivion for the very name of Whitney than that you by chance should accomplish. . . .

Now for more than a decade the Whitney Museum has changed the course of every one of the bigger trustee-run museums in their acceptance of American art. And you have made a national reputation. Fatal error! Did you inherit a fortune? If not what right have you to be a personality? How do you suppose Gertrude escaped? The story of a family in quest of oblivion, anything to save the effort of thinking. I suppose if you keep everyone with energy away from you, you can cheat yourself into thinking that you have some energy. One can live perhaps on the smirking of the sycophants.

There's still a lot to do for art. And the thing for you is to conquer again as you did before. . . .

I could go on and on but I shall be seeing you next week. Apparently wealth beyond one's capacity to use it not only creates pus on the brain but pus on the heart.

Enough of raving. Up and at 'em!

Love,
Forbes

These letters, plus the many others she received, meant much to Juliana, for she saved them, contrary to practice. Nonetheless there was no choice for her but to start arranging Gertrude's memorial show—the museum's final public offering. The opening was as jolly as a burial service, and the artists were conspicuous by their baleful expressions and funereal bearing as they trooped through the galleries full of Gertrude's Pans, Neptunes, and Daphnes, taking their last looks at the brave old rooms about to be dismantled. Juliana presided with a stoic demeanor, but Henry McBride reported that he and the other party goers felt that the occasion was marking "a helpless submission to doom." Juliana's friends "maintain[ed] a shocked air of defeatism as they wandered through the rooms . . . looking upon the collapse of her project as their own special collapse."

After the memorial exhibition opened, Juliana did collapse. She caught a cold that that developed into what she thought was a grippe. By the middle of February, she had pneumonia and had to be hospitalized for the rest of the month. When she left the hospital, Gertrude's show was over, and the Whitney was out of business. Juliana bought $75 worth of war bonds for each employee to mark the end.

Her convalescence was not restful. Along with shutting down the museum, the trustees said that the apartment above the galleries would have to be vacated because Flora had plans for selling the building. Juliana had to move out of her gorgeous salon, where she had plotted, schemed, and done so much for American art, and find a new place to live. "Juliana was like an animal who had been hit and didn't know why," Elizabeth Bart Gerald said. "She had so much to do with not much warning. She turned to me and said, 'Where will I go?' " The

eviction was yet another enactment of the Bucks County dispossession—the child disinherited from her rightful home—and Juliana was heartsick at leaving West Eighth Street. "It was an awful shock for her," said Eugene Ludins. "The whole damn art world fell into her lap there and she made the most of it. She lived like a queen in her *gemütlich* little castle." More than that, observed Gordon Washburn, Juliana's actually residing in the building was crucial to its essence. "She presided over the Whitney by living in it like a house," he said. "It was what made the museum so intimate. She loved good living, and she made those rooms something of a rallying point for the museum world, especially in American art."

Any future apartment would lack the rambling eccentricity and color of the old rooms, so Juliana would have no space for her collections of pictures, furniture, and bric-a-brac. She consigned over 200 pieces of Victoriana to Parke-Bernet, to be sold on April 30, 1943. Most of her best furniture was sent to that sale, including her Aubusson carpets, her Venetian blackamoors, her Minton porcelain, her lacquered papier-mâché tables and cabinets with mother-of-pearl insets, and her Regency side chair shaped like a shell and upholstered in eggshell-colored satin. The contents of Juliana's library followed her furniture to the auction block, and they were sold on May 17. Among the rare books she owned were early editions of the works of Byron, Voltaire, Dickens, and Longfellow; a Shakespeare Second Folio; first editions, often signed, of Poe, James Fenimore Cooper, Mary Wollstonecraft, Dreiser, Jack London, Conrad, Hardy, Thackeray, Whitman, Booth Tarkington, Twain, Crane, Theodore Roosevelt, and Eugene O'Neill; seventeenth- and eighteenth-century albums of hand-colored botanicals and herbals; and finely printed and illustrated art books.

Because the Victoriana was advertised as being owned by Juliana, who had legendary status among collectors of nineteenth-century furniture, the pieces fetched good prices. The sale grossed over $20,000, and the net proceeds came to $15,193. The check was sent to Crocker, who passed it on to Juliana with a note saying, "Please put this in your bank and leave it there. Don't give it away, and don't forget that there is hard sledding ahead." The library sale brought Juliana $1,309.

Scarcely had the contents of the apartment been packed and trucked away to Parke-Bernet when Juliana received grave news from Chatham. Months before, Mary Rieser was discovered to have cancer of the liver and stomach, and as the disease wasted her, she was in horrible pain. She died on April 7, 1943, and was buried in Doylestown two days later. After the funeral, Juliana attended to the onerous detail of finding a new place to live in Manhattan. She rented an apartment on the twelfth floor of 825 Fifth Avenue, at 64th Street, overlooking the Arsenal. The fancy address was not the attraction, but the location of the building was a consideration. It was near the Metropolitan, her future place of work. Mary Rieser's death, compounded by the demise of the museum, the sale of her possessions, and her own removal from her beloved rooms, plunged Juliana into a grief that came close to breaking her. She mixed up some transactions in dealing with Edith Halpert, and was so disturbed about it that she admitted, "That [the confusion] I suppose *was* my fault, but I cannot tell you what awful

things I've been through the last five weeks. My sister's terrible illness & death was just the burden I could not stand."

At a time like this, the last thing Juliana would do was to listen to Crocker and salt away her money. She did not merely want to spend it, she wanted to spend it *fast*. What would mend her spirits was an exuberant splash of home improvement that defied all practicalities. Juliana threw herself into getting her new house in Woodstock, which she named Laughing Water, in shape for the gay times she would have after her arrival in the summer. Carl Walters's plain little cottage was no residence for Juliana, who ordered the addition of a second floor and dormers. She also wanted a terrace and gardens laid out before she moved in, and the trees at the edge of the property had to be topped off to expose the sight of Overlook Mountain in the distance and the foreground view of the village and church steeple. If she was to recover her strength and her appetite for combat at Laughing Water, it had to be grand enough to sustain the hospitality she loved to serve up. And if nothing else, Juliana was not going to look defeated. Nan Mason, a Woodstock artist hired to supervise the contractors and lay out the gardens, said that Juliana put nearly $30,000 worth of work (the money was probably what Gertrude left to her) into her $5,000 house.

Before Juliana returned to Woodstock on June 15, she and the Whitney received a real gift—a reprieve from absorption by the Met. The Millers, Crocker, Juliana, and George Francis convened in late May in reaction to the details of the coalition agreement, which had recently been prepared by the Met's attorneys. The Met had gotten greedy, and the imprint of Taylor, a champion bargainer and horse trader who was never averse to trying a bluff, is visible. The first agreement, of January 18, was only a list of vague assurances; the second, dated May 19, was an attempt to extract new concessions and take away what had been previously offered.

The Whitney trustees were united in thinking that they had been handed a mess of pottage for Gertrude's birthright. In a material departure from the January statement, the new contract neglected to make provisions for Juliana, More, Goodrich, or the Whitney trustees, for the Whitney collection's access to the Hearn or other purchase funds, or for the continuation of the American Art Research Council. The Met also reneged on its promise that all American art would be under the direction of the Whitney wing. The attorneys were suddenly angling to keep them separated, and at the discretion of the Met's staff. Taylor attempted to wriggle out of naming the addition built by Gertrude's money the Whitney wing; it would just be a section of the Metropolitan in which the Whitney collection was housed. Crocker, the Millers, and Juliana felt that the Met was trying to press an advantage because they had closed their building and were embarked irrevocably on the road to incorporation. Rejecting the May contract, they drafted a rejoinder that read in part, "In other words, there is nothing in the agreement to assure that the ideals and policies of the Whitney Museum will be continued after the coalition. There are general statements to that effect, but no means of implementing them."

By June 14, the next time the Whitney board and Juliana met, the Met's architects had submitted their renderings for the transplanted Whitney, and

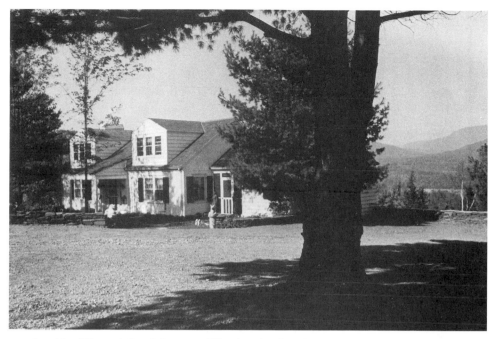

Laughing Water, Juliana's house in Woodstock, after she got through with it. Before, it was a simple, one-story cottage.

neither the Millers nor Juliana liked them. Two unpleasant surprises had been introduced, confirming their impression that the Met had not listened to their dissatisfaction with the coalition agreement as it now stood. First, an auditorium for the benefit of the entire museum, but near enough to the future Whitney galleries that Gertrude's money was supposed to be applied to pay for it, had been added to the blueprints. Second, instead of moving the art collection uptown for storage as planned, the Met wanted Flora to leave everything where it was and hand over the Eighth Street buildings "to supplement its activities"!

Then there was the important matter of the proposed galleries themselves. The overall design failed to retain, as had been promised, the intimate character of West Eighth Street. Nor was it a separate wing at all, but a harsh, anonymous space within an expanded main building. Juliana said that the long, dour, and almost windowless structure reminded her of Alcatraz. (Robert Moses, not to be outdone, would soon refer to the Whitney addition as "another wart" on the face of Central Park, and independently reject the preliminary architectural plans.) The penitential look of the wing, which would have to be altered to gain the Millers' and Robert Moses's approval, plus the wartime prohibitions on use of labor and materials for nonessential civilian purposes, made it impossible to fix a date for completion, but both sides concurred that a wing would take two years from start to finish after ground was broken during peacetime.

The Met's arrogance gave the Whitney trustees pause—it was time to reconsider at leisure. Not only should the construction of the wing be postponed,

they proposed, but the final terms of the coalition agreement should not be determined in the near future. The Millers and Crocker rethought how they might carry on the Whitney and best perpetuate Gertrude's memory, and they acted creditably. They agreed, although still among themselves and in confidence, to contemplate reopening the museum at the end of the year for one exhibition—the annual, which was the show that meant the most to young artists. And even if the differences with the Metropolitan were disregarded, it was apparent that the war was not going to be over soon, and perhaps the trustees were haunted by a patriotic resolution made by most of the country's museum directors in December of 1941, in which they pledged to keep their galleries open as a community service. The public, they declared, needed a refuge from world events, and Gertrude herself had stated in 1939 that the Whitney's work should not be deterred by the outbreak of war. Gertrude's name and ideals were not being served by the Met, and on that subject Flora, Crocker, and Juliana were as one. With that shred of hope to cling to, Juliana wrote a check for $5,697.96 for the back taxes she owed for 1942 (because of the war, extra taxes had been imposed), and was gone.

Nan Mason had done an excellent job of keeping the builder and the other contractors on schedule, and Laughing Water was ready for its owner. Even the flowers cooperated, and long rows of dazzling white lilies greeted Juliana. She loved to watch them wave in the breeze, and when the stalks were tossed by the wind, she would say, "That's my white wash." Still, the scenery lacked something, so she installed some garden figures of George and Martha Washington that she bought from the Downtown Gallery. There was still not quite enough statuary, so she asked the sculptor Paul Fiene, a Woodstock resident who was known for his carvings of animals, for one of his pieces for her garden. Fiene and Juliana went back a long way—the brother of Ernest Fiene, he had sculpted a portrait of McTaggart, one of her Scotties, in the late 1920s—and although he did not want to sell it, he let her buy a life-size sculpture of a kneeling deer in pinkish stone for the lawn. Fiene didn't want to let the piece go because he couldn't guarantee that the stone could take extremes of heat and cold, but Juliana loved it, had to have it, promised to cover it up in the winter, and offered him $500 for it. Fiene gave in—after all, she was the angel of Woodstock, the patron the artists always counted on. It looked as if a good summer were in store for Juliana, full of parties and friends and laughter.

Being in Woodstock provided Juliana with the chance to become closer to Bradley Walker Tomlin, who owned a big Victorian house. Like Juliana, he was partial to nineteenth-century furniture and paintings, and in general she trusted his taste and judgment. (In 1942, she commissioned him to research and write a catalog on contemporary Brazilian painters, but he never finished it.) Tomlin's house was so large that a friend, the painter Antoinette Schulte, used one of the rooms as a studio. Juliana would often come over for lunch or elegant English teas—Tomlin was as Anglophilic as she. One day while Juliana was there, Schulte broke her wrist and wanted to go to a local physician for

treatment. "Nonsense!" Juliana insisted. "I'm going to drive you back to New York right away for the best care." And off they went, Juliana driving at breakneck speed.

Juliana did her share of visiting and party giving during her first summer in Woodstock, but living in an art colony was not the idyll she had envisioned. Severe gas rationing cut down on drives and errands, and daily life was unlike those Woodstock weekends of yore, when she was entertained around-the-clock. On the weekdays the artists were working in their studios and unwilling to loaf with her. At the end of the day, when they were free, the rationing restricted the number of social calls they could make. Juliana was hurt by this because she wanted to see more of everyone, and the artists weren't as manageable (or as worshipful) as she would have liked. Used to having everything her way in Woodstock, she was confident that these inconveniences would pass.

The coming autumn was looking as gloomy as the previous spring. Because the Whitney was closed, some employees were fired, and the ones who stayed had to take a pay cut. Sonny Whitney, said Crocker, demanded that money spent on salaries be cut in two. Juliana's salary was reduced from $30,000 to about $24,000 or $25,000. She learned what it was like to be at home at 825 Fifth Avenue on an everyday basis, and she hated the isolation. The artists were still in brownstones in the Village, and she was stuck in a correctly appointed but boring apartment house among the rich and stodgy.

But Juliana's sense of humor had not deserted her, and she was still capable of seeing the ridiculous in people, including herself, and laughing about it. Living on Fifth Avenue during a period of wartime constrictions led Juliana into some humorous commerce at those times when she was caught between her old largesse and her new reality, as in one story she liked to tell on herself. With taxis at a premium on account of gas rationing and her access to Whitney cars and chauffeurs a thing of the past, Juliana now had to use the Fifth Avenue bus to get to West Eighth Street. The first time Juliana took the bus, she didn't know the bus's route or the amount of the fare, lacked the right change, had to get it from another rider, and ended up causing a great deal of confusion. After she paid her fare, Juliana apologized to the driver by way of saying that she hadn't been on a bus in years. "Lady," he answered, "we missed you."

Juliana had just about steeled herself to the bus when she encountered the subways, which she regarded as a frightening descent into the underworld. Juliana had gone to a party with Andrée Ruellan and her husband, John Taylor, and they said they would escort her home. It was late at night, and the only way to go was by subway. "Juliana was so nervous," said Andrée Ruellan. "She had probably never been in a subway, and she was shaking as we went underground past some drunks and disreputables. To divert her, I said, 'Doesn't this scene look just like a Reginald Marsh?' 'No,' she shot back, 'It's more like a Cadmus.' "*

---

*This was a prescient remark as well as a witticism. Many years later, Cadmus painted a horrific satire of a New York subway as hell.

Juliana was the director of a ghost museum. She had so much less work to do that she was in a state of involuntary semiretirement. For the first time in forty years, she was not organizing a full calendar for the Whitney; she was not heading a vital institution, but only an attenuated version of its former self; she was not racing gloriously from place to place. She was less busy, too, because there was no longer Gertrude's career to manage and promote. Juliana was intent on filling in the spaces of her once-jammed appointment book: She accepted invitations to speak, to judge exhibitions, and to be on the boards of various institutions with a frequency that would have been impossible in the past. Juliana was determined not to disappear, as Taylor or Crocker would have wished.

She became an increasingly active trustee of the American Federation of Arts, a national body that circulated art exhibitions. This meant frequent meetings and travel. The federation's journal, the *Magazine of Art*, was about to go under, and she made saving it a personal crusade. One meeting on the fate of the publication took place in Washington, and it was attended by Peppino Mangravite, a painter who was involved with art education and fond of Juliana. The meeting, he said, became "a tempestuous experience," after someone nominated a museum director to fill one place on a committee. Mangravite objected violently, saying that theoreticians and administrators shouldn't be running everything. Juliana, who was leading the discussion, asked, "Who would you have?" in a voice dripping with venom. When Mangravite answered, "Artists," she slammed the book she was holding onto the table, said, "That can't be done," and went into a long tirade about how wrong he was. Later, they found themselves in the same car on the train going back to New York. Both had been drinking, and both lost their tempers. Mangravite said, "She was still enraged about the meeting, and I thought she was tyrannical, so we started arguing, and we went on insulting each other all the way up to New York. But the next day, she wrote me a long, apologetic letter saying I was right, so we made it up."

Following up on her remorse, Juliana then did try to get some artists to go on the AFA's board. However, her wish to make amends didn't work out in practice because, more often than not, artists didn't want their time eaten up that way. Katherine Schmidt, one of the painters asked to serve, said, "Mrs. Force wanted me to go on the board of the American Federation of Arts. Of all the boresome ways for an artist to spend her life, it seems to me, is to be with the American Federation of Arts. Well, she didn't like that at all, and she would complain to my husband about me. I suppose she wanted people who agreed with her on the board, or who would be more apt to agree with her. But they never asked me again, and that was the end of that."

In the last three months of 1943, Juliana traveled extensively on crowded wartime trains. In October she went to Minneapolis and then to Chicago. On November 7, 1943, she returned to Minnesota to judge the Minneapolis Art Institute's annual of contemporary painting. From there, she went to the Art Gallery of Toronto to open Americans 1943: Realists and Magic Realists, a show organized by the Museum of Modern Art. In the speech she delivered in Canada, Juliana inserted her perennial message of "Pictures must be bought," but during an interview beforehand, Juliana tellingly spoke her mind on other matters that

were concerning—and disturbing—her. Asked if her work was finished because American art had gained in acceptance, Juliana replied, "No, for I fear a boom in native art which may be a boomerang because discrimination is lacking." Well, then, did she feel like an old and seasoned campaigner? Once more the answer was contradictory, but this time it was not tinged with the caution of a prediction, but worldly cynicism born of bitter experience. "No; I feel like a new pioneer," Juliana said. "There is always new work, and it is always the same: ridicule, criticism and then applause, and by the time the applause comes you don't care."

Juliana's words were certainly applicable to herself, but they were also germane to someone else in her thoughts who had been treated more callously and unjustly than she. This was the man whom she had replaced in Toronto—in fact, the man who had asked her to take his place. Just a month before Juliana's trip to Canada, Alfred Barr, who had written such a kind and understanding letter to her at her nadir, had been asked to resign as director of the Modern. Barr could either leave the museum or accept the board's alternative—a demotion to something called "advisory director." This job, which consisted of unspecified duties and no responsibilities, was akin to being a research assistant. Even his office was taken from him. Barr was allotted a small desk in the museum library and a salary of $6,000 a year. The trustees were trying to push Barr out by demeaning him, but he refused to be ejected. He moved himself and his research into a tiny cubicle and began working on his books. Juliana knew firsthand what agonies the embattled director was feeling, and after Barr's plight was made public, they purposely escorted each other to several art-world affairs—the two museum directors, discarded and deposed, partners in misfortune—as a tacit commentary on their situations. Their linked presence challenged others to draw their own moral as to the judgment obtaining in museums and the trustworthiness of trustees, and it occurred to Dorothy Miller, who was then the curator of painting and sculpture at the Modern and Barr's closest associate there, that their dismissals smacked of conspiracy and menace. In "the same year that Alfred Barr was fired," she recalled, "[Juliana's] museum was given away to the Met by a couple of trustees . . . and it was very peculiar that both . . . directors had their throats cut by the trustees. . . . It was Francis Taylor . . . who once said, 'I will absorb all the museums in New York City.' He didn't say the Metropolitan would, he said I would absorb."

Taking the measure of these tensions and discontents was Fiske Kimball. Kimball, who had been director of the Philadelphia Museum of Art since 1925, was responsible for propelling his institution from a provincial depot for local holdings into a respected fine arts institution. He found it a gargantuan shell of a building—seven acres of floor space had been allotted for galleries—standing half empty and unfinished on its promontory above the Schuylkill, and he left it a completed and furnished museum whose halls were filled with great treasures and unduplicatable collections. A stocky, barrel-chested man with a head shaped like a cannonball and a drive to match, Kimball was one of the unquenchable

freebooters of the museum world, but his raids were just an aspect of his single-minded and unflagging mission to fill, furnish, and finish the Philadelphia Museum of Art.

Building a great museum in a city that was smug about its lethargy was not a task for the timid, and Kimball was an irascible, domineering, ruthless, and restless executive. He prowled around the galleries like a lion tamer minus a whip. That temperament was suppressed in the presence of superiors, for Kimball had a trick of turning into a humble courtier when he socialized with potential donors. To his staff, he was fond of quoting a La Rochefoucauld maxim that he modified to suit himself: "Gratitude is the lively sense of future benefits to come." Kimball had little money—his museum nearly went broke during the Depression—and he had to accomplish everything with a minimum of cash outlays and a maximum of his own initiative and statecraft. Fortunately for Philadelphia, the latter two were in large supply.

Within a few weeks of becoming director, Kimball had solicited advice on what he should do. When told "to see the widow Eakins," Kimball, "displaying an alacrity to be repeatedly associated with him in the years to come," sought out Susan Eakins in her house on Mount Vernon Street. A year later, during the Philadelphia Sesquicentennial Exposition, he bought Eakins's *Wrestlers* for his personal collection for $400. Mrs. Eakins was impressed by this, and Kimball's purchase led her and Mary Adeline Williams, who was left a share of Eakins's estate, to make the priceless gift of seventy of his works to the Philadelphia Museum in 1929 and 1930. When asked why she did this, Mrs. Eakins said, "Other museum directors came and admired the pictures, Mr. Kimball came and bought one."

Kimball had miles of halls yet to furnish in his post-and-lintel fortress on Fairmount, and his readiness to bend to collectors netted him a string of munificent acquisitions. The most recent—and one of the most astonishing—occurred in December of 1942. At that time, Albert Gallatin, whose Gallery of Living Art had been housed at New York University since 1927, was unceremoniously told to find another place for his collection of early twentieth-century avant-garde art so that the university could have more space for library books. Masterworks by Picasso, Léger, Miró, Mondrian, de Chirico, Braque, and Arp were suddenly left homeless, and Kimball did not hesitate. On the day he heard that Gallatin was evicted, he telephoned the distraught collector and offered him exhibition space for the entire collection, which contained about 170 objects. Kimball reeled in the Gallatin pictures, and they were moved to Philadelphia in early 1943.

In October of 1943, Kimball scented another prize. His antennae had been stirred by a routine letter from Crocker on the twenty-sixth asking him to certify that his museum, the recipient of the tapestries and ceiling from 871 Fifth Avenue, was a charitable and tax-exempt educational institution. With that letter came a copy of the residuary clause from Gertrude's will, which stated that the remainder of her estate constituted a charitable trust. Kimball excitedly realized that the Whitney children were trustees of a sizable fund and empowered to distribute the income and principal. This meant that he might tap the trust

again. On October 29, Kimball asked for an appointment with Crocker as soon as possible, while writing blandly, "The clause from Mrs. Whitney's will which you quote is of extreme interest to this institution, and I am eager to have an opportunity of speaking with you regarding other aspects of this matter." In the journal he kept for chronicling his adventures in the museum game, Kimball wrote, "I could imagine Francis Taylor smacking his lips over this fund also, and determined to cut in on it if possible." Kimball and Taylor were mentor and protégé, which did not preclude them from being cutthroat professional rivals. Zigrosser described the two of them as buccaneers who had no compunction about raiding each other's territories.

Kimball was prompted to test just the one provision of Gertrude's will at first, but always a man of opportunity, he broadened his pursuit beyond a portion of the residuary trust. He was going after part or all of the $2.5 million legacy and the permanent collection of the Whitney Museum. How much Kimball knew beforehand about the Whitney trustees' misgivings concerning the merger is only to be surmised, but he did learn of the snag while he was in New York and exploited it. Talking to Crocker, Kimball used the ploy that had worked so effectively with Gallatin. The Met, Kimball contended, could never show the whole Whitney collection even within the area assigned to a Whitney wing— if and when it was ever erected. Why not transfer some or even, dare one say it, all of the holdings elsewhere? Philadelphia, now that Kimball mentioned it, already had halls ready and waiting to receive the Whitney collection. His wing was built but not finished on the inside. If the Whitney trust would make over $500,000 to complete the interior—a big saving, as anyone could see, over the $2.5 million the Met required—Kimball would open a Gertrude Vanderbilt Whitney Wing of American Art in Philadelphia, thus spreading that great lady's name and influence ever more widely.

Kimball was a genius at feeding people this sort of line, but it was not his persuasiveness alone that hooked Crocker. Crocker was prone to Kimball's blandishments because he was still smarting from the Met's inept and peremptory handling of him and the Millers. On September 30, 1943, just a month before Kimball had his brainstorm, Crocker wrote in a confidential memo that analyzed a Whitney press release, "We are by no means sure that the coalition can be effected, and we must not put ourselves in a position where the Metropolitan can say that we have committed ourselves to the public." Philadelphia stood to benefit from Crocker's doubts, and Kimball wrote in his journal that Crocker

received this very well, though he said they had not yet thought of branches of the Whitney Museum.* So far as the money went, the trustees could spend two million tomorrow if they wished. He said Mrs. Miller's attitude would be the most important; Mrs. Henry was inactive, but Colonel Whitney would have also to be persuaded. He was absorbed in Washington and a new wife—he had divorced Gwladys Hopkins of Philadelphia [wife number two] for Eleanor Searle, a beautiful airline receptionist and choir singer of New Rochelle—and it would be hard to go into it with him. We were welcome to try.

* Nor would anyone, until 1973, when the Whitney's first branch museum opened.

Kimball dropped in on Juliana the morning after his triumph with Crocker to see if he could enlist her. Because of her disaffection with the Metropolitan, Kimball said that she welcomed his pursuit of the Whitney. Juliana recognized that if another suitor joined the dance, his flirtation might bring about more of those diversionary delays and postponements that kept the engagement in limbo and bought the Whitney a few more months of valuable freedom. Taylor and Kimball might knock each other out with their wooing, leaving the Whitney mercifully alone, the bride stripped bare of her bachelors. To help equalize the match, Juliana gave Kimball some suggestions on how to handle Sonny Whitney, and he asked her how things were going with the merger. She replied that "they were crossed up," even though she was allowed to mount an annual on the home grounds. Juliana told Kimball "that there was not Whitney money enough to both hold the exhibition and to buy from it, as they always had and as she insisted was vital. She was trying, so far without success, to get Francis Taylor to finance the exhibition, so that the Whitney money available could be used for purchases." Kimball suggested reversing the financing. The Whitney should use its money to put on the show and ask the Metropolitan for money from the Hearn funds for purchases. Juliana saw at once that this was the solution and rewarded him "with an impulsive kiss."

No sooner was Kimball back in Philadelphia meowing with joy at what he had set in motion when he heard from Taylor, who had become privy to what Kimball had assumed were secret meetings. Taylor wrote, "Keep away from our Whitney friends. Let me remind you in all affection of our being the remaindermen for the Johnson Collection."* To which Kimball retorted, "Everyone for himself. Let me remind you, in equal affection, of our being remaindermen for the Gary pearls, which you folks sold." Taylor was livid and on the defensive, Kimball was spreading dissension and on the attack, the trustees were doubtful and divided, and Juliana had to be smiling at the comedy being played out. Any new proposals for the Whitney's fate meant further waverings and deferrals; in the meantime, the museum would reopen. Kimball, who had long ago learned scheming patience, retreated to wait for the right time to approach Sonny Whitney.

The Whitney's revival in its own quarters went unexplained to the public. A press release merely stated that the Whitney, after being shut eight and a half months, would reopen its galleries on November 23, 1943, in order to mount the annual and have it on its own premises. Juliana brushed off the reporters' queries, causing Rosamund Frost to report tartly in Art News, "Even if Mrs. Force now rather grandly says, 'This is no return, because we never left off,' everyone from press to staff members was frankly taken by surprise."

To ensure that she could hold the Met to its commitment of the purchase money, Juliana inserted a clause in the press release to the effect that the Met's trustees would tap the Hearn funds. Taylor, who read over the draft of the

* A collection Philadelphia coveted and later received.

announcement, did not like the wording but hesitated to change it for fear of scaring off the Whitney for good. He wrote to Roland Redmond, an influential trustee from whom he sought approval, "In view of the delicacy of the situation in other respects, I would recommend taking a chance in putting an OK on this release simply in order not to raise doubts and alarms by pussyfooting." William Church Osborn, the Met's president, doubtless voiced the dim hopes of the board when he wrote to Taylor, "I hope there is something in the show which we would be willing to buy with the Hearn Fund!"

Juliana got $10,000 from the Whitney budget for purchases and $10,000 from the Hearn funds, and split responsibility for acquisition monies became the norm for annuals through 1948. (The division fostered the impression, and correctly so, that works bought by Whitney money were on probation. They would be detained at West Eighth Street until time proved them worthy of passing through the Metropolitan's portals.) This was Juliana's first time advising the Met on contemporary American art, and she seemed to make a special effort to choose carefully. She recommended only six pictures for purchase: oils by Thomas Hart Benton (*July Hay*, one of the artist's best late paintings), Bradley Walker Tomlin (*Burial*, a semiabstraction daringly advanced for the Metropolitan), Eugene Berman, Ernest Fiene, and George Grosz, and *The Coming of Spring*, a watercolor by Charles Burchfield that marked a turning point in the artist's career. These were good choices; in hindsight, the best paintings in the show, along with the Benton and the Tomlin, were those by Davis, Pippin, and Gorky, but the likelihood was low that they would have been approved for purchase. Whitney funds bought a combination of ten sculptures, paintings, and graphic works, the most arresting of which was *Tombstones*, a gouache by Jacob Lawrence. Of the 195 objects in the annual, twenty-eight (14 percent), each by a different artist, found buyers.

Such encouraging figures were but one of many signs of a burgeoning and appreciative audience for contemporary art and a dawning of a new art world in New York. Both North and South America had assumed vital cultural importance as a result of the war, but the pulse of New York in particular was quickened by the European artists in exile and the younger American vanguard. The city was on the verge of something big—the overtaking of Paris as the center for contemporary art. Juliana embraced these changes with caution at first, as can be seen by her comment in Toronto when she wondered if the art boom would become a boomerang. But because buying art was always good for artists, she came around, although not to the forefront of the evolving avant-garde.

One sign of a more ambitious cultural climate was the amassing of corporate art collections, a movement that grew out of the World's Fair. Thomas J. Watson, the president of IBM, was sufficiently moved by what he saw to assemble an art collection owned by his business. In late 1943, the Encyclopaedia Britannica corporation followed IBM's lead and began putting together its own collection of contemporary American art. In January of 1944, Juliana was one of a group of museum directors and curators invited to be on the advisory board of the

Britannica. She was asked to submit a list of artists who should be in the collection, although she was not asked to recommend any specific paintings.

Juliana was also becoming acquainted with several emerging buyers who were making American art the focus of their collections. Through Kuniyoshi, Juliana met Milton and Edith Lowenthal, a New York attorney and his wife who were enraptured by what they saw at the Artists for Victory exhibition and backed their judgment by buying forty paintings—all by living Americans—in 1943. Juliana applauded the Lowenthals' taste and attitude, and they took to her. Edith Lowenthal would later write of Juliana's "strength, courage and unfailing devotion to contemporary American art," and the couple later donated Ben Shahn's *The Passion of Sacco and Vanzetti* to the Whitney in her memory. Juliana also met Roy Neuberger, who had studied art, went into finance, and was heavily buying the work of young Americans. Both the Lowenthals and Neuberger were being guided and encouraged by Edith Halpert, and they, not unnaturally, were among her best clients. In a rare show of humility, Juliana, acknowledging Halpert's success in bringing new collectors along, asked her for the names of people whom she didn't know but who should receive invitations to future Whitney exhibitions.

The dawn of a new cultural age in New York, replete with its peculiar personalities and byzantine conduct, was wryly—and secretly—appraised by Florine Stettheimer in a painting called *Cathedrals of Art*. A catalog of ruling art factions in the guise of a mock-religious processional that also resembles a stage set, the picture contains numerous acerbic and fey caricatures of the cultural elect, one of whom was Juliana. Stettheimer picked only the prominent to be subjects of her mordant gaze, and some of those on her original list were Taylor, Harry Wehle, Chick Austin, Barr, Stieglitz, Valentine Dudensing, McBride, Pierre Matisse, and Juliana. She later added Monroe Wheeler, Pavel Tchelitchew, and the photographer George Platt Lynes. To Stettheimer, these people were "Art in America"—the phrase she sometimes used as a title when referring to the painting and which appears prominently in the picture itself.

Most of *Cathedrals of Art*'s population are lining up to greet the arrival of an infant who symbolizes Art and heralds a new epoch. The image of a baby lying bathed in light—the light coming from the flashbulbs of Lynes's camera —satirically embroiders on the fabric of thousands of religious paintings portraying the birth of Christ. The idea of Art as a welcomed infant may also have occurred to Stettheimer because she started the painting on or close to New Year's Day. The canvas, which is dated 1942, was first mentioned in her diary on January 1, 1942. The picture was unfinished at her death on May 11, 1944.

During her two years of work on *Cathedrals of Art*, Stettheimer made special visits to the museums and galleries to spy out her subjects. Besides recording her victims' likenesses, she slyly, obliquely, and unerringly incorporated much of the fact and gossip—as an extremely knowing painter and unquenchable party giver who had dozens of highly placed friends in the art world, not much escaped her—of their lives as well. Only an insider like Stettheimer could have known how to ridicule Harry Wehle, the Met's curator of paintings, so wickedly. He is shown with his arms around a pretty young girl wearing a sash that says

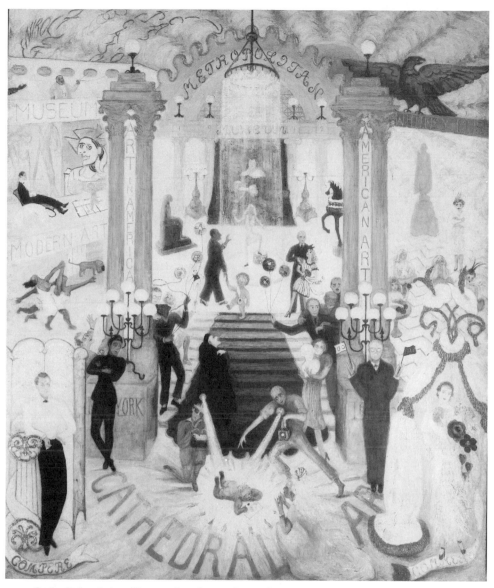

Cathedrals of Art, Florine Stettheimer's mocking distillation of art-world politics, 1942–1944. Juliana stands inconspicuously off to the right, and Alfred Barr sits in the upper left balcony. In contrast, Francis Taylor, with infant in tow, is in the center of the picture.

"PRIZE." This was a doubly adroit thrust, for the caricature broadcasts Wehle's reputation as an nonentity of art officialdom in two ways. It reminded viewers of his penchant for selecting pictures of pretty girls, his favorite subject matter, for the Met, and of his faith in the prize system and other bogus honors.

Cathedrals of Art is very appropriately in the collection of the Metropolitan, for its action takes place on the museum's grand staircase. After the infant Art is photographed, he is received at the top of the long flight of stairs by Francis Taylor, the bishop of the cathedral, who guides him to the high altar. That is, the consummation of an artist's career and the consecration of a work of art are marked by the entrance of an object into the permanent collection of the Metropolitan Museum of Art.

Stettheimer divided the painting into three vertical parts, in imitation of the central area and two sides of the Metropolitan's Great Hall. Within each side, as an adjunct, are representations of the Modern and Whitney museums. The tripartite composition works successfully, as it should, on artistic grounds, and it contributes to the witty message by fostering the impression of the art world as a three-ring circus. The threefold division also establishes the Metropolitan and Taylor as the dominant art institution and leading museum man of the prophesied new age. Stettheimer was too aware an artist not to be commenting on the altered positions of Barr and Juliana by their placing and poses. Whereas Taylor is active and depicted in midstep, Barr, a floor above the noise on the staircase, sits quietly off to the side reading. He is removed from the action— a shorthand for his recent removal from responsibilities. As befitting her personality, Juliana is not made to look as contemplative as Barr, but she too is put in a spot peripheral to the main goings-on. She stands in front of *Chinoise*, one of Gertrude's early sculptures. The ghostly looking statue is a full-length female figure and can be taken as a stand-in for Gertrude, who assumes the form of both an apparition watching over Juliana and a patron saint being guarded by her. Like Barr, Juliana is stationary. She is standing, not doing. Her arms are crossed, indicating that her hands are tied. She is an onlooker who is too far away to join the homage to Art or hobnob with Taylor. If art-world politics are a three-ring event, Francis Taylor is the proprietor of the central arena, leaving the ex-directors of the Modern and Whitney with the sideshows.

The Whitney galleries were closed after the 1943 annual ended on January 4, 1944. The local artists were thrilled by the museum's resurrection—"[i]t was as though," they would say, "we adventitiously found ourselves back in a home which we thought we had lost." Katherine Schmidt and Henry Schnakenberg, as friends of Juliana and die-hard Whitney stalwarts who knew about the friction between her and Crocker, took it on themselves to lobby for the museum's independence. They started what might be called an informal Whitney Defense League to garner support for Juliana and the museum as she ran it. Picking artists who were close to Juliana or had grown up with the Whitney Studio Club, they invited Peter Blume, Louis Bouché, Jo Davidson, Stuart Davis, Philip Evergood, Leon Kroll, Yasuo Kuniyoshi, Julian Levi, Reginald Marsh, George

Picken, Raphael Soyer, Eugene Speicher, and William Zorach to be part of their group.

The committee decided to marshal a massive vote of confidence for Juliana. In the form of a letter to Flora Miller, Schmidt and her husband, Irvine Shubert, composed a testimonial dwelling on the large debt that American artists owed the Whitney and Gertrude. The Whitney, they proclaimed, had been so much a part of their lives that its future was of overwhelming importance to them, and they were distressed to see it change. The writers did not say it directly, but they were urging Flora Miller not to go on with the merger. Juliana's partisans circulated the letter, and 174 artists, well-known and obscure, traditional and avant-garde, signed it, from Peggy Bacon and Alexander Calder to Arshile Gorky and Edward Hopper to David Smith, Georgia O'Keeffe, Isamu Noguchi, and Charles Sheeler. The letter, dated February 3, 1944, was sent first to Flora Miller and then published in the *Herald Tribune* and the *Magazine of Art*.

Flora, who was moved by the appeal, got a true inkling of her institution's seminal place in New York life and its meaning to the local artists, but she turned to Crocker for advice on how to answer the letter. Flora replied non-committally, writing that the trustees would carry on her mother's museum "wherever it may be finally located." Yet the Whitney was permitted to reopen and sponsor a limited exhibition program. The artists were pleased to think that they had affected the trustees' deliberations, but the turnaround had more to do with the war, with Crocker and the Millers' misgivings about the terms of the coalition agreement, and with the avid attention being paid to the Millers by Fiske Kimball, who popped up at the end of January with renewed energy for carving off part of the Whitney from the Met. He was writing fawning letters to Flora and Crocker, and leaning on every connection—mutual friends and old school ties—he could muster. On March 2, 1944, the trustees and Juliana gathered to go over the Whitney's future exhibition schedule. The galleries, if they had their way, would reopen in the fall.

This made for brittle relations between Juliana and Taylor. In the ensuing contest of wills, exactly the kind of battle Juliana was not accustomed to losing, Taylor would be the one to impose his point of view. Peppino Mangravite had a drink with Juliana after her exit from one of these confrontations, and he remembered:

> When I asked what happened, she started to sob. At first she said she would rather not say, but then she told me, "We met to talk about who would be the director of the whole enterprise when everything quieted down. And he said to me, 'Remember that when everything is settled, there is only going to be one director of this museum, and that's me.' " Then Juliana talked about the beginnings of the museum and she got sentimental. She mentioned Mrs. Whitney and at the thought of her, tears appeared in Juliana's eyes.

As evidence of her subdued posture, Juliana had to submit the exhibition plan for the 1944–1945 season for Taylor's approval. When the director pronounced it "excellent," Crocker felt obliged to write, "In these times of uncer-

tainty, it is very pleasing to receive such assurance at approval from our friends at the Metropolitan."

Other friends, not content with assurances, made obeisances. Kimball resurfaced in May to court Flora Miller. He lunched with her and Crocker and promised to visit her at Old Westbury in the fall. After these very agreeable conversations, Kimball said it was time "to draw in" Sonny and Eleanor Whitney. He addressed Sonny as one of the distributors of Gertrude's estate and acknowledged that his view would be determining. Kimball wrote, "We know, of course, of the linkage of the Whitney Museum of American Art with the Metropolitan, and the specific provision made for it. We are in hopes that those residuary benefactions may be spread more widely, and would like a chance to explain what could be done in her memory, and for American art, at the Philadelphia Museum." When George Francis, who was still acting for Sonny while he was away, responded positively, Kimball was emboldened enough to compare the bargain that Philadelphia represented with the profligacy of the Metropolitan's proposal. Kimball's letter of July 26, 1944, was the closest to a flat statement that he ever made on the subject.

> The wing which should be devoted to American art . . . is entirely complete externally, with its floors, at a cost of say $2,000,000, but undivided and unfinished internally. To finish the interior, with about 25 galleries for American painting and sculpture, is estimated to cost $500,000. If that sum could be made available from the Whitney residue it could become a Whitney Wing of American Art, which would further Mrs. Whitney's objectives in another great city and museum.
>
> Compared to related possibilities elsewhere, this is a very economical one, as all the facades are already built and it is only a matter of fitting up the interior. I believe there would be no difficulty in filling it worthily with suitable examples of American art, whether from our own collections or by deposit of certain works among the great number acquired by Mrs. Whitney through the Whitney Museum.

Kimball thought he was on the brink of another dazzling coup, but he was thwarted. Sonny could not be pinned down and was difficult to reach, but more detrimental to his cause was the existence of a previous competitor. Before Kimball could draw in the remaining Whitneys, a far superior spinner of webs had wound himself around them first.

Eleanor Searle had been a voice major for a year at Florida Southern College, an obscure, debt-ridden school in the orange groves of Lakeland. As Eleanor Searle Whitney, she had enough money to do something for Florida Southern. "Something" had one meaning for Eleanor and another for its president, a Dr. Ludd Spivey. Spivey was as hard-charging as Kimball, but lacked his social graces. In 1938 Spivey invited Frank Lloyd Wright to design the school's campus, which would consist of eighteen buildings and extensive landscaping. Money to fuel this spree was nonexistent, but Spivey was undeterred. When he fell in with Eleanor Whitney, he saw a gold mine to be quarried for his school's enrichment and his own posterity.

Florida Southern had no facilities for holding concerts or other musical activities, and in 1942, the second year of Eleanor's marriage to Sonny, Spivey

talked her into donating money for a building that would be called the Eleanor Searle Whitney School of Music. After Gertrude died, Spivey suggested that the structure become a memorial to Eleanor's recently deceased mother-in-law and renamed accordingly. He must have calculated, as did Fiske Kimball, that a bigger gush of Whitney money would flow in his direction.

Eleanor Whitney was amenable to a memorial to Gertrude and ready to look at detailed sketches, but Wright dragged his feet in preparing them. His contribution was way overdue, but practically speaking, it didn't matter much when the plans were drawn up since nonmilitary construction was prohibited during wartime. In late November of 1943, Wright wrote to Spivey in response to his pleading, "I have a good scheme—(a remarkable one really) for Gloria Vanderbilt Whitney [sic]. How much is she willing to pay?" Conflating Gertrude, Gloria, and Eleanor as interchangeable moneybags, Wright was in haste to expand the one modest Whitney-endowed building into an art complex whose size would dwarf the acreage within the Philadelphia Museum of Art.

In early 1944, presentation drawings were completed that delineated not only a music building, but galleries for painting and sculpture, artists' residences, arts and crafts workshops, classrooms, a lecture hall, a library, a theater, and a children's center called The Little Dipper. Here was the temple of culture Gertrude deserved to have. It was also a temple Wright was sure he was destined to build, as he neglected to consult Eleanor about these inflations.

Wright's feat of derring-do paid off, for Eleanor Whitney proved to be extremely suggestible: She did not veto the new scheme. In return, she felt she was owed steady attention and prompt replies, but Wright, just when he should have been piling on the blarney, fell perversely silent. On August 21, 1944, Spivey admonished his truant architect—only Wright's magic could keep their patron spellbound.

> Doubtless you have received the letter from Mrs. Whitney. Now that we have her in a good mood I hope you will do everything you can to keep her in this state. You are the key to the whole matter. See what miracles your letter accomplished. . . .
> I just had a letter from the Foundation, which means that our Art Project is going through providing we can please Mrs. Whitney in this present project.
> I wish I could say something else to impress upon you the high importance of your keeping in touch with Mrs. Whitney. Otherwise this Music Building, and the whole art scheme will come to naught.

This was the state of affairs when Fiske Kimball came calling in the summer of 1944. Sonny was absent, and Eleanor was engrossed in Frank Lloyd Wright, who was in line to pocket a sizable share of Gertrude's trust, since the foundation Spivey mentions must have been the one deriving from the residuary estate. (Eleanor, who would have known about the Whitney trust, probably told Spivey that grants could be made available for Florida Southern.) But Spivey and Wright overreached themselves, and their predatory fantasies of a Gertrude Vanderbilt Whitney art complex faded. Wright ignored Eleanor's suggestions and her need for attention, and in 1946 the project shrank back to a music building.

The music building itself was never executed because of a quarrel between

Eleanor Whitney and Frank Lloyd Wright. They disagreed over who knew better about planning a concert hall. "Wright was not willing to modify his unworkable interior," Eleanor Whitney later wrote. "He placed the orchestra in the right hand balcony. No musician—pianist, violinist or singer—nor oratorio nor opera could give a unified performance with the conductor and orchestra way up on a faraway balcony." When she inquired how the singers would be able to see the conductor, Wright replied that the conductor would use a baton with a big light on the end of it. Eleanor Whitney also balked at the prodigality of bathrooms—a dozen toilets were supposed to be installed. "I really hope the music won't be that bad," she said, and withdrew her support altogether. Her final verdict on Wright was that he was a four-flusher, a scoundrel who swaggered around the school with his cape and stick, and a bad architect.

During the ascent and crash of Florida Southern's fortunes, Juliana evidently was not informed that a memorial to Gertrude was threatening to rise out of the orange groves of Lakeland. Carl Rieser said that in early 1946, when he was at the museum with his aunt, Frank Lloyd Wright was seen strolling around the galleries and Juliana invited him upstairs. As far as Carl Rieser could tell, the two did not know each other. They indulged in some raillery about architectural styles, but Wright never mentioned his involvement with a memorial to Gertrude or his relationship to Sonny and Eleanor Whitney, and Juliana seemed completely unaware of his past or present connections to the Whitney family. Carl Rieser was certain that if his aunt had been familiar with the art complex at Florida Southern, she would have brought it up.

Although Kimball didn't get far with Eleanor and Sonny, his Whitney efforts were not useless. For the pains he took over the summer, he did extract $7,490, the amount it would cost to install the Italian ceiling he received from 871 Fifth Avenue, from the residuary trust. How it came about provides an enlightening glimpse of what art professionals like Kimball and Juliana were up against when they depended upon the rich to help them. Kimball formally applied to Crocker for the money, but he heard nothing. One day in the summer of 1944, the publisher Thomas (Tim) Coward, who was a friend of Kimball and the Millers, chanced to be at Old Westbury playing gin rummy with Flora when Crocker dropped by to discuss some estate matters, including the request for Philadelphia. Tim Coward said nonchalantly, "Oh, do that," and Kimball got his money.

As for Juliana, she was in Woodstock and not cognizant of Kimball and Spivey sweetening their traps for the Whitneys. She felt good enough about Laughing Water and detached enough about Shaker Hollow, which she had not lived in much lately, to get rid of the latter. Ever since she stumbled into the nest of Nazis in South Salem, Juliana felt queasy about going there, and at one point she rented out the property. On July 29, 1944, Juliana sold Shaker Hollow; for the first time in decades she was the owner of only one house.

Juliana was pleased about being in Woodstock because of the renewed proximity to artists who admired her, but she found herself somewhat isolated. Juliana had no car, so if an artist couldn't come to her, she was dependent on the town's

one-man taxi service. As opposed to her first summer in Woodstock, when she expected nonstop socializing, Juliana had accepted the reality that most of the artists were in their studios all day and didn't want to be interrupted. But during the evenings they could certainly take an hour out and have a drink with her. Juliana complained to Arnold Blanch that here she was, sitting up on the hill by herself, and no one invited her over. She didn't need or want expensive dinners. She just wanted to be invited casually or on the spur of the moment. Blanch informed Juliana that some artists felt it prudent to see her in moderation. Friends of the longest standing, like Dorothy Varian, Hermon More, or Eugene Speicher, were above suspicion and might see Juliana without being reproached, but artists who were less well ensconced believed that if they hung around her too much, they would be accused of playing up to her. There also were the artists who felt they did not know Juliana well enough to have her over and were timorous about pushing themselves forward. Juliana understood what Blanch had to say, but she reassured him that the artists, who she felt were being a tad ultra-nice, need not fear for their integrity. She was lonely, she hated being by herself for any length of time, and she just wanted to have people—preferably, creative ones—around her.

Juliana hoped that her life in Woodstock would improve, but she had had enough of 825 Fifth Avenue. A conflict arose because Juliana employed two black servants, whom she treated as companions as much as employees. This made some of the other tenants uncomfortable. The managing agents spoke to Juliana about her breach of protocol, but when she ignored them and refused to change, they backed down. Then a few tenants began to complain again that she was allowing her servants "too much freedom." Her reaction was succinct. "I'm getting the hell out of here," she announced to her friends. Juliana went apartment hunting in the Village with John Frear, John Gerald's former assistant, who was now on his own as a designer. They found a small railroad flat at 42 West Ninth Street. The place was unprepossessing when compared with her grand rooms of old, but Juliana didn't mind. "I like it better than Fifth Avenue," she proclaimed.

Juliana wanted some of her furniture reupholstered, but because of wartime shortages, there was no fabric to be had, so she and Frear covered everything in the only material they could get—pure white sheets from B. Altman's, which the two of them decided was tremendously chic. The decor also made a flamboyant contrast to Juliana's latest couture. After the Whitney closed and she had to move away, she had taken to wearing dead-black clothes as a sartorial statement of bereavement. Katherine Schmidt said of the Ninth Street apartment, "It was a dreadful kind of flat for her to be in, but as always, she had made it charming. She had beautiful Biedermeier furniture, and there again she was always original. The curtains were made of white ruffled sheeting with ruffles that fell in the most beautiful way, and her face was so white and her position so insecure, but she did her best. Irvine and I went over there sometimes to spend the evening with her—she'd call us when she was lonely." Irvine Shubert added, "It was sad to see her there. We used to go over and hold her hand. We were always

friendly, but she wanted more from us than we could give because we were busy with other people and activities."

The Met doled out $5,000 from the Hearn funds for each of the 1944 annuals—the Whitney was allowed to have two again. From the first one, Juliana recommended four paintings for purchase, one of them being *The Portentous City* by Julio de Diego. Before he knew that she had earmarked it for the Met, Duncan Phillips asked Juliana to reserve it for him. She answered, "I will be very glad to have the de Diego painting set aside but I have recommended it for purchase to the Metropolitan. That, as you know, may mean nothing." To Juliana's surprise, the Met accepted all the pictures, but the process did not always run that smoothly. During the run of another annual, as she escorted Taylor through the Eighth Street galleries and pointed out the Met's future acquisitions, Juliana asked, "What do you think your trustees will feel about these purchases?" "I think they will puke," Taylor replied.

Juliana, said Charles Sawyer, was "deeply offended" by that answer. "It was my own impression," he wrote, "which I tried to convey to her without much success, that Francis was really referring to the notoriously conservative views of some of his trustees, a subject on which he could be eloquent among his friends." Sawyer's reading of the exchange was probably correct, but Juliana discounted literal accuracy here. Her feud with Taylor was too violent for her to extend him much credit, and it would be like him to represent his sentiments as coming from the trustees. For his love of a riposte, he couldn't restrain a gibe that was sure to hurt and infuriate her.

The second section of the annual, devoted to sculpture and graphic work, opened on January 2, 1945. The Lowenthals were guests at the party, and their celerity as collectors earned them a rap on the knuckles from Juliana. "We bought a Kuniyoshi drawing [*Murdered*] from the show," Edith Lowenthal said. "Juliana Force had it in the back of her mind that she wanted the Whitney to buy it, so she was a little sore at us. The following year we went to the opening, and she was standing in front of a Ben Shahn picture [*Reconstruction*]. She said to us, 'You're not going to get this one!' The Whitney has it."

Juliana could hardly stay peeved at the Lowenthals for buying pictures and supporting the same artists she did, and not long after the couple bought the Kuniyoshi drawing they invited her to dinner. Unfortunately, their well-meaning gesture was doomed to failure, for the Lowenthals' other guest was Edith Halpert, who had irked Juliana yet again. The collector Wright Ludington, another Downtown Gallery client, wanted *Pertaining to Yachts and Yachting*, the early Sheeler drawing that Juliana owned, and he asked Halpert to get it for him. Halpert approached Juliana, who asked $3,000 for it. Ludington didn't want to go any higher than $2,000, and Halpert worked the price down to $2,500. Juliana said that $2,000 was out of the question, but Halpert persisted. The two women were testy toward each other, and Halpert reminded Ludington that Juliana was "temperamental."

There had been another run-in that was also distasteful to Juliana. Daniel Catton Rich wanted to buy *The River*, a painting by O. Louis Guglielmi, an artist also represented by the Downtown Gallery, for the Art Institute. The Whitney had shown it in the 1943–1944 annual. The picture was not sold, but Flora Miller later decided that she wanted to buy the picture and put a hold on it. In February of 1945 Juliana interceded on Rich's behalf to get Flora to relinquish the picture, but Halpert took the credit for it. On April 4, 1945, Rich wrote to Juliana about Halpert, "Happy ending! . . . I greatly appreciate your advice and interest in the matter. Meanwhile I am going to keep my fingers crossed on the lady's future business activities."

The Lowenthals had no idea that Juliana and Halpert were on bad terms. "They hated each other," Milton Lowenthal said, "and they each brought their dog." Juliana had Comet alongside her, and Edith Halpert arrived with Adam, a nasty, unhousebroken little dachshund from whom she was inseparable. Juliana sat on one side of the room, Halpert sat on the other, and their dogs growled at each other the whole night.

Although Katherine Schmidt was repelled by the boresome duties entailed in governing the American Federation of Arts, she was an unshirking activist when it came to the advancement of her fellow artists. As the wife of a corporation lawyer, she was now a well-off woman, but she never forgot that the majority of her peers teetered on the brink of indigence. (In 1944, Elizabeth McCausland compiled an income survey of 500 American artists who had practiced professionally for at least twenty years. Of the 200 who answered her questionnaire, the average annual income for men was $4,144, with $1,154 of that sum earned from sales of work; the average annual income for women artists was $2,131, with an average of $548 resulting from sales.)

In late January of 1945, Schmidt and Irvine Shubert got the idea of creating legislation providing for the state of New York to acquire work by contemporary artists who were residents of New York, for use in public buildings within the state. A commission of nine experts, serving three-year terms without compensation, would buy paintings, sculpture, and graphic works. The New York State Museum in Albany would have jurisdiction over the resulting collection and be responsible for its storage and circulation to other institutions, such as museums, libraries, and government buildings. It was a lean, well-reasoned purchasing program, but the Shuberts knew that it would go nowhere without vigorous backing. They asked Juliana to join them in formulating a bill. Since the proposal was not a relief measure or an intermittent fund based on need, but a direct, ongoing, and straightforward plan of buying meritorious art, she was for it— provided she could be the boss. That was exactly the response Schmidt and Shubert wanted and, said the artist Elizabeth Olds, who also served on the committee, Juliana became the "chairman and dominant figure."

Most of the groundwork on the bill was done by a core group composed of Juliana, the Shuberts, James Thrall Soby, a curator at the Modern (who was named vice-chairman), Barr, Goodrich, Edwin Burdell, who was the president

of the Cooper-Hewitt (then the Cooper Union) Museum, and Hudson Walker, an art patron, dealer, collector, and staunch supporter of American art. No one from the Metropolitan was on the executive committee, or on the bigger list of more than 100 distinguished New York State residents in the arts, sciences, and humanities who lent their names to the project and were willing to lobby for it and write letters to their local representatives.

The first few months of work were spent in hammering out the language of a bill that might be sent to the legislature the following winter. Juliana, said Irvine Shubert, "relied on Hudson Walker and myself for political wisdom. In terms of the discussions, she was useful because she could get everyone together and push a point forward. Besides, she knew what the artists needed, and she could express that well." Meanwhile, the auguries were good. The measure had bipartisan support in New York City, and no one, either upstate or downstate, voiced any opposition. Shubert was a friend of Paul Lockwood, the press secretary of Gov. Thomas E. Dewey, so the committee automatically had privileged access to the Statehouse.

In March of 1945, the Whitney presented a vital, laudable, and somewhat controversial show called European Artists in America. Many of the artists who had come to the United States since the outbreak of war were not exhibiting much in New York, and in their native countries their work was banned by the Nazis. Since these men had been prevented from full professional participation as artists through extraordinary and horrific circumstances, Juliana broke a big rule and asked them to show at her museum, which of course was expected to be 100 percent American. She characteristically classified her action not as a violation of policy but an extension of hospitality. Nearly forty refugee artists then living in New York accepted Juliana's invitation, among them Max Ernst, Léger, Mondrian, Chagall, Dali, Duchamp, André Masson, Kurt Seligmann, Jacques Lipchitz, Yves Tanguy, and André Breton. They each were represented by three or four works, which filled the museum.

The majority of the liberal critics were delighted by the exhibition and baldly stated that the Europeans were producing work superior to their American counterparts. Similarly, there were a great many American artists who were as tender-hearted as Juliana toward the artists in exile, but the ones she heard from were the jealous few. They grumbled loudly about aliens who had already gotten too much play at the Modern invading the one place that was theirs. Nor could Juliana have been cheered much at the opening when Sonny Whitney walked in and asked, "What are all those funny-looking pictures doing here?"

His question was only the beginning of a suitably surreal episode that evening. After a bad experience or two with party crashers who had stolen food and liquor, the museum required guests at openings to come with invitation in hand, and the guards were following their instructions to the letter. Ben and Bernarda Shahn arrived at the door to see a curator from a museum in Georgia turned away by the guard because she was without a written invitation. The woman was temporarily in town, had heard about the opening, and tried to get in. The Shahns said she could go in with them, and the guard was pacified.

Just as the three of them were about to disappear inside, there arrived a

handsome, grizzled older man in a cape. With him was a younger man, who was obviously a friend. They had no invitation, and the guard would not let them past the entrance. The older man became indignant and planted himself there, putting his hands on his hips and refusing to move. He then began shouting at the windows, behind which a party was very definitely in progress. Juliana heard the commotion, came to the window, and looked down on the scene. The man's words rushed up to her—"C'est Chagall! C'est Chagall!" She threw up her hands in embarrassment, ran downstairs, and personally brought Chagall into the building, all apologies. The guard, the Shahns ascertained, thought Chagall was a derelict who would make off with the food and drink by hiding it under his cloak.

Juliana challenged the detractors of European Artists in America, characterizing her foes as selfish, petty, and untrue to the principles of a democratic society. To emphasize her conviction, she invited Ernst, Léger, Chagall, Seligmann, and other resident foreign artists to the succeeding annuals. For a young painter then, having a picture hang in the same gallery as one of those masters was a thrilling honor. Stephen Greene, who first exhibited at the Whitney in those days, wrote:

> In 1945, while I was a graduate student in a midwestern university, my mother, at my request, brought to the Whitney . . . a portfolio of drawings and gouaches of which a gouache was invited for their annual. The following year I crated a number of paintings for viewing and they invited a painting for the 1946 annual. I knew no one at the Whitney. The process was truly democratic, and it gave me a start in the art world and helped me to mature inasmuch as I was able to hang next to a truly accomplished artist. In the 1946 annual I hung next to what I thought was a wonderful work, a large Chagall, and that simply spurred me on. That annual also helped me in being asked to join Durlacher Bros., a then powerful and fascinating gallery.

As the 1944–1945 season drew to a close, Juliana stepped up her rounds of jurying, speaking, and committee sitting. She was one of a group of dignitaries who were supposed to select works of art for a deluxe edition of American paintings to be published by Macmillan. (The company had cash to burn—that is, to invest in prestige—because of the runaway financial success it enjoyed the year before with *Forever Amber*, a trash romance that still makes money.) Unfortunately, Macmillan was so hooked on prestige that only the curators and directors most in demand were invited—Juliana (who insisted on having More and Goodrich, too), Hyatt Mayor of the Metropolitan, Dorothy Miller and her husband, Holger Cahill, and Jack Baur of the Brooklyn Museum. "It was the most harmonious group of people," Dorothy Miller said, and plenty of fascinating information was being traded, but it was impossible to get everyone together at once, so the meetings—and the book—dragged on for years. (It would eventually be dumped, because the *Forever Amber* money had gone elsewhere.) But at the book's inception, everyone involved was optimistic.

On June 4, Juliana chaired a meeting on the New York State art legislation, in which it was decided that a draft bill would be completed and a fall publicity campaign mapped out by the end of the summer. She then went to Woodstock, with expectations of returning to the city briefly in July to organize some grass-roots support for the bill. A week or so later, both Juliana and the Whitneys received a shock that brought her back downstate. On June 16, Frank Crocker dropped dead of a heart attack. His death would not alter matters with the Metropolitan, but as Juliana would discover, her own position would be improved. Thomas Regan, the Whitney business manager, would handle the museum's finances again, and he and Juliana could get along. Walter Dunnington, who had been Crocker's law partner, took on more legal responsibilities related to the museum, and Juliana had no history of quarreling with him.

Juliana was under the impression that she would be doing a lot of commuting between Woodstock and West Ninth Street to hold extra meetings on the art bill. But conditions in the Catskills were just as discouraging as before. Gas rationing was still in effect, and she could not arrange to have a car take her to the city when she wished. At one point Juliana was frantic about the inconvenience. She told Nan Mason that if she could not go back and forth to work on the pending legislation, she would have to give up on Woodstock. Juliana was also feeling querulous because she was having persistent stomach cramps that she chalked up to indigestion. Her digestive and intestinal tract gave her trouble whenever she was tense, and if she was not careful, her spastic colon flared up. Nan Mason remembered seeing Juliana so overcome by abdominal pain that she would have to lie down. Moreover, Juliana ate little—she had coffee for breakfast, nothing for lunch, and a light meal later, and the food she did eat was finicky and mild.

Persistent indigestion would never have pushed Juliana out of Woodstock, but a final disillusionment with life in the art colony did. On July 22, 1945, Juliana, Harry Wehle (who also had a place in Woodstock), and Albert Heckman, a local painter, juried a show put on by the Woodstock Art Association. About 100 entries were submitted, and the judges threw out sixty-four of them. One of the rejects was a painting by Paul Burlin. He denounced the proceedings, and cried loudly enough for *Art Digest* and *Newsweek* to hear him. But before any stories saw print, Arnold Blanch and Doris Lee, to whom Blanch was then married, acted unreasonably. They thought that Juliana should have protected Burlin. After the jury's decision was known, they drove up to Juliana's house, told her she had no basis for rejecting the picture, and asked her to defend herself. Juliana blew up at their cheek, and the three fought it out. Juliana felt mightily ill-used, especially by Blanch, who owed her so much. She could no longer see a future for herself in Woodstock, and she put Laughing Water up for sale at the end of the summer.

Juliana's leave-taking of Woodstock was not traumatic because she was looking forward to putting over her committee's art bill. Her job would be to make speeches and win converts, and she and Goodrich, Shubert, and Soby were also scheduled to go to Albany to seek advice from Dewey's counsel on how to steer

the bill through the assembly and senate. When Juliana wrote to Carl Rieser, who had just been discharged from the army, her mood was positive.

Dear Carl. "Nothing stays, not the sun, not man's concept of God, not the sovereignty of nations." Not Woodstock, not the Army. It comforted Darwin & me & should you, because it spells movement & sometimes progress. We used to sing in church "I'm nearer my home today, today, than I've ever been before.". . .

I have, too, undertaken a new piece of work which will take me away from New York from next month[?] until November & am up to my head top in research & preparation. It's keeping me alive and grateful. I shall sorely miss Woodstock but my conversations with Comet convince me that there's something somewhere else, and I am glad indeed that I'm not "2 old" as you told me yrs ago!

Love,
Aunt J.

NB. 1. This is moving day up here, very dank, very lonely & very busy.

NB. 2. The house isn't sold yet & I am leaving enough to housekeep in case you get here before the finals.

Before Juliana's speaking tour commenced, she had one more round of jurying to fulfill, but it was prize giving of a much higher order than what went on in Woodstock. Dan Rich had invited her to Chicago for the Art Institute's annual of American paintings. She would be there from October 11 to 13, and the other judges were Raphael Soyer and Reginald Marsh. In a write-up of the show, *Time* referred to Juliana as the Whitney's "doughty duenna," which, in vintage *Time*-ese, was a thesaurus-thumbing substitution for *Newsweek*'s epithet of two months before. Then she was "Mrs. Juliana Force, imperious dowager of American art," for throwing out the Burlin painting.

Juliana stayed in Chicago briefly, because a buyer had appeared for Laughing Water, and she needed to get back to New York. William Pachner, a young painter, had seen the property a few weeks before, but the two couldn't settle on a price. Because he was an artist and Juliana liked him, she gave away the house, which was in perfect, move-in condition, and inhabitable all year round, for $15,000. On October 18, the day of the closing, Pachner and Juliana rode up from New York to Kingston, the county seat, on a sparkling fall morning. Juliana told Pachner that she regretted selling the house, but it couldn't be helped. She also touched on the cold self-interest of some of the Woodstock artists. Pachner, looking out the window, said that the magnificent gold of the leaves drifting off the trees reminded him of an early Italian painting, and Juliana was soothed. "I'm so glad that someone connected with art, someone aesthetic, is going to have this house," she said.

The unsinkable Fiske Kimball was back. In July he had called Flora Miller to nudge her about "the big proposition," but she had not lifted a finger or signed a check. With the advent of the fall art season, he launched his biggest strike. By an irony, it grew out of a conversation Kimball had with Juliana the previous spring. She happened to suggest that he organize a show in honor of

John Sloan; Kimball, elaborating on the idea, conceived an exhibition called Artists of the Philadelphia Press, which focused on Sloan, Glackens, Luks, and Shinn. Whereas Juliana had envisaged an innocent homage to Sloan, Kimball saw the group show as a demonstration of how neatly the Whitney's permanent collection (significant examples from which had been borrowed for the occasion) would mesh with Philadelphia's.

The show opened on October 14, 1945, and the night before, the Millers came down from New York with Tim Coward and his wife for the private preview. Kimball went all out for the Millers, and his showmanship would have earned him a nod of approval from Ziegfeld. The first gallery was set up as a replica of McSorley's Bar, the inspiration for several of Sloan's paintings and prints. There was a period bar, a potbellied stove, and men in handlebar mustaches and long aprons. The second gallery, in which a "free lunch" was served, had tables covered with checked tablecloths. Sitting at an upright piano was a "professor" in tails and cutaway whose job it was to tickle the ivories. The Millers and the Cowards joined in and warbled the old-time tunes. Kimball, his mouth watering from the pictures he could already see being loaded into the truck for Philadelphia, would write, "Our alcove was hung with Whitney paintings, and Flora went through everything with close interest. She almost wilted, on her little clogs, before we got to the far end of the building and let them into the empty loft. 'What is this?' 'The Whitney Wing, we hope.' 'And this?' as we went to the floor below. 'Whitney Hall.' " These tantalizing sights were followed by a succulent dinner at Kimball's house. "[T]he whole occasion," he said, "was the greatest success. At least we could continue to hope for the future."

Even after his wonderful party, Kimball was unable to conquer. The Whitney collection and trust slipped away from him, but not because he committed an error. With the death of Crocker, Kimball's most active and interested partisan, also died Philadelphia's claim. Kimball's bid for the Whitney was not so much defeated as eroded by Flora's passivity. She was content to drift along, letting the management of the trust slide or leaving it to others. And since others were no longer Crocker, but Dunnington, a lawyer still unfamiliar with the complexities of Gertrude's estate and the Met's merger, so much the better to leave well enough alone. Francis Taylor outlasted and wore out Fiske Kimball through the power of Flora's inertia.

Having a cause always invigorated Juliana, and as she and her delegation traveled around New York State in behalf of legislation to buy art, she was firmly convinced that she was not "2 old." And what amounted to a minor miracle confirmed her belief. It will be remembered that Crocker was the one who made the most fuss about Juliana moving her office out of the 8 West Eighth Street building, and he must have been instrumental in tossing her out of her apartment. Flora was softer-hearted than Crocker, and had lately discovered that most of his financial advice had been bad. Flora, in a conciliatory gesture, decided that if the Eighth Street galleries were open on a regular basis, it made little sense to keep the upstairs locked up. Juliana was invited to return to her quarters

above the galleries. Only the restoration of the museum to its old, sovereign self could have pleased her more, and she moved back to her beloved apartment in the late autumn of 1945.

Juliana's return to Eighth Street meant that her hand was strengthened, and not the least important aspect of that strength was the perpetuation of her personality through the maintaining of appearances. The writer and art collector Eloise Spaeth, then living in Dayton, Ohio, was invited to be on the board of the American Federation of Arts in 1945, and came to New York for her first meeting, which was held at the Whitney. "Juliana was always extremely nice to me, and made a little speech at the first meeting I attended," Eloise Spaeth wrote, "saying that what we needed at the A.F.A. was more women on the Board." After business, she continued, "we repaired to Juliana's outstandingly attractive apartment on top of the Museum for cocktails and luncheon. I felt I had arrived on the New York art scene when I was invited to this inner sanctum." Eloise Spaeth would have retained a different impression if her introduction to Juliana had occurred in the railroad flat on West Ninth Street.

At war's end, abstract artists and the New York School had arrived, even at the Whitney. Both sections of the 1945–1946 annuals had a host of new exhibitors: William Baziotes, Romare Bearden, Louise Bourgeois, Hans Hofmann, Carl Holty, Louise Nevelson, Jackson Pollock, Robert Motherwell, Mark Rothko, Leon Polk Smith, Theodoros Stamos, and Dorothea Tanning. There was much twitter in the papers about the museum "going completely modern," although Greenberg, in a toughly argued dissent, charged the Whitney with "affable timidity," "eclectic conformity," and a lack of "strongmindedness" as it picked and chose among trends hit-or-miss. He also stated, "The best painting at the present show is Jackson Pollock's 'Two.' Those who think that I exaggerate Pollock's merit are invited to compare this large vertical canvas with everything else in the Annual." The Whitney would not go so far as to buy a Pollock, but it would stretch to Rothko and Louis Schanker, two alumni of the Whitney Dissenters.

The Whitney had shifted its orientation, and to accommodate the fifty newcomers, a like number of regulars were dropped. Hermon More, who made the more experimental choices, must have taken a drubbing from the excluded older artists, especially the ones who were his neighbors in Woodstock. Forbes Watson saw the first section of the annual, was contemptuous of it, attributed what he considered a "submissive falling in with the abstract" to Juliana, and made some mean-spirited remarks to Alice Sharkey, who demanded to know his opinion of the show. "I first jollied her by saying it looks like 53rd Street provincialism," Watson wrote, "a timid copy of Modern Museum exhibitions. . . . I told her that one had only to look at the pictures in order to discover exactly whom Mrs. Force was playing with socially. Then asked her if Mrs. Force had been seeing much of Sweeney because it looked more like a Sweeney show than a Force show."

Forbes was talking about James Johnson Sweeney, the brilliant curator and

critic who was briefly the director of painting and sculpture at the Modern. To have one's work taken for a Sweeney show, even if one were being thrashed for it, was inversely congratulatory, as Sweeney had a piercing grasp of European modernism and was known for his bold pronouncements. Forbes, in his catty but perceptive way, bit on a kernel of truth. He was correct in guessing that Juliana had taken up with Sweeney and was influenced by him in trying to adjust her taste to the New York School. This was an adjustment Juliana was only fractionally capable of making, but if she were to open herself to the new, she would do so through the method that came best to her—through socializing, talking, and looking, just as twenty-five years before, by playing with Forbes socially, she had absorbed what he had to teach her. (Juliana would write, only half facetiously, to a colleague who wanted her to lecture on the sprawling subject of the state of art in American life in 1945, "I have been too busy with pictures and people all these years to think much about art and . . . therefore, I am incapable of talking on this subject.")

Juliana often assured Carl Rieser that she knew what she had missed by not possessing the technical and professional training of some of her college-educated peers. She repeated to him over the last decade of her life her deep regrets about not having the background she would have liked. By now, Juliana had spent many hours in the company of men like Sweeney, Barr, Rich, Soby, and Goodrich, and she could not help but observe the degree to which disciplined instruction and connoisseurship burnished and augmented their native intelligence. Of course, when Juliana was a tyro, such concerns did not exist. Her own liveliness and vivacity, moored in the solidity of Gertrude's trust, and not the quality or thoroughness of her formal education, brought about her success. To have chosen other than what she did, Juliana would have had to have been a clairvoyant.

Forbes and Nan Watson were about to move back to the New York area, and as can be gathered from the tenor of his writing, Forbes was miffed that Juliana was listening to someone else even though he was available again for counsel. He did have one avid and credulous listener, however. Alice Sharkey seconded everything he said about the exhibition, and went on to heap abuse on Juliana and Hermon More's handling of it, but she was not strictly accountable for her spiteful remarks. Mrs. Sharkey was in the initial stages of arteriosclerosis, and her speech was a reflection of her mental deterioration. As she became less rational, she entertained fantasies of becoming the director of the Whitney and savaged More and Juliana's qualifications with a view to exalting her own. At this stage, her conduct, although unbecoming, was still harmless, and everyone at the museum protected her. She was liked and appreciated at the Whitney, and when her condition did not affect her, she performed impeccably. The real unpleasantness would come later.

The new direction the Whitney was charting in its annuals was not at all plausible for the Metropolitan, so Juliana chose only one painting for uptown, which was *Off Cape Split, Maine*, by Marin. Stieglitz was asking $6,000, but Juliana thought that was a ridiculous price, and got it for $4,700. She also picked out seven graphic works, including examples by Baziotes, Mark Tobey, Andrew

Wyeth, and Jacob Lawrence. (Lawrence was an artist whom Juliana greatly admired. In December of 1945, in her role as head of the exhibitions committee for the AFA, she arranged for his *John Brown* series,* a group of twenty-two gouaches portraying the life and death of the abolitionist, which she had just seen at the Downtown Gallery, to be given a two-year tour.)

The Metropolitan could not spend the Hearn funds on sculpture, and its trustees would not appropriate other money for it, so any sculpture entering either collection had to be acquired by the Whitney. The prohibition was a source of future fortune for the Whitney, for not a few of the acquisitions of most interest today were made in sculpture. For example, in 1946 Juliana bought *Cockfight—Variation* by David Smith, and in 1947 she would buy *Humpty Dumpty*, one of Noguchi's finest slate sculptures. But the record was not without blemishes, some of which may be laid to the Whitney's having an annual budget of $5,000 to $10,000 for *all* art, and some to a lingering taste for traditional figurative sculpture. Alexander Calder wanted the Whitney to buy a work, and he wrote to Juliana that he had been waiting "hopefully, but in vain" for the honor. She, too, wanted to purchase a Calder, but the budget had restricted her. Juliana wrote to the artist:

> Our budget, as you know, is a very small one and sculpture is necessarily so expensive that we have made few purchases in recent years. This is not at all a criticism of your work because, as you very well know, we think that you are one of the foremost sculptors of the day and have always looked at your work with interest and also the conviction that we sometime must acquire a selection of your work.
>
> You ask if something couldn't be done? That is not the question; we have done what we could and hope to do better in the future.

Her letter rings less true than it reads if one knows that the future did not come during Juliana's lifetime. Calder was a regular exhibitor in the annuals, but the Whitney didn't buy a sculpture until 1950.

Juliana spent the first months of 1946 lobbying for her art legislation, which was introduced in the new session of the New York State senate and assembly. She and her fellow committee members amassed signatures, wrote letters, and talked to local politicians in both parties. Juliana called a press conference on March 5 that got national coverage and secured an emphatic *Times* editorial in her favor, but the bill died in committee because, according to Charles Breitel, the governor's counsel, the idea was still too new. Juliana was disappointed, but not crushed. By April, she was intensifying her activities to get the bill reintroduced in 1947.

Juliana was also at the helm of another crusade in early 1946. The issue was unpopular and it had nothing to do with American art or artists, but if she did not take up this cause, she would have lost that self-respect she esteemed as a

---

* The entire series was bought out of the gallery's show by Milton Lowenthal, who later donated it to the Detroit Institute of Art.

fierce necessity. As one writer said about Juliana's definite stands, "She first made sure she was right, then poured all of her gallant spirit into the battle." Loving to lead, she also recognized that the power to lead carried its own responsibility.

On April 7, 1945, 202 Old Master paintings were found in a salt mine near Merkers, Germany, by American soldiers of the Third Army. Most of the paintings, which were stored in the mine to protect them from aerial bombing, were the property of the Kaiser Friedrich Museum* in Berlin, but a few came from the Deutsches Museum. None of the pictures—irreplaceable examples of Giotto, Masaccio, Fra Angelico, Fra Lippo Lippi, Botticelli, Sassetta, Mantegna, Dürer, Raphael, Rembrandt, Vermeer, Velázquez, Rubens, Caravaggio, Titian, Holbein, Poussin, and Watteau—had been looted by the Nazis from occupied countries. All of the evacuated art had been in the permanent collections of German museums before Hitler came to power.

After the pictures were found in the salt mine, a special containment center was built in Wiesbaden to house them. There the paintings were supposed to sit until they could be returned to the Kaiser Friedrich Museum or its new incarnation, because the old building was destroyed. For reasons never made clear, except for the obvious one that he assumed he might get away with the deed, Lt. Gen. Lucius Clay, the military governor of Germany under Eisenhower, ordered the 202 paintings transferred from Wiesbaden to Frankfurt for eventual shipment to the United States for safekeeping until "the German people earned the right to have them."

Clay's order was unconscionable and illegal on two grounds. First, as has been said, the pictures legitimately belonged to two German museums. Neither institution received the paintings through Nazi looting or other dubious avenues of ownership. Second, under an article of the Hague Convention, to which the United States was a signatory, the property of institutions dedicated to the arts, even when they are state property, were to be treated as private property, which meant that *any seizures whatsoever* were forbidden.

After Clay ordered the German pictures into "protective custody" on September 26, 1945, thirty-two of the thirty-five officers—three were unreachable —with the Monuments, Fine Arts and Archives section in Germany published an open letter urging Clay to rescind the transfer order. (To help ensure that the cultural treasures of Europe would be preserved during and after the war, the Roosevelt government created a Monuments, Fine Arts and Archives section and solicited many of the country's top museum men to staff it as civilian officers. They were charged with preserving museums, private collections, archives, and historic monuments in the European theater.) Because the paintings were carefully packed and adequately cared for, the letter alleged that the general's motives were questionable and established a precedent neither morally tenable nor ethically trustworthy. All of the officers in the American Zone were acknowledged art experts, and many of them have since become eminent. Some of the signers of the letter, later nicknamed the Wiesbaden Manifesto, were the future museum

* Now the State Museums.

directors Andrew C. Ritchie, Charles Parkhurst, James Rorimer, Thomas Carr Howe, the conservator Sheldon Keck, and Lincoln Kirstein. When Parkhurst refused to move the paintings, he was threatened with a court-martial.

No line of argument would sway the general, so the worried monuments officers modified their request. If Clay truly believed the pictures were at risk in Germany, then, they begged him, please send the collection to the Louvre for safekeeping. Under no circumstances should most of the paintings, which were on fragile wood panels sensitive to the minutest movement or change in climate, be moved around, shaken, and exposed to lengthy travel, especially across the ocean. But on November 25, 1945, the Kaiser Friedrich pictures started across the Atlantic.

They reached the United States on December 7, 1945. As a consequence of a sea journey and a sharp change of climate, some of the Italian Renaissance paintings were reported to be brittle and cracking. The art, still in "protective custody," was taken to the National Gallery of Art and sequestered there.

The chief monuments officer in Berlin when the Kaiser Friedrich pictures were discovered was Calvin Sutliffe Hathaway, a curator at the Cooper Union Museum before the war. Hathaway was furious at the seizure of the German pictures and their exposure to incalculable harm. He wanted the pictures returned to Wiesbaden and the care of the Kaiser Friedrich Museum's head curator, who was left in Germany. But he was having a difficult time convincing anyone he was right, because the American government was not doing anything to dispel the popular opinion that commandeering Old Master paintings was deserved punishment for the Germans as opposed to the scandalous illegal maneuver it was. How to get justice done? Realizing that he didn't have the name or connections to get some action on his own, Hathaway turned to an old friend of clout and conscience after he returned to New York at the end of 1945. He went to Juliana, briefing her on the physical hazards and moral ambiguities at issue. What Clay had said, although later whitewashed, was that although the paintings he seized were bona fide German property, the Germans had to behave themselves or the United States had the right to keep them. Almost as outrageously, some of the paintings were receiving conservation treatment in Washington. Was it right for American restorers to do this without the knowledge or consent of the rightful owners? If Old Master paintings belonging to the National Gallery had been worked on, let alone seized, by another museum, how would our art officials feel?

Juliana jumped into the row with her usual zest and promised to lead the protest against the government and the National Gallery. She naturally recognized that because of her identification with American art, her intrusion might not look relevant. Accordingly, she asked Frederick Mortimer Clapp, the director of the Frick Collection, to join her, and for the next two years Juliana, Clapp, and Hathaway would be an unflagging team. As a power in the AFA, Juliana quickly got the federation behind her. The *Magazine of Art* published a cross section of articles and letters about the affair in the February issue, and on February 7, 1946, the *Times* ran a story acknowledging that the transfer of the art raised a valid question of ethics.

In April Juliana, Clapp, and Hathaway drafted a resolution eventually destined for President Truman. They decried the current status of the German paintings and urged that they be returned to their rightful owners in Germany. They collected the signatures of 111 leading art authorities around the nation. The letter they sent to their colleagues declared the protest "to be our plain and simple duty, for it is our considered judgment that no explanation or excuse acceptable to the public conscience can be found for sending old masters across the sea to this country." Another pressing reason for going forward with the resolution, Juliana and Clapp said, was that they had received reports that further shipments of art might be undertaken. If scholars and administrators were silent, the excuse of "protective custody" could be invoked again. Charles Sawyer, who was then in Washington, wrote to Clapp that the marshaling of opposition to the government's protective custody "had considerable weight in discouraging further shipments."

Every important museum director in the country approved the letter and agreed to sign the resolution, save two. One, as would be expected, was David Finley, the director of the National Gallery, the repository for the Kaiser Friedrich pictures. The other was Francis Taylor. Thomas Parker, the editor of the *Magazine of Art*, wrote to Juliana and Hudson Walker that Taylor "carried the ball" for the National Gallery and the State Department.

In standing up for Clay's action in print, Taylor, who was enjoying the scrap as much as Juliana, constructed his arguments in a galling framework of innuendo and inference. He portrayed his opponents—those who had signed the Wiesbaden Manifesto or who were about to sign the Truman resolution—as art radicals in the foolish minority. Juliana and her cohorts were denounced in the letters columns of several art magazines as Communist sympathizers for criticizing the army and the federal government. Associate Justice Owen Roberts, a trustee of the National Gallery and the chairman of a presidential committee on the protection and salvage of monuments, condemned their dissent as "deplorable" and "without justification."

The baseness of these accusations did not shake Juliana because she knew from her first meetings with Calvin Hathaway that she would be a lightning rod for enemy thunderbolts. Lincoln Kirstein acknowledged that in a letter to her touching upon her position vis-à-vis Taylor:

> Due to your outstanding position as a protector and aid to American art, and the present situation of the Museum which you direct, I am certain that you will be the focus of an attack both by the leading national and the largest metropolitan museum. This attack is an honor, and there are a great many people, not only in New York but all over the country who will realize what this fight means. . . .
> I am, dear Mrs. Force, always at your disposal.

On May 9, 1946, the resolution was mailed to Harry Truman and Dean Acheson, the acting Secretary of State, with the addition of the provocative lines, "many, including the Germans themselves, may find it hard to distinguish between the resultant situation and the 'protective custody' used by the Nazis as a camouflage for the sequestration of artistic treasures of other countries." Juliana

and Clapp received official answers—vague, uninformative, and noncommittal—on May 22, from Acheson and from Truman's secretary. Juliana then advised Clapp that although he need take no notice of Justice Roberts's fusillade, both he and she had to write personal notes of acknowledgment to Truman and Acheson. In her letter to Acheson, Juliana tried again. She reiterated that the high-handedness of confiscating the Kaiser Friedrich collection was detrimental to the country's reputation as well as to the physical health of the pictures. She received no satisfaction from this letter either, but responsible people in art circles applauded her courage. On June 11, 1946, Juliana wrote to a colleague that the wrongdoers were unequal to the outcry they provoked.

> Your appreciation of the work that was done on the resolution has been a great comfort to me. The job was not pleasant, but I have private and reliable information that the resolution has been effective, but the opposition has not had the courage to be frank about this any more than they have been from the beginning.

Confident that the protest had succeeded in its aims and that the Kaiser Friedrich paintings would shortly be on their way to Berlin, Juliana left the Truman Administration to itself and its conscience and caught up on her work for the New York State art legislation. She held several meetings to assign responsibilities for the fall campaign, which was aimed at getting a bill passed in early 1947. Several of Dewey's aides and friends were invited to her apartment for enlightenment. Over cocktails, the committee members did their best to convince them that the bill would benefit other constituencies than artists, that it was free of boondoggling features, and that it was not a continuation of the WPA. As before, everyone had high hopes.

Juliana was working on these two projects until the middle of June, and she had given no thought to where she would spend the summer. John Frear had already taken a house near Rhinebeck, New York, and he was enchanted by the middle portion of the Hudson River valley, where the descendants of Dutch patroons and English Tories still dwelled genteelly in the Greek Revival mansions and Italianate villas of their founding progenitors. He talked with Juliana about his love for the area, and she asked, "Isn't there something up there for me?"

Happy to oblige, Frear looked into rentals for her, and thought that one of the smaller houses scattered over the grounds of Sylvania, a 400-acre estate in Barrytown, would suit her well. Sylvania belonged to Chanler Chapman, who was a direct descendant of the American writer John Jay Chapman and a nephew of Juliana and Gertrude's raucous artist-friend, Bob Chanler. Frear correctly guessed that she would like the dower house, a cottage painted barn red with pink trim. It had a terrace that looked west to the Hudson and a resident ghost. The latter was the ultimate draw for Juliana, who had retained her strong fin-de-siècle interest in the supernatural.

Juliana wanted to look at the cottage at once, and she and Carl Rieser drove to Barrytown from Manhattan. When Carl saw how ravishing the house was, the first words out of his mouth were, "Now, don't let my aunt buy anything." Juliana had lunch with the Chapmans to discuss the rental, about which Frear

said, "I thought Juliana was shrewd until I heard how much Olivia Chapman had charged her for the cottage. But she came out of there saying, 'I took it, Jack! I took it!'" Juliana was set for the season, and she retrieved the furniture she had stored in Woodstock.

Juliana called on the Livingstons, Aldriches, and some of the other established families in the valley, but their abstemious habits dismayed her. Mrs. Aldrich was a teetotaler, and after a dry evening at the Aldrich house, she complained to Frear, "What do you think I had at dinner? Nothing!" and made it a point not to go there again.

Seeing so much of Juliana that summer, Frear could not help but notice that she was pained sporadically by indigestion. She had seen a physician about her malady because he gave her some kind of medicine. However, she stopped taking it after a while, she told Frear, because it never seemed to do any good. Instead, she drank martinis, which did kill the pain.

The painter Edward Powis Jones said that Juliana was lonely in Barrytown and craved companionship. To be nice to her, he took her to meet his grandmother, Mrs. Andrew C. Zabriskie, who owned a house in the area. It proved to be an excellent match, because the two women had much in common, with the prospect of more visits in the offing. Juliana wrote to Carl about her new acquaintance:

> I had a completely delicious time with his grandmother, Mrs. Zabriskie, a martinet if there ever was one, but with a divine sense of humor & a fabulous house full of Hudson River paintings, sofas, rugs, views and solid silver. Lunch accordingly. The pool is a mile from the house & you are free to swim any time there. For me, I was content to swim in the luxury of bygone days & talk about Prague and Vienna & the baroque of prewar days.

Back at the dower house, Juliana entertained young Jones with a string of English ghost stories, which she told with practiced relish. She loved having a local ghost in tow—any company was better than none—and she was waiting eagerly for the entrance of her guest from the spirit world.

With or without benefit of an apparition, Juliana went to Cornish, New Hampshire, in the middle of July to infuse some spirit into yet another languishing cause that she had adopted earlier in the year. Cornish had been a thriving art colony in the late nineteenth century, and its central presence then was Augustus Saint-Gaudens, who built an attractive house and studio there. After the sculptor's death, his family had been partially successful in preserving the property as a public site, but in 1944 a fire destroyed the studio, and the other buildings were in disrepair. Since Juliana and Homer Saint-Gaudens, the artist's son, were great chums, she agreed without hesitation to become a trustee of the Saint-Gaudens Memorial in February of 1946. Her enterprise was desperately needed in any money-raising and publicity drive for getting the house and studio refurbished and noticed, as in those days Saint-Gaudens was not the revered figure that he is now.

An ardent admirer of Saint-Gaudens, Juliana was a vocal trustee at the July meeting. The only other credible professionals on the board were Homer Saint-

Gaudens and Margaret French Cresson, who was Daniel Chester French's daughter and likewise a sculptor. The rest were good-hearted but hopelessly sentimental amateurs whose ideas, as Juliana made clear, were inane. Her chief mission was to block the suggestion that Saint-Gaudens's studio be converted into a tearoom and/or showcase for local artists. She then laid down the law: Exhibitions, if held, had to meet the high standards of Saint-Gaudens himself. Juliana laboriously explained the need for setting strict criteria for shows and resisting the temptation to hold any until a proper place was completed for them.

With September came the resumption of lobbying for the New York State art bill; the executive committee had done its work, and the legislation now had the support of every museum and library in the state. The campaign climaxed with a back-slapping dinner at the Hotel Utica on January 17, 1947. The politicians were receptive and jovial, and Juliana and her henchmen thought that passage of the legislation was secure. But as they were shortly to see, the bill went down to defeat for the second and last time. They had been vanquished by the legislators' choosing salary raises for teachers over sales for artists, and by the political ambitions of Gov. Thomas E. Dewey, whose eyes were on the White House. Irvine Shubert said the bill was doomed because "it was bad politics for Dewey. He would say to us, 'What would the farmers say if they knew we were wasting money on artists?' " The bill didn't stand a chance without Dewey's support, and it was not resuscitated again until Nelson Rockefeller became governor. The work Juliana and her committee did was the seed of the New York State Council on the Arts.

Losing vexed Juliana, especially after her steady travail. Her resistance was low, and she came down with a long siege of flu. As soon as she could get out of bed, she threw herself into the trenches again. She was battling for the artists' welfare and against censorship; for the umpteenth time, her adversary was the federal government and its knee-jerk response that art was a waste of the taxpayers' money. Or, as she put it, her quarrel was with "arrogance appearing in official disguise."

In May and June 1946, a State Department employee purchased seventy-nine contemporary American oils and thirty-eight watercolors for a government program of circulating exhibitions. The selections were a liberal and judicious mix of older and younger painters—examples by O'Keeffe, Dove, Davis, Shahn, Sheeler, Kuniyoshi, Bearden, Baziotes, Adolph Gottlieb, Guston, Motherwell, and Ralston Crawford were in the collection. In October, as a prelude to an overseas tour to improve cultural relations, the seventy-nine paintings were shown at the Metropolitan to favorable reviews in the art press.

A month later, the Hearst syndicate ran three reactionary attacks on the State Department collection. Modern art was linked to communism and called junk; the paintings were the work of "the lunatic fringe," and the artists with foreign-sounding names were defamed for having foreign-sounding names. A reproduction of an oil by Guglielmi bore the caption, "If you contemplate adding to the suicide rate, we recommend this picture for the guest room." Even for a

Hearst paper, these broadsides were ignorant. They were all too reminiscent of the vilification and scare headlines of Nazi propaganda, but congressmen, radio commentators, and *Look* magazine slung as much mud as the Hearst columnists and screamed about good American dollars being thrown away. They demanded that the State Department justify this "artistic flim-flam." After Harry Truman characterized modern art as "the vaporings of a half-baked, lazy people," and said of the Kuniyoshi painting, "If that's art, I'm a Hottentot," the State Department knew it was licked. In early 1947, the man who bought the art resigned, the circulating exhibitions program was canceled, and the collection was reclassified as war surplus in order to sell it off. Watching in disbelief, Juliana, More, and Goodrich could not abide any more. They could not halt the sale, but they could and did arrange to give the unjustly maligned collection a dignified exhibition—scheduled for May of 1948—before the government got rid of it.

The controversy over the State Department pictures and the ignominious end of its exhibition program led directly to the establishment of the Artists Equity Association, an organization formed to lobby for artists' rights and protect its members against unscrupulous practices, in April of 1947. Artists Equity's first action was to petition, albeit futilely, the State Department to reinstate its overseas tour. Kuniyoshi was the first president, and Henry Schnakenberg was made one of the vice-presidents. Because of their reputation as artists' champions, Schnakenberg asked Juliana, Sweeney, and Watson to help launch the group. Juliana gave freely of her energies to promote Artists Equity, and she, Schnakenberg, and Sweeney met several times during March and April. Francis Taylor joined them at the first meetings in April and May to speak out against the dispersal of the State Department's art collection. The Met, because it had shown the paintings, was also a target of the reactionary obloquies.

Juliana and Taylor were allied against these stupidities, but a short time later sparks were struck between them again. Taylor was consummating the second phase of the plan that Dorothy Miller heard him foretell: the absorption of the other museum in New York. In 1947, after some years of wrangling and waiting, he was maneuvering delicately through a sweetheart deal for the Met that was more neutrally known as the Three Museum Agreement. This was a pact dividing up the territory of the New York art world among the Met, the Modern, and the Whitney in such a fashion that the apportioning would eliminate confusion and repetition. The Met would confine itself to classic and historical art, refraining from collecting twentieth-century works, the Whitney would limit itself (as usual) to American art, and the Modern would attend only to strains of twentieth-century modernism in America and abroad. After a work in the Modern's collection passed from the controversially modern to the safely historical or classic, it would go to the Metropolitan; in return, the Met would give the Modern acquisition funds for these purchases. To start the sorting out, the Modern would *sell* the Metropolitan twenty-six works of art, among them, works by Cézanne, Picasso, Matisse, Seurat, Rouault, and Daumier, and the Met would *lend* the Modern a Maillol bronze and Picasso's portrait of Gertrude Stein.

Taylor must have been pirouetting around his office in a high state of glee after the preliminary contract was made in March of 1947. The new arrangement,

to last for five years, effectively reduced the Modern and the Whitney to vassals of the Metropolitan, slowly but inexorably feeding all their best pieces into its uptown maw. The Whitney was already a satrapy of 82nd Street, but the Modern was not. The treaty had the added boon of relieving the Met of the responsibility of buying any twentieth-century art at all. For all the negotiating, the Met merely agreed not to enter a field which it had never understood or wanted to be in, and the Whitney promised not to leave a field which it had no intention of departing from. The Whitney and the Modern would be pitted against each other, and the Modern would slowly be skimmed of the cream of its collection after doing the hard and experimental job of obtaining it.

Juliana, More, and Goodrich were angered by this cunning deal and the preferential treatment accorded the Modern. The plan had been gestating for some time, but the Whitney had been consulted as an afterthought. Most galling of all, Taylor was going to hand over $25,000 a year to the Modern for acquisitions, whereas the Whitney had to fight for every dime of its annual $10,000. Juliana, on the warpath, wanted to discuss the Whitney's potential loss of leadership in the American field with Roland Redmond, who had recently succeeded William Church Osborn as the president of the Met. In preparation for her meeting, Goodrich drafted a stinging memo setting forth the Whitney's position.

> The policy of acquisitions raises a serious question. As I understand it, the Metropolitan pays $25,000. a year to the Modern to buy contemporary art, which will remain in the Modern Museum until it becomes respectable enough to hang in the Metropolitan. As the Modern already has a large number of American objects in its collection, and presumably will continue to add to them, does this mean that the Metropolitan is ready to expend annually an amount larger than is put at the disposal of the Whitney to build up the Modern Museum's collection of contemporary American art? It seems strange to me that the Metropolitan is willing to trust the judgment of the Modern Museum in its purchases of contemporary art, which generally are of the most advanced order, while it mistrusts any recommendation of ours from the Hearn fund unless the painting comes from the walls of the Academy.
>
> It is true that consultation on acquisitions is required among all three Museums, but I cannot believe that the Modern will make any concessions, even though the Metropolitan furnishes the funds. The Whitney should have equal freedom in choosing additions to its collections.
>
> Consultation is presumably advised to prevent duplication, but Mr. Barr with more funds at his disposal could purchase more examples and could thus almost monopolize the field of modern American art by proposing that the Whitney refrain from purchasing the works of certain artists because of their inclusion in the Museum's collection. We would then be forced to forego [sic] purchases of works that might be shown in our Museum for many years until time and the Metropolitan Trustees made them classics, suitable to hang among the masterpieces.

In their talks with Redmond, Juliana and Barr raised enough questions requiring legal resolution that the agreement, which was supposed to go into effect in June of 1947, could not be enacted for several more months.

Juliana was also harsh with Carl Rieser, who was guilty of proposing marriage to Edith Lewis, a young woman he had known for about a year. As with Allan

before him, Juliana did everything in her power to discourage women from becoming too attentive to Carl. At a party, she saw him talking most of the evening with an attractive woman, and suspecting the latter's impure designs on him, Juliana, through a mutual friend, warned her to stay away from her nephew.

Edith Lewis met Juliana in the first months of 1947, shortly after she became engaged to Carl. The encounter and the setting were high drama for her. The feeling of entering the world of the stage began from the moment the little red elevator took her upstairs to Juliana's apartment and mounted after she laid eyes on the Biedermeier chairs, the gessoed bed by Max Kuehne, and the handmade bookshelves tapering to tiny Gothic arches and filled with first editions of English classics. Edith Lewis (now Edith Nolder) recalled:

> This woman is out of a storybook, I thought. She was one of a kind, and she had whatever she wanted when she wanted it. She acted in character all the time, but not like any other character I had ever met. She said what she pleased, and she would crumple the ordinary person. When I met Carl's mother, she threw her arms around me and gave me a present, but Aunt Juliana displayed a lack of affection. The first thing she said to me was "Do you read?" Then I knew why Debs [Deborah Rieser] used to hide in the kitchen to get up her nerve when she came to call. . . . She was a very tiny eater, and later on when I had her to dinner, I gave her a lot of food. She wheeled on me and said, "I am not a garbage can."
>
> Juliana was a very disciplined person, and she ran her life very neatly. She made things work and they did. She never put a foot wrong when it came to etiquette. The first time I visited her, I was wearing little white gloves and I left them there. They were returned to me pressed and laundered. She would never be rude or gauche or cruel by mistake. She would be rude by design.

Edith Lewis was right to regard Juliana as a rival, although as she said, "There was no winner in that battle. It was a standoff." Juliana almost persuaded Carl to break off with Edith, but they made plans to marry in the fall.

In the midst of her meddling with Carl and Edith, Juliana's better nature asserted itself elsewhere. Alice Sharkey's behavior and mental state deteriorated sharply as her disease progressed, and her extreme forgetfulness made it very difficult to cover for her at the museum. Mrs. Sharkey's daughters, Anne and Margaret, were also cognizant of the situation, and they begged their mother to quit her job. But the poor woman was too ill to know that she was not rational, and she said cruel things to them for their perceived disloyalty. At wit's end, the Sharkey children secretly made an appointment with Juliana. They told her that their mother was no longer responsible for her actions, and that she needed to be cared for at home. The Sharkeys asked Juliana if she would spare them by playing the villain and dismissing their mother. Juliana was extremely sympathetic to their plight and said yes at once. She fired Alice Sharkey in the spring of 1947 and gave her a check for $1,500 in severance pay. Mrs. Sharkey did blame Juliana for getting rid of her, and her daughters faced one less anxiety during their trials.

Before Juliana closed the museum, she toured the Saint-Gaudens Memorial again, and then made her first and only application to the Whitney trust, the elusive grail of Kimball, Spivey, Wright, and Taylor. The estate awarded her

$5,000 for the refurbishing of the site. Saint-Gaudens's studio could now be restored, and the grant also provided enough money to underwrite centennial exhibitions of the sculptor's work in New York and New Hampshire in 1948. Then Juliana was off to spend a few weeks with Guy Pène du Bois and his family at Linden Hall, their Victorian manor in Stonington, Connecticut. Du Bois ran an art school during the summer, and he was busy with his work as administrator, teacher, and tame bohemian. Over the summer Juliana and du Bois's daughter, Yvonne, became very close. Juliana confided to Yvonne that something was wrong with her intestinal tract and that her monthly visits to New York were for medical treatments, as opposed to the pressing business matters she cited as the reason for her absences to the rest of the family. Yvonne, sufficiently alarmed by what she intuited to be a serious illness, told Juliana how much she had meant to the du Bois family all through the years. The two women looked at each other and burst into tears.

Juliana was back in harness, and agreeably so, by Labor Day. On August 29 and 30, 1947, she was a featured panelist at the first Woodstock Art Conference, a symposium cosponsored by the Woodstock Art Association and Artists Equity. The subject of the conference was that well-chewed yet indigestible chestnut, "The Contemporary Artist in Relation to Society," but the speakers were provocative and varied. Joining Juliana, who represented the museum profession, were Harold Clurman, who spoke for the theater, Milton Lowenthal for the collector, Heywood Hale Broun and Howard Devree for the press, Kuniyoshi for the painter, and David Smith, who was also active in Artists Equity, for the sculptor.

Kuniyoshi opened the conference, and after his and Smith's speeches he introduced Juliana. She was given all of fifteen minutes to explain the function of the museum in American society, but she made do with a sentence or two. An American art museum had a twofold duty, Juliana stated: to be constantly involved with the artistic life that was going on around it while also demonstrating that this same art had a heritage, a proud tradition in which the public could take pride. Dispensing with the pronouncements expected of her, she then wryly enumerated the qualities that an ideal art museum and its director should possess. Juliana's satire was light, yet it had been conditioned by the bitter lessons of the last few years. In the best of all possible worlds, a museum would be free of trustees. It would employ instead "a good honest bookkeeper whose accounts shall be open to public inspection." Nor would this museum have to plead with trustees or other benefactors for financial aid; it would be supported entirely by taxation. As for the director, Juliana proclaimed, "His tenure of office will only be ten years. He must undergo eye and heart examinations, because if he has not sensibility and love for art, he should not be eligible. His ears should be examined so that he can hear what the walls are saying, and lastly, his head should be examined, to see if he is crazy enough to take the position." Everyone laughed with Juliana, but her jokes had been earned.

The mood of the symposium changed after Smith, speaking during a ques-

tion-and-answer period, dwelled on the economic hardships that sculptors faced, among them the discounts on purchases that museums insisted on taking. He then advocated the necessity of state sponsorship of art, a topic in which he was not well-versed. As he talked on, long on bombast and short on facts, he unwittingly criticized the New York State art legislation, which had consumed two years of Juliana's life. Smith should have approached Juliana with caution, as she could be depended on to punish him for his chance denigration of a pet project. Juliana asked Smith if the failure of the state to sponsor art could be traced to a lack of understanding on the part of the public. Unaware of the legislation's terms or history, Smith rushed ahead and declared that a bill for a state art program should be introduced at once.

The trap had been laid and sprung, and Smith was caught fast in it. Juliana took Smith to task, pointing out that the very legislation he wanted was defeated twice in Albany, and no wonder, if the artists didn't trouble to familiarize themselves with a bill that should have been of deepest concern to them. Smith confessed his ignorance of the bill and, obviously flustered, could summon up nothing better than a weak reply. "I'd rather be judged on my work than my memory," he said, "but I'm afraid I don't know about the bill." He then retreated, wretchedly embarrassed at being caught out.

Juliana had trounced Smith unequivocally in public, and he could not let it go. In the days and weeks to come, he became obsessed with persuading everyone involved with the conference that the bill's existence had merely slipped his mind. Smith even sent an excuse-filled letter of apology to Juliana; he could back down, yet he could not admit to plain ignorance, especially to the formidable authority that Juliana represented. The sculptor then went on to ask the organizers of the conference if they would expunge his exchange with Juliana from the published transcript of the proceedings. They complied, and the edited booklet on the conference contains no hint of the debate.

September brought the wedding of Carl Rieser and Edith Lewis. Juliana accepted the marriage because it was going ahead for better or worse, and the wedding reception was held in her apartment. In full fettle as hostess and head of the family, she was in the role she required, but the atmosphere was frosty. "She spoke of separating the sheep from the goats, meaning her family from mine," Edith Nolder said.

Adding to Juliana's general discontent with the world, the Three Museum Agreement was signed on September 15, 1947. In this case, the sheep and the goats were not separated, but thrown in among the foxes, yet Juliana and her staff were gratified to see that their objections had carried weight. The contract contained an important alteration—the Met was still going to buy twenty-six objects from the Modern, but 53rd Street would not be given an annual purchase fund. The Modern's curators were to buy as usual, and if and when the Met was ready to allow a work into its collection, an offer would be made for it. The Whitney still chafed at the pact, but the Modern's competitive edge had been eliminated.

Anne and Margaret Sharkey had a childhood friend named Jane Wasey who was introduced to Juliana during her art student days. An accomplished carver and modeler, Wasey began exhibiting in the sculpture annuals in the early 1940s, and in September of 1947, she wanted to make a portrait bust of Juliana. "She was ugly, but distinguished-looking," Wasey remembered, "so I thought of her as handsome. She had one of the most interesting faces I had ever seen, so I asked if I could do a head of her. 'I'd love you to do it,' she said. 'Let's start it right away.' "

For the next few weeks, the two women retired to the Benton room two or three afternoons a week. Wasey encouraged her sitter to talk because she wanted to observe the movement of Juliana's neck and facial muscles. Both enjoyed their sessions together immensely: Juliana because she looked on the time as a relaxing interlude, and Wasey because she had such an animated sitter to work with. Wasey esteemed Juliana because she was sophisticated and tolerant about the portrait, as it was to be an unidealized likeness. Wasey modeled a face that was as stern and monumental as an ancient lawgiver, a face that had endured much and knew its own hardihood. "Juliana was a realist, and she could take the head I did," Wasey said, although others at the museum disapproved of its severity.

Juliana liked the sculpture enough to throw a cocktail party in Wasey's honor, to take place just before the clay version was cast in bronze. Until it was necessary to take it to the foundry, Wasey left the bust upstairs in the Benton room and didn't check it until the afternoon of the party. When she went into the room, the head was not on its stand. Wasey rushed over there and found her sculpture in pieces on the floor. One of the night watchmen had evidently knocked the bust off its pedestal while making his rounds, but didn't tell anyone. Wasey screamed when she saw the damage, and Juliana ran in to see what had happened. She stayed calm and took command. "Look, we're going to start a fresh head tomorrow, and we're going to have a party today just the same," she told her distraught friend. Juliana was so positive that Wasey took heart and was in fit spirits by the time the guests arrived for her party. The next day, they started over. Wasey modeled another bust that was cast in bronze and later entered the Whitney's collection.

Juliana never saw the finished version of her portrait. In modeling her sitter's appearance as accurately as she did, Wasey depicted a woman in a ravaged physical condition. The bronze shows not the puffy countenance of a few years before, but a face worn by pain. On October 6, 1947, Henry Schnakenberg noted in his diary that he went to see Juliana, who was ill. Later in the month, her complaints were so serious and frequent that no amount of medicine or other quackish regimens would allow her to keep neglecting them. (Her fondness for health fads notwithstanding, Juliana, who had always scorned her mother's weakness in using real and feigned sickness for sympathy, ignored illness whenever possible, preferring the consequences of a foolish stoicism. She had a further horror of giving way to illness in public.) She was admitted to Harkness Pavilion at Columbia Presbyterian Hospital for tests and the diagnosis was an advanced

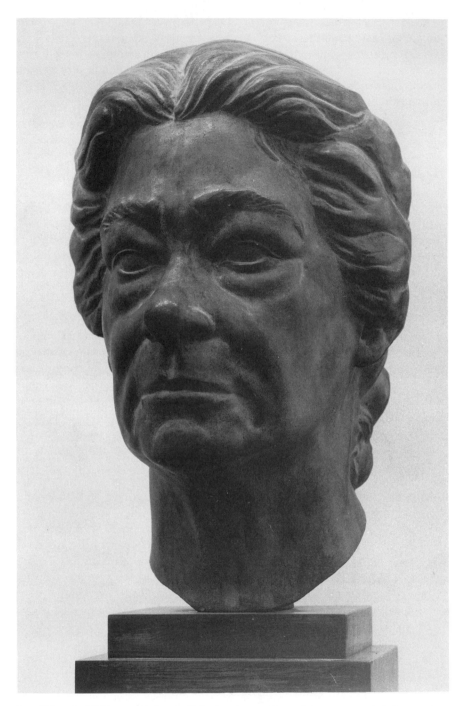

Jane Wasey's 1947 portrait bust of Juliana, stern and pared down, recorded the wasting effects of the cancer that would kill her.

state of stomach cancer. A colostomy was performed, but she was not expected to live for more than a few weeks.

Once Juliana accustomed herself to her fate, she began winding up her professional obligations. She resigned her post at the AFA and sent word to Eloise Spaeth, whom she asked to step in for her. Then she turned to the museum. On November 2, Juliana wrote to Flora Miller:

> Dear Flora. The surgeon has at last told me everything. It has taken me two days to get over the verdict. I must tell some one & I want that some one to be you. Besides you are the only one who has any right to know. I do hope you will not mind & that you will call me soon.
> With love & many thanks for everything—J.

At this point, Juliana could not bring herself to use the word "cancer," which was then a taboo subject in polite society. The disease was spoken about in whispers, if at all, and more often than not, physicians did not inform their patients of the true nature of their condition. Juliana was told—and probably demanded—the facts, but, then again, she was no stranger to cancer: It had claimed Mary Rieser four years earlier.

Juliana's mood of acceptance and euphemism did not last long. It is characteristic of mortally ill patients to cry out in despair, How can this be happening to me? In Juliana's case, the anguish was suffused with fury, and her question —How *dare* this happen to me?—was more like an imprecation, as if death were an unruly artist or an inept government official. She was so angry about dying that she insisted she was going to live. Juliana simply made up her mind that she would treat cancer as she had every other adversary in her life—she would fight it until it backed down. To begin with, she would submit to any operation that held out a hope of a cure, and in November, she underwent a second operation for the removal of two-thirds of her stomach and part of her colon.

The extraordinary measures Juliana insisted upon meant that she was hospitalized from late October through mid-December of 1947. (Juliana was discharged for three days in November, but her going home was premature, and she had to return to Harkness.) The Whitney, being the small, family-run place that it was, had no financial provisions for an employee's retirement, disability, or catastrophic illness, and Juliana was overextended. She lived from check to check, and her one cash reserve was earmarked for the maintenance of Clara Rieser, whom she still supported, in her house in Chatham. Two months' worth of hospital, doctors' and nurses' bills had to be paid out of Juliana's own pocket. To help her manage, she was given her October and November salary in October, and her December salary in November, but these advances were not sufficient. Flora Miller, wanting to be helpful, then had the museum's accountant pay Juliana $2,500 in "additional compensation" on November 24. After Juliana received the gift, she wrote to Flora from Harkness:

> My dear Flora. You realize of course that this is a fight for my life & will take all of my money for some time to come. That does not worry me, but it would kill my pride & my self-respect if I should be forced to have you *give* me that money. It is

not an uncommon custom in educational institutions to grant a sabbatical year with full pay in advance & sometimes a bonus. This is what I thought you meant to do. I am now only a month ahead of my salary & I never for a moment dreamed of any other idea, until you spoke to me this afternoon & practically asked what I had done with that last salary cheque. It made me quite ill when I realized that you must have considered my advance salary as a gift. I would not accept this from anybody in the world. I have assets & wd sell my books & my pictures at once if I were able to get around. I must have money to help out until I am well enough to face such an issue. There was no money in the bank today & I sold my mink coat for 200.00 to my charwoman!! I give her 8.00 a day & it looks very funny indeed & at least made me laugh once.

Please understand me. You must not do anything for me per se. You can & have made things easier & I am very grateful, but I can not ever be a charity patient. It would kill me quicker than this black horror hanging over me day & night. You must not get cross. I am serious & very unhappy. JRF

Juliana thought about her impetuous reaction to Flora's kindness, and rushed her an apology in another letter.

I am very much ashamed & hope you will forgive me. It was a dreadful morning, dreadful to look back upon & dreadful to contemplate. . . . I was so helpless and forlorn no more effort seemed possible. But after a day in bed I went through everything quite well. I have been flat on my back & doped every four hours. Your roses came & I open my eyes on them regularly. Then tonight I read yr card & yr letter & for the first time in my life I feel like a mutt.

But the reality of paying for Juliana's medical care did not disappear, and when Flora left for South Carolina in December, Walter Dunnington kept her informed. Visiting Juliana at Columbia Presbyterian, Dunnington was extremely surprised to learn that she had left the hospital for a few hours on the evening of December 5 to attend the opening of the 1947 painting annual. Edith Lowenthal, who was at the Whitney that night, remembered how astonished everyone at the museum was that Juliana, in the toils of fatal illness, had risen from her hospital bed to say hello to the artists. She stayed at the Whitney only about twenty minutes, but she had made an appearance.

Dunnington wrote to Flora again on December 19, telling her of a way to advance Juliana money without hurting her pride. The accountant would give her $1,400 in bonuses, and a check for the next three months of her salary could be sent to her on January 1, 1948. Dunnington also reported what the specialists had told him. "Mrs. Force has a cancer in the stomach and another cancer in the intestines," he wrote. "She has been having internal hemorrhages although she may not realize it. These hemorrhages will probably grow worse. She is, however, anxious to go home and if two good nurses can be obtained the doctors are going to let her go as they feel she should do whatever will make her happiest for the few weeks that they think she will last."

Two experienced nurses were found and put on the Whitney payroll, and just before Christmas Juliana was permitted to go home. She was thin and wan and could barely keep any food down, but she was no more amiable about death than she had been in October. "I want to live!" Juliana cried to Schnakenberg,

a steadfast visitor that winter. "I don't want to leave life!" Dunnington, who visited Juliana on December 23, reported to Flora:

> Of course, she looks quite badly and is weak. It was pathetic to see her but she displayed a lot of courage and talked about getting well. Her main topic of conversation was about you, Sonny and your mother. She is devoted to all of you and cried from time to time as she became a little sentimental. I do not think any visit was ever more appreciated than the one Sonny paid her on Sunday.
>
> She wants me to come to see her again which I shall do in a few days. She wants to discuss with me her plans for her Sabbatical year.

Two days after Dunnington's visit, Juliana tried to keep a promise she made to Schnakenberg. Knowing that the prospect of a party would cheer her, he invited Juliana to spend Christmas Eve with him and his niece. She said she would if she could, and summoned up all her stamina for the occasion. She got as far as putting on her clothes and makeup, but she collapsed before she could get downstairs.

Carl and Edith Rieser were living in an apartment in the Village, which made it convenient for them to see Juliana often. Carl stopped by nearly every night after work, and Edith saw her about once a week. Juliana had trouble digesting most foods, and Edith thought that home-made custards, soft and bland, might be something she could eat. She began baking custards, taking them round to West Eighth Street, and staying for a visit with the patient. Juliana valued the trouble Edith took over her, and a gruff rapproachment developed between the two women as each grew to appreciate the other. "Being ill made her a bit vulnerable," Edith Nolder remembered,

> and I was willing to be obliging. She liked the custards, and she liked our Christmas present to her, a subscription to *The Manchester Guardian*. When she introduced me, she would say, "This is Carl's wife. I didn't like her at first, but she's all right now," and looked around to see what effect she had. Sometimes she was like a precocious child—it tickled her to see what she could get away with.
>
> She was gutsy. She didn't disintegrate when she learned she was going to die—I never saw her break down. She had great self-control when she cared to use it.
>
> As I got to know her better, I realized that she had done something seminal in American art, but she was not a braggart and never blew her horn about it. Even when she was ill, she was very stimulating. She was never boring—she was the *reverse* of boring.

In the middle stages of Juliana's illness, when she was resting at home with her nurses, her fury was tempered by depression or hope, depending on how well she felt and how efficacious the therapy of the moment was. Psychologically, her vow to stay alive carried her longer than anyone had a right to expect, but she had great trouble adjusting to the aftermath of the colostomy. She hated the pouch she had to wear; the appliance was repulsive and mortifying to her, representing as it did an invasion of privacy and a gruesome loss of control. Juliana told Elizabeth Bart Gerald that the colostomy was the most humiliating

procedure she had ever experienced and that she felt robbed of her human dignity. She, who had been so fastidious all her life, was apprehensive about odors escaping from the appliance. Juliana also made things worse for herself because she kept drinking, though she switched from Scotch to brandy. She insisted that her doctors said that it was all right for her to drink brandy as long as it was in a glass of milk. Her statement was probably true because a total withdrawal from alcohol might have delivered a harmful shock to her body.

Juliana's sickness was excruciating because it was prolonged by her will to continue, which was as unwavering as her fortitude in public. Allan Rieser said, "Her illness was terrible, dragged out, I believe, by her fierce struggle to live, which urged the doctors on to extreme and hideously painful efforts. This was thrown into relief by intervals of wild euphoria, during which she had allowed herself to think that some cure had been found." Lloyd Goodrich, whose office was below Juliana's bedroom, said that sometimes he would hear her screaming with pain from the cancer. At other times, when the disease was temporarily in remission, Juliana was valiant and gay, and flashes of her old humor reappeared. For one of her operations, the surgeon used gold in the repair, and Edith Nolder remembered Juliana joking with her, "Now that I'm filled with gold, do you think some man will want to marry me for it?"

Much to the astonishment of her caretakers, who had not expected her to survive, Juliana revived enough to visit her office and give orders. As she wrote to Flora Miller, she would accept no more gifts, so she sold some of her pictures for cash, most notably *Pertaining to Yachts and Yachting*, which the Whitney bought for $2,500.

Nothing, least of all cancer, was going to keep Juliana from recommending selections from the painting annual to the Met. Just two of her choices were accepted, and Juliana, who had long been fed up with the Met, certainly had nothing to lose by being impolitic. For once in her long battle, she made death her accomplice—if she could not say what she felt now, what good had it all been? On February 20, 1948, she resigned as adviser to the Met, writing irately to Taylor, "Considering the difference in the point of view between the Metropolitan Museum and the Whitney Museum, I feel that it is useless for me to continue as 'Art Advisor.' I am sure you will be able to find some expert whose point of view does agree with yours and your board."

Juliana's resignation was also fueled by her rage at a direct assault Taylor made on the Whitney just three days before. It took place at the Brook Club, and the incident has attained an almost iconic status in Whitney annals. The Three Museum Agreement was not working out to anyone's satisfaction—the Met and the Whitney still could not concur on a design for the wing, and Barr resented surrendering on demand objects in the Modern's collection. Hoping that bruised feelings would heal over the expansiveness of food and wine and cigars, the Met's president, Roland Redmond, invited the policymakers from all three institutions to have dinner with him at the Brook Club on the seventeenth. Juliana was too ill to go, and she was steeling herself for a few weeks' stay at Memorial Hospital, which she would enter on February 23. Therefore, More and Goodrich were deputized for the Whitney, Barr and Soby represented the

Modern, and Taylor and Horace Jayne, one of the museum's vice-presidents, spoke for the Met.

Everything rolled pleasantly along until about 10:00 P.M., when dessert was served and Taylor chose to provoke his dinner partners. He brought up the Whitney's purchasing policies, opining that the curators were excessively partial to abstract art and New York artists. Goodrich and More, he and Jayne asserted, didn't know what went on in the hinterlands and weren't in touch with the broadest spectrum of American art. The Whitney men naturally disputed this evaluation of their competence, and Barr and Soby sided with them against Taylor and Jayne. The six men argued back and forth for hours. At one point, Taylor expressed disdain for all those visitors in blue jeans and rumpled clothes who were a fixture at Whitney openings—more care would be taken in sending out invitations when the museum moved uptown. More and Goodrich gave Taylor a level look. "Those are the artists," they said. The debate went on until 2:00 A.M., when everyone gave up and departed.

The next day, Barr and Soby dropped by the Whitney and raised the subject of the Met's antagonism toward contemporary American art with More and Goodrich. All four grew more and more perturbed by it, and they decided to report what had transpired at the dinner to Juliana, who "was enraged" at Taylor's highfalutin attitudes. She and the others concluded that because of the deep divisions of opinion between the Met and the Whitney, the merger would have to be dissolved. The Whitney could not join an institution that was hostile to contemporary American art and snobbish toward artists. After all, the whole atmosphere of the Whitney depended on the artist—that was the reason the place existed. Juliana, More, and Goodrich reminded themselves that no written agreement had ever been signed. However, they would have to persuade Flora Miller, Sonny Whitney, and Walter Dunnington that irreconcilable differences existed between the two museums and then get the trustees to reverse their decision and assume fiscal responsibility for the Whitney again. Flora was not in New York in February, so the consultations would move slowly, but the primacy of the artist was the still the lodestar by which the Whitney would be guided.

Knowing that the Whitney's fortunes were tied partially to her own stamina and appetite for combat, Juliana entered Memorial Hospital with the intention of preserving herself. She received excellent care there and felt better than she had in months. Her bowel was too inflamed for the colostomy to be closed, but she thought she had vanquished the malignancy. Her physicians told her that she was going to live. In any event, the disease had gone into remission in March, and Juliana was jubilant. She wrote to Dan Rich in Chicago from Memorial Hospital on March 15:

> Dear Dan. I am cured. The operation was extensive & a complete success. I owe my life to a Dr. Brunswegger [sic] & he came to this hospital from *Chicago*! So I am twice blest. I am too weak to write much less think, but I want you to know at once. Love
>
> J.

Rich sent a telegram by return mail reading, WONDERFUL NEWS MY DEAR. YOU DONT KNOW HOW HAPPY IT MAKES ME.

With the possibility of recovery, Juliana's pride in her appearance was resuscitated. While undergoing treatment, she was fed intravenously, and because she had not been able to get to her hairdresser in many weeks, the hair framing her face was pure white. Juliana did not want people to see her looking anything less than her usual fashionable self, and she forbade many of her friends to visit her.

Juliana left Memorial Hospital on March 22 in order to participate in an important first at the museum. The Whitney had finally overruled itself on the policy of not giving retrospectives to living artists, and the first such survey was to open on March 25. There had been talk of awarding the show to either Sloan or Kuniyoshi, and the staff settled on the latter. Their choice was also a statement of social concern, because Kuniyoshi, a native of Japan, was not permitted to become a United States citizen. Whereas the Metropolitan abided by the letter of American law and refused to let the Hearn funds be spent on Kuniyoshi's work, the Whitney, in honoring Kuniyoshi, gave him his citizenship papers in the world of art. Sara Kuniyoshi, the artist's widow, said of Juliana:

> It seemed to me astoundingly bold, also courageous, for her to consent to giving the first retrospective of an American artist at the Whitney Museum to Kuniyoshi. . . . It was an amazing gesture and Kuniyoshi was well aware of the singular honor.
>
> Perhaps I should explain that of the utmost importance to my late husband was the fervent desire to become an American citizen. However, the opportunity for a Japanese to become a citizen came too late for him. He died very shortly after the ruling was passed by our government.

The opening of the Kuniyoshi retrospective was Juliana's last public appearance at the museum. As always, she was there to greet the throng of guests, and she insisted on standing up. Appearing at the entrance of the museum and supported by a nurse at each side, Juliana caused a sensation. "We knew she was going to die," said Raphael Soyer, "but she insisted on greeting every artist who came in. Then she had to be taken upstairs." Katherine Schmidt, who remembered Juliana's attempts at vivacity, said, "Her hair was dyed and she was playing gay. 'Oh, I'm going to Europe this summer,' she said. 'I think that I'll go to England for a while, and I have some friends in Italy I'm going to meet.' She knew darn well that's not where she was going." George Biddle, who was also at the party, noted, "Poor Juliana Force looked very frail but I thought lovely. . . . Her illness has given her a look of spiritual serenity which I have never noticed. How I should love to do a painting of her." Forbes Watson, charged with keeping a friend in Italy abreast of the news, went to the opening and wrote:

> About Mrs. Force: Several months ago she was reported to be dying. . . . I was told that she could not stand another operation and everyone of course declared it was cancer. She came home and Nan happened to see her: an old woman with white hair and scarcely able to speak. Well she has had another operation which has been completely successful and she is said to be completely out of danger. No one with less courage or less will to live could possibly have gone through what she has. We

were flabbergasted to see her at the Kuniyoshi opening. But there she was smiling, weak and dignified. I was struck of a heap by her courage. She was very cordial and kissed us both but of course she did not stay long. She smiled at me briskly and said: "I'm going to live." I was overflowing with admiration.

Juliana had reason to be smiling. Flora Miller, after hearing the account of the Brook Club dinner, was shocked by Taylor's attack and wanted to pull out of the merger. Dunnington, writing to Sonny Whitney on March 29, 1948, said:

> Mrs. Force . . . is now at the Museum and is making satisfactory progress. She is still quite weak and has some bad days but the doctors feel she will recover. I saw her on Friday and thought she looked better than she did in December. It is almost miraculous to me that she is still here and it is due, as I see it, to two factors—the exceptional treatment she received at the Memorial Hospital and her unusual will power.
>
> Flora and I had a long conference with Roland Redmond last week and suggested that we abandon the idea of the coalition with the Metropolitan. We covered the subject very thoroughly. Roland said he felt we were unduly disturbed and that he naturally would like to see the coalition effected. I tried to point out that, as I see it, there is a conflict of purpose in the two museums, the Metropolitan being interested primarily in works of art by recognized artists, whereas the Whitney Museum is primarily interested in encouraging young and unknown artists and affording them an opportunity to display their works. I told him that I felt the merger would lead to misunderstanding and that it was better to give up the whole idea. It was left that we would have a further talk when Flora gets back from Aiken toward the end of April.

Juliana, having been declared alive and almost well by herself and others, took up the swords and pistols again, aiming them directly at the custodians of the Kaiser Friedrich collection. Calvin Hathaway, Frederick Mortimer Clapp, and Juliana had relied on the Truman Administration to return the art promptly to Germany in 1947, but in March of 1948 the confiscated pictures had been held illegally by the United States for exactly three years. Even worse, the National Gallery put the pictures on display, although the museum had no right whatsoever to exhibit or otherwise make free with another institution's property. This new outrage spurred the three authors of the resolution to a fresh round of protests, and in April of 1948, Senate hearings were held on the fate of the Berlin pictures.

The hearings, which were being conducted by Sen. J. William Fulbright, revealed the opportunism of some prominent museum men. John Walker engaged in some masterly fence straddling, testifying that although he could advance no opinion on the ongoing exhibition in Washington, it was certainly too dangerous to send the 202 paintings, especially the 140 that had been executed on wood panel, on tour. Francis Taylor did not appear in person, but he wanted those Old Master paintings at his museum, and for the services he rendered to the government, he felt he deserved them. Instead, four other Metropolitan employees packed the witness box. Each duly swore that the pictures could be transported to New York and then exhibited at the Met without risk.

After reminding Senator Fulbright that Truman and Acheson had pledged a prompt return of the Kaiser Friedrich pictures, Hathaway, Juliana, and Clapp tried polling the museum directors who had been their allies in 1946. But that base of support disintegrated after the directors saw that the Senate would bow to the wisdom of the Met's staff and let them have the Berlin pictures for New York. Even friends and former stalwarts such as Dan Rich and William Edgell, the director of the Museum of Fine Arts in Boston, ignored the ethical questions in their eagerness to get the show for their own institutions. Then, as various senators woke up to the prestige of having a world-famous cache of Old Master paintings visit their home state, they rushed to tack more stops on to the itinerary. By the time everyone was finished cutting himself in, the Kaiser Friedrich pictures were shipped to fourteen museums. The pictures traveled over 11,000 miles in thirteen months and were unpacked and repacked at each destination. (If such an exhibition were ever organized today, it would go to three places, at most.)

Juliana was crushed by the voracity of the art museums on the tour. Paintings belonging to no one involved with their handling were being paraded all over the continent and subjected to a host of dangers. The collection would be traveling for at least a year, meaning that it would not be returned to Berlin until, at best, April of 1949, a full four years after its seizure.* Nor were any of the parties circulating or exhibiting the collection expressing any concern about indemnifying the rightful owners for damages should an accident occur. A thirteen-month tour made the government's promise of safekeeping a travesty.

Shortly after receiving this blow, Juliana acknowledged that her health was not improving, and she checked into Memorial Hospital on May 1 for another stay. Dunnington, writing to Sonny Whitney on May 12, again prefaced his summary of relations between the Met and the Whitney with a description of Juliana's prognosis.

> I am sorry that I have very bad news for you about Mrs. Force. She has left the Memorial Hospital and has now returned to the Museum. It was impossible to operate again and the doctors do not feel there is any chance for her. The disease has spread very rapidly through her system. She is not aware of this condition and thinks that after she has recuperated this summer she will go back in the autumn for another operation. The longer she fails to realize it the easier it will be for her.
>
> Flora and I have had a good many discussions with reference to the abandonment of the idea of the coalition with the Metropolitan Museum. On yesterday afternoon we had a conference with Roland Redmond and he could not have been nicer about the whole problem. It was agreed that there was no obligation on either Museum to consummate the coalition but if and when the Metropolitan Museum's building project became feasible we would consider anew the possibility of working out a coalition satisfactory to both, unless in the meantime other plans had been made for the development of the Whitney Museum.

To defer the coalition was a face-saving out for everyone, and although the breakup was not yet firm, Juliana was relieved and comforted by such assurances of the Whitney's reemergence as an independent institution. She was not through

---

*Indeed, the pictures did not go back until the spring of 1949.

fighting, but the ordeal to come was made more tolerable because the museum was no longer imperiled and American artists—her first and truest cause—would have their stronghold again. As Juliana's own life ebbed, the Whitney Museum moved out of danger, and there was a sense of finality in many of the things she said and did. She pretended to believe her physicians, but there were no more illusions about recovery. Lloyd Goodrich recalled the last time he saw Juliana:

> I took her out to dinner in the summer of 1948 and she never said a word about her health. But when I went up to get her and take her out to a restaurant, she burst into tears and said, "Lloyd, I've been so mean to you." I said, "I always think of the happy times we had." And we went out to dinner, and she was just her old self. It was a very hot night and right afterwards we dropped in on the Hermon Mores and I took her home.

The museum world had not seen the last of Juliana's old self, either. The committee for the art book to be published by Macmillan was still meeting, and Juliana, who had missed a good many of the recent sessions, wanted to have a final say in the book's composition before the season ended. In observing her on the committee over the years, Hyatt Mayor had come to admire her "intuitive accuracy of judgment, her no-nonsense warmth of heart." When he visited Juliana in the hospital, he found her "all-seeing and unflinching." Yet no word or image topped Mayor's memory of Juliana's entrance into the inner chambers of Macmillan that spring. The meeting had already begun, when the door swung open. The curators sitting in the room could only gape at what they saw. Juliana had risen "from her death bed," Mayor wrote, "put her war paint over the hideous yellow of her illness, armed herself in electric blue silk, with a plumed hat to match, and stormed into the meeting, half way through, under the brutalizing glare of a ceiling spotlight. None of us expected ever to see her again when she burst into the room, gathering the last of her life to fling at our remembrance. Her ghost could not have startled us more."

It became increasingly apparent that the summer of 1948 would be Juliana's last, and Harry and Bernice Farmer invited her to spend the next three months with them in Roxbury, Connecticut. The Farmers' country house had a small wing consisting of a separate little apartment called the "mother-in-law house." The arrangement promised a combination of friends, rural surroundings, and privacy, and Juliana accepted their invitation. The lodgings would also be free, which, for once, was a consideration. By July, the museum had advanced Juliana her salary through November of 1948—which came to about $1,300 a month after taxes. That money was consumed by hospital, nursing, and other medical bills because she had no insurance. In addition, she was still making the mortgage payments on Clara Rieser's house in Chatham. Max Rieser now lived there, too, but he did not help pay for the house.

Before leaving for Roxbury in June, Juliana conferred with Calvin Hathaway about drafting another resolution addressed to Harry Truman. She remained

devastated by the affair, but Hathaway persuaded her to try again, and the letter went out on June 7, 1948. Through early August, whenever she could summon up her dwindling energies, Juliana assisted Clapp and Hathaway in trying to liberate the German pictures from their American captivity.

Just as Juliana was about to depart for Connecticut, she received emphatic word that the merger between the Whitney and the Met had definitely been called off. The announcement of the break would not be made until the fall and the trustees' change of heart was supposed to be kept a secret, but Juliana could not contain herself. She had to tell someone, and when John and Elizabeth Bart Gerald invited her to have drinks with them and John Frear, she confided the joyous news to these trusted friends. "Juliana felt dreadful and she was very ill," Frear remembered, "but she said, 'This is the happiest day of my life. The Met is not getting the Whitney. I've done my work.' She was wonderful company that night, and I like to remember her that way."

She then moved into her rooms in the Farmers' house, but she didn't like the accommodations after all. The Farmers had a new grandchild with them, and the baby's crying disturbed Juliana's rest. Furthermore, there was less privacy than she had been led to believe. Juliana quipped to Carl Rieser, "If there is a summer in Heaven it's just like this—only Saints cd stand it."

There was solace, however, in the Connecticut countryside, and Henry Schnakenberg soon came to the rescue. Juliana gladly alternated her stay in Roxbury with long drives and visits with Henry Schnakenberg in nearby Newtown. Elizabeth Navas spent a few days with Edith Halpert, who also had a house in Newtown, in July of 1948, and saw Juliana at Schnakenberg's on the eleventh. Navas said, "Juliana fought to the last inch. It was terribly hard on Henry, because she fought and fought, and she hated dying so much. He was so upset that he went away on a trip after her death."

At times Juliana's spirits were good, and in her last letter to Carl Rieser, she could look at herself with unimpaired egotism and humor.

My life has been more wonderful than, I'm afraid, yours will ever be & I'm sorry for you. A lifetime of spending—money, energy, brains and that precious gift, time for others. Now that it is all gone I am very happy, & need no pity. Kindness appears to me now as the only quality—since imagination today is just a shabby remnant of gracious living.

Too bad if you laugh but I am for the first time (& entirely too late) quite pleased with myself. My inferiors have taught me so much (there are so many of them) my superiors . . . too, & I have never met my equal! Don't you think I could run for President? On the commutation ticket perhaps?

In this letter, Juliana also told Carl that she would return to New York for some intellectual stimulation as soon as the weather permitted. But she left Connecticut because she was in too much pain to do without professional nursing anymore.

On August 7, Schnakenberg wrote one word in his diary about Juliana— "Failing." Two days later, she was admitted to Doctors Hospital for terminal care. The cancer had metastasized throughout the entire abdominal cavity, and

it was accompanied by heavy internal bleeding. Juliana's treatment mainly consisted of administering drugs for the unremitting pain, changing her dressings, and doing anything else that would make her comfortable, such as letting her have a ritual brandy-and-milk every afternoon.

Each day Juliana grew weaker, but not less gregarious. She liked holding court if she felt up to it, and her ability to extract comic mileage from a story remained intact. One day she regaled John Gerald with tales of the nurse who hid her painkillers instead of letting her have access to them. "What does she think I am going to do," Juliana asked Gerald with dramatic nonchalance, "kill myself?" But this indignity was nothing compared to the nurse's ultimate silliness. "And then, of course," wailed Juliana, "where does she put the pills? She hides them in the teapot!" Juliana was more irked—and amused—by her keeper's poverty of imagination than her lack of trust.

By August 15, the narcotics were not doing their work. They did not eradicate Juliana's pain—they only made her confused and irrational. She was unable to sleep, and sank into a depression. On the seventeenth, she told Schnakenberg and her nurses that the drugs were making an idiot of her. On the nineteenth, she was crying uncontrollably and demanded to be allowed to die at home.

The idea of home gave Juliana a real focus for her emotions, and it helped stop the crying jags. She became fixated on spending her last moments in the place she loved best—in her own apartment on Eighth Street, within the protective walls of the Whitney Museum. On August 24, Juliana said she felt better and lost no time in throwing off her bedclothes, sitting up, and hauling herself over to the side of the bed as a prelude to her eventual exit. She was too weak to do more, but for the next two days she refused painkillers and talked about going home.

On the afternoon of August 26, John Gerald stopped by Doctors Hospital, and he wondered if there was anything he could do for Juliana. She had deteriorated too much to make further attempts to go home, so she asked him to run down to her apartment, pick out some pictures from her personal collection, and bring them back. Gerald then had to locate Flora Miller to get permission to enter the building and remove Juliana's property. He was overjoyed when Flora said, "Mrs. Force can have anything she wants." He was let into the apartment and removed six paintings from the walls.

At the sight of her pictures, Juliana was more cheered than she had been in days. "I have my friends around me," she said. "Now I feel at home." Gerald had not reappeared at the hospital until the early evening, and by the time he realized that he had forgotten to bring a hammer, the hardware stores were closed. Unfazed, this faithful friend went rummaging around the hospital for a substitute until he was finally able to cadge a meat cleaver from the kitchen, which was on the floor below Juliana's room. When Gerald triumphantly brandished the fatal instrument of countless murder mysteries, she said with appreciative emphasis, "*That* will fix them." Gerald hung the pictures as Juliana instructed. From her bed, she directed him to move each one a little higher or a little lower, a little to the right or a little to the left. As Gerald banged a nail in with the cleaver, Juliana cradled one picture after another in her arms and

wrote something on the back of each one. Every painting was inscribed to its future owner—one of the doctors or nurses who had taken care of her. John Gerald did not leave Juliana until 9:30 that night. From then on, whenever she opened her eyes, they rested on objects she cherished.

Over the next two days, Juliana had long sieges of excruciating restlessness relieved occasionally by less fitful periods of rest. Her brothers were at the hospital on Saturday, August 28, and they carried out an urgent request. The second Woodstock Art Conference was being held then, and that morning Kuniyoshi disclosed the gravity of Juliana's condition to a hushed crowd. The audience voted to send a telegram of greeting to Doctors Hospital, and after Juliana received it, she insisted that a return message of good wishes be forwarded.

The communication was the last to be sent out under her name. While her family went to do her bidding, Juliana's pulse rate dropped, and she struggled to breathe, but the long battle was over. She was pronounced dead at 2:55 P.M., an hour or so before her telegram reached Woodstock and was read to several hundred artists who did not know she had died. To the last, Juliana remained their friend and champion.

Later in the afternoon of August 28, Woodstock learned of Juliana's death. Kuniyoshi was one of the first to hear the bulletin, whereupon he broke down and cried. At the Sunday session of the conference, the death was announced to a suddenly grieving assembly. Elsewhere, artists who had loved Juliana expressed their reactions on paper. In Connecticut, Henry Schnakenberg could not bear to say more in his journal than "Poor dear she should not have suffered so." In Philadelphia, George Biddle also mourned, writing, "Juliana Force died last night. Another landmark washed away. Who is there in New York who can begin to replace her?" In Santa Fe, John Sloan reflected, "She has been a good friend of mine for nearly 40 years. I have never frequented her office nor sought her out but in the past she always could be depended on."

The funeral service took place on the morning of August 31, 1948, and it was held at the First Presbyterian Church at Fifth Avenue and Twelfth Street. The heat was intense, but the church was packed as all segments of the art world came to pay their respects. The pallbearers were as distinguished as Juliana could have wished: Hermon More, Lloyd Goodrich, Alfred Barr, Hardinge Scholle, Hudson Walker, Frederick Mortimer Clapp, Sonny Whitney, Henry Schnakenberg, Eugene Speicher, John Gerald, and Guy Pène du Bois attended the coffin. Forbes Watson, loyal and waspish, was saddened by Juliana's death, and "by the fact that a lot of artists who should have been there even if benefactions had been followed by fights were not." Hyatt Mayor remembered that the church was "filled with artists. One had a notebook, and was writing in it all the time. One family of two painters had come with their little baby strapped to the husband's back and of course the baby began to mewl and fume and cry and had to be taken out. But it was touching . . . people came because they had loved Juliana and wanted to say good-bye to her." Genevieve Rindner, the seamstress who became a sculptor at Juliana's urging, attended the service, and

she marveled at all the famous and sophisticated people who were in tears. When she said as much to Dorothea Denslow, who was also there, Miss Denslow replied, "You have no idea how many artists she has helped." Kathryn McHale of the American Association of University Women noticed that the artists at the service "looked stricken. Something in their vocational life was broken. Most of them were younger than she, but they felt that they were burying their youth."

At the close of the service, the body was taken to the Doylestown Cemetery for burial in the Rieser family plot. Bucks County, which had scarcely recovered from the selling of Barley Sheaf Farm to a Jew, was newly offended because the more elaborate ceremony had been reserved for New York, and the funeral procession had taken several hours to wind through New Jersey, whereas the native heath had to be content with a quick and unprepossessing interment. The day after the burial, the *Doylestown Daily Intelligencer* ran a page-one story indignantly headlined JULIANNA [*sic*] FORCE BURIED IN 2 MINUTE CEREMONY, and twenty years later, certain residents were still exercised about this profound oversight. The Riesers were sorry to disappoint the funeral buffs of Doylestown, but the one who would have most savored the kerfuffle was absent. How delighted Juliana would have been by it all—even in death she had outraged the local gossips and entertained everyone else.

Doylestown, expecting to appropriate the fame of one of its daughters, could not understand that Juliana had no use for the easy pieties of eulogies and wreath layings. As someone who steered clear of reminiscing and was unable to recall the facts of her life with any accuracy, she cared little for posterity and never showed the slightest interest in self-memorialization. Instead, her life was based on ready sympathy, unfailing generosity, merry friendships, indulgent play, doughty advocacy, strong opinions, creative labor, and the interactions of people and pictures. Wherever these things are understood and valued, Juliana Force's spirit is there.

EPILOGUE

On October 1, 1948, the Whitney and the Metropolitan formally announced that their engagement was broken. Hermon More was appointed to be the next director of the Whitney, and Lloyd Goodrich became associate director. In 1949, seven years after the offer was originally made, the Whitney accepted the Museum of Modern Art's donation of a plot of real estate at 22 West 54th Street —precisely because there were no strings attached to the gift—with the aim of erecting a new museum building to replace the one on West Eighth Street, which no longer had adequate gallery or storage space. Also during 1949, the Whitney family, against the advice of the staff, chose to liquidate the museum's nineteenth-century holdings. The proceeds were to be spent on contemporary art, but the sale didn't realize much money for two reasons. First, at that time, nineteenth-century American art was vehemently out of fashion. Second, before the collection was offered for public sale, Gertrude's children had first choice of the deaccessioned paintings and sculptures. Some of the best works were snapped up at noncompetitive prices by Sonny and Eleanor Whitney.

The Whitney Museum left West Eighth Street at the end of 1953. The property was rented out to indifferent tenants and fell into disrepair. (It is now in friendly hands: The Village building has been the home of the New York Studio School, which took it over in 1967. The place is still run-down, but it is filled with artists, art students, and paint again—a deserving denouement Gertrude and Juliana would have liked.) Before the Whitney moved to 54th Street, More, Goodrich, and John I. H. Baur, who had since joined the Whitney as a curator, sorted through the permanent collection and removed or exchanged a number of works purchased by Juliana.

The Whitney, now in more modern facilities, reopened on October 26, 1954, but being on 54th Street in the shadow of the Modern was not an ideal situation. The museum, although independent as ever, surrendered some of its identity by being within the compound of another fine arts institution, and the new building was not flexible enough to display contemporary art—the scale of painting and sculpture, as well as the New York art scene itself, had expanded radically since Juliana's day. Once more, the museum decided to move uptown, this time to a plot of land at 75th Street and Madison Avenue, the up-and-coming center of the Manhattan art world. Marcel Breuer, the innovative modernist architect associated with the Bauhaus, was commissioned to design the building.

A two-year fund-raising campaign for a bigger and better Whitney was high-lighted by a luncheon at the Plaza Hotel on December 14, 1964. The affair, attended by 175 people, was billed as a tribute to Gertrude Whitney. The December date was specially chosen because it was the fiftieth anniversary of the Whitney Studio's first shows, which Juliana had organized because Gertrude was in France.

The event naturally was an occasion for much speechifying and reminiscing about the museum's early history, and after Lloyd Goodrich (director of the museum since 1958) and Henry Schnakenberg invoked both Gertrude and Juliana in their speeches, there was a discernible shift in emphasis as the afternoon proceeded. Gertrude was beatified as the only begetter of all Whitney art activities, and Flora—and then other members of the Whitney family—increasingly came in for the rest of the credit for everything else that had transpired in the fifty-year span. Ethel Renthal, Helen Appleton Read, and John and Elizabeth Bart Gerald, who were seated near each other, exchanged progressively more horrified glances as the glorification of the uninvolved rolled on. At the end of the meal, Helen Read and Ethel Renthal commiserated with each other about the niggardly attention paid to Juliana's place in Whitney annals. "Well, you and I know the truth," they said to each other.

On September 27, 1966, after a solid month of press coverage, the newest Whitney, a gray granite fortress startlingly cantilevered over Madison Avenue, was dedicated by Jacqueline Kennedy and Flora Miller. Every New York paper, as well as almost every other newspaper in the country, carried interviews with Flora Miller and Marcel Breuer, photo spreads of the permanent collection, the ribbon cutting and the string of glittering parties, and long appraisals of the museum's past, present, and future. All of these stories had one fact in common—Juliana Force's name was never mentioned.

NOTES

To avoid confusion in citing documents from the often overlapping papers of Juliana Force, Gertrude Vanderbilt Whitney, and the Whitney Museum of American Art, I have provided their microfilm reel numbers in the Archives of American Art. For collections with less multitudinous reels of microfilm, I have not listed the reel and/or frame numbers unless they are required by individuals, institutions, or their assigns.

The following abbreviations are used throughout the notes:

AAA — Archives of American Art
FWP — Forbes Watson Papers
GV — Gertrude Vanderbilt
GVWP — Gertrude Vanderbilt Whitney Papers
GW — Gertrude Whitney
JF — Juliana Force
JFAA — *Juliana Force and American Art*
JFP — Juliana Force Papers
JR — Juliana Rieser
LC — Manuscript Division, Library of Congress
MMAA — The Metropolitan Museum of Art Archives
RFC — Rieser Family Collection
WMAA — Whitney Museum of American Art, New York, N.Y.
YU — Collection of American Literature, Beinecke Rare Book and Manuscript Library, Yale University

INTRODUCTION

4 "Juliana . . . Metropolitan Museum of Art." Telephone interview with Allene Talmey.

4 "Handsome, auburn . . . Renaissance." Peggy Bacon, *Off With Their Heads!* (New York, 1934), unpaged.

4 "Before . . . carefully culled few." Allene Talmey, "Whitney Museum," *Vogue*, February 1, 1940, p. 131.

5 "We . . . artistic failure." John Sloan, quoted in *Juliana Force and American Art* (New York: Whitney Museum of American Art, 1949), p. 34.

5 "What do you mean . . . notice." Avis Berman, "The Making of a Collection," *Portfolio*, 2 (September 1980), p. 63.

5 "Outlaw salons" " 'The Eight' Exhibit New Art Realism," *New York American*, February 4, 1908.

6 "What with . . . world." Forbes Watson, unpublished lecture, 1949, FWP, AAA.

7 "Our desire . . . doing." JF to Julian Levi, October 28, 1935, Julian Levi Papers, AAA.

7 "If . . . buy it." Jane Watson, "Whitney Museum Holds to Policy of Art by Consistent Buying," *Washington Post*, January 16, 1944.

7 "Do not . . . heard!" "Think for Yourself!" *Art Digest*, 6 (February 1, 1932), p. 13.

7 "Juliana . . . without any fuss." Telephone interview with Allene Talmey.

8 "Dependably . . . stand." Talmey, "Whitney Museum," p. 94.

8–9 "Up to that moment . . . Whitney." *Ibid.*, p. 131.

9 "The story . . . investigate." Telephone interview with Allene Talmey.

9–10 "Educated . . . abroad." Entry forms, Reel 2396, JFP, AAA; *Who's Who In America*, 1944–1945 (Chicago, 1944), p. 701.

9–10 "It seemed incredible . . . anything else." Alexander Brook, quoted in *JFAA*, p. 47.

10 "We were all gathered . . . yourself." Interview with Allan Rieser.

10 "She . . . actresses of the age." Telephone interview with Edmund Archer.

CHAPTER ONE

For the picture of Doylestown, Pennsylvania, and the documentation of the Riesers' life there, I am indebted to the extensive records of the Bucks County Historical Society and the Bucks County Courthouse, both in Doylestown. I also benefited enormously from numerous conversations with the Rieser family.

13 "Spent . . . company." "Death of Julius Kuster," *Doylestown Democrat*, July 30, 1867.

17 "Mad . . . nobby neckties" *Doylestown Democrat*, April 28, 1874.

17 "In one . . . ruffian" Charles Rieser, undated, unpublished reminiscence, RFC.

18 "She was . . . private school." Interview with W. Lester Trauch.

18 "Though . . . them." *Bucks County Intelligencer*, December 4, 1880.

18 "Was not needed." W. W. H. Davis, Alfred Paschall, and Mary Higgins to John L. Dubois, January 1, 1881, Bucks County Historical Society.

19 "Our former townsman . . . New York." *Doylestown Democrat*, May 12, 1885.

21 "Left . . . eyes of his children." Charles Rieser, unpublished reminiscence.

21 "Cursed . . . essentials." *Ibid.*

22 "The whole family . . . disappear." Interview with Beverly Rieser Smock.

23 "You . . . respect." Carl Rieser, "Juliana Rieser Force: A Memoir," unpublished manuscript, 1977, RFC.

24 "Grandmother Rieser . . . falling down.' " Interview with Marjorie Rieser.

24 "Her temper . . . captive audience." Charles Rieser, unpublished reminiscence.

24 "I won't . . . be poor!" Interview with Beverly Rieser Smock.

25 "Under socialism . . . change." Interviews with Allan and Carl Rieser.

26 "Rob . . . pest of himself." Interview with Marjorie Rieser.

28–29 "I want . . . echo's sake." JR, application form for Northfield Seminary, 1896. Courtesy of Northfield Mount Hermon Archives, Northfield, Mass.

29 "The central book . . . Christian.' " Burnham Carter, *So Much to Learn: The History of Northfield Mount Hermon School for the One Hundredth Anniversary* (Northfield, Mass., 1976), p. 14. I am beholden to Carter's book for my descriptions of Northfield while Juliana was a student. Any facts not directly referenced below are based on his account.

29 "Practically . . . yes." JR, application form for Northfield Seminary, 1896.

29–30 "She is . . . so?" William Willcox to Dwight L. Moody, May 20, 1896, Northfield Mount Hermon Archives.

30 "Miss . . . brilliant woman." C. J. Brower to Evelyn Hall, March 5, 1896, *ibid.*

30 "Love . . . tongue." JR, application form for Northfield Seminary, 1896, *ibid.*

30 "Father . . . comfortable." *Ibid.*

30 "I am sure . . . so?" JR to Evelyn Hall, January 31, 1896, *ibid.*

30 "And would you . . . eighteen." JR to Hall, February 13, 1896, *ibid.*

31 "I was . . . my place." JR to Nellie Starr, July 20, 1896, *ibid.*

31–32 "Contacts . . . chaperoned." Carter, p. 53.

32 "Lives . . . Christ." Carter, p. 101.

33 "In order . . . $100." *Ibid.*

33 "Remembered . . . classes." Carl Rieser, "Juliana Rieser Force: A Memoir."

33 "She . . . school." Talmey, p. 131.

34 "I think we should all . . . wall-eyed?" Interview with Lloyd Goodrich.

35 "A Window . . . Middle Class." Interview with Yvonne Pène du Bois McKenney.

35 "My aunt . . . Coward." Interview with Allan Rieser.

35 "Her courage . . . it." Lloyd Goodrich to Lura Beam, September 15, 1948, WMAA; Archives (H.3/f74).

35 "She had . . . knew." *Ibid.*

35 "I can still see . . . like that." Interview with Lloyd Goodrich.

35–36 "She might know nothing . . . done." Hermon More and Lloyd Goodrich, quoted in *JFAA,* p. 33.

36 "Such a gusto . . . quietude." Forbes Watson, quoted in *JFAA,* p. 55.

36 "To personify . . . encouragement." Julius Bloch to JF, January 16, 1933, WMAA; Library.

CHAPTER TWO

I have taken many details about Gertrude Whitney's background and early life from the biography *Gertrude Vanderbilt Whitney,* written by B. H. Friedman, with the research collaboration of Flora Miller Irving. Their book is an invaluable mine of information on the Vanderbilts and Whitneys, and I am indebted to their industry.

38 "Slightest . . . public opinion." Gustavus Myers, *History of the Great American Fortunes* (Chicago, 1909), 1:226.

38 "The Vanderbilts . . . live." Quoted in Grace Mayer, *Once Upon a City* (New York, 1958), p. 30.

38 "Everything . . . did or said." GV, "My History," undated manuscript, ca. 1893, Reel 2371, GVWP, AAA.

39 "If I thought . . . nature again." GV to Ann Winsor, April 16, 1893, Reel 2369, *ibid.*

39 "I look . . . unhappy." B. H. Friedman, *Gertrude Vanderbilt Whitney* (Garden City, N.Y., 1978), p. 48.

39 " 'A Vanderbilt . . . on." *Ibid.,* p. 62.

40 "All the brains . . . family" GV, "The Story of a Child," undated manuscript, Reel 2371, GVWP.

40 "G.V. is dull." GV, diary, April 7, 1893, Reel 2369, *ibid.*

40 "My childhood . . . incident." GV, "My History."

40 "The Four . . . Frenchman." Mrs. Winthrop Chanler, *Roman Spring: Memoirs* (Boston, 1934), p. 238.

42 "I think . . . Vanderbilts." Allen Churchill, *The Upper Crust: An Informal History of New York's Highest Society* (Englewood Cliffs, N.J., 1970), p. 126.

42 "Supreme . . . appeals." Ward McAllister, quoted in Matthew Josephson, *The Robber Barons* (New York, 1962), p. 329.

42–44 "Bristling . . . reasons." Henry James, *The American Scene* (Bloomington, Ind., 1968), p. 162.

44 "Prefer a room . . . null!" Charles Henry Caffin, *American Masters of Sculpture* (Freeport, N.Y., 1969), pp. 196–97.

44 "Gilt panels . . . trees." Allen Churchill, *The Splendor Seekers: An Informal Glimpse of America's Multimillionaire Spenders—Members of the $50,000,000 Club* (New York, 1974), p. 75. See also Mrs. Gloria Vanderbilt, with Palma Wayne, *Without Prejudice* (New York, 1936), pp. 93–94.

46 "Did not continue . . . important." Wayne Andrews, *The Vanderbilt Legend* (New York, 1941), p. 224.

47 "Fresh . . . incredibly dull." Nathalie Dana, *Young in New York: A Memoir of a Victorian Girlhood* (Garden City, N.Y., 1963), p. 84.

48 "Crazy . . . out." Friedman, p. 51.

49 "Interesting . . . seen." GV, "People" Book, June 16, 1895, Reel 2369, GVWP.

49 "You have . . . blues." January 22, 1896, Reel 2369, *ibid.*

50–51 "I'm having . . . his life for me?" GV, diary, September 2, 1894, Reel 2369, *ibid.*

50–51 "Why . . . sport." Friedman, p. 140.

52 "The house . . . that . . ." GW, "Beginning of Autobiography," undated manuscript, ca. 1912, Reel 2371, GVWP.

52 "For social reasons," Friedman, p. 159.

52n. "The American . . . Man." Henry Adams, *The Education of Henry Adams* (Boston, 1961), p. 353.

53 "The more I tried . . . satisfaction." GW, "Beginning of Autobiography."

53 "If one has been surrounded . . . spread." Friedman, p. 188.

53 "A sort of protégé" *Ibid.*, p. 160.

53 "Secret Society"; "privilege . . . acquiring." GW, "Beginning of Autobiography."

54 "Would rather die . . . feelings." Friedman, p. 188.

56 "No art . . . America." Daniel Robbins, "Statues to Sculpture: From the Nineties to the Thirties," in *200 Years of American Sculpture* (New York, 1976), p. 115.

57 Although . . . money." Dana, p. 141.

58 "So . . . master-thumb. . . ." Henry James to Hendrik C. Andersen, October 23, 1899, Hendrik Christian Andersen Papers, LC.

58 "I am not over anxious . . . trumps!" Hendrik C. Andersen to Andreas M. Andersen, May 5, 1900, *ibid.*

59 "Faith in my own capacity" GW, "Beginning of Autobiography."

59 "It makes little difference . . . well-intended suggestions." Hendrik C. Andersen to GW, December 1, 1900, Reel 2357, GVWP.

59 "About Mrs. Whitney . . . surprisingly quick." Andreas M. Andersen to Hendrik C. Andersen, September 22, 1901, Hendrik Christian Andersen Papers.

59 "In expression . . . joy, etc." Hendrik C. Andersen to Helena and Arthur Andersen, July 16, 1905, *ibid.*

59 "Mania . . . huge" James to Hendrik C. Andersen, April 14, 1912, *ibid.*

60 "I hope . . . those we love!" Alice Gwynne Vanderbilt to GW, September 3, September 19, and October 4, 1900, Reel 2357, GVWP.

60 "Mood of deviltry . . . in my life." Friedman, pp. 178, 182, 187.

60 "I pity . . . the dregs of humanity." *Ibid.*, p. 181.

61 "If I could not . . . very close." GW to Harry Payne Whitney, Autumn 1903, Reel 2357, GVWP.

62 "The arranging . . . surroundings" *Ibid.*

62 "Positively . . . attitude to combat." GW, "Beginning of Autobiography."

62 "You have known . . . at all." GW, journal, July 2, 1905, Reel 2369, GVWP.

64 "Your real power . . . pass." GW, journal, June 27, 1904, Reel 2369, *ibid.*

64 "To see . . . artists . . ." *Ibid.*

CHAPTER THREE

65 "Too vulgar"; "I know . . . indecent." Bruce St. John, ed., *John Sloan's New York Scene, From the Diaries, Notes and Correspondence, 1906–1913* (New York, 1965), p. 33.

66 "Is it . . . sores?" "Palette and Brush," *Town Topics*, 59 (February 6, 1908), p. 16.

67 "An obnoxious . . . painting." John Sloan, verbatim notes, 1944–1951, John Sloan Archives, Delaware Art Museum, p. 102. Courtesy of Helen Farr Sloan.

68 "Had never . . . mentioned." Nancy Hale and Fredson Bowers, eds., *Leon Kroll: A Spoken Memoir* (Charlottesville, 1983), p. 20.

68 "Funeral . . . coffins." Edith DeShazo, *Everett Shinn, 1876–1953: A Figure in His Time* (New York, 1974), p. 64.

68 "The pictures . . . poets." Wallace Stevens, *Letters of Wallace Stevens* (New York, 1966), p. 116.

68 "Inanities . . . space." Quoted in Bennard B. Perlman, *The Immortal Eight: American Painting from Eakins to the Armory Show, 1870–1913* (Westport, Conn., 1979), p. 125.

68 "Feeling . . . back in again" Robert Henri, *The Art Spirit* (Philadelphia and New York, 1960), p. 241.

69 "Henri . . . artist." Sloan, verbatim notes, p. 153.

71 "Be willing . . . picture." Henri, p. 200.

71 "We found . . . honest." Sloan, verbatim notes, p. 104.

71 "Interest . . . things." Henri, p. 200.

71 "Did not do . . . again." *Ibid.*, pp. 206–7.

71 "Peer . . . American life." Lloyd Goodrich, *Thomas Eakins* (Cambridge, Mass., 1982), 2:269.

72 "Respectability . . . appalling." Goodrich, *Thomas Eakins*, 1:185.

72 "An element . . . him" Van Wyck Brooks, *Days of the Phoenix: The Nineteen-Twenties I Remember* (New York, 1957), p. 102.

73 "The American man . . . pretty." Samuel Isham, *The History of American Painting* (New York, 1936), p. 500.

74 "Eaten up" Ira Glackens, *William Glackens and The Eight: The Artists Who Freed American Art* (New York, 1983), p. 54.

74 "Today Mrs. Harry . . . decoration." Henri, diary, March 30, 1906, Robert Henri Papers, AAA. I thank Bennard B. Perlman, who shared this information with me.

74 "Disturbs . . . enlightens" Henri, *The Art Spirit*, p. 15.

74 "A rock . . . lace." Guy Pène du Bois, *Artists Say the Silliest Things* (New York, 1940), p. 86.

75 "There is . . . unrest." Lloyd Goodrich, "The Whitney's Battle for U.S. Art," *Art News*, 53 (November 1954), p. 38.

76 "Array . . . wobble." Malvina Hoffman, *Yesterday is Tomorrow* (New York, 1965), p. 73.

77 Dubiousness of Kitson: Blendon Campbell to Rosalind Irvine, July 1949, WMAA; Archives (H.1/f38).

77 "Mrs. Harry . . . purpose." St. John, p. 199.

77–78 Architectural League controversy: "Mrs. H. P. Whitney Wins Prize in Art," *New York Herald*, February 1, 1908, and "Row Over Award to Mrs. H. P. Whitney," *New York Times*, February 6, 1908.

78 "Mrs. Aitch . . . orders." "Social Artistry," *Town Topics*, 59 (February 6, 1908), pp. 12–13.

78–79 *Paganisme Immortel* incident: Interview with Karl Gruppe; "American Fakirs Ready with Exhibition," *New York Times*, April 11, 1910; "Fine Prices for Prize Art Fakes," *New York Times*, April 15, 1910; "The Fakirs Satirize the Work of National Artists," *New York Times*, April 17, 1910; "Mrs. Harry Payne Whitney Stimulates Latent Genius in Art," *New York Times*, May 22, 1910.

79 O'Connor's role: Interviews with Karl Gruppe, Edward Laning, and Carl Rieser.

80 "I was very interested . . . deal." Daniel Chester French to Andrew O'Connor, April 15, 1914, Daniel Chester French Papers, LC.

80 "I went . . . your return." John Gregory to GW, September 23, 1919, Reel 2361, GVWP.

81 "Peace . . . sought." Du Bois, p. 178.

81–82 "About six . . . booming." Louis Bouché, unpublished, undated memoirs, Louis Bouché Papers, AAA.

82 "A Gargantua . . . colossal." Du Bois, p. 176.

82 "Says live . . . conversations." GW, journal, April 2, 1906, Reel 2370, GVWP.

83 "No more . . . Company." John Sloan, *Gist of Art: Principles and Practise Expounded in the Classroom and Studio* (New York, 1977), p. 28.

83 "The advisability . . . impossible." St. John, p. 112.

83 "Mr. Fraser. . . . true beauty." Arthur B. Davies to GW, April 10, 1907, Reel 2358, GVWP.

83 "Shows . . . stupidity." "National Academy Elects 3 Out Of 36," *New York Times*, April 12, 1907.

84 News clippings saved by Gertrude: see Reel 2373, GVWP.

84 "An amazing creature." Jo Davidson, interview with Rosalind Irvine, June 3, 1949, WMAA; Archives (H.1/f38).

84 "So jolly and nice." Blendon Campbell, interview with Rosalind Irvine, March 22, 1949, WMAA; Archives (H.1/f38).

85 "Of course . . . some of it." JR to GW, undated, Reel 2358, GVWP.

85 "The little . . . book of wisdom could." GW, "White Voices," unpublished manuscript, 1911, unmicrofilmed GVWP, AAA, Washington, D.C.

85–86 "The general economic . . . supporting themselves." GW, unpublished essay, ca. 1920–1924, Reel 2372, GVWP.

86 "Take what . . . themselves." GW, diary, April 2, 1906, Reel 2370, *ibid.*

87 "A personal . . . sensation." More and Goodrich, quoted in *JFAA*, p. 12.

90 "Willful . . . obstinate" Divorce petition of Willard and Mary Grace Barnes Force, January 8, 1911, New Jersey Supreme Court records.

90 "Running around"; "What . . . herself." Interview with Marjorie Rieser.

91 "Unadulterated . . . nausea." "Palette and Brush," *Town Topics*, 59 (February 6 1908), p. 16.

91 "As significant . . . American art." William Innes Homer, *Robert Henri and His Circle*, (Ithaca and London, 1969), pp. 145–46.

92 "At that time . . . them." Sloan, quoted in *JFAA*, p. 34.

92 "Sits . . . past." Henri, pp. 131–32.

93 "Collection . . . artist." Watson, quoted in *JFAA*, p. 63.

94–95 "Your copy . . . . sooner." JR to GW, August 2, 1911, Reel 2358, GVWP.

95–96 "In New York . . . quick." "Mrs. Whitney's Sec'y And Architect Delighted With Plinth of Cody Statue," *The Cody Enterprise*, April 2, 1924.

CHAPTER FOUR

I owe much of this reconstruction to the unpublished reminiscences of Forbes Watson, written in 1949 and now in the Archives of American Art. I have borrowed heavily from Watson's phrasing and point of view.

97 "Artists . . . remain." Van Wyck Brooks, *John Sloan: A Painter's Life* (New York, 1955), p. 198.

98 "I didn't . . . astonished." Talmey, p. 131.

98 "Contained . . . highlights." Watson, reminiscences, 1949, FWP.

98 "She could sell . . . anybody." Campbell, interview with Rosalind Irvine.

100 "Splendid as a temple" Arthur Lee to GW, July 11, 1912, Reel 2358, GVWP.

100–101 "In 1913 . . . picture." Ben Hecht, *A Child of the Century* (New York, 1954), p. 330.

101 "The most vital . . . stage." Milton W. Brown, *The Story of the Armory Show* (New York, 1963), p. 28.

102 "Nightmare of sculptured rhetoric" *Ibid.*, p. 78.

103 "But she . . . side." Bernard Karfiol, interview with Rosalind Irvine, February 11, 1949, WMAA; Archives (H. 1/f38).

104 "I was very glad . . . in our art." GW, draft of speech, ca. 1914–1915, unmicrofilmed GVWP.

106 "Umbilical staircase" Talmey, p. 132.

106 "Mrs. Whitney . . . 1930." Stuart Davis, transcript of radio broadcast, 1953, WMAA; Archives (H. 1/f 42).

106 "Georgian . . . chateauette." James A. Wright, "A History of Barley Sheaf Farm," unpublished paper, August 25, 1977. Courtesy of Don F. Mills, Holicong, Pa.

108 "Aunt Jule . . . have"; "We learned . . . people"; "We were told . . . like it." Interviews with Beverly Rieser Smock and Marjorie Rieser.

109 "You said . . . sculptor . . ." Friedman, p. 335.

109 "In the face . . . truth." GW, diary, December 4–5, 1913, Reel 2370, GVWP.

109 "I do not wish . . . produced!" Friedman, p. 343.

111 "By the fact . . . for it." GW, diary, November 29, 1914, unmicrofilmed GVWP.

111 "I know . . . responsibilities." GW, diary, December 18, 1914, Reel 2370, GVWP.

112 "A full-length . . . seaweed" "Aid War Sufferers by Whitney Studio Show," *New York World*, December 3, 1914.

112 "Pictures . . . upstairs." Invitation to "50–50" sale, December 17, 1914, Van Dearing Perrine Papers, AAA. I thank Arleen Pancza for pointing out this and other related materials.

113 "I was . . . my door again." William Zorach, *Art Is My Life* (Cleveland, 1967), p. 70.

114 "Is there any . . . nude figure?" Margaret Two (?) to JF, November 28, 1914, Reel 2359, GVWP.

115 "It is one . . . repays a visit." "Another Art Relief Show," *American Art News*, 13 (February 6, 1915), p. 3.

115 "Neo-classical . . . gold." Frank Crowninshield, "The World of Warren Davis," in *Memorial Exhibition of Paintings, Pastels and Etchings by Warren Davis* (New York, 1928), unpaged.

115 "The youngest . . . for a year." "Young Painters Competition," *American Art News*, 13 (July 17, 1915), p. 3.

116 "The wholesale encouragement . . . lasting achievement." Watson, "Art Notes," *New York Post*, May 1, 1915.

118 "Never . . . boss." Watson, quoted in *JFAA*, p. 55.

118–120 Roosevelt's visit: "Art Judges Awry Roosevelt Declares," *New York Tribune*, December 8, 1915; "Colonel's Big Stick Batters Cubist Art," *New York Times*, December 3, 1915.

120–121 "Juliana . . . whisked me off." Sylvia Winsor Dudley to author, November 8, 1978 and November 16, 1978.

121 "Three fine marbles" William Macbeth to GW, December 17, 1915, Macbeth Gallery Papers, AAA.

122 "Our own time . . . something.' " Watson, "In The Art Galleries," *Evening Post Saturday Magazine*, January 15, 1916.

123 "May I . . . favored." Sloan to GW, January 7, 1916, WMAA; Archives (H. 1/f4).

123 "He is . . . American art." Watson, "One Man Show," *Evening Post Saturday Magazine*, January 29, 1916.

123 "Presents . . . themes." "Comprehensive Exhibit of John Sloan at Mrs. Whitney's," *New York Globe*, January 26, 1916.

124 "For it . . . Whitney Show.' " Sloan to GW, June 1916, Reel 2359, GVWP.

124 "Sloan was . . . so gay." Watson, reminiscences, 1949, FWP.

124 "Tabasco tongue" Brooks, *John Sloan: A Painter's Life*, p. 205.

124 "A romantic little girl." Watson, interview with Rosalind Irvine, February 18, 1949, WMAA; Archives (H. 1/f38).

126 "Too deep-seated . . . cured." St. John, p. xvi.

126–128 John Butler Yeats: unless otherwise stated, details about Yeats's life in New York are from William M. Murphy's biography, *Prodigal Father: The Life of John Butler Yeats (1839–1922)*. I am grateful to William Murphy for the extra information he has provided about Yeats, Sloan, and JF.

126 "Hopeful penury," "hopeless penury" Sloan, biographical information sheet, 1951, WMAA; Library.

126 "Yeats . . . succeeded." James C. Young, "Yeats of Petitpas'," *New York Times Book Review & Magazine*, February 19, 1922.

126 "His Penelope's web." Helen Vendler, "J.B.Y.," *The New Yorker*, January 8, 1979, p. 66.

126–127 "I am off . . . delightful." John Butler Yeats to John Quinn, April 21, 1916, John Quinn Memorial Collection, Rare Books and Manuscripts Division, The New York Public Library, Astor, Lenox, and Tilden Foundations.

127 "There . . . people." Yeats to John Quinn, April 24, 1916, *ibid.*

127 "I had one . . . sketch." *Ibid.*

128 "Don't daunten youth," Margaret French to author, May 5, 1978.

128 "Sloan was . . . jail." Glackens, p. 136.

128 "The serious . . . boredom." Watson, quoted in *JFAA*, p. 57.

129 "Was not to be bored . . . necessary." Watson, reminiscences, 1949, FWP.

130 "I should . . . amusing myself." "Mrs. Whitney Services Will Be Tomorrow," *New York Herald Tribune*, April 19, 1942.

131 Bellows "was . . . subtle." Watson, reminiscences, 1949, FWP.

132 "Paris in . . . of New York." Louise Varèse, *Varèse: A Looking-Glass Diary, Vol. 1 (1883–1928)* (New York, 1972), p. 127.

132 "A document . . . nations." Helen Farr Sloan, ed., *John Sloan: New York Etchings* (New York, 1978), unpaged.

133 Friedman estimates: Friedman, pp. 380–81.

133 "Arranged . . . background." JF, exhibition layout, July–August 1916, Reel 2369, GVWP.

134 "Sloan started . . . were." William M. Murphy, *Prodigal Father*, p. 457.

134 "She believed . . . women." Carl Rieser, "Juliana Rieser Force: A Memoir."

136 Contributions to Society of Independent Artists: Clark S. Marlor, *The Society of Independent Artists: The Exhibition Record, 1917–1944* (Park Ridge, N.J., 1984), pp. 4, 15, 28, 76.

136 "Perhaps . . . Artists." Sloan, quoted in *JFAA*, p. 39.

137 "The annual exhibitions . . . great art." Jeanne Bertrand, "Young Artists to Show Work," *Morning Telegraph*, February 19, 1917.

138 "Extend from . . . flatter the truth." "Notes of the Studios and Galleries," *Arts and Decoration*, 7 (January 1917), p. 142.

138–139 Meeting Forbes Watson: Watson, transcript of speech given at WMAA, November 12, 1931; Watson, reminiscences, 1949, both in FWP.

139 "Protest . . . imagination." Edith W. Powell, "The Introspectives," *International Studio* 61 (May 1917), p. 92.

140 "It was . . . afternoon affair." Winifred Ward to GW, March 12, 1917, Reel 2360, GVWP.

CHAPTER FIVE

142 "We formed . . . destinies." Jerome Myers, "Confidences of an Errant Artist," *Arts and Decoration* 7 (June 1917) p. 419.

143–144 Change in direction: Watson, reminiscences, 1949, FWP.

144 "We have always . . . exhibiting." Anabel Parker McCann, "Mrs. Juliana Force, Friend of Artists," *New York Sun*, January 23, 1934.

144 "It's . . . appreciation." Telephone interview with David Eisendrath.

145 "She did not view . . . fine art." Robert Bishop, *American Folk Art: Expressions of A New Spirit* (New York, 1982), p. 6.

147 "Freshness of the primitives" Henry Schnakenberg, interview with Wanda M. Corn, May 22, 1965. I thank Dr. Corn for giving me a transcript of her interview.

148 "An air . . . happen." Gloria Vanderbilt, *Once Upon a Time* (New York, 1985), p. 225.

148 "In the foreground . . . Aunt J." Allan Rieser, unpublished memoir, 1978, RFC.

148 "Aunt J. . . . Philadelphia." *Ibid.*

149 "The exhibition . . . this year." Helen Appleton Read, "Landscapes at the Whitney Studio," *Brooklyn Daily Eagle*, December 22, 1917.

149 Dolly Sloan: Interview with Helen Farr Sloan; Sloan, verbatim notes, p. 330.

150 "Possibly . . . personality" Daty Healy, "A History of the Whitney Museum of American Art, 1930–1954" (Ph.D. diss., New York University, School of Education, 1960), p. 53.

150 "No one will . . . reach her." Sloan, quoted in *JFAA*, pp. 35–36.

150–151 "Raised . . . humor." Du Bois, p. 190.

151–152 Davis and Luks: Davis, transcript of radio broadcast; Davis, interview with Harlan Phillips, 1962. Courtesy of Earl Davis, New York City.

151 "An old rounder . . . lily." Du Bois, p. 191.

151 Identification of Glenn O. Coleman: Davis, interview with Harlan Phillips.

152 "Oh, that's . . . along." Sloan, quoted in *JFAA*, p. 40.

152 "To any casual . . . columns." Du Bois, p. 190.

152–153 Luks at opening: Davis, interview with Harlan Phillips; Campbell, interview with Rosalind Irvine.

153 "The Exhibition . . . painters." Robert Chanler to GW, February 11, 1918, Reel 2361, GVWP.

153 "It costs . . . cheque to him." JF to GW, February 1918, Reel 2361, *ibid.*

153 "Erected in admiration . . . therefrom." "Mrs. H. P. Whitney 'Interns' Sculptors; Much Work Done," *New York Herald*, March 3, 1918.

153–154 "The Exhibition . . . deal." Jo Davidson to GW, March 1918, Reel 2361, GVWP.

154 "Not only . . . are respected." "Cuban Ways Shown in Randall Davey's Recent Sketches," *The Touchstone*, 5 (May 1919), pp. 123–24.

154 "Chilly . . . Museum." Henry McBride, "News and Comments in the World of Art," *New York Sun*, January 20, 1918.

154n. "Gertrude . . . sculpture." Lincoln Kirstein, *Gaston Lachaise* (New York, 1947), p. 4.

155 "I have often asked . . . capacities." GW, essay, 1917, Reel 2372, GVWP.

155 "For the present . . . achieve." "The Whitney Studio Club," *Greenwich Village Spectator*, February 1918.

155 "Everybody here . . . come!" JF to GW, March 1918, Reel 2361, GVWP.

156 "Hiked . . . over." Frank Crowninshield to GW, April 8, 1918, Reel 2361, *ibid.*

156 "Have you heard . . . least." JF to Carl Zigrosser, April 11, 1918, Carl Zigrosser Papers, Special Collections, Van Pelt Library, University of Pennsylvania.

157 "The most pure . . . handled." Millia C. Davenport, "Greenwich Village Interiors," *The Quill*, June 1918, p. 11.

157 "To play . . . ideas." Jo Davidson, *Between Sittings: An Informal Autobiography of Jo Davidson* (New York, 1951), p. 126.

158 "She was someone . . . identified with." Interview with Katherine Schmidt.

158 "Protective . . . war." "Thayer Camouflage Pictures," *American Art News*, 16 (July 13, 1918), p. 2.

158 "Wretched . . . wonderful!" Interview with Dorothy Varian.

159 "He can't . . . ready." Brook, quoted in *JFAA*, p. 50.

160–161 "My dearest Becky . . . Sedley." Rockwell Kent to JF, November 22, 1918, WMAA; Library.

161–162 "Best Christmas . . . this data." Kent to JF, December 1918, *ibid.*

162 "I do not think . . . know." Zigrosser to Kent, January 27, 1919, Rockwell Kent Papers, AAA.

162 "She compelled . . . entertaining one." Kent to Zigrosser, March 8, 1919, Carl Zigrosser Papers.

162 "A woman . . . looks." Rockwell Kent, *It's Me O Lord: The Autobiography of Rockwell Kent* (New York, 1955), p. 313.

162–163 "Always felt . . . pretty face.' " Allan Rieser, unpublished memoir, 1978.

163 "Oh, that face!" Interview with Edith Goodrich.

163 "A typically . . . winds." George Palmer Putnam, *Wide Margins: A Publisher's Autobiography* (New York, 1942), p. 87.

163 "Kent . . . account." David Traxel, *An American Saga: The Life and Times of Rockwell Kent* (New York, 1980), p. 120.

163 "The deadliest . . . created" Watson, interview with Rosalind Irvine.

164 "Went to school . . . backyard." Watson to Van Wyck Brooks, May 25, 1953, FWP.

165 "Omaha . . . like it." Watson, U.S. Treasury Department report, 1937, *ibid.*

165 "My first visit . . . security." Watson, unpublished manuscript, 1946, *ibid.*

166 "Forbes . . . chat." Telephone interview with Maria Ealand.

167 "[Mrs. Force] was . . . bounds." Florence Ballin Cramer, diary, October 26, 1933. Courtesy of Aileen Cramer, Woodstock, N.Y.

168 "All my life . . . this!" Lawrence Campbell, ed., *"Chris": Reminiscences by Christian Buchheit as told to Lawrence Campbell* (New York, 1956), p. 26

168 "Now the bottom . . . names. . . ." Harry Payne Whitney to GW, August 1919, Reel 2361, GVWP.

168–169 "Mrs. . . . knock." GW, undated limericks, Reel 2372, *ibid.*

169 "A tea . . . smile." Du Bois, diary, January 13, 1920. Excerpt provided by Betsy Fahlman.

169 "Wonderful . . . people." Katherine Schmidt, interview with Rosalind Irvine, February 10, 1949, WMAA; Archives (H.1/f38).

169–170 "The Club . . . Academy." Interview with Katherine Schmidt.

171 "Terrible . . . well-earned lunch." Watson, "Prince, Bourgeois and Bolshevist," *Arts and Decoration* 13 (September 1920), p. 228.

171 "I am distressed . . . hotel room." Auguste Jaccaci to JF, December 5, 1920, Reel 2396, JFP.

172 "A special . . . April 15th." Lizzie P. Bliss et al. to Robert de Forest, January 26, 1921, MMAA.

173 "Well, I was up there . . . Quinn." B. L. Reid, *The Man from New York: John Quinn and His Friends* (New York, 1968), p. 499.

173–174 "I do not . . . *Journal.*" Quoted in John R. Lane, *Stuart Davis: Art and Art Theory* (New York, 1978), p. 94.

174 "Encouraged . . . making" Davis, transcript of radio broadcast.

174 "Piano nightmare" Varèse, p. 155.

174–175 "The composer . . . individual." *Ibid.*, pp. 166–67.

176 "Then she would . . . growl." Interview with Patra Cogan.

178 "The most vivid . . . show.' " Edward L. Bernays to author, August 21, 1979.

179 "Mrs. . . . officer." Friedman, p. 439.

179 "No one will . . . through." Allan Rieser to author, September 30, 1978.

179 "My mother . . . chosen." C. V. Whitney, *High Peaks* (Lexington, Ky., 1977), pp. 91–92.

179–180 "She was . . . acquainted." Friedman, p. 447.

179–180 "Directed . . . profanity." Zigrosser, *My Own Shall Come To Me: A Personal Memoir and Picture Chronicle* (Philadelphia, 1971), p. 171.

179–180 "The audience . . . season." Varèse, p. 174.

181 "A wonderful . . . on my side." Kent to JF, August 8, 1922, WMAA; Library.

181 "A young savage . . . friends again later." Interview with Reuben Nakian.

CHAPTER SIX

183 "It seems . . . Club." McBride, "National Academy's Concession to Modernism Seems Hardly a Complete Success," *New York Sun*, March 26, 1927.

183–184 "As . . . months." Varèse, p. 194.

184 "I am enclosing . . . summer." JF to Ernest Fiene, May 13, 1926, Ernest Fiene Papers, AAA.

184 Whitney Studio Club invitation: Townsend Ludington, ed., *The Fourteenth Chronicle: Letters and Diaries of John Dos Passos* (Boston, 1973), p. 353.

184 "I didn't ask . . . show.' " Interview with Reuben Nakian.

184–185 *"Come and bring . . . Dos"* Ludington, pp. 353–54.

186–187 "A mouthpiece . . . the outside." Watson, "Editorial," *The Arts*, 3 (January 1923), p. 1.

186n. "Almost anyone . . . belonged to it." William Schack, *Art and Argyrol* (New York, 1963), pp. 133, 182–83.

188 "In some places . . . this moment." John Dos Passos, *The Best Times: An Informal Memoir* (New York, 1966), p. 138.

188 "Like a fire engine" Alexander Brook, interview with Paul Cummings, July 7–8, 1977, AAA.

188 "You'll hang for this." Brook, quoted in *JFAA*, p. 48.

188 "You felt . . . were." Allan Rieser, unpublished memoir.

188 "The social . . . room." Interview with Lloyd Goodrich.

189 "There was always . . . new ground." Interview with Katherine Schmidt.

189–190 "Juliana boiled . . . his hands." *Ibid.*

190–191 "I KNOW . . . because you want to!" Whitney Studio Club advertisements, *The Arts*, 4 (July and September 1923) and 9 (June 1926).

191 "Radically . . . universal." Douglas Hyland, *Marius de Zayas: Conjuror of Souls* (Lawrence, Kans., 1981), p. 13.

191 "The Picasso . . . taken" GW to Davidson, undated [May 1923], Jo Davidson Papers, LC.

192 "A barometer . . . women." "Random Impressions in Current Exhibitions," *New York Tribune*, April 8, 1923.

195 "About the only way . . . that!" Kent to JF, September 30, 1923, WMAA; Library.

195 "If you didn't . . . missed." "Interview: Katherine Schmidt Talks with Paul Cummings," *Archives of American Art Journal*, 17 (1977), p. 18.

195 "Sunless chamber" Brook, "Myself and Others," unpublished memoir, 1979, Firestone Library, Princeton University. Courtesy of John Graves.

195 "When . . . Now." Brook, interview with Paul Cummings.

195 "Without . . . questions" Brook, quoted in *JFAA*, p. 48.

195–196 "And preferably unknown"; "was a glorious . . . wishing for." Brook, "Myself and Others."

196 "Missed . . . *Gemütlichkeit*." Vàrese, p. 186.

197 "Was human . . . glad." Kent, p. 314.

197 "Seduction . . . affair" Traxel, p. 150.

199 "Mr. Sheeler . . . last year." Interview with Lloyd Goodrich.

201 "We'll see about that." Interview with William Lane.

201 "The ideal . . . plan" "A Unique Experiment" (advertisement), *The Arts*, 4 (November 1923), inside front cover.

202 "Cigar-store . . . art." Henry Schnakenberg, unpublished speech, December 14, 1964, WMAA; Archives (H.1/f35).

202 "Odds and ends . . . Studio Club." "The World of Art: Art in Exhibitions and Books," *New York Times Magazine*, February 17, 1924; "Art Exhibitions of the West," *New York Times*, February 17, 1924.

202 Folk art and primitivism: Schnakenberg, interview with Wanda M. Corn.

203 "The air . . . serious." McBride, "Art News and Reviews," *New York Herald*, March 9, 1924.

203 "Next year . . . hope." Brook to Florence Cramer, February 5, 1924, Florence and Konrad Cramer Papers, AAA.

204 "The ladies . . . career." Brook, "Myself and Others."

204 "[Mrs. Whitney's] statue . . . subject." Quoted in Friedman, p. 456.

204 "The happiest . . . Cody." "Buffalo Bill Memorial Assured Mrs. Whitney Dedicated To Task," *Northern Wyoming Herald*, July 4, 1923.

206 "I have never . . . has made." "Buffalo Bill Memorial is an Expression of American Life Well Interpreted by Gertrude V. Whitney, The Sculptor," *Park County Herald*, April 2, 1924.

207 "Speaking . . . make it." JF, transcript of speech, March 1924, Reel 2365, GVWP.

207 "Isn't it strange . . . fail." Franklin Watkins to JF, April 24, 1924, Reel 2365, *ibid*.

208 "The Whitney . . . caught on." McBride, "Lively Exhibit Ends Season for the Whitney Studio Club," *New York Sun*, May 17, 1924.

208 "I asked you . . . done so." Brook to Konrad Cramer, August 1924 [dated incorrectly by recipient as April 5, 1925], Florence and Konrad Cramer Papers.

209 "Since I left . . . 1860." Watson to GW, Summer 1924, Reel 2361, GVWP.

209 "Went storming . . . envelope." Brook, "Myself and Others."

210 "Barely. . . . times." *Ibid*.

210–211 "The years . . . circumvent." Zigrosser, pp. 172–74.

211 "It sounded . . . gears" Interview with Lloyd Goodrich.

211 "Life . . . polite statement." Du Bois, quoted in *JFAA*, p. 47.

211–212 "I had . . . triumphant smile." Rebecca West to author, July 6, 1978.

212 "Sir . . . Judgment Day." Allan Rieser, unpublished memoir.

212–213 "Occasional difference . . . for it." Davis, transcript of radio broadcast; Davis, interview with Harlan Phillips.

213 "Stolen" jewelry incident: interview with Eleanor Lambert Berkson.

213–214 "No portrait . . . oddity." Allan Rieser, unpublished memoir.

214 "She . . . odd." Interview with Katherine Schmidt.

216 "Of her former . . . heroine." Brook, "Myself and Others."

216 "But in the whole . . . first time." Fernand Ouellette, *Edgard Varèse* (New York, 1966), pp. 82–83.

218 "[In New Jersey] I used to . . . reading." Carl Rieser to JF, August 9, 1934, RFC.

218 "If Aunt . . . her way." Interview with Beverly Rieser Smock.

218 "She thought . . . artists." Interview with Allan Rieser.

218–219 "Told us . . . Fletcherizing a glass of milk." *Ibid.*

219 "A group . . . monogrammed.' " Interview with Dorothy Varian.

221 "Special . . . policies." Robert J. Forsyth, "John B. Flannagan: His Life and Works" (Ph.D. diss., University of Minnesota, 1965), p. 20.

223 "Met Mrs. Force . . . being done." Henri, diary, January 25, 1926, Robert Henri Papers.

224 "Time . . . useful." Virginia Woolf, "How It Strikes a Contemporary," *The Common Reader*, First Series (New York and London, 1980), p. 245.

224 "Had . . . Americans?' " Herbert J. Seligmann, *Alfred Stieglitz Talking: Notes on Some of His Conversations, 1925–1931, with a Foreword* (New Haven, 1966), p. 122.

224 "The life . . . to me." Watson, unpublished lecture, 1949, FWP.

225 "Enemy" Quoted in Sasha M. Newman, *Arthur Dove and Duncan Phillips: Artist and Patron* (New York, 1981), p. 34. This catalog sets forth the Stieglitz-Dove-Phillips relationship in detail, and I have gratefully used its documentation to support my own argument.

225–226 "Stieglitz . . . conversation." Watson, unpublished memoirs, April 28, 1946, FWP.

226 "He does . . . well known." Watson, "Galleries in the News," *New York World*, March 8, 1925.

226 "One must . . . so much." Watson, unpublished memoirs, 1946, FWP.

226 "I went to a show . . . things.' " Inslee Hopper, interview with Robert Brown, July 28, 1981, AAA.

227 "That he is the one . . . commercial venture." Watson, unpublished memoirs, 1946, FWP.

227 "The first days . . . 37 years." Seligmann, p. 120.

227 "I must see to it . . . unspeakable crowd." Quoted in Newman, p. 32.

227–228 "Field Marshall . . . powers." Duncan Phillips to Watson, March 21, 1927, The Phillips Collection Papers, AAA, Smithsonian Institution, Reel 1937:447.

228 "I am a bit amused . . . make up." Quoted in Newman, p. 33.

228 "Hartley . . . cash!" *Ibid.*

228 "It was . . . art." Quoted in Cynthia Jaffee, "Reuben Nakian" (Master's thesis, Columbia University, 1967), p. 25.

229 "Once said . . . at that time." Sloan, quoted in *JFAA*, p. 39.

229 "When Mrs. Force . . . sensible and just." Brook, quoted in *JFAA*, pp. 51–52.

230 "To the map . . . Woodstock." Quoted in Karal Ann Marling, *Woodstock: An American Art Colony, 1902–1977* (Poughkeepsie, N.Y., 1977), unpaged.

230 "In those days . . . best of it." Interview with Hannah Small.

231 "She bought . . . for it." Arnold Blanch, interview with Dorothy Seckler, June 13–August 3, 1963, AAA.

231 "She took to us . . . may have been." Interview with Lucile Blanch.

231 "Mrs. Force . . . Whitney." Interview with Eugenie Gershoy.

231 "While Woodstock . . . support." Marling.

231 "Very familiar . . . 'professional.' " *Ibid.*

CHAPTER SEVEN

233 "Vigorous . . . Academy visitors." Bryson Burroughs to Reginald Marsh, March 28, 1926, Reginald Marsh Papers, AAA.

233 "These parties . . . greetings." Louis Bouché, unpublished memoirs.

233 "Leaving so. . . . life there." Interview with Lloyd Goodrich.

233–234 History of Saint-Nazaire monument: Saint-Nazaire file, American Battle Monuments Commission Papers, National Archives and Records Service.

234 "With a crusader's . . . eagle." Subscription brochure, Saint-Nazaire Association, American Battle Monuments Commission Papers.

235 "Golden age of gallery trotting." Joseph Cornell to John I. H. Baur, May 4, 1957, WMAA; Library.

236 "Did you ever . . . name." "THE BARREN PERIOD," *The Arts*, 9–12. This advertisement ran consecutively in the May–September 1927 issues.

236 "I saw . . . nothing about it." Davidson to Yvonne Davidson, November 5, 1926, Jo Davidson Papers.

236 "SAW . . . PROGRESS." JF to Davidson, November 18, 1926, *ibid.*

236–237 "Handsomely . . . 14th Street." Davis, transcript of radio broadcast.

237 "Genuine talent for painting" McBride, "Retrospective Show of Stuart Davis," *New York Sun*, December 11, 1926.

237 "Laboratory work" Watson, "Art Notes," *New York World*, December 13, 1926.

237 "Right . . . year." Davis, transcript of radio broadcast.

237 "Nailed . . . egg beater idea." Quoted in James Johnson Sweeney, *Stuart Davis* (New York, 1945), pp. 16, 18.

237–238 "He wore an overcoat . . . twice more." Brook, "Myself and Others."

238 "Thereafter . . . my pictures." Raphael Soyer, *Diary of an Artist* (Washington, D.C., 1977), p. 218.

238 "An exhibition . . . excellent drawings." McBride, "Portraits of Women as Seen by Men," *New York Sun*, January 8, 1927.

239 "It is impossible . . . town." McBride, "National Academy's Concession to Modernism Seems Hardly a Complete Success," *New York Sun*, March 26, 1927.

239–240 "Delightful . . . She was . . . admiration for her." Brook, interview with Paul Cummings.

240 "Despite hazards . . . Juliana Force." Brook, "Myself and Others."

240 "Mr. Robb . . . immediately!" Interview with William Robb.

240 "No two days . . . holder." Interview with Ethel Renthal.

240 "The winter . . . Lloyd." Interview with Edith Goodrich.

242 "I realized . . . paint." Interview with Dorothy Varian.

242 "The sensation . . . beautiful." "New York's Statues Called 'Ridiculous,' " *New York Times*, October 3, 1926.

243 "Kitchen . . . supplies." Edward Steichen, unpublished speech, December 14, 1964, WMAA; Library (Special Collections). See also Edward Steichen, *A Life in Photography* (Garden City, N.Y., 1963), unpaged.

243 "Objects . . . only." "Empirical," *Art Digest*, 1 (March 1, 1927), p. 2.

243 "Well . . . handle it." Steichen, unpublished speech.

244 "Based . . . art" Watson, "Editorial," *The Arts*, 9 (March 1927), p. 113.

244 "I . . . to be a part." JF to Aline Solomons, April 6, 1927, Reel 2366, GVWP.

245 "Would be accepted if offered." Burroughs to JF, June 15, 1927, WMAA; Archives (H.1/f31).

245 "As usual . . . conquered." Solomons to JF, October 24, 1927, Reel 2366, GVWP.

246 "If questioned . . . nothing." GW to JF, March 23, 1927, Reel 2362, *ibid.*

246 "Thank goodness . . . ocean." GW to JF, July 15, 1927, Reel 2362, *ibid.*

247 "You told me . . . yrs." JF to GW, September 1, 1927, Reel 2362, *ibid.*

247 "CONGRATULATIONS . . . YOU." JF to GW, September 4, 1927, Reel 2366, *ibid.*

247 "Of having . . . impossible." Du Bois, pp. 245–46.

248 "Read of . . . sculptor." Robert Aitken and Thomas Jones, testimony, transcript of stenographic minutes, *C. Brancusi* v. *United States*, October 21, 1927, Museum of Modern Art Library.

248–249 "As a valid . . . euthanasia" Varèse, pp. 210, 258.

249 "I think I succeeded . . . trivial." JF to Solomons, November 29, 1927, Reel 2366, GVWP.

250 "Tell me . . . instead of a name." JF to Herndon Smith, May 22, 1928, WMAA; Archives (H.1/f13).

250 "I believe . . . Studio." JF to Herbert Fleishhacker, March 13, 1928, *ibid.*

250 "I think . . . at this time." JF to Beulah Stevenson, February 17, 1928, Beulah Stevenson Papers, AAA.

250 "As though miraculously . . . ending." Alma M. Reed, *Orozco* (New York, 1956), pp. 38–39.

251 "The credit . . . Force." Phillips to Sloan, February 3, 1928, The Phillips Collection Papers, Reel 1937:96.

251 "Judging . . . Whitney." Marya Mannes, "Gallery Notes," *Creative Art*, 2 (April 1928), p. viii.

251 "Declarations of love." Watson, unpublished lecture, 1949, FWP.

251 "Her lines . . . everything." Watson, quoted in *JFAA*, p. 61.

252 "If there is a moment . . . process." JF to Royal Cortissoz, December 1926, Royal Cortissoz Papers, YU.

252 "What with a little . . . came back." Davis, transcript of radio broadcast; Davis, interview with Harlan Phillips.

253–254 "In the belief . . . disbanding." JF, press release, September 1928, WMAA; Library (microfilm).

254 "I will show . . . inspired." "Hail and Farewell!" *Art Digest*, 3 (October 1, 1928), p. 16.

254 "Mrs. . . . people." Interview with Ethel Renthal.

255 "I am so happy . . . extent." Julius Bloch, diary, January 5, 1932, Philadelphia Museum of Art. Courtesy of Benjamin D. Bernstein, Philadelphia.

255 "Everyone . . . Watson." John Flannagan, *Letters of John B. Flannagan* (New York, 1942), p. 20.

255 "I am distressed . . . better. . . ." JF to Harry Gottlieb, December 18, 1928, WMAA; Archives (H.1/f2).

256–257 "Should promptly . . . circus pictures." McBride, "Whitney Studio Club [*sic*] Arranges a 'Circus in Paint' and Does It Most Successfully," *New York Sun*, April 6, 1929.

257 "Yes . . . gratitude." Edward Alden Jewell, "Sawdust and Peanuts," *New York Times*, April 7, 1929.

258 "Running away . . . time." Du Bois, p. 245.

259 "Constantly calm . . . proceeding." *Ibid.*

259 "Of the American . . . chimneys" Interview with Katie Harris.

260–261 "I was particularly . . . days." Du Bois, p. 258.

261 "I feel . . . collection." Daniel Chester French to William Church Osborn, February 28, 1916, Daniel Chester French Papers.

261 "For six years." JF to Glenn O. Coleman, December 5, 1929, WMAA; Library.

262 "Amazing gap" McBride, "The Palette Knife," *Creative Art*, 6 (February 1930), supp. 33.

263 "So far . . . 1913." "A Hearn Protest," *Art Digest*, 1 (February 15, 1927), p. 6.

263 "Was old school . . . behavior." Watson, unpublished draft of essay for *JFAA*, 1949, WMAA; Library; unpublished lecture, 1949, FWP.

263 "What will we do . . . already." Interview with Lloyd Goodrich.

264 "Pontifical . . . gift." Watson, unpublished lecture, 1949, FWP; unpublished draft of essay for *JFAA*.

264 "Why don't you . . . art?" Interview with Lloyd Goodrich.

264 "Dr. Robinson . . . American art." Watson, unpublished draft of essay for *JFAA*.

264 "I'll never forget . . . *American* Art.' " Telephone interview with Maria Ealand.

265 "The great advantage . . . artists." Watson, quoted in *JFAA*, pp. 55–57.

265 "Forbes . . . middle of it.' " Interview with Lloyd Goodrich.

CHAPTER EIGHT

267 "One day . . . Depression." Quoted in Barbara Goldsmith, *Little Gloria . . . Happy at Last* (New York, 1980), p. 230.

267 "The little flurry downtown." Quoted in Michael L. Lawson and Frederick S. Voss, *The Great Crash* (Washington, D.C., 1979), p. 7.

268 "Artists . . . else." Margaret French to author, May 5, 1978.

268 "I was one of . . . your best." Interview with R. Buckminster Fuller.

268 "You've been patient . . . arguments." Joseph Pollet to JF, December 28, 1930, WMAA; Library.

268–269 "Had looked . . . anyone to take notice." Emlen Etting, "Studio in Paris, 1930," unpublished memoirs, 1970s, pp. 95, 102. Courtesy of Emlen Etting, Philadelphia, Pa.; interview with Emlen Etting.

269 "Even my old friend . . . out." Oscar Bluemner to Anna Freeman, February 14, 1930, WMAA; Library.

269 "I told him." Bluemner, catalog cover for exhibition at Marie Harriman Gallery, January 2–26, 1935. Courtesy of John Davis Hatch, Lenox, Mass. I thank Mr. Hatch for calling this item to my attention.

269 "Grand lady" Bluemner to Freeman, February 14, 1930.

269n. "Mrs. Force . . . Museum." Bluemner, annotated Whitney Studio Galleries catalog, 1929, Oscar Bluemner Papers, AAA.

272 "Kansas has found her Homer." Quoted in Laurence E. Schmeckebier, *John Steuart Curry's Pageant of America* (New York, 1943), p. 62.

272 "Not a recognition . . . period." *Ibid.*, p. 165.

272 "The best delver . . . French." McBride, "Work of Four American Painters," *New York Sun*, November 30, 1929.

272–273 "In speaking . . . understand." Davis to McBride, *Creative Art*, 6 (February 1930), supp. 34–35.

273–274 "On account . . . conditions." JF to Hobson Pittman, December 12, 1929, WMAA; Archives (H.1/f4).

274 "All compulsive smokers" Interview with Donn Mosenfelder.

275 "Since Mrs. Force . . . matters." Freeman to Edith Halpert, March 10, 1931, WMAA; Archives (H.2/F30).

275 "Mrs. Force . . . for it." Interview with Lloyd Goodrich.

276 "Except for . . . American." McBride, "Work of Four American Painters," *New York Sun*, November 30, 1929.

277 "If you will have . . . present." JF to Coleman, December 5, 1929, WMAA; Library.

277 "You have . . . deserves." George William Eggers to JF, December 17, 1929, WMAA; Archives (H.1/f8).

277 "If you ever want . . . sell me a Rousseau!" Interview with Lloyd Goodrich.

278 "Ever since . . . museum." "Mrs. Whitney Plans Art Museum Here," *New York Times*, January 4, 1930.

278 "The word . . . pronounces it so." JF, "The Whitney Museum of American Art," *Creative Art*, 9 (November 1931), p. 388.

278 "A very interesting scheme." "Mrs. Whitney Plans Art Museum Here," *New York Times*, January 4, 1930.

279 "Had no . . . professional." Watson, unpublished reminiscences, 1949, FWP.

280 "While this museum . . . collection." "Whitney Museum Opens in Fall," *Art News*, 28 (March 29, 1930), p. 9.

281 "To prove . . . generation." Alfred H. Barr, Jr., *An Exhibition Of Work Of 46 Painters & Sculptors Under 35 Years Of Age* (New York, 1930), p. 2.

281 "Art, like . . . records." JF, "The Whitney Museum of American Art," p. 388.

282 "We have not . . . a course." Hermon More to Edward Weston, March 10, 1936, WMAA; Archives (H.2/f35).

283 "Is it too much . . . face?" JF, "The Whitney Museum of American Art," p. 389.

283 "I used . . . at all." Interview with Lloyd Goodrich.

284 "They . . . impersonal." Watson, quoted in *JFAA*, p. 63.

284 "Seem to have studied . . . Woodstock." McBride, "The Palette Knife," *Creative Art*, 10 (March 1932), p. 178.

285 "From its founding . . . art." Henry Geldzahler, *New York Painting and Sculpture, 1940–1970* (New York, 1969), p. 25.

285 "We send out . . . party." Jewell, "Paintings Shown By 153 Americans," *New York Times*, November 28, 1934.

285 "Broadminded . . . Mrs. Force's reception." Bluemner, "An Open Letter and a Private Opinion," unpublished manuscript, December 1932, Oscar Bluemner Papers.

286 "It was . . . century." John I. H. Baur, interview with Paul Cummings, January 22–February 19, 1970, AAA.

286–287 "In 1931 . . . pictures." Charles Sawyer to author, January 20, 1978.

287 "I look forward . . . you." Alfred H. Barr, Jr. to JF, November 7, 1930, WMAA; Archives (H. 2/f30).

287 "With its problems . . . supporters." Alfred H. Barr, Jr. to A. Conger Goodyear, September 25, 1934, Museum of Modern Art Archives, Alfred H. Barr, Jr., Papers; AAA microfilm 2165:350.

287 "Juliana . . . exploit." Interview with C. Adolph Glassgold.

287–288 "I think . . . time." "Interview: Katherine Schmidt Talks with Paul Cummings," p. 19.

288 "A full-time . . . log fires." Ernest Small to author, April 23 and June 16, 1979.

288 "A fast woman" Interview with Katie Harris.

289 "It looks . . . ever!" Daniel Chester French to George S. Keyes, July 15, 1930, Daniel Chester French Papers.

289 "It's . . . grand!" Charles Demuth to JF, October 4, 1931, WMAA; Registrar's Dept.

291 "It means . . . multiple sides." GW to Cortissoz, December 11, 1930, Royal Cortissoz Papers.

293 "She got teary . . . her." Interview with Allen Saalburg.

294 "Everything . . . dinner party." Interview with Lloyd Goodrich.

294 "That . . . again!" *Ibid.*

295 "Before . . . everybody." JF to Sloan, April 22, 1931, John Sloan Archives.

295 "Mrs. Force . . . folding." Interview with William Robb.

295 "I couldn't . . . to me." Interview with Lloyd Goodrich.

296 "She was . . . cry." Interview with Ethel Renthal.

296 "Much use . . . intimate banter." Allan Rieser, unpublished memoir.

296 "Bitter" "frustrated" George Biddle, interview with Harlan Phillips, 1963, AAA.

297 "No feelings . . . stand." Bacon, *Off With Their Heads!*, unpaged.

297 "A chic . . . tempered." Interview with Peggy Bacon.

297 "Peggy . . . show." Cramer, diary, April 27, 1931.

299 "I cannot . . . gratifying." Cecil Beaton to author, January 25, 1978.

300 From a childhood . . . alive." "Force, Juliana," *Current Biography: Who's News and Why* (New York, 1941), p. 296.

300 For definitions, symptoms, and causes of phobias, see Paul G. Emmelkamp, *Phobic and Obsessive-Compulsive Disorders* (New York and London, 1982); Joy Melville, *Phobias and Obsessions* (New York, 1977); and Stanley Rachman, *Phobias: Their Nature and Control* (Springfield, Ill., 1968).

300 "Juliana . . . buying." Interview with Dorothea Greenbaum.

301 "Marsh . . . person." Interview with Lloyd Goodrich.

301 "Mrs. Force . . . made." Minutes of staff meeting, January 14, 1931, WMAA; Archives (H. 2/f40).

302 " 'Control' . . . Rockefeller." Sue Davidson Lowe, *Stieglitz: A Memoir/Biography* (New York, 1983), p. 331. I am grateful to Ms. Lowe for providing me with extracts from two pertinent Stieglitz letters.

302 "The politics . . . any kind." Quoted in Russell Lynes, *Good Old Modern: An Intimate Portrait of the Museum of Modern Art* (New York, 1973), p. 156.

303 "Mr. Stieglitz . . . conditions." Minutes of staff meeting, December 16, 1931, WMAA; Archives (H. 2/f40).

303–304 "My dear . . . you." Alfred Stieglitz to JF, February 5 (?), 1932, WMAA; Registrar's Dept. Copyright 1990 Estate/Foundation of Georgia O'Keeffe.

304 "Naturally . . . one." Stieglitz to JF, February 15, 1932, *ibid*. Copyright 1990 Estate/Foundation of Georgia O'Keeffe.

304 "Please . . . July 1/32." Stieglitz to JF, June 21, 1932, *ibid.* Copyright 1990 Estate/ Foundation of Georgia O'Keeffe.

304 "How much . . . businesswoman." Interview with Lloyd Goodrich.

305 "Even if . . . generation." Mary Fanton Roberts, "Upstairs in a Museum," *Arts and Decoration,* 41 (June 1934), p. 44.

305 "What . . . claustrophobia!" Interview with Lloyd Goodrich.

306 "One . . . amusing." Glackens, p. 234.

306 "Those parties . . . drawingroom." Interview with Lloyd Goodrich; More and Goodrich, quoted in *JFAA,* p. 32.

308 "It is interesting . . . pieces." Augusta Owen Patterson, "The Decorative Arts," *Town & Country,* 85 (February 15, 1931), p. 83.

308 "An opportunity . . . ensemble." Helen Appleton Read, "An Experiment in the Rococo," *House & Garden,* October 1932, p. 62.

308 "Produced . . . effects." Stanley Walker, *Mrs. Astor's Horse* (New York, 1935), p. 136.

308 "My wife . . . liveable." Interview with Lloyd Goodrich.

308 "We stayed . . . hers." Interview with Edith Goodrich.

309 "Depression . . . turn to." Moses Soyer, "Three Brothers," *Magazine of Art,* 32 (April 1939), p. 207.

310 "In what. . . the day." Sidney Geist, "Prelude: The 1930's," *Art in America,* 30 (September 1956), p. 49; telephone interview with Sidney Geist.

310 "I had . . . note." Interview with Eugene Ludins.

310 "I cannot . . . go ahead." Abby Aldrich Rockefeller to JF, April 16, 1931, Reel 2396, JFP.

310 "With . . . self-respect." JF to Rockefeller, December 14, 1932, WMAA; Archives (H.2/f31).

311 "Artist's . . . suttee." Interview with Lloyd Lózes Goff.

311 "Here . . . talents." Christopher Morley, "The Bowling Green," *Saturday Review of Literature* 8, (December 5, 1931), p. 347.

311 "In . . . hence." McBride, "Enthusiasm for Native Work Is Suddenly Quite à la Mode," *New York Sun,* November 21, 1931.

311 "The Whitney . . . hesitancy." JF, "The Whitney Museum of American Art," p. 389.

312 "Mrs. Whitney . . . wonders." Bloch, diary, November 19, 1931.

312 "It has . . . mind." Bertha Horn to GW, November 18, 1931, WMAA; Archives (H.2/f30).

312 "Dear Gertrude, A crown . . . Juliana." JF to GW, December 1931, Reel 2363, GVWP.

312 "My fears . . . groundless." McBride, "The Palette Knife," *Creative Art,* 10 (January 1932), p. 13.

313 "The vogue . . . wane." Jewell, "American Art Comes of Age: The Opening of a New Epoch," *New York Times Magazine,* November 22, 1931, p. 12.

313 "The bulk . . . to it." Cortissoz, "A New Landmark in Our Museum History," *New York Herald Tribune,* November 22, 1931.

313 "Trudging . . . their work." Samuel M. Kootz, "America Uber Alles," *New York Times,* December 20, 1931.

313 "There . . . them." Jewell, "The Whitney Museum of American Art Opens Its Doors," *New York Times,* November 22, 1931.

313 "Bought with . . . pompous doors." Paul Rosenfeld, "The Whitney Museum," *The Nation,* 133 (December 30, 1931), pp. 731–32.

313 "Was much . . . brick-bats." More to K. LeVan, February 25, 1932, WMAA; Archives (H.2/f31).

313–314 "Miracle . . . common movement." A. Hyatt Mayor, "Art Chronicle," *Hound & Horn,* 5 (January–March 1932), pp. 289–91.

314 "The severely . . . Whitney." James Michener, "The Collector: An Informal Memoir," in *The James A. Michener Collection,* edited by Earl A. Powell III (Austin, 1977), pp. x–xi.

314 "Organization . . . world." Healy, p. 167.

314 "Mr. Luks . . . rich!" Lawrence Campbell, p. 26. The story also crops up in the unpublished memoirs of Louis Bouché as well as in "George Luks," a memoir by Everett Shinn, published in the April 1966 issue of the *Archives of American Art Journal.*

315 "Endless guests" Bloch, diary, May 5, 1932.

315 "Hoped . . . strength." Rockefeller to JF, September 23, 1932, WMAA; Archives (H. 2/f31).

315 "Horrified" Interview with Allan Rieser.

315 "Such . . . to us." Cramer, diary, January 1933.

316 "Junk dealers" Faith Andrews, interview with Robert Brown, January 14–April 23, 1982, AAA.

316 "Most people . . . doing." Interview with Faith Andrews.

316 "She saw . . . to us." *Ibid.*

316 "Mrs. Force . . . their work." Edward Deming Andrews, in Edward Deming Andrews and Faith Andrews, *Fruits of the Shaker Tree of Life: Memoirs of Fifty Years of Collecting and Research* (Stockbridge, Mass., 1975), p. 147.

316 "The Whitney . . . work." Faith Andrews, interview with Robert Brown.

316 "The first place . . . given her." *Ibid.*

316 "Loved meeting . . . culture." Interview with Faith Andrews.

317 "It [her visit] . . . she needed." Faith Andrews, interview with Robert Brown.

317 "A round table . . . winter." JF to Vernon Porter, November 1932, Washington Square Outdoor Exhibit Papers, AAA. I thank Francis V. O'Connor for calling my attention to JF's part in the Washington Square show.

317 "Down with private capital!" Watson, "Gallery Explorations," *Parnassus*, 4 (December 1932), p. 4.

318 "It ought . . . will." Quoted in Ann Lee Morgan, ed., *Dear Stieglitz, Dear Dove* (Newark, Del., 1988), pp. 256, 260.

318–319 "I was . . . like cordwood." Harry Sternberg to author, October 1982; Sternberg to Thomas N. Armstrong III, September 22, 1980, WMAA; Library.

319 "Was outspoken . . . them." Thomas Hart Benton, *An Artist in America.* (Columbia, Mo., 1983), p. 248.

320 "Benton . . . pants." Interview with Maynard Walker.

321 "Was profoundly . . . profession." Benton, p. 12.

322 "One highball . . . off." Avis Berman, "Thomas Hart Benton: American Images," *Art & Antiques*, 4 (September–October 1981), p. 59.

322 "I'll paint . . . eggs." Emily Braun and Thomas Branchick, *Thomas Hart Benton: The America Today Murals* (New York, 1985), p. 15.

322 "In contrast . . . spirituality." Benton, *The Arts of Life in America: A Series of Murals by Thomas Benton* (New York, 1932), pp. 4, 5.

323 "As I stated . . . work. . . ." JF to Benton, May 25, 1932, WMAA; Library.

323 "Parties . . . Museum." Benton, *An Artist in America*, pp. 250–51.

324 "The Museum . . . misunderstanding." JF to Benton, December 8, 1932, WMAA; Library.

324 "Alas . . . jobs." Anita Brenner, "Art and American Life," *The Nation*, 130 (January 18, 1933), p. 72.

324 "Try to get . . . to me." Benton to JF, February 26, 1933, WMAA; Library.

324–325 "After the incident . . . will.' " Interview with Edward Laning.

325 "She felt . . . on me.' " Interview with Eugene Ludins.

325 "I don't . . . an artist." Interview with Lloyd Goodrich.

325n. "Was . . . in fact." Benton, interview with Paul Cummings, July 23–24, 1973, AAA.

CHAPTER NINE

326 Out of town." Minutes of staff meeting, January 12, 1933, WMAA; Archives (H. 2/f42).

326 "We have . . . bleachers." "33 Dallas Artists Comment on Whitney Loan Collection on View At Dallas Museum," *Dallas Times-Herald*, December 10, 1933.

326 "This artist . . . epic." Interview with Dorothy Varian.

327 "A ceaseless . . . work." JF, "Mrs. Force Discusses Changed Attitudes Toward American Art And Tells Whitney Museum Aims," *Dallas Times-Herald*, December 10, 1933.

327 "The aims . . . exhibitions. . . ." *Ibid.*

327 "At one . . . predicament." Thomas Carr Howe to author, August 27, 1979.

328 "It was . . . city." Theodore Roszak to More, September 25, 1949, WMAA; Registrar's Dept.

328 "Did lead . . . to me." Roszak, interview with Harlan Phillips, 1963, AAA.

328 "An exciting . . . ever since." Roszak to Thomas N. Armstrong III, March 18, 1980, WMAA; Library.

328 "At the opening . . . museum." Bloch, diary, December 16, 1932.

329 "She and Hermon . . . swan." Aaron Bohrod to author, January 8, 1979; interview with Aaron Bohrod.

329 "Poison . . . gold" Gerald Kelly to JF, September 17, 1932, Reel 2396, JFP.

329–330 "Juliana . . . passed around." Interview with Marchal Landgren.

330 "First . . . better now." Richmond Barthe to JF, January 17, 1933, WMAA; Registrar's Dept.

332 "Private . . . check" Marchal E. Landgren, in "A Dialogue," in Francis V. O'Connor, ed., *The New Deal Art Projects: An Anthology of Memoirs* (Washington, D.C., 1972), p. 314.

332 "Hopes . . . cloth." Delmore Schwartz, *The World is a Wedding* (Norfolk, Conn., 1948), p. 11.

332 "A vital national expression." George Biddle to Franklin D. Roosevelt, May 9, 1933, quoted in George Biddle, *An American Artist's Story* (Boston, 1939), p. 268.

332 "DEAR . . . work." Roosevelt to Biddle, May 19, 1933, quoted in Biddle, p. 269.

332 "As I read . . . excitement." *Ibid.*

333 "Frail . . . path." *Ibid.*

333 "Controversy," "embarrassment" Charles Moore to Roosevelt, July 28, 1933, George Biddle Papers, LC.

333 "On July 28 . . . suggestion." Watson to Biddle, September 7, 1951, *ibid.*

333 "I think . . . experiences." Moore to Roosevelt, July 28, 1933, *ibid.*

333 "The mephitic . . . Commission." Biddle to Edward Bruce, November 16, 1933, *ibid.*

333 "We have . . . art?" Henry T. Hunt to L. W. Robert, October 25, 1933, *ibid.*

334 "As . . . bricklayer." Biddle, diary, November 8, 1933, *ibid.*

334 "There are . . . outside in." Biddle, diary, November 9, 1933, *ibid.*

335 "Done more . . . museum." Bruce to Robert, November 17, 1933, Reel 2396, JFP.

335 "As you might . . . operative." JF to Bruce, November 25, 1933, *ibid.*

336 "OVER THREE . . . TO ME." Quoted in Belisario R. Contreras, "The New Deal Treasury Department Art Programs and the American Artist: 1933 to 1943" (Ph.D. diss., American University, 1967), p. 12.

336 "A fine old warhorse of a woman." Interview with James Thomas Flexner.

336 "Very fine" Gaston Lachaise to Ernest Fiene, November 26, 1927 or 1928, Ernest Fiene Papers.

336 "Did not . . . sitter." Gerald Nordland, *Gaston Lachaise: The Man and His Work* (New York, 1974), p. 95; also, Gerald Nordland to author, May 8, 1985.

336 "All . . . valiant stand" Isabel Lachaise to More, November 28, 1948, WMAA; Registrar's Dept.

336 "The interest . . . work." Gaston Lachaise to JF, January 25, 1934, WMAA; Registrar's Dept.

336–337 "Unbelievable . . . fullest." Quoted in Richard D. McKinzie, *The New Deal for Artists* (Princeton, 1973), p. 10.

337 "The only lady present" Martha Blair, "These Charming People," *Washington Herald*, December 11, 1933.

337 "Mrs. Force . . . life." Interview with Lloyd Goodrich.

337 "I imagine . . . other." *Ibid.*

337 "For the first time . . . me." Juliana Force, Federal Emergency Relief Administration press release, December 11, 1933, Records of the Public Buildings Service, Record Group 121, PWAP, National Archives and Record Service, Reel DC 3 in AAA. (Hereafter referred to as RG 121, plus AAA microfilm reel number.)

337n. "You . . . candidate." Interview with Lloyd Goodrich.

338 "Boiling . . . swill." Biddle, diary, December 11, 1933.

338 "I do not . . . Art. . . . ." Leon Kroll to Bruce, December 1933, Leon Kroll Papers, AAA.

338 "That I am . . . academicians." "Art Conservatives Attack CWA Plan," *New York Times*, December 13, 1933.

338 "We are interested . . . employment?" "CW Artists," *Time*, December 25, 1933, p. 19.

338 "You understand . . . walls or not." Arthur F. McCullough, "Artists to Bury the Temperament Hatchet—Honestly," *New York Post*, December 16, 1933.

339 "This trouble . . . flying." "Mural Art Group Backs CWA Board," *New York Times*, December 14, 1933.

339 "If the people . . . fighting." *Ibid.*

339 "If conditions . . . mine." JF to Watson, January 31, 1934, RG 121, Reel DC 113.

339 "He would have . . . Whitney." Interview with Karl Gruppe.

339 "Teach . . . lesson." Quoted in Robert A. Caro, *The Power Broker: Robert Moses and the Fall of New York* (New York, 1975), p. 185. Background information on Moses, the Northern State Parkway, and the rehabilitation of Central Park is also drawn from Caro's biography.

340 "Already . . . jobs. . . . ." Cramer, diary, December 16, 1933.

340 "I was stuck . . . at once." Interview with Dorothy Varian.

340 "Suddenly . . . why." Ben Shahn, interview with Harlan Phillips, October 3, 1965, AAA.

340 "Amazed . . . exist." Davis, interview with Harlan Phillips.

340 "I write . . . hold you." Raphael Soyer to JF, December 20, 1933, RG 121, Reel DC 114.

341 "Every day . . . there." Interview with Lloyd Goodrich.

341 "I believe . . . so little." "80 Jobless Artists Already at Work," *New York Times*, December 22, 1933.

341 "Oh, this . . . Czar." "80 Idle Artists Begin Designing C.W.A. Projects," *New York Tribune*, December 22, 1933.

341 " 'We'll . . . sometimes." Interview with Lloyd Goodrich.

342 "My instructions . . . unemployed." "80 Jobless Artists Already at Work," *New York Times*, December 22, 1933.

342 "I appreciate . . . Government." JF to Edith Halpert, December 18, 1933, WMAA; Archives (H.2/f32).

342 "Our enemies . . . money." Interview with Lloyd Goodrich.

343 "I am deeply . . . projects." "Decries Art Job Row," *New York Times*, December 19, 1933.

343 "Need . . . vocabulary." Quoted in McKinzie, p. 15.

343 "You admit . . . questions." *Ibid.*

343 "Thoroughly . . . assigned." "356 Artists Get Jobs on Buildings Here," *New York Times*, January 8, 1934.

343 "THE WORD . . . SYSTEM." "Idle Artists March in Protest on CWA," *New York Times*, January 8, 1934. See also McKinzie, p. 16.

343 "It was a matter . . . PWAP." Ilya Bolotowsky, interview with Paul Cummings, March 24–April 7, 1968, AAA.

344 "The majority . . . art." JF to Bruce, February 19, 1934, Reel 2396, JFP.

344 "I felt . . . great artist." JF to Lincoln Kirstein, January 21, 1947, WMAA; Registrar's Dept.

345 "Thanks . . . free." Sloan, "Can the Artist Be Independent?," radio talk with Gertrude Weil, 1934, John Sloan Archives.

346 "Impressions . . . Citizen." Harry Holtzman to JF, December 13, 1933, RG 121, Reel DC 113.

346 "An abstract . . . them." Ibram Lassaw, progress report, January 1934, *ibid.*

346 "If you feel . . . do so." Goodrich to Jan Matulka, February 14, 1934, *ibid.*

346 "Should . . . based." JF to Horace Day, January 19, 1934, RG 121, Reel DC 112.

346 "Had . . . dimension." Quoted in Paul Cummings, *Artists In Their Own Words* (New York, 1979), p. 104.

346 "Pure sculpture" Goodrich to JF, April 13, 1934, RG 121, Reel DC 114.

347 "Impractical." *Ibid.*

347 "Moses . . . Department." Quoted in Cummings, p. 104.

347 "Noguchi . . . thumb nails." Watson to Goodrich, February 28, 1934, RG 121, Reel DC 114.

347 "May . . . C.W.A." Isamu Noguchi to JF, February 28, 1934, *ibid.*

348 "You then . . . timid hope." Noguchi to JF, April 12, 1934, *ibid.*

348–349 Flannagan on PWAP: RG 121, Reel DC 113, plus documents provided by Francis V. O'Connor.

349 "Extremely . . . lost." JF to Biddle, February 26, 1934, George Biddle Papers.

349 "Mrs. Force . . . Club." Biddle, diary, February 9, 1934, *ibid.*

350 "We would . . . pretty tough." Interview with Lloyd Goodrich.

351 "The thought . . . new pair." Allan Rieser, unpublished memoir.

351 "His political . . . Republicans!" JF to editor of *New York Herald Tribune*, March 16, 1934, RG 121, Reel DC 113.

351 "Complete with placards . . . feet!' " Edward Laning, "The New Deal Art Projects," in O'Connor, ed., pp. 89–90.

351 "Dear Museum . . . painters." Bluemner to Whitney Museum, January 9, 1934, WMAA; Library.

352 "FIND CHIEF/CLERK . . . DEMOCRAT." JF to Cecil Jones, March 30, 1934, RG 121, Reel DC 10.

353 "Arsenic and Old Face." Laning, "The New Deal Art Projects," in O'Connor, ed., p. 106.

353 "Great rivalry . . . interference." Audrey McMahon, interview with Harlan Phillips, November 18, 1964, AAA.

353 "The Whitney . . . museums." Bruce to JF, November 17, 1933, Reel 2396, JFP.

353 "We had an armed . . . coordination." Audrey McMahon, in "A Dialogue," in O'Connor, ed., p. 314.

353 "I wouldn't . . . Museum." Ben Shahn, interview with Harlan Phillips.

353–354 "Mrs. Force . . . angry at her." Interview with Bernarda Bryson Shahn.

354 "Had the unprecedented . . . city." Audrey McMahon, "A General View of the WPA Federal Art Project," in O'Connor, ed., p. 71.

354 "Mrs. Whitney's almoner." Holger Cahill, interview with Joan Pring, April–June 1957, Oral History Research Office, Columbia University.

355 "We are not a detective agency." "Sloan Revealed As Public Works Art Beneficiary," *New York Herald Tribune*, March 18, 1934.

355 "During . . . way . . ." Alexander Stirling Calder to JF, March 26, 1934, Reel 2396, JFP.

355 "If I have . . . on it." Hayley Lever to JF, March 24, 1934, *ibid.*

355 "I certainly . . . it." A. S. Baylinson to JF, March 23, 1934, RG 121, Reel DC 112.

355 "Boy . . . trouble." Zorach, p. 100.

356 "The consumption . . . skillful." "Sloan Revealed As Public Works Art Beneficiary," *New York Herald Tribune*, March 18, 1934.

356 "I have here . . . week." *Ibid.*

356 "We got . . . artists." Zorach, p. 100.

357 "Of callous . . . artists." Artists Union to JF, March 17, 1934, Reel 2396, JFP.

357 "We want . . . useful" Biddle, interview with Harlan Phillips.

357 "When I started . . . sometimes!" "Official Reports on Artists' Relief Work," *Art News*, 30 (April 7, 1934), p. 11.

358 "Our surprise and delight" Goodrich, in Philip Eliasoph, *Paul Cadmus, Yesterday and Today* (Oxford, Ohio, 1981), p. 7.

358 "A minor . . . guts" Lewis Mumford, "The Art Galleries," *The New Yorker*, June 2, 1934, p. 38.

358–359 "The New Yorker . . . to talk about." JF, draft of letter to Mumford, June 11, 1934, Reel 2396, JFP. The letter is not in the Mumford Papers at the University of Pennsylvania, so it may not have been sent or received.

360 "West Point . . . mural." Thomas Loftin Johnson, "The Washington Hall Mural," *Assembly*, 2 (January 1944), p. 1. Other details about Johnson's mural are drawn from his unpublished

essay, "Art out of Eggs," in the West Point Museum, West Point, N.Y. I thank Richard Kuehne for calling this paper to my attention.

360 "I could only say . . . it." JF to Kroll, May 23, 1934, Leon Kroll Papers.

361–362 "Dear Gertrude. Here in this twilight . . . Lovingly, J." JF to GW, May 31, 1934, Reel 2363, GVWP.

363–366 William Randolph Hearst incident: interview with Eleanor Lambert Berkson; W. A. Swanberg, *Citizen Hearst* (New York, 1961).

364 "He is a marvelous . . . job." Quoted in Swanberg, p. 430.

365 "So far . . . sent." "Styka's Davies," *Time*, July 2, 1934, p. 36.

365 "In justice . . . exhibition." "Marion Davies Portrait Shifted to End Dispute," *Bronx Home News*, June 24, 1934.

365 "You certainly . . . happen." Bruce to JF, July 21, 1934, RG 121, Reel DC 4.

366 "Graduate . . . meet." JF to GW, July 28, 1934, Reel 2363, GVWP.

366 "Dear Mrs. Whitney . . . will be?" JF to GW, September 1, 1934, Reel 2363, *ibid*.

367 "That same . . . tender." Mrs. Gloria Vanderbilt with Palma Wayne, *Without Prejudice* (New York, 1936), p. 114.

367–372 Gloria Vanderbilt custody trial: background information has been drawn from *Once Upon a Time* by Gloria Vanderbilt (New York, 1985), *Little Gloria . . . Happy at Last* by Barbara Goldsmith (New York, 1980), *Without Prejudice*, and *Double Exposure: A Twin Autobiography* by Gloria (Morgan) Vanderbilt and Thelma Lady Furness (New York, 1958).

368 "She was capable . . . later." Vanderbilt, *Once Upon a Time*, p. 7.

368 "Elder . . . newspapers." Geoffrey T. Hellman, "The Man Who Is Not His Cousin," *The New Yorker*, June 21, 1941, pp. 24–25.

370 "The *Matter* . . . out." Goldsmith, p. ix.

370 "Ripped away" Vanderbilt, *Once Upon a Time*, p. 70.

370 "Aunt J.'s . . . character." Allan Rieser, unpublished memoir.

370 "Thereupon . . . daughter" "Socialities' Solomon," *Time*, November 26, 1934, p. 49.

370 "Straight . . . happening" Vanderbilt, *Once Upon a Time*, p. 73.

371 "Down . . . Gertrude!" *Ibid.*, p. 98.

371 "('A man's . . . child')" Goldsmith, p. 431.

371 "A mural . . . leapfrog" "Art Photos Shown In Vanderbilt Case," *New York Times*, November 8, 1934.

371 "The judge . . . up." "Socialites' Solomon," p. 51.

371–372 "I was . . . perfect." Vanderbilt and Furness, *Double Exposure* p. 270.

372 "Fridolyn . . . suggestion." Interview with Marchal Landgren.

372–373 "When I . . . yield." Bloch, diary, November 26, 1934.

373 Hitchhiking anecdote: interviews with Marchal Landgren, Marjorie Rieser, and Beverly Rieser Smock.

373 "Her sense . . . me." Interview with Lloyd Goodrich.

373–374 "There must have been . . . figure." Interview with Marchal Landgren.

374 "The production . . . painting." "New York Woman Lauds Gimbel Art Galleries," *Philadelphia Inquirer*, November 29, 1934.

374 "She believed . . . did." Interview with Emlen Etting.

375 "The need . . . matter." Minutes of staff meeting, February 13, 1933, WMAA; Archives (H.2/f42).

376 "You must analyze . . . about it." Interview with Lloyd Goodrich.

376 "One of . . . movement." Foreword, *Abstract Painting in America* (New York, 1935), unpaged.

377 "One did . . . group." David Smith, *David Smith by David Smith*, edited by Cleve Gray (New York, 1968), pp. 18, 35.

377 "Why are so many . . . art." Watson, "The Innocent Bystander," *American Magazine of Art*, 28 (March 1935), pp. 168–69.

377 "Persuasive beauty" McBride, "Abstract Art in America," *New York Sun*, February 16, 1935.

378 "She looked . . . clothes." Interview with Edward Laning.

378 "A zest . . . ugly." Interview with Horace Day.

378 "Was a distressing . . . changing." Interview with Charles Sawyer.

378–379 "She was always . . . completely." Interview with Faith Andrews.

379 "I liked . . . knife." Interview with Hannah Small.

379 "This so-called . . . where?' " Lloyd Lózes Goff to author, March 18, 1978.

379 "A tasteless . . . view." Mumford, "The Art Galleries," *The New Yorker*, April 6, 1935, pp. 95, 96.

379 "I could not . . . harboring" JF to Mumford, April 8, 1935, and J. O. Whedon, April 15, 1935, Lewis Mumford Papers, Special Collections, Van Pelt Library, University of Pennsylvania.

380 "Juliana . . . equity." Interview with Charles Sawyer.

380 "With a few . . . artist." Katherine Schmidt, "The Rental Policy," in *First American Artists' Congress* (New York, 1936), p. 87.

380–381 Gertrude's worth and income: Reel 2363, GVWP.

382 "Mrs. Force . . . me.' " Interview with Ethel Renthal.

383 "Dear Carl . . . a bit." JF to Carl Rieser, September 1, 1935, RFC.

384 "Bloomingdale . . . told." Flannagan to JF, October 7, 1935, WMAA; Archives (H. 2/f34).

385 "It was a real . . . left us." Interview with Faith Andrews; Faith Andrews, interview with Robert Brown.

386 Museum expenses and budget: Administrative files, WMAA.

CHAPTER TEN

387 Insurance squabble: letters of JF, Harry Farmer, and Frank L. Crocker, 1935–1936, Administrative files, WMAA; Archives.

388 "We have decided . . . prints." JF to Davis, January 2, 1936, Stuart Davis Papers, AAA.

388 "Yes . . . Deluge!" JF to F. A. Whiting, Jr., November 20, 1935, WMAA; Archives (H. 2/f35).

388 "Outweighed. . . producer." Barr to J. Arthur MacLean, May 4, 1936, Museum of Modern Art Archives: Alfred H. Barr, Jr. Papers; AAA microfilm 2165:673.

388 "I wish . . . painters." Ward Lockwood to JF, April 1, 1936, WMAA; Archives (H. 2/f35).

390 "But really . . . do." JF to Carl Rieser, January 19, 1936, RFC.

391–392 "There was a fair . . . rid of him." Allan Rieser, unpublished memoir.

392 "Many . . . ecstasy." *Thorpe v. Astor*, *Time*, August 17, 1936, p. 42.

392 "And . . . Astor." Allan Rieser, unpublished memoir.

392 "A grand . . . Salem." Irene Rieser to Carl Rieser, October 13, 1936, RFC.

393 "Here . . . best days." JF to Carl Rieser, September 30, 1936, *ibid.*

393 "Your letter . . . ill." JF to Carl Rieser, October 30, 1936, *ibid.*

393 "Don't . . . if you were." JF to Carl Rieser, November 16, 1936, *ibid.*

393 "No doubt . . . begun." Allan Rieser, unpublished memoir.

393 "She wanted . . . be." Carl Rieser to author, undated.

394 "Had . . . understanding." Interviews with Lloyd Goodrich and John and Elizabeth Bart Gerald.

394 "I want . . . did." Jared French to author, February 25, 1978.

395 "Cloud of futility" Anita Brenner, "New York Painters and English Architecture," *Brooklyn Eagle*, February 14, 1937.

395 "Juliana . . . much about." Interview with Charles Sawyer.

396 "The Whitney . . . it was." Interview with Jacob Kainen.

396 "Too . . . ago." Talmey, p. 131.

396 "What I would *not* . . . prominent." Allan Rieser, unpublished memoir.

396–397 "Mayer . . . vituperation." *Ibid.*

397 "Oh, . . . artist." Hudson Walker and Elizabeth McCausland, "Marsden Hartley," *Journal of the Archives of American Art*, 8 (January 1968), p. 10.

397 "To help . . . life." Quoted in Barbara Haskell, *Marsden Hartley* (New York, 1980), p. 102.

397 "Wrote . . . teeth fixed." Interview with Lloyd Goodrich.

398 "Won't . . . impossible." GW to JF, undated (but designated as June 1937 on the basis of external evidence), Reel 2363, GVWP.

399 "I have . . . J." JF to Carl Rieser, June 9, 1937, RFC.

400 "I told . . . etc." Friedman, p. 619.

400 "I was sorry . . . every thing." Clara Rieser to Carl Rieser, August 9, 1937, RFC.

400 "We went . . . soul." JF to Carl Rieser, August 25, 1937, *ibid.*

400 "More foreign than in Europe." JF to Carl Rieser, September 15, 1937, *ibid.*

400–401 "It takes . . . late." JF to Carl Rieser, October 5, 1937, *ibid.*

401 "Wasn't . . . kiss it." Quoted in Goldsmith, p. 581.

401 "It was . . . Gilchrist." Gloria Vanderbilt, *Black Knight, White Knight* (New York, 1987), p. xiv.

401–402 "Like Aunt . . . banquet!" Vanderbilt, *Once Upon a Time*, pp. 225–28.

402 "Felt a surge of hope" Vanderbilt, *Black Knight, White Knight*, p. xiv.

402 "It was . . . she did." Interview with John Davis Hatch.

403 "Will . . . 1939." "Whalen Warned on 'Neglect' of U.S. Art at Fair," *New York Evening Post*, January 27, 1938.

403 "Art . . . artist." June Provines, "Front Views and Profiles," *Chicago Tribune*, April 24, 1941.

403 "You know I collect eagles." Interview with Edward Laning.

403 "Mrs. Force . . . investment" Anna Freeman to Faith Andrews, February 8, 1938, WMAA; Archives (H.2/f78).

404 "We must have the drawings!" Interview with Faith Andrews; also, Freeman to Faith Andrews, January 12, 1938, WMAA; Archives (H.2/f78).

404 "I can tell you . . . tradition. . . ." Edith Halpert to Blanchette Rockefeller, February 28, 1938, unmicrofilmed Downtown Gallery Papers, AAA, Washington, D.C.

404 "I hope . . . permit." Frank L. Crocker to JF, February 7, 1938, WMAA; Archives (H.2/f38).

405 "Looking . . . future" "Wings on Statue Fool the Mayor," *New York Times*, May 26, 1939.

406 "Aunt . . . Rights." Allan Rieser to Carl Rieser, August 16, 1938, RFC.

406 "Was about as . . . it." JF to Emlen Etting, September 19, 1938. Courtesy of Emlen Etting.

406 "Humiliation" Margaret Scolari Barr, "Our Campaigns: Alfred H. Barr, Jr., and the Museum of Modern Art: A Biographical Chronicle of the Years 1930–1944," *The New Criterion*, Summer 1987, p. 52n.

406 "Thinking . . . NY." JF to Carl Rieser, August 29, 1938, RFC.

406 "Be what . . . banality!" *Ibid.*

407 "Life . . . Art!" JF to Etting, September 19, 1938.

407 "Score 1 . . . wedding." Irene Rieser to Carl Rieser, November 8, 1938, RFC.

407 "The Ten . . . Nine" Diane Waldman, *Mark Rothko, 1903–1970: A Retrospective* (New York, 1978), p. 31.

407–408 "We were . . . duty." Joseph Solman, interview with Avis Berman, May 6–8, 1981, AAA.

408 "The reputed . . . art." Joseph Solman, "The Easel Division of the WPA Federal Art Project," in O'Connor, ed., p. 128.

409 "Extreme tolerance" Ilya Bolotowsky, interview with Ruth Gurin, November 5, 1963, AAA.

409 "The New . . . approval." JF to Mercury Galleries, November 1, 1938, WMAA; Archives (H.2/f37).

409 "I believed . . . standards." Interview with Betty Parsons.

409 "She was . . . about that." Telephone interview with Maud Morgan.

410 "Courageous . . . show it." Noguchi to author, 1978 and November 24, 1982; telephone interview with Isamu Noguchi.

410 "I just wrote . . . art world." Interview with Elizabeth Navas.

411 "Haven't . . . blame her." Irene Rieser to Carl Rieser, December 9, 1938, RFC.

411 "It just . . . tell." *Ibid.*

411 "You say . . . money." Friedman, p. 635.

412 "I think . . . do." Interview with Elizabeth Navas.

412 "Taxes . . . jail." JF to Carl Rieser, February 26, 1938, RFC.

413 "Condemnation . . . fantastic." Zorach, p. 114.

414 "Juliana . . . death." Interview with Gertrude Henry Conner.

415 "I'm not . . . thing." Interview with Edith Goodrich.

415 Gift to Hardinge Scholle: Interview with Simmons Persons.

415 "Gratitude . . . quality." JF to Carl Rieser, February 9, 1939, RFC.

415 "American . . . adequate." "20th Century Art Displayed," *New York Sun*, September 13, 1939.

415–416 "That . . . everything." Watson, "The Growth of the Whitney Museum," *Magazine of Art*, 32 (October 1939), p. 558.

416 "To . . . spirit." "War Held No Curb to Artists' Work," *New York Times*, September 13, 1939.

416 "When . . . you." Jewell, "The Whitney Dedicates Itself Anew," *New York Times*, September 17, 1939.

416 "You cannot . . . blessed." "Think for Yourself!" *Art Digest*, 6 (February 1, 1932), p. 13.

416 "What about . . . adore it." Interviews with John Gerald and John Frear.

416 " 'Can't' . . . it." Interview with John Gerald.

417 "Was . . . up" Interview with John Frear.

417 "I fell . . . Gertrude." Vanderbilt, *Once Upon a Time*, pp. 260–61.

417 "You could . . . time." Davis to JF, September 13, 1939, WMAA; Library.

417 "I want . . . self-supporting." JF to Davis, October 10, 1939, *ibid.*

417–419 "It's outrageous . . . outrageous!" McBride to JF, October 26, 1939, Reel 2396, JFP.

419 "I had hoped . . . beginning." Flannagan, pp. 67–68.

419–420 "She had . . . expose him." Interview with Edward Laning.

420 "Juliana . . . principles." Telephone interview with Allene Talmey.

420 "Despite . . . Art." *Ibid.*

421 "Was such . . . boy." George Biddle, interview with Harlan Phillips, 1963.

421 "Had . . . judgment." Charles Sawyer to author, April 17, 1978; interview with Charles Sawyer.

421 "I'm delighted . . . hand." Calvin Tomkins, *Merchants and Masterpieces: The Story of the Metropolitan Museum of Art* (New York, 1973), p. 293.

421 "Francis . . . ass." Interview with Monroe Wheeler.

421 "There's . . . hands with." "Custodian of the Attic," *Time*, December 29, 1952, p. 48.

421–422 "With the exception . . . on it." Audrey McMahon, in "A Dialogue," in O'Connor, ed., p. 308.

422 "The proper . . . ultra-modern art." Francis Henry Taylor to Davis and Harry Wehle, May 22 and May 23, 1940, Stuart Davis Papers.

422 "Genuinely . . . friends." Watson to Alice Sharkey, March 29, 1940, FWP.

422–423 "Oh, Mrs. Force . . . here!" Lloyd Lózes Goff to author, March 18, 1978.

423 "He thought . . . angrier." Interview with Edward Laning.

423–424 Bund incident: Interviews with Eugenie Prendergast and Marchal Landgren; Jan Pirzio-Biroli to author, April 18 and August 10, 1980.

425 "I have visited . . . harmony." JF to GW, August 4, 1940, Reel 2364, GVWP.

425 "How . . . present?" "The Whitney Museum," clipping of unidentified magazine interview with JF, winter 1940–1941, Reel N594, WMAA Papers, AAA.

425–426 "I am sorry . . . with you." JF to Crocker, October 1, 1940, WMAA; Archives (H.3/f62).

427 "I had . . . steam.' " Interview with Stanton Catlin.

427 "She wasn't . . . Outhouse.' " Interview with Aaron Bohrod.

429 "Don't . . . themselves." Jared French to author, February 25, 1978.

429 "The Government . . . knowledge." Mary Williams, "WPA Art Works Litter Basements, Says Former Head of City Project," *New York Sun*, April 8, 1941; "Mrs. Force Attacks WPA Project Art," *Art Digest*, 15 (May 1, 1941), p. 9.

429 "She never . . . ammunition." Margaret French to author, May 5, 1978.

430 "Anyone . . . memory." Kathryn McHale, "Notes on the Arts," *General Director's Letter* [American Association of University Women], 16 (February 1949), pp. 47–48.

431 "The firm . . . certain!" Allan Rieser to author, December 4, 1988.

431–432 "Yesterday . . . friend." Cortissoz to GW, October 7, 1941, Reel 2364, GVWP.

432 "A strain . . . possible." Cramer, diary, November 13, 1941.

432 "When . . . it went." Genevieve Rindner to author, September 11, 1979.

432 "Thanks . . . have." Flannagan, p. 96.

433 "We have . . . personally." Duncan Phillips to JF, January 2, 1942, The Phillips Collection Papers, Reel 1959:984.

433 "She has . . . miracle." Zigrosser, notes of unpublished speech, March 1941, Carl Zigrosser Papers.

433 "Although . . . wanted to do." Interview with Lloyd Goodrich.

434 "We ended . . . interests." *Ibid.*

434 Whitney and Museum of Modern Art affiliation: John D. Rockefeller, Jr. to Stephen Clark, March 11, 1942, The Rockefeller Family Collection, RG 2, Office of the Messrs. Rockefeller, Cultural Interest Series, Box 23, Rockefeller Archive Center.

434 "I remember . . . commitments." Zigrosser, *My Own Shall Come To Me*, p. 175.

435 Gertrude Whitney's medical condition: Friedman, pp. 659–60.

CHAPTER ELEVEN

436 "Outside . . . control." Friedman, p. 660.

436 "Everyone . . . there." Interview with Lloyd Goodrich.

437 "Smaller . . . Hortense." Friedman, p. 664.

437 "Be devoted . . . deserving." *Ibid.*; "Whitney Will Is Made Public," *New York Sun*, May 4, 1942.

437–438 "The museums . . . items." Fiske Kimball, unpublished memoirs, Fiske Kimball Papers, Philadelphia Museum of Art Archives.

438 "Here . . . Francis." Interview with Gordon Washburn.

438 "A pair . . . wainscoting." Kimball, unpublished memoirs.

438 "Reliance . . . heart." Cortissoz to JF, May 9, 1942, Reel 2365, GVWP.

439 "At a very reasonable charge" Hobart Nichols to JF, May 5, 1942, National Academy of Design Archives.

440 "This club . . . 1900." Robert Moses, *Public Works: A Dangerous Trade* (New York, 1970), p. 43.

440 "Your list is extremely like mine!" JF to Barr, November 11, 1942, Museum of Modern Art Archives: Alfred H. Barr, Jr., Papers; AAA microfilm 2170:1254.

441 "She knew . . . gouache.' " Interview with Rosella Hartman.

441 "Mrs. Force . . . at all." Interview with Hananiah Harari.

441–442 "For the tenth time . . . think not." Clement Greenberg, "Art," *Nation*, 156 (January 2, 1943), p. 32.

442 "Dull and unimaginative." Robert M. Coates, "The Art Galleries," *The New Yorker*, December 5, 1942, p. 67.

442 "Some . . . Metropolitan." Tomkins, p. 301.

443 "She and I . . . acquired." Interview with Charles Sawyer.

443 "I want . . . generous." JF to Stieglitz, December 9, 1942, WMAA; Archives (H. 3/f63).

443 "I have . . . watercolors." Stieglitz to JF, December 15, 1942, Alfred Stieglitz Collection, YU. Copyright 1990 Estate/Foundation of Georgia O'Keeffe.

444 "Good Christ . . . you?" Interview with Lloyd Goodrich.

444 "Was that . . . resented." Interview with Charles Sawyer.

444 "That . . . trustees." Interview with Lloyd Goodrich.

444 "Selling . . . river." Interview with Elizabeth Bart Gerald.

444 "She felt . . . understood." Interview with Charles Sawyer.

444 "I am not . . . discussion." Gordon Washburn to JF, February 18, 1943, WMAA; Archives (H. 3/f64).

444 "It was . . . Taylor." Kimball, unpublished memoirs.

446 "An appendage . . . winter." Lee Simonson to JF, January 28, 1943, WMAA; Archives (H. 3/f64).

446 "Believing . . . Museum." JF to Crocker, January 6, 1943, WMAA; Archives (H. 3/f4).

446 "The deadliest . . . Whitney." Coates, "The Art Galleries," *The New Yorker*, January 30, 1943, p. 59.

447 "You . . . right" Brook to JF, January 20, 1943, WMAA; Archives (H. 3/f64).

447 "I express . . . Metropolitan." Philip Evergood to JF, February 1943, *ibid*.

447 "The Museum . . . artist." Yasuo Kuniyoshi to JF, February 9, 1943, *ibid*.

447 "I just want . . . shudders." Herbert Meyer to JF, February 2, 1943, *ibid*.

447–448 "Like every-one . . . straw." Charles Burchfield to JF, February 20, 1943, WMAA; Library.

448 "Dear Juliana . . . Alfred." Barr to JF, undated [1943], WMAA; Archives (H. 3/f65A).

448–449 "Dear . . . Forbes." Watson to JF, January 12, 1943, WMAA; Archives (H. 3/f64).

449 "A helpless . . . collapse." McBride, "Gertrude Whitney Memorial," *New York Sun*, January 29, 1943.

449 "Juliana . . . go?' " Interview with Elizabeth Bart Gerald.

450 "It was . . . castle." Interview with Eugene Ludins.

450 "She presided . . . art." Interview with Gordon Washburn.

450 "Please . . . ahead." Crocker to JF, June 2, 1943, Reel 2396, JFP.

450–451 "That . . . stand." JF to Halpert, undated [May 1943], unmicrofilmed Downtown Gallery Papers.

451 "In other words . . . them." Whitney trustees' statement, May 1943, WMAA; Archives (H. 3/f4).

452 "To supplement its activities" Crocker, minutes, Whitney board of trustees, June 14, 1943, *ibid*.

452 "Another wart" Tomkins, pp. 302–3.

453 "That's my white wash." Interview with Nan Mason.

454 "Nonsense! . . . care." Antoinette Schulte to author, March 8, 1978.

454 "Lady, we missed you." Interview with Carl Rieser.

454 "Juliana . . . Cadmus.' " Interview with Andrée Ruellan and John W. Taylor.

455 "A tempestuous . . . made it up." Interview with Peppino Mangravite.

455 "Mrs. Force . . . that." Interview with Katherine Schmidt.

455–456 "Pictures . . . care." Pearl McCarthy, "Famous Art Personality Opens Gallery Exhibit," *Toronto Globe and Mail*, November 13, 1943.

456 "The same . . . absorb." Dorothy Miller, interview with Paul Cummings, May 26, 1970–June 16, 1971, AAA.

456–457 Sketch of Fiske Kimball is drawn from Carl Zigrosser's eponymous essay in his *A World of Art and Museums* (Philadelphia, 1975), pp. 218–38.

457 "Gratitude . . . come." *Ibid*., p. 222.

457 "To . . . Eakins" Kimball, unpublished memoirs.

457 "Displaying . . . come" Evan H. Turner, in Theodor Siegl, *The Thomas Eakins Collection* (Philadelphia, 1978), p. 7.

457 "Other museum . . . one." Kimball, unpublished memoirs.

458 "The clause . . . matter." Kimball to Crocker, October 29, 1943, Fiske Kimball Papers.

458 "I could imagine . . . possible." Kimball, unpublished memoirs.

458 "We are . . . public." Crocker to Whitney trustees, September 30, 1943, WMAA; Archives (H. 3/f4).

458 "Received . . . try." Kimball, unpublished memoirs.

459 "They were . . . purchases." *Ibid*.

459 "With . . . sold." *Ibid*.

459 "Even . . . surprise." Rosamund Frost, "Encore by Popular Demand: The Whitney," *Art News*, 42 (December 1, 1943), p. 21.

460 "In view . . . pussyfooting." Francis Henry Taylor to Roland L. Redmond, September 24, 1943, MMAA.

460 "I hope . . . Fund!" William Church Osborn to Taylor, September 27, 1943, *ibid.*

461 "Strength . . . art" Edith Lowenthal to Hermon More, December 22, 1949, WMAA; Registrar's Dept.

463 "It was . . . lost." Henry Schnakenberg, Katherine Schmidt, et al. to Flora Miller, February 3, 1944, WMAA; Archives (H.3/f4).

464 "Wherever . . . located." Flora Miller to Henry Schnakenberg, February 10, 1944, *ibid.*

464 "When . . . eyes." Interview with Peppino Mangravite.

464–465 "Excellent . . . Metropolitan." Taylor to JF, May 23, 1944; Crocker to JF, May 25, 1944, WMAA; Archives (H.3/f66).

465 "We know . . . Museum." Kimball to C. V. Whitney, July 7, 1944, Fiske Kimball Papers.

465 "The wing . . . Museum." Kimball to George M. Francis, July 26, 1944, Fiske Kimball Papers.

465–466 Whitney-Wright-Florida Southern affair: Besides drawing on the citations given below, I am grateful to Randolph C. Henning, Bruce Brooks Pfeiffer, William Wesley Peters, Indira Berndtson, and Eleanor Searle McCollum for their many helpful insights.

466 "I have . . . pay?" Handwritten response by Frank Lloyd Wright at the bottom of a letter from Ludd Spivey to Wright, November 15, 1943. Copyright © The Frank Lloyd Wright Foundation, 1990. Courtesy The Frank Lloyd Wright Archives.

466 "Doubtless . . . come to naught." Spivey to Wright, August 21, 1944, *ibid.*

467 "Wright was not . . . bad." *Of Fact and Fancy . . . At Florida Southern College*, edited by Charles T. Thrift, Jr. (Lakeland, Fla., 1979), p. 53, and Eleanor Searle Whitney, *Invitation to Joy* (New York, 1971), pp. 80–81; interview with Eleanor Searle Whitney McCollum. I thank Randolph C. Henning for furnishing me with these references.

467 "Oh, do that." Kimball, unpublished memoirs.

467–468 JF in Woodstock: interviews with Dorothy Varian, Nan Mason, Andrée Ruellan, John Taylor, Eugene Ludins, Hannah Small, Mary Earley, Raoul Hague, and William Pachner.

468 "Too much freedom . . . Avenue." Interviews with John Frear, John and Elizabeth Bart Gerald, and Betty Bartlett Madden.

468–469 "It was . . . activities." Interviews with Katherine Schmidt and Irvine Shubert.

469 "I will . . . nothing." JF to Duncan Phillips, November 29, 1944, The Phillips Collection Papers, Reel 1965:1124.

469 "What do you . . . puke." Lloyd Goodrich, interview with Harlan Phillips, 1962–1963, AAA.

469 "Deeply offended . . . friends." Charles Sawyer to author, April 17, 1978.

469 "We bought . . . has it." Interview with Edith and Milton Lowenthal.

469 "Temperamental" Halpert to Wright Ludington, February 21, 1945, unmicrofilmed Downtown Gallery Papers.

470 "Happy . . . activities." Daniel Catton Rich to JF, April 4, 1945, Daniel Catton Rich Papers, Art Institute of Chicago Archives.

470 "They hated . . . dog." Interview with Edith and Milton Lowenthal.

470 McCausland survey: Elizabeth McCausland, "Why Can't America Afford Art?" *Magazine of Art*, 39 (January 1946), p. 18.

470 "Chairman and dominant figure." Elizabeth Olds to author, January 28, 1978.

471 "Relied . . . that well." Interview with Irvine Shubert.

471 "What . . . here?" Interview with Lloyd Goodrich.

471–472 Chagall incident: Interview with Bernarda Bryson Shahn.

472 "In 1945, . . . gallery." Stephen Greene to author, April 3, 1978.

472 "It was the most . . . people" Dorothy Miller, interview with Paul Cummings.

473 Paul Burlin incident: "Are Grazing Asses Art?" *Newsweek*, August 13, 1945, p. 98; interviews with Nan Mason, Dorthy Varian, Andrée Ruellan, and William Pachner.

474 "Dear Carl . . . finals." JF to Carl Rieser, September 17, 1945, RFC.

474 "Doughty duenna" "Artists' Choices," *Time*, November 5, 1945, p. 57.

474 'Mrs. Juliana . . . art" "Are Grazing Asses Art?" p. 98.

474 "I'm . . . house" Interview with William Pachner.

474 "The big proposition" Kimball, unpublished memoirs.

475 "Our alcove . . . future." *Ibid.*

476 "Juliana . . . sanctum." Eloise Spaeth to author, January 14, 1978.

476 "Going completely modern." McBride, "The Whitney Museum," *New York Sun*, December 1, 1945; also, Jewell, "Modernism Marks Whitney Art Show," *New York Times*, February 5, 1946.

476 "Affable . . . Annual." Greenberg, "Art," *Nation*, 163 (December 28, 1945), p. 767.

476 "Submissive . . . show." Watson, unpublished reminiscences, December 18, 1945, FWP.

477 "I have . . . subject." JF to John Hartell, April 18, 1945, Reel 2396, JFP.

478 "Hopefully . . . vain" Alexander Calder to JF, February 3, 1945, WMAA; (H.3/f12).

478 "Our budget . . . future." JF to Calder, February 6, 1945, *ibid.*

478–479 "She first . . . battle." "In Memoriam," *Art Digest*, 22 (September 15, 1948), p. 9.

479–482 Kaiser Friedrich collection: A large scrapbook and correspondence file on the "protective custody" issue was collected by JF, who followed the conflict for four years. After her death, one of her secretaries presented the material to Calvin Sutliffe Hathaway, who in turn gave it to Columbia University.

481 "To . . . country." JF to Rich, April 22, 1946, Daniel Catton Rich Papers.

481 "Had considerable . . . shipments." Charles Sawyer to Frederick Mortimer Clapp, April 29, 1946, Box 2, Calvin Sutliffe Hathaway Papers, Rare Book and Manuscript Library, Columbia University.

481 "Carried the ball" Thomas Parker to JF and Hudson Walker, February 14, 1946, Box 2, Calvin Sutliffe Hathaway Papers.

481 "Deplorable . . . justification." "Roberts Hits Back on Looting Charge," *New York Times*, June 11, 1946.

481 "Due to your . . . disposal." Lincoln Kirstein to JF, April 30, 1946, Box 1, Calvin Sutliffe Hathaway Papers.

481 "Many . . . countries." JF et al. to Harry Truman and Dean Acheson, May 9, 1946, Box 2, *ibid.*

482 "Your . . . beginning." JF to Charles Nagel, June 11, 1946, Box 2, *ibid.*

482–483 "Isn't . . . nothing!" Interview with John Frear.

483 "I had . . . prewar days." JF to Carl Rieser, July 4, 1946, RFC.

484 "It was bad . . . on artists?' " Interview with Irvine Shubert.

484 "Arrogance . . . disguise." "Artists to Protest Halting Art Tour," *New York Times*, May 6, 1947.

484 "The lunatic fringe" *Advancing American Art: Politics and Aesthetics in the State Department Exhibition, 1946–48* (Montgomery, Ala., 1984), p. 19.

484 "If you . . . guest room." *Advancing American Art*, p. 19.

485 "Artistic flim-flam" "Uncle Sam Loser on This Art Deal," *New York Journal American*, May 28, 1948.

485 "The vaporings . . . Hottentot." *Advancing American Art*, p. 20.

486 "The policy . . . masterpieces." Goodrich to JF, April 4, 1947, WMAA; Archives (H.3/f4).

487 "This woman . . . standoff." Interview with Edith Nolder.

488 "A good . . . position." "Juliana Force," *Art Digest*, 22 (September 15, 1948), p. 15.

489 David Smith's discomfort: Stanley E. Marcus, *David Smith: The Sculptor and His Work* (Ithaca and London, 1983), pp. 83–84; Stanley E. Marcus to author, August 27, 1979.

489 "I'd rather . . . bill." David Smith, transcript, First Woodstock Art Conference, August 1947, David Smith Papers, AAA.

489 "She spoke . . . from mine." Interview with Edith Nolder.

490 "She was . . . the same." Interview with Jane Wasey.

492 "Dear Flora . . . J." JF to Flora Miller, November 2, 1947, author's collection. Courtesy of Flora Miller Biddle, New York City.

492–493 "My dear Flora . . . JRF." JF to Flora Miller, November 28, 1947, *ibid.*

493 "I am very much . . . mutt." JF to Flora Miller, November 1947, *ibid.*

493 "Mrs. Force . . . last." Walter G. Dunnington to Flora Miller, December 19, 1947, WMAA; Archives (H. 3/f32).

493–494 "I want . . . life!" Interview with Lloyd Lózes Goff; interview with Betty Bartlett Madden.

494 "Of course . . . Sabbatical year." Dunnington to Flora Miller, December 23, 1947, WMAA; Archives (H. 3/f32).

494 "Being . . . boring." Interview with Edith Nolder.

495 "Her illness . . . found." Allan Rieser, unpublished memoir.

495 "Now that . . . it?" Interview with Edith Nolder.

495 "Considering . . . board." JF to Taylor, February 20, 1948, MMAA.

496 "Those are the artists." Interview with Lloyd Goodrich; interview with Helen Farr Sloan.

496 "Was enraged" Lloyd Goodrich, interview with Harlan Phillips.

496 "Dear Dan . . . J." JF to Rich, March 15, 1948, Daniel Catton Rich Papers.

497 "WONDERFUL . . . ME." Rich to JF, March 17, 1948, *ibid.*

497 "It seemed . . . government." Sara Kuniyoshi to author, April 5, 1978.

497 "We knew . . . upstairs." Interview with Raphael Soyer.

497 "Her . . . going." Interview with Katherine Schmidt.

497 "Poor . . . her." Biddle, diary, March 25, 1948.

497–498 "About Mrs. Force: . . . admiration." Watson to Concetta Scaravaglione, March 27, 1948, Concetta Scaravaglione Papers, AAA.

498 "Mrs. Force . . . April." Dunnington to C. V. Whitney, March 29, 1948, WMAA; Archives (H. 3/f32).

499 "I am sorry . . . Museum." Dunnington to C. V. Whitney, May 12, 1948, *ibid.*

500 "I took her out . . . home." Interview with Lloyd Goodrich.

500 "Intuitive . . . more." A. Hyatt Mayor to author, January 20, 1978.

501 "Juliana . . . way." Interview with John Frear.

501 "If there is a . . . it." JF to Carl Rieser, undated [June 1948], RFC.

501 "Juliana . . . her death." Interview with Elizabeth Navas.

501 "My life . . . perhaps?" JF to Carl Rieser, undated [June–July 1948], RFC.

501 "Failing." Henry Schnakenberg, diary, August 7, 1948, Henry Schnakenberg Papers, AAA.

501–503 Stay in Doctors Hospital: JF medical records, Doctors Hospital, August 1948.

502 "What . . . teapot!" Interview with John Gerald.

502 "Mrs. Force . . . fix them." *Ibid.*

503 "Poor dear . . . suffered so." Schnakenberg, diary, August 28, 1948.

503 "Juliana . . . replace her." Biddle, diary, August 29, 1948.

503 "She . . . depended on." Sloan, diary, September 2, 1948, John Sloan Archives.

503 "By the fact . . . not." Watson to Concetta Scaravaglione, October 4, 1948, Concetta Scaravaglione Papers.

503 "Filled with . . . her." A. Hyatt Mayor, interview with Paul Cummings, March 21–May 5, 1969, AAA.

504 "You have no idea . . . helped." Genevieve Rindner to author, September 11, 1979.

504 "Looked stricken . . . youth." [Kathryn McHale] "Juliana Force, 1881–1948," *Journal of the American Association of University Women,* 42 (Winter 1949), p. 103.

504 "JULIANNA . . . CEREMONY" "Julianna [*sic*] Force Buried in 2-Minute Ceremony," *Doylestown Daily Intelligencer,* September 1, 1948. In addition, a report prepared in 1967 by a librarian at the Bucks County Free Library in Doylestown for a biographical sketch of Juliana Force for *Notable American Women* cited recent interviews with residents who still bore a grudge about the minor part Doylestown played in the funeral arrangements.

SELECTED BIBLIOGRAPHY

UNPUBLISHED MATERIALS

PRINCIPAL MANUSCRIPT COLLECTIONS CONSULTED

1. *Archives of American Art*
Papers: Alfred H. Barr, Jr., Oscar Bluemner, Louis Bouché, Konrad and Florence Cramer, John Steuart Curry, Stuart Davis, Downtown Gallery, Emlen Etting, Ernest Fiene, Juliana Force, Albert Gallatin, Lloyd Goodrich, Harry Gottlieb, Dorothea Greenbaum, Karl Gruppe, Leon Hartl, Robert Henri, Rockwell Kent, Leon Kroll, Gaston Lachaise, Edward Laning, Julian Levi, Macbeth Gallery, Henry McBride, Elizabeth McCausland, Reginald Marsh, F. Luis Mora, Elizabeth Navas, Guy Pène du Bois, Van Dearing Perrine, The Phillips Collection, Public Works of Art Project, Helen Appleton Read, Mary Fanton Roberts, Concetta Scaravaglione, Katherine Schmidt, Henry Schnakenberg, Ben Shahn, Charles Sheeler, David Smith, Joseph Solman, Raphael Soyer, Eugene Speicher, Beulah Stevenson, Dorothy Varian, Maynard Walker, Carl Walters, Washington Square Outdoor Exhibit, Forbes Watson, Gertrude Vanderbilt Whitney, Whitney Museum of American Art.
Oral Histories: Faith Andrews, Mildred Baker, John I. H. Baur, Thomas Hart Benton, George Biddle, Arnold Blanch, Ilya Bolotowsky, Alexander Brook, Olin Dows, Lloyd Goodrich, Inslee Hopper, Audrey McMahon, A. Hyatt Mayor, Dorothy Miller, Isamu Noguchi, Fairfield Porter, Theodore Roszak, Katherine Schmidt, Ben Shahn, Joseph Solman.

2. *Rieser Family Collection*
Papers: Memoirs by Allan, Carl, and Charles Rieser; Juliana Rieser, holograph notebook; Juliana Force, address book, will, estate papers; letters of Juliana Force and Allan, Carl, Clara, Irene, and Mary Rieser; photographs of Juliana Force, her family, and her residences. All materials are in the author's possession.

3. *Whitney Museum of American Art*
Papers: Administrative files; bills of sale; artists' vertical files; chronological correspondence; exhibition catalogs and records; minutes of staff meetings; photographs; registrar's office notes; reproductions; salary registers; scrapbooks of clippings; stock books and cash receipts; summaries of interviews by Rosalind Irvine with Blendon Campbell, Jo Davidson, Bernard Karfiol, Max Kuehne, Katherine Schmidt, and Forbes Watson in 1949, and with Stuart Davis in 1953; memoir by Samuel Wood Gaylor, 1954.

OTHER MANUSCRIPT COLLECTIONS CONSULTED

Art Institute of Chicago (Robert Harshe, Daniel Catton Rich papers); Brooklyn Museum (Delia Akeley, American Art Research Council, William Henry Fox, George

Thayer files); Bucks County Courthouse; Bucks County Historical Society; Columbia University (Calvin Sutliffe Hathaway, Florine Stettheimer papers; Holger Cahill oral history); Delaware Art Museum (Everett Shinn papers, John Sloan Archives, Society of Independent Artists papers); Solomon R. Guggenheim Museum (Hilla von Rebay Foundation Archives); Library of Congress (Hendrik Christian Andersen, George Biddle, Margaret French Cresson, Jo Davidson, Daniel Chester French, Waldo Peirce, William Zorach papers); Metropolitan Museum of Art (directors, Whitney Museum of American Art files); National Academy of Design; National Archives and Records Service (American Battle Monuments Commission papers); Newberry Library (Sherwood and Tennessee Mitchell Anderson papers); New York Genealogical and Biographical Society; New-York Historical Society; New York Public Library (Mitchell Kennerley papers, John Quinn Memorial Collection); Northfield Mount Hermon School; University of Pennsylvania (Lewis Mumford, Carl Zigrosser papers); Philadelphia Museum of Art (Julius Bloch, Fiske Kimball papers); Princeton University (Alexander Brook memoirs); Rockefeller Archive Center; University of Texas at Austin, Humanities Research Center (Christopher Morley papers); Wadsworth Atheneum (A. Everett Austin papers); West Point Museum; Frank Lloyd Wright Memorial Foundation; Yale University (Royal Cortissoz, William Adams Delano, Florine Stettheimer papers, Alfred Stieglitz Collection).

PAPERS IN PRIVATE HANDS

Cramer, Florence Ballin. Diaries. Courtesy of Aileen Cramer, Woodstock, N.Y.

Davis, Stuart. Interview with Harlan Phillips. 1962. Courtesy of Earl Davis, New York City.

Etting, Emlen. "Studio in Paris, 1930." Memoir, 1970s. Courtesy of Emlen Etting, Philadelphia, Pa.

Schnakenberg, Henry. Interview with Wanda M. Corn. May 22, 1965. Courtesy of Wanda M. Corn, Stanford University, Stanford, Calif.

Whitney, Gertrude Vanderbilt. Journals, letters, and drawings. Courtesy of Flora Miller Biddle, New York City.

Wright, James A. "A History of Barley Sheaf Farm, Holicong, Bucks County, Pennsylvania." August 25, 1977. Courtesy of Don Mills, Holicong, Pa.

Yeats, John Butler. Letters. Courtesy of William M. Murphy, Union College, Schenectady, N.Y., and Donald Torchiana, Northwestern University, Evanston, Ill.

DISSERTATIONS AND THESES

Contreras, Belisario R. "The New Deal Treasury Department Art Programs and the American Artist: 1933 to 1943." Ph.D. dissertation, American University, 1967.

Forsyth, Robert J. "John B. Flannagan: His Life and Works." Ph.D. dissertation, University of Minnesota, 1965.

Healy, Daty. "A History of the Whitney Museum of American Art, 1930–1954." Ph.D. dissertation, New York University, 1960.

Jaffee, Cynthia. "Reuben Nakian." Master's thesis, Columbia University, 1967.

LEGAL DOCUMENTS

C. Brancusi v. *United States*. Transcript of court case, October 21, 1927, Museum of Modern Art Library.

Divorce petition of Willard and Mary Grace Barnes Force, January 8, 1911, New Jersey Supreme Court, Trenton.

PUBLICATIONS

BOOKS AND CATALOGS

Note: In addition to the Whitney Studio, Club, Galleries, and Museum publications specifically cited, every extant Whitney catalog published between 1914 and 1949 was consulted.

Abstract Painting in America. New York: Whitney Museum of American Art, 1935.

Adams, Henry. *The Education of Henry Adams.* Boston: Houghton Mifflin, 1961.

Advancing American Art: Politics and Aesthetics in the State Department Exhibition, 1946–48. Montgomery, Ala.: Montgomery Museum of Art, 1984.

The American Renaissance, 1876–1917. New York: Brooklyn Museum, 1979.

Andrews, Edward Deming, and Andrews, Faith. *Fruits of the Shaker Tree of Life: Memoirs of Fifty Years of Collecting and Research.* Stockbridge, Mass.: Berkshire Traveller Press, 1975.

Andrews, Wayne. *The Vanderbilt Legend.* New York: Harcourt, Brace & Co., 1941.

Appleton's Annual Cyclopaedia and Register of Important Events of the Year 1876. New series, vol. 1. New York: D. Appleton & Co., 1877.

Bacon, Peggy. *Off With Their Heads!* New York: Robert McBride & Co., 1934.

Baigell, Matthew. *The American Scene: American Painting of the 1930s.* New York and Washington, D.C.: Praeger, 1974.

Balsam, Consuelo. *The Glitter and the Gold.* New York: Harper & Bros., 1952.

Barr, Alfred H., Jr. *An Exhibition Of Work Of 46 Painters & Sculptors Under 35 Years Of Age.* New York: Museum of Modern Art, 1930.

Beaton, Cecil. *The Wandering Years: Diaries, 1922–1939.* Boston: Little, Brown & Co., 1962.

Benton, Thomas Hart. *The Arts of Life in America: A Series of Murals by Thomas Hart Benton.* New York: Whitney Museum of American Art, 1932.

——. *An Artist in America,* 4th rev. ed. Columbia, Mo.: University of Missouri Press, 1983.

Biddle, George. *An American Artist's Story.* Boston: Little, Brown & Co., 1939.

Bishop, Robert. *American Folk Art: Expressions of A New Spirit.* New York: Museum of American Folk Art, 1982.

Bradley Walker Tomlin: A Retrospective View. Garden City, N.Y.: Whaler Press, 1975.

Braun, Emily, and Branchick, Thomas. *Thomas Hart Benton: The America Today Murals.* New York: Equitable Life Assurance Company of the United States, 1985.

Brooks, Van Wyck. *The Confident Years, 1885–1915.* New York: E.P. Dutton & Co., 1952.

——. *Scenes and Portraits: Memories of Childhood and Youth.* New York: E. P. Dutton & Co., 1954.

——. *John Sloan: A Painter's Life.* New York: E. P. Dutton & Co., 1955.

——. *Days of the Phoenix: The Nineteen-Twenties I Remember.* New York: E. P. Dutton & Co., 1957.

Brown, Milton W. *The Story of the Armory Show.* New York: Joseph Hirshhorn Foundation, 1963.

Caffin, Charles Henry. *American Masters of Sculpture,* reprint of 1903 edition. Freeport, N.Y.: Books for Libraries Press, 1969.

Campbell, Lawrence, ed. *"Chris": Reminiscences by Christian Buchheit as told to Lawrence Campbell.* New York: Art Students League, 1956.

Caro, Robert. *The Power Broker: Robert Moses and the Fall of New York.* New York: Random House, 1975.

Carter, Burnham. *So Much to Learn: The History of Northfield Mount Hermon School for the One Hundredth Anniversary.* Northfield, Mass.: Northfield Mount Hermon School, 1976.

Catalogue of an Exhibition of Early American Art. New York: Whitney Studio Club, 1924.

Chanler, Mrs. Winthrop. *Roman Spring: Memoirs.* Boston: Little, Brown & Co., 1934.

Charles Sheeler. Washington, D.C.: Smithsonian Institution Press, 1968.

Churchill, Allen. *The Upper Crust: An Informal History of New York's Highest Society.* Englewood Cliffs, N.J.: Prentice-Hall, 1970.

————. *The Splendor Seekers: An Informal Glimpse of America's Multimillionaire Spenders—Members of the $50,000,000 Club.* New York: Grosset & Dunlap, 1974.

The Circus in Paint. New York: Whitney Studio Galleries, 1929.

Clark, Eliot. *History of the National Academy of Design, 1825–1953.* New York: Columbia University Press, 1954.

Cortissoz, Royal. *John La Farge: A Memoir and a Study.* Boston: Houghton Mifflin, 1911.

Cummings, Paul. *Artists In Their Own Words.* New York: St. Martin's Press, 1979.

Dana, Nathalie. *Young in New York: A Memoir of a Victorian Girlhood.* Garden City, N.Y.: Doubleday & Co., 1963.

David Park (1911–1960). New York: Salander-O'Reilly Galleries, 1987.

Davidson, Jo. *Between Sittings: An Informal Autobiography of Jo Davidson.* New York: Dial Press, 1951.

Davis, W. W. H. *History of Doylestown, Old and New.* Doylestown: Doylestown Intelligencer Press, 1905.

DeShazo, Edith. *Everett Shinn, 1876–1953: A Figure in His Time.* New York: Clarkson Potter, 1974.

Dos Passos, John. *The Best Times: An Informal Memoir.* New York: New American Library, 1966.

The Edith and Milton Lowenthal Collection. New York: Brooklyn Museum, 1981.

Eliasoph, Philip. *Paul Cadmus, Yesterday and Today.* Oxford, Ohio: Miami University Art Museum, 1981.

Emmelkamp, Paul G. *Phobic and Obsessive-Compulsive Disorders.* New York and London: Plenum Press, 1982.

Evers, Alf. *The Catskills: From Wilderness to Woodstock.* Garden City, N.Y.: Doubleday & Co., 1972.

Exhibition of Modern Paintings by American and Foreign Artists. New York: Mrs. H. P. Whitney's Studio, 1916.

Exhibition of Twenty New Oil Paintings on Panels by Oscar Bluemner. New York: Whitney Studio Galleries, 1929.

Fahlman, Betsy. *Guy Pène du Bois: Artist About Town.* Washington, D.C.: Corcoran Gallery of Art, 1980.

First American Artists' Congress. New York: American Artists' Congress, 1936.

First Biennial Exhibition of Contemporary American Painting. New York: Whitney Museum of American Art, 1932.

Flannagan, John. *Letters of John B. Flannagan.* New York: Curt Valentin, 1942.

Force, Juliana. "The Function of the Museum in Our Society." In *The First Woodstock Art Conference.* Edited by John D. Morse. New York: Woodstock Art Association & Artists Equity Association, 1947.

"Force, Juliana." In *Current Biography: Who's News and Why.* New York: H. W. Wilson, 1941.

Foster, Edward Halsey, and Clark, Geoffrey W., eds. *Hoboken: A Collection of Essays.* New York: Irvington Publications, 1976.

Friedman, B. H., with the research collaboration of Flora Miller Irving. *Gertrude Vanderbilt Whitney.* Garden City, N.Y.: Doubleday & Cò., 1978.

Gallatin, Albert E. *Certain Contemporaries: A Set of Notes in Art Criticism.* New York: John Lane, 1916.

Garvan, Beatrice B., and Hummel, Charles F. *The Pennsylvania Germans: A Celebration of Their Arts, 1683–1850.* Philadelphia: Philadelphia Museum of Art, 1982.

Geist, Sidney. *Brancusi: A Study of the Sculpture,* rev. 1968 ed. New York: Hacker Art Books, 1983.

Geldzahler, Henry. *New York Painting and Sculpture, 1940–1970.* New York: E. P. Dutton & Co., 1969.

Glackens, Ira. *William Glackens and The Eight: The Artists Who Freed American Art.* New York: Horizon, 1983.

Goldsmith, Barbara. *Little Gloria . . . Happy At Last.* New York: Alfred A. Knopf, 1980.

Goldstein, Malcolm. *George S. Kaufman: His Life, His Theater.* New York and Oxford: Oxford University Press, 1979.

Goodrich, Lloyd. *Yasuo Kuniyoshi.* New York: Whitney Museum of American Art, 1948.

———. *John Sloan.* New York: Whitney Museum of American Art, 1952.

———. "Force, Juliana Rieser." In *Notable American Women, 1607–1950.* 3 vols. Edited by Edward T. James. Cambridge, Mass.: Harvard University Press, Belknap Press, 1971.

———. *Thomas Eakins.* 2 vols. Cambridge: Harvard University Press, 1982.

Hale, Nancy, and Bowers, Fredson, eds. *Leon Kroll: A Spoken Memoir.* Charlottesville: University Press of Virginia, 1983.

Hapgood, Hutchins. *A Victorian in the Modern World.* New York: Harcourt, Brace & Co., 1939.

Haskell, Barbara. *Marsden Hartley.* New York: Whitney Museum of American Art/New York University Press, 1980.

Hecht, Ben. *A Child of the Century.* New York: Simon & Schuster, 1954.

Henri, Robert. *The Art Spirit.* Philadelphia and New York: Lippincott, 1960.

Hills, Patricia. *Turn-of-the-Century America: Paintings, Graphics, Photographs, 1890–1910.* New York: Whitney Museum of American Art, 1977.

Hills, Patricia, and Tarbell, Roberta K. *The Figurative Tradition and the Whitney Museum of American Art: Paintings and Sculpture from the Permanent Collection.* Newark: Whitney Museum of American Art/University of Delaware Press, 1980.

Hiss, Priscilla, and Fansler, Roberta. *Research in Fine Arts in the Colleges & Universities of the United States.* New York: Carnegie Corporation, 1934.

Hoboken Board of Trade. *History of Hoboken.* Hoboken: Inquirer Press, 1907.

Hoffman, Malvina. *Yesterday is Tomorrow.* New York: Crown, 1965.

Holroyd, Michael. *Augustus John: A Biography.* Middlesex and New York: Penguin Books, 1976.

Homer, William Innes, with the assistance of Violet Organ. *Robert Henri and His Circle.* Ithaca and London: Cornell University Press, 1969.

Homer, William Innes. *Alfred Stieglitz and the American Avant-Garde.* Boston: New York Graphic Society, 1977.

Houseman, John. *Run-Through.* New York: Simon & Schuster, 1972.

Hoyt, Nancy. *Elinor Wylie: The Portrait of an Unknown Lady*. New York: Bobbs-Merrill, 1935.

Hyland, Douglas. *Marius de Zayas: Conjuror of Souls*. Lawrence: University of Kansas, 1981.

Isham, Samuel. *The History of American Painting*, rev. ed. New York: Macmillan, 1936.

James Earle Fraser: American Sculptor. New York: Kennedy Galleries, 1969.

James, Henry. *The American Scene*. Bloomington: Indiana University Press, 1968.

John Sloan, 1871–1951. Washington, D.C.: National Gallery of Art, 1971.

Josephson, Matthew. *The Robber Barons*. New York: Harcourt Brace Jovanovich, 1962.

Juliana Force and American Art. New York: Whitney Museum of Art, 1949.

The Juliana Force Victorian Collection. New York: Parke-Bernet Galleries, 1943.

Karlstrom, Paul. *Louis Michel Eilshemius*. New York: Harry N. Abrams, 1978.

The Katherine Schmidt Shubert Bequest and A Selective View of Her Art. New York: Whitney Museum of American Art, 1982.

Kelder, Diane, ed. *Stuart Davis: A Documentary Monograph*. New York: Praeger, 1971.

Kent, Rockwell. *It's Me O Lord: The Autobiography of Rockwell Kent*. New York: Dodd, Mead & Co., 1955.

Kirstein, Lincoln. *Gaston Lachaise*. New York: M. Knoedler & Co., 1947.

Landgren, Marchal E. *Years of Art: The Story of the Art Students League of New York*. New York: Robert McBride & Co., 1940.

Lane, John R. *Stuart Davis: Art and Art Theory*. New York: Brooklyn Museum, 1978.

Lane, John R., and Larsen, Susan C., eds. *Abstract Painting and Sculpture in America, 1927–1944*. Pittsburgh: Museum of Art, Carnegie Institute/Harry N. Abrams, 1983.

Lately, Thomas. *The Astor Orphans: A Pride of Lions: The Chanler Chronicle*. New York: William Morrow & Co., 1971.

Lawson, Michael L., and Voss, Frederick S. *The Great Crash*. Washington, D.C.: Smithsonian Institution Press, 1979.

Levy, Julien. *Memoir of an Art Gallery*. New York: G. P. Putnam's Sons, 1977.

Lowe, Sue Davidson. *Stieglitz: A Memoir/Biography*. New York: Farrar, Straus & Giroux, 1983.

Ludington, Townsend, ed. *The Fourteenth Chronicle: Letters and Diaries of John Dos Passos*. Boston: Gambit, 1973.

Lynes, Russell. *Good Old Modern: An Intimate Portrait of the Museum of Modern Art*. New York: Atheneum, 1973.

McKinzie, Richard D. *The New Deal for Artists*. Princeton: Princeton University Press, 1973.

Marcus, Stanley E. *David Smith: The Sculptor and His Work*. Ithaca and London: Cornell University Press, 1983.

Marin, John. *The Selected Writings of John Marin*. Edited with an introduction by Dorothy Norman. New York: Pellegrini & Cudahy, 1949.

Marling, Karal Ann. *Woodstock: An American Art Colony, 1902–1977*. Poughkeepsie, N.Y.: Vassar College Art Gallery, 1977.

Marlor, Clark S. *The Society of Independent Artists: The Exhibition Record, 1917–1944*. Park Ridge, N.J.: Noyes Press, 1984.

May, Henry F. *The End of American Innocence: A Study of the First Years of Our Time, 1912–1917*. New York: Alfred A. Knopf, 1969.

Mayer, Grace. *Once Upon a City*. New York: Macmillan, 1958.

Melville, Joy. *Phobias and Obsessions*. New York: Coward, McCann & Geoghegan, 1977.

Memorial Exhibition of Paintings, Pastels and Etchings by Warren Davis. New York: Harlow, McDonald & Co., 1928.

Meyerowitz, Theresa Bernstein. *William Meyerowitz: The Artist Speaks.* Philadelphia: Art Alliance Press, 1986.

Morgan, Ann Lee, ed. *Dear Stieglitz, Dear Dove.* Newark, Del.: Associated University Presses, 1988.

Moses, Robert. *Public Works: A Dangerous Trade.* New York: McGraw-Hill, 1970.

Murphy, William M. *Prodigal Father: The Life of John Butler Yeats (1839–1922).* Ithaca and London: Cornell University Press, 1978.

Myers, Gustavus. *History of the Great American Fortunes.* 2 vols. Chicago: Charles H. Kern & Co., 1909.

Myers, Jerome. *Artist in Manhattan.* New York: American Artists Group, 1940.

Naylor, Maria, comp. & ed. *The National Academy of Design Exhibition Record, 1861–1890.* 2 vols. New York: Kennedy Galleries, 1973.

Newman, Sasha M. *Arthur Dove and Duncan Phillips: Artist and Patron.* New York: The Phillips Collection/George Braziller, 1981.

Nordland, Gerald. *Gaston Lachaise: The Man and His Work.* New York: George Braziller, 1974.

Norman, Dorothy. *Alfred Stieglitz: Introduction to an American Seer.* New York: Duell, Sloan and Pearce, 1960.

O'Connor, Francis V. *Federal Support For The Visual Arts: The New Deal and Now,* 2d ed. Greenwich: New York Graphic Society, 1971.

———, ed. *The New Deal Art Projects: An Anthology of Memoirs.* Washington, D.C.: Smithsonian Institution Press, 1972.

———, ed. *Art for the Millions: Essays from the 1930s by Artists and Administrators of the WPA Federal Art Project.* Boston: New York Graphic Society, 1975.

Ouellette, Fernand. *Edgard Varèse.* Translated by Derek Coltman. New York: Orion Press, 1966.

Pach, Walter. *Queer Thing, Painting: Forty Years in the World of Art.* New York: Harper & Bros., 1938.

Parry, Albert. *Garrets and Pretenders.* New York: Covici-Friede, 1933.

Pène du Bois, Guy. *Artists Say the Silliest Things.* New York: American Artists Group, 1940.

Perlman, Bennard B. *The Immortal Eight: American Painting from Eakins to the Armory Show, 1870–1913.* Westport, Conn.: North Light Publishers, 1979.

Powell, Earl A. III, ed. *The James A. Michener Collection.* Austin: University of Texas Press, 1977.

Putnam, George Palmer. *Wide Margins: A Publisher's Autobiography.* New York: Harcourt, Brace & Co., 1942.

Rachman, Stanley. *Phobias: Their Nature and Control.* Springfield, Ill.: Charles C Thomas, 1968.

Read, Helen Appleton. "Force, Juliana Rieser." In *Dictionary of American Biography.* Supplement 4, 1946–1950. New York: Charles Scribner's Sons, 1974.

Reed, Alma M. *Orozco.* New York: Oxford University Press, 1956.

Reid, B. L. *The Man from New York: John Quinn and His Friends.* New York: Oxford University Press, 1968.

Rich, Daniel Catton, ed. *The Flow of Art: Essays and Criticisms of Henry McBride.* New York: Atheneum, 1975.

Rorimer, James J., with the collaboration of Gilbert Rabin. *Survival: The Salvage and Protection of Art in War.* New York: Abelard Press, 1950.

Rothenstein, William. *Men and Memories: Recollections of William Rothenstein.* 3 vols. London: Faber & Faber, 1932.

St. John, Bruce, ed. *John Sloan's New York Scene, From the Diaries, Notes and Correspondence, 1906–1913.* New York: Harper & Row, 1965.

Schack, William. *And He Sat Among the Ashes.* New York: American Artists Group, 1939.

———. *Art and Argyrol.* New York: A. S. Barnes and Co., 1963.

Schmeckebier, Laurence E. *John Steuart Curry's Pageant of America.* New York: American Artists Group, 1943.

Schwartz, Delmore. *The World is a Wedding.* Norfolk, Conn.: New Directions, 1948.

Seligmann, Herbert J. *Alfred Stieglitz Talking: Notes on Some of His Conversations, 1925–1931, with a Foreword.* New Haven: Yale University Library, 1966.

Shaker Handicrafts. New York: Whitney Museum of American Art, 1935.

Sheridan, Clare. *My American Diary.* New York: Boni and Liveright, 1922.

Shinn, Earl [Edward Strahan]. *Mr. Vanderbilt's House and Collection.* 10 vols. Holland ed., privately printed. New York, Boston, and Philadelphia: 1883–1884.

Siegl, Theodor. *The Thomas Eakins Collection.* Philadelphia: Philadelphia Museum of Art, 1978.

Sims, Patterson. *Charles Sheeler: A Concentration of Works from the Permanent Collection of the Whitney Museum of American Art.* New York: Whitney Museum of American Art, 1980.

Sloan, Helen Farr, ed. *John Sloan: New York Etchings.* New York: Dover, 1978.

Sloan, John. *Gist of Art: Principles and Practise Expounded in the Classroom and Studio,* rev. ed. New York: Dover, 1977.

Smith, David. *David Smith by David Smith.* Edited by Cleve Gray. New York: Holt, Rinehart & Winston, 1968.

Smith-Rosenberg, Caroll. *Disorderly Conduct: Visions of Gender in Victorian America.* New York: Oxford University Press, 1986.

Soyer, Raphael. *Diary of an Artist.* Washington, D.C.: New Republic Books, 1977.

Spring Exhibition 1930. New York: Whitney Studio Galleries, 1930.

Steichen, Edward. *A Life in Photography.* Garden City, N.Y.: Doubleday & Co., 1963.

Stevens, Wallace. *Letters of Wallace Stevens.* Selected and edited by Holly Stevens. New York: Alfred A. Knopf, 1966.

Swanberg, W. A. *Citizen Hearst.* New York: Charles Scribner's Sons, 1961.

———. *Whitney Father, Whitney Heiress.* New York: Charles Scribner's Sons, 1980.

Sweeney, James Johnson. *Stuart Davis.* New York: Museum of Modern Art, 1945.

Tarbell, Roberta. *Peggy Bacon: Personalities and Places.* Washington, D.C.: Smithsonian Institution Press, 1975.

Thrift, Charles T., Jr., ed. *Of Fact and Fancy . . . At Florida Southern College.* Lakeland: Florida Southern College Press, 1979.

Tomkins, Calvin. *Merchants and Masterpieces: The Story of the Metropolitan Museum of Art.* New York: E. P. Dutton & Co., 1973.

Traxel, David. *An American Saga: The Life and Times of Rockwell Kent.* New York: Harper & Row, 1980.

Troyen, Carol, and Hirshler, Erica E. *Charles Sheeler: Paintings and Drawings.* Boston: Museum of Fine Arts, 1987.

200 Years of American Sculpture. New York: Whitney Museum of American Art/David Godine, 1976.

Tyler, Parker. *Florine Stettheimer: A Life in Art.* New York: Farrar, Straus & Co., 1963.

U.S. Bureau of the Census. *Historical Statistics of the United States, Colonial Times to 1957.* Washington, D.C.: U.S. Government Printing Office, 1960.

Vanderbilt, Gloria. *Once Upon a Time.* New York: Alfred A. Knopf, 1985.

———. *Black Knight, White Knight.* New York: Alfred A. Knopf, 1987.

Vanderbilt, Mrs. Gloria, with Palma Wayne. *Without Prejudice.* New York: E. P. Dutton, 1936.

Vanderbilt, Gloria (Morgan), and Lady Furness, Thelma. *Double Exposure: A Twin Autobiography.* New York: David McKay, 1958.

Varèse, Louise. *Varèse: A Looking-Glass Diary, Vol. 1 (1883–1928).* New York: W. W. Norton, 1972.

Waldman, Diane. *Mark Rothko, 1903–1970: A Retrospective.* New York: Solomon R. Guggenheim Museum, 1978.

Walker, Stanley. *Mrs. Astor's Horse.* New York: Frederick A. Stokes, 1935.

Wheeler, Monroe. *20th century Portraits.* New York: Museum of Modern Art, 1942.

Whitney, C. V. *High Peaks.* Lexington: University Press of Kentucky, 1977.

Whitney, Eleanor Searle. *Invitation to Joy.* New York: Harper & Row, 1971.

Whitney, Gertrude [L. J. Webb]. *Walking the Dusk.* New York: Coward-McCann, 1932.

———. *A Love Affair.* New York: Richardson & Snyder, 1984.

Whitney Museum of American Art. *Whitney Museum of American Art, Catalogue of the Collection.* New York: Whitney Museum of American Art, 1931.

———. *Whitney Museum of American Art: History, Purpose and Activities, With a Complete List of Works in its Permanent Collection to June, 1937.* New York: Whitney Museum of American Art, 1937.

———. *Supplement To Catalogue of the Collection, July 1937–June 1942.* New York: Whitney Museum of American Art, 1942.

———. *Catalogue of the Collection.* New York: Whitney Museum of American Art, 1973.

Who's Who in America, 1944–1945. Chicago: A. N. Marquis, 1944.

Woolf, Virginia. *The Common Reader: First Series.* New York and London: Harcourt Brace Jovanovich, 1980.

Yasuo Kuniyoshi. New York: Whitney Museum of American Art at Philip Morris, 1986.

Zigrosser, Carl. *My Own Shall Come To Me: A Personal Memoir and Picture Chronicle.* Philadelphia: Casa Laura, 1971.

———. *A World of Art and Museums.* Philadelphia: Art Alliance Press, 1975.

Zilczer, Judith. *"The Noble Buyer": John Quinn, Patron of the Avant-Garde.* Washington, D.C.: Smithsonian Institution Press, 1978.

———. *Oscar Bluemner: The Hirshhorn Museum and Sculpture Garden Collection.* Washington, D.C.: Smithsonian Institution Press, 1979.

Zorach, William. *Art Is My Life.* Cleveland: World Publishing Co., 1967.

NEWSPAPERS AND PERIODICALS

Because hundreds of articles and reviews about Juliana Force, Gertrude Whitney, and their art enterprises were used and already have been listed in the Notes, only those by or materially about Juliana Force are repeated below.

"Antiques in Domestic settings." *Antiques* 29 (April 1936), pp. 152–153.

Berman, Avis. "Pioneers in American Museums: Juliana Force." *Museum News* 55 (November–December 1976), pp. 45–49, 59–62.

———. "A Pictorial History of the Whitney Museum." *ARTnews* 79 (May 1980), pp. 54–59.

————. "Juliana Force: Visionary Champion of American Art." *Architectural Digest*, February 1988, pp. 78, 80, 86–87, 92.

"Buffalo Bill Memorial is an Expression of American Life Well Interpreted by Gertrude V. Whitney, The Sculptor." *Park County Herald*, 2 April 1924.

Force, Juliana. "The Whitney Museum of American Art." *Creative Art* 9 (November 1931), pp. 387–89.

————. "Mrs. Force Discusses Changed Attitudes Toward American Art And Tells Whitney Museum Aims." *Dallas Times-Herald*, 10 December 1933.

————. "Whitney Getting Annual in Shape." *New York World Telegram*, 30 October 1942.

————. Foreword to "Research in American Art." *Art in America* 33 (October 1945), p. 176.

————. "The Whitney Museum of American Art." *American Magazine of Art* 39 (November 1946), pp. 271, 328.

Frankfurter, Alfred M. "Juliana R. Force." *Art News* 47 (October 1948), p. 13.

"In Memoriam." *Art Digest* 22 (15 September 1948), p. 9.

"Juliana Force." *Art Digest* 22 (15 September 1948), pp. 14–15.

"Juliana Force Dies, Whitney Museum Head." *New York Herald Tribune*, 29 August 1948.

"Juliana Force, Friend of Woodstock, Is Dead." *Woodstock Times*, 2 September 1948.

McBride, Henry. "The Reaper, Death!" *New York Sun*, 22 October 1948.

McCann, Anabel Parker. "Mrs. Juliana Force, Friend of Artists." *New York Sun*, 23 January 1934.

McCarthy, Pearl. "Famous Art Personality Opens Gallery Exhibit." *Toronto Globe and Mail*, 13 November 1943.

[McHale, Kathryn.] "Juliana Force, 1881–1948." *Journal of the American Association of University Women* 42 (Winter 1949), p. 103.

McHale, Kathryn. "Notes on the Arts." *General Director's Letter* [American Association of University Women] 16 (February 1949), pp. 47–48.

"Mrs. Force Dead; Assisted Artists." *New York Times*, 29 August 1948.

"Mrs. Whitney's Sec'y And Architect Delighted With Plinth of Cody Statue." *Cody Enterprise*, 2 April 1924.

"New York Woman Lauds Gimbel Art Galleries." *Philadelphia Inquirer*, 29 November 1934.

Patterson, Augusta Owen. "The Decorative Arts." *Town & Country*, 15 February 1931, pp. 50–53, 83.

Read, Helen Appleton. "An Experiment in the Rococo." *House & Garden*, October 1932, pp. 36–37, 62.

Roberts, Mary Fanton. "Upstairs in a Museum." *Arts and Decoration* 41 (June 1934), pp. 42–44.

Talmey, Allene. "Whitney Museum." *Vogue*, 1 February 1940, pp. 94–95, 131–33.

"Think for Yourself!" *Art Digest* 6 (1 February 1932), p. 13.

Watson, Forbes. "The Growth of the Whitney Museum." *Magazine of Art* 32 (October 1939), pp. 558–67, 606–607.

INDEX

In this index the initials JF stand for Juliana Force and GW for Gertrude Vanderbilt Whitney. Page numbers in *italics* indicate illustrations.

Beaux-Arts sculptors, 131. *See also specific artists*
Becker, Maurice, 250
Bellows, Emma, 311
Bellows, George, 72, 78, 132, 144, 170n.; and Armory Show, 103; *Dempsey and Firpo*, 311; *Floating Ice*, 122 and n.; and JF, 131, 311; in Henri circle, 71, 72, 128; and Indigenous Exhibition (1918), 150–151, 152; Metropolitan Museum memorial exhibition, 263; *Nude with Parrot*, 122; *Stag at Sharkey's*, 395 and n.; in Whitney Museum shows and collection, 166, 311, 395; and Whitney Studio Club shows, 153n.; in Whitney Studio shows, 113, 117, 122 and n., 137, 199; in Woodstock, 229
Benn, Ben, 222, 310, 340
Benton, Rita, 319, 324, 325
Benton, Thomas Hart, 8, 187, 270, 271, 273; *American Historical Epic* murals, 271 and n., 319; and JF, 271, 288, 319–325; *July Hay*, 460; *The Lord Is My Shepherd*, 288; in Metropolitan collection, 460; New School murals, 292, 293 and n., 301, 319, 322; photograph of, *320*; Whitney Museum mural commissions, 319–325; in Whitney Museum shows and collection, 166, 288, 301, 460; in Whitney Studio Club and shows, 216, 222, 271 and n.
Berg, Alban, 248
Berkshire Museum, 316
Berkson, Seymour, 363, 364, 366
Berman, Eugene, 460
Bernays, Doris, 178
Bernays, Edward L., 178, 199
Bernstein, Theresa, 115–116
Besnard, Albert, 121
Between Two Wars: Prints by American Artists, 1914–1941 (1942, Whitney Museum), 433
Bianco, Pamela, 222
Biddle, George, 187, 296, 421; and JF, 328, 497, 503; and New Deal art projects, 332–338, 349, 352, 357
Biennials, Whitney. *See* Whitney Museum of American Art, **shows**
Bierstadt, Albert, 45
Bilotti, Salvatore, 158
Bingham, George Caleb, 389
Bingham, Robert Worth, 392 and n.
Biomorphic abstraction, Whitney preference for, 375, 376
Bishop, Isabel, 318; in Whitney Studio Club and shows, 169, 208, 222, 233
Bishop, Robert, 145
Blakelock, Ralph Albert, 262
Blanch, Arnold, 252; in Woodstock, 230, 231, 468, 473

Blanch, Lucile, 231, 252
Blanche, Jacques-Emile, 121
Blashfield, Edwin, 113
Bliss, Lillie P., 172, 262; collection of, 101, 170
Bloch, Julius, 312, 374; and JF, 255, 328, 372–373
Bloch, Lucienne, 352
Bluemner, Oscar, 8, 351; *Composition*, 318; death of, 402; and JF, 269 and n., 270, 277, 402; *Last Evening of the Year*, 269 and n.; *Old Canal Port*, 269 and n.; in Stieglitz circle, 269; Whitney Galleries show (1929), 269, 277; on Whitney Museum biennials, 285; in Whitney Museum shows and collection, 166, 269 and n., 318, 375
Blume, Peter, 284, 301, 443, 463; *The Light of the World*, 318, 363
Blumenthal, George, 440
Bohrod, Aaron, 329, 427
Bolotowsky, Ilya: on PWAP, 343, 346; in The Ten, 407–409
Bonheur, Rosa, *The Horse Fair*, 46
Boothe, Clare, 428
Borglum, Gutzon, 6, 102, 112
Boston, 56, 102, 166, 253
Boswell, Peyton, Sr., 271
Bouché, Louis, 81, 116, 220, 299, 306–307, 463; *Arrangement, 280*; and Whitney Galleries, 256, 280; and Whitney Studio Club, 169, 233, 236
Bouguereau, Adolphe William, 46, 47
Bourdelle, Antoine, 55, 187
Bourgeois, Louise, 476
Bourgeois Gallery, 154
Boyer, Philip, 328, 372–373, 374, 419
Boyer Galleries, 328, 374
Brancusi, Constantin, 101, 105, 121, 165, 186, 222, 287, 306; *Bird in Space*, and trial over, 243–244, 248 and n., 369; Brummer Gallery show (1926), 243, 244; *Prometheus*, 191, 307
Brangwyn, Frank, 121
Braque, Georges, 114, 199, 202, 262, 272, 457
Breakers, The (Newport, R.I.), 38, 44, 51, 52
Brenner, Anita, 324, 395
Breton, André, 471
Breuer, Marcel, 505, 506
Brevoort Hotel, 132, 142, 166, 242
Brook, Alexander, 188, 202, 247, 253, 297, 447; criticism of GW's work, 239, 243–244; in Downtown Gallery, 253; and JF, 9–10, 188, 195–196, 208–210, 212, 215, 219–222, 229, 233, 239–240, 242–243, 256; and John Graham, 209–210; photograph of, *203*; as Whitney Studio Club assistant director, 195–196, 201–

Conner, Gertrude (Gerta) Henry, 414–415
Constructivism, 114, 375
Contemporary North American Painting
(1941), 427
Cook, George Cram, 132
Coolidge, Calvin, 233, 242
Cooper-Hewitt (Cooper Union) Museum, 471,
480
Copley, J. S., 273, 389
Corcoran Gallery of Art, 56, 270, 321, 395*n*.;
1934 PWAP show, 357–359
Cornell, Joseph, 235
Corporate art collections, 1940s growth of,
460–461
Cortissoz, Royal, 104 and *n*., 105, 165, 252,
291, 431; on Whitney Museum, 311,
313, 431–432, 438
Couture, Thomas, 46
Covarrubias, Miguel, 201
Coward, Noël, 8, 35
Coward, Thomas (Tim), 467, 475
Craig, Martin, 340
Cramer, Florence, 297, 340, 432
Cramer, Konrad, 203, 229; in Whitney
Museum shows, 318, 375; in Whitney
Studio Club and shows, 208, 214,
222
Craven, Thomas, 271
Crawford, Ralston, 484
Creative Art, 272
Cresson, Margaret French, 484
Criss, Francis, 317, 345
Crocker, Frank L., 369; death of, 473; vs. JF,
380–382, 385–390, 394, 397, 398, 404–
405, 414, 423, 425–426, 433, 436–437,
442, 444, 463, 473; and Fiske Kimball,
457–459, 464, 465, 475; and little Gloria
custody battle, 369, 371, 372; and GW,
372, 380–382, 385–386, 390, 394, 397,
398, 401, 404, 414, 426, 431, 437; and
Whitney merger agreements, 442, 446,
451–453, 458, 464–465, 473; as Whitney
Museum trustee, 386, 439, 440
Cropsey, Jasper, 45
Crowninshield, Frank, 145, 156, 248
Cubism, 68, 69, 71, 102, 104, 105, 119, 120,
173, 185, 202, 270, 272, 375, 377
Cubism and Abstract Art (1936, MOMA),
248*n*., 377
Curran, Charles C., 439
Curran, Mary, 373 and *n*.
Curry, John Steuart, 8, 270–271; *Baptism in
Kansas*, 270, 272, 363; *The Flying
Codonas*, 318; and JF, 270 and *n*., 271,
272; *The Ne'er-Do-Well*, 272; and
Regionalism, 271 and *n*., 272, 273; *The
Stockman*, 272; Whitney Galleries show
(1930), 272; in Whitney Studio Club,
270
Curtis, Edward L., 170

Cushing, Howard, 57, 58, 59, 60, 61, 63, 92,
178; in Whitney Studio shows, 112, 122
Cushing, Olivia, 58, 59

Dabo, Leon, 156
Dada, 202, 256
Daily Worker, 351, 426
Dali, Salvador, 427, 471
Dallas Museum of Fine Arts, 327
Dana, Nathalie, 47, 57
Daniel Gallery, 198, 225–226, 253
Dasburg, Andrew, 75, 187, 214, 222, 229,
282, 375, 425
Daumier, Honoré, 71, 115, 186, 192, 199,
257, 485
Davenport (Iowa) Municipal Gallery, 274
Davey, Randall, 72, 113, 131
Davidge, Clara S., 101, 103
Davidson, Jo, 8, 75, 102, 144, 158, 209, 256,
399, 427, 463; and Indigenous Exhibition
(1918), 151–154; in MacDougal Alley,
167; and GW, 167, 168, 179, 235, 236,
258, 361*n*., 438–439; in Whitney
Museum shows and collection, 336; in
Whitney Studio Club and shows, 157,
192, 222, 251; in Whitney Studio shows,
137
Davidson, Morris, 375
Davidson, Yvonne, 209, 361*n*.
Davies, Arthur B., 72, 74, 78, 82, 83, 139,
144, 172, 221, 313, 371; and Armory
Show, 101–104; and The Eight show
(1908), 83–84; and JF, 112; and GW, 83,
121; in Whitney Museum shows and
collection, 166, 374–375; and Whitney
Studio Club, 156; in Whitney Studio
shows, 113, 199
Davis, Stuart, 8, 72, 78, 132, 282, 314, 326,
352, 377, 379, 395, 396, 405, 411, 428,
434, 463, 484; *Bull Durham*, 173 and *n*.,
237 and *n*.; *Cigarette Papers*, 237 and *n*.;
in Downtown Gallery, 253; *Early
American Landscape*, 252 and *n*.;
Eggbeater, Number 2, 252 and *n*.;
Eggbeater, Number 4, 212 and *n*., 213;
Eggbeater series, 212 and *n*., 213, 237;
and JF, 173–174, 212–213, 236–237,
252, 277, 376, 417, 422, 427–428; *House
and Street*, 428; and Indigenous
Exhibition (1918), 15, 152; *Lucky Strike*,
173 and *n*., 237 and *n*.; in Metropolitan
collection, 422 and *n*., 440; in MOMA
show, 283; *Multiple Views*, 151; and
National Academy, 239; 1926
retrospective, 236–237; *Place Pasdeloup*,
252 and *n*., 363; on PWAP, 340, 345,
357; *Radio Tubes*, 417 and *n*., 418; on
Regionalism, 272–273; *Sweet Caporal*,
237 and *n*.; on GW, 106; in Whitney
Studio Galleries shows, 272–273; in

Davis, Stuart (*cont.*)
    Whitney Museum and collection, 318,
    375, 388, 427–428, 460; in Whitney
    Studio Club and shows, 159, 173–174,
    182, 192, 201, 212–213, 222, 236–237;
    in Whitney Studio shows, 148
Davis, Warren, 115, 122, 123
Day, Horace, 378
de Chirico, Giorgio, 457
de Diego, Julio, *The Portentous City*, 469
de Forest, Robert, 263
Degas, Edgar, 115, 172, 187, 192, 257
De Kooning, Willem, 377
Delacroix, Eugène, 187, 199
Delaney, Beauford, 279
Delano, Frederic A., 337
Delano, William Adams, 100, 386, 390
de Lanux, Eyre, 362 and *n.*
Delaware Art Museum, 138*n.*
DeMenil Collection, 237*n.*
de Meyer, Baron Adolf, 109, 138
Deming, Edward, 76, 77, 82
Demuth, Charles, 8, 132, 186, 199, 202,
    289, 314, 433; and JF, 198, 328, 374;
    From the Garden of the Chateau, 328,
    374; illustrations for *Nana*, 177; *My
    Egypt*, 301, 363; and Stieglitz circle, 223,
    225, 302; in Whitney Museum shows and
    collection, 166, 301, 302, 328, 375, 428;
    in Whitney Studio Club and shows, 222,
    225, 238; in Whitney Studio shows, 148,
    198
Denver Art Museum, 249, 286
Depression, 266, 267, 281, 385, 395; effects
    on Whitney-Force operations, 266, 273–
    274, 309–311, 329, 330–332, 380–382,
    386; impact on artists, 309–311, 330–
    332, 355; relief programs for artists, *see*
    Public Works of Art Project; Works
    Progress Administration's Federal Art
    Project
Derain, André, 121, 172, 173, 199
de Rivera, José, 345
de Rosales, Emanuele, 109
Despiau, Charles, 187
de Strelecki, Jean, 138
Detroit Institute of Art, 434, 478*n.*
Devree, Howard, 444, 488
Dewey, Thomas E., 471, 473, 482, 484
de Zayas, Marius, 191, 198, 202; collection
    of, 170; as organizer of Whitney Studio
    shows, 191, 192, 198–200, 203, 210,
    223; and Stieglitz, 225
d'Harnoncourt, Rene, 448
Dial, The, 181, 227
Dickinson, Edwin, 376
Dickinson, Preston, 1, 198 and *n.*, 306
Diederich, Hunt, 153
Diller, Burgoyne, 317, 346, 357
Dirks, Rudy, 222
Dos Passos, John, 8, 187, 188, 222; and JF,

181–182, 184–185; Whitney Studio Club
    shows (1923–1925), 184–185
Dougherty, Paul, 82, 151, 152, *152*, 172
Dove, Arthur, 69, 73, 284, 440, 484; *Red
    Barge, Reflections*, 318; in Stieglitz circle,
    223, 225, 227, 228, 302, 318; in
    Whitney Museum shows and collection,
    302, 318, 375, 428
Downtown Gallery, 34, 253, 277, 297, 302,
    303, 309, 317, 328, 331, 374, 453, 469,
    470, 478
Doylestown, Pa., 11, 17–19, 106, 163; JF
    buried in, 504; JF's roots in, 11–19, 20,
    27–28, 106–108; social snobberies of,
    17–18, 108
Draper, Charles, 247 and *n.*, 258, 314
Dreiser, Theodore, 69, 73, 132–133, 450
Drewes, Werner, 345, 375
Driggs, Elsie, 199, 222, 340; *Pittsburgh*, 198
    and *n.*
Duchamp, Marcel, 101, 132, 471; *Apropos
    of Little Sister*, 202 and *n.*; *Chocolate
    Grinder, No. 2*, 202 and *n.*; *Fountain*,
    135 and *n.*, 141; *The King and Queen
    Surrounded by Swift Nudes*, 202 and *n.*;
    *The King and Queen Traversed by Swift
    Nudes*, 202 and *n.*; 1924 Whitney Studio
    Club show, 202–203, 204; *Nude
    Descending a Staircase*, 202 and *n.*, 203,
    204; and Society for Independent Artists,
    135, 141
Dudensing, Valentine, 419, 420, 461
Dudensing Gallery, 253
Duffy, Edmund, 236
Dulac, Edmund, 121
Dunnington, Walter G., 473, 493, 494, 496,
    498, 499
Durand, Asher B., 389
Durand-Ruel, Paul, 199
Durand-Ruel Galleries (Paris), 1923 exhibition
    of American art, 199
Duveneck, Frank, 389
Dwight, Mabel, 116; caricature of Club's life
    class, *196*; on PWAP, 340; in Whitney
    Studio Club and shows, 157, 158, 159,
    196, 232

Eakins, Thomas, 47, 105, 187, 273, 275,
    389, 410; *Between Rounds*, 170*n.*; *The
    Biglin Brothers Racing*, 329 and *n.*; *The
    Concert Singer*, 170*n.*; death of, 170; *The
    Gross Clinic*, 11; influence on New York
    Realists, 71–72; in Overseas Exhibition
    (1920), 170 and *n.*, 171; in Philadelphia
    Museum collection, 457; *Portrait of Riter
    Fitzgerald*, 300 and *n.*, 301; and GW,
    73, 100; *William Rush Carving His
    Allegorical Figure of the Schuylkill River*,
    170*n.*; *Wrestlers*, 457
Early American Art (1924, Whitney Studio
    Club), 201–202

140–141, 216; reform of prize system, 136–137, 141; shows and competitions, 113–116, 135, 140–141; Ward sabotage of, 140–141, 142
Frieseke, Frederick Carl, 121; *Before Her Appearance*, 122; in Whitney Studio shows, 122
Frost, Rosamund, 459
Fry, Roger, 271
Fuller, R. Buckminster, 8, 267–268, 405; and JF, 267–268, 293
Futurism, 185, 377

Gallatin, Albert Eugene, 114–115, 261, 262 and *n.*, 457, 458
Gallatin Collection, 457; in Gallery of Living Art, 262 and *n.*; in Philadelphia Museum of Art, 457; Whitney Studio show of, 114–115, 123
Gallery of Living Art, 262 and *n.*, 457
Ganso, Emil, 252, 255, 432
Gatch, Lee, 407
Gauguin, Paul, 121, 172, 173, 186, 276
Gaylor, Wood, 238
Geist, Sidney, 309–310
Geldzahler, Henry, 284–285
Genthe, Arnold, 138
Geometric abstraction, Whitney resistance to, 375, 376
George, Waldemar, 187
Gerald, Elizabeth Bart, 439, 449, 494, 501, 506
Gerald, John, 416, 417, 439, 501, 502–503, 506
Germany, 406; and Kaiser Friedrich collection controversy, 479–482, 498–499, 500–501; WWII, 415, 423, 433
Gérôme, Jean Léon, 46
Gershoy, Eugenie, 231
Gifford, Sanford, 45
Gilchrist, Thomas, 367, 369, 401
Gimbels Galleries, 372
Givenwilson, Irene, 117–118, 129, 133, 140
Glackens, Edith, 131, 222
Glackens, Ira, 128, 296, 306
Glackens, William, 8, 69, 72, 73, 83, 128, 132, 144, 152, 186, 209, 282, 475; and Armory Show, 101; *Cafe Lafayette*, 122 and *n.*; *Chez Mouquin*, 74 and *n.*; and The Eight show (1908), 83–84, 91; and JF, 131; in Metropolitan collection, 173, 263; *Nude with Apple*, 124 and *n.*; and Society for Independent Artists, 135; in Whitney Museum collection and shows, 301, 395; in Whitney Studio Club and shows, 179, 192, 222; in Whitney Studio shows, 113, 115, 122 and *n.*, 137
Glassgold, Cooke, 287, 340, 375
Gleizes, Albert, 135
Godey's Magazine, 56
Goff, Lloyd Lózes, 379

Goldbeck, Walter D., 138
Goldman, Emma, 8, 81, 128
Goodrich, Edith, 163, 240, 300, 308
Goodrich, Lloyd, 163, 186*n.*, 187, 221, 240, 264, 305, 329, 337*n.*, 436, 451, 470, 472, 485; on American Art Research Council, 433–435; as *The Arts* contributing editor, 257, 258, 265, 275, 293, 295; and Alfred Barr, 337 and *n.*; and JF, 35–36, 188, 257–258, 275–276, 283, 294, 295, 300, 308, 325, 350, 373, 415, 495, 500, 503; and Gorky, 376; as Metropolitan adviser, 440; photograph of, *276*; on PWAP committee, 337, 339, 340–342, 344, 364, 347, 349–350, 357–358; and Stieglitz circle, 226–227, 304; as Whitney Museum associate director, 505; as Whitney Museum curator, 275–276, 277, 283, 285, 294, 301, 304, 325, 375–376, 394, 397, 409, 428, 444, 486, 495–496; as Whitney Museum director, 506
Goodyear, A. Conger, 405, 413
Gorky, Arshile, 284, 377, 464; *Painting*, 376; on PWAP, 345, 357, 376; in Whitney Museum shows and collection, 375, 376, 460
Gottlieb, Adolph, 407, 409, 484
Gottlieb, Harry, 222, 252; and JF, 255; in PWAP, 340; in Whitney Galleries shows, 255, 256
Grafly, Charles, 139
Graham, John, 209, 284, 377, 407, 408; on PWAP, 340, 345; in Whitney Museum shows, 318, 375; in Whitney Studio Club and shows, 209–210, 222
Greenbaum, Dorothea, 251, 300
Greenberg, Clement, 441, 442 and *n.*, 476
Greene, Balcomb, 375, 442
Greene, Stephen, 472
Greenwich Village, 61, 80–81, 151, 177, 178, 261, 278, 371, 447; 1910–1920, 132–133, 141, 167; GW moves her studio to, 75–76. See also MacDougal Alley
Greenwich Village Spectator, The, 155
Gregg, James, 91
Gregory, John, 75, 80, 86, 144, 153, 167, 289, 317, 405
Gropper, William, 208, 222, 352, 440; on PWAP, 351; *The Senate*, 394
Gross, Chaim, 382; on PWAP, 340
Grosz, George, 442, 460
Gruppe, Karl, 79, 80, 339–340; *Manicure Artistic*, 79
Guggenheim, Peggy, 409
Guggenheim, Solomon R., 262
Guggenheim Fellowships, 221, 330, 346, 385, 433
Guggenheim (Solomon R.) Museum, 202*n.*
Gugler, Eric, 384, 389, 405
Guglielmi, O. Louis, 484; *The River*, 470
Guiffrey, Jean, 171 and *n.*

Guston, Philip, 484
Guy, Seymour J., 45; *The William Henry Vanderbilt Family*, 45 and *n*., 46

Hackett, Frances Goodrich, 227
Hague, Raoul, 346
Halpert, Edith Gregor, 34, 170*n*., 192, 253, 275, 309, 317, 328, 374, 450, 501; and JF, 330–331, 342, 404, 461, 469–470
Halpert, Samuel, 222, 253, 301
Hamilton, Carl, 355–356
Hammond, Ogden, 246 and *n*., 258
Harari, Hananiah, 441, 442; *Diagrams in Landscape*, 441 and *n*.
Harris, Louis, 407
Harriton, Abraham, 139
Harshe, Robert, 327–328, 329, 380
Hart, George ("Pop"), 159
Hartl, Leon, 178; and JF, 221; in Whitney Studio Club shows, 178, 221, 238
Hartley, Marsden, 69, 73, 395, 411, 440, 443; *The Old Bars, Dogtown*, 397; in Stieglitz circle, 223, 225, 228, 302, 397; in Whitney Museum shows and collection, 166, 228, 301, 302, 318, 375, 397, 443
Hartman, Bertram, 156
Hartman, Rosella, 441
Haseltine, Herbert, 75
Hassam, Childe, 104, 115, 167, 170*n*.
Hastings, Thomas, 113
Hathaway, Calvin Sutliffe, 480, 481, 498, 499, 500, 501
Hawthorne, Charles, 77, 121, 122
Hayden, Palmer, 317
Hearn, George A., 262–263
Hearst, William Randolph, 8; his headlining of little Gloria custody battle, 370–371; and 1934 Venice Biennale controversy, 363–366, 370; State Department collection attacked by his syndicate, 484–485
Hecht, Ben, 100–101
Held, John, Jr., 222
Heliker, John, 442
Henri, Marjorie Organ, 127; caricature by, *127*
Henri, Robert, 8, 68, 72, 73, 126, 128, 131, 132, 229, 311; and Armory Show, 101, 103; caricature of, *127*; his circle and influence, 69–75, 82, 113, 143, 223, 313; and Eakins, 71–72; and The Eight show (1908), 83–84, 91–93; and Exhibition of Independent Artists (1910), 78; on exhibition procedure reform, 135, 143; and JF, 112, 143, 223; *Herself*, 122 and *n*.; and Indigenous Exhibition (1918), 150–151, 153 and *n*.; *Laughing Child*, 92 and *n*., 93, 122 and *n*.; in Metropolitan collection, 263; vs. National Academy, 74, 78, 83–84, 91, 92; photograph of, *70*; GW's relations with

his circle, 73–75, 82–84, 91–93, 102, 113, 117, 122, 131, 143, 158, 170, 178, 223, 313, 395; in Whitney Museum shows, 395; and Whitney Studio Club shows, 153*n*.; in Whitney Studio shows, 122 and *n*., 137
Henry, Barbara Whitney, 62, *63*, 117, 118, 179, 368, 414, 437
Henry, Barklie, 414
Henry, E. L., 201
Herald Tribune, 263, 354, 356, 464
Hering, Harry, 232
Hersey, Brig. Gen. Mark L., 179, 234
Higgins, Eugene, 115, 116, 152
Hill, W. E., 201, 212, 222
Hine, Lewis, 69
Hirsch, Stefan, 318, 375
Hirshhorn Museum and Sculpture Garden, 122*n*.
Hitchcock, Henry-Russell, 187
Hitler, Adolf, 364, 423, 424, 479
Hoboken, N.J., 20, 87, 155–156; JF's early life in, 20, *20*, 21–36, 88–90, 96
Hoffman, Malvina, 76, 112, 113, 145
Hofmann, Hans, 414, 439, 476
Hogarth, William, 257, 358
Holty, Carl, 375, 476
Holtzman, Harry, 340, 345, 346
Homer, Winslow, 45, 187, 389, 394
Hoover, Herbert, 267, 311
Hopkins, Harry L., 334
Hopper, Edward, 8, 72, 78, 179, 187, 282, 314, 410, 411, 434, 464; *The Circle Theatre*, 394; *Early Sunday Morning*, 288, *363*; and JF, 169, 233, 288; in Metropolitan collection, 440; in MOMA show, 283; and Regionalism, 271 and *n*.; in Whitney Museum shows and collection, 166, 288, 318, 394; in Whitney Studio Club and shows, 159, 169, 170, 179, 182, 192, 195, *196*, 199, 222, 238, 244
Hopper, Inslee, 226
Horter, Earl, 375, 428
Hound & Horn, 313
House & Garden, 308
Howard, Cecil, 214, 258, 259, 260, 273, 274
Howe, Thomas Carr, 327, 480
Howells, William Dean, 67, 69
Hudson River School, 187
Huneker, James, 84, 91
Hunt, Henry T., 333
Hunt, Richard Morris, 38

Ickes, Harold, 333, 334
Immigrant in America show (1915, Whitney Studio), 117, 118–*120*, 131
Immigration and the arts, 68–69, 117
Impressionism, 68, 71, 102, 114, 170, 172–173, 199; American, 84, 114, 122, 170
Independents, 223; Independent Show (1910),

Laning, Edward, 79, 324, 340, 351, 352, 353, 378, 403, 419, 423
Lassaw, Ibram, 342, 343, 345, 346
La Touche, Gaston, 121
Laurent, Robert, 140, 156, 185, 192, 220, 222, 301, 371; *The Awakening, 290*
Lavery, John, 121
Lawrence, Jacob, 478; *John Brown* series, 478 and *n.; Tombstones,* 460
Lawson, Adelaide, 181–182, 184
Lawson, Ernest, 72, 74, 77, 82, 83, 84, 144; and Armory Show, 101; and The Eight show (1908), 83–84, 92, 93, 178; and GW, 92, 178; in Whitney Museum shows, 395; in Whitney Studio Club and shows, 156, 222; in Whitney Studio shows, 112, 113, 115, 121, 122 and *n.; Winter on the River,* 92 and *n.,* 93, 122 and *n.,* 178, 363
Lay, Charles Downing, 263
Lazzari, Pietro, 345–346
Lechay, Myron, 252
Le Corbusier (Charles Edouard Jeanneret), 309
Lee, Arthur, 75, 153
Lefebvre, Jules Joseph, 46
Léger, Fernand, 114, 262, 273, 287, 376, 427, 457, 471, 472
Lentelli, Leo, 405
Lescaze, William, 208, 222
Lever, Hayley, 355
Levi, Julian, 463
Levy, Edgar, 377, 407, 408
Lewis, Martin, 208, 222
Lewisohn, Adolph, collection of, 170
Lie, Jonas, 82, 156
Life magazine, 373
Lindbergh, Charles, 251
Lipchitz, Jacques, 471
Lippmann, Walter, 333
Literary Digest, The, 128
Little Galleries of the Photo-Secession, 69, 113
Little Gallery of Contemporary Art, Phila., 373*n.*
Little Review, The, 132
Loan Exhibition of Impressionist and Post-Impressionist Paintings (1921, Metropolitan Museum), 172–173
Locher, Robert, 202, 220, 225, 307, 314, 341, 347
Locke, Alain, 187
Locke, Charles, 305
Lockwood, Ward, 425
Look magazine, 485
Louvre, 171*n.*
Lowenthal, Milton and Edith, 461, 469–470, 478*n.,* 488, 493
Lozowick, Louis, 222, 340, 352
Luce, Molly, 214, 425
Ludington, Wright, 469

Ludins, Eugene, 325, 354, 450; *Landscape,* 310 and *n.*
Luhan, Mabel Dodge, 187
Luks, George, 8, 69, 72, 78, 83, 151*n.,* 410, 433, 475; and Armory Show, 101; and The Eight show (1908), 83–84, 92, 93; and Indigenous Exhibition (1918), 151, 152, *152,* 168; in Metropolitan collection, 173, 263; *Mrs. Gamley,* 301, *315; The Spielers,* 122 and *n.,* 395 and *n.;* and GW, 92, 152–153, 168, 314; in Whitney Museum shows and collection, 166, 301, 395; in Whitney Studio shows, 115, 121, 122 and *n.,* 137, 138; *Woman with Goose,* 92 and *n.,* 93
Lusitania, 111, 115
Lynes, George Platt, 461

Macbeth, William, 66, 112, 113, 121
Macbeth Gallery, The Eight show (1908), 83, 91–93
Macdonald-Wright, Stanton, 375
MacDougal Alley, 61, 123, 131, 288, 416; Alley Festa (1917), 144–145; No. 19 (GW's studio), 75–77, 80–81, 84, 86, 92, 98–100, 105–106, 167–168, 178, 192, *412,* 437; 1919–1921 gatherings, 167–169; photographs of, *76, 412;* No. 23, 167–168. *See also* Whitney Studio
MacDougal Alley sculpture show, 162
Macmillan, 472, 500
MacMonnies, Frederick, 248
MacRae, Elmer, 101, 102
Madison Gallery, 101, 103
Magazine of Art, 455, 464, 480, 481
Mager, Gus, 301
Magic Realism, 375
Maillol, Aristide, 176, 187, 199, 485
Mancini, Antonio, 121
Manet, Édouard, 71, 102, 115, 199
Mangravite, Peppino, 455, 464
Mannes, Marya, 251
Manship, Paul, 144, 145, 154, 248, 403, 405, 427, 434; in Whitney Studio Club and shows, 222; in Whitney Studio shows, 113, 153
Marceau, Henri, 443
Marin, John, 69, 71, 314, 344, 363; *Deer Island, Maine,* 303; *Off Cape Split, Maine,* 477; in Stieglitz circle, 223–228, 302, 303, 443; *Sunset,* 303; in Whitney Museum shows and collection, 228, 301, 303, 375, 428, 442, 443; *The Woolworth Building,* 303
Marsh, Reginald, 8, 233, 275, 282, 358, 411, 454, 463, 474; in Whitney Museum collection, 166, 301; in Whitney Studio Club and shows, 159, 169, 208, 214, 222, 238, 270; *Why Not Use the "L"?,* 301, 363
Martiny, Philip, 77

Masses, The, 132
Masson, André, 471
Master Institute of United Artists, 220
Matisse, Henri, 69, 103, 104, 121, 165, 173, 186, 199, 287, 485
Matisse, Pierre, 362 and *n.*, 461
Matulka, Jan, 252; on PWAP, 345, 346; in Whitney Museum shows, 375; in Whitney Studio Club and shows, *196*, 222, 232
Maurer, Alfred, 75, 102, 2~8, 375, 433
Maxwell, Elsa, 145
Mayer, Arthur, 396
Mayor, A. Hyatt, 313–314, 472, 500, 503
McAdams, Edgar, 75
McBride, Henry, 136, 139, 154, 186, 187, 227, 244, 248, 262, 311, 318, 449, 461; on decline of National Academy, 239; and JF, 417, 419; on MOMA, 276; on Whitney shows, 183, 203, 208, 237, 238, 256–257, 272–273, 276, 285, 312, 377, 395
McCausland, Elizabeth, 397, 470
McFee, Henry Lee, 229
McKim, Charles, 64
McLane, Laura, 130–131
McMahon, Audrey, 352, 357; vs. JF, 352–354, 421, 426; on Francis Taylor, 421–422
Mears, Helen Farnsworth, 130
Meissonier, Jean, 46
Mellon, Andrew, 267
Mellon Galleries, 328
Mercury Galleries, The Whitney Dissenters Show (1938), 407–409
Metropolitan Museum of Art, 4, 38, 46, 58, 75, 186*n.*, 228, 284, 313, 318, 326, 351*n.*, 356*n.*, 379, 389, 419*n.*, 420, 427, 434, 437, 463, 471; American art in, 173, 202, 245, 251, 261, 262–263, 422 and *n.*, 440, 443; Artists for Victory show (1942), 443; conservative exhibition policies, 154, 172–173, 262–264, 278, 422, 440, 496; Hearn funds, 262–263, 440, 443, 444, 446, 451, 459–460, 469, 478, 486, 497; incorporation of, 56; Loan Exhibition of Impressionist and Post-Impressionist Paintings (1921), 172–173; merger agreements, and abandonment of, 431, 437–438, 451–453, 458–460, 464–465, 475, 485–486, 489, 495–496, 498, 499, 501, 505; modern art ignored by, 5, 46, 172–173, 262–264, 278, 422, 440, 496; National Academy affiliations, 144, 172; 1918 American sculpture exhibition, 154; Stettheimer's *Cathedrals of Art* in, 462, 463; Francis Taylor as director of, 420–422, 440, 442–444, 451, 459, 464–465; Whitney-Force relations with, 128, 173, 261–264, 278, 420–422, 431, 437–448, 451–453, 458–460, 464–465, 485–

486, 489, 495–496; GW's collection first offered to (1929), 261–265, 278; GW's work in, 128, 261
Meyer, Agnes, 172
Meyer, Herbert, 447
Milch Gallery, 329
Millay, Edna St. Vincent, 211
Miller, Dorothy, 472, 485
Miller, Flora Whitney Tower, 52, 53, 62, 117, 118, 133, 211–212, 234, 258, 289, 211–212, 234, 258, 289, 362*n.*, 438, 440, 446, 470, 506; Eighth St. buildings inherited by, 437, 449, 452; and JF's illness, 492–493, 495, 502; Whitney-Metropolitan merger agreements, and abandonment of, 444, 447, 449, 451–453, 458, 464–465, 475, 496; as Whitney Museum trustee, 386, 437, 439
Miller, G. Macculloch, 258, 289; as Whitney Museum trustee, 439, 440, 451
Miller, George, 236
Miller, Kenneth Hayes, 157, 169, 252, 289
Milliken, William, 335
Milwaukee Art Museum, 122*n.*
Minneapolis Institute of Arts, 249, 250, 455
Miró, Joan, 262, 287, 376, 457
Modernism, 69–75, 170; and American art, divisions between, 271–273, 377–378; and Armory Show, 100–105; and customs regulations, 243–244, 248 and *n.*; expansion of commercial galleries and public institutions, 253–254, 260, 261–262; ignored by Metropolitan Museum, 5, 46, 172–173, 262–264, 278, 422, 440, 496; New York Realists vs. Stieglitz circle, 69–73, 223–228, 313; and PWAP, 338, 341, 345–346, 357; vs. Regionalism, 271–273; Whitney Museum's changing tastes in, 375–378, 476–478; GW's reluctant acceptance of, 101–105, 121–122, 243. *See also* European modernism; *specific artists and movements*
Modern Paintings by American and Foreign Artists (1916, Whitney Studio), 121–122
Mondrian, Piet, 262, 375, 376, 457, 471
Monet, Claude, 172, 199
Montross Gallery, 215
Moody, Dwight L., 29, 32, 33, 89
Moore, Alexander P., 245–247, 249, 258
Moore, Charles, 333, 334
Moore, James B., 74, 84
Moore, Marianne, 73, 344
Mora, F. Luis, 152, 153
More, Edna, 274, 275, 309
More, Hermon, 261, 274, 309, 428, 434, 451, 472, 485; and JF, 274–275, 300, 468, 503; as Whitney museum curator, 274–275, 282, 283, 291, 292, 301, 304, 310, 328–329, 375, 396, 404, 409, 441, 476, 477, 486, 495–496; as Whitney Museum director, 505

Morgan, Anne, 246, 247
Morgan, Herbert, 309
Morgan, J. Pierpont, 138, 246
Morgan, Laura Kirkpatrick, 368–370
Morgan, Maud, 409
Morley, Christopher, 8, 293, 311
Morris, George L. K., 442
Morris, Newbold, 428
Moses, Robert, 339–340, 347, 389, 428, 440, 452
Motherwell, Robert, 476, 484
Motley, Archibald, 329
Mumford, Lewis, 358, 359 and n., 379
Mungo-Park, Eirene, 214–216, 217, 221–223, 244, 275
Municipal Art Society, 56
Munsey, Frank, 165
Murdock Collection (Wichita), 410–411
Murphy, Gerald, 376n.
Musée d' Orsay (Paris), 172
Museum of American Folk Art, 145
Museum of Fine Arts, Boston, 56, 171n., 217n., 356, 499
Museum of Modern Art, 173n., 192n., 228, 265, 326, 389, 404, 405, 406, 421, 427, 448, 463, 470, 477; Barr fired from, 456; Cubism and Abstract Art (1936), 248n.; emphasis on international modernism, 101, 278, 287, 338; opening of (1929), 186, 262, 266, 276; origins in the Armory Show, 101; policies on American art, 278, 281, 283, 287, 302, 377, 394; and PWAP, 338, 344; retrospectives of 1930s and 1940s, 283, 287; and Stieglitz, 302; and the Three Museum Agreement, 485–486, 489, 495–496, 498, 499, 501; Whitney-Force relations with, 286, 287–288, 344, 394, 431, 434, 446, 505
Museum of the City of New York, 286, 389, 415
Music, modern, Whitney-Force patronage of, 174–175, 177, 180, 193–194, 196–197, 216, 248–249
Mussolini, Benito, 363, 364
Myers, Ethel, 156, 222
Myers, Jerome, 72, 78, 82, 83; and Armory Show, 101, 103; on JF, 142; on PWAP, 342; in Whitney Studio Club and shows, 156, 192, 222

Nadelman, Elie, 153, 248
Nakian, Reuben, 8, 182, 282, 344; in Downtown Gallery, 253; and JF, 181, 184, 219–220, 228, 235; The Lap Dog, 235; Pastorale, 235; in Whitney Museum collection, 181n., 235, 301; in Whitney Studio Club and shows, 181, 184, 192, 222, 235, 251
Nast, Thomas, 314
Nation, The, 311, 324, 333, 441
National Academy of Design, 74, 143, 154,

228, 242, 253; conservatism of, 5, 68, 69, 147, 170, 438–439; 1874 exhibition, 45–46; vs. Henri circle, 74, 78–79, 83–84, 91, 92, 408; Metropolitan Museum affiliations, 144, 172; 1907 annual, 83; 1910 annual, 78–79; 1927 annual, 239; post-Armory Show decline of, 101, 144, 239; and PWAP, 337–338, 349; Forbes Watson on, 165; Whitney-Force relations with, 78–79, 80, 92, 99, 239, 438–439
National Commission of Fine Arts, 234
National Gallery of Art, 286, 329n., 428, 448; and Kaiser Friedrich collection controversy, 480, 481, 498
National Sculpture Society, 80, 154, 242
Navas, Elizabeth Stubblefield, 410–411, 501
Nazis, 208, 315, 406, 415, 423–424, 467, 471, 479
Neel, Alice, 317
Nelson-Atkins Museum of Art, 271n.
Neo-Plasticism, 114, 375, 376, 377
Neuberger, Roy, 461
Neumann, J. B., 376
Nevelson, Louise, 352, 476
Newark Museum, 279, 286, 337
New Britain Museum of American Art, 322n.
New Deal, 4, 34, 332, 337, 346, 348, 354, 358. See also Public Works of Art Project (PWAP); Works Progress Administration
Newman, Robert Loftin, 374–375
New Orleans Arts and Crafts Club, 249, 250
Newport, R.I., 38, 48, 49, 50, 51, 52, 57, 58, 75, 129, 133; GW's studio in, 58, 59, 60, 61
Newport Art Association, 133, 144
Newport Art Museum, 133
New Republic, The, 333
New School for Social Research, 293, 322
Newsweek, 473, 474
New York American, 91
New York art scene, 141; and Armory Show, 100–105; early conservatism of, 4–5, 46–47, 65–69, 74, 78–79, 83–84; early modernism, 69–75; and The Eight show (1908), 91–93; expansion of commercial art galleries and public institutions, 253–254, 260, 261–262; late-nineteenth-century growth of, 56; mid-1940s growth of, 460–461; New York Realists vs. Stieglitz circle, 69–73, 223–228, 313; post-JF changes in, 505–506; and WWII, 141. See also specific artists, galleries, movements, museums and shows
New York City Parks Department, 339–340, 347, 389
New Yorker, The, 227, 235, 358, 368, 379, 441
New York Herald, 77, 123
New-York Historical Society, 145 and n., 413
New York Post, 338, 403; Forbes Watson as art critic for, 116, 123, 138, 165, 225

New York Public Library, 113, 319
New York Realists, 72, 222, 394–395; and
Armory Show, 101–105; Eakins's
influence on, 71–72; as early modernists,
69–75; The Eight show (1908), 72, 83–
84, 91–93, 223; and exhibition procedure
reform, 135, 136, 143; Henri's circle and
influence, 69–75; in Metropolitan
collection, 173, 263; vs. National
Academy, 74, 78–79, 83–84, 91, 92,
408; in Overseas Exhibition (1920), 170
and n., 171; Whitney Museum founded
on, 92 and n., 101, 223, 287, 313, 394–
395; GW's relations with, 73–75, 82–84,
91–93, 102, 113, 117, 122–124, 131,
143, 170, 178, 223, 313, 395. See also
Eight, The; specific artists
New York Realists: 1900 to 1914 (1937,
Whitney Museum), 394–395
New York School, 209, 396, 476–478
New York State art legislation, 5, 489; JF
lobbies for, 470–471, 473–474, 475, 478,
482, 484, 489
New York State Council on the Arts, 484
New York State Museum in Albany, 470
New York Studio School, 505
New York Sun, 91, 94n., 123, 136, 139, 227
New York Times, 79, 83, 120, 202, 227n.,
242, 243, 257, 272, 285, 313, 371, 444,
478, 480
New York Tribune, 104n., 192, 201
New York University, 262, 457
New York World, 120, 127; Forbes Watson as
art critic for, 165, 185, 226, 296
New York World's Fair (1939), 384, 389,
402–403, 405, 411, 413, 415, 422, 423,
460
Nichols, Hobart, 439
Noel & Miller, 289, 384
Noguchi, Isamu, 8, 301, 464; and JF, 346–
348, 410; Humpty Dumpty, 478;
Monument to Ben Franklin, 346, 347
and n.; Monument to the Plough, 346,
347 and n.; Play Mountain, 346, 347
and n.; on PWAP, 346–348; Radio
Nurse, 410
Nolder, Edith Lewis, 486–487, 489, 494, 495
Norris, Frank, 73; Blix, 65
Norton Gallery and School of Art, 304n.

O'Connor, Andrew, 75, 77, 86, 109, 153,
158, 167; Head of Lincoln, 290; and
GW, 79–80, 109, 178, 234, 235, 247,
258
O'Day, Caroline, 163
O'Keeffe, Georgia, 434, 464, 484; in MOMA
shows, 302; The Mountain, New Mexico,
303–304, 363; 1917 show at 291, 141;
Pelvis with the Moon, New Mexico, 304
and n.; Skunk Cabbage, 303 and n.; and
Stieglitz, 141, 223, 224, 225, 226, 227,

302–304; White Flower, 303–304; in
Whitney Museum shows and collection,
166, 228, 303–304, 318, 375, 428
Olds, Elizabeth, 470
Old Westbury, Long Island, 49, 52, 75, 117,
129, 291, 339, 467; little Gloria
Vanderbilt in, 367, 368–369, 370; GW's
studio in, 100, 105, 108, 178
O'Neill, Eugene, 132, 450
Orozco, José Clemente, 201 and n., 250,
359n.
Orpen, Sir William, 121
Osborn, William Church, 460, 486
Overseas Exhibition (1920–1921), 170–172,
175, 176, 177, 199, 406
Ozenfant, Amédée, 427

Pach, Walter, 135, 187, 375
Pachner, William, 474
Page, William H., 245–247, 258
Panama-Pacific Exposition (1915), 118, 121,
122, 130
Pan-American Exposition (1901, Buffalo), 60
Paris, 47, 132, 399; American artists in, 75,
252; Beaux-Arts training in, 54; 1923
Durand-Ruel show of American art, 199;
Three Centuries of American Art (1938),
406; GW in, 75, 80, 86, 171; WWI,
111, 112. See also specific artists and
museums
Paris Salon, 135, 170; of 1924, 80
Paris, School of, 101, 103, 121, 199, 210,
242, 270, 313. See also specific artists
Parke-Bernet Galleries, 411, 413, 450
Parker, Thomas, 481
Parkhurst, Charles, 480
Parrish, Maxfield, 82, 122
Parsons, Betty, 7, 409
Pascin, Jules, 222, 238
Pène du Bois, Guy, 1, 8, 34–35, 72, 78, 91,
135, 139, 158, 170n., 187, 209, 247,
256, 282, 427; on Bob Chanler, 81, 82;
on expansion of commercial galleries,
260–261; and JF, 131, 143, 169, 175–
176, 211, 258, 488, 503; on Henri, 74;
and Indigenous Exhibition (1918), 151,
152, 152; Juliana Force at the Whitney
Studio Club, 175 and n., 175, 176; in
MacDougal Alley, 167–168; in
Metropolitan collection, 173; The Three
Hour Portrait: A Comedy by George Luks
in Six Acts, 168 and n.; and GW, 167,
168, 169, 235, 258, 259; in Whitney
Museum shows and collection, 301, 395;
in Whitney Studio Club and shows, 157,
182, 192, 222, 238; in Whitney Studio
shows, 113, 139; A Window in the
Union Club, 151 and n.; work of, 241
Pennsylvania Academy of the Fine Arts, 72
Pereira, I. Rice, 375
Perkins, Frances, 333

Rieser, Irene Grosel, 107, 176, 197, 382, 400, 407, 411
Rieser, Joseph, 17, 28, 413
Rieser, Julia Schmutz Kuster, 12, 13 and *n.*, *14*, *23*, 26–28, 96, 107, 217, 490; financial and social decline, 17–22, 33, 88, 217; first marriage of, and widowhood, 13–17; and JF, 22–24, 89–90, 213, 217; marriage to Max Rieser, 15–17, 21–22, 88; Sheeler's painting of, 217 and *n.*
Rieser, Louis, 17, 22, 24, 28, 32
Rieser, Marjorie, 24, 26, 90, 121
Rieser, Mary, 10, 17, 22, *23*, 25, 28, 89, 148, *149*, 392, 450–451, 492; supported by JF, 22, 24, 25, 108, 382
Rieser, Mathias, 15–16
Rieser, Maximilian (brother of JF), 12, 17, 25–*26*, 28, 134, *149*, 500
Rieser, Maximilian (father of JF), 11, 15–16, 28, 96, 107; financial and social decline, 16–22, 33, 88; and JF, 24, 30; marriage to Julia Kuster, 15–17, 21–22, 88
Rieser, Robert, 17 and *n.*, 25, 28, 155–156
Rindner, Genevieve, 432, 503
Ritchie, Andrew C., 480
Rivera, Diego, 187; Rockefeller Center mural controversy, 352
Robb, William, 240
Robert, Lawrence W., 333, 335
Roberts, Laurance, 405, 434, 448
Roberts, Mary Fanton, 128, 305
Roberts, Owen, 481, 482
Robinson, Boardman, 132, 179, 199, 222, 301
Robinson, Edward, 261; as Metropolitan director, 261, 263–264, 278, 327, 440
Robinson, Edward Arlington, 69, 74
Robinson, Theodore, 170*n.*, 262
Rockefeller, Abby Aldrich, 145, 262, 295, 302, 309, 315, 404, 413, 446; aid to Depression artists, 310, 317, 331, 372
Rockefeller, Blanchette, 404
Rockefeller, Nelson, 330, 352, 427, 484
Rockefeller Center, 330; Rivera mural controversy, 352
Rockefeller family, 262, 352
Rodin, Auguste, 55, 115
Rodzinski, Artur, 249
Roesen, Severin, 147*n.*; *Nature's Bounty*, 147
Rohland, Paul, 255, 256, 272; *Peonies*, *305*
Rollins, Lloyd, on PWAP, 341, 347
Romney, George, 47
Roosevelt, Eleanor, 333, 336–337, 358, 394
Roosevelt, Franklin D., 87, 134, 267, 332, 335, 427, 429; and New Deal art projects, 332–333, 341, 352, 358, 394, 426
Roosevelt, Theodore, 8, 61, 118–*120*, 131, 134, 450
Rorimer, James, 480

Rosen, Charles, 230
Rosenborg, Ralph, 345
Rosenfeld, Paul, 248; on Whitney Museum, 313
Roszak, Theodore, 318, 328, 329, 375, 442
Roth, Frederick G. R., 130
Rothko, Mark, 396, 407, 409, 476
Rouault, Georges, 173, 187, 485
Rourke, Constance, 407*n.*
Rousseau, Henri, 135, 192, 277, 306; *Mauvais Surprise*, 200 and *n.*; Whitney Studio show, 199–200, 202
Rubens, Peter Paul, 47, 273
Ruellan, Andrée, 252, 454
Ruggles, Carl, 8; "Vox Clamans in Deserto," 193, *194*, 197; Whitney-Force patronage of, 177, 180, 182, 193, 197, 425
Rumsey, Mary Harriman, 389
Ruskin, John, 34, 112, 229
Russell, Morgan, 75, 86, 103
Russman, Felix, 140
Ryder, Albert P., 47, 104, 105, 139, 170*n.*, 301, 329, 389, 433

Sachs, Paul J., 252–253
Saint-Gaudens, Augustus, 44, 55, 57, 77, 130, 483, 488; *The Pilgrim*, 290
Saint-Gaudens, Homer, 335, 483–484
Saint-Gaudens Memorial, 483, 487–488
Salzedo, Carlos, 174, 175, 180, 197
San Francisco, 327, 406; Panama-Pacific Exposition (1915), 118, 121
Sanger, Margaret, 69
Sargent, John Singer, 47, 77, 82, 389; Metropolitan memorial exhibition, 263; portrait of GW, 109, *110*; *Portrait of the Wyndham Sisters*, 263; in Whitney Studio shows, 122, 139
Satie, Erik, 248
Sawyer, Charles, 395, 416, 421, 443, 444, 469, 481; and JF, 286–287, 378, 380, 440
Schack, William, 186*n.*, 419
Schamberg, Morton, 78, 135, 375
Schanker, Louis, 346, 375, 407, 409, 476; Whitney Dissenters poster, *408*
Schapiro, Meyer, 187
Schary, Saul, 301
Schmidt, Katherine, 202, 214, 287–288, 380, 425, 470–471; and JF, 158, 169–170, 188–189, 190, 195, 216, 455, 463–464, 468, 497; and GW, 158, 169; in Whitney Studio Club and shows, 158, 159, 169–170, 188–189, 192, 216, 222
Schmutz, Elisabetha Schuler, 12
Schmutz, Hermann, 12–13, 15, 17
Schmutz, Maria, 15
Schnakenberg, Henry, 135, 147, 177, 187, 193, 195, 199, 201–202, 239, 258, 485, 506; and JF, 131, 143, 463, 490, 493–494, 501, 503; *Still Life*, *305*; in

Museum, 285, 311, 327, 415–416, 476–477; on Whitney Studio shows, 116, 121–122, 138–139; as *World* art critic, 164, 165, 185, 226, 296

Watson, Thomas J., 460

Weber, Max, 69, 170, 314, 440; *Chinese Restaurant*, 301, 363; in Whitney Museum shows and collection, 166, 283, 301, 318, 375, 442

Wehle, Harry, 422, 461, 463, 473

Weir, Julian Alden, 101, 104, 112, 113, 139

West, Benjamin, 389

West, Rebecca, 8, 211–212, 353

Weston, Edward, 282

West Point PWAP-WPA mural, 359–360

Weyhe Gallery, 221, 253, 303

Wharton, Edith, 40, 42, 54

Wheeler, Monroe, 421, 461

Whistler, J. A. M., 47, 82, 105, 114, 273, 389

White, Clarence, 113, 138

White, Stanford, 57, 64, 75

Whitney, Cornelius Vanderbilt (Sonny), 52, 53, 61, 62, 179, 368, 471, 503, 505; *High Peaks*, 179, 180; and JF's illness, 494, 498, 499; marriage to Eleanor Searle, 465–467; as Whitney Museum trustee, 386, 437, 439, 454, 458–459, 465, 496, 498

Whitney, Dorothy, 77

Whitney, Eleanor Searle, 465–467, 505

Whitney, Flora Payne, 49, 234

Whitney, Gertrude Vanderbilt, 4, 37–64, 446, 494, 505, 506; birth of, 37; childhood and family relations, 37–51; courted by Harry Whitney, 49–51; and Frank Crocker, 372, 380–382, 385–386, 390, 394, 397, 398, 401, 404, 414, 426, 431, 437; custody battle for Gloria Vanderbilt, 367–372, 381, 401; death of, and estate settlement, 5, 434–439, 457–458, 467, 487–488; early plans for the museum, 264–266, 280–281; education of, 47, 48; effects of wealth and social prominence on, 37–40, 42, 49, 51–52, 57, 60–62, 73, 85, 129–130, 158, 207; in Europe, 46–47, 48, 60, 75, 234–235, 244; extramarital affairs of, 55, 62, 86, 168; married life of, 51–53, 57, 60–64, 75, 77, 88, 111, 168–169, 235, 267, 291; as a mother, 52, 53, 61, 62, 133, 179, 368, 401; photographs of, *48*, *63*, *130*, 298, *412*; physical appearance of, 49; portrait of, by Sargent, *110*; promiscuity of her husband, 51, 53, 57, 61–62, 168; and PWAP, 335, 361, 362; rebelliousness of, 40, 62–64, 92, 95, 102, 129–130; her role in the Whitney Museum, 282, 291, 312, 416, 431–432, 434; 438; writings of, 37–40, 52–54, 61, 62, 85–86, 93–96,

99, 103–105, 109, 168–169, 426, 431; WWI relief effort, 109, 111–115, 142, 144–145

artwork of, 37, 222, 282, 289, 438; Architectural League award, 77–78, 106; Arlington Fountain, 80, 99, 109, 280; *Aspiration*, 59, 60; assistance with her commissions, 55, 79–80, 109; *Buffalo Bill*, 80, 179–180, 204–205, 205, 206–208; *Chinoise*, *462*, *463*; Colony Club shows, 82–84, 91; Columbus monument, 245–247, 249, 251, 258–259; criticism of, 77–80, 109, 128, 234, 249; DAR commission, 244, 245, 249; early career, 73–96; effects of modernism on, 105; Foch memorial, 278; Fourth Division memorial, 179, 180; *Head of a Spanish Peasant*, 109, 112, 128, 261; in Independent Show vs. Academy annual (1910), 78–79; mediocrity of, 54, 55, 79–80, 109, 128, 234, 405; memorial exhibition (1943), 446, 449; in Metropolitan Museum, 128, 261; *Paganisme Immortel*, 78–79; in Panama-Pacific Exposition (1915), 118, 121; Pan-American Building commission, 99, 109; in Paris Salon (1924), 80; pseudonymous exhibition of, until 1910, 57, 77; retrospectives, 123, 128, 176; Rumsey memorial, 389; Saint-Nazaire monument, 208, 233–235, 245; vs. social obligations, 40–41, 55, 57, 60–64, 75, 81, 85–86, 129–130, 133, 179, 207; Stuyvesant statue, 389; *Titanic* memorial, 99, 108–109, 135, 234; *To The Morrow*, 384, 389, 405, 413, 424; training, 54, 64, 77; war sculptures, 169, 171

collection of, 137, 149, 166, 178, 198, 221, 235; blasted in little Gloria trial, 371; confused with JF's collection, 178–179, 201*n*., 261, 269*n*., 277*n*.; donated to other museums, 173, 177, 193, 245, 252; offered to the Metropolitan in 1929, 261–265, 278; her patronage and collecting patterns, 63, 75, 78, 84, 91–93, 99–103, 111–116, 122, 130–131, 136–137, 149, 172, 177–179, 262, 269 and *n*., 270, 281; pooled with JF's collection, 277 and *n*. See also *specific artists, institutions*; Whitney Museum of American Art, collection of

relationship with JF, *see* Force, Juliana, relationship with GW

relations with the art world, 53, 72, 109, 131–132, 178, 278; and Armory Show, 100–105, 170; and Brancusi trial, 243–244, 248, 369; Bob Chanler, 81–82, 158, 178; John Steuart Curry, 270*n*.; Jo Davidson, 167, 168, 178, 235, 236, 258, 361*n*., 438–439; Arthur B. Davies, 83,

PERMISSIONS AND ACKNOWLEDGMENTS

Grateful acknowledgment is made to the following: Doubleday, a division of Bantam, Doubleday, Dell Publishing Group, Inc., for excerpts from *Young in New York* by Nathalie Dana, copyright © 1963 by Nathalie Dana, used by permission; Harcourt Brace Jovanovich, Inc., for excerpts from "Whispers of Immortality" from *Collected Poems, 1909–1962* by T. S. Eliot, copyright 1936 by Harcourt Brace Jovanovich, Inc., copyright 1964, 1963 by T. S. Eliot, used by permission; Gunther Stuhlmann, Author's Representative, for excerpts from *Gertrude Vanderbilt Whitney*, copyright © 1978 by B. H. Friedman, all rights reserved, used by permission; Vogue Magazine, for excerpts from "Whitney Museum," copyright © 1940 (renewed 1968) by The Condé Nast Publications Inc., used by permission; Alfred A. Knopf, Inc., for excerpts from *Once Upon a Time* by Gloria Vanderbilt, copyright © 1985 by Gloria Vanderbilt, used by permission; the Collection of American Literature, Beinecke Rare Book and Manuscript Library, Yale University, for excerpts from the Royal Cortissoz Papers: Juliana Force, letter to Cortissoz, December 1926; Gertrude Whitney, letter to Cortissoz, December 11, 1930, and excerpts from the Alfred Steiglitz Collection: letter to Juliana Force, December 15, 1942, used by permission.

ABOUT THE AUTHOR

AVIS BERMAN was born in Hartford, Connecticut, and is a graduate of Bucknell and Rutgers universities. A freelance writer and critic in the arts, she has written extensively on painting, sculpture, photography, architecture, and museum history for many magazines and newspapers. She also heads the oral history program for the New York branch of the Archives of American Art. She lives in Manhattan.